Handbook of Experimental Pharmacology

Continuation of Handbuch der experimentellen Pharmakologie

Vol. 50/I

Inflammation

Contributors

A. C. Allison · K. F. Austen · I. L. Bonta · P. Davies
D. T. Fearon · W. S. Feldberg · S. H. Ferreira · R. J. Flower
R. van Furth · J. Garcia Leme · L. E. Glynn · J. V. Hurley
K. Krakauer · L. M. Lichtenstein · A. S. Milton · S. Moncada
J. Morley · A. Nicholson · M. Plaut · M. Rocha e Silva
S. E. Smith · J. L. Turk · J. R. Vane · P. C. Wilkinson
A. L. Willis · D. A. Willoughby · L. J. F. Youlten · R. B. Zurier

Editors

J. R. Vane · S. H. Ferreira

Springer-Verlag Berlin Heidelberg New York 1978

Dr. JOHN R. VANE, The Wellcome Research Laboratories, Langley Court, Beckenham, Kent BR3 3BS, UK

Dr. SERGIO H. FERREIRA, Universidade de São Paulo, Faculdade de Medicina de Ribeirão Preto, CEP 14.100, São Paulo, Brazil

With 95 Figures

ISBN-13: 978-3-642-66890-6 e-ISBN-13: 978-3-642-66888-3
DOI: 10.1007/978-3-642-66888-3

Library of Congress Cataloging in Publication Data. Main entry under title: Inflammation. (Handbuch der experimentellen Pharmakologie: New series; v. 50/1) Includes bibliographies and indexes. 1. Inflammation. 2. Anti-inflammatory agents. I. Allison, Anthony, 1925-. II. Vane. John R. III. Ferreira, S. H., 1934-. III. Title. QP905.H3 vol. 50/1. [RB131]. 615'.1'08s. [616.07'2]. 78-2393.

Softcover reprint of the hardcover 1st edition 1978

Preface

Throughout the centuries, inflammation has been considered as a disease in itself. This misconception arose from the inability to distinguish between inflammatory changes and the insults which induce them. The understanding of the distinction between the genesis of inflammation and the tissue reactions that follow is attributed to JOHN HUNTER, who, at the end of the 18th century, substantially contributed to the analysis of inflammation in objective terms. Today, however, we are still trying to find explanations for Celsus' Signs in terms of structural and functional changes occurring in the inflamed tissue. There are drugs which modulate these signs but, without a detailed knowledge of the basic physiopathological events, it is impossible to understand their mechanism of action. Notwithstanding, the effects of anti-inflammatory drugs provided new knowledge of the relevance of the signs and symptoms to the sequence of biochemical and morphological changes occurring in inflammation.

When we accepted the invitation to edit a Handbook on Inflammation and Anti-Inflammatory Drugs, we were aware of the magnitude of the task. We knew the impossibility of covering the whole field in detail, especially taking into account the rapid accumulation of experimental knowledge which would, in all likelihood, overtake the process of publication. But we accepted the challenge because we thought it would be useful to bring together the experience of many different experts, in the hope that this would crystallise the present state of knowledge, and ease the way for scientists who are being attracted to the area. We tried to organize a book that could be of help in the evaluation of background knowledge, and to identify the inconsistencies of different expert opinions in order to stimulate the search for new anti-inflammatory agents.

The Handbook reflects the concept that control of inflammation may be achieved successfully by interfering with the synthesis, release or action of the inflammatory mediators. Many drugs available today interfere with the synthesis, release or action of some receptor-type mediators such as histamine or prostaglandins. But these drugs, although of great benefit to the patient, modulate symptoms, apparently without affecting the ultimate progression of the disease. Furthermore, all these drugs have side effects which frequently limit their usefulness.

As discussed in the book, the future in anti-inflammatory therapy may lie in the discovery of:

a) agents capable of minimizing the side effects of presently existing drugs;

b) development of similar anti-inflammatory agents but devoid of side effects;

c) agents which can block the evolution of chronic inflammatory diseases either by blocking the effects of the trauma or by acting on some step of the inflammatory reaction which is responsible for irreversible lesions, such as the release or action of the enzymes responsible for the deterioration of tissue structure. We hope the book will stimulate the search for such agents.

We are indebted to Mrs. J. REELEY, Mrs. C. BRIERLEY and Miss M. VANE for invaluable help in the handling and editing of the manuscripts and to all the authors for their outstanding contributions.

Beckenham/São Paulo, July 1978 J. R. VANE · S. H. FERREIRA

Contents

CHAPTER 3

Mononuclear Phagocytes in Inflammation. R. VAN FURTH. With 14 Figures

CHAPTER 4

The Adhesion, Locomotion, and Chemotaxis of Leucocytes. P. C. WILKINSON. With 1 Figure

CHAPTER 6

Regeneration and Repair. L. E. GLYNN. With 1 Figure

CHAPTER 7

Immunological and Para-Immunological Aspects of Inflammation. J. L. TURK and D. A. WILLOUGHBY. With 2 Figures

CHAPTER 8

The Release of Hydrolytic Enzymes From Phagocytic and Other Cells Participating in Acute and Chronic Inflammation. P. Davies and A. C. Allison. With 6 Figures

CHAPTER 9

Lysosomal Enzymes. R. B. Zurier and K. Krakauer

CHAPTER 10

Lymphokines. J. Morley. With 8 Figures

Inflammatory Mediators Generated by Activation of Plasma Systems

CHAPTER 13

Complement. A. NICHOLSON, D. T. FEARON, and K. F. AUSTEN

CHAPTER 14

Bradykinin-System. J. GARCIA LEME. With 3 Figures

CHAPTER 15

Endogenous Modulators of the Inflammatory Response. I. L. BONTA. With 5 Figures

Contribution of the Inflammatory Mediators to the Signs and Symptoms of Inflammation

CHAPTER 16

Inflammatory Mediators and Vascular Events. L. J. F. YOULTEN

CHAPTER 17

Pain and Inflammatory Mediators. S. MONCADA, S. H. FERREIRA, and J. R. VANE. With 4 Figures

CHAPTER 18

Prostaglandins and Body Temperature. W. S. FELDBERG and A. S. MILTON. With 2 Figures

Contents
Part II: Anti-Inflammatory Drugs

Screening and Toxicity of Anti-Inflammatory Drugs

Pharmacology of the Anti-Inflammatory Agents

List of Contributors

A. C. ALLISON, Medical Research Council, Clinical Research Centre, Division of Cell Pathology, Watford Road, Harrow, Middlesex HA1 3UJ, UK

K. F. AUSTEN, Harvard Medical School, The Seeley G. Mudd Bldg., 250 Longwood Ave., Boston, Massachusetts 02115, USA

I. L. BONTA, Department of Pharmacology, Erasmus Universiteit Rotterdam, Postbus 1738, Rotterdam, Holland

P. DAVIES, Merck Institute for Therapeutic Research, Rahway, New Jersey 07065, USA

D. T. FEARON, Harvard Medical School, Department of Medicine, Robert B. Brigham Hospital, 125 Parker Hill Avenue, Boston, Massachusetts 02120, USA

W. S. FELDBERG, Laboratory of Neuropharmacology, National Institute for Medical Research, The Ridgeway, Mill Hill, London NW7 1AA, UK

S. H. FERREIRA, Universidade de São Paulo, Faculdade de Medicina de Ribeirão Preto, CEP 14, 100 Ribeirão Preto, São Paulo, Brazil

R. J. FLOWER, Department of Prostaglandin Research, The Wellcome Research Laboratories, Langley Court, Beckenham, Kent BR3 3BS, UK

R. VAN FURTH, Department of Microbial Diseases, University Hospital, Rijnburgerweg 10, Leiden, Holland

J. GARCIA LEME, Universidade de São Paulo, Faculdade de Medicina de Ribeirão Preto, CEP 14,100 Ribeirão Preto, São Paulo, Brazil

L. E. GLYNN, The Mathilda and Terence Kennedy Institute of Rheumatology, Bute Gardens, Hammersmith, London W6 7DW, UK

J. V. HURLEY, Department of Pathology, University of Melbourne, Parkville, Victoria 3052, Australia

K. KRAKAUER, Division of Rheumatic Diseases, Department of Medicine, University of Connecticut, Farmington, Connecticut, 06032, USA

L. M. LICHTENSTEIN, The John Hopkins University, Division of Clinical Immunology, The Good Samaritan Hospital, 5601 Loch Raven Boulevard, Baltimore, Maryland, 21239, USA

A. S. MILTON, University of Aberdeen, Department of Pharmacology, Medical Buildings, Aberdeen AB9 2ZD, UK

S. MONCADA, Department of Prostaglandin Research, The Wellcome Research Laboratories, Langley Court, Beckenham, Kent BR3 3BS, UK

J. MORLEY, Department of Clinical Pharmacology, Cardiothoracic Institute, Fulham Road, London SW3 6HP, UK

A. NICHOLSON, Harvard Medical School, Robert B. Brigham Hospital, 250 Longwood Ave., Boston, Massachusetts 02120, USA

M. Plaut, The John Hopkins University, Division of Clinical Immunology, The Good Samaritan Hospital, 5601 Loch Raven Boulevard, Baltimore, Maryland 21239, USA

M. Rocha e Silva, Universidade de São Paulo, Faculdade de Medicina de Ribeirão Preto, CEP 14, 100 Ribeirão Preto, São Paulo, Brazil

S. E. Smith, The Wellcome Research Laboratories, Langley Court, Beckenham, Kent BR3 3BS, UK

J. L. Turk, Department of Pathology, The Royal College of Surgeons of England, 35–43 Lincoln's Inn Fields, London WC2A 3PN, UK

J. R. Vane, The Wellcome Research Laboratories, Langley Court, Beckenham, Kent BR3 3BS, UK

P. C. Wilkinson, Department of Bacteriology and Immunology, University of Glasgow, Western Infirmary, Glasgow G11 6NT, UK

A. L. Willis, Syntex Corps, Department of Physiology, Stanford Industrial Park, 3401 Hillview Avenue, Palo Alto, California 94304, USA, and University Department of Medicine, Leeds General Infirmary, Leeds, Yorks., UK

D. A. Willoughby, The Rheumatology and Experimental Pathology Department, St. Bartholomew's Hospital Medical School, London EC1A 7BE, UK

L. J. F. Youlten, Department of Medicine, Guy's Hospital Medical School, London Bridge, London SE1 3RT, UK

R. B. Zurier, Division of Rheumatic Diseases, Department of Medicine, University of Connecticut, Farmington, Connecticut 06032, USA

List of Abbreviations

AA	adjuvant arthritis
Aa	arachidonic acid
ACI	anti-inflammatory cyclo-oxygenase inhibitors
ACTH	adrenocorticotrophic hormone
ADCC	antibody-dependent cellular cytotoxicity
ADP	adenosine diphospate
AH	anterior hypothalamus
AI	anaphylatoxin inactivator
AID	anti-inflammatory drug
ALG	antilymphocyte globulin
ALS	antilymphocyte serum
ANTU	alphanaphthyl thiourea
AThP	azathioprine
ATP	adenosine triphosphate
BAL	dimercaptopropanol
$BaSO_4$	Barium sulphate
BCG	Bacille Calmette-Guerin
BGG	bovine γ globulin
Bk	bradykinin
BK-A	basophil kallikrein of anaphylaxis
Bkg	bradykininogen
BP	bacterial pyrogen
BPF	bradykinin potentiating factor
BSA	bovine serum albumin
BSV	bovine seminal vesicle
cAMP	cyclic adenosine 3′,5′-monophosphate
CB	cytochalasin B
CBC	chlorambucil
C3bINA	C3b inactivator
C3NeF	C3 nephritic factor
C3PA	C3 proactivator
CBH	cutaneous basophil hypersensitivity
CFC	citrus flavonoid complex
cGMP	cyclic guanosine 3′,5′-monophosphate
CH_{50}	haemolytic complement
CiSLs	circulating sensitized lymphocytes
CNDO	complete neglect of differential overlap
Col	colchicine
Con-A	concanavalin A
CP	cyclophosphamide
CPA	N-(Z-carboboxyphenyl)-phenoxyacetamides
CP-CPK	creatinine phosphate-phosphokinase
CPPD	calcium pyrophosphate dihydrate
CR	capillary resistance
CRF	corticotrophin releasing factor
CTL	cytolitically active T-lymphocytes
CVF	cobra venom factor
CVP	citrus vitamin P
CY	cyclophosphamide
DAS	depressor active substance
Db-cAMP	dibutyryl derivative of cAMP
DES	diethylstilboestrol
DFP	diisopropylphosphofluoridate
DH	delayed hypersensitivity
DHM	dehydromonocrotaline
DMSO	dimethyl sulphoxide

$DNBSO_3$	dinitrobenzene sulphonic acid
DNCB	2,4,-dinitrochlorobenzene
DNP	dinitrophenylated
DPP	diphloretin phosphate
EACA	epsilon-aminocaproic acid
ECF	eosinophil chemotactic factor
ECF-A	eosinophil chemotactic factor of anaphylaxis
EDTA	ethylenediaminetetra-acetic acid
EFA	essential fatty acid
EGTA	ethylene gycol tetraacetic acid
ER	endoplasmic reticulum
ESR	erythrocyte sedimentation rate
ETA	eicosatetraynoic acid
FA	fluocinolone acetonide
FCA	Freund's complete adjuvant
FIA	Freund's incomplete adjuvant
GBG	glycene-rich β-glycoprotein
GFR	glomerular filtration rate
HAO	hereditary angio-oedema
HETE	12-L-hydroxy-5,8,10,14-eicosatetraenoic acid
HGPRT	hypoxanthine-guanine phosphoribosyltransferase
HMW	high molecular weight
HNA	heparin-neutralising activity
HPETE	12-L-hydroperoxy-5,8,10,14-eicosatetraenoic acid
HPF	human plasma factor
HSA	human serum albumin
5-HT	5-hydroxytryptamine
HTT	12-L-hydroxy-5,8,10-heptadecatrienoic acid
IAP	intra-articular pressure
IDS	inhibitor of DNA synthesis
IF	initiating factor
ITAIF	irritated tissue anti-inflammatory factor
KAF	C3b inactivator
KDO	2-beta-3 deoxyoctonic acid
LASS	labile aggregation stimulating substance
LDH	lactate dehydrogenase
LMW	low molecular weight
LoSLs	locally sensitized lymphocytes
LPF	lymph node permeability factor
LSD	lysergic acid diethylamide
MAF	macrophage activating factor
MCDP	mast cell degranulating peptide
MDA	malondialdehyde
MED	minimal erythemal dose
MEM	minimal essential medium
MF	mitogenic factor
MIF	migration inhibitory factor
MNI	methylnitroimidazole
6MP	6-mercaptopurine
MPGN	membranoproliferative glomerulonephritis
MPI	monocyte production inhibitor
MSU	monosodium urate mono-hydrate
MTX	methotrexate
NCF	neutrophil chemotactic factor
NEM	N-ethylmaleimide
NSAID	nonsteroid anti-inflammatory drug
OAF	osteoclast activating factor
P	properdin
PAF	platelet-activating factor

PCA	passive cutaneous anaphylaxis
pCPA	p-chlorophenyl-alanine
PCZ	procarbazine
PDE	phosphodiesterase
PF3	platelet factor 3
PF/dil	permeability globulin factor
PF/Glob	high molecular permeability factors
PG	prostaglandin
for example:	
PGE_1	prostaglandin E_1
PHA	phytohaemagglutinin
PHD	8-(1-hydroxy-3-oxo-propyl)-9, 12S-dihydroxy-5-cis, 10-transhepta-decadienoic acid
PMA	phorbol myristate acetate
PMN	polymorphonuclear leucocytes
PNP	pyroninophilic
PPD	protein-purified derivative of tuberculin
PPG	C-mucopolysaccharide-peptidoglycan
PPLO	mycoplasmas
PPP	polyphloretin phosphate
PPS	pain-producing substance
PVP	polyvinylpyrrolidone
PVPNO	polyvinyl pyridine N-oxide
R	rectus
RA	rheumatoid arthritis
RCS	rabbit aorta contracting substance
RCS-RF	RCS-releasing factor
RES	reticulo-endothelial system
RF	rheumatoid factor
RPA	reverse passive Arthus reaction
SBTI	soybean trypsin inhibitor
SGOT	serum glutamic oxaloacetic transaminase
SGPT	serum glutamic-pyruvic transaminase
SLE	systemic lupus erythematosus
SPD	storage pool deficient
SRS	slow-reacting substance
SRS-A	SRS of anaphylaxis
SRS-C	SRS from cobra venom
SSV	sheep seminal vesicle
TAMe	p-tosyl-arginine methyl ester
TBA	thiobarbituric acid
THFN	tetrahydrofurfuryl nicotinate
TNP	trinitrophenylated
TYA	eicosatetraynoic acid
UPD	uridine diphosphate
UDPG	uridine diphosphate glucose

Historical Survey of Definitions and Concepts of Inflammation

S. E. Smith

The Egyptian medical texts had a number of terms, apparently referring to inflammatory conditions, which were all derived from the hieroglyphic for "fire". According to Blersch (1973) they had terms which distinguished local from generalised inflammation, and regarded the condition as a superficial heating arising from outside the body, and not internally generated.

Florey (1962) says that papyri of the 2nd millenium describe "pus as related to the demon of disease."

The term "phlegmone", again a fiery heat, was used in the early Greek Hippocratic writings to describe a variety of conditions which were thought to be due to an influx of blood into parts which normally did not contain it (Hippocratic treatise on "Head Wounds") (Talamonti, 1968). In the Hippocratic treatise on "Ulcers" it is noted that the ease of healing is inversely related to the degree of inflammation.

Erasistratus (about 250 BC), of the Alexandrian school, also regarded inflammation as due to an influx of blood. In keeping with the current humoral theories, he thought that the veins normally contained blood and the arteries "pneuma," and that in inflammation the blood forced its way via interconnections from vein to artery, driving out the pneuma. He regarded the excess of blood as the cause of the malady, giving rise to inflammation and secondarily to fever (Talamonti, 1968).

Celsus, in the 1st century AD, was a Roman medical compiler drawing from Greek sources. He gave the classical definition regularly quoted: "The characteristics of inflammation are four: redness and swelling, with heat and pain" ("Notae vero inflammationes sunt quattuor: rubor et tumor cum calore et dolore;" in De Medicina, Liber 3, Cap. 10). Galen (129–200 AD)attributed essentially this definition to Erasistratus:

> But this tumor, assuming a pulsation and fiery heat, answers then properly to the ancient title of phlegmone. But the ancients do not thus distinguish it; for they called any heat or inflammation a phlegmone, as I have frequently demonstrated. But from the time of Erasistratus it has been customary to term those tumors phlegmones, in which there is not only an inflammatory heat but also a resistance and pulsation; they have also of necessity a redness so-called ...

(in Liber Hippocrat. de Fracturis) (von Swieten, 1776). Galen followed the simpler Hippocratic idea of an influx of blood, which he believed effused into spaces between the vessels. In accordance with a more developed humoural theory, he classified inflammations according to the humours involved, e.g. pure blood gave rise to a phlegmone, blood mixed with "phlegm" to oedema, with "yellow bile" to erysipelas, with "black bile" to cancers, and so on (Talamonti, 1968). He accorded a central function to pain which, perhaps by weakening the locality, allowed the influx of humours. He correlated the degree of sensibility to pain of a region with its proneness to inflammation (Niedyl, 1971).

BARTHOLOMEW PARDOUX (1641), a 16th century Galenist, gave what might be considered the ultimate classical definition, supported by references to GALEN: "... phlegmone can be defined as a hot, prominent and circumscribed tumor, derived from an afflux of blood, with redness, tension, resistance, pulsation and pain joined thereto."

RATHER (1971) argues that the "fifth cardinal sign: loss of function," attributed to GALEN by modern textbooks, does not appear in Galenic writings, or indeed anywhere until after the 17th century.

VAN HELMONT (1577–1644) elaborated a mystical concept of disease based on the inflammatory response. He exemplified the external cause of disease by a thorn or splinter in response to which the vital principle, the "Archeus," mounted an inflammatory response which was the disease process. He generalised from this to metaphorical humoural thorns leading to disease. He regarded the inflammatory response as essentially harmful and to be regarded as the main target for treatment (NIEBYL, 1971).

HERMANN BOERHAAVE (1663–1738) heralds the beginning of modern developments. He focussed attention on blood and other body fluids, and at first regarded inflammation as due to a rupture of blood vessels and the escape of blood into the tissues. He listed various causes, including viscidity of the blood causing obstruction, and "acrimony" by which the blood could damage the blood vessels. Later he developed the idea that blood became obstructed in smaller vessels, the lumen of which was reduced, and that heat was generated by the friction between obstructed and flowing blood. This obstructive stagnation could then resolve by dilution and loosening of the obstruction, or subsequent putrefraction of varying degrees could occur, leading to suppuration or gangrene. BOERHAAVE introduced the modern concept that inflammation arises in the small blood vessels (JARCHO, 1970a, b). ALBRECHT VON HALLER (1708–1777), a pupil of BOERHAAVE, disagreed with the theory of impaction and argued from observations that the blood must be exuded from the vessels into surrounding spaces, coinciding with the view of GALEN (JARCHO, 1970c).

JOHN HUNTER (1728–1793) introduced an essentially modern concept of inflammation. He regarded it as a response to disease or injury, not a disease in itself; local inflammation, for example, might be a response to fever: "... but from whatever cause inflammation arises, it appears to be nearly the same in all, for in all it is an effect intended to bring about a reinstatement of the parts nearly to their natural functions." He made no fundamental distinction between healing and inflammation, and regarded the latter as involved in all healing other than by first intention. Extravasation from the blood vessels he saw as the primary event, with coagulation of blood and lymph as the first stage of healing, the "adhesive" phase of inflammation. Suppuration and ulceration were more extreme phases: increasingly violent efforts to drive out the extraneous irritant. He was impressed by the violence of apparently spontaneous inflammations such as boils and, of course in "pre-bacteriological" times, they puzzled him. Although he accorded the blood vessels a central role in inflammation and regarded their obstruction as a possible cause, he disagreed with BOERHAAVE's theory that such obstruction was a first stage in the process, or that it could lead to increased flow and impaction of blood (JARCHO, 1970d).

JAMES MACARTNEY (1770–1843), denied any positive connection between inflammation and healing, and maintained that it impeded healing. Suppuration, to him, was always an evil, and the consequences of inflammation were injurious. He believed that inflammation was a reaction of arterial vessels and developed a neurogenic doctrine, the disturbance of the arterial vessels being the result of stimuli transmitted by the nervous system. From experiments on ligation of vessels and from observation of erectile tissues he concluded that congestion must be distinguished from inflammation (JARCHO, 1971 a, b).

WILLIAM ADDISON (1802–1881) ushered in the period of microscopical studies of inflammation. He described the presence of colourless, lighter globules as well as heavier, red globules in the buffy coat which was known to be a striking feature of blood drawn from inflammatory cases. He observed the flow of blood and its corpuscles in the web of the frog's foot and also, in response to an irritant, the engorgement of the vessels and obstruction of blood flow, with stagnation of the white corpuscles. He observed the extravascular appearance of the white corpuscles in pus, and finally he observed that white cells in the inflamed foot web could be seen immobilised along the insides of the vessels and also lying outside the capillary walls (JARCHO, 1971c, 1971d). AUGUSTUS VOLNEY WALLER (1816–1870) carried these observations one stage further. In the living frog's tongue, he described the actual passage of white cells through the vessel walls (diapedesis) and reported that pus originated "from the extravasation of the colourless or spherical corpuscles from the capillaries" (JARCHO, 1971e).

JULIUS COHNHEIM (1839–1884) put together the preceding concepts in his classic essay on inflammation. He gave detailed descriptions of the vascular and cellular processes and affirmed once again the importance of the blood vessels. "Without vessels there is no inflammation." He also drew attention to connective tissue, pointing out that "suppuration remains associated first and last with connective tissues" since it is the one tissue with space for the accumulation of white cells. He was puzzled by the ultimate causes of the inflammatory behaviour of vessels and white cells and the absence, for example, of diapedesis in ordinary venous stasis (JARCHO, 1972a, b). These later developments accorded well with VIRCHOW's elevation of the importance of cells in pathology (VIRCHOW, 1871), while a vital concept for the interpretation of inflammation was supplied by METCHNIKOFF with his theory that phagocytosis was the central phenomenon and that the inflammatory process was centred on the white cell as a defence against microbial invasion (METCHNIKOFF, 1892).

Modern definitions of inflammation are once again simple, although functional rather than descriptive, and would probably not have surprised HUNTER:

Sir J. BURDON-SANDERSON (1962): "The succession of changes which occurs in a living tissue when it is injured, provided that the injury is not of such a nature as to at once destroy its structure and vitality."

V. MENKIN (1962): "The complex vascular, lymphatic and local tissue reaction elicited in higher animals by the presence of microorganisms or of non-viable irritants."

BOYD's Textbook of Pathology (1970): "The reaction of living tissue to injury."

References

Bersch, H. V.: Wärme bei Fieber und Entzündung in den altägyptischen medizinischen Texten. (smm und srf). Med. Hist. J. **8**, 35—52 (1973)

Boyd's Textbook of Pathology: 8th ed., p. 77. London: Henry Kimpton 1970

Burdon-Sanderson, Sir J.: In: Florey, H. (Ed.): General Pathology, 3rd ed. London: Lloyd-Luke 1962

Florey, H. (Ed.): General Pathology, 3rd ed. London: Lloyd-Luke 1962

Jarcho, S.: Boerhaave on inflammation I. Amer. J. Cardiol. **25**, 244—246 (1970a)

Jarcho, S.: Boerhaave on inflammation II. Amer. J. Cardiol. **25**, 480—482 (1970b)

Jarcho, S.: Albrecht von Haller on inflammation. Amer. J. Cardiol. **25**, 707—709 (1970c)

Jarcho, S.: John Hunter on inflammation. Amer. J. Cardiol. **26**, 615—618 (1970d)

Jarcho, S.: Macartney on inflammation I. Amer. J. Cardiol. **27**, 212—214 (1971a)

Jarcho, S.: Macartney on inflammation II. Amer. J. Cardiol. **27**, 433—435 (1971b)

Jarcho, S.: William Addison on blood vessels and inflammation (1840—1841). Amer. J. Cardiol. **27**, 670—672 (1971c)

Jarcho, S.: William Addison on blood vessels and inflammation (1841—1843). Amer. J. Cardiol. **28**, 223—225 (1971d)

Jarcho, S.: Augustus Volney Waller on blood vessels and inflammation. Amer. J. Cardiol. **28**, 475—477 and 712—714 (1971e)

Jarcho, S.: Cohnheim on inflammation I. Amer. J. Cardiol. **29**, 247—249 (1972a)

Jarcho, S.: Cohnheim on inflammation II. Amer. J. Cardiol. **29**, 546—547 (1972b)

Menkin, V.: In: Florey, H. (Ed.): General Pathology, 3rd ed. London: Lloyd-Luke 1962

Metchnikoff, E.: In: Masson, G. (Ed.): Leçons sur la Pathologie Comparée de l'Inflammation. Paris: 1892

Niebyl, P. H.: The Helmontian thorn. Bull. Hist. Med. **45**, 570—595 (1971)

Pardoux, B. (Ed.): Universa Medicina, 2nd ed. Paris: 1641

Rather, L. J.: Disturbance of function (functio laesa): the legendary fifth cardinal sign of inflammation, added by Galen to the four cardinal signs of Celsus. Bull. N.Y. Acad. Med. **47**, 303—322 (1971)

Talamonti, R.: Evoluzione storica del concetto di infiammazione da Ippocrate a John Hunter. Pagine Storia Med. **12**, 102—108 (1968)

Virchow, R. (Hrsg.): Die Cellularpathologie, 4th ed. Berlin: 1871

Von Swieton, Baron G.: Commentaries on Boerhaave's aphorisms concerning the knowledge and cure of diseases. Translated, Edinburgh 1776 and quoted in: Bull. N.Y. Acad. Med. **47**, 303—322 (1971)

CHAPTER 1

A Brief History of Inflammation

M. Rocha e Silva

A. From the Origins to the 19th Century

Though there are records of pus formation in Egyptian papyri dating from the 2nd millenium B.C. (Encyclopaedia Britannica 1970), the first coherent description of the phenomenon was presented by Celsus, a Roman physician of the 1st century A.D., who described the classic signs of inflammation: *rubor* (redness), *tumor* (swelling), with *calor* (heat) and *dolor* (pain). However, formation of pus with heat, redness and pain are characteristic of the phenomenon as it develops in the highest phyla of the animal kingdom. It seems the term inflammation (*phlogosis*, in Greek) from the Latin word *flamma* for fire, was intended to cover the most complex manifestations of the

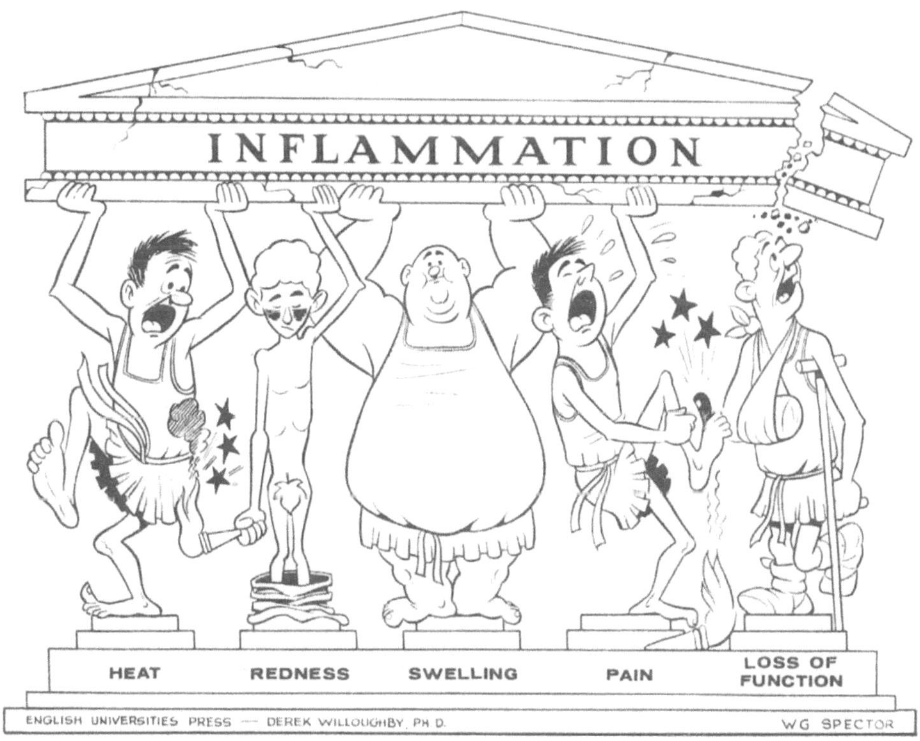

Fig. 1. *Ex libris* of the International Inflammation Club, designed by Willoughby and Spector. To the four signs by Celsus *(calor, rubor, tumor et dolor)*, the fifth characteristic of the inflammatory process, *loss of function*, gives a forceful idea of the situation

The Inflammatory Reaction

phenomenon, as it occurs in man, as a defence mechanism against aggression or injury. Under this connotation, the phenomenon was recognized by Galen (3rd century, A.D.) as a reaction of the body against injury, as well as by JOHN HUNTER (1794), an English doctor of the 18th century. An interesting wealth of historical information about that period can be found in the series of papers by JARCHO (1970–1972).

The phenomenon was not scientifically studied, however, until our knowledge of the agents of injury had developed. This occurred from the XIX century onwards, with the timely discoveries by PASTEUR, KOCH, and LISTER that many infections are caused by germs or viruses, and also with the development of some of the fundamental phenomena of physiological regulations by CLAUDE BERNARD, LUDWIG, DUBOIS-RAYMOND and many others. Among these founders of scientific medicine, the name of VIRCHOW as the initiator of cellular pathology (VIRCHOW, 1871), completes the roster of those who tried to establish on a sound basis our understanding of the elementary functions of the living cell: sensibility, irritability, movement (response), degeneration, and death (necrosis). As we shall see, the inflammatory reaction involves, in differing degrees according to species and phyla, these elementary reactions of the cell as a defensive mechanism against injury.

It has commonly been found that a biological phenomenon cannot be fully understood unless it is analysed into its basic components. In this sense, the classic description by Celsus could be considered a masterpiece of programming to study the phenomenon, that is according to its four main signs. Up until now, no better definition of inflammation in birds and mammals could be found, and it actually became the *Leitmotiv* or *Ex Libris* of the Inflammation Club, as reproduced in Figure 1. I know of no other biological phenomenon that has been so aptly commented upon by an ancient doctor as the description given by Celsus in the 1st century A.D. However, during the latter half of the 19th century A.D., the phenomenon was widely questioned as a biological entity by several influential pathologists.

In 1889, ZIEGLER attempted a definition of inflammation:

> "The notion of 'inflammation' comprises a series of phenomena occurring partly in the circulatory apparatus, partly in the tissues, in varied proportions. As the phenomenon is not unique, a brief and precise definition of inflammation is altogether impossible. Even if one considers as characteristic of the inflammatory process only phenomena taking part in the circulatory apparatus, their definition would not exhaust the notion of inflammation."

For RECKLINGHAUSEN (1883), "it would be impossible to determine the *primum movens*, the starting point of the alteration, i.e. the site of the first lesion;" for him the only acceptable attitude would be for the pathologist to describe in detail, and with precision, the inflammatory phenomena. A similar view was sponsored by CORNIL and RANVIER, in their *Manuel d'Histologie Pathologique* (1881).

In the face of all such difficulties in defining the phenomenon, THOMA (1886) proposed a pure and simple rejection of the term 'inflammation,' an attitude that has been common among pathologists even in recent times. In fact by that time, and even to-day, the notion of inflammation was defined in purely operational terms, as appears in the definition proposed by NEUMANN (1889), "Under this name we have to understand the series of local phenomena developing as the result of primary lesions of the tissues *(lesio continui* or *necrose)* and that tend to restore their health." In spite of such pessimistic views among pathologists, there were some attempts to

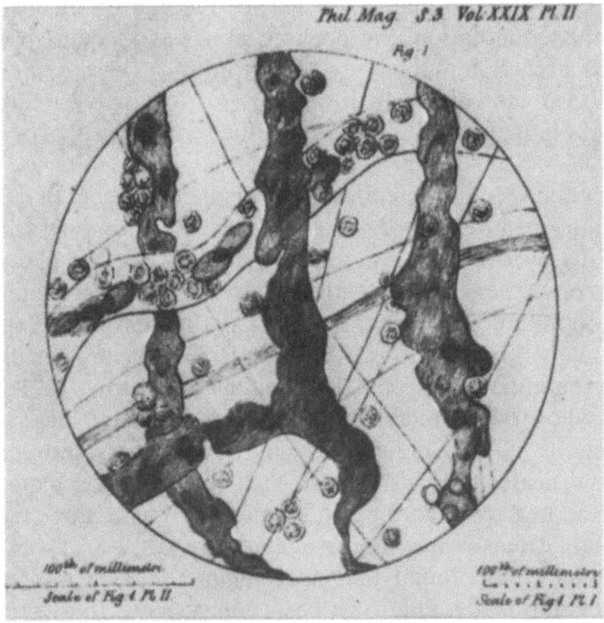
Phil Mag S.3 Vol XXIX Pl II
Fig 1
100th of millimetre
Scale of Fig 1 Pl II
100th of millimetre
Scale of Fig 1 Pl I

a

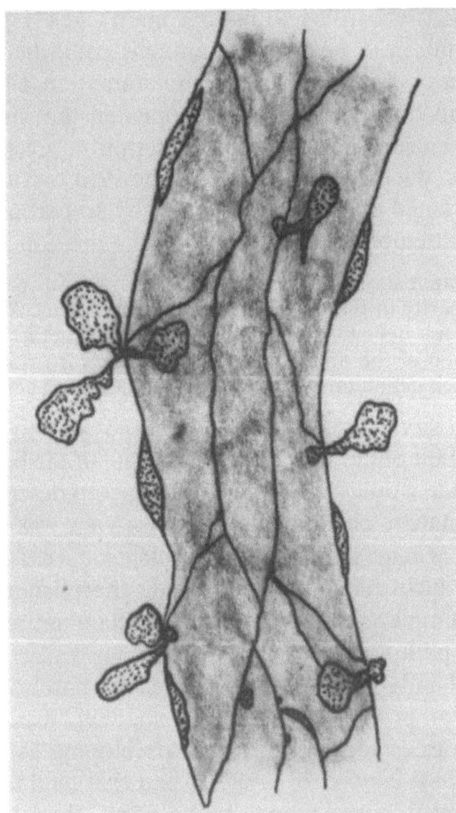

b

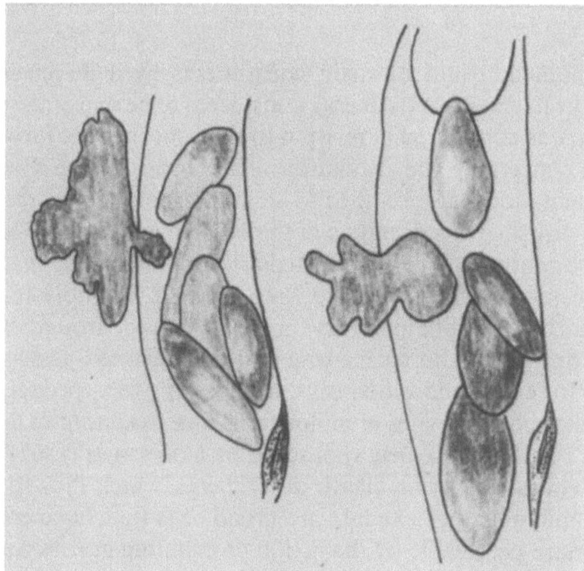

c

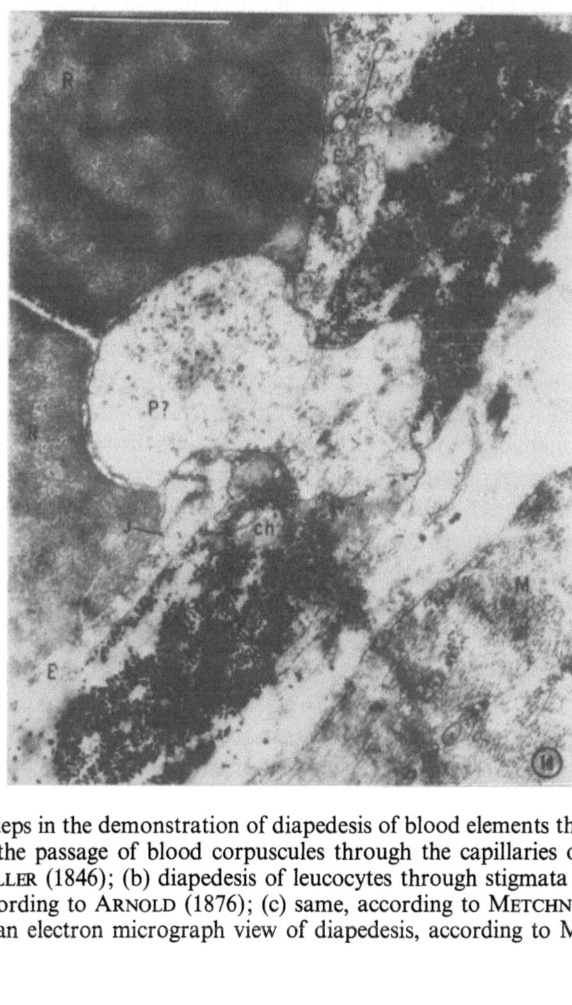

d

Fig. 2a–d. Four steps in the demonstration of diapedesis of blood elements through vessel walls. (a) A scheme of the passage of blood corpuscules through the capillaries of the frog tongue, according to WALLER (1846); (b) diapedesis of leucocytes through stigmata of the walls of the small vessels, according to ARNOLD (1876); (c) same, according to METCHNIKOFF (1892); (d) a modern version, an electron micrograph view of diapedesis, according to MAJNO and PALADE (1961)

analyse the phenomenon into its main constituents by a direct experimental approach. Firstly, the hyperaemia (redness), considered to be one of the cardinal signs of the phenomenon, was considered in relation to the concepts put forward by CLAUDE BERNARD (1872) concerning the regulation of the tonus of the small vessels, "The theories on inflammation were confined to an analysis of the hyperaemia, considered by some as a consequence of a paralysis of the vaso-motor nerves *(paralytic theory)*, or by a spasmodic contraction of the affected arteries *(spasmodic theory)*, with afflux of blood from the neighborhood" (METCHNIKOFF, 1892). Secondly, for SAMUEL (1867) the cardinal point of the inflammatory process centred around "a lesion of the vessels, by irritating agents, in such a way that the inflamed vessels were rendered more permeable to liquids and blood cells, in a passive way, producing the exudate that would be collected at the sites of minor resistance, resulting in the inflammatory tumor (swelling)." This was the view sponsored by COHNHEIM (1867a, 1867b; 1873a, 1873b; 1877) and expanded by his classic experiments, which showed that the cells to be found in any inflammatory exudate are blood cells that have crossed the vessel walls, rendered more permeable by the action of irritating agents. Such experiments by COHNHEIM were carried out in frogs, and showed that even when the circulation of the tongue was interrupted, the inflammatory reaction was still observed, with passage of leucocytes into the interstitial spaces: "I consider indisputable that the cause of inflammation must be found in the vessels themselves, everything that occurs outside of the vessels gives the impression of secondary phenomena that cannot constitute an explanation" (COHNHEIM, 1873b). Therefore, for COHNHEIM, the hyperaemia was not to be considered the cause, but a consequence of the lesion of the vessels. In favour of COHNHEIM'S views one of his disciples, the famous histologist WEIGERT (1889), identified the cells to be found in inflammatory exudates as being of blood origin. Greatly and decisively supporting such a view was the demonstration by ARNOLD (1875) of the phenomenon of diapedesis (see Fig. 2)[1].

A third view of the phenomenon was put forward by the founder of cellular pathology, VIRCHOW (1871), who postulated that any inflammatory process derives from the increased activity (nutritive irritability) of the cell in order to find the appropriate source of food in the surrounding tissues; thus, "The inflammatory reaction is the consequence of an excessive intake by the interstitial cells, of food provenient from the liquid part of the blood, filtering through the vessel walls." The end result would be hypertrophy or degeneration (mucous, fatty, amyloid, hyaline) of the cells that would multiply to form the inflammatory tumor. This view was, of course, in opposition to that sponsored by COHNHEIM and his pupils, that the cells appearing in the inflamed area are derived from blood cells. To VIRCHOW, the other signs of the process, such as hyperaemia and afflux of blood cells following lesion of the vessels, would constitute secondary events resulting from malnutrition of the interstitial cells.

It is of course this tendency to emphasize one of the signs of the process as the main event that characterizes the earliest theories of the inflammatory process. We

---

[1] Though descriptions of the passage of blood corpuscles from the interior of the vessels to the interstitial spaces, when blood stagnated in the frog's tongue, already appear in papers by WALLER (1846a, 1846b), the discovery of the phenomenon of diapedesis is generally attributed to ARNOLD (1875).

may say, in retrospect, that each one partly explained the four signs suggested by Celsus. The main argument to consider such views as only partial explanations of the phenomenon came from the work by a Russian zoologist, ELIE METCHNIKOFF, working at the Pasteur Institute in Paris, who started a new line of research on what may be defined as "comparative pathology of inflammation" (METCHNIKOFF, 1892).

We may call METCHNIKOFF'S view a fourth line of approach to the phenomenon since, in spite of his broad comparative outlook, his main interest focussed on the migration of leucocytes and phagocytosis:

"The *primum movens* of the inflammatory reaction is a digestive action of the protoplasma toward the noxious agent. This action, characteristic of the whole organism in protozoa, is also performed by the whole plasmodic mass of myxomycetes, but from the sponges on, it is restricted to the mesoderma. The phagocytic cells of this layer move toward, englobe and destroy the noxious agent in the case when the invaded organism becomes victorious. This phagocytic reaction, at first slow since the means of the phagocytes to get near the noxious agent consists mainly in ameboid movements, becomes accelerated in the higher forms of organization by the appearance of a blood and vessel system. Through the blood circulation, the organism at any moment can dispatch to the menaced locale a considerable number of phagocytes to stop the illness. When the circulation is done in a lacunar system, the afflux of phagocytes operates without special difficulties. But, when the defenders of the organism are contained in closed vessels, they cannot attain their objective without a special adaptation, namely diapedesis across the walls" (METCHNIKOFF, 1892).

Nevertheless, with such a definition extending the inflammatory process from amoeba and Infusoria to man, some of the connotations previously implied in the definition of inflammation became inappropriate, and the four signs of Celsus lost part of their meaning. The term "inflammation," meaning increase in temperature, the Latin from *flamma* (fire) or the Greek *phlogosis* (heat), could not be applied to the defence reaction exhibited by organisms from protozoa to the lowest vertebrates without a thermoregulatory system (fish, amphibia, and reptiles). Actually, for METCHNIKOFF, the essence of the inflammatory process was one of intracellular digestion, following phagocytosis either by the whole unicellular organism, or by special cells that would wander through vessel walls and interstitial spaces to digest in loco the noxious agent (mainly bacteria). Consequently, reduced to its elementary function—namely intracellular digestion—the process became an object of natural history studies (ROCHA E SILVA and GARCIA-LEME, 1972).

Nevertheless, the retention of the term "inflammation" for the whole field would not meet with difficulties, especially in an introduction to a volume of *Heffter's Handbook*, intended to be used mainly be medical men, or at least by research workers in the field of inflammation in vertebrates, particularly mammalian species. Given that limited connotation, the phenomenon can be understood as one of co-operative reactions of many functions of the body toward injury by physical, chemical or biological (not only bacteriological) agents. What appears to be characteristic of such "pattern reactions" is that they do not depend as much on the nature of the aggressive (or noxious) agent, but mainly on the manner by which the organism can mobilize its defensive resources. Along such lines, all of the views developed in the last century by CLAUDE BERNARD, COHNHEIM, VIRCHOW and METCHNIKOFF, with the four signs of Celsus in the background, constituted major leads to understanding the whole pattern developed by the body to fight aggression.

B. Earlier 20th Century

At the beginning of this century, an interesting view of the phenomenon was developed by immunologists, who have introduced the concept of antibody production—phagocytic stimulation (opsonization), which renders the noxious agents (germs, or foreign bodies) more vulnerable to the englobing and digestion by phagocytes. Furthermore, from the work of physiologists and immunologists an entirely new class of events (specific inflammation) became the object of intensive experimental attack. In 1902, PORTIER and RICHET (1902a, 1902b) described the phenomenon of anaphylaxis in dogs receiving extracts of poisonous sea animals (anemones and actinias). In 1903, ARTHUS and BRETON, described serum anaphylaxis in the rabbit, the local manifestation of which was further studied by ARTHUS (1909) and became known as the Arthus reaction. In 1902, THEOBALD SMITH had described phenomena of intoxication of guinea pigs reinjected with anti-diphtheria therapeutic sera, and attributed the symptoms to residues of the toxin still present in the therapeutic sera. As late as 1906–1907, OTTO in Germany, and ROSENAU and ANDERSON in the United States, affiliated the phenomenon described by SMITH to anaphylaxis, as previously described by RICHET and PORTIER, and ARTHUS. One year before, v. PIRQUET and SCHICK (1905) published the classic book on similar phenomena observed after injection of sera (serum disease), and abnormal reactions produced in humans by noxious agents. These phenomena were called allergic and later on were classified as belonging to the group of anaphylactic reactions as described for guinea pigs, dogs, and rabbits. Such phenomena of anaphylaxis and allergy appeared to belong to the broad scheme of patterned biological reactions embodied in the general concept of inflammation (specific inflammation).

To establish a bridge between the earliest views of the inflammatory process and the modern concept of 'chemical mediators,' which will be the object of the last part of this survey, nothing is more suitable than the concept of pattern reaction already explicit in Celsus' four signs.

The whole phenomenon acquired a new meaning with the notion of *autopharmacology*, introduced by SIR HENRY DALE (1933), to describe phenomena that depend upon formation, synthesis or release of endogenous active substances, the so-called mediators of physio-pathological phenomena. According to this view, most of the physiological phenomena of synaptic transmission, as well as many pathological events such as anaphylaxis, allergy and some kinds of shock and inflammatory reactions, are mediated by the release of acetylcholine, catecholamines, histamine and so forth. At the time DALE (1929) formulated his autopharmacological concept, the number of such agents that had been identified in the mammalian body was small and there was a tendency to assume that any symptom resistant to atropine, characterized by fall in blood pressure or spasm of the smooth musculature of the guinea pig ileum or uterus, might be due to histamine.

Such a broad idea of the participation of histamine came of course from the successful demonstration of a release of histamine to explain many features of anaphylaxis and allergy. It is not easy, however, to determine the origin of this idea that histamine or a histamine-like agent (H-substance) would be the agent released in many forms of injury. It is to be stressed first that DALE and LAIDLAW (1910, 1911) assumed that histamine was the main agent in anaphylaxis based on the striking similarity of its physiological or pharmacological effects. Histamine (β-imidazolethylamine) was synthesized as a chemical curiosity by WINDAUS and VOGT (1907) and extracted from putrefying mixtures by ACKERMANN (1910) and KUTSCHER (1910) and by BARGER and DALE (1910) from officinal preparations of ergot, the so-called *Ergotinum dialysatum*. But its presence in the mammalian body was not established beyond doubt before the work by BEST et al. (1927). However, we might say that the arguments put forward by DALE and his colleagues about histamine being the cause of smooth muscle spasm in in vitro anaphylaxis, were so forceful that histamine became the basis of the so-called cellular theory of anaphylaxis, in opposition to be "anaphylatoxin or humoral theory" proposed by FRIEDBERGER (1909, 1911), FRIEDEMANN (1909), and BORDET (1913). Since the work by DALE and KELLAWAY (1922), showing that the effects of anaphylatoxin on the smooth muscle were not very constant, the humoral theory entered into a decline, being defended only by immunologists. Later on, however, it was shown that both theories were not so mutually exclusive, since anaphylatoxin was shown to act through a release of histamine (ROCHA E SILVA and ARONSON, 1952; ROCHA E SILVA et al., 1951; ROCHA E SILVA, 1952, 1954) and besides, anaphylatoxin shock was prevented by mepyramine (Neo-Antergan), the most specific antihistamine agent known at that time (HAHN and OBERDORF, 1950). For a review see GIERTZ and HAHN (1966).

From a historical point of view, it is pertinent to say that EPPINGER (1913) was the first to demonstrate that histamine (ergamine) produced a typical flare in human skin indistinguishable from that produced by insect bites and other irritating agents, including the antigen or allergen in allergic individuals. This histamine reaction in human skin was exhaustively studied by LEWIS and his colleagues. (LEWIS and GRANT, 1924; LEWIS and ZOTTERMANN, 1926, 1927) and became generally known as the Lewis' triple response. Owing to the analogy with the reaction by the antigen in allergic individuals, LEWIS (1927) postulated that either histamine itself or an H-substance might be released from the skin in many forms of injury, such as insect bites, and allergic reactions produced by physical agents. Although histamine had not been identified as such in skin extracts, the possibility of an analogous substance (H-like) was cautiously postulated by LEWIS (1927). Likewise, KROGH (1929) studying the production of erythema in the skin by ultraviolet radiation, observed that the agent responsible for the redness was either slowly released or belonged to a class of large molecular weight compounds, travelling a few millimeters in 24 h as a consequence of a single exposure to ultraviolet radiation. Consequently, KROGH (1929) postulated the release of a large molecular (colloidal) substance to which he gave the name H-colloid. A similar slow-diffusing substance was postulated by LEWIS and ZOTTERMAN (1926) as the mediator of the erythema produced in human skin by the same kind of irradiation. Later on, MITCHELL (1938) attempted to give a chemical basis to KROGH's idea by showing that among the products of degradation of skin proteins by direct exposure to ultraviolet radiation, a material similar to KROGH's H-colloid might be generated.

Then came the substantial evidence of the release of histamine in anaphylaxis of the guinea pig (BARTOSCH et al., 1932; SCHILD, 1936, 1939; CODE, 1939), dog (DRAGSTEDT and GEBAUER-FUELNEGG, 1932; CODE, 1939) and rabbit (KATZ, 1940; ROSE, 1941). For a review see ROCHA E SILVA (1966).

In spite of such indirect and direct evidence of the participation of histamine in the so-called specific inflammation (anaphylaxis and allergy), allergists and clinicians in general, were not convinced that histamine played a major role in the production of symptoms in humans. They had to wait until the 1940's when specific and powerful synthetic antihistamine agents were introduced by BOVET and STAUB (1837), STAUB (1939), HALPERN (1942), BOVET and WALTHERT (1944), LOEW (1947; LOEW et al., 1945) and many others, for the histamine theory to have a fair trial in clinical medicine through the use of Antergan, mepyramine, Benadryl, and so forth. For a review see ROCHA E SILVA (1978).

Though the use of antihistamine drugs demonstrated beyond doubt that certain forms of allergic symptoms and anaphylactic shock in the guinea pig were mainly due to release of histamine, it also became evident that histamine was not the sole or even the main mediator in all anaphylactic and allergic reactions. Human asthma, for instance, was resistant to the most potent antihistamine drugs; furthermore, some physiological functions that were attributed to the release of histamine, such as reactive hyperaemia and gastric secretion, were not blocked by the classic antihistamine drugs. Even some of the symptoms of anaphylaxis, such as fall in blood pressure in dogs and rabbits, were only slightly affected by the most potent antihistamine drugs.

C. Chemical Mediators: Further Development

One might say that the advent of such powerful and specific antihistamine drugs gave the tool needed to test the participation of histamine in many forms of physiological and pathological reactions, stimulating the search for the other endogenous principles that have since been discovered. One of the reasons for the failure of classic antihistamine drugs to prevent the effects of histamine on gastric secretion, on the mammalian heart and perhaps on blood pressure, became evident through the work of ASH and SCHILD (1966) who described two different histamine receptors: H_1 in the guinea pig gut and lung, and H_2 in the guinea pig atria and acting in gastric secretion. This suggestion was recently confirmed by BLACK et al. (1972) who found a number of compounds with a specific antagonistic action upon H_2-receptors—the burimamide, metiamide, and cimetidine series. However, the forecast that the effects of histamine on blood pressure might depend upon H_2-receptors, was not fully confirmed, and apparently both types of receptors mediate the effects of histamine on blood pressure and vascular permeability (OWEN and PARSONS, 1974; OWEN, 1975).

The other reason for the failure of antihistamine drugs in many reactions that were attributed to the release of histamine was the possible participation of other endogenous agents still unknown in the earliest days of anaphylaxis and allergy. As said above, any reaction involving a fall in blood pressure and spasm of the smooth musculature, and resistant to atropine, was tentatively attributed to histamine or to an H-like substance. Actually, a series of papers in the 1930s and 1940s were dedicated to demonstrating the release of histamine in many forms of injury, following the lead of LEWIS (1927) who demonstrated the release of histamine by noxious agents. For reviews see VUGMAN (1966) and BERALDO and DIAS DA SILVA (1966).

The discovery of other autopharmacological agents greatly reduced the importance of histamine in many reactions to injury, with the exception of specific inflammation (anaphylaxis and allergy). Into this category fell the symptoms induced by toxins and animal venoms, proteolytic enzymes, ultraviolet radiation, trauma, and certain forms of allergy, such as asthma, eczema and shock. The effects of trypsin and other proteases, as well as of venoms and toxins, deserves a special mention. Trypsin was found to release histamine (ROCHA E SILVA, 1939, 1940a) and to act upon smooth muscle in a way strikingly similar to that of in vitro anaphylaxis. It also produced a fall in blood pressure in rabbits, cats, and dogs (ROCHA E SILVA, 1940a, b). The perfusion of the guinea pig lung with trypsin (ROCHA E SILVA, 1939, 1940a) was shown to release histamine; a similar releasing effect was shown by ARELLANO et al. (1940) from the liver of the dog, and from cells into plasma in samples of rabbit blood (DRAGSTEDT and ROCHA E SILVA, 1941; MCINTIRE and SPROULL, 1950).

The pharmacological effects of trypsin, similar to those produced by venoms, were shown to be surprisingly resistant to the newly available antihistamine drugs. Incidentally, it was also found that in vitro anaphylaxis, and the lung spasm in guinea pig anaphylaxis, were more resistant to antihistamine agents than similar effects produced by histamine itself or by anaphylatoxin, a typical releaser of endogenous histamine (see GIERTZ and HAHN, 1966). The possibility of other endogenous agents contributing to the symptoms of anaphylaxis, and injury, was first represented by 5-hydroxytryptamine (5-HT) and almost simultaneously by bradykinin (Bk). 5-HT was shown to be 200 times more potent than histamine in producing increased vascular permeability (ROWLEY and BENDITT, 1956). Unfortunately, 5-HT was active in rats and mice, and ineffective in guinea pigs and rabbits. In humans, it was suggested that 5-HT might act as a histamine releaser; as a consequence, the hopes that 5-HT might constitute a universal mediator of inflammatory reactions fell to a low level of credibility. Nonetheless, the participation of 5-HT in some forms of inflammatory reactions occurring in rats, and the possibility of its participation in anaphylaxis in rats and mice, became an attractive hypothesis (FINK, 1956; UDENFRIEND and WAALKES, 1959). We have also to limit our claims of histamine as a universal mediator of inflammation, not only because of the limitations described above, but also owing to the fact that in some species (rabbit and mouse) histamine is an extremely inefficient agent in producing changes typical of the inflammatory process. Nonetheless, we had shown in the early 1940s that kallikrein (Padutin) would act strongly in the skin of the immature (200 g) rabbit, increasing permeability to trypan blue in situations where histamine (and an inflammatory agent such as turpentine) would be unable to increase vascular permeability (ROCHA E SILVA, 1940c).

The search for new mediators of the inflammatory reaction became a main concern when MENKIN published a series of papers on the *dynamics of inflammation* (MENKIN, 1938, 1939, 1940, 1941) describing new agents, such as "leukotaxine" and "necrosin," on the basis of specific effects of exudates obtained from the rabbit peritoneal cavity by injection of irritating agents, especially turpentine. According to MENKIN (1938, 1940) leukotaxine, a new principle isolated in crystalline form from inflammatory exudates, produced both increased vascular permeability and leucocytic migration. The increased vascular permeability was studied with the trypan blue test on the rabbit's skin. On the basis of such a test, MENKIN undertook purification and crystallization of a material claimed to be a polypeptide. The material had no effect on the isolated ileum of the guinea pig, though producing a strong blue test and attracting leucocytes. The criticism formulated by BIER and ROCHA E SILVA (1930b) and ROCHA E SILVA and BIER (1939), and presented to the 3rd International Congress of Microbiology (1939), centred on the lack of evidence of the purity of the material, and since a great number of substances can produce a positive blue spot, including many of the solvents used by MENKIN, the biochemical individuality of 'leukotaxine' was strongly questioned. However, a few years later DUTHIE and CHAIN (1939) and SPECTOR (1951) described the isolation from inflammatory exudates and hydrolysates of fibrin by pepsin, of polypeptide fractions, some of which were active in producing a positive blue test. Concomitantly, MILES and MILES (1952) questioned the separate identity of leukotaxine, assuming that MENKIN'S extracts might act in the blue test by releasing histamine. In fact histamine itself, when injected intracutaneously in rabbits and guinea pigs, produced a peculiar blue halo surrounding a central area of ischaemia (BIER and ROCHA E SILVA, 1939a), but if histamine is released from the skin by many basic substances, it may produce a more homogenous blue area, than that described by MENKIN as typical of leukotaxine (MILES and MILES, 1952; ROCHA E SILVA and DRAGSTEDT, 1941; BIOZZI et al., 1948; MILES and WILHELM, 1960; WILHELM, 1962, 1969). All kinds of histamine releasing agents (basic compounds, ovomucoid, compound 48/80 and so forth), when injected intradermally, elicit a strong positive blue test. Furthermore, as mentioned above, many of the solvents used by MENKIN (pyridine, xylene, chloroform, and so forth) would also produce a blue test and since, according to MENKIN, leukotaxine had no other observable biological activity, its existence became highly questionable.

Nonetheless, according to FELDBERG (personal communication) the merit of MENKIN'S work resided in the fact that he called attention to the possibility of participation of polypeptides in the inflammatory process, especially in the increase of vascular permeability. In fact, by the time MENKIN was having problems with leukotaxine, the possibility of a polypeptide material derived from a precursor in plasma by the action of the venom of *Bothrops jararaca* and by trypsin, was described with the name of bradykinin, by ROCHA E SILVA et al. (1949) and ROCHA E SILVA and BERALDO (1949).

Bk and bradykininogen (Bkg) became possible mediators of some of the signs of inflammation ever since ROCHA E SILVA (1955), VAN ARMAN (1955) and SCHACHTER (1960, 1961) indicated that Bk might have strong vascular permeability activity, and since a correlation could be established between its effects on blood pressure, on the ileum of the guinea pig and its effect of increasing vascular permeability (blue test), it became quite possible that Bk might be a strong candidate as a mediator of inflammatory reactions. This was confirmed when Bk was obtained in pure form (ANDRADE and ROCHA E SILVA, 1956; ELLIOTT et al., 1960a, 1960b, 1961) and synthesized by the SANDOZ group (BOISSONNAS et al., 1960; BOISSONNAS, 1962).

Even before Bk was isolated and synthesized, strong evidence was put forward by KEELE and ARMSTRONG that Bk might be identical with the pain-producing substance (PPS) obtained by shaking normal human plasma with glass ballottini (ARMSTRONG et al., 1954, 1957; JEPSON et al., 1956). For reviews, see KEELE and ARMSTRONG (1964, 1968) and ARMSTRONG (1970). Using an entirely different technique, LIM and his colleagues showed that the so-called pseudo-affective phenomenon, could be elicited by injecting Bk into the artery of the spleen (see LIM et al., 1962, 1964; GUZMAN et al., 1964; LIM, 1968).

Therefore, being a vasodilating, oedema-forming and pain-producing agent, Bk could account for the four cardinal signs of inflammation: (1) increase of blood flow, producing erythema *(rubor)*; (2) increase in vascular permeability causing afflux of the blood constituents into the interstitial spaces *(tumor)*; (3) producing pain *(dolor)*, and (4) increase in local temperature *(calor)* caused by the increase in blood flow as demonstrated by plethysmographic methods by EHRINGER et al. (1961) and KONZETT (1962).

For an endogenous material to be considered a chemical mediator in any physiological or physio-pathological phenomenon, it should—

1. be found in the tissues in amounts that can explain the observed symptoms or effects;
2. be capable of being endogenously released, by the stimulus which produces the observed phenomenon;
3. have the same universality (or versatility) of actions as the phenomenon itself, in difference species;
4. usually be destroyed in the place of its release in the interstitial or circulating fluid, in order to avoid undue accumulation in the reacting body.
5. Furthermore, inhibitors of the natural physio-pathological phenomenon should block directly or indirectly the action of the chemical mediator, or its mechanism of release.

Bk derived from a large pool of Bkg in blood and tissues by an endogenous enzymatic system that can be activated spontaneously or under the action of noxious agents (heat, acid pH, sulphated polysaccharides, peptone, dilution, and so forth), reproduces the four signs of inflammation in all mammalian species so far tested and, being destroyed by kininases present in blood and tissues, fulfils the first four requirements for a chemical mediator. Concerning the fifth requirement, there is some correlation between the action of anti-inflammatory drugs and anti-Bk actions (ROCHA E SILVA and ANTONIO, 1960; COLLIER, 1961, 1962; COLLIER et al., 1960; COLLIER and SHORLEY, 1960; GUZMAN et al., 1964; LIM, 1968) but owing to the lack of specific anti-Bk agents, the fifth requirement is still open to discussion and further experimentation, which will be the object of specific contributions to this volume (GARCIA-LEME) (see ROCHA E SILVA, 1970; ROCHA E SILVA and ROTHSCHILD, 1974).

Histamine would pass requirements 1, 2, and 4, but would only pass 3 and 5 in certain animal species, and only for the so-called specific inflammation (anaphylaxis and allergy).

5-HT would hardly comply with more than requirements 1 and 2, being able to explain inflammatory reactions in some species of rodents only (rats and mice), though it may have co-operative actions by potentiating Bk and histamine in the production of inflammatory symptoms (for instance it has been shown that 5-HT potentiates pain production by Bk, and contributes to the effects of histamine in rats, by mast cell destruction). For reviews see MOTA (1966), ROCHA E SILVA (1966), SICUTERI (1968, 1970).

Other putative mediators, such as *prostaglandins* (COLLIER, 1971; CRUNKHORN and WILLIS, 1971a, 1971b; HORTON, 1969, 1971; VANE, 1971, 1972; FERREIRA et al., 1971, 1973a, 1973b; and many others in other chapters of this volume), *high molecular permeability factors* (PF/Glob), *lymph node permeability factor* (LPF) and others, will be presented in other sections of this book. They all belong to the history of inflammation *in the making*, and many undecided peculiarities have to be solved before they go into a general framework of the history of inflammation.

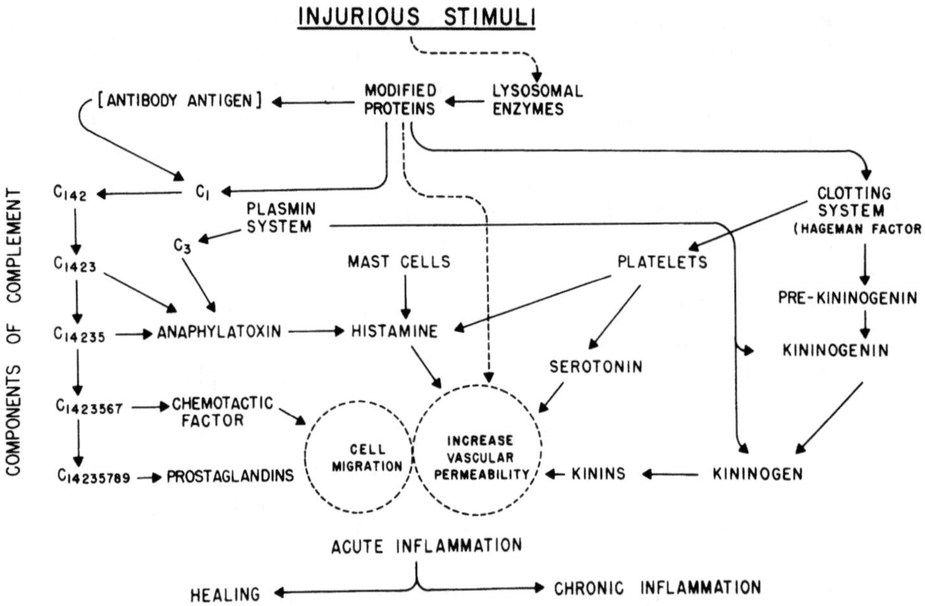

Fig. 3. Operational scheme of the multimediated inflammatory reaction (modified from WILLOUGHBY, 1970)

We have left to other sections of this book analysis of the participation of complement, leucocytic migration, chemotaxis, phagocytosis and so forth, which have lately been the object of advanced immunological techniques by KAPLAN and AUSTEN (1970, 1971), KAPLAN et al. (1972), WUEPPER (1972, 1973), WEISSMANN et al. (1973, 1975), WEISSMANN (1975), WARD (1975a, 1956b), COCHRANE (1975) and many others, and the subject of books and symposia (LEPOW and WARD, 1972; ROCHA E SILVA and ROTHSCHILD, 1973; KATONA and BLENGIO, 1975; PISANO and AUSTEN, 1976). We are also leaving to others the analysis of the participation of the so-called suicide bags of lysosomes, put forward by COHN and HIRSCH (1960), DE DUVE (1964), WEISSMANN (1975), and DOUWES (1975). This is a concept to be historically affiliated to VIRCHOW'S and METCHNIKOFF'S views that the inflammatory reaction is dependent upon misbehaviour of cells derived from the connective tissues or from blood (polymorphonuclear granulocytes, eosinophils and the macrophages or monocytes and lymphocytes) (see SPECTOR, 1975).

Our main concern in this brief historical survey has been to present the developments of the participation of the so-called chemical mediators of the acute inflammatory reaction, namely histamine, kinins, permeability factors, 5-HT, and prostaglandins, and their possible interaction in the production of the signs of inflammation. Some of the most authoritative contributors in each field will amplify the above mentioned subjects in other sections of this book.

If we consider such mediators of the acute inflammatory reaction, we obtain a definition of inflammation as a multi-mediated phenomenon, of a *pattern* type, in which all mediators come and go at the appropriate moment to play their roles in increasing vascular permeability, attracting leucocytes, producing pain, local oedema, and necrosis, and in which the extent of involvement of any one would be incidental or dependent upon its specific properties in producing symptoms—some directly, some indirectly, some by potentiating or by releasing other agents. As an illustration, I am presenting the interesting scheme of Figure 3 proposed by WILLOUGHBY (1970). "I am sure of interpreting the feelings of all contributors to this volume that it would be very unfortunate if any of the above mentioned mediators might constitute the final answer to the problem, because that would mean to shut our laboratories, or do something else" (ROCHA E SILVA, 1973). It is a known historical fact that the discovery of any new factor or scientific event, instead of closing doors, opens up new lanes to which the old ones converge amplifying views and landscapes to the future of scientific achievement.

References

Ackermann, D.: Über den bakteriellen Abbau des Histidins. Z. physiol. Chem. **65**, 504—510 (1910)

Andrade, S. O., Rocha e Silva, M.: Purification of bradykinin by ion-exchange chromatography. Biochem. J. **64**, 701—705 (1956)

Arellano, M.R., Lawton, A.H., Dragstedt, C.A.: Liberation of histamine by trypsin. Proc. Soc. exp. Biol. (N.Y.) **43**, 360—361 (1940)

Armstrong, D.: Pain. In: Erdös, E.G. (Ed.): Bradykinin, Kallidin, and Kallikrein. Handbook of Experimental Pharmacology, Vol. XXV, pp. 434—481. Berlin-Heidelberg-New York: Springer-Verlag 1970

Armstrong, D., Jepson, J.B., Keele, C.A., Stewart, J.W.: Pain-producing substance in human inflammatory exudates and plasma. J. Physiol. (Lond.) **135**, 350—370 (1957)

Armstrong, D., Keele, C.A., Jepson, J.B., Stewart, J.W.: Development of pain producing substance in human plasma. Nature (Lond.) **174**, 791—792 (1954)

Arnold, J.: Über das Verhalten der Wandungen der Blutgefäße bei der Emigration weißer Blutkörper. Virchows Arch. path. Anat. **62**, 487—503 (1875)

Arthus, M.: La séro-anaphylaxie du lapin. Arch. int. Physiol. **7**, 471—526 (1909)

Arthus, M., Breton, M.: Lésions cutanées produites par les injections de serum de cheval chez le lapin anaphylactisé. C.R. Soc. Biol. (Paris) **55**, 1478—1480 (1903)

Ash, A.S.F., Schild, H.O.: Receptors mediating some actions of histamine. Brit. J. Pharmacol. **27**, 427—439 (1966)

Barger, G., Dale, H.H.: β-Iminazolylethylamine and the other active principles of ergot. J. chem. Soc. **97**, 2592—2595 (1910)

Bartosch, R., Feldberg, W., Nagel, E.: Das Freiwerden eines histaminähnlichen Stoffes bei der Anaphylaxie des Meerschweinchens. Arch. ges. Physiol. **230**, 129—153 (1932)

Beraldo, W.T., Dias da Silva, W.: Release of histamine by animal venoms and bacterial toxins. In: Rocha e Silva, M. (Ed.): Histamine and Antihistaminics, Handbook of Experimental Pharmacology, Vol. XVIII/1, pp. 334—366. Berlin-Heidelberg-New York: Springer-Verlag 1966

Bernard, C.: Leçons de Pathologie Experimentale. J.B. Boullières et Fils, Paris 1872

Best, C.H., Dale, H.H., Duddley, H.W., Thorpe, W.V.: The nature of the vasodilator constituents of certain tissue extracts. J. Physiol. (Lond.) **62**, 397—417 (1927)

Bier, O.G., Rocha e Silva, M.: Untersuchungen über Entzündung. I. Mechanismus der Erhöhung der Capillarpermeabilität bei der Entzündung, mit besonderer Berücksichtigung der Rolle des Histamins. Virchows Arch. path. Anat. **303**, 325—336 (1939a)

Bier, O.G., Rocha e Silva, M.: Histamine as the primary cause of the increased capillary permeability in inflammation. Proc. III Int. Congr. Microbiol., p. 767. New York: 1939b

Biozzi, G., Mené, G., Ovary, Z.: L'histamine et la granulopexie de l'endothelium vasculaire. Rev. Immunol. (Paris) **12**, 320—334 (1948)

Black, J.W., Duncan, W.A.M., Durant, G.J., Ganellin, C.R., Parsons, M.E.: Definition and antagonism of histamine H_2-H_1 receptors. Nature (Lond.) **236**, 385—390 (1972)

Boissonnas, R.A.: Synthesis of bradykinin. Biochem. Pharmacol. **10**, 35—38 (1962)

Boissonnas, R. A., Guttmann, St., Jaquenoud, P. A., Konzett, H., Stürmer, E.: Synthesis and biological activity of peptides related to bradykinin. Experientia (Basel) **16**, 326 (1960)
Bordet, J.: Gélose et anaphylatoxine C.R. Soc. Biol. (Paris) **74**, 877—878 (1913)
Bovet, D., Staub, A. M.: Action protectrice des éthers phénoliques au cours de l'intoxication histaminique. C.R. Soc. Biol. (Paris) **124**, 547—549 (1937)
Bovet, D., Walthert, F.: Structure chimique et activité pharmacodynamique des antihistaminiques de synthèse. Ann. pharm. franc. **2**, 1—43 (1944)
Cochrane, C. G.: The Hageman factor: its characterization and potential participation in inflammation. In: Katona, G., Blengio, J. R. (Eds.): Inflammation and Antiinflammatory Therapy. International Symposium, Mexico 1974, pp. 119—128. New York: Spectrum Publications Inc. 1975
Code, C. F.: The histamine content of the blood of guinea pigs and dogs during anaphylactic shock. Amer. J. Physiol. **127**, 78—93 (1939)
Cohn, Z. A., Hirsch, J. G.: Isolation and properties of the specific cytoplasmic granules of rabbit polymorphonuclear leukocytes. J. exp. Med. **112**, 983—1004 (1960).
Cohnheim, J.: Über Entzündung und Eiterung. Virchows Arch. path. Anat. **40**, 1—79 (1867a)
Cohnheim, J.: Über venöse Stauung. Virchows Arch. path. Anat. **41**, 220—238 (1867b)
Cohnheim, J.: Die embolischen Processe. In: Metchnikoff, E. (Ed.): 1892
Cohnheim, J.: Neue Untersuchungen über die Entzündung. Berlin: Hirschwald 1873b
Cohnheim, J.: Vorlesung über allgemeine Pathologie. Berlin: Hirschwald 1877
Collier, H. O. J.: La bradykinine et ses antagonistes. Actualités pharmacol. **14**, 53—74 (1961)
Collier, H. O. J.: Antagonists of bradykinin. Biochem. Pharmacol. **10**, 47—56 (1962)
Collier, H. O. J.: Prostaglandins and aspirin. Nature (Lond.) **232**, 17—19 (1971)
Collier, H. O. J., Holgate, J. A., Schachter, M., Shorley, P. G.: The bronchoconstrictor action of bradykinin in the guinea-pig. Brit. J. Pharmacol. **15**, 290—297 (1960)
Collier, H. O. J., Shorley, P. G.: Analgesic antipyretic drugs as antagonists of bradykinin. Brit. J. Pharmacol. **15**, 601—610 (1960)
Cornil, V., Ranvier, L.: In: Alcan, F. (Ed.): Manuel d'Histologie Pathologique, 2nd ed. Paris: Germer-Ballière, 1881
Crunkhorn, P., Willis, A. L.: Cutaneous reaction to intradermal prostaglandins. Brit. J. Pharmacol. **41**, 49—56 (1971a)
Crunkhorn, P., Willis, A. L.: Interaction between prostaglandins E and F given intradermally in the rat. Brit. J. Pharmacol. **41**, 507—512 (1971b)
Dale, H. H.: Some chemical factors in the control of the circulation. Croonian Lectures II and III. Lancet 1929/I, 1233—1237; 1285—1290 (1929)
Dale, H. H.: Progress in auto-pharmacology. Bull. Johns Hopk. Hosp. **53**, 297—312; 312—329; 329—347 (1933)
Dale, H. H., Kellaway, C. H.: Anaphylaxis and anaphylatoxins. Phil. Trans. B **211**, 273—315 (1922)
Dale, H. H., Laidlaw, P. P.: The physiological action of β-iminazolylethylamine. J. Physiol. (Lond.) **41**, 318—344 (1910)
Dale, H. H., Laidlaw, P. P.: Further observations on the action of β-iminazolylethylamine. J. Physiol. (Lond.) **43**, 182—195 (1911)
De Duve, C.: Lysosomes and cell injury. In: Thomas, L., Uhr, J. W., Grant, L. (Eds.): Injury, Inflammation and Immunity, pp. 283—311. Baltimore: Williams and Wilkins Co. 1964
Douwes, F. R.: Metabolic deviation of polymorphonuclear leukocytes in rheumatological diseases. In: Katona, G., Blengio, J. R. (Eds.): Inflammation and Antiinflammatory Therapy. International Symposium, Mexico 1974, pp. 19—29. New York: Spectrum 1975
Dragstedt, C. A., Gebauer-Fuelnegg, E.: Studies in anaphylaxis. I. The appearance of a physiologically active substance during anaphylactic shock. Amer. J. Physiol. **102**, 512—519 (1932)
Dragstedt, C. A., Rocha e Silva, M.: Effect of trypsin upon blood histamine of rabbits. Proc. Soc. exp. Biol. (N.Y.) **47**, 420—422 (1941)
Duthie, E. S., Chain, E.: A polypeptide responsible for some of the phenomena of acute inflammation. Brit. J. exp. Path. **20**, 417—429 (1939)
Ehringer, H., Herzog, P., Konzett, H.: Über die Wirkung von synthetischem Bradykinin auf die Durchblutung der Extremitäten des Menschen. Helv. physiol. pharmacol. Acta **19**, C66 (1961)

Elliott, D. F., Horton, E. W., Lewis, G. P.: Actions of pure bradykinin. J. Physiol. (Lond.) **153**, 473—480 (1960a)
Elliott, D. F., Horton, E. W., Lewis, G. P.: The isolation of bradykinin from ox blood. Biochem. J. **78**, 60—65 (1961)
Elliott, D. F., Lewis, G. P., Horton, E. W.: The structure of bradykinin—A plasma kinin from ox blood. Biochem. biophys. Res. Commun. **3**, 87—91 (1960b)
Encyclopaedia Britannica: Vol. **12**, Inflammation. The University of Chicago: William Benton 1970
Eppinger, H.: Über eine eigentümliche Hautreaktion, hervorgerufen durch Ergamin. Wien. med. Wschr. **63**, 1414 (1913)
Erdös, E. G. (Ed.): Bradykinin, Kallidin, and Kallikrein. Handbook of Experimental Pharmacology, Vol. XXV. Berlin-Heidelberg-New York: Springer-Verlag 1970
Ferreira, S. H., Moncada, S., Vane, J. R.: Indomethacin and aspirin abolish prostaglandin release from the spleen. Nature (New Biol.) **231**, 237—239 (1971)
Ferreira, S. H., Moncada, S., Vane, J. R.: Further experiments to establish that the analgesic action of aspirin-like drugs depends on the inhibition of prostaglandin biosynthesis. Brit. J. Pharmacol. **47**, 629P (1973a)
Ferreira, S. H., Moncada, S., Vane, J. R.: Prostaglandins and the mechanism of analgesia produced by aspirin-like drugs. Brit. J. Pharmacol. **49**, 86—97 (1973b)
Fink, M. A.: Anaphylaxis in the mouse: Possible relation of the Schultz-Dale reaction to serotonin release. Proc. Soc. exp. Biol. (N.Y.) **92**, 673—675 (1956)
Friedberger, E.: Kritik der Theorien über die Anaphylaxie. Z. Immun.-Forsch. **2**, 208—224 (1909)
Friedberger, E.: Die Anaphylaxie mit besonderer Berücksichtigung ihrer Bedeutung für Infektion und Immunität. Dtsch. med. Wschr. **37**, 481—487 (1911)
Friedemann, U.: Weitere Untersuchungen über den Mechanismus der Anaphylaxie. Z. Immun.-Forsch. **2**, 591—641 (1909)
Giertz, H., Hahn, F.: Makromolekulare Histaminliberatoren. In: Rocha e Silva (Ed.): Histamine and Antihistaminics, Handbook of Experimental Pharmacology, Vol. XVIII/I, pp. 481—568. Berlin-Heidelberg-New York: Springer-Verlag 1966
Guzman, F., Braun, C., Lim, R. K. S., Potter, G. D., Rogers, D. W.: Narcotic and non-narcotic analgesics which block visceral pain evoked by intra-arterial injection of bradykinin and other analgesic agents. Arch. int. Pharmacodyn. **149**, 571—588 (1964)
Hahn, F., Oberdorf, A.: Antihistaminica and anaphylaktoide Reaktionen. Z. Immun.-Forsch. **107**, 528—538 (1950)
Halpern, B. N.: Les antihistaminiques de synthèse. Essais de chimiothérapie des états allergiques. Arch. int. Pharmacodyn. **68**, 339—408 (1942)
Horton, E. W.: Hypothesis on physiological roles of prostaglandins. Physiol. Rev. **49**, 122—161 (1969)
Horton, E. W. (Ed.): Prostaglandins. In: International Encyclopaedia of Pharmacology Therapeutics: Pharmacology of Naturally Occurring Polypeptides and Lipid-Soluble Acids, Vol. I, pp. 1—28. London: Pergamon Press 1971
Hunter, John: A treatise on the blood, inflammation and gun-shot wounds. 1794 Cited In: Encyclopaedia Britannica, Vol. II, p. 881, 1970
Jarcho, S.: Boerhaave on inflammation I. Amer. J. Cardiol. **25**, 244—246 (1970a)
Jarcho, S.: Boerhaave on inflammation II. Amer. J. Cardiol. **25**, 480—482 (1970b)
Jarcho, S.: Albrecht von Haller on inflammation. Amer. J. Cardiol. **25**, 707—709 (1970c)
Jarcho, S.: Ganbius on inflammation I. Amer. J. Cardiol. **26**, 192—195 (1970d)
Jarcho, S.: Ganbius on inflammation II. Amer. J. Cardiol. **26**, 406—408 (1970e)
Jarcho, S.: John Hunter on inflammation. Amer. J. Cardiol. **26**, 615—618 (1970f)
Jarcho, S.: Macartney on inflammation I. Amer. J. Cardiol. **27**, 212—214 (1971a)
Jarcho, S.: Macartney on inflammation II. Amer. J. Cardiol. **27**, 433—435 (1971b)
Jarcho, S.: William Addison on blood vessels and inflammation (1840—1841). Amer. J. Cardiol. **27**, 670—672 (1971c)
Jarcho, S.: Cohnheim on inflammation I. Amer. J. Cardiol. **29**, 247—249 (1972a)
Jarcho, S.: Cohnheim on inflammation II. Amer. J. Cardiol. **29**, 546—547 (1972b)
Jarcho, S.: Simon Samuel (1867) on inflammation I. Amer. J. Cardiol. **29**, 860—862 (1972c)
Jarcho, S.: Simon Samuel (1867) on inflammation II. Amer. J. Cardiol. **30**, 274—276 (1972d)

Jepson, J. B., Armstrong, D., Keele, C. A., Stewart, J. W.: Pain-producing substance and human bradykinin. Biochem. J. **62**, 3P (1956)

Kaplan, A. P., Austen, K. F.: A pre-albumin activator of prekallikrein. J. Immunol. **105**, 802—811 (1970)

Kaplan, A. P., Austen, K. F.: A pre-albumin activator of prekallikrein. II. Derivation of activators of prekallikrein from active Hageman factor by digestion with plasmin. J. exp. Med. **133**, 696—712 (1971)

Kaplan, A. P., Schreiber, A. D., Austen, K. F.: A fibrinolytic pathway of human plasma. Isolation and characterization of the plasminogen proactivator. J. exp. Med. **136**, 1378—1396 (1972)

Katona, G., Blengio, J. R. (Eds.): Inflammation and Antiinflammatory Therapy. International Symposium, Mexico 1974. New York: Spectrum 1975

Katz, G.: Histamine release from blood cells in anaphylaxis in vitro. Science **91**, 221 (1940)

Keele, C. A., Armstrong, D.: Substances Producing Pain and Itch. London: Edward Arnold 1964

Keele, C. A., Armstrong, D.: Mediators of Pain. In: Lim, R. K. S. (Ed.): Pharmacology of Pain. Proceedings III International Pharmacol. Meeting, São Paulo 1966, Vol. IX, pp. 3—24. Oxford: Pergamon Press 1968

Konzett, H.: Some properties of synthetic bradykinin-like polypeptides. Biochem. Pharmacol. **10**, 39—45 (1962)

Krogh, A.: Anatomy and Physiology of Capillaries, 2nd ed. New Haven: University Press 1929

Kutscher, F.: Die physiologische Wirkung einer Secalebase und des Imidazolyläthylamins. Zbl. Physiol. **24**, 163—165 (1910)

Lepow, I. H., Ward, P. A. (Eds.): Inflammation Mechanisms and Control. New York: Academic Press 1972

Lewis, T.: Blood Vessels of the Human Skin and Their Responses. London: Shaw and Sons Ltd. 1927

Lewis, T., Grant, R. T.: Vascular reactions of the skin to injury. II. Liberation of a histamine-like substance in injured skin. Heart **II**, 209—265 (1924)

Lewis, T., Zottermann, Y.: Vascular reactions of the skin to injury. VI. Some effects of ultraviolet light. Heart **13**, 203—217 (1926)

Lim, R. K. S.: Neuropharmacology of pain and analgesia. In: Lim, R. K. S. (Ed.): Pharmacology of Pain. Proceedings III Internat. Pharmacol. Meeting, São Paulo 1966, Vol. IX, pp. 169—217. Oxford: Pergamon Press 1968

Lim, R. K. S., Guzman, F., Rodgers, D. W., Gotto, K., Braun, C., Dickerson, G. D., Engle, R. J.: Site of action of narcotic and non-narcotic analgesics determined by blocking bradykinin evoked pain. Arch. int. Pharmacodyn. **152**, 25—58 (1964)

Lim, R. K. S., Liu, C. N., Guzman, F., Braun, C.: Visceral receptors concerned in visceral pain and the pseudo-affective response to intra-arterial injection of bradykinin and other algesic agents. J. comp. Neurol. **118**, 269—293 (1962)

Loew, E. R.: Pharmacology of anti-histamine compounds. Physiol. Rev. **27**, 542—573 (1947)

Loew, E. R., Kaiser, M. E., Moore, V.: Synthetic benzhydryl alkamine ethers effective in preventing fatal experimental asthma. J. Pharmacol. exp. Ther. **83**, 120—129 (1945)

Majno, G., Pallade, G. E.: Studies on inflammation. I. The effect of histamine and serotonin on vascular permeability. An electron microscope study. J. biophys. biochem. Cytol **11**, 571—605 (1961)

McIntire, F. C., Sproull, M.: In vitro histamine release from sensitized rabbit blood cells. Evidence against participation of fibrinolysin. Proc. Soc. exp. Biol. (N.Y.) **73**, 605—609 (1950)

Menkin, V., The role of inflammation in immunity. Physiol. Rev. **18**, 366—418 (1938)

Menkin, V.: A note on the differences between histamine and leukotaxine. Proc. Soc. exp. Biol. (N.Y.) **40**, 103—106 (1939)

Menkin, V.: Dynamics of Inflammation. New York: Macmillan 1940

Menkin, V.: Note concerning the mechanism of increased capillary permeability in inflammation. Proc. Soc. exp. Biol. (N.Y.) **47**, 456—460 (1941)

Metchnikoff, E.: Leçons sur la Pathologie Comparée de l'Inflammation. Masson, G. Paris: 1892

Miles, A. A., Miles, E. M.: Vascular reactions to histamine, histamine-liberator and leukotaxine in the skin of guinea-pigs. J. Physiol. (Lond.) **118**, 228—257 (1952)

Miles, A. A., Wilhelm, D. L.: The activation of endogenous substances inducing pathological increases of capillary permeability. In: Stone, H. B. (Ed.): The Biochemical Response to Injury, pp. 51—83. Oxford: Blackwell 1960
Mitchell, J. S.: The origin of the erythema curve and the pharmacological action of ultraviolet radiation. Proc. roy. Soc. B **126**, 241—256 (1938)
Mota, I.: Release of histamine from mast cells. In: Rocha e Silva, M. (Ed.): Histamine and Antihistaminics, Handbook of experimental Pharmacology, Vol. XVIII/I, pp. 569—659. Berlin-Heidelberg-New York: Springer-Verlag 1966
Neumann, E.: Über den Entzündungsbegriff. Beitr. path. Anat. **5**, 347—364 (1889)
Otto, R.: Das Theobald-Smith Phänomenon der Serumüberempfindlichkeit. Gedenkschr. Rud. Leuthold, Berlin 1906
Otto, R.: Zur Frage der Serumüberempfindlichkeit. Münch. med. Wschr. **34**, 1665—1670 (1907)
Owen, D. A. A., Parsons, M. E.: Histamine receptors in the cardiovascular system of the cat. Brit. J. Pharmacol. **51**, 123 P—124 P (1974)
Owen, D. A. A.: The effects of histamine and some histamine-like agonists on blood pressure in the cat. Brit. J. Pharmacol. **55**, 173—179 (1975)
Pirquet, C. v., Schick, B.: Serumkrankheit. Leipzig-Vienna 1905
Pisano, J., Austen, K. F. (Eds.): International Conference on Chemistry and Biology of the Kallikrein-Kinin System in Health and Disease. Reston (Virginia) 1974. Fogarty Intern. Center Proc. No. **27**, DHEW Publication No. (NIH) 76-791
Portier, P., Richet, C.: De l'action anaphylactique de certains venins. C.R. Soc. Biol. (Paris) **54**, 170—172 (1902a)
Portier, P., Richet, C.: Nouveaux faits d'anaphylaxie ou sensibilization aux venins par doses réitérées. C.R. Soc. Biol. (Paris) **54**, 548—551 (1920b)
Recklinghausen, F. D. v. (Hrsg.): In: Handbuch der allgemeinen Pathologie des Kreislaufs und der Ernährung. Stuttgart: Enke 1883
Rocha e Silva, M.: Libération de l'histamine par la perfusion du poumon du cobaye au moyen de la trypsine. C.R. Soc. Biol. (Paris) **130**, 186—188 (1939)
Rocha e Silva, M.: Beiträge zur Pharmakologie des Trypsins. I. Wirkung des Trypsins auf die glatten Muskeln des Dünndarms und die Gebärmutter von Säugetieren. Die Freisetzung von Histamin nach Durchströmung der Meerschweinchenlunge mit Trypsin. Naunyn-Schmiedeberg's Arch. exp. Path. Pharmak. **194**, 335—350 (1940a)
Rocha e Silva, M.: Idem II. Wirkung des Trypsins auf den Blutkreislauf bei Katze, Kaninchen und Hund. Naunyn-Schmiedeberg's Arch. exp. Path. Pharmak. **194**, 351—361 (1940b)
Rocha e Silva, M.: Kallikrein and Histamine. Nature (Lond.) **145**, 591 (1940c)
Rocha e Silva, M.: Concerning the mechanism of anaphylaxis and allergy. Brit. med. J. **1952/I**, 779—784
Rocha e Silva, M.: Anaphylatoxin and histamine release. Quart. Rev. Allergy **8**, 220—238 (1954)
Rocha e Silva, M.: Bradykinin: occurrence and properties. In: Gaddum, J. H. (Ed.): Polypeptides Which Stimulate Plain Muscle, p. 45. Edinburgh-London: E. & S. Livingstone 1955
Rocha e Silva, M.: Release of histamine in anaphylaxis. In: Rocha e Silva, M. (Ed.): Histamine and Antihistaminics, Handbook of Experimental Pharmacology, Vol. XVIII/2, pp. 431—480. Berlin-Heidelberg-New York: Springer-Verlag 1966
Rocha e Silva, M.: Kinin Hormones. With special reference to bradykinin and related kinins. Springfield, Ill.: Charles C. Thomas 1970
Rocha e Silva, M.: Opening remarks. Agents Actions **3**, 265—266 (1973)
Rocha e Silva, M. (Ed.): Antihistaminics. Handbook of Experimental Pharmacology, Vol. XVIII/2. Berlin-Heidelberg-New York: Springer-Verlag 1978
Rocha e Silva, M., Antonio, A.: Release of bradykinin and the mechanism of production of a "thermic edema (45° C)" in the rat's paw. Med. exp. (Basel) **3**, 371—382 (1960)
Rocha e Silva, M., Aronson, M.: Histamine release from the perfused lung of the guinea pig by serotonin. Brit. J. exp. Path. **33**, 577—586 (1952)
Rocha e Silva, M., Beraldo, W. T.: Um novo principio auto-farmacologico (Bradicinina) liberado do plasma sob a ação de venenos de cobra e da tripsina. Cienc. Cult. **1**, 32—35 (1949)
Rocha e Silva, M., Beraldo, W. T., Rosenfeld, G.: Bradykinin, a hypotensive and smooth muscle stimulating factor released from plasma globulin by snake venoms and by trypsin. Amer. J. Physiol. **156**, 261—273 (1949)

Rocha e Silva, M., Bier, O. G.: Untersuchungen über Entzündung. II. Zusätzliche Versuche über die Beziehung von Menkinschen Leukotaxin zum Histamin. Virchows Arch. path. Anat. **303**, 307—345 (1939)
Rocha e Silva, M., Bier, O. G., Aronson, M.: Histamine release by anaphylatoxin. Nature (Lond.) **168**, 465—466 (1951)
Rocha e Silva, M., Dragstedt, C. A.: Observations on the trypan blue capillary permeability test in rabbits. J. Pharmacol. exp. Ther. **73**, 405—411 (1941)
Rocha e Silva, M., Garcia-Leme, J.: Chemical Mediators of the Acute Inflammatory Reaction. Oxford: Pergamon Press 1972
Rocha e Silva, M., Rothschild, H. A. (Eds.): Inflammation and anti-inflammatory drugs. Internat. Symp. Ribeirão Preto, Agents Actions **3**, 265—386 (1973)
Rocha e Silva, M., Rothschild, H. A. (Eds.): A Bradykinin Anthology. São Paulo: Hucitec 1974
Rose, B.: Studies on the histamine content of the blood and tissues of rabbit during anaphylactic shock. J. Immunol. **42**, 161—180 (1941)
Rosenau, M. J., Anderson, J. F.: A study of the cause of sudden death following the injection of horse serum. U.S. Hyg. Lab. Bull. **29**, 95 (1906)
Rosenau, M. J., Anderson, J. F.: Further studies upon hypersusceptibility and immunity. U.S. Hyg. Lab. Bull. **36** (1907)
Rowley, D. A., Benditt, E. P.: 5-Hydroxytryptamine and histamine as mediators of the vascular injury produced by agents which damage mast cells in rats. J. exp. Med. **103**, 399—412 (1956)
Samuel, S.: Versuche über die Blutzirculation in der akuten Entzündung. Virchows Arch. path. Anat. **40**, 213—224 (1867)
Schachter, M.: Some properties of kallidin bradykinin and wasp venom kinin. In: Schachter, M. (Ed.): Polypeptides Which Affect Smooth Muscle and Blood Vessels, pp. 232—246. Oxford: Pergamon Press 1960
Schachter, M.: Bradykinin and other capillary active factors. Biochem. Pharmacol. **8**, 178 (abs.) (1961)
Schild, H. O.: Histamine release and anaphylactic shock in isolated lungs of guinea pigs. Quart. J. exp. Physiol. **26**, 165—179 (1936)
Schild, H. O.: Histamine release in anaphylactic shock from various tissues of the guinea pig. J. Physiol. (Lond.) **95**, 393—403 (1939)
Sicuteri, F.: Sensitization of nociceptors by 5-hydroxytryptamine in man. In: Lim, R. K. S. (Ed.): Pharmacology of Pain, Proc. III Internat. Pharmacol. Meeting, São Paulo 1966, Vol. IX, pp. 57—86. Oxford: Pergamon Press 1968
Sicuteri, F.: Bradykinin and intracranial circulation in man. In: Erdös, E. G. (Ed.): Bradykinin, Kallidin and Kallikrein. Handbook of Experimental Pharmacology, Vol. XXV, pp. 482—515. Berlin-Heidelberg-New York: Springer-Verlag 1970
Smith, Theobald: (1902) Cited In: Otto (1906)
Spector, W. G.: The role of some higher peptides in inflammation. J. Path. Bact. **63**, 93—110 (1951)
Spector, W. G.: Cellular events in inflammation. In: Katona, G., Blengio, J. R. (Eds.): Inflammation and Antiinflammatory Therapy. Internat. Symp. Mexico 1974, pp. 153—156. New York: Spectrum 1975
Staub, A. M.: Recherches sur quelques bases synthétiques antagonistes de l'histamine. Ann. Inst. Pasteur **63**, 400—436; 485—524 (1939)
Thoma, R.: Über die Entzündung. Berl. klin. Wschr. **6** (1886)
Udenfriend, S., Waalkes, T. P.: On the role of serotonin in anaphylaxis. In: Mechanisms of Hypersensitivity. Henry Ford Hospital International Symposium, pp. 219—226. Boston-Toronto: Little, Brown and Co. 1959
Van Arman, C. G.: Interrelationship among some peptide precursors. In: Gaddum, J. H. (Ed.): Polypeptides Which Stimulate Plain Muscle, p. 103. Edinburgh: E. & S. Livingstone 1955
Vane, J. R.: Inhibition of prostaglandin synthesis as a mechanism of action for aspirin-like drugs. Nature (New Biol.) **231**, 232—235 (1971)
Vane, J. R.: Prostaglandins and aspirin-like drugs. In: Proceedings V. International Congress on Pharmacology, pp. 24—25. San Francisco, Basel: Karger 1972
Virchow, R.: Cellularpathologie, 4th ed. Berlin: A. Hirschwald 1871

Vugman, T.: Release of histamine by noxious physical agents, organic compounds and by metals. In: Rocha e Silva, M. (Ed.): Histamine and Antihistaminics. Handbook of Experimental Pharmacology, Vol. XVIII/1, pp. 367—385. Berlin-Heidelberg-New York: Springer-Verlag 1966

Waller, A. V.: Microscopic examination of some of the principal tissues of the animal frame, as observed in the tongue of the living frog, toad. Philosophical Magaz. (London, Edinburgh, Dublin) **29**, 271—287 (1846a)

Waller, A. V.: Microscopic observations on the perforation of the capillaries by the corpuscles of the blood and on the origin of mucus and pus globules. Philosophical Magaz. (London, Edinburgh, Dublin) **29**, 397—405 (1846b)

Ward, P. A.: The inflammatory mediators of 1974. In: Katona, G., Blengio, J. R. (Eds.): Inflammation and Antiinflammatory Therapy. International Symposium, Mexico 1974, pp. 99—109. New York: Spectrum 1975a

Ward, P. A.: Complement dependent phlogistic factors in synovial fluids. Ann. N.Y. Acad. Sci. **256**, 169—174 (1975b)

Weigert, C.: Fortschritte der Medizin, **15** and **16** (1889). Cited in: Metchnikoff (1892)

Weissman, G.: Leukocytes, lysosomes and inflammation. In: Katona, G., Blengio, J. R. (Eds.): Inflammation and Antiinflammatory Therapy. International Symposium, Mexico 1974, pp. 3—13. New York: Spectrum 1975

Weissman, G., Goldstein, T., Hoffstein, S., Chauvet, G., Robineaux, R.: Yin/Yang modulation of lysosomal enzymes release from polymorphonuclear leukocytes by cyclic nucleotides. Ann. N.Y. Acad. Sci. **256**, 222—231 (1975)

Weissman, G., Zurier, R. B., Hoffstein, S.: Leukocytes as secretory organs in inflammation. Agents Actions **3**, 370—379 (1973)

Wilhelm, D. L.: The mediation of increased vascular permeability in inflammation. Pharmacol. Rev. **14**, 251—280 (1962)

Wilhelm, D. L.: The pattern and mechanism of increased vascular permeability in inflammation. In: Bertelli, A., Houck, J. C. (Eds.): Inflammation, Biochemistry and Drug Interaction, pp. 136—144. Amsterdam: Excerpta Medica 1969

Willoughby, D. A.: Prostaglandins are added to list of key mediators. Inflammation **3**, 1 (1970)

Windaus, A., Vogt, W.: Synthese des Imidazolylethylamins. Ber. dtsch. chem. Ges. **40**, 3691—3695 (1907)

Wuepper, K. D.: Biochemistry and biology of components of the plasma kinin-forming system. In: Lepow, I. H., Ward, P. A. (Eds.): Inflammation Mechanisms and Control, pp. 93—114. New York: Academic Press 1972

Wuepper, K. D.: Prekallikrein deficiency in man. J. exp. Med. **138**, 1345—1355 (1973)

Ziegler, E.: In: Lehrbuch der pathologischen Anatomie, 6th ed., **I**. Jena: G. Fischer 1889

CHAPTER 2

The Sequence of Early Events

J. V. HURLEY

A. Introduction

When living tissues are injured, a characteristic series of changes follows in the small vessels and related tissues within the damaged area. The reaction in the first few hours is more or less independent of the nature of the noxious agent, the response being very similar after widely diverse types of injury. The sequence and interrelation of the complex dynamic changes that occur in the first few hours after injury can be appreciated fully only by examination of living transparent tissues. The changes seen in living preparations are the basic frame of reference with which information acquired by all other techniques—histological, ultrastructural, biochemical or pharmacological—must be compared in order to determine its relevance to the morphology and mechanisms of the tissue response to injury.

More than 100 years ago, ADDISON, WALLER, COHNHEIM and others described in detail the essential features of the early stages of inflammation as seen in living transparent tissues, and subsequent studies using more sophisticated techniques have added little to their findings. The reactive changes that occur in the first few hours after sublethal injury involve, in varying degree, three processes:

1. Changes in the calibre of and flow in small blood vessels.

2. Increased vascular permeability, which leads to the formation of protein-rich exudate and to local oedema. There is a consequential increase in the volume and protein content of the lymph that drains from the injured area.

3. Escape of leucocytes from circulating blood into extravascular tissues. Erythrocytes may accompany the emigrating white blood cells. In milder injuries only a few red cells escape but after more severe stimuli there may be gross haemorrhage into the damaged tissues.

Once this initial reaction to injury has developed, subsequent changes within the area of damaged tissue depend upon the severity, nature and duration of action of the injurious agent. If this is of brief duration or is rapidly and successfully overcome by the defence mechanisms of the host, the inflammatory changes will either resolve completely or subside leaving a variable amount of scar tissue within the injured area. However, many irritant stimuli are of much longer duration and tissue injury may continue beyond the period necessary for full development of the initial stages of the inflammatory reaction. In these circumstances the later changes within the injured area depend upon the nature of the noxious agent. Some types of persistent stimulus lead to massive continued polymorph migration and to suppuration (i.e. pus formation) within the damaged area; with other types of long-acting stimulus the initial stages of inflammation are succeeded by a chronic granulomatous reaction.

In the first part of the present chapter current knowledge of each of the three processes which together make up the early stages of the inflammatory reaction will be reviewed. This will be followed by an account of the phenomena involved in resolution of an area of inflammation and in pus formation. Granulomatous inflammation and the formation of scar tissue will be dealt with in Chapters 3 and 6 respectively.

B. The Phenomena of the Initial Response to Injury

I. Changes in Vascular Calibre and Flow

1. The Normal Microcirculation

a) Structure

Although the detailed pattern of the microcirculation varies in different tissues, there is a common basic anatomical arrangement of small blood vessels throughout the body. This was first described in detail by CHAMBERS and ZWEIFACH (1944). Blood enters the microcirculation via a vessel with a thick muscular wall, the arteriole, and leaves by way of a larger thin-walled venule. Arterioles and venules are joined to one another by metarterioles, which have a structure midway between arterioles and capillaries, and by capillaries. No smooth muscle fibres are present in the capillary wall, but at their origin muscle fibres encircle the metarteriole to form a precapillary sphincter. Some capillaries are large and are called preferential channels; others are small—the true capillaries.

b) Function

Blood flow through capillaries is not continuous, but occurs in a series of spurts caused by intermittent contraction of metarterioles and precapillary sphincters. Erythrocytes pass along the capillaries in single file because of the small diameter and may be deformed during their passage along the smaller vessels. Not all capillaries are patent at any one time in resting tissues, and the proportion of red cells to plasma varies in different patent capillaries—a condition known as plasma skimming.

Within larger vessels, both arterioles and venules, blood flow is divided into two zones—a peripheral zone of almost cell-free plasma, and a central stream of closely packed red and white corpuscles. This pattern is a consequence of the laminar or streamline flow in all blood vessels larger than capillaries. In laminar flow, velocity increases and lateral pressure decreases progressively from the vascular wall to the centre of the stream. As a result particles such as blood corpuscles accumulate in the central low pressure part of the stream of flowing blood, producing so-called axial flow.

Total blood flow through different tissues varies widely in different physiological states. Increased tissue activity—whether it be muscular exercise, glandular secretion or intestinal absorption—is generally accompanied by increased blood flow through the active area. The details of the regulation of this increased flow are beyond the scope of the present chapter, but it is generally agreed that the intrinsic myogenic activity of the vascular wall, and nervous and humoral factors, are the major controls of flow in arterioles and venules. However, these factors appear to be of minor importance in the intrinsic regulation of flow within the terminal vascular bed. Capillary flow appears to be modulated largely by locally released by-products of tissue activity.

2. The Changes Seen After Injury

a) Morphology

These changes can be observed only in living transparent tissue and whilst elegant and sophisticated techniques, such as rabbit ear chambers and cine-microphotography, have been used to study them in recent years, relatively little has been added to the detailed observations made last century by COHNHEIM (1882) and his contemporaries.

Immediately after injury there may be a transient constriction of arterioles. As COHNHEIM realized, this initial vasoconstriction does not always occur, and most authorities regard it as being of little importance. It is a prominent feature of mild thermal burns (ALLISON et al., 1955) and of mechanical stroking of the skin (LEWIS and GRANT, 1924), but is not seen after injuries of more gradual onset, such as ultraviolet light (GRANT et al., 1962). The next stage is a widespread dilatation of arterioles and venules and the opening up of many small blood vessels which had previously been carrying little or no blood. Blood flow through the injured area may increase as much as tenfold (ASCHEIM and ZWEIFACH, 1962). Initially, flow through the dilated vessels is extremely rapid, and as a consequence axial flow in both arterioles and venules is accentuated so that cells become packed more tightly into the central part of the rapidly flowing blood. This stage of rapid flow is of variable duration. After mild stimuli, such as the application of histamine, rapid flow lasts 10–15 min and then gradually returns to normal. After more severe injury, increased flow may last for hours and be followed by a gradual decrease in the rate of flow through still dilated vessels. As flow slows, the axial column of packed cells widens and the outer plasmatic zone shrinks progressively until flow may finally cease entirely in some vessels, which now form distended immobile columns of tightly packed cells. Stasis may persist and end in death and disintegration of the affected vessel, but in many instances flow gradually begins again and eventually returns to normal (FLOREY, 1970).

As the rate of flow decreases, leucocytes begin to appear in the marginal plasma stream of venules in the injured area and impinge from time to time on the venular wall. At first these leucocytes stick momentarily to the wall and then fall back into the flowing blood, but when the injury is sufficiently severe progressively more leucocytes pass to the periphery, hit the venular wall and adhere to it. The luminal aspect of the wall of most venules in the injured area soon becomes covered with a layer of living adherent leucocytes, an appearance which COHNHEIM described graphically as pavementing of leucocytes.

Some of the adherent cells may subsequently pass out through the venular wall into extravascular tissues. This process, leucocytic emigration, is discussed below. In injuries of mild or moderate severity, pavementing may last for several hours then gradually cease, and the affected venules return to their normal appearance.

Certain aspects of these early vascular changes require further comment.

α) Vasoconstriction and Vasodilatation

Arteriolar constriction, when present, appears to be due to a direct response of the arteriolar smooth muscle to the damaging agent. Local release of an adrenaline-like substance may also be involved (SPECTOR and WILLOUGHBY, 1960).

More is known about the mechanism of the subsequent vasodilatation. The important features of this phase of the response may be summarized as follows:

1. Both nervous and humoral factors participate in the vasodilatation seen after injury to human skin. This was first shown by LEWIS (1927) in his description of the so-called triple response to injury which is described in Chapter 20. To what extent LEWIS's findings can be applied to other tissues is not certain. Similar reflexes occur in the cornea (BRUCE, 1910) and the tongue (KROGH, 1920) but have not been identified in other tissues. It is well established that all features of acute inflammation may occur in completely denervated tissues (CHAPMAN and GOODELL, 1964).

2. Most, if not all, of the substances found in damaged tissues—which will be considered in later chapters as possible mediators of increased vascular permeability—are vasodilators. However, vasodilatation in itself does not cause increased escape of protein from the dilated vessels. Widespread and prolonged vasodilatation may occur, as for example in exercising muscle, without any concurrent increase in vascular permeability to protein. The time course of vasodilatation and increased permeability differ widely in many types of inflammation. After crush injury to muscle, for example, prominent vasodilatation persists for many hours after the permeability of vessels within the injured area has returned to normal (HURLEY and EDWARDS, 1969) and similar temporal separation of the two effects occurs after chemical injury (STEELE and WILHELM, 1966).

β) Slowing of Flow and Stasis

The cause of the slowing of flow and eventual stasis of the dilated vessels in areas of inflammation is not altogether clear. Stasis can appear very rapidly before any of the phenomena of leucocytic emigration have had time to occur (FLOREY, 1970), and the main factor causing stasis is thought to be the increase in permeability of the wall of the injured vessel. This allows plasma to escape but retains erythrocytes within the injured vessel, and the consequent rise in haematocrit leads to an increase in blood viscosity. More force is then required to drive blood through small blood vessels so that slowing of flow and, in extreme cases, stasis results. It is supposed that re-establishment of flow in static vessels is made possible by concurrent recovery of the vascular wall towards its normal state. Detailed experimental confirmation of this hypothesis is not available. Blood viscosity and the factors which govern blood flow through tubes of capillary size constitute a complex field in which theoretical predictions do not fully agree with experimental findings.

As will be described below, changes may occur in the endothelium of injured vessels, but there is no evidence that these changes are important in slowing blood flow. An auxiliary cause of stasis may be the rise in tissue pressure which follows rapid escape of fluid into extravascular spaces. This may slow blood flow by external compression of venules and small veins.

γ) Leucocytic Adherence and Pavementing

This is discussed below under the heading Leucocytic Emigration.

II. Increased Vascular Permeability

The wall of small blood vessels in most tissues is fully permeable to water and crystalloids but only very slightly permeable to plasma proteins. In the context of acute inflammation, increased vascular permeability means an increase in permeability to plasma proteins. To understand the basis of this increased permeability it is necessary to review briefly the structure and behaviour of normal small blood vessels.

1. Normal Structure of Small Blood Vessels

The thickness of the wall of blood capillaries is at the limit of resolution of the light microscope and it is only since the introduction of electron microscopy that the complex structure of the capillary wall has become apparent. The electron microscope appearance of a small blood vessel of the type found in skin or muscle is shown in Figure 1. Endothelial cells contain all the usual types of cytoplasmic organelles and in addition an extensive system of intracytoplasmic vesicles, the so-called pinocytotic vesicles, some of which appear to be continuous with the cell membrane and to open either into the lumen or into extravascular tissues. Similar vesicles are present in the periendothelial cells which partially surround the smallest capillaries, and in the smooth muscle cells in the wall of larger vessels. Adjacent endothelial cells are joined to one another by intercellular junctions of varying complexity and of approximately 15–20 nm width. Within these junctions are localized areas where the cell membranes of adjacent endothelial cells come very close together. Early studies

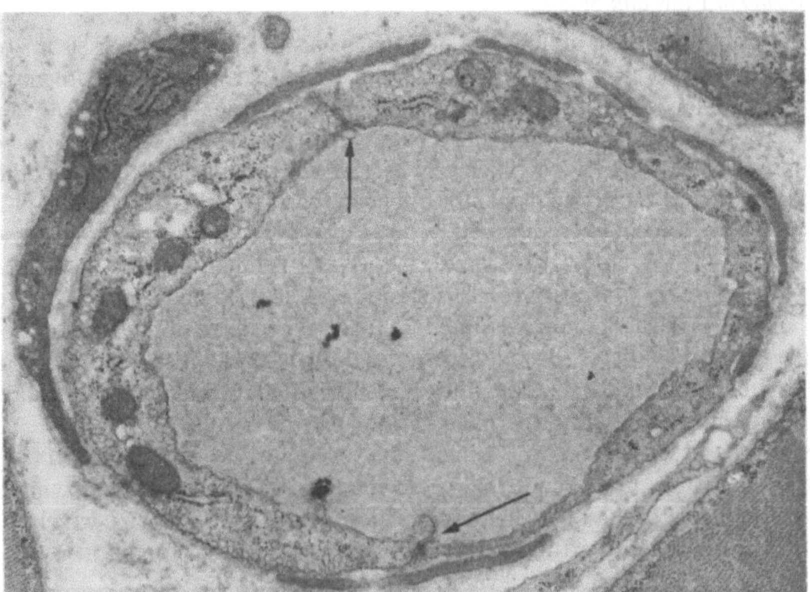

Fig. 1. Electron micrograph (EM) of capillary in cremaster of rat. Note closed intercellular junctions (↗) and numerous pinocytotic vesicles within endothelial cell cytoplasm. x 18000

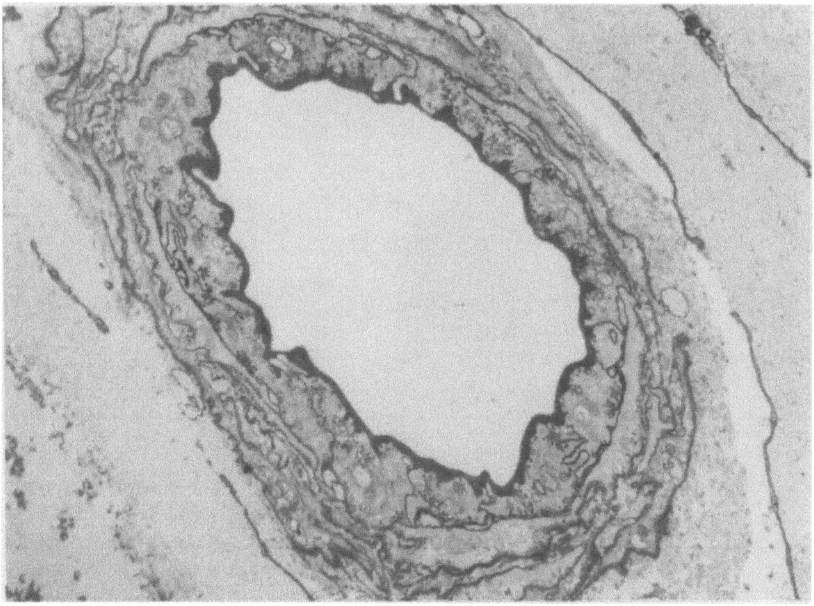

Fig. 2. EM of small blood vessel in cremaster of rat stained by alcian blue lanthanum technique of SHEA (1971). A thick darkly stained layer of amorphous material covers the luminal aspect of the endothelium. x 7000

suggested that at these sites the outer membranes of two endothelial cells have fused with one another to form a pentalaminar membrane which acts as a tight seal across the junction (FARQUHAR and PALADE, 1963). More recent studies have shown that the fusion is not as complete as was at first thought and that in fact fusion occurs at discrete spots, or maculae, and not as a complete belt, or zonule, around the endothelial cell. The only vessels in which true zonulae occludentes are present appear to be those of cerebral and retinal capillaries where the zonulae form the anatomical basis of the blood-brain barrier.

Early electron microscope studies revealed no evidence of a layer of material in the luminal aspect of endothelial cells, as was postulated by CHAMBERS and ZWEIFACH (1947), but recently it has been shown that a layer is present which can be stained with ruthenium red (LUFT, 1973), colloidal iron (JONES, 1970) or alcian blue (SHEA, 1971) (Fig. 2). Deep to the endothelium is a basement membrane which invests the vessel completely and which splits to pass on either side of the deeper layer of periendothelial cells. There is biochemical evidence that the basement membrane contains collagen but electron microscopy has failed to reveal any fibrils with the banding characteristic of collagen.

Vessels of the type just described are found in skin, cardiac, smooth, and skeletal muscle, the lung and loose connective tissues. Two other types of small blood vessel also occur in human and animal tissues. In many areas, including endocrine and exocrine glands, the kidney and the intestinal mucosa, the capillaries and some small venules are of the fenestrated type (Fig. 3). The endothelium of these vessels contains numerous thin areas or fenestrae, 0.5 1.0 μm in diameter. Here the vascular wall is

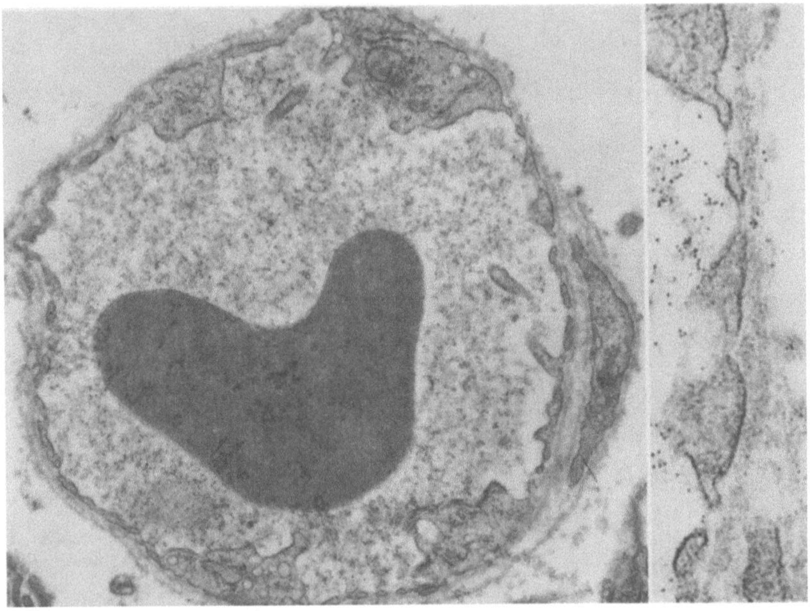

Fig. 3. EM of small blood vessel of fenestrated type in mucosa of small intestine of rat. x 16600 Insert: Fenestrae are occluded by a thin membrane. Ferritin particles in large numbers are visible in the vascular lumen and a few have escaped into extravascular space. x 50000

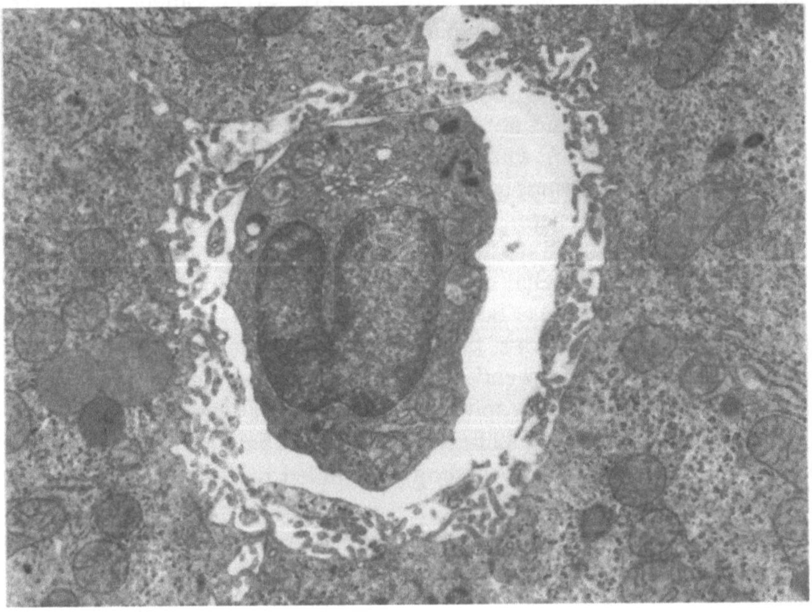

Fig. 4. EM of sinusoid in rat liver. Endothelium contains numerous deficiencies and there is free communication between the vascular lumen and the underlying space of Disse which contains microvilli of adjacent hepatocytes. x 7500

reduced to a thin membrane which appears to be continuous with the plasma membrane of the endothelial cell. After some years of dispute it is now generally agreed that fenestrae in most situations are occluded by a membrane, but those in glomerular vessels appear to be patent. Fenestral membranes are hard to stain and to visualize, so that it is not possible to say with certainty that there are no open fenestrae within a predominantly closed population. A complete basement membrane is present deep to the fenestrated endothelium.

The third type of small blood vessel is the sinusoid, found in liver, spleen, bone marrow and some other tissues (Fig.4). Here the endothelium contains deficiencies so large as to form no effective barrier to even the largest molecules. The basement membrane in sinusoids is either incomplete or entirely absent.

2. Exchanges Across the Wall of Normal Small Vessels

Materials may pass across the vascular wall by two distinct mechanisms. First molecules may move by diffusion. This will cause nett transfer of a substance only when there is a difference in the concentration of that substance on the two sides of the vascular wall. For small molecules diffusion is extremely rapid and during a single passage through the capillaries of skeletal muscle nearly all the water and 60% of the potassium ions exchange (RENKIN, 1968). Secondly bulk transfer of water and small solute molecules may occur by ultrafiltration. The mechanism responsible for this type of exchange was first described by STARLING (1896) who conceived fluid exchange across the capillary wall as a dynamic balance between the hydrostatic pressure in the capillaries tending to force fluid out and the osmotic pressure of plasma colloids tending to draw fluid into the vessels. Under normal circumstances fluid would be lost from the high pressure arterial end of capillaries and resorbed again at their low pressure venular end. STARLING's hypothesis has been fully substantiated by later workers. In 1927, LANDIS demonstrated its validity for frog capillaries by direct measurement and PAPPENHEIMER and SOTO RIVERIA (1948) did likewise for mammalian muscle.

Physiologists have made extensive quantitative studies of the behaviour of the capillary wall towards molecules of varying size. It was established early on that the overall permeability of the capillary wall to water is many times that of cell membranes, but very much less than a collodion membrane of similar thickness. In a now classic paper PAPPENHEIMER et al. (1951) established that the passage of water and dissolved solutes takes place by passive processes which require no expenditure of energy by the endothelial cells, and that the observed rate of escape could be explained by the presence in the capillary wall of either pores of mean radius 30 Å or slits of half width 18.5 Å, which in total occupied only a small fraction of the area of the capillary wall. GROTTE (1956) suggested that to explain the small but significant leakage of molecules of mol wt >40000 from capillaries in skeletal muscle, a second system of pores of diameter about 10 times that of the small pores must also exist. As intestinal vessels leak much more protein than vessels in muscle many more large pores must be present in intestinal vessels. MAYERSON et al. (1960) confirmed and extended GROTTE's findings.

As soon as electron microscopic examination of biological tissues became possible, attempts were made to identify the two sets of pores in the capillary wall which seemed necessary to explain the findings of the physiologists. After years of argument and disagreement, a general consensus as to the morphological equivalent of the small pore system has now been established. It is agreed "that the transport of small hydrophilic molecules takes place through the free space between the endothelial cells" (CRONE, 1970), and that intercellular junctions of the maculae occludentes type are the site of the small pore system in capillaries in skeletal muscle. In fenestrated capillaries additional small pores appear to be present in the fenestral membranes (CLEMENTI and PALADE, 1969).

Unfortunately there is as yet no similar agreement with regard to the large pore system. In fenestrated intestinal vessels there is good evidence that fenestral diaphragms hold back large marker particles like ferritin (FLOREY, 1961; CLEMENTI and PALADE, 1969), but are permeable to the smaller molecules of horseradish peroxidase, and it is widely believed that the large pore system in these vessels lies in the fenestrae. Whether all fenestrae are involved or only a small minority in which the diaphragm is temporarily absent, as CLEMENTI and PALADE suggest, is not clear. There is even less agreement concerning capillaries lined with continuous type endothelium. Some, of whom PALADE and BRUNS (1968) are the strongest advocates, believe that active transport of large molecules across endothelial cells occurs via pinocytotic vesicles. However, most authorities (JENNINGS and FLOREY, 1967; LUFT, 1973) believe that pinocytosis plays no role in capillary permeability. Others, impressed by the finding that horseradish peroxidase seeps through apparently unaltered intercellular junctions (KARNOVSKY, 1967), believe that these are also the site of the large pore system. A third possibility is that transient gaps, of the type known to occur in large numbers at intercellular junctions in venules stimulated by histamine-type permeability factors, appear from time to time in non-inflamed vessels. The findings of ROUS et al. (1930), LANDIS (1964), and HURLEY and MCCALLUM (1974) support this hypothesis, which would both account for the large pores required by the physiologists and be in full accord with the known functional capacity of endothelial cells. It appears that further technical advances are required before the morphological equivalent of the large pore system can be identified with certainty.

3. The Effects of Histamine-Type Permeability Factors—Vascular Labelling

The structural changes in the vascular wall which are responsible for the increased permeability induced by histamine-type permeability factors were first described by MAJNO and PALADE (1961), who found that these agents cause transient opening of the junctions between adjacent endothelial cells to form gaps 0.1–0.4 μm wide (Fig. 5). There is no evidence of concurrent damage to endothelial cell cytoplasm, and when leakage ceases the cells come together again to reform a morphologically normal junction (Fig. 6).

MAJNO and PALADE located these gaps by injecting large marker particles of carbon or colloidal mercuric sulphide intravenously before applying the permeability factor. When gaps form, plasma and circulating marker particles are forced out through the gap by the hydrostatic intravascular pressure. The plasma passes out through the basement membrane but carbon or mercuric sulphide particles are too large to do likewise and accumulate against the luminal surface of the basement membrane. The marker particles in circulating blood are removed within 30–60 min

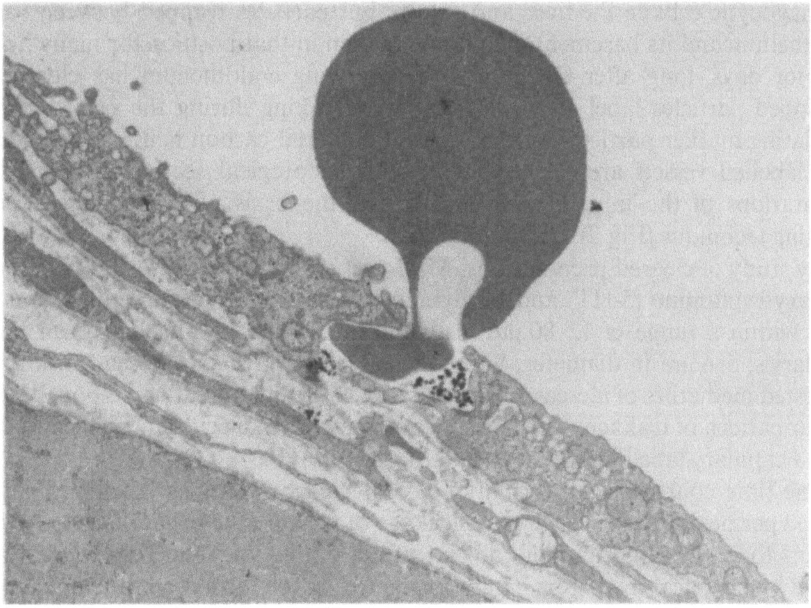

Fig. 5. Venule in cremaster of rat killed 2 min after application of histamine solution. A large gap is visible in endothelium of normal appearance. Carbon particles and portion of an erythrocyte lie within the gap. Note pinocytotic vesicles in endothelial cell cytoplasm. x 13800

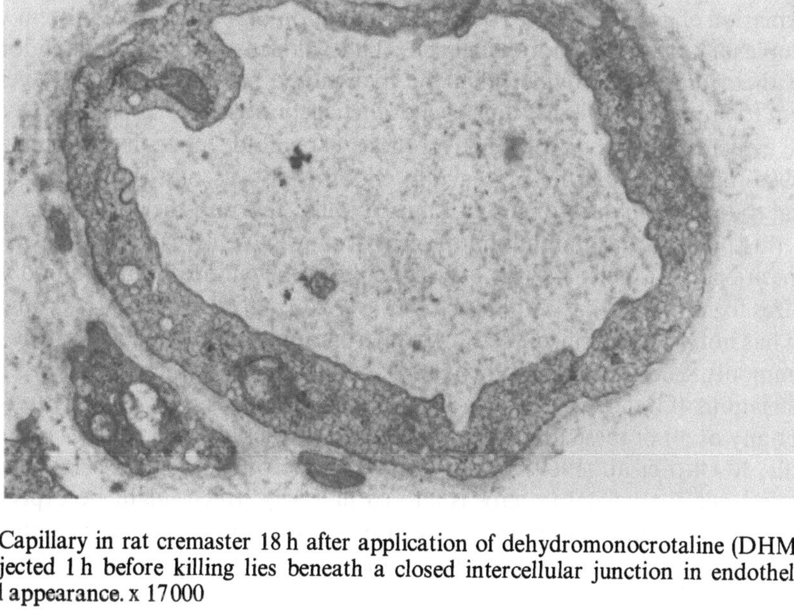

Fig. 6. Capillary in rat cremaster 18 h after application of dehydromonocrotaline (DHM). Carbon injected 1 h before killing lies beneath a closed intercellular junction in endothelium of normal appearance. x 17000

by phagocytic cells in the liver and spleen, but particles trapped between vascular endothelium and its basement membrane remain in that position for many hours or even for days, long after the gap in the overlying endothelium has closed. Such entrapped particles label all vessels that were leaking during the period in which circulating marker particles were present. If colloidal carbon is used as the marker, such labelled vessels are easily seen in both histological sections and in cleared preparations of the injured area, and this is the basis of the so-called vascular labelling technique (Fig. 7).

By study of cleared preparations, MAJNO et al. (1961) showed that histamine, 5-hydroxytryptamine (5-HT) and bradykinin cause leakage from venules and small veins within a range of 12–80 μm in diameter, but are without effect on the true capillaries, 5–6 μm in diameter. Subsequent studies have shown that all known or suggested mediators of increased permeability in the inflammatory response induce a similar pattern of leakage, with the sole exception of lysolecithin which causes widespread capillary labelling (COTRAN and MAJNO, 1964 b).

The time course of gap formation as detected by vascular labelling and of increased permeability as measured by leakage of trypan blue or ^{131}I labelled albumin appears to be the same, and all known features of the type of increased permeability caused by chemical mediators can be explained by the formation of temporary gaps in normally continuous vascular endothelium. There is no evidence that any other mechanism is concerned in the escape of protein induced by permeability factors of this type.

Further details of several features of the response to histamine-type mediators merit discussion.

a) The Cause of Gap Formation

The formation of gaps appears to be due to activation of a contractile protein within the cytoplasm of vascular endothelial cells. This will cause separation of endothelial cells at their junctions provided that the hydrostatic pressure within the vessel is sufficient to prevent its collapse during endothelial contraction.

The evidence in support of this hypothesis is twofold. First, BECKER and MURPHY (1969) demonstrated the presence in endothelial cells of a protein apparently identical to the actomyosin of smooth muscle cells. Several other groups have confirmed this finding, and immunofluorescent studies have revealed that proteins of this type are present in many types of cell, including the endothelium of blood vessels of all sizes from the aorta to capillaries (MAJNO et al., 1972). To date this contractile protein has not been identified in electron micrographs. Large numbers of fine fibrils are commonly seen within endothelial cells and sometimes these show prominent cross striations (GIACOMELLI et al., 1970; GABBIANI et al., 1975, and Fig. 8), but whether any or all of these fibrils are the actual contractile apparatus is not known. Secondly, MAJNO et al. (1969) showed that in electron micrographs the shape of endothelial nuclei adjacent to gaps is altered in a way which might be expected to follow active cell contraction, and more recently JORIS et al. (1972) demonstrated similar nuclear changes during in vivo examination of the effects of histamine on mesenteric blood vessels.

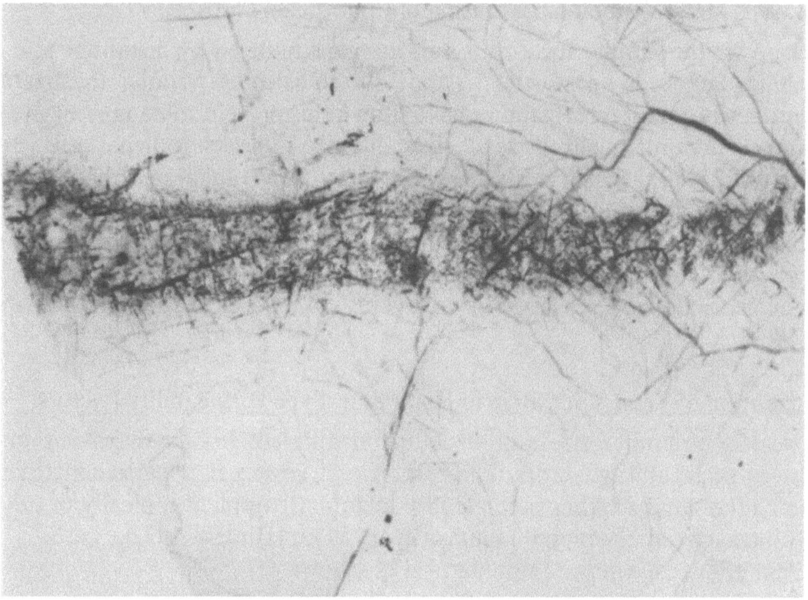

Fig. 7. Cleared specimen of cremaster of rat. Muscle was crushed with artery forceps, injected with carbon 10 min later and killed 2 h after carbon injection. Carbon deposits outline almost completely the microcirculation within the injured area. x c. 6

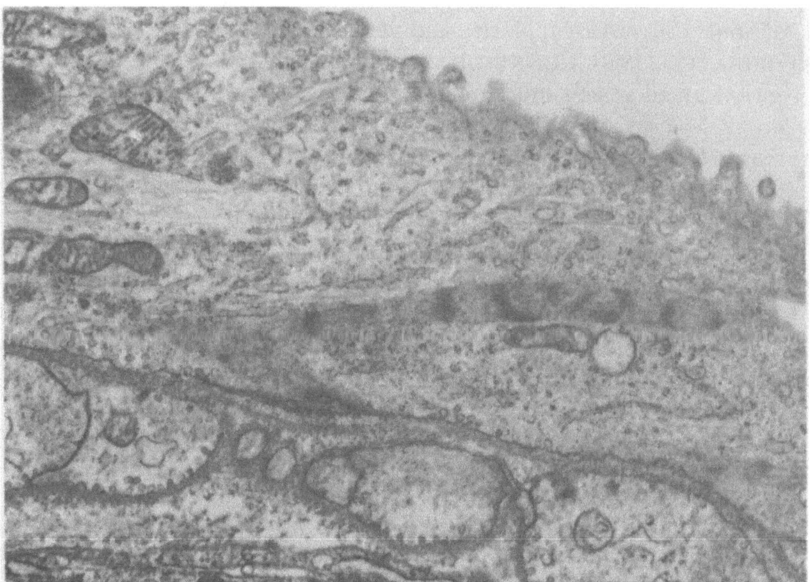

Fig. 8. Portion of wall of small blood vessel in rat skin. Endothelial cell cytoplasm contains a localized bundle of microfibrils which show prominent cross-striations. x 12000

b) The Basis of the Venular Localization of Endothelial Gaps

The reason for the venular localization of the gaps induced by histamine and other permeability factors is unknown. It is not due to selective venular localization of actomyosin, since fluorescent studies have shown this protein to be present in apparently similar amounts in vessels of all sizes and also in periendothelial cells (BECKER and MURPHY, 1969; MAJNO et al., 1972). ROWLEY (1964) suggested that gap formation might be due to local rise in intravenular pressure caused by constriction of veins distal to the area of leakage, but subsequent studies of the effects of permeability factors on living transparent tissues showed that carbon labelling develops without any constriction of either venules or veins (MAJNO et al., 1967; BUCKLEY and RYAN, 1969).

c) Distribution of Vessels Sensitive to Histamine-Type Permeability Factors

Blood vessels of similar size and structure in different tissues may vary in their response to permeability factors. The response of vessels in a particular tissue appears to be the same whether permeability factors are applied topically or administered by intraarterial injection (GABBIANI et al., 1970; HURLEY, 1972).

Present knowledge may be summarised as follows:

1. Venules adjacent to many surfaces of the body and in loose tissues are sensitive to histamine and similar agents. Such tissues include skin and subcutaneous tissues, skeletal muscle, serous membranes including pleura, peritoneum and mesentery, lip, conjunctiva and the mucosa of the trachea and large bronchi.

2. Venules in solid organs including testis, kidney, salivary gland and CNS, and vessels in the mucosa of the small intestine (HURLEY and MCQUEEN, 1971) fail to respond. However, pituitary vessels are sensitive to histamine.

3. Pulmonary alveolar capillaries and venules are insensitive to histamine-type agents (PIETRA et al., 1970; CUNNINGHAM and HURLEY, 1972).

4. Newly formed vessels in granulation tissue are unresponsive to permeability factors until 2–3 weeks after their formation (HURLEY et al., 1970).

The reason for this variable response to permeability factors is not clear, but does not appear to reflect variations in the distribution of actomyosin in endothelial cells in different organs. Whatever its cause, the phenomenon is of great practical importance in laboratory studies of inflammation. It is clear that it may be grossly misleading to draw generalized conclusions as to the mechanism of any particular type of injury from the study of its effects on only one tissue; vessels of apparently identical structure in other tissues may respond in a quite different way to the same type of injury.

4. Increased Permeability in Other Types of Inflammation

a) Endothelial Changes

Since MAJNO and PALADE'S paper was published, acute inflammation caused by many different types of injury has been studied by the combined use of the vascular labelling technique and of electron microscopy. Although findings differ in detail, the main features have been found to be similar in all types of injury, and may be summarised as follows:

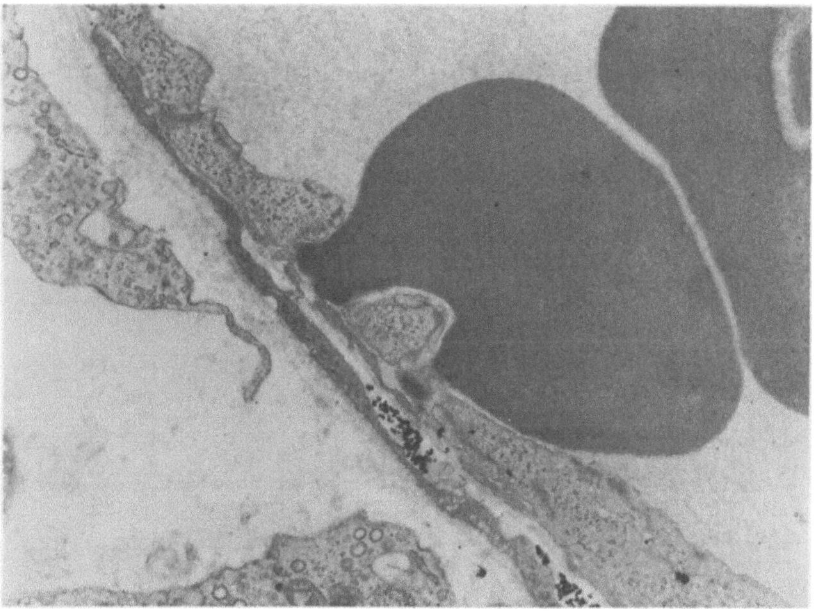

Fig. 9. Rat cremaster 23 h after injection of DHM. Portions of an erythrocyte project into two large gaps (one not quite in plane of section) in the endothelium of this venule. Extravascular carbon is visible close to the gap. Rosettes of RNA are prominent in endothelial cell cytoplasm. x 10000

1. The essential morphological abnormality in leaking vessels in all types of inflammation is the presence of deficiencies or gaps in vascular endothelium (Figs. 9–11). Deficiencies can always be found by adequate examination of the injured area during the period when vascular permeability is increased. The endothelial defects may range in size from gaps similar to those induced by histamine to total absence of endothelium over part of the circumference of the vessel.

It is important to realize that the combined use of vascular labelling and electron microscopy is a vastly more sensitive way of detecting the presence of gaps than is unaided electron microscopy. The volume of tissue that can be examined by electron microscopy is so tiny that it is impossible to exclude the presence of gaps by this technique used alone. However, even very small deposits of carbon can be detected by careful examination of cleared specimens. When subsequent electron microscope studies are made of carbon-labelled areas it is easy to determine whether the carbon lies deep to the vascular endothelium. When intramural carbon deposits are identified, this is conclusive evidence that gaps are, or have been, present, as all authorities agree that carbon particles are too large to escape through continuous vascular endothelium in any other way. Careful search will invariably reveal gaps in a proportion of the labelled vessels.

To prove that increased permeability in a particular type of injury was due to a mechanism other than gap formation it would be necessary to establish the presence of a significant increase in leakage of protein in the absence of a comparable amount

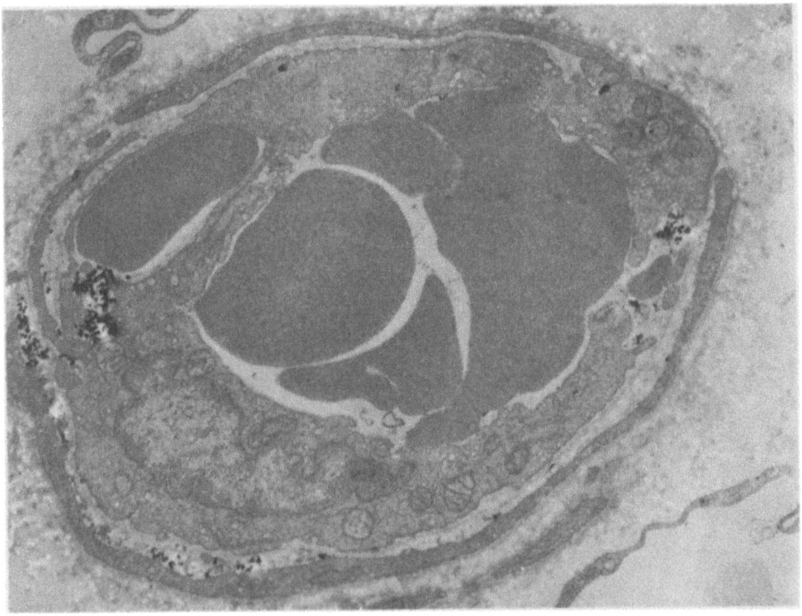

Fig. 10. Rat cremaster 24 h after injection of DHM. A large gap is present at one end of this capillary and at the opposite end an erythrocyte and aggregates of carbon particles lie under a closed intercellular junction. x 8000

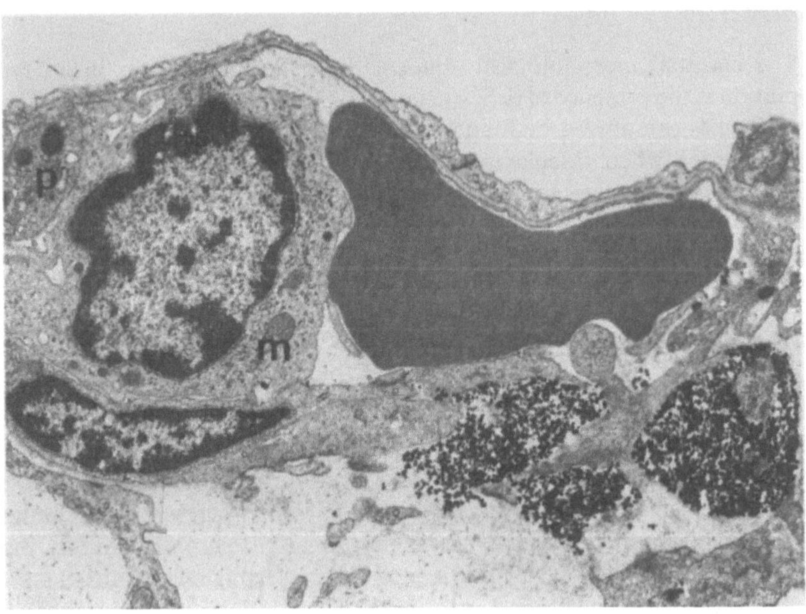

Fig. 11. Lung of rat killed 19 h after i.v. injection of 30 mg/kg DHM. A large extravascular deposit of carbon lies beneath a gap in capillary endothelium of normal appearance. A monocyte (*M*), platelet (*P*) and an erythrocyte are visible in the vascular lumen. x 9000

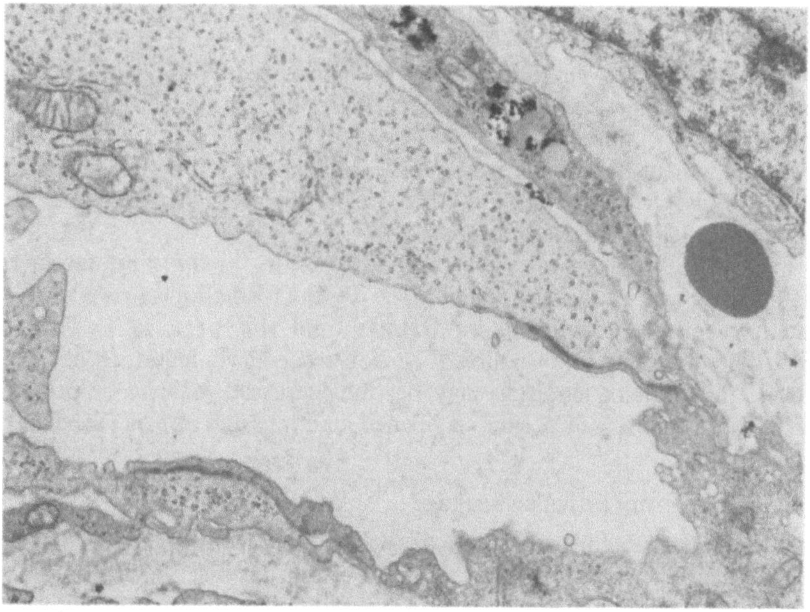

Fig. 12. Rat cremaster 53 h after injection of DHM. The cytoplasm of two endothelial cells in this venule shows well developed regenerative activity and contains many RNA rosettes. The intervening cell is little altered. Carbon injected 5 h before killing is visible in extravascular tissues and in a periendothelial cell. x 11000

of carbon labelling in cleared specimens. There is no published study which fulfils this criterion, and on the evidence available it appears that gap formation is the invariable basis of increased vascular permeability in inflammation.

2. There may or may not be ultrastructural evidence of damage to the endothelium of the leaking vessels. Severe injuries such as thermal burns or turpentine may cause early gross changes in endothelial cells. In less severe injuries ultrastructural evidence of damage may increase progressively over several hours. Examination of the later stages of many types of injury shows that even gross changes in the appearance of endothelial cells are compatible with cell survival. During the process of recovery, the injured endothelium comes to resemble closely that seen in young growing vessels, such as those in granulation tissue (Fig. 12). In mild injuries these later changes are a more sensitive index of damage than is the appearance during the first few hours after injury (HAM and HURLEY, 1968).

Recently GABBIANI and BADONNEL (1975) described irregular dilatations within the interendothelial clefts of small vessels—arterioles, capillaries, and venules—which they claim develop in the first 5–10 min after mild thermal burns. Increased permeability did not begin until several hours later. Similar changes apparently occur in the early stages of the response to intoxication with cadmium salts (GABBIANI et al., 1974), and GABBIANI and BADONNEL suggest that these changes in interendothelial clefts may be the earliest morphological equivalent of delayed increase in small vessel permeability. Further work is required to determine whether this change is an invariable precursor of delayed-prolonged leakage, and if so, what is its significance.

3. Individual vessels, the endothelium of which appears little damaged, may leak for many hours (HURLEY and EDWARDS, 1969) and prolonged leakage may also occur from severely injured vessels.

4. The basement membrane is extremely resistant to injury and may remain as an apparently effective barrier to erythrocytes and carbon particles long after the overlying endothelium has been destroyed.

5. Fenestrated vessels appear to respond to injury in the same manner as do vessels lined by continuous endothelium, i.e. by the formation of reversible gaps at the junctions between endothelial cells (HURLEY and MCQUEEN, 1971). There was no evidence that either ferritin or colloidal carbon escaped via fenestrae, and whatever the normal function of fenestrae may be, the increased leakage of protein from inflamed fenestrated vessels occurs via opened junctions and not via fenestrae.

b) The Topography of Vascular Leakage

When the vascular labelling technique was applied to different types of inflammation it at once became apparent that not all types of injury cause the venular pattern of leakage which is seen after application of histamine or similar permeability factors. Capillary labelling was first described in the delayed response to mild thermal injury by WELLS and MILES (1963) and COTRAN and MAJNO (1964a), and subsequent studies have shown that vascular labelling patterns vary widely in different types of injury and even in different stages of the response to a single damaging agent. In some instances labelling is purely venular, in others it is virtually restricted to capillaries and in others still it involves vessels of all sizes within the area of injury.

Several aspects of this variable pattern of vascular labelling require more detailed discussion.

α) The Nature of Capillary Labelling

Whilst electron microscope studies have shown that, with very rare exceptions, the carbon in all labelled venules is intramural and thus a true indicator of increased vascular permeability, three distinct types of carbon labelling of capillaries have been identified, which can be distinguished definitely only by electron microscopy or careful study of 1 μm sections:

1. Intramural carbon deposits similar to those found in venules. These must reflect protein leakage from capillaries, but this type of deposit is found in only a minority of labelled capillaries in many types of injury, including the delayed response to thermal injury (COTRAN, 1965; HAM and HURLEY, 1968) or X-irradiation (HURLEY, HAM and RYAN, 1969) and the immediate response to crushing injury (HURLEY and EDWARDS, 1969). In a few instances, however, virtually all labelled capillaries contain intramural deposits of this type—for example with pulmonary oedema induced by either alphanaphthyl thiorurea (ANTU) (CUNNINGHAM and HURLEY, 1972) or dehydromonocrotaline (DHM) (HURLEY and JAGO, 1975) and with the effects of DHM on cremasteric vessels (HURLEY and JAGO, 1976) (Fig. 6).

2. Intraluminal plugs of carbon which either alone or admixed with platelets and fibrin entirely occlude capillaries (Fig. 13). These were first described in turpentine-

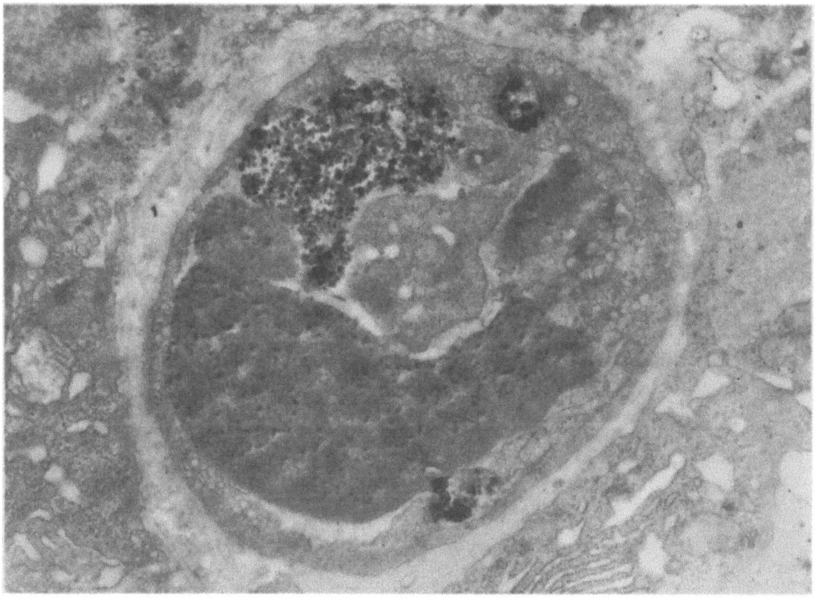

Fig. 13. Capillary in rat cremaster killed 24 h after severe crush injury. Carbon injected 22 h before killing is visible in vacuoles in endothelial cell cytoplasm, and together with platelets and an erythrocyte forms a plug which occludes the vascular lumen. x 20000

induced pleurisy by HURLEY and SPECTOR (1965) who found that the degree and time course of capillary labelling in this system bore no apparent relationship to the time course of increased vascular permeability. Despite prolonged search, HAM and HURLEY (1965) were unable to find a single instance of a defect in the capillary endothelium in relation to these plugs, which appear to reflect endothelial injury and in no way to be related to increased capillary permeability.

3. Carbon labelled capillaries in which intraluminal plugs are associated with obvious defects in the vascular endothelium (Fig. 14) and sometimes with intramural carbon deposition as well (Fig. 15). This is the most common form of capillary labelling in many types of injury, including mild thermal burns, X-ray and chemical injuries and crushing injury, and there has been disagreement about its significance. Many, including the present writer, feel that such labelled capillaries are a valid index of increased capillary permeability, but others, notably COTRAN (1967) and SHEA et al. (1973) consider that such labelled capillaries contribute little or nothing to fluid leakage which they believe occurs mainly from the much smaller number of labelled venules also present within the area of injury.

Recently WELLS (1971, 1972) has provided important new evidence as to the significance of this kind of capillary labelling. WELLS made a detailed histological study of the capillary labelling that follows local injection of *Cl. perfringens α toxin* or mild thermal injury to the rat cremaster, and reported a close correlation between the duration of exposure to circulating carbon and the proportion of labelled capillaries plugged with carbon. When the interval between injection of carbon and killing the animal was 1 h or more, most carbon appeared as intraluminal plugs;

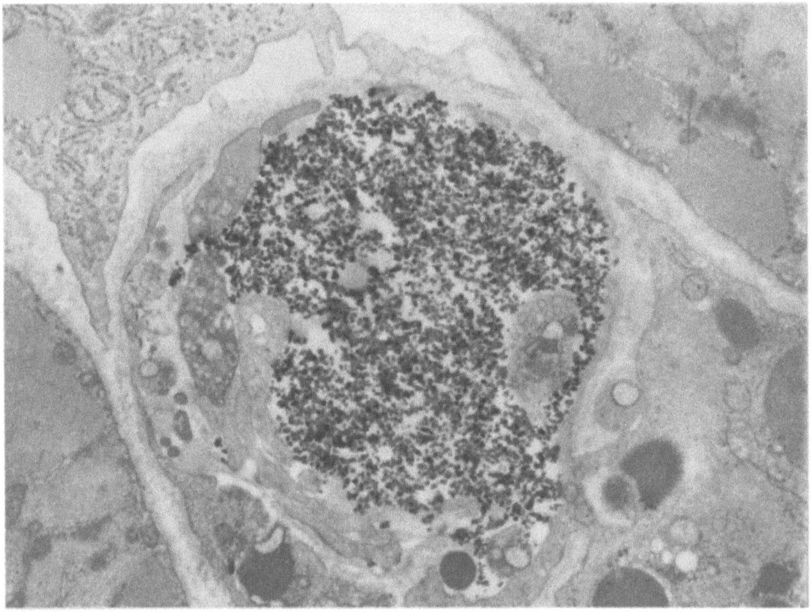

Fig. 14. Capillary in rat cremaster 23 h after injection of DHM. Carbon injected 1 h before killing. Multiple gaps are present in severely damaged endothelium. Lumen is filled with carbon and some has spread into extravascular tissues. x 12000

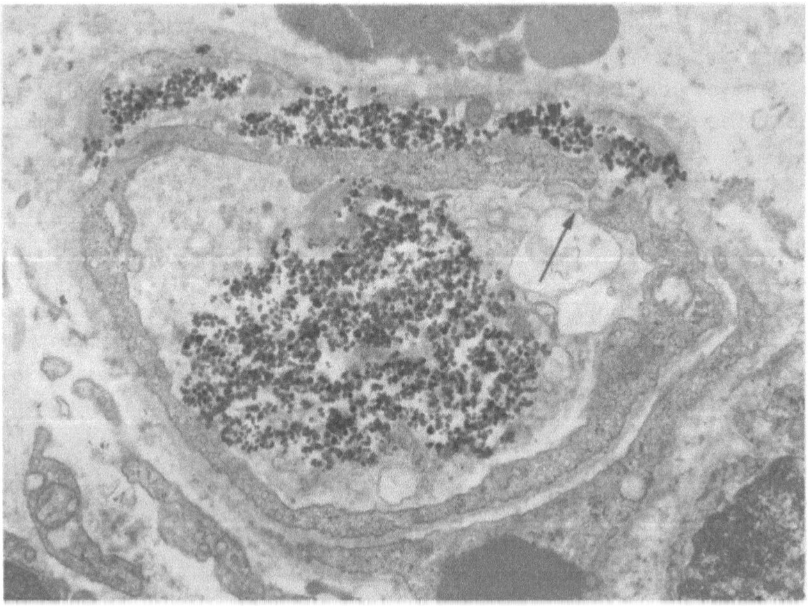

Fig. 15. Rat cremaster 20 h after injection of DHM. Carbon injected 1 h before killing. Endothelium of this capillary appears normal apart from presence of a gap (↗). Carbon is present in the vascular wall beneath gap and as a plug in the lumen. x 20000

when exposure to carbon was restricted to 10 min, the intensity of carbon labelling was less and the carbon in most labelled capillaries formed a well-defined layer superimposed on the vascular wall. WELLS considers that carbon in plugged capillaries may accumulate by accretion to pre-existing intramural deposits trapped by an inelastic capillary basement membrane at a gap proximal to the line of flow and hence not seen by electron microscopy. WELLS's studies were made on 5 µm paraffin-embedded sections where it is often not possible to be sure of the precise relationship of carbon deposits to the wall of vessels as small as capillaries. In as yet unpublished experiments, we have confirmed WELLS's findings in both 1 µm sections and by electron microscopy for thermal burns and for injury due to *Cl. perfringens α toxin.* It appears probable that WELLS's hypothesis is of general application and that the contribution of leakage from capillaries to increased vascular permeability has been grossly underestimated by both COTRAN and SHEA, but further work is needed to decide this issue finally.

β) The Significance of Variations in Vascular Labelling Patterns

The two outstanding findings of the vascular labelling studies outlined above are:

1. The action of all known or suggested mediators of increased vascular permeability in inflammation is restricted to venules and small veins.

2. Leakage in many of the types of injury examined involves both capillaries and venules, the apparent relative contributions to total leakage of the two types of vessel showing wide variation in different types of injury.

There would appear to be only three possible explanations of these findings:

1. That mediators as yet unidentified, exist that are capable of increasing the permeability of capillaries.

2. That the circumstances of a single injection into healthy tissues are not comparable to those of continuing production of an endogenous permeability factor during the course of inflammation, and hence in other circumstances known mediators might be able to affect capillaries as well as venules. The evidence available does not support this possibility. For example, the phase of leakage that follows immediately after many types of injury is believed to be mediated by release of histamine (SPECTOR and WILLOUGHBY, 1963), and the time course and labelling pattern of this phase of leakage are identical with those following a single injection of histamine into the injured tissue.

3. That some mechanism other than the release of endogenous chemical mediators plays a role in increased vascular permeability in inflammation. The only real possibility here is some type of direct vascular response to the injurious stimulus.

c) The Role of Direct Vascular Injury in Increased Permeability

It is well established that bacterial, chemical or physical injury of sufficient severity can damage the vascular wall directly. For example, it has been known for many years that the major part of the fluid loss in severe thermal burns is caused in this way. The characteristics of this type of leakage were described by COTRAN and MAJNO (1964b): leakage begins instantly after injury and affects all small vessels, arterioles, capillaries, and venules within the damaged area; individual vessels may leak for 24 h or more and, electron microscope examination shows obvious and severe damage to endothelial cells.

Lesser degrees of injury by the same agents produce leakage with a quite different time course. There may be a brief initial phase of increased permeability which appears to be histamine-mediated, but the major phase of leakage does not begin for some time after injury, and once started persists for several hours. This type of increased permeability is commonly called delayed-prolonged leakage. It was first described in mild thermal injury by SEVITT (1958), and subsequently has been shown to occur, with a variable time course, after injuries due to cold, ultraviolet light, X-irradiation and certain bacterial toxins and other chemical agents. Carbon labelling studies have shown that the labelling pattern in the delayed-prolonged response varies with both the damaging stimulus and with the tissue which is injured. In a few instances, leakage occurs only from venules as in turpentine-induced pleurisy (HURLEY and SPECTOR, 1965) or after injection of carrageenin (HURLEY and WILLOUGHBY, 1973), but more commonly capillaries are also involved—either almost alone as in mild thermal injury (COTRAN and MAJNO, 1964a; WELLS and MILES, 1963), or together with venules as in X-ray injury (HURLEY, HAM and RYAN, 1969) or in the delayed response to clostridial toxins (COTRAN, 1967) or DHM (HURLEY and JAGO, 1976). As discussed above, it is now certain that in at least some of these types of injury, capillary labelling in the delayed-prolonged response is a valid index of leakage from capillaries, which cannot be explained by the action of any known endogenous chemical mediator.

After studying the different vascular patterns of mild thermal injury to skin and to muscle, HURLEY, HAM and RYAN (1967) suggested that the delayed phase of leakage in this type of injury was due to a delayed manifestation of direct vascular damage, and gave detailed evidence in support of this hypothesis. After several further types of delayed-prolonged response had been examined by the same techniques as those used for thermal burns, HURLEY (1972) suggested that direct vascular injury played a more important role in increased permeability in inflammation than had been thought by previous workers, and laid down criteria by which leakage due to direct vascular injury could be identified.

1. Labelling should be confined strictly to the injured area.

2. The pattern of leaking vessels should reflect not vascular calibre but the intensity of injury to which individual vessels are exposed. The pattern of labelling will depend upon the anatomy of the microcirculation in the injured area and the degree of penetration of the damaging agent. The same type of injury may cause different patterns of labelling in different tissues.

3. There should be electron microscopic evidence of damage to endothelial cells. These changes take time to develop and may be more apparent at 24–28 h than in the first few hours after injury.

If these criteria be accepted, the present state of knowledge may be summarized as follows:

1. The delayed-prolonged response in many types of injury is due to direct vascular damage. Thermal burns, X-ray injury, ultraviolet injury, and the delayed effects of clostridial toxins and certain other chemical substances fall into this category, as do those types of pulmonary oedema induced by ANTU or DHM.

2. The delayed phase of leakage after intrapleural injection of turpentine or other irritants (HURLEY and RYAN, 1967) or of injection of carrageenin, has the characteristics of a mediated type of response.

3. Too little is known of the morphological aspects of many widely used experimental models of acute inflammation to assess the relative roles of endogenous chemical mediators and direct vascular injury in these types of inflammation.

Knowledge of the mechanisms responsible for increased vascular permeability after injury might advance more rapidly if, in future experiments, attention is paid to the relative roles of direct vascular injury and endogenous chemical factors, rather than to the search for still other potential permeability mediators.

d) The Nature of Direct Vascular Injury

Little is known of the intimate nature of direct vascular injury. The electron microscope appearances of the leaking vessels show that a mechanism is required which will cause separation of injured endothelial cells at their intercellular junctions. In severe injuries, total destruction of some endothelial cells may occur. However, in the majority of leaking vessels in severe injuries and in all leaking vessels after milder degrees of injury which evoke a delayed-prolonged form of increased permeability, the degree of endothelial injury is slight—in some instances so slight that it is hard to recognize by electron microscopy in the first hours after injury.

If histamine-type permeability factors induce endothelial cells to separate by stimulation of a contractile protein within endothelial cell cytoplasm, then direct vascular injury might also cause contraction of intracellular actomyosin. Smooth muscle fibres will respond to a direct pinch in the same way as to application of acetylcholine, hence vascular endothelium might respond similarly to direct injury and to histamine-type mediators. Such direct stimulation could account for leakage that begins immediately after injury, but some additional hypothesis is required to explain leakage that is due to direct vascular injury but which does not begin for hours or even days after injury.

The situation is analagous to the reaction of liver cells to chemical toxins. Whilst the initial lesion liver cells produced by carbon tetrachloride has still not been identified for certain, it is well established that there is an interval of some hours between the time at which the damaging agent reaches the liver and the time at which functional and ultrastructural abnormalities are first detectable in liver cells (McLEAN et al., 1964). A further similarity between carbon tetrachloride-induced liver injury and increased vascular permeability due to direct injury to the endothelium is the finding by RYAN and HURLEY (1968) that drugs which protect liver cells against toxic chemicals also suppress the vascular leakage which follows mild thermal injury to skin or muscle. In more severe burns, 56° for 27 s, suppression of fluid leakage by drugs was significant but not complete, indicating that there is an upper limit to the protective action of the drugs used.

If changes basically similar to those in damaged liver cells occur in injured endothelium it is possible that when disturbance of some aspect of cell metabolism reaches a critical level, activation of intracellular actomyosin may occur. Alternatively, the delayed type of increased permeability due to direct endothelial injury might not be due to activation of actomyosin but result from a quite different change in endothelial cells. For example, injury might cause damaged endothelial cells to swell and to assume a more spherical shape. This change in shape, perhaps assisted by some loosening of intercellular junctions, might result in separation of adjacent endothelial cells. Against this suggestion is the absence of any apparent correlation in electron micrographs of individual vessels between the degree of endothelial swelling and leakage of marker particles. In either of the above hypotheses, the disturbance of endothelial cell metabolism would have to be reversible and not such as to cause later death of the injured cell.

Although we have as yet no knowledge of the metabolism of injured endothelial cells, enough is known of the time course of injury to other types of cell to make it certain that there is nothing unusual about the existence of an interval of several hours between injury to endothelium and the appearance of its functional consequence—increased permeability. When more is known of the intracellular consequences of injury, the way in which damage to endothelial cells causes the delayed phase of increased vascular permeability in acute inflammation may become clear.

III. Leucocytic Emigration

Observation of living transparent tissue shows that following injury there is a striking and consistent pattern of behaviour of leucocytes passing through the small blood vessels of the damaged area. This was first described in detail by COHNHEIM (1882).

Soon after injury, leucocytes begin to leave the axial column of blood cells, to appear in the marginal plasma stream and to impinge from time to time on the venular wall. At first the leucocytes stick momentarily to the wall, may roll along it for a short distance and then fall back into the passing stream of blood. As the reaction progresses, more leucocytes pass to the periphery of the stream, hit the venular wall and adhere to it for longer periods, until before long the luminal surface of many venules within the inflamed area becomes covered with a layer of living adherent leucocytes—an appearance described as pavementing by COHNHEIM.

With injuries of moderate severity, many of the adherent leucocytes subsequently pass out through the venular wall into the extravascular tissues by a process known as leucocytic emigration. Having reached the extravascular space these cells may wander about at random or move in an apparently directed manner towards a focus of damaged tissue or a clump of bacteria. This directed movement is believed to occur under the influence of chemical concentration gradients and is known as chemotaxis.

It is convenient to discuss the details of the three stages of leucocytic behaviour—pavementing, emigration, and chemotaxis—in turn.

1. Pavementing of Leucocytes

This aspect of leucocytic behaviour can be studied only in living tissues, and many aspects of the phenomenon are still obscure. Impingement of leucocytes on the venular wall occurs not only in inflammation but also from time to time in undamaged tissues. In normal vessels, the leucocytes bounce off the wall again back into the blood stream. Leucocytic sticking in inflamed vessels depends upon some alteration in the vascular wall and not in the adhering leucocytes. This can be shown by localizing injury to one side of a venule in an ear chamber, when cells are seen to adhere only to the damaged side of the vessel (ALLISON et al., 1955), or by using a stimulus such as ultraviolet light (FLOREY and GRANT, 1961). In this type of injury leucocytic sticking does not begin until several hours after exposure to the damaging agent has ceased. It is inconceivable that the few leucocytes present in vessels within the ear chamber during the brief exposure to ultra-violet light are the same cells that adhere to the damaged venules some hours later.

However, the nature of the endothelial change responsible for leucocytic sticking is not known. CLARK et al. (1936) made a careful and prolonged study of vessels in the tadpole's tail and concluded that sticking of leucocytes was seen so frequently after mild, often unrecognized, stimuli that the causative change in the vascular wall must be a normal and reversible one which is not accompanied by damage to endothelium. Prior to the advent of electron microscopy, both CHAMBERS and ZWEIFACH (1940, 1947) and McGOVERN (1955, 1956a, b) suggested that endothelial cells secrete a gelatinous material on their inner surface, and that alterations in this material might account for the adherence of leucocytes to inflamed venules. Early electron microscopists found no evidence of such a layer inside endothelial cells, but it is now clear that an endocapillary layer does exist, which, as described above, can be stained by several different methods. The chemical nature of this layer is not known but it has similar staining characteristics to the glycocalyx which surrounds most, if not all, cells. Unfortunately the change, if any, in this layer that is responsible for leucocytic sticking is not known. The only published study of inflamed vessels stained to demonstrate this layer (JONES, 1970) showed no change in it in relation to adhering leucocytes, and our own unpublished studies of inflamed vessels stained with lanthanum and alcian blue support JONES's findings (Figs. 16, 17). Further work is needed to clarify the role, if any, of this endocapillary layer in leucocytic sticking.

It has been suggested by several writers that electrostatic forces may be responsible for leucocytic sticking. BANGHAM (1964) made a detailed study of the forces that might be involved in such a process. He claimed that the surface anions of leucocytes and erythrocytes are different, and that this might explain why white cells adhere whereas red cells do not. He also suggested that leucocytes were more likely to be able to come close enough to the similarly charged vascular wall to enable chemical bonding between the two if the first approach was made by a pseudopod and not by the whole cell. There is no experimental confirmation of this hypothesis, but there is evidence that divalent cations, probably calcium ions, are essential for leucocytic adherence. THOMSON et al. (1967) showed that the chelating agent ethylene diamine tetra acetic acid (EDTA) can reverse existing sticking and prevent adherence of further cells to venules in ear chamber preparations. Using a new, semi-quantitative method, ATHERTON and BORN (1972, 1973a) confirmed this finding. They also showed that leucocytic sticking could occur without any concurrent slowing of the rate of flow of blood through the affected venule and that certain factors known to be chemotactic to polymorphs actively promoted leucocytic adherence. The significance of this last finding is discussed further below.

Although the mechanisms responsible are still unknown, adherence of different elements of circulating blood to vascular endothelium appears to be a highly specific phenomenon. The cells that adhere to acutely inflamed venules are predominantly

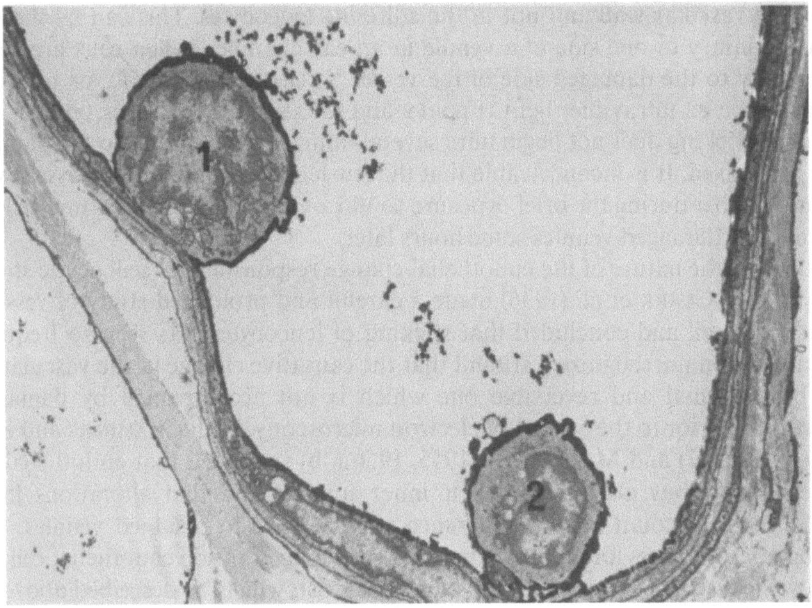

Fig. 16. Venule in rat cremaster 3 h after local injection of normal rat serum, stained with alcian blue lanthanum technique. Deeply stained material covers endothelium and surrounds lower polymorph (*2*). Similar material covers upper adherent polymorph (*1*) but is not visible between this cell and the underlying endothelium. x 3000

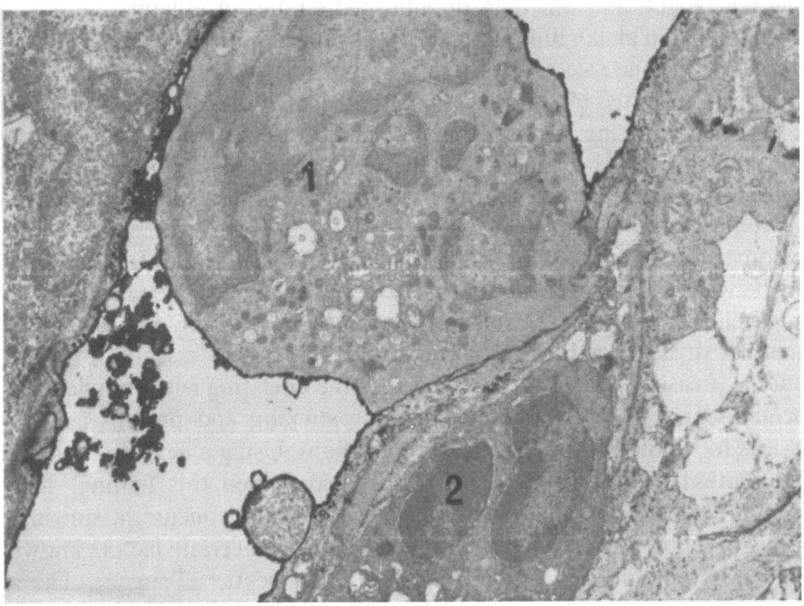

Fig. 17. Portion of another venule in same cremaster as in Figure 16. The advancing edge of polymorph (*1*) has passed entirely through the endothelium and another cell (*2*) which has escaped lies in the venular wall. Alcian blue-stained material covers the endothelium and the luminal aspect of cell (*1*), but is absent where the cell penetrates the venular wall. x 7500

neutrophil polymorphs together with some eosinophils and monocytes. Lymphocytes are not involved. By contrast, lymphocytes adhere selectively to the endothelium of postcapillary venules in normal lymphoid tissue (MARCHESI and GOWANS, 1964), which fails to attract other types of leucocytes. In still other circumstances, platelets stick to the vascular wall in the early stages of thrombosis whereas leucocytes do not, and ATHERTON and BORN (1973b) have provided direct evidence to support the long-held belief that the factors causing platelet adherence are quite distinct from those responsible for leucocytic sticking.

2. Leucocytic Emigration

a) Morphology

The main features of this process are well established. Escape of cells occurs from venules and small veins; only very occasionally do cells escape from capillaries. Observation of living transparent tissue shows that leucocytes emigrate by active amoeboid movement, polymorphs taking 2–9 min to pass through the venular wall and thereafter moving in tissues at up to 20 μm per min (CLARK et al., 1936). In addition to white cells, some red cells escape especially in severe types of injury. Escape of erythrocytes is entirely passive, the cells being seen to be pushed by intravascular pressure through tiny, apparently transient, breaches in the vascular wall.

Electron microscope examination of semiserial sections has shown that some leucocytes at least escape by dissecting down intercellular junctions, the junction reforming apparently unaltered behind the escaping cell (MARCHESI and FLOREY, 1960; MARCHESI, 1961; HURLEY and XEROS, 1961) (Fig. 18). It appears almost certain that all neutrophils, eosinophils and monocytes escape in this way, but the work necessary to produce and examine serial sections of large numbers of emigrating leucocytes has prevented full proof of this hypothesis. It is of interest that as early as 1875 ARNOLD claimed that leucocytes left vessels via areas stained by silver nitrate—i.e. intercellular junctions—and gave clear drawings of his observations.

In the first electron microscope study of the escape of lymphocytes from the postcapillary venules of lymphoid tissue it was claimed that, in contrast with other types of leucocytes, lymphocytes migrate through the cytoplasm of endothelial cells, and a special immunological significance was postulated for this route of escape (MARCHESI and GOWANS, 1964). Subsequently, a similar transcellular passage of lymphocytes was claimed, but not proven, to occur in areas of delayed hypersensitivity (WIENER et al., 1967) and of graft rejection (WIENER et al., 1969). However, in a most meticulous serial section and reconstruction study of lymphocyte emigration across postcapillary venules by SCHOEFL (1972), every escaping lymphocyte examined was shown to be passing down an intercellular junction. Unpublished electron microscope studies employing lanthanum staining support SCHOEFL's conclusion. This tracer is confined to intercellular spaces and does not penetrate within cells, and in postcapillary venules of sections stained with lanthanum the tracer is clearly visible around emigrating lymphocytes (Figs. 19, 20). Until a study as carefully conducted as SCHOEFL's provides contrary evidence it must be concluded that lymphocytes cross the vascular wall by the same route as other types of leucocyte.

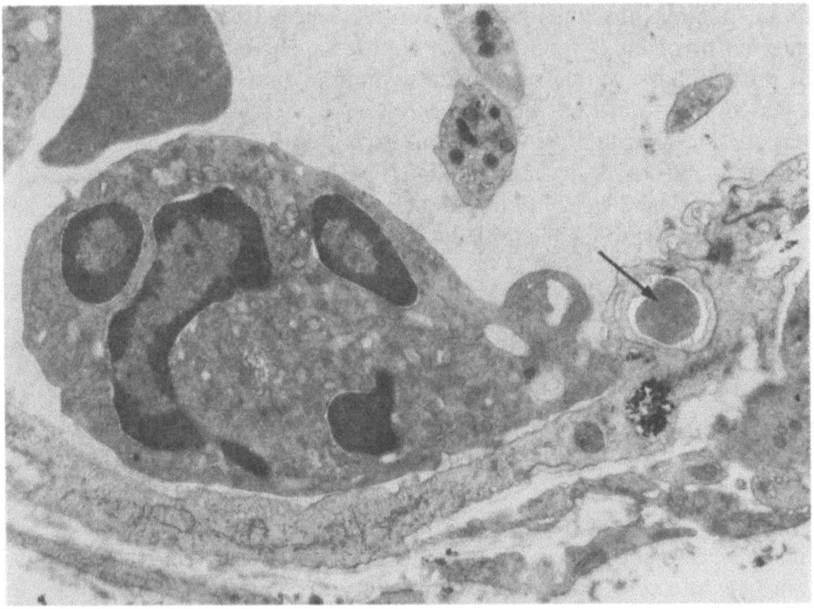

Fig. 18. Rat cremaster 6 h after local injection of carrageenan. A polymorph has inserted a pseudopod (↗) into an intercellular junction in the endothelium of this venule. Endothelial cell cytoplasm appears normal and contains a large carbon filled vacuole. x 9700

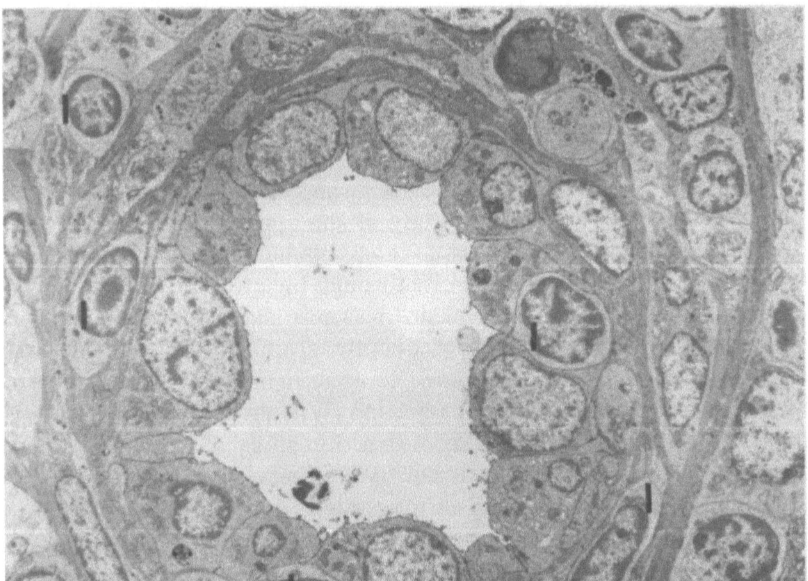

Fig. 19. Post-capillary venule in Peyer's patch of rat fixed by perfusion and stained with alcian blue lanthanum. Numerous lymphocytes (l) are embedded at different levels in the vascular wall which is lined by columnar type endothelium. x 2100

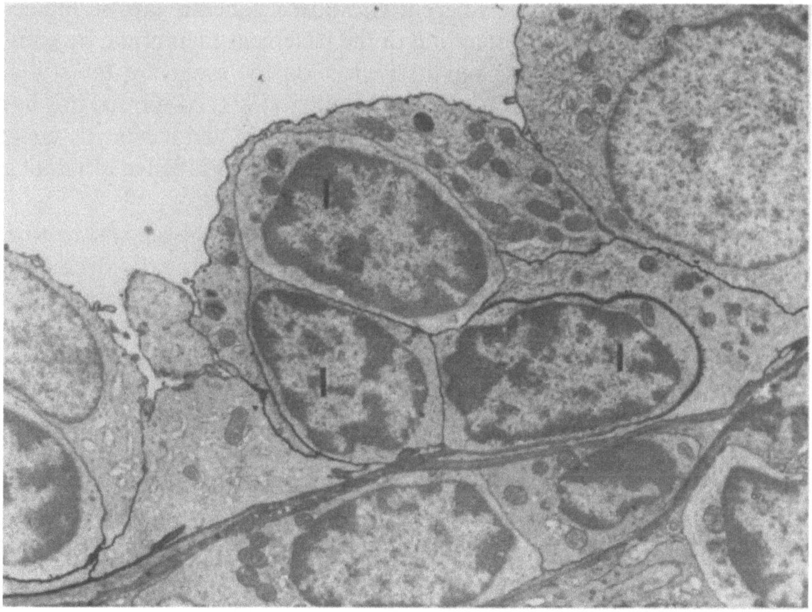

Fig. 20. Higher power view of portion of wall of a post-capillary venule stained as in Figure 19. Dark deposits of lanthanum surround lymphocytes (l) which appear to be embedded in endothelial cell xytoplasm. x 4500

It is commonly assumed that the venular wall plays a purely passive role in the escape of leucocytes. However, after studying leucocytic emigration in rabbit ear chambers, CLARK et al. (1936) reported that "following the period of emigration, the endothelium of blood vessels underwent reversal of consistency to a phase in which no more leucocytes penetrated the wall. The reversal occurred so abruptly that migrating cells were frequently caught in the wall and remained for hours half inside and half outside the capillary." This observation appears hardly consistent with purely passive behaviour of the venular wall.

In all electron microscope studies of leucocytic emigration, escaping cells are seen much more frequently between the endothelium and its basement membrane than in the process of passing between endothelial cells. Although the basement membrane appears insubstantial, it seems to offer more resistance to emigrating cells than does the much thicker endothelium. The basement membrane is also an effective barrier to large marker particles like carbon, this property forming the basis of the vascular labelling technique. However, when vessels from which large numbers of leucocytes are escaping are stimulated by permeability factors such as histamine, the emigrating cells disrupt the basement membrane and allow carbon to escape freely into extravascular tissues (HURLEY, 1964a). Whether this phenomenon is due to mechanical disruption of the basement membrane by escaping leucocytes or to some more subtle, possibly enzymic, change is not known. The change is a reversible one and when leucocytic emigration ceases the basement membrane once more becomes impermeable to carbon particles. Small marker particles like ferritin pass freely through the basement membrane where it is exposed beneath gaps in the endothelium of leaking vessels, so that disruption of the basement membrane by emigrating leucocytes might be expected to have little effect on the escape of the still smaller molecules of plasma protein. MCQUEEN and HURLEY (1971) confirmed this hypothesis and found that neither concurrent nor recently completed leucocytic emigration had any detectable effect on the rate of accumulation of ^{131}I labelled albumin at sites of i.d. injection of histamine.

However, the wall of blood vessels in thermal burns has been shown to exert a sieving effect on large lipoprotein molecules, the lymph/plasma ratio decreasing with increasing molecular size (COURTICE and SABINE, 1966). This sieving must occur at the level of the basement membrane or even deeper in the vascular wall as the severe degree of thermal injury used in these experiments would certainly have produced large defects in vascular endothelium. It might be anticipated that concurrent leucocytic emigration would increase the escape of the larger lipoprotein molecules, but no evidence is available on this point.

Lymph draining from peripheral tissues contains a higher proportion of smaller protein molecules like albumin than does plasma. This implies the presence of a sieving mechanism in the normal vascular wall or in extravascular tissues, but at what level sieving occurs is not known. If protein seeps down unaltered intracellular junctions, as does horseradish peroxidase (KARNOVSKY, 1967), sieving might occur at this level. If, however, as suggested above, gaps similar to those induced by histamine appear from time to time in the endothelium of normal venules under physiological conditions, such gaps would be too large for restricted diffusion to occur at the endothelial level and sieving must then take place at the basement membrane, at some deeper layer of the vascular wall or in the extravascular space.

b) Increased Vascular Permeability and Leucocytic Emigration as Separable Phenomena

It has been known for many years that there is a poor correlation between the time course and magnitude of increased vascular permeability and leucocytic emigration after different types of injury. For example, GRANT and WOOD (1928) showed that the massive increased permeability that follows injection of histamine is not accompanied by significant leucocytic emigration, and HURLEY and SPECTOR (1961) found a similar lack of correlation between the two phenomena after injection of a variety of tissue extracts.

It can be shown by simple experiments that increased permeability and leucocytic emigration are completely separable phenomena. When various solutions are injected intradermally into rats, a delayed emigration of leucocytes begins 2–3 h later and lasts for several hours. In this system, the degree of leucocytic emigration induced by a particular solution is unrelated in both time and extent to an increase in permeability caused by the material injected. Furthermore, with all solutions examined, permeability has returned to normal before leucocytic emigration begins, and no detectable increase in permeability accompanies the escape of cells from the vessels (HURLEY, 1964b). When the carbon labelling technique is used as the indicator of increased permeability in this system, study of histological sections shows that massive escape of leucocytes can occur without any accompanying carbon labelling of the affected vessels. Even at the greater resolution obtainable by electron microscopy, leucocytes may pass through the vascular wall with no detectable concurrent escape of either carbon or ferritin particles (HURLEY, 1963). When carbon labelling technique is applied to different types of inflammation, it can be shown that dissociation of leucocytic emigration and increased permeability in individual vessels is a common finding in all types of tissue injury. In histological sections some vessels are blackened, indicating increased vascular permeability; in others active leucocytic emigration is in progress but not carbon is visible in the vascular wall, yet other vessels show both leucocytic emigration and carbon labelling. Extravascular carbon is visible adjacent to labelled vessels from which leucocytes are escaping, but not elsewhere. The two processes of increased permeability and leucocytic emigration appear to occur at least as frequently from separate but adjacent vessels as concurrently from the same vessel.

3. Chemotaxis

This aspect of leucocytic emigration is described in detail in Chapter 4.

4. Mediators of Leucocytic Emigration

This topic is dealt with in detail in later chapters. However, several features of the process of leucocytic emigration described above are especially important in this regard, and must be borne in mind in any explanation of this process. These features are as follows:

1. Since increased permeability and leucocytic emigration are separable phenomena, at least some mediators of leucocytic emigration must exist which are distinct from the factors responsible for increased vascular permeability.

2. Leucocytic emigration cannot be assessed in vitro, but only by the ability of suspected active principles to cause early and massive escape of leucocytes within a short time (40 min) after injection into living tissues. The time is important as many solutions, including physiological saline, will cause leucocytic emigration after an interval of several hours.

3. Leucocytic emigration and chemotaxis are separate phenomena each with its own method of assessment and not necessarily mediated in the same way.

4. Present evidence suggests that many, perhaps all, known chemotactic factors for polymorphs are active in inducing leucocytic emigration after local injection (WARD, 1968). Apart from the observations of CLARK et al. (1936), mentioned above, no evidence exists that changes in the venular wall, other than those caused by chemotactic factors, are concerned in leucocytic emigration. Chemotaxis offers a simple and sufficient explanation for all other phenomena of leucocytic emigration once leucocytes have stuck to the inflamed epithelium.

5. Whilst the basis of leucocytic adherence is still unknown, the findings of ATHERTON and BORN (1972) that some chemotactic factors are able to induce leucocytic sticking, whereas permeability factors like histamine are unable to do so, raise the possibility that chemotactic factors may be responsible, at least in part, for leucocytic adherence. If these findings are confirmed and if it is found that other

chemotactic factors possess similar activity, it may well emerge that all three stages of leucocytic behaviour in acute inflammation depend on the same chemical mediators.

C. Subsequent Course of the Inflammatory Reaction

After the initial stages of inflammation, described above, have developed, subsequent changes within the area of injury may follow one of four possible courses:

1. Resolution
2. Healing by scar with or without regeneration of lost parenchymal cells.
3. Suppuration
4. Chronic inflammation.

The later course of any particular injury depends upon the nature and duration of the injurious stimulus, the type of tissue injured and the degree of destruction of tissue caused by the damaging agent.

The basic features of the processes involved in resolution and suppuration are outlined below; more details of some of these processes are given in later chapters. Healing by scar and chronic inflammation are described in detail in later chapters and will not be discussed here.

I. Resolution

Resolution is the process of complete restoration of the injured area to the normal state. It can only occur if the damaging agent does not cause areas of dead tissue above a certain critical size. In many tissues, single cells or a small group of cells can be killed, their remains removed and the defect filled by division of neighbouring cells of the same kind. However, local defects in tissue larger than a few cells in size become filled with newly formed scar tissue and complete resolution is then no longer possible.

Resolution is the usual sequel to mild chemical and physical injuries of brief duration, and to many types of infection in which the causative organism does not induce large areas of tissue destruction. Cellulitis, many viral infections and some types of pneumonia, including most strikingly lobar pneumonia, fall into this category.

Resolution involves not only the subsidence of vascular changes, such as vasodilatation and increased permeability, but also the removal of all abnormal material from the extravascular spaces of the injured area. The material to be removed includes inflammatory exudate, polymorphs, fibrin and dead tissue cells and their breakdown products. It is convenient to discuss the removal of these several elements separately.

1. Inflammatory Exudate

As vasodilatation subsides, the balance of hydrostatic and osmotic forces across the wall of small blood vessels in the inflamed area returns to its normal resting state. As a result, some of the fluid part of the inflammatory exudate is resorbed into the venous end of the capillaries. However, the bulk of the fluid and all the protein of the exudate is removed via lymphatics. To understand how this occurs it is necessary to review briefly the structure and function of lymphatics in normal and inflamed tissues.

a) Lymphatic Vessels

α) Structure

Terminal lymphatics are blind thin-walled tubes present in nearly all tissues in numbers comparable to blood capillaries. As they contain colourless fluid and are commonly collapsed they tend to be overlooked in histological sections and it is only after perfusion studies that their true frequency can be appreciated. Terminal lymphatics drain into collecting lymphatics which, after passage through one or more lymph nodes, finally discharge either via the right lymph duct or the thoracic duct into the veins at the root of the neck. Valves are present in all collecting lymphatics, so arranged that fluid can flow only towards the final point of discharge into the venous system.

Electron microscope studies have shown that lymphatic capillaries are similar in structure to blood capillaries. However, lymphatic endothelium is thinner and more irregular and its basement membrane tenuous and often absent (Fig. 21). Junctions between adjacent cells are simpler in form than those in blood vascular endothelium and it seems that gaps are present in some normal lymphatics (CASLEY-SMITH and FLOREY, 1961). Fine fibrils join the outer surface of the endothelial cells of terminal lymphatics to adjacent collagen fibres and other connective tissue structures. These

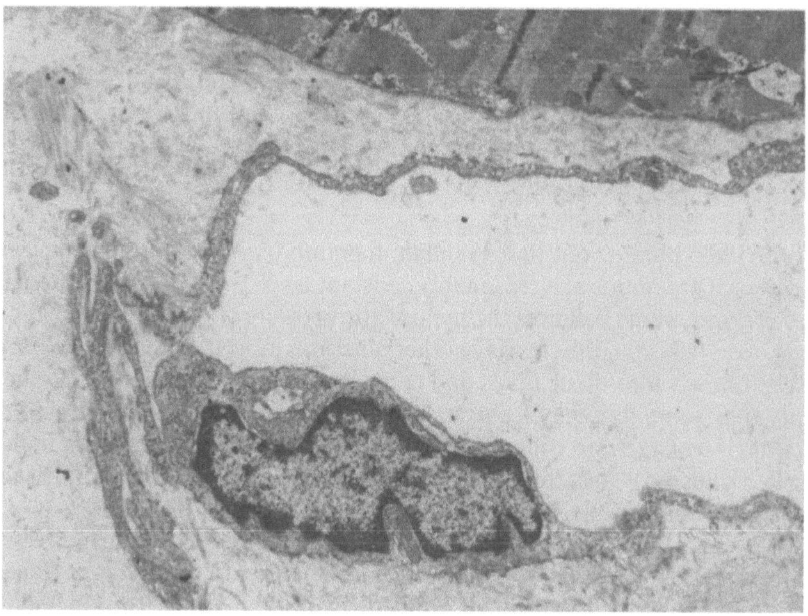

Fig. 21. Terminal lymphatic in cremaster muscle of rat. Endothelium is lower and much more irregular than that lining blood vessels of similar calibre. x 6000

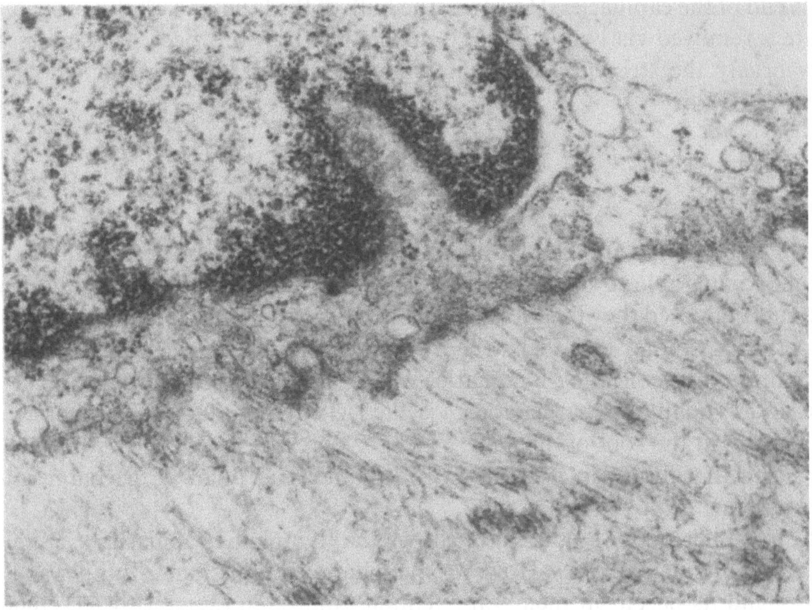

Fig. 22. Higher power of portion of lymphatic shown in Figure 21. Numerous fine fibrils radiate out into adjacent tissues from outer aspect of lymphatic endothelial cell. x 40000

fibres were first described in a light microscope study of inflammation in the mouse ear by PULLINGER and FLOREY (1935) and their presence has been confirmed by electron microscopy by LEAK and BURKE (1967, 1968) and by CASLEY-SMITH (1967) (Fig. 22). The origin and composition of these fibres is not known.

Larger collecting lymphatics have a complete endothelium and a more distinct basement membrane, and smooth muscle cells are present in the outer part of their wall.

β) Function in Normal Tissues

COURTICE (1969) pointed out that the main function of plasma proteins is to maintain intravascular volume at a reasonably constant level. They do this by exerting an osmotic pressure which balances the hydrostatic pressure within small blood vessels. However, many plasma proteins have other functions as well, and it is necessary that they escape slowly into tissue fluids and come into contact with tissue cells, i.e., it is necessary that some leakage of plasma proteins into normal tissues should occur. The extent of leakage into different normal tissues varies greatly. It is highest in organs with sinusoidal small blood vessels such as the liver and lowest in tissues like skeletal muscle whose vessels are lined by continuous-type endothelium.

Once proteins have reached extravascular tissues they cannot return directly into small blood vessels. Such return would require the presence of an energy-dependent pump to move proteins against the gradient of protein concentration that exists between plasma and tissue fluids. There is no such mechanism. Instead the lymphatic system of vessels developed, the structure of which is especially adapted to take up extravascular proteins and return them to the blood stream. Electron microscope study has shown that when large marker particles like carbon are injected into extravascular tissues they readily enter lymphatics. Entry occurs via intercellular junctions, a proportion of which appear to be open in normal tissues, and others to open after trivial physiological stimuli. Pinocytosis does not appear to be involved. The wall of collecting lymphatics is much less permeable and dyes injected into them do not spread out into surrounding tissues (HUDACK and MCMASTER, 1933).

Once extravascular fluid and protein has entered terminal lymphatics, the passage of lymph along collecting lymphatics is largely a passive process that occurs by the combined action of lymphatic valves and pressure from adjacent tissues, especially contracting muscle, assisted in some parts of the body by variations in intrathoracic pressure. Active contraction of lymphatics may play an auxiliary role: the frog has lymph hearts, lymphatics in the bat wing contract rhythmically and lymph in unanaesthetized sheep is propelled by regular contraction of lymphatic trunks (HALL et al., 1965). Little is known of the capacity for contraction of human lymphatics.

γ) Lymphatics in Acute Inflammation

When tissues swell due to accumulation of inflammatory exudate, the fine anchoring filaments described above, which join the outer surface of lymphatic endothelial cells to adjacent extravascular structures, exert an outward pull on the lymphatic wall. As a result, terminal lymphatics in areas of inflammation are widely dilated and much more prominent than in normal tissues. An increased number of gaps is present in the endothelium of the distended vessels. Whether these gaps are due to the action of endogenous permeability factors with an action on lymphatic endothelium similar to that which causes gap formation in inflamed venules, or are merely a consequence of the outward pull of anchoring filaments on the wall of the distended vessel, is not known.

The exudate that escapes from inflamed blood vessels enters terminal lymphatics via these gaps, and as a consequence lymph drainage from the area of inflammation increases greatly in both volume and total protein content. Due to its high fibrinogen content, such lymph usually clots after removal from the body.

Thus in all types of inflammation, exudate is removed from the injured area via lymphatics by acceleration of normal lymphatic function. Local oedema will only arise in an area of inflammation when the rate of formation of exudate from small blood vessels exceeds the capacity of the lymphatics to remove it from the extravascular tissues. This concept has important practical consequences for the experimental study of inflammatory processes. The rate of accumulation of labelled protein, whether labelled by "bluing" or isotopically, is not an accurate measure of increased vascular permeability unless allowance is made for the amount of exudate removed from the inflamed area via lymphatics. In a recent study, WILLIAMS and MORLEY (1974) have shown that for short term leakage, such as that induced by intradermal injection of histamine, this error is negligible, but in experiments of longer duration an appreciable difference may exist between the rates of vascular leakage and of local oedema formation.

The greatly increased volume of lymph that drains from an area of inflammation indicates that no significant "fibrin barrier" of the type suggested by MENKIN (1940) can be present around damaged tissues. MILES and MILES (1958) showed that lymphatic blockage does not occur in acute infections and that lymphatic channels are occluded only when they lie within areas of coagulative necrosis at the centre of the infected area.

2. Polymorphs

Polymorphs are end cells incapable of further division. In blood they have a life span which has been estimated variously as 3–13 days. The duration of survival of polymorphs after escape into extravascular tissues appears to be less than in circulating blood since observations in both ear chambers and histological sections show that when emigration of polymorphs ceases in areas of resolving inflammation most polymorphs disappear from the injured area within 24–48 h. Some polymorphs leave the damaged area either via lymphatics or tissue spaces and finally die at some distance from the site of inflammation. However, most die locally, disintegrate and liberate their granules and cytoplasmic enzymes into adjacent tissue spaces. The remnants of the dead cells are then engulfed by macrophages. Factors that may be released from living or disintegrating polymorphs and the role that such factors may play in tissue injury and in the causation of later stages of the inflammatory response are discussed in later chapters.

As polymorphs disappear, mononuclear cells come to form an ever-increasing proportion of the extravascular cells within the injured area, and as resolution proceeds an infiltrate composed initially almost exclusively of polymorphs is transformed to an accumulation of mononuclear cells. The origin, kinetics and behaviour of these mononuclear cells is described in detail in the next chapter, and only one aspect of macrophage behaviour which is especially relevant to resolution of an area of acute inflammation will be discussed here. This is the question why macrophages appear within an area of resolving inflammation somewhat later than do polymorphs. For many years it was accepted that this phenomenon was due to later emigration of mononuclear cells from vessels coupled with a relatively short period of survival of polymorphs in extravascular tissues. However, PAZ and SPECTOR (1962), after counting perivascular cells in histological sections at various times after intradermal injection of irritants, claimed that emigration of polymorphs and mononuclear cells began at the same time after injury. They suggested that in the early stages of the inflammatory reaction the more numerous polymorphs obscured the mononuclear cells, but that as the short-lived polymorphs died and disappeared the mononuclear cells with their longer life span became the predominant cell within the injured area. On this hypothesis one substance could mediate the escape of both types of leucocyte. HURLEY et al. (1966) re-examined this problem by counting the total number and type of leucocytes present in the pleural cavity of rats at different stages of experimental pleurisy. The response to a variety of stimuli showed that, at least in this system, polymorphs and mononuclear cells emigrate independently, and with non-viable stimuli, they emigrate successively from subpleural vessels. Successive escape of polymorphs and mononuclear cells has been described in quantitative studies of both experimental peritonitis (FRUHMAN, 1964) and of simple skin abrasions (RYAN, 1967). On this evidence it appears almost certain that in simple types of resolving inflammation the traditional concept of successive emigration of polymorphs and mononuclear cells is correct. The simplest explanation of this pattern of behaviour would be the existence of separate factors governing the escape of different types of leucocyte. A number of such factors have been described in the last few years, and are discussed in detail below in Chapter 4.

However, the cellular changes that follow persistent stimuli of the type that induce chronic inflammation are much more complex, and in different types of chronic inflammation it has been clearly established that both successive and concurrent escape of different types of leucocyte may occur over a period of several weeks (SPECTOR et al., 1967).

3. Fibrin

Most fibrin that forms in inflamed extravascular tissue is lysed and the soluble breakdown products removed via lymphatics. A small amount of fibrin may be engulfed by macrophages as fibrin is visible within vacuoles in the cytoplasm of some macrophages in areas of resolving inflammation.

Fibrinolytic enzymes from three sources play a role in removal of fibrin from areas of inflammation. First and most important is plasmin. The inactive form of this enzyme, plasminogen, is normally present in plasma and may be activated by material released from damaged tissue or leucocytes. Clotting factors XII and XI, activated by surface contact, may also be concerned in plasmin activation (MACFARLANE, 1970). Secondly, all granular leucocytes contain one or more fibrinolysins (JANOFF, 1970), which may be released from either living or dead leucocytes in areas of inflammation. Details of these enzymes are given in later chapters. Thirdly, certain bacteria produce powerful fibrinolysins which may play an important role in infections caused by these microorganisms.

4. Dead Tissue Cells

Most cells possess enzymes contained within special cytoplasmic organelles, the lysosomes, which are capable of causing degradation and liquefaction of the cell if it dies. In areas of inflammation, breakdown is assisted by enzymes derived from leucocytes. In polymorphs the prominent cytoplasmic granules are lysosomes (HIRSCH and COHN, 1960). When polymorphs die they release their granules into surrounding tissues; the enzymes within the granules are liberated and aid in the digestion of adjacent dead tissue cells. The more polymorphs that are present, the more rapidly does digestion of dead tissue take place, the extreme example of this process occurring within an area of suppuration. The many enzymes that may be released from polymorphs and their possible role in the inflammatory process are described in later chapters. When dead tissue produces material which cannot be broken down either by its own enzymes or by enzymes derived from leucocytes, it is ingested and slowly removed by macrophages. Details of this process are described in Chapter 3.

II. Suppuration

A common sequel to the early stages of acute inflammation is suppuration or pus formation. Suppurative lesions are characterized by an inflammatory exudate which contains very large numbers of polymorphs, which, together with dead tissue cells, break down to form a thick creamy or yellow fluid called pus. Pus may form diffusely in loose tissues or body cavities or be localized in discrete foci which are known as abscesses.

The conditions necessary for acute inflammation to proceed to suppuration are two—the stimulus must persist and must be of a type which evokes massive emigration of polymorphs. The common cause of suppuration is infection by certain so-called pyogenic microorganisms, the most important of which are staphylococci, certain types of streptococci, gonococci, meningococci, and *Escherichia coli* and related bacilli. Injection of certain chemicals such as croton oil and turpentine, which cause marked local tissue destruction and evoke massive polymorph emigration, may also cause abscess formation.

Pus consists of living polymorphs, of polymorphs in all stages of death and disintegration, of living and dead microorganisms and of the debris of dead leucocytes and dead tissue cells, all suspended in inflammatory exudate. The high concentration of nucleic acids, both DNA and RNA, derived from cell breakdown is responsible for the high viscosity which is characteristic of pus.

When local accumulation of pus occurs to form an abscess, the collection becomes separated with time from adjacent tissues by the development of a surrounding zone of granulation tissue, which subsequently matures to form dense fibrous tissue. These processes are described in Chapter 6.

When an area of inflammation proceeds to suppuration, the cells that escape from inflamed vessels around the area of pus formation are all polymorphs; the later emigration of mononuclear cells seen in areas of resolving inflammation and in many types of chronic inflammation does not take place. The situation can be mimicked experimentally by injection of living *Klebsiella pneumoniae* into the pleural cavity of rats (HURLEY et al., 1966). After injection of these organisms, the total number of polymorphs increases rapidly and progressively until by 24 h the massive exudate present is turbid and resembles thin pus. At no stage of the reaction does the total number of mononuclear cells in the pleural cavity rise above the level present in control animals, i.e., no mononuclear cells emigrate into the exudate in this type of inflammation.

Thus at all stages of abscess formation, all the living host cells in pus are polymorphs, and this remains the case even in very long-standing abscesses like those in chronic osteomyelitis or the lesions of actinomycosis.

References

Allison, F., Jr., Smith, M. R., Wood, W. B., Jr.: Studies in the pathogenesis of acute inflammation. I. The inflammatory reaction to thermal injury as observed in the rabbit ear chamber. J. exp. Med. **102**, 655—668 (1955)

Arnold, J.: Über das Verhalten der Wandungen der Blutgefäße bei der Emigration weißer Blutkörper. Virchows Arch. path. Anat. **62**, 487—503 (1875)

Ascheim, E., Zweifach, B. W.: Quantitative studies of protein and water shifts during inflammation. Amer. J. Physiol. **202**, 554—558 (1962)

Atherton, A., Born, G. V. R.: Quantitative investigations of the adhesiveness of circulating polymorphonuclear leucocytes to blood vessel walls. J. Physiol. (Lond.) **222**, 447—474 (1972)

Atherton, A., Born, G.V.R.: Relationship between the velocity of rolling granulocytes and that of blood flow in venules. J. Physiol. (Lond.) **233**, 157—165 (1973a)
Atherton, A., Born, G.V.R.: Effects of neuraminidase and N-acetyl neuranimic acid on the adhesion of circulating granulocytes and platelets in venules. J. Physiol. (Lond.) **234**, 66—67 (1973b)
Bangham, A.D.: The adhesiveness of leukocytes with special reference to Zeta potential. Ann. N.Y. Acad. Sci. **116**, 945—949 (1964)
Becker, C.G., Murphy, G.E.: Demonstration of contractile protein in endothelium and cells of the heart valves, endocardium, intima, arteriosclerotic plaques and Aschoff bodies of rheumatic heart disease. Amer. J. Path. **55**, 1—37 (1969)
Bruce, A.N.: Über die Beziehung der sensiblen Nervenendigungen zum Entzündungsvorgang. Naunyn-Schmiedeberg's Arch. exp. Path. Pharmak. **63**, 424—433 (1910)
Buckley, I.K., Ryan, G.B.: Increased vascular permeability. The effect of histamine and serotonin on rat mesenteric blood vessels in vivo. Amer. J. Path. **55**, 329—347 (1969)
Casley-Smith, J.R.: Electron microscopical observations on the dilated lymphatics in oedematous regions and their collapse following hyaluronidase administration. Brit. J. exp. Path. **48**, 680—686 (1967)
Casley-Smith, J.R., Florey, H.W.: The structure of normal small lymphatics. Quart. J. exp. Physiol. **46**, 101—106 (1961)
Chambers, R., Zweifach, B.W.: Capillary endothelial cement in relation to permeability. J. cell. comp. Physiol. **15**, 255—272 (1940)
Chambers, R., Zweifach, B.W.: Topography and function of the mesenteric capillary circulation. Amer. J. Anat. **75**, 173—205 (1944)
Chambers, R., Zweifach, B.W.: Intercellular cement and capillary permeability. Physiol. Rev. **27**, 436—463 (1947)
Chapman, L.F., Goodell, H.: The participation of the nervous system in the inflammatory reaction. Ann. N.Y. Acad. Sci. **116**, 990—1017 (1964)
Clark, E.R., Clark, E.L., Rex, R.D.: Observations on polymorphonuclear leukocytes in the living animal. Amer. J. Anat. **59**, 123—173 (1936)
Clementi, F., Palade, G.E.: Intestinal capillaries. I. Permeability to peroxidase and ferritin. J. Cell Biol. **41**, 33—58 (1969)
Cohnheim, J.: Lectures on General Pathology, 2nd Ed. (translated from 2nd German Ed.), Vol. I. London, 1889. The New Sydenham Society (1882)
Cotran, R.S.: Delayed and prolonged vascular leakage in inflammation. II. An electron microscopic study of the vascular response after thermal injury. Amer. J. Path. **46**, 589—620 (1965)
Cotran, R.S.: Studies on inflammation. Ultrastructure of the prolonged vascular response induced by *Clostridium oedematiens* toxin. Lab. Invest. **17**, 39—60 (1967)
Cotran, R.S., Majno, G.: The delayed and prolonged vascular leakage in inflammation. I. Topography of the leaking vessels after thermal injury. Amer. J. Path. **45**, 261—281 (1964a)
Cotran, R.S., Majno, G.: A light and electron-microscope analysis of vascular injury. Ann. N.Y. Acad. Sci. **116**, 750—763 (1964b)
Courtice, F.C.: The biological basis of organ transplantation. Aust. J. Sci. **32**, 215—221 (1969)
Courtice, F.C., Sabine, M.S.: The effect of different degrees of thermal injury on the transfer of protein and lipoproteins from plasma to lymph in the leg of the hypercholesterolaemic rabbit. Aust. J. exp. Biol. med. Sci. **44**, 37—44 (1966)
Crone, C.: In: Crone, C., Lassen, N.A. (Eds.): Capillary Permeability, p. 29. New York: Academic Press 1970
Cunningham, A.L., Hurley, J.V.: Alpha-naphthyl-thiourea-induced pulmonary oedema in the rat: a topographic and electron microscope study. J. Path. **106**, 25—35 (1972)
Farquhar, M.G., Palade, G.E.: Junctional complexes in various epithelia. J. Cell Biol. **17**, 375—412 (1963)
Florey, H.W.: The structure of normal and inflamed small blood vessels of the mouse and rat colon. Quart. J. exp. Physiol. **46**, 119—122 (1961)
Florey, Lord: General Pathology. London: Lloyd-Luke (Medical Books) 1970
Florey, H.W., Grant, L.H.: Leucocyte migration from small blood vessels stimulated with ultraviolet light: an electron-microscope study. J. Path. Bact. **82**, 13—17 (1961)

Fruhman, G.J.: Extravascular mobilisation of neutrophils. Ann. N.Y. Acad. Sci. **113**, 968—1002 (1964)
Gabbiani, G., Badonnel, M.C., Majno, G.: Intra-arterial injection of histamine, serotonin or bradykinin: a topographic study of vascular leakage. Proc. Soc. exp. Biol. (N.Y.) **135**, 447—452 (1970)
Gabbiani, G., Badonnel, M.C.: Early changes in endothelial clefts after thermal injury. Microvasc. Res. **10**, 65—75 (1975)
Gabbiani, G., Badonnel, M.C., Mathewson, S.M., Ryan, G.B.: Acute cadmium intoxication. Early selective lesions of endothelial clefts. Lab. Invest. **30**, 686—695 (1974)
Gabbiani, G., Badonnel, M.C., Rona, G.: Cytoplasmic contractile apparatus in aortic endothelial cells of hypertensive rats. Lab. Invest. **32**, 227—234 (1975)
Giacomelli, I., Wiener, J., Spiro, D.: Cross striated arrays of filaments in endothelium. J. Cell Biol. **45**, 188—192 (1970)
Grant, L.H., Palmer, P., Sanders, A.G.: The effect of heparin on the sticking of white cells to endothelium in inflammation. J. Path. Bact. **83**, 127—133 (1962)
Grant, R.T., Wood, J.E.: Histamine and leucocyte emigration. J. Path. Bact. **31**, 1—7 (1928)
Grotte, G.: Passage of dextran molecules across the blood-lymph barrier. Acta chir. scand. Suppl. **211**, 1—84 (1956)
Hall, J.G., Morris, B., Wooley, G.: Intrinsic rhythmic propulsion of lymph in the unanaesthetized sheep. J. Physiol. (Lond.) **180**, 336—349 (1965)
Ham, K.N., Hurley, J.V.: Acute inflammation: an electron-microscope study of turpentine-induced pleurisy in the rat. J. Path. Bact. **90**, 365—377 (1965)
Ham, K.N., Hurley, J.V.: An electron-microscope study of the vascular response to mild thermal injury in the rat. J. Path. Bact. **95**, 175—183 (1968)
Hirsch, J.G., Cohn, Z.A.: Degranulation of polymorphonuclear leucocytes following ingestion of microorganisms. J. exp. Med. **112**, 1005—1014 (1960)
Hudack, S., McMaster, P.D.: The lymphatic participation in human cutaneous phenomena. A study of the minute lymphatics of the living skin. J. exp. Med. **57**, 751—774 (1933)
Hurley, J.V.: An electron microscopic study of leucocytic emigration and vascular permeability in rat skin. Aust. J. exp. Biol. med. Sci. **41**, 171—186 (1963)
Hurley, J.V.: Acute inflammation: the effect of concurrent leucocytic emigration and increased permeability on particle retention by the vascular wall. Brit. J. exp. Path. **45**, 627—633 (1964a)
Hurley, J.V.: Substances provoking leukocytic emigration. Ann. N.Y. Acad. Sci. **116**, 918—935 (1964b)
Hurley, J.V.: Acute Inflammation. Edinburgh-London: Churchill-Livingstone 1972
Hurley, J.V., Edwards, B.: Acute inflammation: a combined light- and electron-microscope study of the vascular response to incisional and crushing injury of skeletal muscle in the rat. J. Path. **98**, 41—52 (1969)
Hurley, J.V., Edwards, B., Ham, K.N.: The response of newly formed blood vessels in healing wounds to histamine and other permeability factors. Pathology **2**, 133—145 (1970)
Hurley, J.V., Ham, K.N., Ryan, G.B.: The mechanism of the delayed prolonged phase of increased vascular permeability in mild thermal injury in the rat. J. Path. Bact. **94**, 1—12 (1967)
Hurley, J.V., Ham, K.N., Ryan, G.B.: The mechanism of the delayed response to X-irradiation of the skin of hairless mice and of rats. Pathology **1**, 3—18 (1969)
Hurley, J.V., Jago, M.: Pulmonary oedema in rats given dehydromonocrotaline. A topographic and electron microscope study. J. Path. **117**, 23—32 (1975)
Hurley, J.V., Jago, M.: Delayed and prolonged vascular leakage in inflammation: the effect of dehydromonocrotaline on blood vessels in the rat cremaster. Pathology **8**, 7—20 (1976)
Hurley, J.V., McCallum, N.E.W.: The degree and functional significance of the escape of marker particles from small blood vessels with fenestrated endothelium. J. Path. **113**, 183—196 (1974)
Hurley, J.V., McQueen, A.: The response of the fenestrated vessels of the small intestine of rats to application of mustard oil. J. Path. **105**, 21—29 (1971)
Hurley, J.V., Ryan, G.B.: A delayed prolonged increae in venular permeability following intrapleural injections in the rat. J. Path. Bact. **93**, 87—99 (1967)
Hurley, J.V., Ryan, G.B., Friedman, A.: The mononuclear response to intrapleural injection in the rat. J. Path. Bact. **91**, 575—587 (1966)

Hurley,J.V., Spector,W.G.: Endogenous factors responsible for leucocytic emigration in vivo. J. Path. Bact. **82**, 403—420 (1961)
Hurley,J.V., Spector,W.G.: A topographical study of increased vascular permeability in acute turpentine-induced pleurisy. J. Path. Bact. **89**, 245—254 (1965)
Hurley,J.V., Willoughby,D.A.: Acute inflammation—a combined topographical and electron microscope study of the mode of action of carrageenan. Pathology **5**, 9—21 (1973)
Hurley,J.V., Xeros,N.: Electron microscopic observations on the emigration of leucocytes. Aust. J. exp. Biol. med. Sci. **39**, 609—623 (1961)
Janoff,A.: Mediators of tissue damage in human polymorphonuclear neutrophils. Ser. Haematol. **3**, 96—130 (1970)
Jennings,M.A., Florey,H.: An investigation of some properties of endothelium related to capillary permeability. Proc. roy. Soc. B **167**, 39—63 (1967)
Jones,D.B.: The morphology of acid mucosubstances in leukocytic sticking to endothelium in acute inflammation. Lab. Invest. **23**, 606—611 (1970)
Joris,I.: In: Lepow,I.H., Ward,P.A. (Eds.): Inflammation—Mechanisms and Control, pp. 13—27. New York-London: Academic Press 1972
Joris,I., Majno,G., Ryan,G.B.: Endothelial contraction in vivo: a study of the rat mesentery. Virchows Arch. B **12**, 73—83 (1972)
Karnovsky,M.J.: The ultrastructural basis of capillary permeability studied with peroxidase as a tracer. J. Cell Biol. **35**, 213—236 (1967)
Krogh,A.: Studies on the capillariomotor mechanism. I. The reaction to stimuli and the innervation of the blood vessels in the tongue of the frog. J. Physiol. (Lond.) **53**, 399—419 (1920)
Landis,E.M.: Micro-injection studies of capillary permeability. II. The relation between capillary pressure and the rate at which fluid passes through the walls of single capillaries. Amer. J. Physiol. **82**, 217—238 (1927)
Landis,E.M.: Heteroporosity of the capillary wall as indicated by cinematographic analysis of the passage of dyes. Ann. N.Y. Acad. Sci. **116**, 765—773 (1964)
Leak,L.V., Burke,J.F.: Special filaments associated with the lymphatic capillary. Anat. Rec. **157**, 276 (1967)
Leak,L.V., Burke,J.F.: Ultrastructural studies on the lymphatic anchoring filaments. J. Cell Biol. **36**, 129—149 (1968)
Lewis,T.: The blood vessels of the human skin and their responses. London: Shaw and Sons 1927
Lewis,T., Grant,R.T.: Vascular reactions of the skin to injury. Part II. The liberation of a histamine-like substance in injured skin: the underlying cause of factitious urticaria and of wheals produced by burning; and observations upon the nervous control of certain skin reactions. Heart **11**, 209—265 (1924)
Luft,J.H.: In: Zweifach,B.W., Grant,L., McCluskey,R.T. (Eds.): The Inflammatory Process, 2nd Ed., Ch. 2. New York: Academic Press 1973
MacFarlane,R.G.: In: Lord Florey (Ed.): General Pathology, p. 226. London: Lloyd-Luke 1970
McGovern,V.J.: Reactions to injury of vascular endothelium with special reference to the problem of thrombosis. J. Path. Bact. **69**, 283—293 (1955)
McGovern,V.J.: Mast cells and their relationship to endothelial surfaces. J. Path. Bact. **71**, 1—6 (1956a)
McGovern,V.J.: The effect of antazoline (antistin) on endothelial surfaces. J. Path. Bact. **72**, 143—147 (1956b)
McLean,A.E.M., Ahmed,K., Judah,J.D.: Cellular permeability and the reaction to injury. Ann. N.Y. Acad. Sci. **116**, 986—989 (1964)
McQueen,A., Hurley,J.V.: Aspects of increased vascular permeability following the intradermal injection of histamine in the rat. Pathology **3**, 191—202 (1971)
Majno,G., Gilmore,V., Leventhal,M.: On the mechanism of vascular leakage caused by histamine-type mediators: a microscopic study in vivo. Circulat. Res. **21**, 833—847 (1967)
Majno,G., Palade,G.E.: Studies in inflammation. I. The effect of histamine and serotonin on vascular permeability: an electron microscopic study. J. biophys. biochem. Cytol. **11**, 571—605 (1961)
Majno,G., Palade,G.E., Schoefl,G.I.: Studies in inflammation. II. The site of action of histamine and serotonin along the vascular tree: a topographic study. J. biophys. biochem. Cytol. **11**, 607—626 (1961)

Majno, G., Shea, S. M., Leventhal, M.: Endothelial contraction induced by histamine-type mediators. J. Cell Biol. **42**, 647—672 (1969)
Marchesi, V. T.: The site of leukocytic emigration during inflammation. Quart. J. exp. Physiol. **46**, 115—118 (1961)
Marchesi, V. T., Florey, H. W.: Electron micrographic observations on the emigration of leukocytes. Quart. J. exp. Physiol. **45**, 343—348 (1960)
Marchesi, V. T., Gowans, J. L.: The emigration of lymphocytes through the endothelium of venules in lymph nodes: an electron microscope study. Proc. roy. Soc. B **159**, 283—290 (1964)
Mayerson, H. S., Wolfram, C. G., Shirley, H. H., Jr., Wasserman, K.: Regional differences in capillary permeability. Amer. J. Physiol. **198**, 155—160 (1960)
Menkin, V.: Dynamics of inflammation. New York: Macmillan 1940
Miles, A. A., Miles, E. M.: The state of lymphatic capillaries in acute inflammatory lesions. J. Path. Bact. **76**, 21—35 (1958)
Palade, G. E., Bruns, R. R.: Structural modulation of the plasma-lemmal vesicles. J. Cell Biol. **37**, 633—649 (1968)
Pappenheimer, J. R., Renkin, E. M., Borrero, L. M.: Filtration, diffusion and molecular sieving through peripheral capillary membranes. A contribution to the pore theory of capillary permeability. Amer. J. Physiol. **167**, 13—46 (1951)
Pappenheimer, J. R., Soto-Riviera, A.: Effective osmotic pressure of the plasma proteins and other quantities associated with the capillary circulation in the hindlimbs of cats and dogs. Amer. J. Physiol. **152**, 471—491 (1948)
Paz, R. A., Spector, W. G.: The mononuclear cell response to injury. J. Path. Bact. **84**, 85—103 (1962)
Pietra, G. G., Szidon, J. P., Leventhal, M. M.: Anatomical basis of histamine-mediated peribronchial interstitial oedema. Lab. Invest. **22**, 508 (1970)
Pullinger, B. D., Florey, H. W.: Some observations on the structure and functions of lymphatics: their behaviour in local oedema. Brit. J. exp. Path. **16**, 49—61 (1935)
Renkin, E. M.: In: Mayerson, H. S. (Ed.): Lymph and the Lymphatic System, p. 68. Springfield, Ill.: Thomas 1968
Rous, P., Gilding, H. P., Smith, F.: The gradient of vascular permeability. J. exp. Med. **51**, 807—830 (1930)
Rowley, D. A.: Venous constriction as the cause of increased vascular permeability produced by 5 hydroxytryptamine, histamine, bradykinin and 48/80 in the rat. Brit. J. exp. Path. **45**, 56—67 (1964)
Ryan, G. B.: The origin and sequence of the cells found in the acute inflammatory response. Aust. J. exp. Biol. med. Sci. **45**, 149—162 (1967)
Ryan, G. B., Hurley, J. V.: The drug inhibition of increased vascular permeability. J. Path. Bact. **96**, 371—379 (1968)
Schoefl, G. I.: The migration of lymphocytes across the vascular endothelium in lymphoid tissue. A re-examination. J. exp. Med. **136**, 568—584 (1972)
Sevitt, S.: Early and delayed oedema and increase in capillary permeability after burns of the skin. J. Path. Bact. **75**, 27—37 (1958)
Shea, S. M.: Lanthanum staining of the surface coat of cells. Its enhancement by the use of fixatives containing Alcian blue or Cetylpyridinium chloride. J. Cell Biol. **51**, 611—620 (1971)
Shea, S. M., Caulfield, J. B., Burke, J. F.: Microvascular ultrastructure in thermal injury: a reconsideration of the role of mediators. Microvasc. Res. **5**, 87—96 (1973)
Spector, W. G., Lykke, A. W. J., Willoughby, D. A.: A quantitative study of leucocyte emigration in chronic inflammatory granulomata. J. Path. Bact. **93**, 101—107 (1967)
Spector, W. G., Willoughby, D. A.: The enzymic inactivation of an adrenaline-like substance in inflammation. J. Path. Bact. **80**, 271—280 (1960)
Spector, W. G., Willoughby, D. A.: The inflammatory response. Bact. Rev. **27**, 117—154 (1963)
Starling, E. H.: On the absorption of fluids from the connective tissue spaces. J. Physiol. (Lond.) **19**, 312—326 (1896)
Steele, R. H., Wilhelm, D. L.: The inflammatory reaction in chemical injury. I. Increased vascular permeability and erythema induced by various chemicals. Brit. J. exp. Path. **47**, 612—623 (1966)

Thompson, P. L., Papadimitriou, J. M., Walters, M. N-L.: Suppression of leucocytic sticking and emigration by chelation of calcium. J. Path. Bact. **94**, 389—396 (1967)
Ward, P. A.: Chemotaxis of polymorphonuclear leucocytes. Biochem. Pharmacol. **17**, Suppl., 99—105 (1968)
Wells, F. R.: The site of vascular response to thermal injury in skeletal muscle. Brit. J. exp. Path. **52**, 292—306 (1971)
Wells, F. R.: The site of vascular response to the α-toxin of *Clostridium perfringens* Type A in skeletal muscle. Brit. J. exp. Path. **53**, 445—456 (1972)
Wells, F. R., Miles, A. A.: Site of the vascular response to thermal injury. Nature (Lond.) **200**, 1015 (1963)
Wiener, J., Lattes, R. G., Pearl, J. S.: Vascular permeability and leukocyte emigration in allograft rejection. Amer. J. Path. **55**, 295—327 (1969)
Wiener, J., Lattes, R. G., Spiro, D.: An electron microscopic study of leukocyte emigration and vascular permeability in tuberculin sensitivity. Amer. J. Path. **50**, 485—521 (1967)
Williams, T. J., Morley, J.: Measurement of rate of extravasation of plasma protein in inflammatory responses in guinea-pig skin using a continuous recording method. Brit. J. exp. Path. **55**, 1—12 (1974)

CHAPTER 3

Mononuclear Phagocytes in Inflammation

R. VAN FURTH

Although METCHNIKOFF (1892) was the first to describe the macrophages and microphages (synonym: granulocytes), HAECKEL (1862) had made the first observation of endocytosis 30 years before. In his book "Die Radiolaren" published in 1862, HAECKEL noted:

> I first observed this phenomenon in May, 1859, in Naples, in a specimen of *Thetis fimbria*, which I had injected with an aqueous suspension of fine Indigo particles in connection with a study of the vascular system. When I put the fine vessels running in the transparent subcutaneous tissues of a loose flap on the animal's back under the microscope, I was more than a little surprised, a few hours later, to find the colourless blood cells filled with fine Indigo particles. These Indigo particles had penetrated the blood cells, sometimes only a few, but sometimes in large numbers, and had formed aggregates, mainly around the slightly oval nucleus.

This was the first observation of the endocytosis of very fine particles, now called pinocytosis, and about 100 years later COHN (1968, 1970) started his extensive studies on this process. METCHNIKOFF (1892) was the first to recognise that phagocytes not only serve as scavengers, but also play an important role in the host defence against micro-organisms. In his classic experiment, in which he infected a tiny transparent fresh-water flea *(Daphnia magna)* with spores of a primitive fungus *(monospora bicuspidata)*, he observed that if the spores were ingested by the phagocytic cells the *Daphnia* remained alive, but when the phagocytes could not deal with the invasion, the fungus started to multiply and eventually killed the host.

The role of the mononuclear phagocytes in various (patho-)physiological processes has been reviewed in a number of monographs during recent years (NELSON, 1969, 1976; VAN FURTH, 1970, 1975a; STUART, 1970; PEARSALL and WEISER, 1970; VERNON-ROBERTS, 1972; CARR, 1973; WAGNER et al., 1974), and the present contribution might seem superfluous. Here, however, no attempt is made to cover the literature exhaustively. Instead, a more selective treatment will be given, and in this connection specific work will be discussed, particularly investigations in areas related to our own research.

A. Nomenclature of Mononuclear Phagocytes

Until recently, macrophages, and monocytes were considered to be the only mononuclear phagocytes, but the relationship between these cells was not always recognised. These cells, present respectively in the tissues and circulation, were often called mononuclear cells, without taking into account that this term also includes the lymphocytes. In addition, cells which are in fact macrophages or fibroblasts are often called dendritic or reticulum cells. Lack of proper characterisation has long hampered correct definition of the cells in the tissues and hence the understanding of the different roles played by the various cell types in pathological processes. A guide for this characterisation is given in Sections B and C.

At present, a number of immature and mature mononuclear phagocytes are distinguished, i.e. monoblasts, promonocytes, monocytes, and macrophages. The specific characteristics of and interrelationships between these cells will be discussed in Sections B, E, and I.

Depending on their localisation, different terms are used to designate macrophages, e.g. histocytes, Kupffer cells, microglial cells, osteoclasts, and synovial A cells.

The epitheloid cell found in tissues during some kinds of chronic inflammatory response is also a transformed macrophage showing a slightly different structure (i.e. an elongated nucleus and cytoplasm with slender extensions, which contains more mitochondria, an increased endoplasmic reticulum and an enlarged Golgi complex, but fewer dense bodies, than macrophages) and a slightly different function from the macrophages (SUTTON and WEISS, 1966; PAPADIMITRIOU and SPECTOR, 1972; SPECTOR, 1974; SPECTOR and MARIANO, 1975). The multinucleate giant cell occurring in some inflammatory lesions, which can be considered a macrophage polykaryon, is formed by the fusion of young and old mononuclear phagocytes (SUTTON and WEISS, 1976; SPECTOR, 1974; SPECTOR and MARIANO, 1975; PAPADIMITRIOU and CORNELISSE, 1975; GILLMAN and WRIGHT, 1966) (see Section F).

B. Approaches to the Characterisation of Mononuclear Phagocytes

An outline for the proper characterisation of mononuclear phagocytes is given in Table 1.

Table 1. Outline for the identification of mononuclear phagocytes

Morphology	Light microscopy
	Phase-contrast microscopy
	Electron microscopy
Cytochemistry	Peroxidase activity
	Esterase activity
Immunology	Specific surface antigens
	Receptors on cell membrane
Function	Immune phagocytosis
	Pinocytosis
Culture	Survival
	Multiplication
Cell proliferation	^{3}H-Thymidine labelling in vitro
	Kinetics of labelled cells in vivo

I. Morphology

The morphological characteristics distinguished by light, phase-contrast and electron microscopy are shown in Table 2. This summary clearly demonstrates that the monoblast is the most immature cell of this cell-line, followed by the slightly more

Table 2. Morphological characteristics of normal mononuclear phagocytes[a]

Characteristics[b]	Bone marrow		Peripheral blood	Tissues	
	Monoblast	Promonocyte	monocytes	Free macrophages	Fixed macrophages
Cell diameter	10–12 μm	14–20 μm	10–14 μm	10–25 μm	
Nuclear to cytoplasmic ratio	>1	≧1	~1	<1	<1
Surface membrane					
Ruffling	±	++	+++	++++	
Microvilli	+	+	++	+++	+++
Nuclear shape	Round or indented	Folded or indented	Reniform	Reniform or oval	Reniform or oval
Nucleoli	+	+	+	+	+
Cytoplasm					
Polyribosomes	++++	+++	+	±	±
Endoplasmic reticulum	±	+	+	++	++
Golgi complex	Small	Large	Smaller	Variable size	Variable size
Mitochondria	++	++	++	++ to +++	++ to +++
Lysosomes	±	+	++	++ to ++++	++ to ++++

[a] Taken from: Bull. Wld. Hlth. Org. **46,** 845–852 (1972); Lab. Invest. **34**, 440–450 (1976)

[b] The greater the number of plus signs shown for each characteristic, the greater its degree of frequency.

mature promonocyte which in turn is less mature than the monocyte in its nuclear and cytoplasmic characteristics. In all its morphological aspects, the macrophage is unquestionably the most mature cell. However, all mononuclear phagocytes share certain morphological properties, such as ruffling of the outer membrane and the presence of pinocytic vesicles and lysosomes, the latter structures occurring sparsely in the immature and abundantly in the mature cells (Table 2).

II. Cytochemical Characterisation

Cytochemical studies on mononuclear phagocytes have shown that all these cells are esterase positive when α-naphthyl butyrate (ANSLEY and ORNSTEIN, 1970; ORNSTEIN et al., 1973; ORNSTEIN et al., 1976; VAN FURTH and DIESSELHOFF-DEN DULK, 1978) is used as substrate (Table 3); α-naphthyl acetate has a similar specificity (YAM et al., 1971). This cytochemical method, which stains the cytoplasm of the mononuclear phagocytes, is very useful for the differentiation between mononuclear phagocytes and other kinds of cells (see Section C). When other substrates are used (BRAUNSTEINER and SCHMALZL, 1970), the characterisation of mononuclear phagocytes must rely on the inhibition of the reaction by sodium fluoride. One point of interest here is that the percentage of positive cells (Table 3) and the intensity of the esterase activity of the murine mononuclear phagocytes increase with the duration of incubation in vitro. Cells just harvested from the mouse are usually weakly positive, irrespective of their maturity, but after 6 or 24 h culture in vitro the esterase activity

Table 3. Characteristics of murine mononuclear phagocytes

	Bone marrow					Peripheral blood		Tissue macrophages				
	Monoblast[a]	Promonocytes		Monocytes		Monocytes		Peritoneum		Lung	Liver	Skin[b]
		6 h	24 h	6 h	24 h	6 h	24 h	6 h	24 h	24 h	24 h	
	%	%	%	%	%	%	%	%	%	%	%	%
Esterase	91.2	30.0	91.2	40.0	97.4	80.5	95.0	92.0	99.3	100.0	99.0	95.0
Peroxidase	78.0[d]	96.3	93.6	90.9	87.0	86.5	59.8	1.0	0.4	0.0	0.0	49.5
Lysozyme	43.0						95.0		100.0			
IgG receptor	96.0	56.4	93.0[c]	56.1	93.0[c]	85.0	99.0	99.0	100.0	90.0	84.3[e]	94.5
C receptor	16.0	31.6	79.5[c]	42.6	79.5[c]	86.4	96.3	100.0	100.0		37.5[e]	95.0
Pinocytosis	21.0	79.0	91.0	87.0	91.0	81.0	98.0	99.0	99.0	93.7	90.4	95.0
Phagocytosis	30.0	69.0	77.0	72.0	74.0	78.0	90.0	99.0	98.0	94.2	84.5	80.0

[a] ⌀ These data pertain to monoblasts in colonies grown for 96 h in vitro (GOUD et al., 1975).
[b] On coverslip left 24 h s.c.
[c] Differentiation between promonocytes and monocytes was not possible.
[d] These data pertain only to mononuclear phagocyte colonies with peroxidase-positive cells; in 50% of the colonies all cells are negative.
[e] This low percentage is due to pronase treatment.

increases considerably, conceivably due to stimulation during incubation. Exceptions are freshly-isolated Kupffer cells and alveolar macrophages that are strongly positive; these cells are most likely already stimulated in vivo. Human mononuclear phagocytes are, however, always strongly esterase positive when α-naphthyl butyrate is used as substrate (VAN FURTH et al., 1978).

Peroxidase staining of the granules (KAPLOW, 1965) only gives positive results in the more immature cells of the mononuclear phagocyte cell-line; the tissue macrophages are all negative (Table 3). The skin macrophages, which can be collected by the subcutaneous insertion of a coverslip, form an exception since 50% of these cells are positive. However, these cells must be considered inflammatory macrophages recently derived from circulating peroxidase-positive monocytes. Similar results have been obtained during an acute inflammatory reaction in the peritoneal cavity (VAN FURTH et al., 1970).

Peroxidase-positive granules are already formed in monoblasts, but mainly in promonocytes and no longer in monocytes and macrophages (NICHOLS and BAINTON, 1975). These granules must be considered primary lysosomes, comparable to the azurophil granules of the neutrophils. The enzyme content of the granules found in mononuclear phagocytes diminishes during maturation, and also during the incubation of immature cells in vitro (VAN FURTH et al., 1970, 1976; VAN FURTH and DIESSELHOFF-DEN DULK 1978), possibly due to degradation of the enzyme or to loss after the fusion of peroxidase-positive granules with pinocytic vesicles. After the first period of granulogenesis in the promonocytes, the new granules formed in these or more mature cells lack peroxidase activity. It is of interest that mononuclear phagocytes can be stimulated, both in vitro and in vivo, to form new enzymes which are packaged in (secondary) lysosomes (GORDON and COHN, 1973, STEINMAN and COHN, 1974), but new synthesis of lysosomal peroxidase does not occur. It is conceivable that the peroxidase activity found in the nuclear envelope and rough endoplasmic reticulum of resident macrophages (FAHIMI, 1970; WIDMAN et al., 1972; WISSE, 1974; DAEMS et al., 1975) is an indication that these cells are still able to synthesize a small amount of peroxidase, but lack the ability to package it in granules.

In addition to peroxidase-positive granules, promonocytes contain peroxidase activity in the nuclear envelope, the rough-endoplasmic reticulum, and the Golgi complex (NICHOLS and BAINTON, 1975) (Table 4). Monocytes exhibit no peroxidase activity at these localizations, and macrophages from the unstimulated peritoneal cavity (DAEMS et al., 1975, 1976) and Kupffer cells (FAHIMI, 1970; WIDMAN et al., 1972; WISSE, 1974) show only peroxidatic activity in the nuclear envelope and endoplasmic reticulum (Table 4). This difference in localization of peroxidatic activity in monocytes and macrophages has been used as evidence that macrophages do not originate from monocytes, because transitional cells with characteristics of both monocytes and macrophages have never been observed in the normal or stimulated peritoneal cavity (DAEMS et al., 1976; OGAWA et al., 1978).

Recently, however, new information throwing more light on this problem was obtained. During in vitro incubation of rabbit, human and rat monocytes, these cells acquire peroxidatic activity in the endoplasmic reticulum (BODEL et al., 1977). Furthermore, a quantitative study on mononuclear phagocytes during an inflammatory reaction in the peritoneal cavity showed that initially, the exudate contained mainly

Table 4. Peroxidatic activity of Mononuclear phagocytes[a]

	Rough endoplasmic reticulum and nuclear envelope	Golgi system	Cytoplasmic granules
Promonocytes	+	+	+
Monocytes	−	−	+
Resident macrophages	+	−	−
Exudate macrophages	−	−	+
Exudate-resident macrophages	+	−	+

[a] Determined by ultrastructural cytochemistry.
From the J. Reticuloendothel. Soc. **23**, 103—110 (1978).

cells with the characteristics of monocytes (Table 4). However, the decline in the number of these cells was accompanied by the appearance of exudate-resident macrophages with peroxidatic activity in the granules, endoplasmic reticulum, and nuclear envelope (Table 4) and there was a concomitant increase in the number of resident macrophages with peroxidatic activity only in the endoplasmic reticulum and nuclear envelope (BEELEN et al., 1978). The finding of these transitional exudate-resident macrophages (Table 4) strongly supports the view that monocytes give rise to macrophages.

Another enzyme formed by the mononuclear phagocytes is lysozyme (GORDON, 1975; MCCLELLAND et al., 1975). In contrast to the peroxidase pattern, the percentage of lysozyme-positive cells increases with increasing maturity of the cells.

III. Functional Characterisation

The presence on monocytes and macrophages of receptors for the Fc part of the IgG molecule and the third factor of complement (C3b) has been firmly established for various animal species and man (HUBER and HOLM, 1975; AREND and MANNIK, 1975; BIANCO, 1976; BIANCO and NUSSENZWEIG, 1976). In the mouse, almost all immature and mature mononuclear phagocytes have an IgG receptor and ingest opsonized red cells. The complement receptor is only present on a minority of the monoblasts, but the percentage of cells with C receptors increase with maturity of the cells (Table 3). However, only a small percentage of complement-(and IgM-)coated red cells is ingested by the monoblasts, promonocytes, monocytes, and macrophages. Apparently, these attached red cells do not trigger ingestion in immature and non-stimulated mononuclear phagocytes (GRIFFIN et al., 1975), although thioglycollate-induced peritoneal macrophages do ingest the complement-coated red cells (BIANCO et al., 1975). IgM receptors are never found on immature or mature mononuclear phagocytes.

The endocytic function also helps to distinguish mononuclear phagocytes from other cells with a similar morphological appearance (see Section C). The main function of the cells of this cell-line is phagocytosis (see Section D), and tests based on the uptake of opsonized red cells or bacteria are easily applied to these cells. The ingestion of opsonized staphylococci increases with the maturation of the cells (Table 3), whereas the ingestion of IgG-coated red cells amounts to 65–70% in immature and 87–100% in mature mononuclear phagocytes. Pinocytosis is another endocytic function providing a good criterion for the characterisation of mononuclear phagocytes, since except for the monoblasts, the majority of the immature and mature cells will pinocytose solutions containing dextran sulphate (Table 3) (COHN, 1970) or horseradish peroxidase as markers (STEINMAN and COHN, 1972; VAN FURTH and DIESSELHOFF-DEN DULK, 1978).

IV. Culture Characteristics

All types of mononuclear phagocytes can survive for periods ranging from days to weeks when cultured, but they do not multiply in vitro. However, when conditioned medium is added to bone marrow cell suspensions, mononuclear phagocyte colonies will grow in vitro (GOUD et al., 1975; GOUD and VAN FURTH, 1975).

C. The Characteristics of Mononuclear Phagocytes in Relation to Those of Other Cells

The main objective of the determination of the characteristics of cells of a given cell-line (e.g. mononuclear phagocytes) is to obtain a basis for the differentiation of such cells from those of other cell-lines. Cells are still too frequently classified according to inadequately determined characteristics and very frequently solely on the basis of morphological similarities. This has given rise to the use of such misleading terms as mononuclear cells and round cell infiltrations, and has perpetuated the erroneous views that macrophages derive from lymphocytes, that macrophages divide, or derive from mesenchymal cells, and that monocytes or macrophages transform into fibroblasts or even vice versa. Recent investigations have shown that the macrophages are non-dividing cells and derive from precursor cells in the bone marrow (see Section E), that lymphocytes cannot transform into macrophages (VAN FURTH and COHN, 1968), and that mononuclear phagocytes are not the precursors of fibroblasts (LEIBOVICH and ROSS, 1975).

For further definition, the derivation of the various types of cell must be taken into consideration. The cells which play a role in an inflammatory process can be classified into cells deriving from the haemopoietic stem cell and from mesenchymal cells (Fig. 1). The cells of the former category originate, divide and mature in the bone marrow compartment and are then transported via the circulation to the tissues, where they exercise their function. There are exceptions to this pattern: lymphoid cells divide mainly outside the bone marrow, i.e. in the lymphoid tissues, and mononuclear phagocytes can differentiate further in the tissues. The cells of the other category, those of mesenchymal origin, do not form a true cell-line, as do the cells deriving from the bone marrow, but divide locally in the tissues.

If the characteristics determined for the various types of cells are considered, it is evident that besides morphological differences which will not be discussed here, there are differences in cytochemical features, in the presence of receptors on the cell surface, and in functional features, as shown in Table 5. It can be seen from this table that esterase staining makes it possible to distinguish between mononuclear phago-

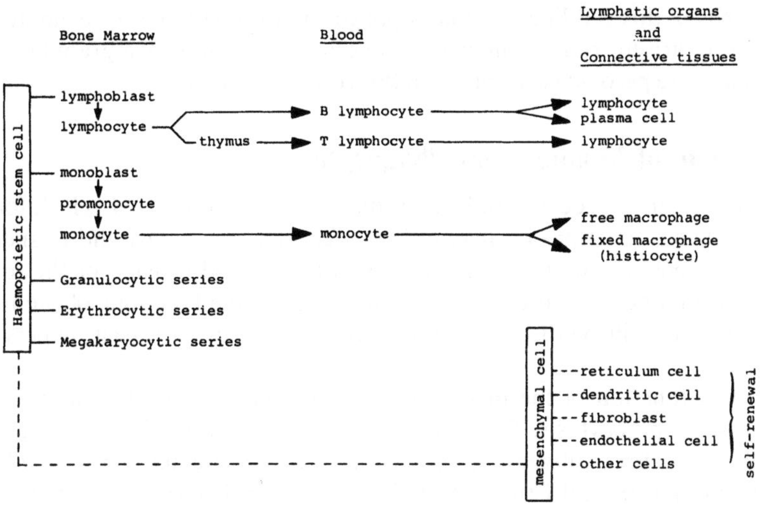

Fig. 1. Differentiation and localisation of cells derived from the haemopoietic stem cell and mesenchymal cells

Table 5. Characteristics of murine macrophages, lymphocytes and fibroblasts

	Macrophages (%)	Lymphocytes (%)	Fibroblasts (%)
Esterase	92–100[c]	0[a]	36[b]
Peroxidase	0– 50	0	0
Lysozyme	100	0	0
IgG receptor	84–100	+[d]	0
C receptor	38–100	+[e]	0
Phagocytosis	85– 99	0	0
Pinocytosis	90– 99[c]	0	99[b]

[a] In T-lymphocytes 1 to 3 positive dots.
[b] Weakly positive.
[c] Strongly positive.
[d] B-lymphocytes and some T-lymphocytes; absent on most T-lymphocytes and nul cells.
[e] B-lymphocytes; absent on T-lymphocytes and nul cells.

cytes and lymphoid cells (almost all mononuclear phagocytes show diffuse staining of the cytoplasm, whereas T-lymphocytes show only one or three positive dots); and although about a third of the fibroblasts are positive, the staining is weak. Fibroblasts also differ from mononuclear phagocytes in their lack of receptors for IgG and C, in their inability to phagocytose, and in the small amount of pinocytosed material found in the fibroblasts. These are reliable criteria for the distinction between lymphoid cells and mononuclear phagocytes, too, since the former are not capable of pinocytosis and phagocytosis and are always peroxidase negative. Monocytes and younger cells of this cell-line and macrophages in an inflammatory exudate—which have recently arisen from monocytes—have peroxidase-positive granules; resident macrophages are peroxidase negative in this respect, however.

D. Functions of Mononuclear Phagocytes

The mononuclear phagocyte can be regarded as a multifunctional cell. Information about the various functions of these cells is accumulating so fast and in such abundance that a separate full-length review could be devoted to each of the functions. Since that would be beyond the scope of this chapter, the functions of the mononuclear phagocytes will be discussed briefly and references to review papers will be given.

The main function of the macrophages is to eliminate deleterious material by phagocytosis or pinocytosis. These cells can ingest microorganisms, neoplastic cells, effete cells, cell debris, antigen-antibody complexes and the like (CARR, 1973; COHN, 1968, 1970; GORDON and COHN, 1973; JONES, 1975a; STEINMAN and COHN, 1974).

Phagocytosis, defined as the uptake of particles larger than 1 µm, can be divided into immune phagocytosis (RABINOVITCH, 1970), which is mediated by IgG and complement receptors on the surface of the phagocytic cells, and the non-immune phagocytosis of non-opsonized particles. Pinocytosis comprises macro-pinocytosis, in which the material is taken up in vacuoles measuring 0.1–1 µm, and micropinocytosis, in which the pinocytic vacuoles are smaller than 0.1 µm (COHN, 1970; CARR, 1973). The divergence between these processes concerns not only the size of the material taken up and of the vacuole formed, but also the metabolic changes occurring during phagocytosis, micro- and macro-pinocytosis. After phagocytosis, microorganisms will be killed intracellularly and eventually digested (MACKANESS, 1960; KARNOVSKY et al., 1970, 1975; KLEBANOFF and HAMON, 1975; ROSSI et al., 1975; VAN FURTH et al., 1978). Obligate intracellular micro-organisms are only killed with some delay or not at all, except when the macrophages are stimulated by the process of cell-mediated immunity (MACKANESS, 1970a, 1970b; MACKANESS et al., 1974; NORTH, 1974; SOLOTOROVSKY and TEWARI, 1974; MAUEL et al., 1974; DRAPER and D'ARCY HART, 1975; JONES, 1975b; MCGREGOR and LOGIE, 1975; DAVID and REMOLD, 1976; BLANDEN et al., 1976).

In addition to this endocytic function, mononuclear phagocytes produce and secrete a great variety of biologically important substances (see Table 6) such as pyrogens, lysosomal hydrolases, lysozyme, complement factors, plasminogen activators, thromboplastin and prostaglandins, as well as collagenase and elastase which are two enzymes that play a role in the healing of a lesion (STECHER, 1970; GORDON, 1975; LAI A FAT, and VAN FURTH, 1975; MCCLELLAND et al., 1975; ALLISON and DAVIES, 1975; DAVIES and ALLISON, 1976a, 1976b; COLTEN, 1976; EPSTEIN, DAVIES et al., 1977; GLATT et al., 1977; RACHMILEWITZ and SCHLESINGER, 1977).

Monocytes and macrophages also produce colony-stimulating factor, which stimulates the proliferation of immature bone marrow mononuclear phagocytes and progranulocytes in vitro (GOLDE and CLINE, 1972; MOORE and WILLIAMS, 1972; GOLDE et al., 1972; CHERVENICK and LOBUGLIO, 1973; RUSCETTI and CHERVENICK, 1974). Furthermore, mononuclear phagocytes play a role in the processes of antibody formation (UNANUE, 1975; FELDMAN et al., 1975; PIERCE and KAPP, 1976;

Table 6. Biologically active products synthetized and secreted by macrophages

Pyrogen
Interferon
Lysosomal hydrolases
Lysozyme
Collagenase
Elastase
Plasminogen activator
Thromboplastin
Prostaglandins (PGE_2, $PGF_{2\alpha}$)
Complement components (C1, C2, C3, C4, C5, C6, factor B and D)
Transferrin
Transcobalamin II
Stimulants of T and B lymphocytes
Inhibitors of T and B lymphocytes
Colony stimulating factor
Tumor growth inhibiting factor
Stimulant of fibroblast proliferation
Stimulant of vascular proliferation
Factor increasing monocytopoiesis

BASTEN and MITCHEL, 1976) and in cell-mediated immunity. In cell-mediated immune reactions, the macrophages have a dual role: they not only participate in the presentation of antigens to T-lymphocytes (OPPENHEIM et al., 1975; ROSENTHAL et al., 1975; OPPENHEIM and SEEGER, 1976; ROSENTHAL et al., 1976; ROSENSTREICH and OPPENHEIM, 1976), which are thus stimulated to proliferate and produce biologically active substances (e.g. lymphokines), but also function as effector cells, which are activated by the lymphokines produced by the T-lymphocytes (DUMONDE et al., 1975). These activated mononuclear phagocytes can deal with micro-organisms much more efficiently than the unstimulated cells, by virtue of the enhanced ingestion and intracellular killing. Another important feature of the multifunctional mononuclear phagocytes is the extracellular cytotoxicity (i.e. cytostatic and cytocidal action) of macrophages against tumour and other cells (EVANS, 1975; LOHMANN-MATTHES and FISCHER, 1975; KELLER, 1975, 1976; REMINGTON et al., 1975; GALLILY, 1975; SELJELID, 1975; LOHMANN-MATTHES, 1976; TEVETHIA et al., 1976; EVANS and ALEXANDER, 1976). Although these effects can be demonstrated in vivo and in vitro, the biochemical mechanisms involved and the way in which macrophages inhibit the growth of other types of cell or kill such cells, are still unknown.

E. Origin and Kinetics of Mononuclear Phagocytes During the Normal Steady State

It has been definitely proven that macrophages do not derive from lymphocytes or originate from mesenchymal cells. Evidence that tissue macrophages originate from monocytes was obtained from chimaera studies demonstrating the bone marrow origin for peritoneal macrophages, liver macrophages and lung macrophages (BALNER, 1963; GOODMAN, 1964; PINKET et al., 1966; VIROLAINEN, 1968; HOWARD, 1970; SHAND and BELL, 1972; GODLESKI and BRAIN, 1972).

Table 7. In vitro and pulse ^{3}H-Thymidine labelling of mononuclear phagocytes

		In vitro labelling[a]	Pulse labelling[b]
		%	%
Monoblasts		92.0–96.0	
Promonocytes		50.3–54.0	68.7
Monocytes:	Bone marrow	0.3– 2.4	1.0
	Blood	2.3	2.3
Macrophages:	Peritoneal	3.6– 4.1	2.4
	Lung	1.5– 3.0	
	Liver	0.8	1.0
	Skin	0.7– 0.9	0.3

[a] In medium with 0.1 μCi/ml ^{3}H-thymidine for intervals of 2–48 h.
[b] 1 or 2 h after 1 × 1 μCi/g ^{3}H-thymidine, given i.v.

Table 8. Effect of hydrocortisone treatment on the ^{3}H-thymidine labelling of peritoneal and liver macrophages

Time after hydrocortisone[a]	Labelling index[b]	
	Peritoneal macrophages	Liver macrophages
h	%	%
0	3.4	0.80
6	2.7	0.75
12	1.4	0.55
18	0.3	0.10
24	0	0.25

[a] 15 mg hydrocortisone acetate s.c.
[b] incubated for 24 h in medium with 0.1 μCi/ml ^{3}H-thymidine.

To obtain more information about the origin of the macrophages, it was first necessary to establish which of the mononuclear phagocytes are actively dividing cells. This question was studied on the basis of the in vitro incorporation of and 1-h pulse labelling with ^{3}H-thymidine. The results of the in vitro labelling studies, shown in Table 7, demonstrate that during the steady state only the monoblasts and promonocytes actively divide and that monocytes and macrophages are in essence non-dividing cells.

The low percentage of ^{3}H-thymidine labelled macrophages could be interpreted as an indication of a slow proliferation of these cells in the tissues. However, during treatment with glucocorticosteroids, which leads rapidly to severe monocytopenia lasting many days, but does not grossly affect the number of macrophages already present in the tissues, the labelling indices of the peritoneal and liver macrophages

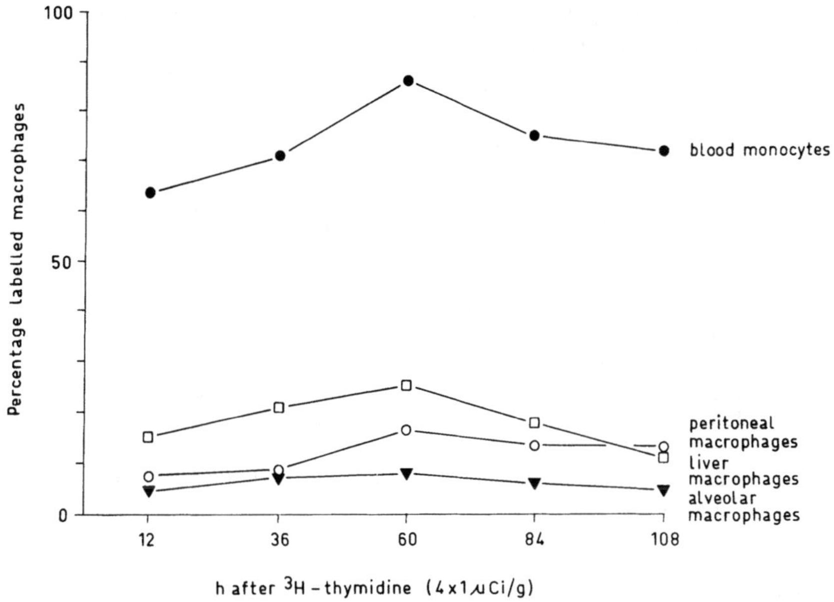

Fig. 2. Course of labelled monocytes, and peritoneal, lung and liver macrophages after four injections of ^{3}H-thymidine prior to zero point

decrease from 3.5% and 0.8%, respectively, to almost nil 18–24 h after the injection of hydrocortisone (Table 8) (VAN FURTH and COHN, 1968; CROFTON et al., 1978). Since glucocorticosteroids do not inhibit the DNA synthesis of promonocytes either in vitro or in vivo (THOMPSON and VAN FURTH, 1970, 1973), but prevent the influx of mononuclear phagocytes into the tissues (see Section G), these findings prove that the DNA-synthesizing mononuclear phagocytes in the tissues derive from the circulation and indicate a bone marrow origin. The rapid decrease in the labelling index of macrophages during hydrocortisone treatment implies that the small percentage of DNA-synthesizing mononuclear phagocytes divide only once, shortly after their arrival in the tissues (within 24 h).

In vivo labelling studies support the bone marrow origin of the macrophages. After a single intravenous injection of ^{3}H-thymidine, the labelling index of the promonocytes is 68.7% at 2 h Table 7) and then decreases in the next 96 h (Fig. 10); the labelling indices of the bone marrow and peripheral blood monocytes are 1.0 and 2.3% after 2 h, respectively (Table 7), and increase to a maximum at 24 or 48 h, after which they decrease again (VAN FURTH and DIESSELHOFF-DEN DULK, 1970). The labelling indices of the peritoneal, lung and liver macrophages are lower than 2.5% 1 h after a single pulse labelling (Table 7), and thereafter show roughly the same course as the labelled peripheral blood monocytes but at a much lower level (VAN FURTH and DIESSELHOFF-DEN DULK, 1970; CROFTON et al., 1978). The labelling indices of the peripheral blood monocytes and of various types of macrophages after four injections of ^{3}H-thymidine show the same course as after a single injection but the values are higher (Fig. 2).

Table 9. Effect of X-irradiation with shielding[a] on the ^{3}H-thymidine labelling[b] index of peritoneal and liver macrophages

Time after labelling	Labelling index			
	Peritoneal macrophages		Liver macrophages	
h	Normal %	X-irradiated %	Normal %	X-irradiated %
12	6.3	0.60	1.4	0.06
36	13.4	0.45	2.0	0.13
60	17.0	1.70	4.0	0.39
84	8.3	2.25	6.4	0.26
152	5.0	1.80	4.1	0.09
156	4.7	0.70	1.9	0.12

[a] 650 R with shielding of both hind limbs and part of pelvis.
[b] 4×1 µCi/g ^{3}H-thymidine i.m.

Proof that peritoneal and liver macrophages derive from the bone marrow was obtained in studies in which the animals received total body irradiation with shielding of both hind limbs and part of the pelvis, and were labelled 24 h later with ^{3}H-thymidine. The results show that in these X-irradiated animals, in which the peritoneal and liver macrophages are also exposed, the labelling indices of these macrophages is about 10% of that in normal animals (Table 9). Since the bone marrow of both hind limbs constitutes about 10% of the total bone marrow mass, the course of these labelling indices agrees well with what could be expected if in normal animals tissue macrophages are continuously replaced by circulating monocytes originating from the bone marrow.

The results of the labelling experiments based on a single injection of ^{3}H-thymidine also provided data about the production of monocytes during the normal steady state, since not only the total number of monocytes in the bone marrow and circulation, but also the half-time of the monocytes in the circulation, is known. The calculations, described in detail elsewhere (VAN FURTH et al., 1973), show that in normal animals 15.6×10^5 labelled monocytes are formed during the first 24 h, after which the production levels off (Fig. 3).

The rate of monocyte production during this period amounts to 0.65×10^5 cells per h (Table 10).

Additional information about monocyte production was obtained from the determination of the cell-cycle time of the promonocytes, which amounts to 16.2 h during the normal steady state (Table 11) (VAN FURTH et al., 1973). From this value and from the total number of promonocytes in the bone marrow, the rate of monocyte production can be calculated, and amounts to 0.62×10^5 cells per h (Table 10). The value for monocyte production calculated according to these two completely independent methods agree very well.

The labelling studies also provided quantitative information about the transit of monocytes through the peripheral blood compartment and their influx into the tissues. These calculations are based on the data obtained during the first 48 h after a

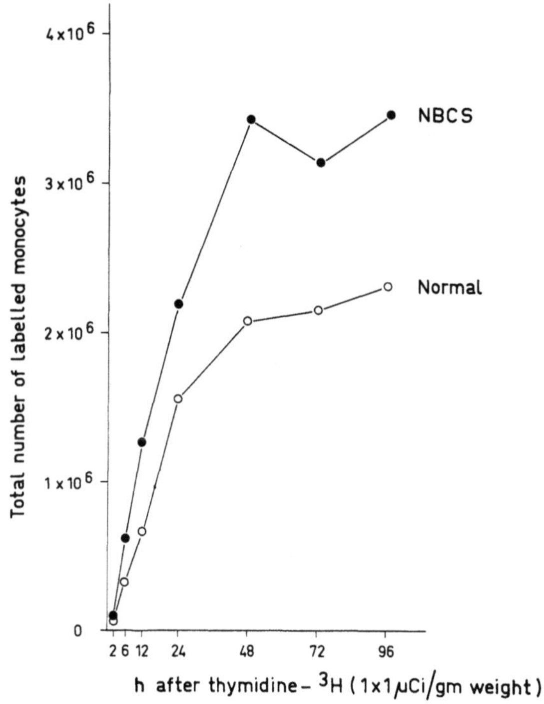

Fig. 3. Total production of labelled monocytes formed after a single injection of ^{3}H-thymidine in normal mice and mice with an acute inflammatory response. (*NBCS* – Newborn Calf Serum). (From J. exp. Med. **138**, 1314, 1973)

Table 10. Monocyte production rate under various conditions

Conditions	Monocyte production	
	Calculation A[a] $\times 10^5$/h	Calculation B[b] $\times 10^5$/h
Normal	0.65	0.62
Inflammation[c] 1–12 h	1.06	
at 12 h		0.96
12–24 h	0.78	
at 24 h		0.70
Azathioprine[d]	0.49	0.49
Azathioprine[d] + Inflammation at 12 h		0.47
1–24 h	0.49	
Glucocorticosteroids[e]		0.50
Glucocorticosteroids[e] + Inflammation at 12 h		0.59

[a] Rate of monocyte production $= \dfrac{\text{total monocyte production in period t}}{\text{t}}$.

[b] Rate of monocyte production $= 2 \times \dfrac{\text{total number of promonocytes}}{\text{cell-cycle time of promonocytes}}$.

[c] 1 ml newborn calf serum injected i.p.

[d] 96 h after daily s.c. injection of 3 mg/kg azathioprine.

[e] 72 h after a s.c. injection of 15 mg hydrocortisone acetate.

Table 11. Cell cycle of promonocytes under various conditions

	Normal	Hydro-cortisone[a]	Azathio-prine[b]	Inflammation 12 h	Inflammation 24 h	Inflammation[c] + Hydro-cortison[a]	Inflammation[c] + Azathio-prine[d]
	h	h	h	h	h	h	h
Cell-cycle time	16.2	14.0	22.8	10.8	16.7	14.1	19.6
DNA-synthesis time	11.8	10.5	18.6	7.6	12.8	10.5	16.0

[a] 15 mg hydrocortisone s.c. 72 h earlier.
[b] daily 3 mg/kg azathioprine s.c.; mean of determinations at 96 and 192 h.
[c] 1 ml newborn calf serum i.p. 12 h earlier.
[d] 3 mg/kg azathioprine daily for 96 h.

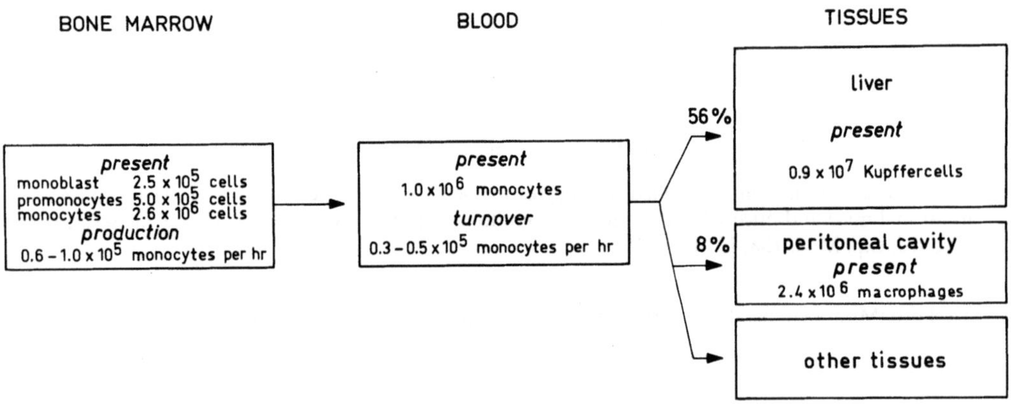

Fig. 4. Data concerning the numbers of mononuclear phagocytes in the bone marrow, circulation, and tissues, and the production and kinetics of monocytes of SPF mice in the normal steady state. The range in the production and turnover rates is due to changes in the general condition of SPF mice over the last 5 years. The percentages shown between the blood and tissue compartments refer to the proportion of the circulating monocytes that arrive in that particular tissue at any given time

single injection of ^{3}H thymidine, since after this period there is almost no production of labelled monocytes. Figure 4 shows the numbers of mononuclear phagocytes in the various compartments of normal mice. The indicated production rate of the monocytes in the bone marrow and the turnover time in the circulation pertain to studies done during the last five years (VAN FURTH et al., 1973; CROFTON et al., 1978) and show a range reflecting a change in the condition of the strain of SPF mice. Nevertheless, these data indicate that half the number monocytes of produced in the bone marrow do not reach the circulation. This must be considered ineffective monocytopoiesis, i.e., the cells die in the bone marrow compartment. Alternative explanations for our kinetic findings, namely another pattern of division of the

Table 12. Characteristics of the production and kinetics of monocytes during the normal steady state

Species	Pro-monocyte cell-cycle time	Monocyte production	Circulating monocytes		Reference
			Pool size	Half-time	
	h	$\times 10^6$ cells/kg/h	$\times 10^6$/kg	h	
Mouse	16.2	2.5	40	22	VAN FURTH and COHN (1968) VAN FURTH et al. (1973)
Rat	18–34	6.9[a]	89	35	VOLKMAN (1967, 1970) VOLKMAN and COLLINS (1974)
Rat	21	0.2[a]		13–14	WHITELAW et al. (1968) WHITELAW and BATHO (1972)
Man	40–82	0.6[a]		71	WHITELAW (1972)
Man	29	7.5[a]	18–25	8.4	MEURET (1974)

[a] The monocyte production estimated from the monocyte turnover in the circulation is too low, because a considerable number of newly formed monocytes remaining in the bone marrow compartment were not taken into account.

promonocytes or a marginating pool of monocytes, would give divergent results for the two ways of calculating monocyte production (VAN FURTH et al., 1973), and therefore cannot be valid.

At present, the destination of about 75% of the monocytes that have left the circulation is known: 8% of these cells arrive in the peritoneal cavity (VAN FURTH et al., 1973), about 10% become lung and alveolar macrophages (BLUSSÉ and VAN FURTH, 1978), and 56% of those which have left the circulation become Kupffer cells (CROFTON et al., 1978) (Fig. 4).

Studies on the production and kinetics of monocytes have also been carried out in normal rats and man. Here, however, information on the production has been obtained indirectly, because the studies did not include the mononuclear phagocytes of the bone marrow and no attempt was made to identify the monocyte precursors. In this respect, the studies of MEURET (MEURET, 1974; MEURET and HOFFMANN, 1973) are difficult to interpret because he refers to all mononuclear phagocytes in the bone marrow as promonocytes; this is misleading, since monocytes account for 85–95% of the mononuclear phagocytes in the bone marrow and 1–2% of the nucleated cells in the bone marrow (VAN FURTH and DIESSELHOFF-DEN DULK, 1970, 1978; VAN FURTH et al., 1976). The data, which in view of the above-mentioned objections should be regarded with some reserve, are shown in Table 12.

F. Origin and Kinetics of Mononuclear Phagocytes During an Inflammatory Response

As already mentioned, the main function of mononuclear phagocytes is to eliminate deleterious material by phagocytosis or pinocytosis, but the number of macrophages occurring in normal tissues is generally much too small to deal effectively with either micro-organisms or non-infectious substances that cause tissue injury. However, the body can resort to circulating phagocytic cells which migrate to the effected tissues and help to eliminate both the inflammatory agents and necrotic tissue, thus contributing to tissue repair. This migration of cells from the circulation to the tissues was described extensively by COHNHEIM as early as 1882 and more recently by EBERT and FLOREY (1939).

I. Acute Inflammation

The kinetics of the mononuclear phagocytes during an acute inflammation has been studied in great detail in the mouse model, the inflammatory stimulus consisting of an intraperitoneal injection of newborn calf serum, polystyrene particles or silica, or an intravenous injection of zymosan (VAN FURTH and COHN, 1968; VAN FURTH et al., 1973; VAN WAARDE et al., 1976, 1976a; CROFTON et al., 1978).

The investigations with newborn calf serum demonstrate that initially granulocytes appear in the peritoneal cavity, and after a short time the number of peritoneal macrophages increases (Fig. 5). Concomitantly, the number of circulating monocytes also increases (Fig. 6).

The problem of whether the increase in number of peritoneal macrophages during an inflammation induced by newborn calf serum is due to local proliferation was studied by in vitro and in vivo pulse labelling with ^{3}H-thymidine. The results gave in vitro labelling indices of 0.2–3% and in vivo labelling of 0.3–4.0% after 1 h (VAN FURTH and COHN, 1968; VAN FURTH et al., 1973), which are the same values as those obtained during the steady state, thus demonstrating that this kind of inflammatory stimulus does not induce proliferation of resident macrophages. After an intravenous injection of zymosan, however, the labelling index of the liver macrophages increased from 0.8% to 9.8 and 11.2% at 24 and 48 h, respectively. When this stimulus was applied to hydrocortisone-treated animals, the labelling index did not increase and even dropped below the normal value (0.3 and 0.6% at 24 and 48 h, respectively) (CROFTON et al., 1978). These results lead to the same conclusion as for the peritoneal and liver macrophages of unstimulated mice (Table 8), i.e. that the DNA-synthesizing cells are recruited from the bone marrow and are not the resident population of liver macrophages.

To obtain further information about the production and kinetics of the mononuclear phagocytes, the animals were first labelled with a single injection of ^{3}H-thymidine and 1 h later received an intraperitoneal injection of newborn calf serum. The results show that during the first 48 h the production of labeled monocytes is 64% greater than in normal mice (Figs. 3 and 7). During that period, the influx of labelled monocytes from the bone marrow into the peripheral blood is twice as high in mice with an acute inflammation as in normal animals; the total efflux of labelled monocytes from the circulation is also twice the normal value during the inflammatory response. The difference between the number of monocytes that have entered the peripheral blood compartment and the number that have left the circulation at 48 h is the number of labelled monocytes still present in that compartment at 48 h. At

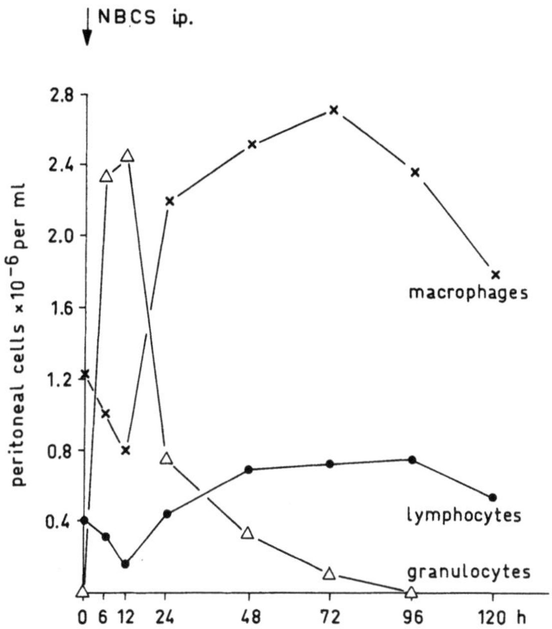

Fig. 5. Course of the numbers of leucocytes in peritoneal cavity during an inflammation induced by an i.p. injection of 1 ml newborn calf serum (*NBCS*)

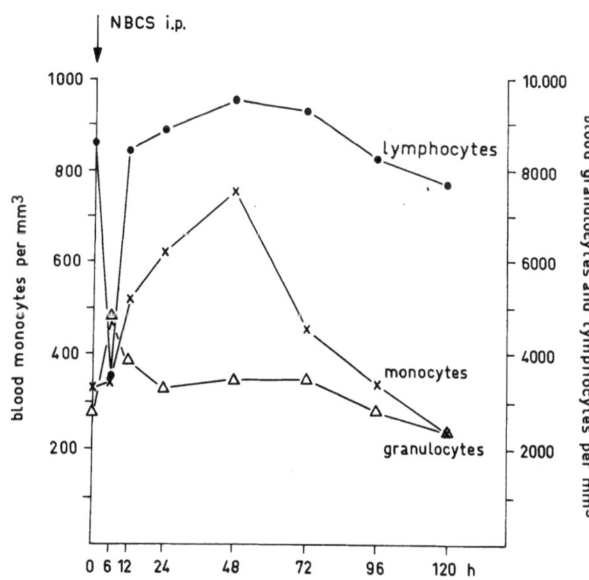

Fig. 6. Course of the numbers of circulating leucocytes during an inflammatory response caused by an i.p. injection of 1 ml newborn calf serum (*NBCS*)

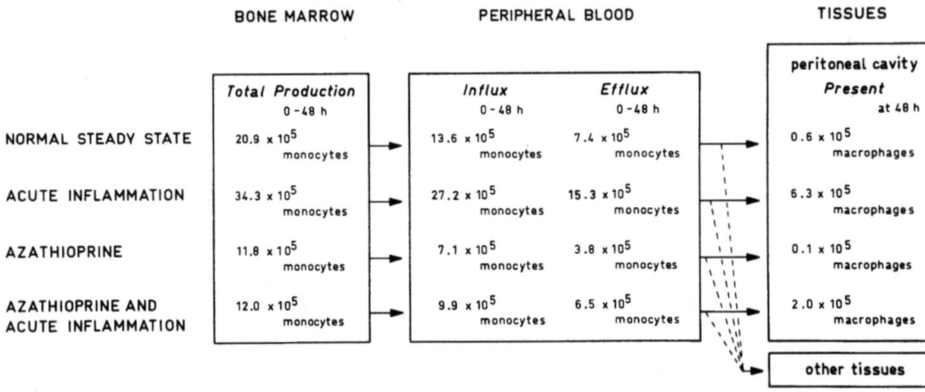

Fig. 7. Total production of labelled monocytes in bone marrow, their transit to peripheral blood compartment and their migration into peritoneal cavity during normal steady state, an acute inflammatory reaction, and treatment with a low dose (3 mg/kg) of azathioprine. (From J. exp. Med. **141**, 531, 1975)

48 h, the inflammatory exudate in the peritoneal cavity contains 41.2% of the labelled monocytes that have left the circulation, whereas in normal mice this value is 7.6%. It is remarkable that about 70% of the extraproduced cells arrive at the site of inflammation (VAN FURTH et al., 1973).

From these experiments, the rate of monocyte production during an acute inflammation could also be calculated; 1.06×10^5 cells were produced during the first 12 h and 0.78×10^5 cells were produced during the next 12–24 h (Fig. 3, Table 10) (VAN FURTH et al., 1973).

The cell-cycle parameters of promonocytes were also determined during an inflammatory response. Initially, 12 h after a newborn calf serum injection, the cell-cycle time is significantly reduced, but later returns to a normal value (Table 11). The values calculated for the monocyte production during the inflammatory response using the promonocyte numbers and the cell-cycle time, are in excellent agreement with those obtained from the labelling experiments (Table 10) (VAN FURTH et al., 1973).

These findings demonstrate that during an acute inflammatory response in the peritoneal cavity, the production of monocytes is augmented and that the majority of the mononuclear phagocytes recruited to the site of the lesions are newly-formed cells. Similar results have been obtained for the liver macrophages, with an intravenous injection of zymosan as the inflammatory stimulus (CROFTON et al., 1978). In the rat, similar studies on the production and kinetics of monocytes carried out during a systemic infection with *Salmonella enteritis* showed a doubling of the monocyte production, an increase of about 3.5 times the number of circulating monocytes and a decrease in the half-time of these cells (15 h instead of 35 h in normal rats) (VOLKMAN and COLLINS, 1974). A comparable pattern of monocyte production was also found in man during certain kinds of inflammation, with or without infection (MEURET, 1974; MEURET and HOFFMANN, 1973).

II. Chronic Inflammation

Chronic inflammatory reactions can be divided into two groups: those with and those without the formation of granulomas, depending on the agent (infectious or non-infectious) responsible for the inflammation. When the irritant cannot be easily disposed of by the mononuclear phagocytes (indigestible material, e.g. mycobacteria, schistosoma, streptococcal cell walls, fibrinogen, Freund's complete adjuvant, silica, carrageenin, paraffin oil), granuloma formation usually occurs (SPECTOR and RYAN, 1970; RYAN and SPECTOR, 1970; SPECTOR, 1974; SPECTOR and MARIANO, 1975; DANNENBERG et al., 1975; GINSBURG et al., 1975; WARREN and BOROS, 1975).

In a simple chronic inflammation, the macrophages at the site of the lesion are bone marrow-derived monocytes, the mechanism underlying cell recruitment being similar to that prevailing during an acute reaction. The granulomatous reaction can be subdivided into two forms: the high-turnover and low-turnover granulomas (SPECTOR and RYAN, 1970; RYAN and SPECTOR, 1970; SPECTOR, 1974; SPECTOR and MARIANO, 1975). Granulomas induced by microbial agents (e.g. mycobacteria, schistosoma, *B. pertussis* vaccine) are usually of the high-turnover type, the cells involved in this inflammatory reaction being recently recruited circulating monocytes and locally proliferating mononuclear phagocytes. The contribution of local proliferation is relatively small; for example, in a tuberculous lesion a third of the recently arrived mononuclear phagocytes divide only once during the first week of residence in the lesion (DANNENBERG et al., 1975). Low-turnover granulomas are highly dependent on the supply of circulating monocytes, and such lesions (induced for example by carrageenin, paraffin oil or talc) show a high proportion of long-lived macrophages virtually without mitotic activity.

Epitheloid cells found in granulomatous lesions are transformed monocytes or macrophages but show much less phagocytic activity than the macrophages; they show a high level of pinocytosis and even more exocytosis. The life span of epitheloid cells is relatively short (on average 1 week, max. 4 weeks) (SPECTOR and MARIANO, 1975).

A striking feature of high-turnover granulomas is the presence of multinucleate giant cells arising from the fusion of mononuclear phagocytes (mainly the conjunction of young, newly arrived monocytes with ageing macrophages) (SPECTOR and MARIANO, 1975) rather than from the nuclear division of macrophages. Once the polykaryon is formed, the nuclei may enter the mitotic cycle in synchrony (PAPADIMITRIOU and CORNELISSE, 1975). Multinucleate giant cells are scarce in low-turnover granulomas.

G. The Effects of Anti-Inflammatory Drugs

The effects of two anti-inflammatory drugs (i.e. glucocorticosteroids and azathioprine) on the formation and kinetics of mononuclear phagocytes during the normal steady state and an inflammatory response, have been studied in more detail.

I. Glucocorticosteroids

The effects of glucocorticosteroids on the kinetics of mononuclear phagocytes, i.e. peripheral blood monocytes and peritoneal macrophages, have been studied in nor-

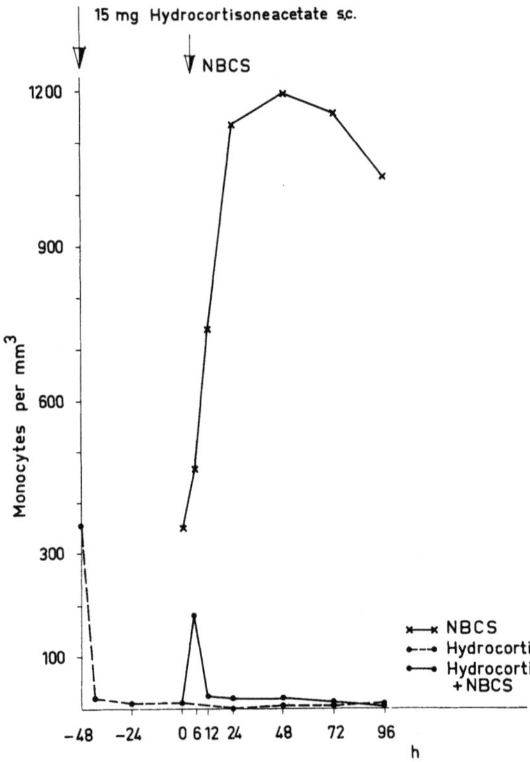

Fig. 8. Effect of an i.p. injection of 1 ml newborn calf serum (*NBCS*) on the number of peripheral blood monocytes of normal mice (×——×), and of mice pretreated 48 h earlier with 15 mg hydrocortisone (●—●). The third line (●----●) shows the effect of an injection of 15 mg hydrocortisone alone. (From J. exp. Med. **131**, 429, 1970)

mal mice as well as in mice with an inflammatory reaction induced in the peritoneal cavity.

The administration of glucocorticosteroids resulted in a rapid decrease (within 3–6 h) in the number of circulating monocytes, the duration of the effect being dependent on the nature and dose of the compound. Water-soluble dexamethasone sodium phosphate is only briefly active (less than 12 h), but hydrocortisone acetate, which forms a subcutaneous depot, reduces the number of monocytes for a period of about 2 weeks (Fig. 8) (THOMPSON and VAN FURTH, 1970). On the basis of the rapid disappearance of the circulating monocytes (in less than the half-time of 22 h) and the exclusion of a lytic effect on mononuclear phagocytes, it was concluded that the cells are (temporarily) sequestered in a compartment of unknown localisation. This effect of glucocorticosteroids, which we studied in mice (THOMPSON and VAN FURTH, 1970), was later shown to occur in the guinea pig, rat, rabbit, and in man (TOMPKINS, 1952; SLONECKER and LIM, 1972; DALE et al., 1974; FAUCI and DALE, 1974), thus showing this action of glucocorticosteroids on the number of circulating monocytes to be common to a number of species.

In normal mice, hydrocortisone does not affect the number of macrophages already present in the peritoneal cavity (Fig. 9), but the transit of mononuclear

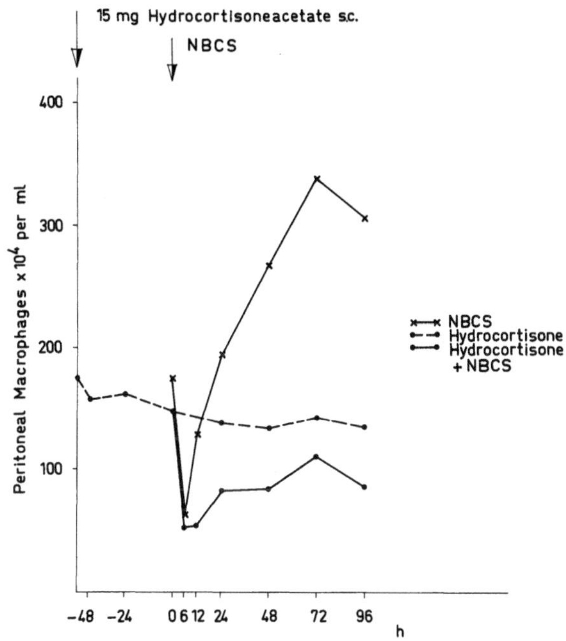

Fig. 9. Effect of an i. p. injection of 1 ml newborn calf serum (*NBCS*) on the number of peritoneal macrophages of normal mice (×——×), and of mice pretreated 48 h earlier with 15 mg hydrocortisone (●——●). The third line (●---●) shows effect of an injection of 15 ml hydrocortisone alone. (From J. exp. Med. **131**, 429, 1970)

phagocytes from the circulation into the peritoneal cavity is arrested. However, during an inflammatory response in the peritoneal cavity, hydrocortisone suppresses the increase in the number of both the monocytes in the peripheral blood and the peritoneal macrophages (Figs. 8 and 9). This reduction appeared to be due to a diminished influx of mononuclear phagocytes from the peripheral blood (THOMPSON and VAN FURTH, 1970).

To elucidate the mechanism underlying the prolonged monocytopenia induced in the peripheral blood of mice during treatment with glucocorticosteroids, the effect of this drug on the production and release of monocytes in and from the bone marrow was studied. The results show that hydrocortisone causes a rapid reduction in the number of bone marrow promonocytes, which falls to about 65% of the normal steady state value, and that the number of monocytes in the bone marrow decreases gradually to 75% of the initial value after 96 h. The mitotic activity of the promonocytes is only slightly diminished, as judged from the in vitro labelling studies and the cell-cycle time (14 h), the latter being only a little shorter than in the normal steady state (16.2 h) (Table 11). With this value and the number of promonocytes, the rate of monocyte production was calculated, giving a value of 0.50×10^5 cells per h (Table 10), which means a reduction of about 20% compared with the normal rate (VAN FURTH, 1975b). The release of monocytes is also retarded by hydrocortisone, since after in vivo labelling the newly formed monocytes remain in the bone marrow longer (Fig. 10) (THOMPSON and VAN FURTH, 1973).

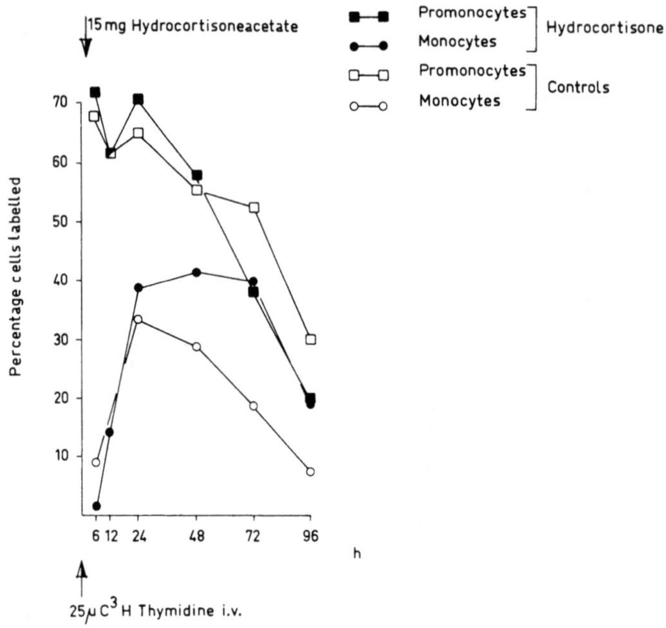

Fig. 10. Effect of a s.c. injection of 15 mg hydrocortisone acetate administered 1 h after 25 μCi of ^{3}H-thymidine i.v. on the percentage of labelled promonocytes and monocytes in bone marrow. (From J. exp. Med. **137**, 10, 1973)

During an inflammatory reaction there is almost no recruitment of monocytes from the bone marrow. Labelling studies showed that in these hydrocortisone-treated mice with an acute inflammation, the cell-cycle time of the promonocytes is not shorter than in mice treated only with glucocorticosteroids (Table 11). However, after the same interval, the number of promonocytes is increased by 20%, and thus the calculated rate of monocyte production during the initial phase of the acute inflammation is 20% higher than in animals treated only with hydrocortisone acetate but still much lower (39%) than in normal animals with an acute inflammation (Table 10) (THOMPSON and VAN FURTH, 1973; VAN FURTH, 1975b).

II. Azathioprine

The effect of azathioprine (Imuran) on the kinetics of peripheral blood monocytes and peritoneal macrophages was studied in normal mice and in mice in which an inflammatory reaction was provoked. The number of peripheral blood monocytes decreases gradually during azathioprine treatment of normal mice, the extent and duration being dependent on the dose and duration of administration. A high dose of 200 mg/kg (which is the maximum tolerated daily dose in mice) administered each day for 9 days, reduces monocyte numbers to almost nil. A low dose of 3 mg/kg (which is roughly equivalent to a non-toxic immunosuppressive, anti-inflammatory dose in man) gave a reduction of about 50% after 9 days (Fig. 11). This effect is reversible, because 24–48 h after treatment is stopped, the number of monocytes starts to increase (GASSMANN and VAN FURTH, 1975).

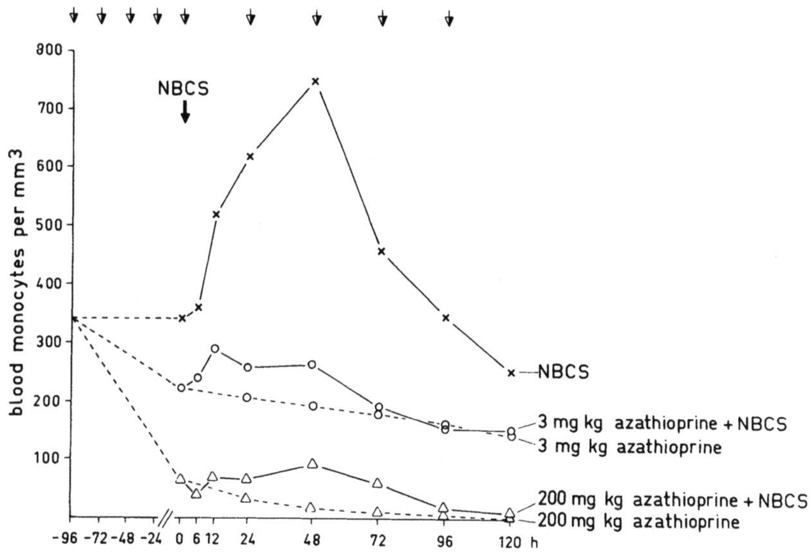

Fig. 11. Effect of azathioprine (daily treatment with 3 or 200 mg/kg) (↓) on the number of peripheral blood monocytes of normal mice and during an acute inflammation in the peritoneal cavity provoked with an injection of 1 ml newborn calf serum (*NBCS*) (↓). For comparison, the course of the number of peripheral blood monocytes in normal mice with a similar acute peritoneal inflammation is shown. (From Blood **46**, 51, 1975)

The number of peritoneal macrophages is only affected when a high dose (200 mg/kg) is given over a long period; a low dose has virtually no effect. Since the macrophages in the tissues are not a static population but are continuously replaced by monocytes from the peripheral blood, the action of a drug affecting the number of tissue macrophages can be interpreted properly only by taking into consideration its effect on the peripheral blood monocytes. Since treatment with a high dose of azathioprine reduces the number of circulating monocytes relatively rapidly, the number of monocytes available to emigrate to the tissues (e.g. peritoneal cavity) is markedly diminished (GASSMANN and VAN FURTH, 1975) (Fig. 11). This results in a decline in the number of peritoneal macrophages after 4 days of treatment with a high dose of azathioprine, the rate of this decline giving an indication of the turnover of tissue macrophages. During the low-dose azathioprine treatment, the number of peritoneal macrophages is only slightly reduced, because sufficient numbers of monocytes are still present in the circulation to replace the loss of macrophages from the peritoneal cavity (Fig. 12).

In mice with an induced inflammatory reaction in the peritoneal cavity, the normally occurring increase in the number of both peripheral blood monocytes and peritoneal macrophages is suppressed, the extent being dependent on the dose of azathioprine administered (GASSMANN and VAN FURTH, 1975) (Figs. 11 and 12). Labelling studies with ^{3}H-thymidine demonstrated that the reduction of peripheral blood monocytes in normal mice and during an inflammatory reaction is due to a diminished monocyte production. As a result, the number of labelled cells arriving in an inflammatory lesion is lower in azathioprine-treated mice than in normal mice

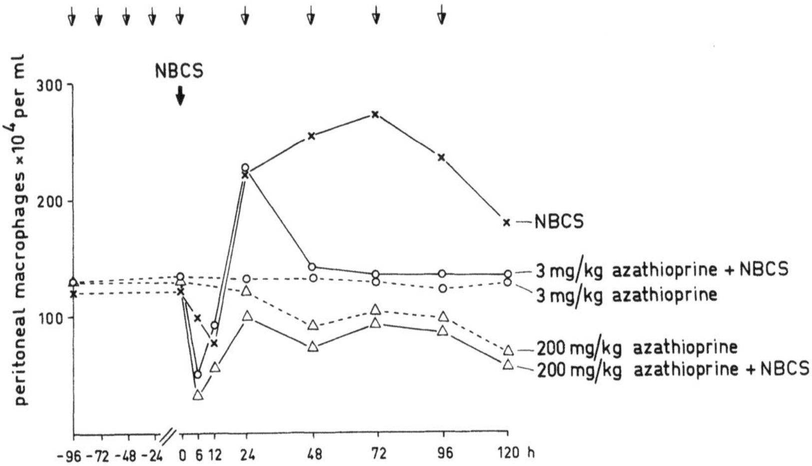

Fig. 12. Effect of azathioprine on the number of peritoneal macrophages in normal mice and during an acute peritoneal inflammation. After daily treatment with 200 mg/kg azathioprine (↓) for 9 days, the number of peritoneal macrophages is reduced by about 50%, whereas daily treatment with 3 mg/kg azathioprine has virtually no effect. An i.p. injection of 1 ml newborn calf serum (*NBCS*) (↓) causes an increase in the number of peritoneal macrophages in normal mice. This effect is considerably smaller in mice treated with azathioprine. (From Blood **46**, 51, 1975)

(Fig. 7), confirming the conclusion drawn from studies without a cell marker. This diminished monocyte production is caused by decreased mitotic activity of the promonocytes. During the treatment with 3 mg/kg azathioprine, the cell-cycle time was 6.6 h longer than in the normal steady state (Table 11), and the rate of monocyte production was reduced by 70% (Table 10). During an acute inflammatory reaction, too, monocyte production in the azathioprine-treated mice was decreased and not increased as normally occurs during an inflammatory response (VAN FURTH et al., 1975a) (Table 10).

On the basis of in vitro and in vivo labelling studies, cytospectrophotometric determination of the Feulgen-DNA content of the promonocytes and determination of the DNA-synthesis time of these cells, it could be concluded that azathioprine arrests the cell-cycle of the promonocytes late in the DNA-synthesis phase or in the postsynthesis (G2) phase and therefore that mitosis does not occur (VAN FURTH et al., 1975a).

H. Humoral Control of Monocytopoiesis During Inflammation

During inflammatory reactions or infections, the number of macrophages at the site of the lesion may increase. Usually, this is due to increased recruitment of monocytes from the circulation, but in some forms of chronic inflammation local proliferation may occur.

The processes locally regulating the transit of circulating leucocytes into the tissues are discussed elsewhere in this volume. Little is known about the factors controlling the proliferation of mononuclear phagocytes in the inflamed tissues. In most instances, it is not the resident macrophages but immature mononuclear phagocytes recruited from the bone marrow that proliferate in the tissues. Factors like the colony stimulating factor but formed locally, for example by fibroblasts (PLUZNIK and SACHS, 1966; BRADLEY and METCALF, 1966; GOUD, 1975) or mononuclear phagocytes (GOLDE and CLINE, 1972; MOORE and WILLIAMS, 1972; GOLDE et al., 1972; CHERVENICK and LOBUGLIO, 1973; RUSCETTI and CHERVENICK, 1974), might stimulate these recruited immature cells to proliferate locally.

Increased recruitment of monocytes into the site of inflammation requires an increased production of these cells in the bone marrow. The processes controlling the production of monocytes in the bone marrow and their release into the circulation remained largely unknown until recently, when more insight into the humoral regulation of these processes was obtained (VAN WAARDE et al., 1976, 1977a, 1977b).

Since the number of monocytes in the normal steady state condition is rather constant, it seems likely that some kind of homeostatic regulatory mechanism controls the production of these cells in the bone marrow. This mechanism is in all probability a more or less complicated homeostatic system in which the demand in the peripheral region (i.e. macrophages in the tissues) determines the rate of production of the macrophages precursors at the source—(i.e. the monocyte production by promonocytes, promonocyte production by monoblasts and possibly even the monoblast production by the (committed) stem cell)—via a (chemical) feedback signal. If a humoral mechanism also controls the extra monocyte production during an inflammatory reaction, a factor increasing monocytopoiesis (FIM) should be demonstrable in the serum during some period of the inflammatory reaction. This possibility was investigated by studying the effect of an intravenous injection into test mice of serum from mice in which an inflammation had been induced.

In an intital study with newborn calf serum as the inflammatory stimulus, a factor increasing monocytopoiesis was demonstrated in mice (VAN WAARDE et al., 1976). To avoid the problem of diffusion of newborn calf serum into the circulation encountered in this study, the inflammatory reaction was subsequently induced in the peritoneal cavity with particulate materials, e.g. polystyrene latex or silica. The course of the number of peritoneal macrophages and circulating monocytes during the inflammatory reaction induced by latex closely resembled that obtained with newborn calf serum; an intraperitoneal injection of silica induced a longer-lasting and stronger reaction in both the peritoneal cavity and the peripheral blood (VAN WAARDE et al., 1976, 1977a).

Sera from mice injected with latex or silica were prepared, and the sera collected during the onset of an inflammatory reaction, proved capable of inducing monocytosis in test mice, whereas normal mouse serum or serum from mice injected with saline did not lead to a higher number of monocytes (VAN WAARDE et al., 1977a). It was evident that the active sera contained a factor that specifically affects the monocytes, because the numbers of granulocytes and lymphocytes remained in the normal range or occasionally showed a small increase (VAN WAARDE et al., 1977a). The course of the activity of the FIM in the serum of mice injected with latex or silica differed (Fig. 13). This activity, expressed in arbitrary units (AU), can be detected 6 h after a latex injection and reaches its peak value at 18 h; the monocytosis-inducing activity then subsides, and from 48 h onward FIM can no longer be demonstrated.

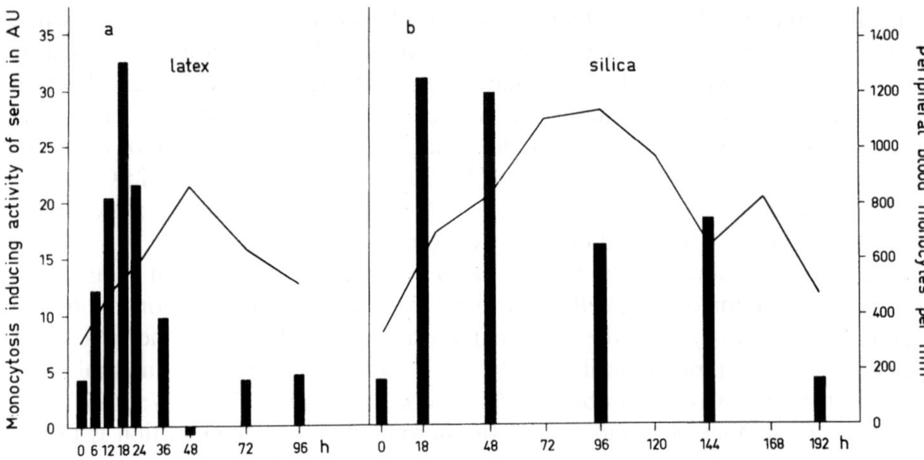

Fig. 13. Course of monocytosis-inducing activity (*bars*) in the serum after an i.p. injection of polystyrene latex (Fig. 13a) or silica (Fig. 13b) compared with the monocytosis induced by these particulates (*line*). Monocytosis-inducing activity (E) of serum obtained at various points after injection of latex or silica is expressed in arbritary units (AU). This value is calculated as difference between area under curve of number of monocytes during period 0–72 h after an i.v. injection of 0.1 ml of a serum (A_e) and product of number of monocytes in corresponding untreated control(N_c) and duration of experiment, i.e. 72 h ($E=A_e-N_c\cdot 72$)

With silica, which induces a more prolonged peritonitis, FIM can be detected for a much longer period (up to 144 h) (Fig. 13). Labelling experiments demonstrated that FIM not only caused release of monocytes from the bone marrow into the circulation, but also increased the monocyte production in the bone marrow (VAN WAARDE et al., 1976, 1977a) by roughly doubling the number of promonocytes and decreasing the cell-cycle time of these cells by 25%.

Information about the site of production of FIM was obtained from studies with extracts of cells from the site of inflammation (i.e. the peritoneal cavity). The extracts of peritoneal cells from normal untreated mice proved to have a high FIM activity, but soon after an intraperitoneal injection of a particulate substance (e.g. latex) this activity drops and then remains low for a period of 12 to 24 h when it increases again to roughly normal values at 96 h (VAN WAARDE et al., 1977a). The courses of the monocytosis-inducing activity of the peritoneal cell extracts and of serum prepared after the intraperitoneal injection of latex, show the reverse pattern. This suggests that FIM is released from the peritoneal cells after the induction of peritonitis and thus controls the number of monocytes (and secondarily the numbers of macrophages, which derive from monocytes) during an inflammatory reaction.

Some of the properties of FIM were determined in serum obtained 18 h after an intraperitoneal injection of latex, as shown in Table 13 (VAN WAARDE et al., 1977b). The FIM molecule is a protein, since the activity was readily destroyed by proteases and FIM was not sensitive to treatment with a mixture of glycosidases, which indicates that a carbohydrate moiety is not needed for its function. Furthermore, immobilised concanavalin-A failed to reduce the activity of a FIM preparation. The latter two findings make it unlikely that FIM is a glycoprotein. The mol wt of FIM,

Table 13. Characteristics of the factor increasing monocytopoiesis (FIM)

Nature: protein, no detectable carbohydrate moieties
Mol wt:
a. 18000–22500 Daltons (ultrafiltration membranes)
b. 18500–24500 Daltons (gelfiltration Sephadex G100)
Stability in serum:
a. 37° C: $t^{1/2}$ 20 min
b. 25° C: $t^{1/2}$ 45 min
c. 4° C: $t^{1/2}$ about 6 h
d. −20° C: stable for more than 3 months
General aspects:
a. no relation to complement factors
b. no relation to clotting factors
c. no chemotactic activity toward macrophages
d. not generated in vitro in normal murine blood by inducers of inflammation

determined with ultrafiltration membranes and by gelfiltration on Sephadex G100, lies between 18000 and 24500 Daltons. Studies in mice deficient in complement (C_5) and in mice treated with cobra venom factor, as well as in vitro treatment of normal murine blood with zymosan or particulate inducers of the inflammatory reaction, ruled out the possibility that FIM is a biologically active fragment of the complement system. Plasma from mice with an acute inflammation showed the same activity as serum or recalcified plasma, which demonstrates that FIM is not one of the clotting factors. Furthermore, active sera had no chemotactic activity toward macrophages. These properties indicate that FIM differs from the colony stimulating factor (a glycoprotein with a mol wt of 45000 Daltons (METCALF, 1973; STANLEY, 1975) and from the known mediators of inflammation (ROCHA E SILVA and LEME, 1972; DOUGLAS, 1975), and is not one of the previously described leucocytosis-inducing or leucocyte-releasing factors (GORDON et al., 1960; BIERMAN, 1964; KATZ et al., 1966; HANDLER et al., 1966; DELMONTE et al., 1968; BOGGS et al., 1968; ROTHSTEIN et al., 1971, 1973; SCHULTZ et al., 1973; DELMONTE, 1974; GOLDE and CLINE, 1974) since these do not induce monocytosis. All this justified the conclusion that FIM is a new factor.

On the basis of the findings with respect to the kinetics, the site of production and mode of action of FIM, the regulation of the mononuclear phagocyte system during an acute inflammatory reaction might be as follows (Fig. 14). During the normal steady state (Fig. 14A), the production of monocytes in the bone marrow is controlled by regulators, i.e. stimulators and inhibitors of monocytopoiesis, which maintain equilibrium in this state. Such mechanisms are common in homeostasis (BULLOUGH, 1965; VERVEEN, 1972), but in normal serum the concentration of these factors is below the detection level of the methods used in the present study. After the induction of an inflammatory reaction (e.g. in the peritoneal cavity), the macrophages at the site of the inflammation phagocytose the inducing substances (Fig. 14B) and the cells at the site of the inflammation release FIM. This is then transported via the circulation to the bone marrow, where it stimulates monocyte production. An increase in the number of promonocytes at 12 h results (Fig. 14C), which indicates that FIM stimulates the monoblast to divide, and hence more pro-

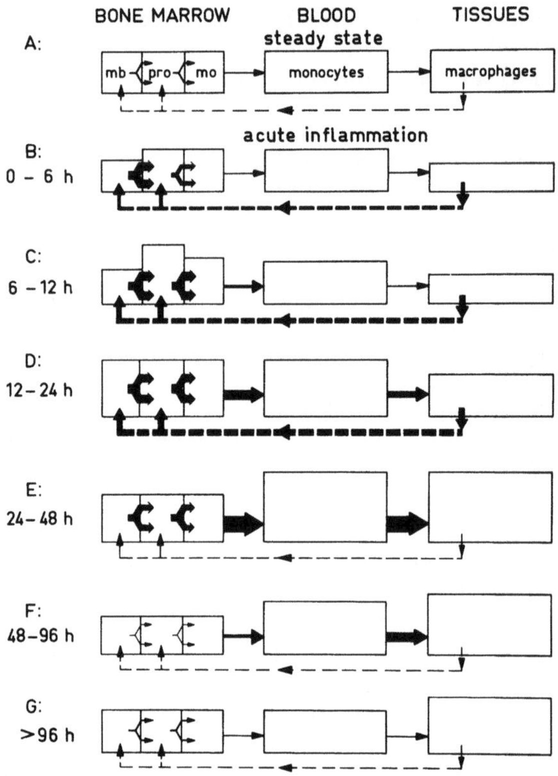

Fig. 14. Schematic representation of reaction of mononuclear phagocyte system to an acute inflammatory stimulus and regulation of this reaction (mb = monoblasts, pro = promonocytes, mo = monocytes)

monocytes are formed. Other effects of the stimulation of monocyte production also become apparent: the cell-cycle time of the promonocytes decreases, giving rise to an increased rate of monocyte production (Fig. 14C). The extra-produced monocytes are released into the circulation, and since more cells enter the blood compartment than leave to go to the tissues, monocytosis develops (Figs. 14D and 14E). Later, more circulating monocytes reach the site of inflammation (Figs. 14E and 14F), but as time proceeds the production of monocytes in the bone marrow and the release of these cells into the peripheral blood both decrease (Fig. 14E) and, as a result, the monocytosis will subside (Fig. 14F). At this point in time (96 h), the cells at the site of the inflammation will again acquire a high FIM content, and after a certain time the mononuclear phagocyte system will return to its normal steady state (Fig. 14G) and be ready to react to a new inflammatory stimulus (VAN WAARDE, 1976).

How the termination of the increased monocyte production is achieved is still unknown. The possibilities to be considered are decreased release and/or production of FIM, and/or increased release of a factor inhibiting monocytopoiesis. Some indications for the existence of a monocyte-production inhibitor (MPI) have been obtained (VAN WAARDE et al., 1977a, 1977b). Such a factor would provide negative feedback.

I. The Mononuclear Phagocyte System and Disease

The information obtained during recent years about the similarities between the morphological, cytochemical, immunological, and functional characteristics of the mononuclear phagocytes (see Section B), and concerning their origin and kinetics (see Sections E and F), has led to a reconsideration of the classification of these cells, which are found among other types of cells in the circulation and tissues. Mononuclear phagocytes have usually been assigned to the reticulo-endothelial system (RES) (ASCHOFF, 1924). According to ASCHOFF (1924), a system is formed by cells sharing a common morphology, origin and function as well as other properties. The RES, however, includes various kinds of cells that do not fulfil the criteria for a system (e.g. endothelial cells, fibrocytes, reticular cells, histiocytes, and monocytes). For example, reticulum cells, dendritic cells, fibroblasts and endothelial cells are of mesenchymal origin (Fig. 1) and proliferate in the tissues, whereas mononuclear phagocytes derive from the haemopoietic stem cell and normally do not multiply outside the bone marrow. In addition, the cytochemical and functional characteristics of mononuclear phagocytes differ from those of the other cells of the RES (see Sections B, C, and E).

Since mononuclear phagocytes do fulfil the criteria for a system, a new classification called the mononuclear phagocyte system was put forward in 1969 (VAN FURTH et al., 1972); the cells assigned to this system are listed in Table 14. This separate classification, which reflects the view that the mononuclear phagocytes form a cell-line distinct from the other cell-lines originating in the bone marrow and are not of mesenchymal origin, should contribute to the understanding of the behaviour of mononuclear phagocytes under normal and pathological conditions.

An attempt to elucidate the participation of mononuclear phagocytes in pathological processes, such as inflammatory reactions, neoplastic processes and storage disorders, is given in Table 15 (VAN FURTH et al., 1975b). The inflammatory reactions include acute, chronic, and chronic granulomatous inflammations caused by

Table 14. Mononuclear Phagocyte System

Stem cell (committed)	Bone marrow
↓	
Monoblasts	Bone marrow
↓	
Promonocytes	Bone marrow
↓	
Monocytes	Bone marrow Peripheral blood
↓	
Macrophages	Tissues Connective tissue (histiocytes) Liver (Kupffer cells) Lung (alveolar macrophages) Lymph nodes (free and fixed macrophages) Spleen (free and fixed macrophages) Bone marrow (macrophages) Serous cavities (pleural and peritoneal macrophages) Synovia? Bone tissue (osteoclasts?) Nervous system (microglial cells)

Table 15. Participation of mononuclear phagocytes in pathological processes

Inflammatory processes	Neoplastic processes	Storage disorders
Acute inflammation	Monocytic leukaemia	Non-digestable substances
Chronic inflammation	Malignant histiocytosis Histiocytic medullary reticulosis Histiocytosis *X*	Enzyme deficiency
Chronic granulomatous inflammation	Histiocytic lymphoma (Reticulum cell sarcoma)	
Destructive granuloma Wegener's granulomatosis Midline granuloma	Malignant Lymphogranuloma (Hodgkin's disease)	

microbial or non-infectious agents. The microbial agents include protista (i.e. bacteria, rickettsiae, chlamydiae, protozoa, fungi) and viruses, as well as multicellular parasites. The participation of the mononuclear phagocyte during the course of an infection can be manifested as monocytosis in the peripheral blood, indicating that an increased number of monocytes is on the way from the site of production (i.e. the bone marrow) to the site of infection (i.e. the tissues).

The non-infectious agents causing an inflammatory reaction, which usually runs a chronic course, are often substances that cannot be degraded by the macrophages—or only partially. Such material is usually stored in the phagocytic cells and therefore these disorders can also be categorised as storage disorders. Thus, mononuclear phagocytes play a role in storage disorders because they are unable to break down ingested material. Two forms can be distinguished, one resulting from the endocytosis of indigestible substances, the other from the accumulation of degradable material in the absence of specific digestive enzymes. The first of these forms includes pneumoconiosis, e.g. anthracosis, silicosis, asbestosis, beryllosis (ZAIDI, 1969; HEPPLESTONE, 1969; ELMES, 1972; MCKERROW, 1972; ALLISON, 1974). The localisation of the lesion in which histiocytes laden with non-digestible material accumulate is determined by the route of entry of the material, e.g. the lung by inhalation of particles in pneumoconiosis, the peritoneal cavity in postoperative talc or starch granuloma (GERMAN, 1943; NEELY and DAVIES, 1971), and the intestinal tract in (pseudo)-melanosis coli caused by absorption of substances that leads to a brownish-black pigmentation in histiocytes (FISHER, 1969). Another group of disorders are the xanthomas, in which macrophages are laden with lipids (cholesterol and phospholipids), which they take up from the plasma but cannot break down (BRAUN-FALCO, 1973).

The second category of storage disorders belongs to the so-called inborn lysosomal disease (HERS, 1973). Because of the deficiency of a lysosomal enzyme, undigested material accumulates in lysosomes of mononuclear phagocytes, for instance glucocerebroside in Gaucher's disease (BRADY and KING, 1973a), sphingomyelin in Niemann Pick's disease (BRADY and KING, 1973b), ganglioside in Tay Sach's disease (O'BRIEN, 1973; SANDHOFF and HARZER, 1973) and galactocerebroside in globoid cell leukodystrophy (Krabbe's disease) (SUZUKI and SUZUKI, 1973).

WEGENER's granulomatosis, a destructive form of granuloma, is a disease of unknown origin characterised by necrotizing granulomatous lesions containing macrophages that proliferate locally or accumulate at the site (WEGENER, 1936, 1939; BLATT et al., 1959; FAUCI and WOLFF, 1973), and can be classified between a reactive inflammation and a neoplastic process.

Mononuclear phagocytes also participate in neoplastic processes, monocytic leukaemia being the most typical neoplastic process of the mononuclear phagocyte system. Histiocytic medullary reticulosis is another malignant disorder of mononuclear phagocytes, characterised by marked erythrophagocytosis by the macrophages (synonym: histiocytes) proliferating in organs (ROBB-SMITH, 1938; SCOTT and ROBB-SMITH, 1939). Histiocytosis comprises a group of related disorders showing proliferation of macrophages but with divergent clinical courses (LICHTENSTEIN, 1953). Histiocytic lymphoma (GALL, 1958) is a form of malignant lymphoma (LUKES, 1968), in which two kinds of cells participate, i.e. lymphoid cells and mononuclear phagocytes. The participating mononuclear phagocytes differ in degree of maturation, and the proliferating cells may contain phagocytosed material such as nucleated cells, cell debris, and erythrocytes. Occasionally, binucleated and multinucleated cells resembling Sternberg-Reed cells are present. The extent to which mononuclear phagocytes participate in malignant lymphogranuloma is not known, but there is evidence indicating that the typical Sternberg-Reed cells are multinucleated macrophages (BRAUNSTEIN et al., 1962; RAPPAPORT, 1966; KAPLAN and GARTNER, 1977).

Further elucidation of the contribution of mononuclear phagocytes to pathological processes will require more investigation of the participating cells found in the lesions. It is essential, however, that the investigation is not restricted to the morphological characteristics. The approach shown in Table 1 is sufficiently wide. When the role of the mononuclear phagocytes in physiological and pathological processes is better understood, we may come to know more about the pathogenesis of certain diseases, which in turn will provide a basis for better and more rational treatment.

References

Allison, A. C.: Pathogenic effects of inhaled particles and antigens. In: Kilburn, K. H. (Ed.): Pulmonary Reactions to Organic Materials. Ann. N.Y. Acad. Sci. 1974, pp. 299—308

Allison, A. C., Davies, P.: Mononuclear phagocyte activation in some pathological processes. In: Wagner, W. H., Hahn, H., Evans, R. (Eds.): Activation of Macrophages, pp. 141—156. New York-Amsterdam: American Elsevier Publishing Co. Inc. 1975

Ansley, H., Ornstein, L.: Enzyme histochemistry and differential white cell counts on the Technicon Hemalog. D. Advanc. Automated Anal. **1**, 5—14 (1970)

Arend, W. P., Mannik, M.: Quantitative studies on IgG receptors on monocytes. In: Van Furth, R. (Ed.): Mononuclear Phagocytes in Immunity, Infection and Pathology, pp. 303—314. Oxford-London-Edinburgh-Melbourne: Blackwell Scientific Publications 1975

Aschoff, L.: Das reticulo-endotheliale System. Ergebn. inn. Med. Kinderheilk. **26**, 1—118 (1924)

Balner, H.: Identification of peritoneal macrophages in mouse radiation chimeras. Transplantation **1**, 217—223 (1963)

Basten, A., Mitchell, J.: Role of macrophages in T-cell-B cell collaboration in antibody production. In: Nelson, D. S. (Ed.): Immunobiology of the Macrophage, pp. 45—90. New York-San Francisco-London: Academic Press 1976

Beelen,R.H.J., Broekhuis-Fluitsma,D.M., Korn,C., Hoefsmit,E.Ch.M.: Identification of exudate-resident macrophages on the basis of peroxidatic activity. J. Reticuloendothel. Soc. **23**, 103—110 (1978)

Bianco,C.: Plasma membrane receptors for complement. In: Day,N.K., Good,R.A. (Eds.): Biological Amplification Systems in Immunity. New York: Plenum Press 1977, pp. 69—84

Bianco,C., Griffin,F.M., Silverstein,S.C.: Studies of the macrophage complement receptor. Alteration of receptor function upon macrophage activation. J. exp. Med. **141**, 1278—1290 (1975)

Bianco,C., Nussenzweig,V.: Complement receptors. In: Contemporary topics in molecular immunology. Porter,R.R. and Ada,G.L. (Eds.) New York: Plenum Press 1977, pp. 145—176

Bierman,H.R.: Characteristics of leucopoietin-G. Ann. N.Y. Acad. Sci. **113**, 753—765 (1964)

Blanden,R.V., Hapel,A.J., Doherty,P.C., Zinkernagel,R.M.: Lymphocyte-macrophage interactions and macrophage activation in the expression of antimicrobial immunity in vivo. In: Nelson,D.S. (Ed.): Immunobiology of the Macrophage, pp. 367—400. New-York-San Francisco-London: Academic Press 1976

Blatt,I.M., Seltzer,H.S., Rubin,P., Furstenberg,A.C., Maxwell,J.H., Schull,W.J.: Fatal granulomatosis of the respiratory tract (lethal midline granuloma—Wegener's granulomatosis). Arch. Otolaryng. **70**, 707—757 (1959)

Blussé,A., Van Furth,R.: Origin and kinetics of lung and alveolar macrophages (in preparation)

Bodel,Ph.T., Nichols,B.A., Bainton,D.E.: Appearance of peroxidase reactivity within the rough endoplasmic reticulum of blood monocytes after surface adherence. J. Exp. Med. **145**, 264—274 (1977)

Boggs,D.R., Chervenick,P.A., Marsh,J.C., Cartwright,G.E., Wintrobe,M.M.: Neutrophil releasing activity in plasma of dogs injected with endotoxin. J. Lab. clin. Med. **72**, 177—185 (1968)

Bradley,T.R., Metcalf,D.: The growth of mouse bone marrow cells in vitro. Aust. J. exp. Biol. med. Sci. **44**, 287—300 (1966)

Brady,R.O., King,F.M.: Gaucher's disease. In: Hers,H.G., Hoof,F. (Eds.): Lysosomes and Storage Diseases, pp. 381—394. New York-London: Academic Press 1973a

Brady,R.O., King,F.M.: Niemann Pick's disease. In: Hers.H.G., Hoof,F. (Eds.): Lysosomes and Storage Diseases, pp. 439—452. New York-London: Academic Press 1973b

Braun-Falco,O.: Origin, structure and function of the xanthoma cell. In: Braun-Falco,O., Keller,Ch., Zilner,N. (Eds.): Xanthoma Formation and other Tissue Reactions to Hyperlipidemias, pp. 68—88. Basel: S. Karger 1973

Braunstein,H., Freiman,D.G., Thomas,W., Gall,E.A.: A histochemical study of the enzymatic activity of lymph nodes. III. Granulomatous and primary neoplastic conditions of lymphoid tissue. Cancer (Philad.) **15**, 139—152 (1962)

Braunsteiner,H., Schmalzl,F.: Cytochemistry of monocytes and macrophages. In: Van Furth,R. (Ed.): Mononuclear Phagocytes, pp. 62—81. Oxford-Edinburgh: Blackwell Scientific Publications 1970

Bullough,W.S.: Mitotic and functional homeostasis: a speculative review. Cancer Res. **25**, 1683—1727 (1965)

Carr,I.: The macrophage: a review of ultrastructure and function. London-New York: Academic Press 1973

Chervenick,P.A., LoBuglio,A.F.: Human blood monocytes: stimulators of granulocytes and mononuclear colony formation in vitro. Science **178**, 164—166 (1973)

Cohn,Z.A.: The structure and function of monocytes and macrophages. In: Dixon,F.J., Kunkel,H.G. (Eds.): Advances in Immunology, pp. 164—214. New York-London: Academic Press 1968

Cohn,Z.A.: Endocytosis and intracellular digestion. In: Van Furth,R. (Ed.): Mononuclear Phagocytes, pp. 121—132. Oxford-Edinburgh: Blackwell Scientific Publications 1970

Cohnheim,J.: Vorlesungen über allgemeine Pathologie. Berlin: Hirschwald 1882

Colten,H.R.: Biosynthesis of complement. In: Dixon,F.J., Kunkel,H.G. (Eds.): Advances in Immunology, pp. 67—118. New York-San Francisco-London: Academic Press 1976

Crofton,R.A., Diesselhoff-den Dulk,M.M.C., Van Furth,R.: Origin and kinetics of liver macrophages. 1978. J. exp. Med. (in press)

Crofton,R.A., Diesselhoff-denDulk,M.M.C., VanFurth,R.: Origin and kinetics of liver macrophages during acute inflammation. 1978 (submitted)

Daems,W.Th., Koerten,H.K., Soranzo,M.R.: Differences between monocyte-derived and tissue macrophages. In: Reichard,S.M., Escobar,M.R., Friedman,H. (Eds.): The reticulo-endothelial system in health and disease. Functions and characteristics pp 27—40. New York-London: Plenum Press 1976

Daems,W.Th., Wisse,E., Brederoo,P., Emeis,J.J.: Peroxidatic activity in monocytes and macrophages. In: Van Furth,R. (Ed.): Mononuclear Phagocytes in Immunity, Infection and Pathology, pp. 57—77. Oxford-London-Edinburgh-Melbourne: Blackwell Scientific Publications 1975

Dale,D.C., Fauci,A.S., Wolff,S.M.: Alternate day prednisone: leukocyte kinetics and susceptibility to infections. New Engl. J. Med. **291**, 1154—1158 (1974)

Dannenberg,A.M., Ando,M., Shima,K., Tsuda,T.: Macrophage turnover and activation in tuberculous Granulomata. In: Van Furth,R. (Ed.): Mononuclear Phagocytes in Immunity, Infection and Pathology, pp. 959—980. Oxford-London-Edinburgh-Melbourne: Blackwell Scientific Publications 1975

David,J.R., Remold,H.G.: Macrophage activation by lymphocyte mediators and studies on the interaction of macrophage inhibitory factor (MIF) with its target cell. In: Nelson,D.S. (Ed.): Immunobiology of the Macrophage, pp. 401—426. New York-San Francisco-London: Academic Press 1976

Davies,P., Allison,A.C.: Secretion of macrophage enzymes in relation to the pathogenesis of chronic inflammation. In: Nelson,D.S. (Ed.): Immunobiology of the Macrophage, pp. 427—461. New York-San Francisco-London: Academic Press 1976a

Davies,P., Allison,A.C.: The macrophage as a secretory cell in chronic inflammation. Agents Actions **6**, 60—72 (1976b)

Davies,P., Bonney,R.J., Dahlgren,M.E., Pelus,L., Kuehl,F.A., Humes,J.L.: Recent studies on the secretory activity of mononuclear phagocytes with special reference to prostaglandins. In: Willoughby,D.A., Girond,J.P., Velo,G.P. (Eds.): Perspectives in inflammation. Future trends and developments. pp. 179—185. Lancaster MTP Press Limited 1977

Delmonte,L.: Hemopoietic cell line specific effects of renal granulopoietic factor (GPF) on transplantable mouse marrow stem cells: comparison with erythrocyte stimulating factor (ESF) and endotoxin. Cell Tiss. Kinet. **7**, 3—18 (1974)

Delmonte,L., Starbuck,W.C., Liebelt,R.A.: Species dependent concentration of granulocytosis promoting factor in mammalian tissues. Amer. J. Physiol. **215**, 768—773 (1968)

Douglas,W.W.: Autacoids. In: Goodman,L.S., Gilman,A. (Eds.): The Pharmacological Basis of Therapeutics, pp. 589—590. New York-Toronto-London: McMillan Publishing Co. Inc. 1975

Draper,P., D'ArcyHart,P.: Phagosomes, lysosomes and mycobacteria: cellular and microbial aspects. In: Van Furth,R. (Ed.): Mononuclear Phagocytes in Immunity, Infection and Pathology, pp. 575—594. Oxford-London-Edinburgh-Melbourne: Blackwell Scientific Publications 1975

Dumonde,D.C., Kelly,R.H., Preston,P.M., Wolstencroft,R.A.: Lymphokines and macrophage function in the immunological response. In: Van Furth,R. (Ed.): Mononuclear Phagocytes in Immunity, Infection and Pathology, pp. 675—699. Oxford London Edinburgh Melbourne: Blackwell Scientific Publications 1975

Ebert,R.H., Florey,H.W.: The extravascular development of the monocyte observed in vivo. Brit. J. exp. Path. **20**, 342—356 (1939)

Elmes,P.C.: In: Muir,D.C.F. (Ed.): Clinical Aspects of Inhaled Particles, pp. 84—129. London: Heineman Medical Books 1972

Epstein,L.B.: The ability of macrophages to augment in vitro mitogen and antigen-stimulated production of interferon and other mediators of cellular immunity by lymphocytes. In: Nelson,D.S. (Ed.): Immunobiology of the Macrophage, pp. 201—234. New York-San Francisco-London: Academic Press 1976

Evans,R.: Macrophage cytotoxicity. In: Van Furth,R. (Ed.): Mononuclear Phagocytes in Immunity, Infection and Pathology, pp. 827—843. Oxford-London-Edinburgh-Melbourne: Blackwell Scientific Publications 1975

Evans, R., Alexander, P.: Mechanisms of extracellular killing of nucleated mammalian cells by macrophages. In: Nelson, D.S. (Ed.): Immunobiology of the Macrophage, pp. 535—576. New York-San Francisco-London: Academic Press 1976

Fahimi, H.D.: The fine structural localization of endogenous and exogenous peroxidase activity in Kupffer cells of rat liver. J. Cell. Biol. **47**, 247—262 (1970)

Fauci, A.S., Dale, D.C.: The effect of in vivo hydrocortisone on subpopulations of human lymphocytes. J. clin. Invest. **53**, 240—246 (1974)

Fauci, A.S., Wolff, S.M.: Wegener's granulomatosis: studies in eighteen patients and a review of the literature. Medicine (Baltimore) **52**, 535—561 (1973)

Feldman, M., Schrader, J.W., Boylston, A.: Macrophage lymphocyte interaction in vitro. In: Van Furth, R. (Ed.): Mononuclear phagocytes in immunity, infection and pathology, pp. 779—791. Oxford-London-Edinburgh-Melbourne: Blackwell Scientific Publications 1975

Fisher, E.R.: Pigmentation of intestinal tract. In: Wolman, M. (Ed.): Pigments in Pathology, pp. 489—506. New York-London: Academic Press 1969

Van Furth, R. (Ed.): Mononuclear Phagocytes. Oxford-Edinburgh: Blackwell Scientific Publications 1970

Van Furth, R. (Ed.): Mononuclear Phagocytes in Immunity, Infection and Pathology. Oxford-London-Edinburgh-Melbourne: Blackwell Scientific Publications 1975a

Van Furth, R.: Modulation of monocyte production. In: Van Furth, R. (Ed.): Mononuclear Phagocytes in Immunity, Infection and Pathology, pp. 161—174. Oxford-London-Edinburgh-Melbourne: Blackwell Scientific Publications 1975b

Van Furth, R., Cohn, Z.A.: The origin and kinetics of mononuclear phagocytes. J. exp. Med. **128**, 415—435 (1968)

Van Furth, R., Cohn, Z.A., Hirsch, J.G., Humphry, J.H., Spector, W.G., Langevoort, H.L.: The mononuclear phagocyte system: a new classification of macrophages, monocytes and their precursor. Bull. Wld Hlth Org. **46**, 845—852 (1972)

Van Furth, R., Diesselhoff-den Dulk, M.M.C.: The kinetics of promonocytes and monocytes in the bone marrow. J. exp. Med. **132**, 813—828 (1970)

Van Furth, R., Diesselhoff-den Dulk, M.M.C.: Characterization of murine mononuclear phagocytes. 1978. in preparation

Van Furth, R., Diesselhoff-den Dulk, M.M.C., Mattie, H.: Quantitative study on the production and kinetics of mononuclear phagocytes during an acute inflammatory reaction. J. exp. Med. **138**, 1314—1330 (1973)

Van Furth, R., Fedorko, M.E.: Ultrastructure of mouse mononuclear phagocytes in bone marrow colonies grown in vitro. Lab. Invest. **34**, 440—450 (1976)

Van Furth, R., Gassmann, A.E., Diesselhoff-den Dulk, M.M.C.: The effect of azathioprine (Imuran) on the cell-cycle of the promonocytes and monocyte production in the bone marrow. J. exp. Med. **3**, 531—546 (1975a)

Van Furth, R., Hirsch, J.G., Fedorko, M.E.: Morphology and peroxidase cytochemistry of mouse promonocytes, monocytes and macrophages. J. exp. Med. **132**, 794—812 (1970)

Van Furth, R., Langevoort, H.L., Schaberg, A.: Mononuclear phagocytes in human pathology—proposal for an approach to improved classification. In: Van Furth, R. (Ed.): Mononuclear Phagocytes in Immunity, Infection and Pathology, pp. 1—15. Oxford-London-Edinburgh-Melbourne: Blackwell Scientific Publications 1975b

Van Furth, R., Raeburn, J.A., Van Zwet, T.L.: Characteristics of human mononuclear phagocytes. 1978, in preparation

Van Furth, R., Van Zwet, T.L., Leyh, P.C.J.: In vitro determination of phagocytosis and intracellular killing by polymorphonuclear and mononuclear phagocytes. In: Weir, D.M. (Ed.): Handbook of Experimental Immunology. Oxford-London-Edinburgh-Melbourne: Blackwell Scientific Publications 1978, chapter 32

Gall, E.A.: The cytological identity and interrelation of mesenchymal cells of lymphoid tissue. Ann. N.Y. Acad. Sci. **73**, 120—130 (1958)

Gallily, R.: The killing capacity of immune macrophages. In: Van Furth, R. (Ed.): Mononuclear Phagocytes in Immunity, Infection and Pathology, pp. 894—909. Oxford-London-Edinburgh-Melbourne: Blackwell Scientific Publications 1975

Gassmann, A.E., Van Furth, R.: The effect of azathioprine (Imuran) on the kinetics of monocytes and macrophages during normal steady state and the acute inflammatory reaction. Blood **46**, 51—65 (1975)

German, W. M.: Dusting powder granulomas following surgery. Surg. Gynec. Obstet. **76**, 501—507 (1943)

Gillman, T., Wright, L. J.: Probable in vivo origin of multinucleated giant cells from circulating mononuclears. Nature (Lond.) **209**, 263—265 (1966)

Ginsburg, I., Mitrani, S., Ne'eman, N., Lahav, M.: Granulomata in streptococcal inflammation: mechanisms of localization transport and degradation of streptococci in inflammatory sites. In: Van Furth, R. (Ed.): Mononuclear Phagocytes in Immunity, Infection and Pathology, pp. 981—1014. Oxford-London-Edinburgh-Melbourne: Blackwell Scientific Publications 1975

Glatt, M., Kälin, H., Wagner, K., Brune, K.: Prostaglandin release from macrophages: an assay system for anti-inflammatory drugs in vitro. Agents and Actions **7**, 321—326 (1977)

Godleski, J. G., Brain, J. D.: The origin of alveolar macrophages in radiation chimeras. J. exp. Med. **136**, 630—643 (1972)

Golde, D. W., Cline, M. J.: Identification of the colony-stimulating cell in human peripheral blood. J. clin. Invest. **51**, 2981—2983 (1972)

Golde, D. W., Cline, M. J.: Regulation of granulopoiesis. New Engl. J. Med. **291**, 1388—1395 (1974)

Golde, D. W., Finley, T. N., Cline, M. J.: Production of colony-stimulating factor by human macrophages. Lancet **1972 II**, 1397—1399

Goodman, J. W.: The origin of peritoneal fluid cells. Blood **23**, 18—26 (1964)

Gordon, A. S., Neri, R. O., Siegel, C. D., Dornfest, B. S., Handler, E. S., Lobue, J., Eisler, M.: Evidence for a circulating leucocytosis-inducing factor (LIF). Acta haemat. (Basel) **23**, 323—341 (1960)

Gordon, S.: The secretion of lysozyme and plasminogen activator by mononuclear phagocytes. In: Van Furth, R. (Ed.): Mononuclear Phagocytes in Immunity, Infection and Pathology, pp. 463—473. Oxford-London-Edinburgh-Melbourne: Blackwell Scientific Publications 1975

Gordon, S., Cohn, Z. A.: The macrophage. In: Bourne, G. H., Danielli, J. F. (Eds.): International Review of Cytology, pp. 171—214. New York-London: Academic Press 1973

Goud, Th. J. L. M.: Identification and characterization of the monoblast. Thesis, Leiden 1975

Goud, Th. J. L. M., Van Furth, R.: Proliferative characteristics of monoblasts grown in vitro. J. exp. Med. **142**, 1200—1217 (1975)

Goud, Th. J. L. M., Schotte, C., Van Furth, R.: Identification and characterization of the monoblast in mononuclear phagocyte colonies grown in vitro. J. exp. Med. **142**, 1180—1199 (1975)

Griffin, F. M., Bianco, C., Silverstein, S. C.: Characterization of the macrophage receptor for complement and demonstration of its functional independence from the receptor for the Fc portion of immunoglobulin G. J. exp. Med. **141**, 1269—1277 (1975)

Haeckel, E.: Die Radiolaren *(Rhizopoda radiaria)*, pp. 104—105. Berlin: Druck und Verlag von Georg Reimer 1862

Handler, E. S., Varsa, E. E., Gordon, A. S.: Mechanisms of leucocyte production and release. V. Studies on the leucocytosis-inducing factor in the plasma of rats treated with thyphoid parathyphoid vaccine. J. Lab. clin. Med. **67**, 398—410 (1966)

Hepplestone, A. G.: Pigmentation and disorders of the lung. In: Wolman, M. (Ed.): Pigments in Pathology, pp. 33—73. New York-London: Academic Press 1969

Hers, H. G.: The concept of inborn lysosomal disease. In: Hers, H. G., Hoof, F. (Eds.): Lysosomes and Storage Diseases, pp. 148—171. New York-London: Academic Press 1973

Howard, J. G.: The origin and immunological significance of Kupffer cells. In: Van Furth, R. (Ed.): Mononuclear Phagocytes, pp. 178—199. Oxford-Edinburgh: Blackwell Scientific Publications 1970

Huber, H., Holm, G.: Surface receptors of mononuclear phagocytes: effect of immune complexes on in vitro function in human monocytes. In: Van Furth, R. (Ed.): Mononuclear Phagocytes in Immunity, Infection, and Pathology, pp. 291—301. Oxford-London-Edinburgh-Melbourne: Blackwell Scientific Publications 1975

Jones, T. C.: Attachment and ingestion phases of phagocytosis. In: Van Furth, R. (Ed.): Mononuclear Phagocytes in Immunity, Infection and Pathology, pp. 269—282. Oxford-London-Edinburgh-Melbourne: Blackwell Scientific Publications 1975a

Jones, T. C.: Phagosome-lysosome interaction with toxoplasma. In: Van Furth, R. (Ed.): Mononuclear Phagocytes in Immunity, Infection and Pathology, pp. 595—607. Oxford-London-Edinburgh-Melbourne: Blackwell Scientific Publications 1975b

Kaplan, H. S., Gartner, S.: Sternberg-Reed giant cells of Hodgkin's disease: cultivation in vitro, heterotransplantation, and characterization as neoplastic macrophages. Int. J. Cancer **19**, 511-525 (1977)

Kaplow, L. S.: Simplified myeloperoxidase stain using benzidine dihydrochloride. Blood **26**, 215—219 (1965)

Karnovsky, M. L., Lasdins, J., Simmons, S. R.: Metabolism of activated mononuclear phagocytes at rest and during phagocytosis. In: Van Furth, R. (Ed.): Mononuclear Phagocytes in Immunity, Infection and Pathology, pp. 423—439. Oxford-London-Edinburgh-Melbourne: Blackwell Scientific Publications 1975

Karnovsky, M. L., Simmons, S., Glass, E. A., Shafer, A. W., D'Arcy Hart, P.: Metabolism of macrophages. In: Van Furth, R. (Ed.): Mononuclear Phagocytes, pp. 103—120. Oxford-London-Edinburgh-Melbourne: Blackwell Scientific Publications 1970

Katz, R., Gordon, A. S., Lapin, D. M.: Mechanisms of leucocyte production and release. VI. Studies on the purification of leucocytosis-inducing factor (LIF). J. reticuloendoth. Soc. **3**, 103—116 (1966)

Keller, R.: Cytostatic killing of syngeneic Tumour cells by activated non-immune macrophages. In: Van Furth, R. (Ed.): Mononuclear Phagocytes in Immunity, Infection and Pathology, pp. 857—868. Oxford-London-Edinburgh-Melbourne: Blackwell Scientific Publications 1975

Keller, R.: Cytostatic and cytocidal effects of activated macrophages. In: Nelson, D. S. (Ed.): Immunobiology of the Macrophage, pp. 487—508. New York-San Francisco-London: Academic Press 1976

Klebanoff, S. J., Hamon, B.: Antimicrobial systems of mononuclear phagocytes. In: Van Furth, R. (Ed.): Mononuclear Phagocytes in Immunity, Infection and Pathology, pp. 507—531. Oxford-London-Edinburgh-Melbourne: Blackwell Scientific Publications 1975

Lai A Fat, R. F. M., Van Furth, R.: In vitro synthesis of some complement components (Cl_9, C_3, and C_4) by lymphoid tissues and circulating leucocoytes in man. Immunology **28**, 359—368 (1975)

Leibovich, S. J., Ross, R.: The macrophage and the fibroblast. In: Van Furth, R. (Ed.): Mononuclear Phagocytes in Immunity, Infection and Pathology, pp. 347—361. Oxford-London-Edinburgh-Melbourne: Blackwell Scientific Publications 1975

Leibovich, S. J., Ross, R.: A macrophage-dependent factor that stimulates the proliferation of fibroblasts in vitro. Amer. J. Path. **84**, 501—514 (1976)

Lichtenstein, L.: Histiocytosis X: integration of eosinophilic granuloma of bone, "Letterer-Siwe disease" and "Schuller-Christian disease" as related manifestations of a single nosological entity. Arch. Path. (Chicago) **56**, 84—102 (1953)

Lohmann-Matthes, M. L.: Induction of macrophage mediated cytotoxicity. In: Nelson, D. S. (Ed.): Immunobiology of the Macrophage, pp. 463—486. New York-San Francisco-London: Academic Press 1976

Lohmann-Matthes, M. L., Fischer, H.: Macrophage-mediated cytotoxic induction by a specific T-cell factor. In: Van Furth, R. (Ed.): Mononuclear Phagocytes in Immunity, Infection and Pathology, pp. 845—855. Oxford-London-Edinburgh-Melbourne: Blackwell Scientific Publications 1975

Lukes, R. J.: The pathological picture of the malignant lymphomas. In: Zarafonetic, C. J. D. (Ed.): Proceedings of the International Conference on Leukaemia-Lymphoma, pp. 333—354. Philadelphia: Lea and Febiger 1968

Mackaness, G. B.: The phagocytosis and inactivation of staphylococci by macrophages of normal rabbits. J. exp. Med. **112**, 35—53 (1960)

Mackaness, G. B.: Cellular Immunity. In: Van Furth, R. (Ed.): Mononuclear Phagocytes, pp. 461—477. Oxford-Edinburgh: Blackwell Scientific Publications 1970a

Mackaness, G. B.: The monocyte in delayed-type hypersensitivity. In: Van Furth, R. (Ed.): Mononuclear Phagocytes, pp. 478—509. Oxford-Edinburgh: Blackwell Scientific Publications 1970b

McClelland, D. B. L., Lai A Fat, R. F. M., Van Furth, R.: Synthesis of lysozyme by human and mouse mononuclear phagocytes. In: Van Furth, R. (Ed.): Mononuclear Phagocytes in Immunity, Infection and Pathology, pp. 475—486. Oxford-London-Edinburgh-Melbourne: Blackwell Scientific Publications 1975

McGregor, D. D., Logie, P. S.: Macrophage-lymphocyte interactions in infection immunity. In: Van Furth, R. (Ed.): Mononuclear Phagocytes in Immunity, Infection and Pathology, pp. 631—651. Oxford-London-Edinburgh-Melbourne: Blackwell Scientific Publications 1975

Mackaness, G. B., Lagrange, P. H., Miller, T. E., Ishibashi, T.: The formation of activated T-cells. In: Wagner, W. H., Hahn, H., Evans, R. (Eds.): Activation of Macrophages, pp. 193—209. Amsterdam: Excerpta Medica. New York: American Elsevier Publishing Co., Inc. 1974

McKerrow, C. B.: Silicosis and coalworkers pneumoniosis. In: Muir, D. C. F. (Ed.): Clinical Aspects of Inhaled Particles, pp. 130—155. London: Heinemann Medical Books 1972

Mauel, J., Noerjasin, B., Behin, R.: Killing of intracellular parasites as a measure of macrophage activation. In: Wagner, W. H., Hahn, H., Evans, R. (Eds.): Activation of Macrophages, pp. 260—268. Amsterdam: Excerpta Medica. New York: American Elsevier Publishing Co., Inc. 1974

Metcalf, D.: Regulation of granulocyte and monocyte-macrophage proliferation by colony stimulating factor (CSF): a review. Exp. Hemat. **1**, 185—201 (1973)

Metchnikoff, E.: Leçons sur la pathlogie comparée de l'inflammation. Paris: G. Masson 1892

Meuret, G.: Monocytopoiese beim Menschen. Blut Suppl. **13** (1974)

Meuret, G., Hoffmann, G.: Monocyte kinetic studies in normal and disease states. Brit. J. Haemat. **24**, 275—285 (1973)

Moore, M. A. S., Williams, N.: Physical separation of colony stimulating cells from in vitro colony-forming cells in hemopoietic tissue. J. cell. Physiol. **80**, 195—206 (1972)

Neely, J., Davies, J. D.: Starch granulomatosis of the peritoneum. Brit. med. J. **1971 III**, 625—629

Nelson, D.: The macrophage in immunology. Amsterdam: North-Holland Publishing Company 1969

Nelson, D.: Immuno-biology of the macrophage. New York-San Francisco-London: Academic Press 1976

Nichols, B. A., Bainton, D. F.: Ultrastructure and cytochemistry of mononuclear phagocytes. In: Van Furth, R. (Ed.): Mononuclear phagocytes in Immunity, Infection and Pathology. pp. 17—55. Oxford-London-Edinburgh-Melbourne: Blackwell Scientific Publications 1975

North, R, J.: T-cell dependent macrophage activation in cell-mediated anti-listeria immunity. In: Wagner, W. H., Hahn, H., Evans, R. (Eds.): Activation of Macrophages, pp. 210—222. Amsterdam: Excerpta Medica. New York: American Elsevier Publishing Co., Inc. 1974

O'Brien, J. S.: Tay-Sachs disease and juvenile Gm2 Gangliodosis. In: Hers, H. G., Hoof, F. (Eds.): Lysosomes and Storage Diseases, pp. 323—344. New York-London: Academic Press 1973

Ogawa, R., Koerten, H. K., Daems, W. Th.: Peroxidatic activity in monocytes and tissue macrophages. Cell and Tiss. Res. 1978 (in press)

Oppenheim, J. J., Elfenbein, G. J., Rosenstreich, D. L.: The role of macrophages in B and T lymphocyte transformation. In: Van Furth, R. (Ed.): Mononuclear Phagocytes in Immunity, Infection and Pathology, pp. 793—812. Oxford-London-Edinburgh-Melbourne: Blackwell Scientific Publications 1975

Oppenheim, J. J., Seeger, R. C.: The role of macrophages in the induction of cell-mediated immunity in vivo. In: Nelson, D. S. (Ed.): Immunobiology of the Macrophage, pp. 111—130. New York-San Francisco-London: Academic Press 1976

Ornstein, L., Ansley, H. and Saunders, A.: Improving manual differential white cell counts with cytochemistry. Blood Cells 1976, 557—585

Ornstein, L., Janoff, A., Sweetman, F., Ansley, H.: Histochemical demonstration of an elastase-like human neutrophil esterase. J. Histochem. Cytochem. **21**, 411 (1973)

Papadimitriou, J. M., Cornelisse, C. J.: A cytophotometric and autoradiographic study of DNA synthesis in macrophages and multinucleate foreign body gain cells. J. reticuloendoth. Soc. **18**, 260—270 (1975)

Papadimitriou, J. M., Spector, W. G.: The ultrastructure of high and low turnover inflammatory granulomata. J. Path. **106**, 37—43 (1972)

Pearsall, N. N., Weiser, R. S.: The macrophage. Philadelphia: Lea and Febiger 1970

Pierce, C. W., Kapp, J. A.: The role of macrophages in antibody responses in vitro. In: Nelson, D. S. (Ed.): Immunobiology of the Macrophage, pp. 1—33. New York-San Francisco-London: Academic Press 1976

Pinket, M. O., Cowdrey, C. M., Nowell, P. C.: Mixed hematopoietic and pulmonary origin of "alveolar macrophages" as demonstrated by chromosome markers. Amer. J. Path. **48**, 859—867 (1966)

Pluznik, D. H., Sachs, L.: The induction of clones of normal mast cells by a substance from conditioned medium. Exp. Cell Res. **43**, 553—563 (1966)

Rabinovitch, M.: Phagocytic recognition. In: Van Furth, R. (Ed.): Mononuclear Phagocytes, pp. 299—313. Oxford-Edinburgh: Blackwell Scientific Publications 1970

Rachmilewitz, M., Schlesinger, M.: Production and release of transcobalamin II, a vitamin B_{12} transport protein, by mouse peritoneal macrophages. Exp. Haematol. 5 (suppl. **2**), 108 (abstract), 1977

Rappaport, H.: Tumors of the haemopoietic system. In: Atlas of Tumor Pathology, Section 3, Fasc 8. Washington: Armed Forces Institute of Pathology 1966

Remington, J. S., Krahenbuhl, J. L., Hibbs, J. B.: A role for the macrophage in resistance to tumor development and tumor destruction. In: Van Furth, R. (Ed.): Mononuclear Phagocytes in Immunity, Infection and Pathology, pp. 869—893. Oxford-London-Edinburgh-Melbourne: Blackwell Scientific Publications 1975

Robb-Smith, A. H. T.: Reticulosis and reticulosarcoma: a histological classification. J. Path. Bact. **47**, 457—480 (1938)

Rocha e Silva, M., Leme, G. J.: Mediators of the inflammatory reaction. In: Alexander, P., Bacq, Z. M. (Eds.): Chemical Mediators of the Acute Inflammatory Reaction. Modern Trends in Physiological Sciences, Vol. XXXVII, pp. 101—197. Oxford-New York: Pergamon Press 1972

Rosenstreich, D. L., Oppenheim, J. J.: The role of macrophages in the activation of T and B lymphocytes in vitro. In: Nelson, D. S. (Ed.): Immunobiology of the Macrophage, pp. 161—199. New York-San Francisco-London: Academic Press 1976

Rosenthal, A. S., Lipsky, P. E., Shevach, E. M.: Macrophage-lymphocyte interaction: morphologic and functional correlates. In: Van Furth, R. (Ed.): Mononuclear Phagocytes in Immunity, Infection and Pathology, pp. 813—825. Oxford-London-Edinburgh-Melbourne: Blackwell Scientific Publications 1975

Rosenthal, A. S., Thomas Blake, J., Ellner, J. J., Greineder, D. K., Lipsky, P. E.: Macrophage function in antigen recognition by T lymphocytes. In: Nelson, D. S. (Ed.): Immunobiology of the Macrophage, pp. 131—160. New York-San Francisco-London: Academic Press 1976

Rossi, F., Zabucchi, G., Romeo, D.: Metabolism of phagocytizing mononuclear phagocytes. In: Van Furth, R. (Ed.): Mononuclear Phagocytes in Immunity, Infection and Pathology, pp. 441—462. Oxford-London-Edinburgh-Melbourne: Blackwell Scientific Publications 1975

Rothstein, G., Hügl, E. H., Bishop, C. R., Athens, J. W., Ashenbrucker, H. E.: Stimulation of granulopoiesis by a diffusable factor in vivo. J. clin. Invest. **50**, 2004—2007 (1971)

Rothstein, G., Hügl, E. H., Chervenick, P. A., Athens, J. W., Macfarlane, J.: Humoral stimulators of granulocyte production. Blood **41**, 73—78 (1973)

Ruscetti, F. W., Chervenick, P. A.: Release of colony-stimulating factor from monocytes by endotoxin and polynosinic-polycytidylic acid. J. Lab. clin. Med. **83**, 64—72 (1974)

Ryan, G. B., Spector, W. G.: Macrophage turnover in inflamed connective tissues. Proc. roy. Soc. B. **175**, 269—292 (1970)

Sandhoff, K., Harzer, K.: Total hexosaminidase deficiency in Tay-Sachs' disease (Variant O). In: Hers, H. G., Hoof, F. (Eds.): Lysosomes and Storage Diseases, pp. 346—356. New York-London. Academic Press 1973

Scott, R. B., Robb-Smith, A. H. T.: Histiocytic medullary reticulosis. Lancet **1939 II**, 194—198

Schultz, E. F., Lapin, D. M., Lobue, J.: Humoral regulation of neutrophil production and release. In: Lobue, J., Gordon, A. S. (Eds.): Humoral Control of Growth and Differentiation, pp. 51—68. New York-London: Academic Press 1973

Seljelid, R.: Cytotoxic effect of macrophages on mouse red cells. In: Van Furth, R. (Ed.): Mononuclear Phagocytes in Immunity, Infection and Pathology, pp. 910—925. Oxford-London-Edinburgh-Melbourne: Blackwell Scientific Publications 1975

Shand, F. L., Bell, E. B.: Studies on the distribution of macrophages derived from rat bone marrow cells in exenogeneic radiation chimeras. Immunology **22**, 549—556 (1972)

Slonecker, Ch. E., Lim, W. Ch.: Effects of hydrocortisone on the cells in an acute inflammatory exudate. Lab. Invest. **27**, 123—128 (1972)

Solotorovsky, M., Tewari, R. P.: Interaction of macrophages with facultative intracellular parasites—Brucella and Salmonella. In: Wagner, W. H., Hahn, H., Evans, R. (Eds.): Activation of Macrophages, pp. 238—248. Amsterdam: Excerpta Medica. New York: American Elsevier Publishing Co., Inc. 1974

Spector, W. G.: Chronic inflammation. In: Zweifach, B. W., Grant, L., McCluskey, R. T. (Eds.): The Inflammatory Process, 2nd Ed., Vol. III, pp. 277—290. New York-London: Academic Press 1974

Spector, W.G., Mariano, M.: Macrophage behaviour in experimental granulomas. In: Van Furth, R. (Ed.): Mononuclear Phagocytes in Immunity, Infection and Pathology, pp. 927—942. Oxford-London-Edinburgh-Melbourne: Blackwell Scientific Publications 1975

Spector, W.G., Ryan, G.B.: The mononuclear phagocyte in inflammation. In: Van Furth, R. (Ed.): Mononuclear Phagocytes. Oxford-Edinburgh: Blackwell Scientific Publications 1970

Stanley, E.R., Hansen, G., Woodcock, J., Metcalf, D.: Colony stimulating factor and the regulation of granulopoiesis and macrophage production. Fed. Proc. **34**, 2272—2278 (1975)

Stecher, V.J.: Synthesis of proteins by mononuclear phagocytes. In: Van Furth, R. (Ed.): Mononuclear Phagocytes, pp. 133—150. Oxford-Edinburgh: Blackwell Scientific Publications 1970

Steinman, R.M., Cohn, Z.A.: The interaction of soluble horseradish peroxidase with mouse peritoneal macrophages in vitro. J. Cell Biol. **55**, 186—204 (1972)

Steinman, R.M., Cohn, Z.A.: The metabolism and physiology of the mononuclear phagocytes. In: Zweifach, B.W., Grant, L., McCluskey, R.T. (Eds.): Inflammatory Process, pp. 450—510. New York-San Francisco-London: Academic Press 1974

Stuart, A.E.: The reticulo-endothelial system. Edinburgh: Livingstone 1970

Sutton, J.S., Weiss, L.: Transformation of monocytes in tissue culture into macrophages, epitheloid cells and multinucleated giant cells. J. Cell Biol. **28**, 303—332 (1966)

Suzuki, K., Suzuki, K.: Globoid cell leukostrophy (Krabbe's disease). In: Hers, H.G., Hoof, F. (Eds.): Lysosomes and Storage Diseases, pp. 395—410. New York-London: Academic Press 1973

Tevethia, S.S., Zarling, J.M., Flax, M.H.: Macrophages and the destruction of syngeneic virus induced tumors. In: Nelson, D.S. (Ed.): Immunobiology of the Macrophage, pp. 509—533. New York-San Francisco-London: Academic Press 1976

Thompson, J., Van Furth, R.: The effect of glucocorticosteroids on the kinetics of mononuclear phagocytes. J. exp. Med. **131**, 429—442 (1970)

Thompson, J., Van Furth, R.: The effect of glucocorticosteroids on the proliferation and kinetics of promonocytes and monocytes in the bone marrow. J. exp. Med. **137**, 10—21 (1973)

Tompkins, E.H.: The response of monocytes to adrenal cortical extracts. J. Lab. clin. Med. **39**, 365—371 (1952)

Unanue, E.R.: The regulation of the immune response by macrophages. In: Van Furth, R. (Eds.): Mononuclear Phagocytes in Immunity, Infection and Pathology, pp. 721—742. Oxford-London-Edinburgh-Melbourne: Blackwell Scientific Publications 1975

Vernon-Roberts, B.: The macrophage. Cambridge: Cambridge University Press 1972

Verveen, A.A.: The application of systems theory in biology. An introduction. Ann. Syst. Res. **2**, 117—139 (1972)

Virolainen, M.: Hematopoietic origin of macrophages as studied by chromosome markers in mice. J. exp. Med. **127**, 943—952 (1968)

Volkman, A.: The production of monocytes and related cells. Haemat. lat. (Milano) **10**, 61—63 (1967)

Volkman, A.: The origin and fate of the monocyte. Ser. Haematol. **3**, 62—90 (1970)

Volkman, A., Collins, F.M.: The cytokinetics of monocytosis in acute Salmonella infection in the rat. J. exp. Med. **139**, 264—277 (1974)

Van Waarde, D.: Humoral regulation of monocytopoiesis. A study on a factor increasing monocytopoiesis during acute inflammatory reactions. Thesis, Leiden 1976

Van Waarde, D., Hulsing-Hesselink, E., Van Furth, R.: A serum factor inducing monocytosis during an acute inflammatory reaction caused by newborn calf serum. Cell Tiss. Kinet. **9**, 51—63 (1976)

Van Waarde, D., Hulsing-Hesselink, E., Van Furth, R.: Humoral regulation of monocytopoiesis during an inflammatory reaction caused by particulate substances (1977a). Blood, **50**, 141—154

Van Waarde, D., Hulsing-Hesselink, E., Van Furth, R.: Properties of a factor increasing monocytopoiesis (FIM) occuring in the serum during the early phase of an inflammatory reaction (1977b). Blood **50**, 727—742

Wagner, W.H., Hahn, H., Evans, R. (Eds.): Activation of macrophages. Amsterdam: Excerpta Medica. New York: American Elsevier Publishing Co. Inc. 1974

Warren, K.S., Boros, D.L.: The schistosome egg granuloma: a form of cell-mediated immunity. In: Van Furth, R. (Ed.): Mononuclear Phagocytes in Immunity, Infection and Pathology, pp. 1015—1028. Oxford-London-Edinburgh-Melbourne: Blackwell Scientific Publications 1975

Wegener, F.: Über generalisierte, septische Gefäßerkrankungen. Verh. dtsch. path. Ges. **29**, 202—210 (1936)
Wegener, F.: Über eine eigenartige rhinogene Granulomatose mit besonderer Beteiligung des Arteriensystems und der Nieren. Ber. path. Anat. allg. Path. **102**, 36—68 (1939)
Whitelaw, D. M.: Observations on human monocyte kinetics after pulse labeling. Cell Tiss. Kinet. **5**, 311—317 (1972)
Whitelaw, D. M., Batho, H. F.: The distribution of monocytes in the rat. Cell Tiss. Kinet. **5**, 215—225 (1972)
Whitelaw, D. A., Bell, M. F., Batho, H. F.: Monocyte kinetics: observations after pulse labelling. J. cell. Physiol. **72**, 65—71 (1968)
Widmann, J. J., Cotran, R. S., Fahimi, H. D.: Mononuclear phagocytes (Kupffer cells) and endothelial cells. Identification of two functional cell types in rat liver sinusoids by endogenous peroxidase activity. J. Cell. Biol. **52**, 159—170 (1972)
Wisse, E.: Observations of the time structure and peroxidase cytochemistry of normal rat liver Kupffer cells. J. Ultrastruct. Res. **46**, 499—520 (1974)
Yam, L. T., Li, C. Y., Crosby, W. H.: Cytochemical identification of monocytes and granulocytes. Amer. J. Path. **55**, 283—290 (1971)
Zaidi, S. H.: Experimental pneumoconiosis. Baltimore: Johns Hopkins Press 1969

CHAPTER 4

The Adhesion, Locomotion, and Chemotaxis of Leucocytes

P. C. WILKINSON

A. Introduction

The earliest cellular responses to injury include margination of leucocytes within small blood vessels at the site of the lesion; adherence of these cells to the vascular endothelium, particularly in postcapillary venules; migration of adherent leucocytes between the endothelial cells and out of the vessel; detachment of the cells and their subsequent homing onto the site of injury (see HURLEY, Chapter 2, this volume). These events require two fundamental properties of cells, adhesion and locomotion, both of which present complex problems as general phenomena as well as in the special context of inflammation. The adhesion of leucocytes to vascular endothelium may result from an enhanced affinity of the surfaces of the two cells for one another which is not understood. The locomotion of leucocytes is difficult to study in vivo but has been much studied in vitro, where it can be shown to be directional or *chemotactic*. The cells of interest in this context are granulocytes, mononuclear phagocytes and lymphocytes. Lymphocyte migration has often been considered to present a special case. It may be, however, that it bears a closer resemblance to the migration of the other cells than was thought a few years ago, and lymphocytes will be considered where appropriate in this chapter.

B. Leucocyte Adhesion

I. General Considerations

It is likely that experimental approaches to the problems of leucocyte adherence to endothelium may be suggested from consideration of the general problems of adhesion in development and in the formation of organs and tissues, and the interested reader is referred to recent reviews on these topics (TRINKAUS, 1969; CURTIS, 1973). Cell-cell adhesions are ubiquitous in tissues. For an organ to have shape and structure it is essential that the cells which form it arrange themselves in regular patterns that are based on the differential adhesion of cells to each other. Blood leucocytes are unusual cells inasmuch as, under physiological conditions, they neither adhere strongly to one another nor to other tissue cells, and they do not form organs. However, certain leucocytes show specific affinities for, and make adhesions to, the cells in particular sites. Examples are the mononuclear phagocytes, such as hepatic Kupffer cells, which adhere to sinusoidal and other cells in a number of organs.

The adhesion of a cell to any object in contact with it is maintained by the interfacial energy of interactions between the cell and that object. These interactions vary according to the nature of the object with which it has come into contact, for instance other cells or fibres in vivo, or glass, plastic or other substrata in vitro. Adhesiveness is not, therefore, an absolute property of cells. This being the case, the fact that neutrophils and macrophages adhere well to glass or nylon fibres may not be relevant to the strength of contact between these cells and vascular endothelium, since different interactions may be involved in the two cases. Moreover, the adhesiveness of cells may show transient or permanent alterations influenced by substances in the environment of the cell or by changes in the detailed structure of its membrane. Adhesion between cells may result from direct interactions between the two cell surfaces, involving a wide variety of noncovalent bonds such as ionic, VAN DER WAALS or hydrogen bonds or hydrophobic interactions, or more permanent covalent attachments. Adhesion would also result from cross-linking or bridging between the two cell surfaces by soluble molecules, as in cell agglutination by antibody.

Membrane glycoproteins are currently popular candidates for a role in cell-cell adhesion. They are the most superficially placed structures on the cell surface and thus well situated to interact with other cells. Since they vary widely in structure they are able to act as recognition units in specific interactions of the cell with other cells or molecules. It has been suggested that cell-cell adhesion could result from complementary bonds between glycoproteins on adjacent cells and that specificity of adhesion could result from the stereochemical affinities between these glycoproteins. As an extension of this idea of stereospecific affinity, ROSEMAN (1970) proposed that glycosyl transferases on the surface of one cell may be able to bind to appropriate sugar substrates on a contiguous cell and that such enzyme-substrate bonding between the two cells leads to adhesion. Once the sugar residue is removed from its chain by the transferase, the enzyme dissociates from its substrate and the adhesion between the two cells is lost. Glycosyl transferases have been demonstrated in the plasma membranes of platelets (JAMIESON et al., 1971) and postulated to play a role in the adhesion of platelets to collagen, but the presence of these enzymes in leucocyte membranes has not been sought.

Another mechanism suggested for adhesion involves the formation of cation bridges between cells. All cells carry a net negative charge and might, therefore, be expected to repel each other. However, physiological media contain divalent cations, and cations containing two or more positive charges might form ionic links with negatively charged groups on the surfaces of apposed cells and thus bind the cells together (BANGHAM, 1964). Divalent cations such as Ca^{2+} or Mg^{2+} would form the simplest of such bridges, but for small cations to act as effective bridges the two negatively charged surfaces would have to approach to within 5 Å of each other (BANGHAM, 1964). Such close contact would be unlikely to occur for physicochemical reasons except at the tips of narrow microvilli. If the bridging molecule were larger, for instance a cationic peptide, close apposition of the negatively charged surfaces would not be necessary. Neuraminic acid on glycoproteins makes a major contribution to the negative surface charge of cells, so that glycoproteins are likely to be of major importance in the cation bridging hypothesis—just as they are in the more direct interactions discussed above.

It has been suggested that cells may control their own capacity to adhere to other cells in their environment by secreting soluble factors which could act as adhesive bridges or, conversely, decrease the adhesiveness of other cells. Leucocytes in inflammation are secreting cells and certain secreted molecules, e.g. the cationic peptides

(JANOFF and ZWEIFACH, 1964), could act as bridges. Conversely, lymphocytes release factors which diminish the adhesiveness of lymphocytes of other types. This has been suggested as a method for the sorting of T- and B-lymphocytes into their respective traffic areas in lymphoid tissue (CURTIS and DE SOUSA, 1973, 1975).

Many other factors affect cell adhesion. For example, the degradation of cell membrane lecithin to lysolecithin (FISCHER et al., 1967) is associated with a decrease in adhesiveness, which suggests that changes in the lipid bilayer as well as in glycoproteins must be considered. An important role for deacylation and reacylation of membrane phospholipids in cell-cell adhesion is suggested by detailed experiments of CURTIS and his colleagues (CURTIS et al., 1975a, b and c).

II. Studies of the Adhesion of Leucocytes

There has been a number of studies of the adhesion of polymorphonuclear leucocytes to glass. GARVIN (1968) found that attachment of these cells to glass beads coated with serum was dependent on the presence of certain divalent cations, e.g. Mg^{2+} but not Ca^{2+}. Cations did not affect the adhesion of leucocytes to uncoated glass. BRYANT and SUTCLIFFE (1972) reported that adhesion to glass was reduced by several factors including lowering the temperature to below 37° C, addition of ethylene glycol tetra-acetic acid (EGTA) or prolonged incubation in the presence of sodium arsenite, an inhibitor of oxidative respiration. Adhesion to glass was enhanced by repeated washing, by moderate hyperosmolarity of the medium and by Mg EGTA.

However, these studies of the adhesion of leucocytes to glass or to nylon fibres may not be relevant to adhesion in vivo. Microtubule-disaggregating agents such as colchicine or vinblastine do not affect the adhesion of fibroblasts to glass (WEISS, 1972) but do inhibit the adhesion of fibroblasts to each other (WADDELL et al., 1974). Aggregation of rabbit polymorphs to one another is also inhibited by microtubule-blocking agents (LACKIE, 1974), as well as by adenosine or methyl xanthines (phosphodiesterase inhibitors).

It is possible, but not proven, that in inflammation there is an increased affinity of the leucocyte for the vascular endothelial cell, following some change in the cell membrane of one or the other cell, and leading to adhesion between the two. However, it is still not excluded that the increased adhesion is simply a result of the slowing of blood flow through the vessel, so that the shearing force preventing adhesion falls below the bonding force between the two cells. Hydrodynamic changes certainly play some part in enhancing the likelihood of adhesion in inflammation.

The study of the adhesion of leucocytes to vascular endothelium has been hampered by the difficulties involved in finding appropriate measurements and suitable experimental models. The observation by ALLISON et al. (1955) that leucocytes adhere preferentially to the side of the vessel nearest to the site of an injury rather than to the opposite side, suggests that the injury may have mediated some change in the endocapillary surface of the endothelial cell increasing its adhesiveness for leucocytes. MARCHESI and FLOREY (1960) and FLOREY and GRANT (1961) studied such vessels by electron microscopy and observed no visible change, although LUFT (1965) suggested, also on electron microscopical evidence, that there was an endocapillary glycoprotein layer which might play a role in endothelium-leucocyte adhesion. There has been recurrent interest in the role of cations in the adhesion of leucocytes to vascular endothelium (BANGHAM, 1964). THOMPSON et al. (1967) reported that ethylene diamine tetra-acetic acid (EDTA) inhibits leucocyte adhesion in experimental inflammation and suggested that divalent cations were required for this adhesion. As mentioned earlier, cationic peptides are released in quantity by leucocytes in inflammatory lesions. The suggestion that they may play a part in mediating leucocyte adhesion (JANOFF and ZWEIFACH, 1964) is only one of several ideas about their function: other suggestions are that they are bactericidal (SPITZNAGEL and CHI, 1963) and that they are vasoactive (MOSES et al., 1964; JANOFF and ZWEIFACH, 1964). These suggestions require further exploration.

ATHERTON and BORN (1972) studied the adhesion of leucocytes to the endothelium of postcapillary venules in spreads of mouse mesentery and in hamster cheek pouch preparations. They quantified this by counting the number of granulocytes rolling along the vessel wall past a selected site on one side of the vessel. Under normal conditions, granulocytes did not roll but flowed down the centre of the vessel. The authors suggested that this was because normally when granulocytes collide with the vessel wall, the collision behaves elastically and the cell bounces off and back into the circulation. However, in inflamed tissue, biochemical changes cause the collisions to behave inelastically and adhesion is increased. As adhesion increases further, rolling is slowed and may be followed by a complete stop and by migration of the cells out of the vessel. The rolling of leucocytes along the side was very much slower (10–20 μm per sec) than the blood flow (200–900 μm per sec). Local application of chemotactic factors, such as casein or a filtrate of *Escherichia coli*, or of plasma permeability factors, caused a reversible increase in the number of rolling cells; the chemotactic factors also caused the leucocytes to leave the vessel and to accumulate in the perivascular tissue. Trypsin and histamine did not affect the rolling cell count, but intravenous injection of neuraminidase (ATHERTON and BORN, 1973) inhibited rolling. Rolling was also abolished in the local presence of EDTA.

Circulating lymphocytes reach their appropriate traffic areas in lymph nodes by migrating across the postcapillary endothelium, probably between the endothelial cells. It has been suggested that this migration results from a specific affinity of the surface glycoproteins of the lymphocyte for the endocapillary membranes of the lymph node endothelium, allowing specific adhesions between them (GESNER and GINSBERG, 1964; WOODRUFF and GESNER, 1968). The evidence for this was based on experiments in which migration of lymphocytes from the blood stream into lymph nodes was abolished by pretreatment of the lymphocytes with trypsin or neuraminidase. However, the interaction between the lymphocyte and the vascular endothelium was not studied directly in these experiments and it now seems that they are open to other interpretations. FORD et al. (1976) showed that neuraminidase-treated thoracic duct lymphocytes perfused directly through isolated mesenteric lymph nodes enter the node normally, and FREITAS and DE SOUSA (1976) showed that enzyme-treated lymphocytes distribute themselves differently from untreated lymphocytes in organs, other than lymph nodes, through which they circulate such as liver, lungs and spleen. They suggested that their redistribution might be due to increased uptake by these organs rather than to any change in affinity for the lymph node vascular endothelium. In any case, experiments with neuraminidase should be interpreted with caution, since commercial samples of this enzyme may differ in biological activity from pure neuraminidase (NOSEWORTHY et al., 1972) and may be contaminated with other membrane-active enzymes such as phospholipases.

C. Leucocyte Locomotion

I. Morphological Observations

The morphological events in moving leucocytes have been described by several groups including ROBINEAUX and FRÉDÉRIC (FRÉDÉRIC and ROBINEAUX, 1951; ROBINEAUX, 1954; ROBINEAUX and FRÉDÉRIC, 1955; ROBINEAUX, 1964), RAMSEY (1972a, b), and ZIGMOND and HIRSCH (1973). The descriptions by these different workers are quite similar in outline. Before the cell begins to move, the anterior end becomes flattened into a hyaline veil or "hyaloplasmic membrane" or "lamellipodium" which extends forwards over the substratum on which the cell is moving. The rear end of the cell forms a tail which may terminate in several adhesive filaments. At first, the anterior lamellipodium may be hyaline and empty of cytoplasmic organelles. There is some difference of opinion about whether there is ruffling at the leading edge. The cell contents then flow forwards into the lamellipodium and the tail breaks away. The cell may then round up and the same series of events happen again at the next translocation. ZIGMOND and HIRSCH (1973), watching horse neutrophils, made the important observation that orientation of the cell to form an anterior lamellipodium and a posterior tail is established before any translocation takes place. ARMSTRONG and LACKIE (1975) have recently described detailed observations of the movement of rabbit polymorphonuclear leucocytes. They distinguished two forms of translocation: (1) lamellipodial movement similar to that described above, and (2) looping movement in which the cell protrudes processes in any plane including away from the substratum. These processes may be hyaline or they may contain organelles. The cells have uropod-like tails with retraction fibres. The tails may act as attachment points since a cell hanging from a coverslip can dangle by its tail and continue to produce cylindrical or lamellar pseudopods with streaming of granules. Thus, the front of the cell does not need to be attached to the substratum for formation of these processes or for streaming. If an anterior process loops over and contacts the substratum it many flatten out and the cellular contents then flow into it and the cell moves forward. The authors suggest that these observations of leucocyte movement might fit best the "rear contraction" model of cell movement which was proposed to explain movement of amoebae by MAST (1926) and more recently by GOLDACRE (1961). In this model, as originally presented, forward movement of the cell resulted from a contraction of "gelated" proteins in the tail of the cell causing forward movement of "solated" endoplasm which then, in its turn, gelated and flowed backwards. By the same token, contractile proteins in the rear end of a leucocyte may initiate forward propulsion of organelles into the lamellipodium. If this is so, leucocyte locomotion may work differently from that of fibroblasts, where contraction may be initiated by filaments in the anteriorly placed lamellipodium. It should be possible to test these ideas experimentally. One group of workers (SENDA et al., 1975) have presented findings on leucocyte movement which are at variance with those of other groups. They suggest that during movement a "contraction wave" passes down the cell from front to back, as in planarian worms.

Locomotion obviously requires the capacity to make and break adhesions rapidly with the substratum and there is electron microscopic evidence that, at the site of contact of mouse macrophages with the substratum, there is local assembly of microfilaments in an ordered network which probably attaches to the cell membrane at the point of adhesion (REAVEN and AXLINE, 1973). It is possible that movement is generated by ordered contraction of microfilaments at sites of adhesion. Presumably, as the cell moves and the point of adhesion changes, there must be rapid assembly and disassembly of these microfilaments since successful movement must entail controlled adhesion and detachment of areas of cell membrane in contact with the substratum. This is supported by the observations of ARMSTRONG and LACKIE (1975), using interference-reflection microscopy, that adherent areas below the cell body of moving neutrophils fluctuate within fractions of a second. The adhesions which neutrophils make with the substratum are weaker than those made by fibroblasts. The latter cells show "black feet"—areas of strong interference coloration indicating close apposition to the substratum—whereas leucocytes show "grey feet"—adherent areas which are less closely apposed to the substratum. These are located below the extending lamellipodia, the cell body, the tail and at the ends of retraction fibres.

The movements of leucocytes in vivo may show modifications of the above description, mediated by their contacts with different tissue cells (but see below). When migrating out of vessels the leucocytes are squeezing through narrow gaps and their anterior extensions are then more like narrow pseudopods (FLOREY and GRANT, 1961) than like the broad lamellipodia seen on glass. It might be imagined that a strong adhesion of the tail of the leucocyte to the endothelial cell allows the untethered anterior extension free movement to find the gap through which the leucocyte is to pass.

II. Contact Inhibition of Movement

ARMSTRONG and LACKIE (1975) also investigated the capacity of leucocytes to show contact inhibition of movement. This phenomenon was first described in fibroblasts (ABERCROMBIE and HEAYSMAN, 1953; ABERCROMBIE, 1967). When a moving fibroblast in tissue culture contacts another fibroblast, there is a cessation of forward extension of pseudopods following the collision and a cessation of ruffling of the membrane at the contact area. This phenomenon may be important in the formation of organized tissues in which it is essential that the cells do not constantly crawl over each other. Certain tumour cells lose contact inhibition of movement and crawl over fibroblasts as readily as over glass (ABERCROMBIE et al., 1957; ABERCROMBIE and AMBROSE, 1962). ARMSTRONG and LACKIE (1975) observed that rabbit neutrophils do not show contact paralysis of pseudopods upon collision with fibroblasts and that they rapidly invade aggregates of fibroblasts. However, they tend not to totally overlap fibroblasts with which they come into contact. Similarly, they do not show contact paralysis when they touch one another (RAMSEY and HARRIS, 1973; ARMSTRONG and LACKIE, 1975). It is, therefore, possible that leucocytes can migrate into the interiors of tissues composed of cells of dissimilar types because they lack contact inhibition.

Their normal function demands that they be invasive cells, and in this respect at least, they resemble certain malignant cells more closely than the cells of normal tissues.

III. Redistribution of Membrane in Moving Cells

It is well known that cross-linking agents such as lectins or antimembrane antibody cause clustering of proteins on the cell membrane and that, when the cell moves, these sites are moved to the rear of the cell to form a cap. RYAN et al. (1974) showed this in polymorphonuclear leucocytes. They also directly labelled membrane protein sites in polymorphs with fluorescein isothiocyanate, which is not a cross-linking agent, and showed that as the cell moved towards a chemotactic stimulus the labelled sites, even though not cross-linked by an external agent, still moved to the tail to form a cap. Such sites may be linked and moved internally, e.g. by microtubules. It seems possible that this redistribution of protein could serve several important functions. (1) These sites may form adhesions with the substratum. If locomotor force is generated from the tail it may be important to concentrate adhesive glycoproteins there. (2) In lymphocytes the tail or "uropod" has been reported to be a specialized structure containing many microvilli (MCFARLAND and SCHECHTER, 1970) which the cell can use to explore its environment. Thus, lymphocytes may attach themselves to macrophages by their uropods (MCFARLAND and HEILMAN, 1965; MCFARLAND et al., 1966) and have been reported to probe the macrophage surface with them (BERMAN, 1966). If the uropod acts as a recognition site, specialized proteins may need to be moved to this site. (3) For certain membrane functions, e.g. membrane fusion, it has been suggested that protein has to be moved out of the way so that fusion can take place between the apposed lipid bilayers (AHKONG et al., 1975). Later in this chapter, I shall discuss the possibility that membrane lipids are involved in chemotactic recognition. It may be that the anterior end of the cell, which is the area of maximum contact with chemotactic factors, is relatively depleted of protein. However, at present all this is speculation. It is known that in phagocytosis the membrane sites included in the phagosome are not random (BERLIN et al., 1974; GRIFFIN and SILVERSTEIN, 1974). For instance, aminoacid transport sites are preferentially excluded from the phagosome and this exclusion is controlled by microtubules (TSAN and BERLIN, 1971; UKENA and BERLIN, 1972). However, the significance of redistribution of membrane sites in moving leucocytes has not been investigated.

D. Chemotaxis

I. Chemotaxis and Chemokinesis

Chemotaxis was defined by MCCUTCHEON (1946) as "a reaction by which the direction of locomotion of cells or organisms is determined by substances in their environment." It must be distinguished from *chemokinesis*, which is a reaction by which the *speed* of migration of cells is determined by substances in their environment but which does not determine the direction of locomotion. For example, KELLER and SORKIN (1966) showed that leucocytes placed in the presence of a chemotactic factor (activated serum) at even concentration, i.e. in the absence of a concentration gradient, migrated randomly but much faster, than the same leucocytes in the absence of a chemoattractant. The distinction between chemotaxis and chemokinesis, which has been ignored, is particularly important in considering how leucocytes react to chemoattractants because, under appropriate conditions, they may show either or both reactions to the same factor. Moreover, the intracellular mechanisms which determine the two reactions are different (see Section D.VI), and it is possible that clinical defects of cell migration may involve specific defects of either reaction.

II. Methods for Measuring Leucocyte Chemotaxis

Two techniques have been widely used for studies of the influence of chemical substances upon leucocyte locomotion in vitro. The first of these is the direct observation of the behaviour of moving cells on a microscope slide in the presence or absence of chemotactic substances. This technique gives information about the locomotion of individual cells and considerable sophistication can be added to it by the use of time-lapse cinematography and various refinements of microscopy. It is time-consuming and not sufficiently quantitative for assessing the activity of different chemotactic factors or for studying the effects of drugs or other environmental factors on the cells' response. Nevertheless, it gives invaluable information about the detailed behaviour of moving cells.

The second method is the familiar micropore filter technique devised by BOYDEN (1962) and adapted in minor ways by other workers. In this technique, cells are placed above a micropore filter which has pores of an appropriate size which allow the cells to squeeze through actively but not to drop through passively. A solution of the chemotactic factor is placed below the filter so that the factor diffuses up, forming a concentration gradient through the filter. The cells then respond by migrating down into the filter. After a given time, the response can be measured by determining the number of cells which have migrated to a given level, e.g. the lower surface of the filter, or more accurately by determining the distance migrated by the leading front of cells (ZIGMOND and HIRSCH, 1973). This method is convenient for rapid investigations, including clinical investigations, to compare cells from different individuals, to identify chemotactic factors, etc. It gives little information about the migration of individual cells or how they reach a given locus.

It has been widely assumed that if cells migrate through a filter towards a chemoattractant, they are migrating by chemotaxis. This is not necessarily so. The cells may be responding to the absolute chemoattractant concentration simply by increasing their speed; they may not be moving directionally or detecting the gradient at all. It is possible to study the influence of gradients on cells migrating in filters (see below). However, in numerous studies during the past decade in which "chemotactic" factors have been isolated, no evidence has been provided that distinguished between the effects of these factors on chemokinesis and chemotaxis. It would be better to call such substances "chemoattractants" unless they have clearly been shown to influence the direction, and not just the speed, of migration of leucocytes.

MCCUTCHEON and his colleagues studied the influence of chemoattractants on the direction of migration of leucocytes (MCCUTCHEON, 1946). If no attractant was present, movement was random. However, cells migrating towards bacterial attractants suspended in plasma on a microscope slide showed clear evidence of directed locomotion. Essentially similar findings were reported by RAMSEY (1972a, b). The most recent exhaustive study was that of ZIGMOND and HIRSCH (1973) who used both the slide and coverslip method and the micropore filter method. The source of attractant in their slide-and-coverslip studies was a streak of aggregated gamma-globulin dried onto a slide. A drop of a suspension of horse neutrophils was added. The leucocytes which settled on the globulin streak flattened out and released substances which attracted other leucocytes that had settled at some distance from the streak. The first thing that happened as the attractants diffused out was that nearby cells became oriented with their anterior lamellipodia facing the streak and their tails away from it. This happened before any translocation of the cells. The oriented cells then showed strong directional locomotion towards the streak. The same workers explored the possibility of distinguishing chemotaxis from chemokinesis in micropore filters by varying the chemoattractant concentration above and below the filter. These experiments showed that (1) when the chemoattractant concentration was the same above and below the filter the cells showed a dose-response to the absolute concentration of the chemoattractant. As the concentration was raised to an optimum, cell migration increased and when raised still further, migration diminished. (2) When there was a positive gradient (higher concentration of chemoattractant below the filter than above), the cells moved further into the filter than would be expected on the basis of chemokinesis alone. (3) When there was a negative gradient (higher concentration of chemoattractant above the filter than below) the cells moved less than would be expected on the basis of chemokinesis alone. This method provides evidence that several factors such as casein, denatured proteins and complement-activated serum are true chemotactic factors, and can be used to distinguish chemotactic and chemokinetic migration in filters (WILKINSON, 1975c; RUSSELL et al., 1975b).

The ability of leucocytes to respond to concentration gradients but also to increase their speed in response to the absolute concentration of attractant in the absence of a gradient, may be of considerable importance in inflammation. Gradients formed in vivo may well be disturbed by movements of the tissues. If this happens, cells at some distance from the source can still accelerate and random migration may bring them close enough to the source to pick up the gradient and respond to it.

III. Methods by Which Cells Detect Gradients

ZIGMOND (1974) has investigated two possible mechanisms by which leucocytes could detect concentration gradients. Firstly, the cell could detect the concentration of attractant at point A, then move to point B, read the concentration there and make its next movement on the basis of the difference between the two readings. This is called *temporal* sensing and is the mechanism used by motile bacteria (BERG and BROWN, 1972). Secondly, provided it has more than one surface receptor capable of detecting the attractant, the cell could detect concentration differences across its own length; this is called *spatial* sensing. ZIGMOND (1974) concluded that leucocytes use spatial sensing, firstly because they take up a correctly oriented morphology in the gradient before making any movement, secondly because the gradient determines the direction of turns which the cell made, but not the frequency of turns as is the case in bacteria.

IV. Chemoattractants

Since BOYDEN (1962) introduced the micropore filter technique, a large number of chemotactic factors have been described, which I have listed elsewhere (WILKINSON, 1974c). Many of these are genuine chemotactic factors on the criteria discussed above; others have not been studied. In this section, therefore, I have used the term "chemoattractants" to cover all such factors, whether or not they have been shown to influence the direction of migration of leucocytes, and "chemotactic factor" where an influence on directional migration has been shown.

Chemoattractants can be classified under several headings based on the type of reaction giving rise to them.

1. Products of Specific Immune Reactions

a) Complement

DELAUNAY et al. (1951) reported that serum complement was necessary for the generation of leucocyte chemotactic activity by starch granules incubated in serum. Since then, the generation of chemotactic activity by antigen-antibody complexes acting through the classical pathway or through the alternate pathway (e.g. guinea pig $7S\gamma_1$-globulin antibody, SANDBERG et al., 1971), or by direct action of proteases on complement components, or by endotoxin, dextran and numerous other complement activators, has been amply confirmed. There has been disagreement about precisely which complement factors are involved. It is generally agreed that C5a is chemotactic for neutrophils (SNYDERMAN et al., 1969, 1970) and macrophages or monocytes (SNYDERMAN et al., 1971b, 1972a), although WISSLER et al. (1972) have crystallized two C5-related peptides, both of which have to be present for chemotactic activity. It is therefore possible that C5a is in fact two substances or that, as WISSLER et al. (1974) suggest, chemotactic activity results from a conformational change in one of the peptides when the other peptide (co-cytotaxin) is present. Two other complement factors, C3a and C567 have been reported to act as chemotactic factors, but there is not general agreement about them.

The chemotactic effects of complement are extremely important. They allow a wide range of substances, including many which are not soluble or diffusible, to exert on leucocytes attractant effects that they could not exert directly. Chemotactic factors have, in fact, been classified on this basis into "cytotaxins" which are directly attractant, and "cytotaxigens" which activate complement or some other endogenous system to exert an indirect attractant effect (KELLER and SORKIN, 1967).

b) Lymphokines

WARD et al. (1969, 1970) described factors released from lymphocytes upon sensitization with antigen, which attract macrophages and neutrophils in vitro, although this attraction has not yet been shown to be chemotactic. These factors are proteins and have been classified as lymphokines. It has been postulated that they attract leucocytes into sites of cell-mediated immune reactions in vivo. This would suggest that the attractants are released by T-lymphocytes, which is so, but they are also released by B-lymphocytes (WAHL et al., 1974). The requirement for antigen-activation is not absolute; mitogens stimulate release of similar factors (ALTMAN and KIRCHNER, 1974; RÜHL et al., 1974). WAHL et al. (1974) reported release of attractants from B-lymphocytes activated with mitogens, antigen-antibody complexes or C3, reacting with different cell surface receptors.

c) Cytophilic Antibody

The attractant effects of complement and lymphokines are exerted from sources at a distance from the responding cells. JENSEN and ESQUENAZI (1975) have recently shown that cell-surface immune reactions also may induce a migratory response in neutrophils. This was shown using neutrophils coated with cytophilic antibody and then exposed to a gradient of specific antigen across a filter. When the antigen became bound to the cell-surface antibody, the cells moved into the filter. This did not happen using unrelated antigens. We have carried out similar experiments using guinea pig macrophages coated with anti-human serum albumin (HSA) and exposed to a gradient of HSA. These results have not been published in detail but are described in brief by WILKINSON (1976).

2. Non-Specific Endogenous Factors

This category includes a variety of factors released in damaged tissues which are not products of specific immune reactions.

a) Cellular Factors

When cells are damaged or die, they release chemotactic factors for leucocytes. This was shown by BESSIS and his colleagues (BESSIS and BURTE, 1964; BESSIS, 1974) who damaged individual cells with a laser beam and showed, using time-lapse cinematography, that leucocytes rapidly home onto the damaged cell. BESSIS named this phenomenon *necrotaxis*. Cytotaxins are released by virus-infected cells (WARD et al., 1972). Cytotaxigens, possibly lysosomal enzymes which hydrolyse complement components, are also released from damaged cells or by secretion of enzymes from healthy cells. Virus-infected cells release C5a-generating factors (BRIER et al., 1970; WARD et al., 1972), and antibody against viruses on the cell surface has similar effects (SNYDERMAN et al., 1972b). Leucocytes engaged in phagocytosis release factors that attract other leucocytes (KELLER and BOREL, 1971). These factors have been localized in the lysosome-rich centrifugal fraction of disrupted cells (BOREL et al., 1969; BOREL, 1970). Contact with chemotactic factors causes fusion of leucocyte lysosomes with the plasma membrane and release of hydrolases from neutrophils (GOLDSTEIN et al., 1973; BECKER and SHOWELL, 1974; BECKER et al., 1974) and macrophages (WILKINSON et al., 1973a).

b) Humoral Factors

It is now clear that chemoattractants are generated by activation of enzyme cascades other than complement in plasma. Kallikrein, activated in the kinin cascade, is one such factor (KAPLAN et al., 1972). Chemoattractants for neutrophils are released during clotting of blood and clot retraction (STECHER et al., 1971) and such activity has been shown in fibrinopeptides (KAY et al., 1973a). Conformationally altered or enzymically digested proteins such as IgG (HAYASHI et al., 1974) and collagen (CHANG and HOUCK, 1970; HOUCK and CHANG, 1971) may have chemoattractant effects which are not shown by the same proteins in the native form. Our own studies on similar lines are discussed below.

A chemotactic protein which is strictly speaking derived from an endogenous source, is milk casein. α-Casein and β-casein, but not κ-casein, are chemotactic for neutrophils and mononuclear phagocytes from a wide variety of sources (WILKINSON, 1972, 1974a). These proteins occur naturally in milk where the Ca^{2+} concentration is very high. Binding of calcium allows the caseins to form very high molecular weight micelles which are not diffusible. In physiological buffers, the caseins form lower molecular weight polymers (NOBLE and WAUGH, 1965) which are diffusible and can form gradients. At physiological Ca^{2+} concentrations, α- and β-casein are strong chemoattractants.

3. Exogenous Chemoattractants

There have been few studies of the actions of bacteria as attractants for leucocytes despite the fact that leucocyte infiltration is the most striking morphological feature of most bacterial infections. Such factors were of considerable interest to METCHNIKOFF (1893) but the first reports about them, using BOYDEN'S method, were those of KELLER and SORKIN (1967) and WARD et al. (1968). A neutrophil attractant which appears to be a protein has been isolated from *E. coli* (SCHIFFMANN et al., 1975b). TAINER et al. (1975) showed activity in lipid and lipoprotein fractions of *E. coli.* We have carried out extensive studies of two groups of organisms, the staphylococci and the anaerobic coryneform bacteria. Staphylococci produce an extremely complex array of activators and inhibitors of leucocyte locomotion: they attract human neutrophils chiefly by activating complement, but they attract human monocytes by a direct action and isoelectric focussing of the chemoattractant material shows multiple peaks of activity (RUSSELL et al., 1976a). Staphylococci produce a number of strong inhibitors of leucocyte migration, including leucocidin (WOODIN, 1972), β-toxin (WILKINSON et al., 1976) and α-toxin (RUSSELL et al., 1976b), so that clearly cellular infiltration into staphylococcal lesions is likely to depend on a complex balance between attraction and inhibition by different factors. The anaerobic coryneform bacteria (*Corynebacterium parvum* group) are of interest as immunostimulants. One of their effects is the attraction of monocytes and macrophages in vitro (WILKINSON et al., 1973a, 1973b)—they have little effect on neutrophils. This chemoattractant has been identified as a lipid, present in capsular material, which is released from the bacteria into their growth medium (RUSSELL et al., 1975b, 1976a). Most leucocyte chemoattractants identified to date have been proteins, and lipids have excited little interest until recently. However, LYNN and his colleagues (TURNER et al., 1975a, 1975b) have suggested that lipids play an important role as attractants. HETE, a 12-hydroxyarachidonic acid derivative produced by platelets had strong activity. Both they and our group have found that a large number of other fatty acids have some chemoattractant activity for leucocytes provided that serum albumin is added to the medium.

V. Possible Modes of Action of Chemoattractants at the Cell Membrane

From the preceding section it is obvious that leucocytes respond to a large number of attractants of widely diverse structure. This poses the question how such a heterogeneous collection of molecules all interact with the leucocyte membrane to initiate an identical locomotor response. This is the central problem of recognition in non-specific immunity; how cells which presumably do not possess large numbers of specific receptors with stereochemical affinities for a wide variety of foreign agents nevertheless respond accurately and rapidly to diverse forms of injury.

We approached the problem of recognition in leucocyte chemotaxis by modifying the structure of proteins such as serum albumin or haemoglobin, which do not act as chemoattractants in the native state, to see which of the various modifications conferred on the proteins the ability to attract leucocytes, and to find whether we could detect any pattern of activity that would give clues as to how these proteins interacted with cell membranes. These experiments have been published in detail. They showed that denaturation of HSA (WILKINSON and MCKAY, 1971, 1974) and of haemoglobin (WILKINSON, 1973) made the protein chemotactic for neutrophils and for monocytes (WILKINSON, 1976). This effect was not due to polymerization of the protein but to the conformational change in protein monomers. The degree of unfolding measured by viscosity (WILKINSON and MCKAY, 1971), by surface activity (WILKINSON, 1974a), and by difference spectroscopy (WILKINSON, 1974b) correlated well with the protein's activity as a leucocyte chemotactic factor. Protein structure was next modified by conjugation of the protein to a number of synthetic side-groups with varying physicochemical properties (WILKINSON and MCKAY, 1972; WILKINSON, 1976). These studies led to the general conclusion that procedures which increased the number of external non-polar side-groups on a protein also made it chemotactic. This could be achieved by denaturation or simply by conjugating such side-groups to the protein. However, bulky non-polar groups such as naphthalene rings were cytotoxic under conditions where less bulky groups such as benzene rings conferred chemotactic activity on the protein.

A possible physicochemical explanation of these findings is that increasing the hydrophobicity of soluble proteins makes them thermodynamically unstable in aqueous solution. In such solutions they find their lowest free energy states under circumstances where their hydrophobic groups can interact in a hydrophobic environment, as for instance in the hydrophobic interior of the lipid bilayer of a cell membrane. Therefore, such proteins would be expected to have an affinity for hydrophobic sites in cell membranes and their interaction at such sites would serve as a signal for a locomotor response in the leucocyte. It is a common feature of denaturation that it increases the number of externally positioned hydrophobic groups on the protein molecule in aqueous solution and this is likely to be true also of damaged proteins found in inflammatory sites. Lipids, mentioned earlier as chemoattractants, might react with cell membranes in a similar way. Other workers also have found hydrophobicity to be an important parameter for chemoattraction (SCHIFFMANN et al., 1975a), as for phagocytosis of particles by leucocytes (VAN OSS and GILLMAN, 1972a, 1972b; THRASHER et al., 1973).

We therefore concluded that the ability of chemoattractants to penetrate into the hydrophobic interior of the phospholipid bilayer of the leucocyte membrane was the factor distinguishing them from non-attractant molecules, and that this penetration acted as a signal, possibly by increasing the permeability of the membrane, for the activation of locomotion. The direction of locomotion might then be determined by the higher number of contacts of the membrane at the front of the cell than at the back with chemotactic molecules.

It is possible that other mechanisms for altering membrane permeability may lead to locomotor responses. The antigen specific migration initiated by interaction of cell-bound cytophilic antibody with antigen (JENSEN and ESQUENAZI, 1975) could result from antigen-induced clustering of cell-bound antibody followed by conformational changes in the Fc fragment which allow it to interact more closely within the bilayer and increase its permeability. This remains to be demonstrated.

Another model for the interaction of chemoattractants with leucocytes is suggested by the recent finding of SCHIFFMANN et al. (1975a) and of SHOWELL et al. (1976) that *N*-formyl-methionyl peptides attract both neutrophils and macrophages. There are several requirements for activity of these peptides. These are *N*-acylation and, in particular, *N*-formylation; activity increases as the molecular weight of the peptide is increased, and evidence has been presented that there is a structural specificity beyond a simple requirement for hydrophobocity. For example the tripeptide f-Met-Leu-Phe is active at concentrations around 10^{-10} M and is a good deal more active than, for instance, the similar tripeptide f-Met-Phe-Leu. It is therefore argued by the above authors that leucocytes possess a specific, high affinity receptor for such tripeptides and further work is in progress to try and establish this. A curious observation is that these peptides and other low-molecular weight attractants only induce cell locomotion if serum albumin is present in the medium (WILKINSON, 1976).

Evidence that chemotactic signals may be transduced at the cell membrane lipid bilayer is derived from recent experiments (Table 1) which showed that highly purified enzymes and toxins (used at non-toxic doses) with specific affinities for membrane lipids can modify the locomotor response of leucocytes to chemoattractants. Phospholipase A enhances the response of neutrophils to such attractants (WILKINSON, 1974a).

Clostridium perfringens θ toxin (a cholesterol-specific toxin) diminishes the locomotor responses of human neutrophils, but not of monocytes, to chemoattractants such as casein, denatured proteins or activated plasma (WILKINSON, 1975a). On the other hand, *C. perfringens* phospholipase C and *Staphylococcus aureus* sphingomyelinase C (sphingomyelin-specific) reduce the responses of human blood monocytes—and mitogen-transformed lymphocytes—to such attractants, but have no effect on neutrophils. All these toxins were used in a high state of purity so that the sites of their action can be pinpointed with precision. These experiments suggest not only that the lipids of leucocyte membranes are closely involved in the initiation of chemically stimulated locomotion but also that the interactions of these lipids with chemotactic molecules must differ in detail in different cell types. Treatment of the cells with enzymes which attack membrane proteins and glycoproteins (e.g. pronase, trypsin, neuraminidase) had only minor effects on the locomotion of neutrophils and macrophages towards casein, activated serum and denatured proteins.

There is not much direct evidence about the role of membrane proteins in the initiation of leucocyte chemotaxis. BECKER and co-workers have suggested that a

Table 1. Effects of membrane-active enzymes and toxins on locomotion of human blood cells towards chemoattractants

Enzyme or toxin and source	Concⁿ per 10^6 cells	Substrate or site of action	Migration of:			
			Neutrophils towards classic chemotactic factors[a]	Monocytes towards classic chemotactic factors[a]	Lymphoblasts (PHA-transformed)	
					towards classic chemotactic factors[a]	towards PHA
Phospholipase A[e] (bee venom, pure)	100 mU	Phospholipids →lysophosphatides	Enhancement	No effect	Variable[b]	*N/T*[c]
Phospholipase C[e] (*Cl. perfringens*: pure)	100 mU	Phospholipids (polar heads)	No effect	Inhibition	Inhibition	No effect
Sphingomyelinase C[e] (*Staph. aureus*: pure)	10^2 HU	Sphingomyelin (polar head)	No effect	Inhibition	Inhibition	No effect
Θ-toxin[e] (*Cl. perfringens*: pure)	0.8 HU	Cholesterol	Inhibition	No effect	No effect	No effect
Pronase® (*Streptomyces grisens* Calbiochem & Sigma)	100 μg[d]	Protein	No effect	No effect	*N/T*[c]	*N/T*[c]
Trypsin (crystalline: bovine pancreas, BDH)	200 μg[d]	Protein	Slight inhibition	Slight inhibition	Slight inhibition	Marked inhibition
α-mannosidase[f] (Canavalia ensiformis, Boehringer)	4–0.5U	α-mannoside	No effect (aggregation)	No effect	No effect	Inhibition
α-Fucosidase (beef kidney, Boehringer)	0.65 U	α-fucoside	No effect	No effect	No effect	No effect
Neuraminidase (Vibrio cholerae: BDH)	4 U	Sialoglycosidases	No effect	No effect	No effect	No effect

[a] Casein 1 mg/ml or endotoxin-activated human serum (10%) or alkali-denatured HSA 1 mg/ml, [b] Enhancement at low doses of chemotactic factor; inhibition at high doses, [c] *N/T*=not tested, [d] Proteases were removed by washing the cells after 15–30 min preincubation (to avoid digestion of the chemotactic factors). The other enzymes were mixed with the cells and the mixture added to the chemotaxis chambers, [e] Lipid-specific enzymes and toxins were highly purified and not derived from commercial sources (*vide* WILKINSON, 1974a, 1975a), [f] Contains concanavalin *A*.

serine esterase, which may or may not be a plasma membrane protein, is activated on contact with chemotactic factors and that this activation is a prerequisite for chemotaxis (WARD and BECKER, 1968). This hypothesis is largely based on the specificity of inhibition of this esterase by a series of organic phosphorus compounds. It has been challenged by WOODIN and WIENEKE (1970a) who argued that the effects of these compounds as serine esterase inhibitors are irrelevant to their actions as chemotaxis inhibitors, and that the latter actions are due to a detergent-like action on membrane phospholipids. It is possible that the membrane proteins likely to be crucially involved in the initiation of message transduction in locomotor responses are ion-pumping enzymes. Potassium and sodium fluxes between the cell and the external medium probably play a role in the activation of leucocyte locomotion (SHOWELL and BECKER, 1976) and K^+ exchange may be regulated by a Na^+K^+ATPase (NACCACHE et al., 1977) or possibly by an acyl phosphatase (WOODIN and WIENEKE, 1970b) and fluxes of Na^+, K^+, and Ca^{2+} are initiated on contact of neutrophils with f-Met-Leu-Phe, 10^{-10} M (NACCACHE et al., 1977).

VI. Motor Mechanisms in Leucocyte Locomotion and Chemotaxis

Actin and myosin have been isolated from polymorphonuclear leucocytes (TATSUMI et al., 1973; STOSSEL and POLLARD, 1973) and alveolar macrophages (HARTWIG and STOSSEL, 1975; STOSSEL and HARTWIG, 1975), and the electron microscopic "arrowhead" formation typical of microfilamentous actin "decorated" by heavy meromyosin can be demonstrated in both neutrophils and macrophages (ALLISON et al., 1971; SENDA et al., 1975). Cytochalasin B reversibly inhibits neutrophil and macrophage migration (BECKER et al., 1972; ALLISON et al., 1971; ZIGMOND and HIRSCH, 1972). These findings furnish some preliminary evidence to suggest that leucocyte locomotion is probably driven by microfilaments. Microtubules also are present in leucocytes (BHISEY and FREED, 1971; ALLISON et al., 1971; REAVEN and AXLINE, 1973). Studies with microtubule disaggregating agents such as colchicine and vinblastine indicate that these drugs do not inhibit chemokinetic locomotion of leucocytes but do diminish the efficiency of chemotactic locomotion (ALLISON et al., 1971; BANDMANN et al., 1974; EDELSON and FUDENBERG, 1973; RUSSELL et al., 1975b). Observations of leucocyte migration even in the absence of a gradient, suggest that cells possess an intrinsic polarity, which may be due to microtubules acting as a cytoskeleton. In chemotactic gradients, a further polarity is imposed from outside the cell. Polarity is not abolished in colchicine-treated cells but direction-finding appears to be less efficient, possibly because the intrinsic polarity is disordered. There is no evidence that microtubules play any direct role in cell locomotion.

One of the unsolved puzzles is how membrane contact with a chemoattractant activates the motile system within the cell. In muscle, contraction requires ATP-derived energy and is controlled by fluxes of Ca^{2+} ions into and out of the cytoplasm, either from outside the cell or from the sarcoplasmic reticulum. Cation influx is initiated by membrane depolarization and calcium is removed by the calcium pump (Ca^{2+} ATPase). We lack information about the role of divalent cations in leucocyte movement. Locomotion is only slightly inhibited in the absence of extracellular Ca^{2+} or Mg^{2+} (BECKER and SHOWELL, 1972; WILKINSON, 1975b) and contact with chemoattractants diminishes uptake of ^{45}Ca by leucocytes (GALLIN and

ROSENTHAL, 1974), rather than augmenting it as would be expected if locomotion were simply activated by increasing the permeability of the plasma membrane to Ca^{2+}. The Mg^{2+} ATPase activity of alveolar macrophage myosin is not dependent on the presence of Ca^{2+} (STOSSEL and HARTWIG, 1975). However, divalent cations probably do play a role, as is suggested by the fact that leucocyte locomotion can be inhibited using the divalent cation ionophore A23187 at concentrations of 10^{-6} M or above (WILKINSON, 1975b). These concentrations of ionophore may increase the cytoplasmic Ca^{2+} concentration sufficiently to induce a "rigor" in the cell. At lower concentrations (10^{-8} to 10^{-9} M), A23187 restores locomotion of leucocytes migrating in divalent cation-depleted media to normal, possibly by assisting the cells to use their own intracellular divalent cation stores for locomotion (WILKINSON, 1975b). Local anaesthetics inhibit leucocyte migration and also diminish ion flow across membranes, but local anaesthetics also inhibit function of membrane-associated contractile proteins (POSTE et al., 1975) so that the site of their action on cell locomotion is uncertain.

VII. Other Biochemical Mechanisms

1. Energy Sources for Locomotion

Chemically stimulated locomotion of leucocytes is accompanied by an increase in metabolic activity (GOETZL and AUSTEN, 1974) manifested as increased hexose monophosphate shunt activity and aerobic glycolysis. These cells accumulate lactate. Inhibitors of anaerobic glycolysis such as iodoacetate (CARRUTHERS, 1966) inhibit leucocyte locomotion. Inhibitors of oxidative phosphorylation such as dinitrophenol cause only a slight decrease in leucocyte locomotion (WARD, 1966; CARRUTHERS, 1967; WILKINSON et al., 1973a) and this effect is reversible on adding ATP to the medium. Ascorbic acid, which stimulates hexose monophosphate shunt activity, enhances leucocyte locomotion (GOETZL et al., 1974). These findings suggest that an increase in metabolism is an essential feature of stimulated locomotion, possibly because ATP necessary for microfilament action is supplied by the metabolic burst.

2. Cyclic Nucleotides

In the recent enthusiasm for cyclic nucleotides as regulators of cellular functions, a number of conflicting reports on their activity in migrating leucocytes have been published. The evidence that extracellular cyclic nucleotides have any effect on leucocyte locomotion is unsatisfactory and unconvincing. On the other hand, the idea that intracellular levels of cyclic nucleotides may play a regulatory role in locomotion, and may themselves be regulated by interactions of extracellular molecules with membrane receptors, is plausible. TSE et al. (1972) reported that a number of compounds which increase intracellular cAMP levels decrease leucocyte migration, and conversely that substances which decrease cAMP levels enhance cell migration. RIVKIN et al. (1975) found that substances which inhibited locomotion raised cAMP levels but did not believe the evidence warranted any suggestion that adenyl cyclase is involved in the regulation of locomotion at the cell membrane. ESTENSEN et al. (1973) reported that substances which increase intracellular cGMP levels enhance migration, a result which we have been unable to confirm. In my view the evidence linking cyclic nucleotides with leucocyte locomotion is insubstantial and further critical experiments are needed.

3. Protein and Nucleic Acid Synthesis

The cell's response to a chemoattractant is an immediate event which appears not to require new synthesis of protein. Inhibitors of protein synthesis have little effect on locomotion (BOREL, 1973; WILKINSON et al., 1973a). Heavily irradiated cells still migrate well (HOLLEY et al., 1974) and even cells which have lost their nuclei can still show chemotactic responses (KELLER and BESSIS, 1975). Increased synthesis of protein or DNA is not associated with enhanced migration. Populations of "activated" macrophages which show such increases in synthetic activity migrate the same distance in Boyden chambers in our hands as unactivated macrophages.

4. Effects of Other Agents

Most workers agree now that vasoactive factors are not chemotactic factors (but see Section VIII.2 for a recent report on histamine). Among other drugs of importance in inflammation, most workers agree with the observations originally made by WARD (1966) that steroids, at doses around 10^{-4} to 10^{-5} M, inhibit leucocyte locomotion. A similar effect was shown with another membrane stabilizer, chloroquine (WARD, 1966).

VIII. Migration of Individual Leucocyte Types

1. Neutrophils and Mononuclear Phagocytes

Both neutrophils and mononuclear phagocytes respond to the majority of the chemoattractants listed earlier. Motile mononuclear phagocytes of many types (exudate macrophages or blood monocytes) all behave in an essentially similar way. Blood monocytes are particularly satisfactory cells for use in routine studies. Neutrophil-specific and macrophage-specific chemotactic factors have frequently been described, by ourselves and others. However, I am not convinced that these factors are completely cell-specific. Most of the substances we have thought to attract only one cell-type, prove on exhaustive testing to have some activity for the other cell-type as well. Monocytes respond better to lipids and other low molecular weight attractants than do neutrophils. An example is the lipid isolated from anaerobic corynebacteria and discussed earlier (RUSSELL et al., 1976a). It seems likely that the interactions between chemotactic factors and the cell membrane differ subtly in neutrophils and monocytes, as is suggested by the cell-specific inhibition of locomotion mediated by different membrane-lipid-specific bacterial toxins (Section D.V).

Neutrophils and monocytes both show brisk responses to chemotactic factors in vitro. If formation of such factors is stimulated in vivo, in the peritoneal cavity for example, neutrophils appear in the exudate in substantial numbers a few hours later (Fig. 1). The ingress of monocytes and lymphocytes is delayed, however, and large

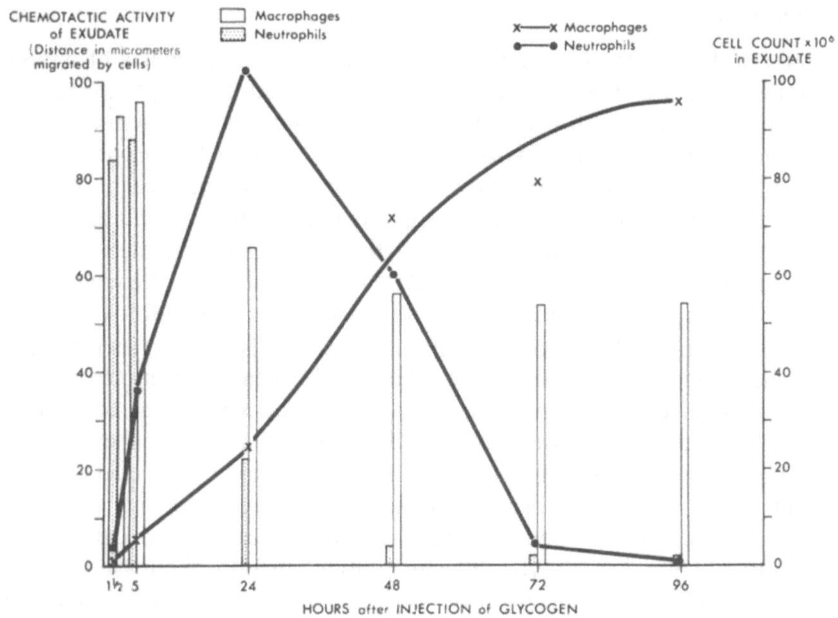

Fig. 1. Production of chemotactic factors in vivo in the guinea pig peritoneal cavity and its relation to cell numbers in the exudate. Histograms show chemotactic activity of the peritoneal exudate at different times after injection of glycogen up to 4 days. Continuous lines show cell counts over same time period. Reproduced from WILKINSON (1974c) by courtesy of Churchill-Livingstone

numbers of these cells appear in the exudate only after 24 to 72 h. Entry of the mononuclear cells is delayed by some mechanism which operates in vivo but not under the simpler conditions which hold in the chemotaxis chamber.

2. Eosinophils

From the nature of the lesions into which eosinophils migrate and of the clinical conditions characterized by blood eosinophilia, it seems likely that eosinophils respond to stimuli different from mononuclear phagocytes or neutrophils. There are indeed eosinophil-specific chemoattractants (though not completely specific—see KAY et al., 1973b) which have not been clearly defined as chemotactic factors. One such factor named eosinophil chemotactic factor of anaphylaxis (ECF-A) is released from chopped lung fragments sensitized with IgE or similar homocytotropic antibodies and then challenged with antigen (KAY et al., 1971; KAY and AUSTEN, 1971). PARISH (1972) showed that basophils or mast cells release this or a similar factor when cell-bound antibody reacts with antigen. A similar ECF is released by neutrophils treated with the ionophore A23187 (CZARNETZKI et al., 1975). Finally, despite a number of previous reports to the contrary, there is a recent well-documented study suggesting that histamine is specifically chemotactic for eosinophils but not other leucocytes (CLARK et al., 1975).

3. Lymphocytes

Over the last decade, there have been several unconvincing reports of lymphocyte chemotaxis and a great many unpublished and unsuccessful attempts to repeat them. We became impressed with evidence from several sources (ASHERSON et al., 1973; MOORE and HALL, 1973; MCGREGOR and LOGIE, 1974) that the lymphocytes which migrate into inflammatory lesions in vivo are blast-transformed cells. We therefore studied the migration of lymphoblasts from human B cell lines maintained in continuous culture. These showed typical chemotactic responses to activated serum, casein and similar factors in Boyden chambers (RUSSELL et al., 1975b). We have since used human blood lymphocytes transformed with mitogens such as endotoxin (B cells), or phytohaemagglutinin (PHA) or concanavalin A (T cells). Both types of blast cell showed chemotactic responses. On the other hand, when we examined the population of lymphoblasts present in the draining lymph nodes following contact sensitization with oxazolone, we were able to demonstrate vigorous chemokinetic responses but no chemotaxis (RUSSELL et al., 1975b). Judged by the effects of enzyme treatment, human PHA-transformed lymphoblasts can respond to chemotactic factors in two ways. Their response to activated serum, casein and denatured HSA resembles that of blood monocytes in being inhibited by phospholipase C and sphingomyelinase C (Table 1) but very little inhibited by trypsin or by α-mannosidase, suggesting that lipids but not glycoproteins are necessary for the response to these factors. In addition, these lymphoblasts migrate towards mitogens such as PHA, which phagocytes do not. This migration is not affected by phospholipases but is inhibited by trypsin and α-mannosidase (Table 1). It is possible that this migration is activated by the permeability change which results from clustering of membrane glycoproteins, and is abolished if these proteins are cleaved by enzymes.

IX. Does Chemotaxis Occur in vivo?

Although leucocyte chemotaxis has been a subject of study ever since LEBER (1891) and METCHNIKOFF (1893) first observed the phenomenon, the direct evidence that it occurs in living tissues or that it accounts for the accumulation of cells in inflammatory loci is still very slender. Workers who have watched cells migrating out of vessels at sites of injury have failed to observe directional migration of the cells (ALLISON et al., 1955; CLIFF, 1966). This is perhaps not surprising considering how difficult it is to set up a stable gradient in vitro, in a slide and coverslip preparation for instance, to say nothing of the disturbances such a gradient may be subject to in living tissues under direct observation. The best evidence for directional migration derived from direct observation of migrating cells in living tissues is that of BUCKLEY (1963) who made microinjuries at a considerable distance from the nearest vessel and, using time-lapse cinematography, watched cells during the subsequent 24 h moving directionally from the vessel to the site of the lesion. However, it could be argued that this was not chemotaxis but some form of contact guidance, and it is difficult to see how such an objection could be overcome.

There is quite a lot of circumstantial evidence for the occurence of chemotaxis in vivo. This is based on many observations that whenever factors which are demonstrably chemotactic in vitro are formed or are injected into any site in vivo, cells can constantly be shown to migrate into the site in response to them. SNYDERMAN et al. (1971a) showed that shortly following injection of endotoxin or glycogen into the peritoneal cavity of guinea pigs or mice, C5a was formed in the peritoneal fluid. After 1 to 2 h, neutrophils were migrating into the peritoneal cavity in large numbers. This infiltration of neutrophils did not occur in C5-deficient animals. We studied the influx of macrophages in similar experiments (Fig. 1) and again observed that macrophages reached the peritoneal cavity following the formation there of macrophage chemotactic factors. These experiments point to conclusions similar to those of ATHERTON and BORN (1972) in which local application of chemotactic factors from *E. coli* or casein to the perivascular tissue in mesenteric spreads or hamster cheek pouch preparations, was followed by emigration of leucocytes from the vessels under observation into the tissues. RYAN and HURLEY (1966) extracted a factor from burned skin which attracted cells in vitro and caused leucocyte emigration in vivo. It is now accepted that cellular emigration can be dissociated from enhancement of vascular permeability (HURLEY, 1963), a point which confused many earlier workers. Most people would now be willing to accept that chemical attractants are identifiable in inflammatory lesions and attract cells into them. The difficulty really arises when it is required to demonstrate that this attraction is due to directional migration. Whether this can or cannot be demonstrated, it will be appreciated that cells may often arrive at a site of injury by chemokinesis in situations where the chemical gradient is poor. The other important point concerning gradients is that when cells reach the source of a gradient, they cannot move away. As soon as a cell moves away from the source, it is attracted back in. This trapping may be an important aspect of chemotaxis in vivo. Nevertheless, it is still important to point out that accumulation of cells at a locus can occur for many reasons and chemotaxis is only one of them. Papers are still published regularly which assume that the two phenomena are identical.

References

Abercrombie, M.: Contact inhibition: the phenomenon and its biological implications. Nat. Cancer Inst. Monogr. **26**, 249—277 (1967)

Abercrombie, M., Ambrose, E. J.: The surface properties of cancer cells. Cancer Res. **22**, 525—548 (1962)

Abercrombie, M., Heaysman, J. E. M.: Observations on the social behaviour of cells in tissue culture. I. Speed of movement of chick heart fibroblasts in relation to their mutual contacts. Exp. Cell Res. **5**, 111—131 (1953)

Abercrombie, M., Heaysman, J. E. M., Karthauser, H. M.: Social behaviour of cells in tissue culture. III. Mutual influence of sarcoma cells and fibroblasts. Exp. Cell Res. **13**, 276—291 (1957)

Ahkong, Q. F., Fisher, D., Tampion, W., Lucy, J. A.: Mechanisms of cell fusion. Nature (Lond.) **253**, 194—195 (1975)

Allison, A. C., Davies, P., Petris, S., de: Role of contractile microfilaments in macrophage movement and endocytosis. Nature (New Biol.) **232**, 153—155 (1971)

Allison, F., Smith, M. R., Wood, W. B.: Studies on the pathogenesis of acute inflammation. I. The inflammatory reaction to thermal injury as observed in the rabbit ear chamber. J. exp. Med. **102**, 655—668 (1955)

Altman, L. C., Kirchner, H.: Mononuclear leucocyte chemotaxis in the chicken. Definition of a phylogenetically specific lymphokine. Immunology **26**, 393—405 (1974)

Armstrong, P. B., Lackie, J. M.: Studies on intercellular invasion in vitro using rabbit peritoneal neutrophil granulocytes (PMNs). I. Role of contact inhibition in locomotion. J. Cell Biol. **65**, 439—462 (1975)

Asherson, G. L., Allwood, G. G., Mayhew, B.: Contact sensitivity in the mouse. XI. Movement of T blasts in the draining lymph nodes to sites of inflammation. Immunology **25**, 485—494 (1973)

Atherton, A., Born, G. V. R.: Quantitative investigations of the adhesiveness of circulating polymorphonuclear leucocytes to blood vessel walls. J. Physiol. (Lond.) **222**, 447—474 (1972)

Atherton, A., Born, G. V. R.: Effects of neuraminidase and N-acetyl neuraminic acid on the adhesion of circulating granulocytes and platelets in venules. J. Physiol. (Lond.) **234**, 66—67 (1973)

Bandmann, U., Rydgren, L., Norberg, B.: The difference between random movement and chemotaxis. Exp. Cell Res. **88**, 63—73 (1974)

Bangham, A. D.: The adhesiveness of leukocytes with special reference to zeta potential. Ann. N.Y. Acad. Sci. **116**, 945—949 (1964)

Becker, E. L., Davis, A. T., Estensen, R. D., Quie, P. G.: Cytochalasin B. IV. Inhibition and stimulation of chemotaxis of rabbit and human polymorphonuclear leukocyte. J. Immunol. **108**, 396—402 (1972)

Becker, E. L., Showell, H. J.: The effect of Ca^{2+} and Mg^{2+} on the chemotactic responsiveness and spontaneous motility of rabbit polymorphonuclear leukocytes. Z. Immun.-Forsch. **143**, 466—476 (1972)

Becker, E. L., Showell, H. J.: The ability of chemotactic factors to induce lysosomal enzyme release. II. The mechanism of release. J. Immunol. **112**, 2055—2062 (1974)

Becker, E. L., Showell, H. J., Henson, P. M., Hsu, L. S.: The ability of chemotactic factors to induce lysosomal enzyme release. I. The characteristics of the release, the importance of surfaces and the relation of enzyme release to chemotactic responsiveness. J. Immunol. **112**, 2047—2054 (1974)

Berg, H. C., Brown, D. A.: Chemotaxis in Escherichia coli analysed by three-dimensional tracking. Nature (Lond.) **239**, 500—504 (1972)

Berlin, R. D., Oliver, J. M., Ukena, T. E., Yin, H. H.: Control of cell surface topography. Nature (Lond.) **247**, 45—46 (1974)

Berman, L.: Lymphocytes and macrophages in vitro. Their activities in relation to functions of small lymphocytes. Lab. Invest. **15**, 1084—1099 (1966)

Bessis, M.: Necrotaxis: chemotaxis towards an injured cell. Antibiot. Chemother. **19**, 369—381 (1974)

Bessis, M., Burte, B.: Chimiotactisme après destruction d'une cellule par microfaisceaux Laser. C.R. Soc. Biol. (Paris) **158**, 1995—1997 (1964)

Bhisey, A. N., Freed, J. J.: Ameboid movement induced in cultured macrophages by colchicine and vinblastine. Exp. Cell Res. **64**, 419—429 (1971)

Borel, J. F.: Studies on chemotaxis: Effect of subcellular leukocyte fractions on neutrophils and macrophages. Int. Arch. Allergy **39**, 247—271 (1970)

Borel, J. F.: Effect of some drugs on the chemotaxis of rabbit neutrophils in vitro. Experientia (Basel) **29**, 676—678 (1973)

Borel, J. F., Keller, H. U., Sorkin, E.: Studies on chemotaxis. XI. Effects on neutrophils of lysosomal and other subcellular fractions from leucocytes. Int. Arch. Allergy **35**, 194—205 (1969)

Boyden, S. V.: The chemotactic effect of mixtures of antibody and antigen on polymorphonuclear leucocytes. J. exp. Med. **115**, 453—466 (1962)

Brier, A. M., Snyderman, R., Mergenhagen, S. E., Notkins, A. L.: Inflammation and herpes-simplex virus: release of a chemotaxis-generating factor from infected cells. Science **170**, 1104—1106 (1970)

Bryant, R. E., Sutcliffe, M. C.: A method for quantitation of human leucocyte adhesion to glass. Proc. Soc. exp. Biol. (N.Y.) **141**, 196—202 (1972)

Buckley, I. K.: Delayed secondary damage and leucocyte chemotaxis following focal aseptic heat injury in vivo. Exp. molec. Path. **2**, 402—417 (1963)

Carruthers, B. M.: Leukocyte motility. I. Method of study, normal variation, effect of physical alterations in environment and effect of iodoacetate. Canad. J. Physiol. Pharmacol. **44**, 475—485 (1966)

Carruthers, B. M.: Leukocyte motility. II. Effect of absence of glucose in medium: effect of presence of deoxyglucose, dinitrophenyl, puromycin, actinomycin D and trypsin on the response to chemotactic substance: effect of segregation of cells from chemotactic substance. Canad. J. Physiol. Pharmacol. **45**, 269—280 (1967)

Chang, C., Houck, J. C.: Demonstration of the chemotactic properties of collagen. Proc. Soc. exp. Biol. (N.Y.) **134**, 22—26 (1970)

Clark, R. A. F., Gallin, J. I., Kaplan, A. P.: The selective eosinophil chemotactic activity of histamine. J. exp. Med. **142**, 1462—1476 (1975)

Cliff, W. J.: The acute inflammatory reaction in the rabbit ear chamber with particular reference to the phenomenon of leukocytic migration. J. exp. Med. **124**, 543—556 (1966)

Curtis, A. S. G.: Cell adhesion. Progr. Biophys. molec. Biol. **27**, 315—386 (1973)

Curtis, A. S. G., Campbell, J., Shaw, F. M.: Cell surface lipids and adhesion. I. The effects of lysophosphatidyl compounds, phospholipase A_2 and aggregation-inhibiting protein. J. Cell Sci. **18**, 347—356 (1975)

Curtis, A. S. G., Chandler, C., Picton, N.: Cell surface lipids and adhesion. III. The effects on cell adhesion of changes in plasmalemmal lipids. J. Cell Sci. **18**, 375—384 (1975)

Curtis, A. S. G., Sousa, M. A. B., de: Factors influencing adhesion of lymphoid cells. Nature (New Biol.) **244**, 45—47 (1973)

Curtis, A. S. G., Sousa, M. A. B., de: Lymphocyte interactions and positioning. I. Adhesive interactions. Cell Immunol. **19**, 282—297 (1975)

Curtis, A. S. G., Shaw, F. M., Spires, V. M. C.: Cell surface lipids and adhesion. II. The turnover of lipid components of the plasmalemma in relation to cell adhesion. J. Cell Sci. **18**, 357—373 (1975)

Czarnetzki, B. M., Konig, W., Lichtenstein, L. M.: Release of eosinophil chemotactic factor from human polymorphonuclear neutrophils by calcium ionophore A23187 and phagocytosis. Nature (Lond.) **258**, 725—726 (1975)

Delaunay, A., Lebrun, J., Barber, M.: Factors involved in chemotactism of leucocytes in vitro. Nature (Lond.) **167**, 774—775 (1951)

Edelson, P. J., Fudenberg, H. H.: Effect of vinblastine on the chemotactic responsiveness of normal human neutrophils. Infect. Immun. **8**, 127—129 (1973)

Estensen, R. D., Hill, H. R., Quie, P. G., Hogan, N., Goldberg, N. D.: Cyclic GMP and cell movement. Nature (Lond.) **245**, 458—460 (1973)

Fischer, H., Ferber, E., Haupt, I., Kohlschütter, A., Modolell, M., Munder, P. G., Sonak, R.: Lysophosphatides and cell membranes. Protides biol. Fluids **15**, 175—184 (1967)

Florey, H. W., Grant, L. H.: Leucocytic migration from small blood vessels stimulated with ultraviolet light. An electron microscope study. J. Path. Bact. **82**, 13—17 (1961)

Ford, W. L., Sedgley, M., Sparshott, S. M., Smith, M. E.: The migration of lymphocytes across specialized vascular endothelium. II. The contrasting consequences of treating lymphocytes with trypsin or neuraminidase. Cell Tiss. Kinet. **9**, 351—361 (1976)

Frédéric, J., Robineaux, R.: Contribution a l'étude de la cytophysiologie de leucocytes par la microcinématographie en contraste de phase. J. Physiol. (Paris) **43**, 732 (1951)

Freitas, A., de Sousa, M. A. B.: Control mechanisms of lymphocyte traffic. Modification of the traffic of ^{51}Cr labelled mouse lymph node cells by treatment with plant lectins in intact and splenectomized hosts. Europ. J. Immunol. **5**, 831—838 (1976)

Gallin, J. I., Rosenthal, A. S.: The regulatory role of divalent cations in human granulocyte chemotaxis: Evidence for an association between calcium exchanges and microtubule assembly. J. Cell Biol. **62**, 594—609 (1974)

Garvin, J. E.: Effects of divalent cations on adhesiveness of rat polymorphonuclear neutrophils in vitro. J. cell. Physiol. **72**, 197—212 (1968)

Gesner, B. M., Ginsburg, V.: Effect of glycosidases on the fate of transfused lymphocytes. Proc. nat. Acad. Sci. (Wash.) **52**, 750—755 (1964)

Goetzl, E. J., Austen, K. F.: Stimulation of human neutrophil leukocyte aerobic glucose metabolism by purified chemotactic factors. J. clin. Invest. **53**, 591—599 (1974)

Goetzl, E. J., Wassermann, S. I., Gigli, I., Austen, K. F.: Enhancement of random migration and chemotactic response of human leukocytes by ascorbic acid. J. clin. Invest. **53**, 813—818 (1974)

Goldacre,R.J.: The role of the cell membrane in the locomotion of amoebae and the source of the motive force and its feedback. Exp. Cell Res. **8**, 1—16 (1961)

Goldstein,I., Hoffstein,S., Gallin,J., Weissmann,G.: Mechanisms of lysosomal enzyme release from human leukocytes. Microtubule assembly and membrane fusion induced by a component of complement. Proc. Nat. Acad. Sci. (Wash.) **70**, 2916—2920 (1973)

Griffin,F.M., Silverstein,S.C.: Segmental response of the macrophage plasma membrane to a phagocytic stimulus. J. exp. Med. **139**, 323—326 (1974)

Hartwig,J.H., Stossel,T.P.: Isolation and properties of actin, myosin, and a new actin-binding protein in rabbit alveolar macrophages. J. biol. Chem. **250**, 5696—5705 (1975)

Hayashi,H., Yoshinaga,M., Yamamoto,S.: The nature of a mediator of leucocyte chemotaxis in inflammation. Antibiot. Chemother. **19**, 296—332 (1974)

Holley,T.R., Van Epps,D.E., Harvey,R.L., Anderson,R.E., Williams,R.C.: Effect of high doses of radiation on neutrophil chemotaxis, phagocytosis, and morphology. Amer. J. Path. **75**, 61—72 (1974)

Houck,J., Chang,C.: The chemotactic properties of the products of collagenolysis. Proc. Soc. exp. Biol. (N.Y.) **138**, 69—75 (1971)

Hurley,J.V.: An electron microscopic study of leucocytic emigration and vascular permeability in rat skin. Aust. J. exp. Biol. med. Sci. **41**, 171—186 (1963)

Jamieson,G.A., Urban,C.L., Barber,A.J.: Enzymatic basis for platelet: collagen adhesion as the primary step in haemostasis. Nature (New Biol.) **234**, 5—7 (1971)

Janoff,A., Zweifach,B.W.: Production of inflammatory changes in the micro-circulation by cationic proteins extracted from lysosomes. J. exp. Med. **120**, 747—764 (1964)

Jensen,J.A., Esquenazi,V.: Chemotactic stimulation by cell surface immune reactions. Nature (Lond.) **256**, 213—215 (1975)

Kaplan,A.P., Kay,A.B., Austen,K.F.: A prealbumin activator of prekallikrein. III. Appearance of chemotactic activity for human neutrophils by the conversion of prekallikrein to kallikrein. J. exp. Med. **135**, 81—97 (1972)

Kay,A.B., Austen,K.F.: The IgE-mediated release of an eosinophil leukocyte chemotactic factor from human lung. J. Immunol. **107**, 899—902 (1971)

Kay,A.B., Pepper,D.S., Ewart,M.R.: Generation of chemotactic activity for leukocytes by the action of thrombin on human fibrinogen. Nature (New Biol.) **243**, 56—57 (1973a)

Kay,A.B., Shin,H.S., Austen,K.F.: Selective attraction of eosinophils and synergism between eosinophil chemotactic factor of anaphylaxis (ECF-A) and a fragment cleaved from the fifth component of complement (C5a). Immunology **24**, 969—976 (1973b)

Kay,A.B., Stechschulte,D.J., Austen,K.F.: An eosinophil leukocyte chemotactic factor of anaphylaxis. J. exp. Med. **133**, 602—619 (1971)

Keller,H.U., Bessis,M.: Migration and chemotaxis of anucleate cytoplasmic leucocyte fragments. Nature (Lond.) **258**, 723—724 (1975)

Keller,H.U., Borel,J.F.: Chemotaxis of phagocytes. Advanc. exp. Med. Biol. **15**, 53—58 (1971)

Keller,H.U., Sorkin,E.: Studies in chemotaxis. IV. The influence of serum factors on granulocyte locomotion. Immunology **10**, 409—416 (1966)

Keller,H.U., Sorkin,E.: Studies on chemotaxis. V. On the chemotactic effect of bacteria. Int. Arch. Allergy **31**, 505—517 (1967)

Lackie,J.M.: The aggregation of rabbit polymorphonuclear leucocytes: Effects of antimitotic agents, cyclic nucleotides and methyl xanthines. J. Cell Sci. **16**, 167—180 (1974)

Leber,T.: Die Entstehung der Entzündung und die Wirkung der entzündungserregenden Schädlichkeiten. Leipzig: Engelmann 1891

Luft,J.H.: The ultrastructural basis of capillary permeability. In: Zweifach,B.W., Grant,L., McCluskey,R.T. (Eds.): The Inflammatory Process, pp. 121—159. New York: Academic Press 1965

McCutcheon,M.: Chemotaxis in leukocytes. Physiol. Rev. **26**, 319—336 (1946)

McFarland,W., Heilman,D.H.: Lymphocyte foot appendage: its role in lymphocyte function and in immunological reactions. Nature (Lond.) **205**, 887—888 (1965)

McFarland,W., Heilman,D.H., Moorhead,J.F.: Functional anatomy of the lymphocyte in immunological reactions in vitro. J. exp. Med. **124**, 851—858 (1266)

McFarland,W., Schechter,G.P.: The lymphocyte in immunological reactions in vitro: ultrastructural studies. Blood **35**, 683—688 (1970)

McGregor,D.D., Logie,P.S.: The mediator of cellular immunity. VII. Localization of sensitized lymphocytes in inflammatory exudates. J. exp. Med. **139**, 1415—1430 (1974)

Marchesi,V.T., Florey,H.W.: Electron micrographic observations on the emigration of leucocytes. Quart. J. exp. Physiol. **45**, 343—348 (1960)

Mast,S.O.: Structure, movement locomotion and stimulation in amoeba. J. Morph. Physiol. **41**, 347—425 (1926)

Metchnikoff,E.: Lectures on the Comparative Pathology of Inflammation. London: Kegan Paul 1893

Moore,A.R., Hall,J.G.: Non-specific entry of thoracic duct immunoblasts into intradermal foci of antigens. Cell Immunol. **8**, 112—119 (1973)

Moses,J.M., Ebert,R.H., Graham,R.C., Brine,K.L.: Pathogenesis of inflammation. I. The production of an inflammatory substance from rabbit granulocytes in vitro and its relationship to leucocyte pyrogen. J. exp. Med. **120**, 57—82 (1964)

Naccache,H.J., Showell,E.L., Becker,E.L., Sha'afi,R.L.: Sodium, potassium and calcium transport across polymorphonuclear leukocyte membranes: Effect of chemotactic factor. J. Cell Biol. **73**, 428—444 (1977)

Noble,R.W., Waugh,D.F.: Casein micelles formation and structure. I. J. Amer. chem. Soc. **87**, 2236—2245 (1965)

Noseworthy,J., Korchak,H., Karnovsky,M.L.: Phagocytosis and the sialic acid of the surface of polymorphonuclear leukocytes. J. cell. Physiol. **79**, 91—96 (1972)

Parish,W.E.: Eosinophilia III. The anaphylactic release from isolated human basophils of a substance that selectively attracts eosinophils. Clin. Allergy **2**, 381—390 (1972)

Poste,G., Papahadjopoulos,D., Nicolson,G.L.: Local anaesthetics affect transmembrane cytoskeletal control of mobility and distribution of cell surface receptors. Proc. Nat. Acad. Sci. (Wash.) **72**, 4430—4434 (1975)

Ramsey,W.S.: Analysis of individual leucocyte behaviour during chemotaxis. Exp. Cell Res. **70**, 129—139 (1972a)

Ramsey,W.S.: Locomotion of human polymorphonuclear leukocytes. Exp. Cell Res. **72**, 489—501 (1972b)

Ramsey,W.S., Harris,H.: Leucocyte locomotion and its inhibition by antimitotic drugs. Exp. Cell Res. **82**, 262—270 (1973)

Reaven,E.P., Axline,S.G.: Subplasmalemal microfilaments and microtubules in resting and phagocytizing cultivated macrophages. J. Cell Biol. **59**, 12—27 (1973)

Rivkin,I., Rosenblatt,J., Becker,E.L.: The role of cyclic AMP in the chemotactic responsiveness and spontaneous motility of rabbit neutrophils. J. Immunol. **115**, 1126—1134 (1975)

Robineaux,R.: Mouvements cellulaires et fonctions phagocytaires des granulocytes neutrophiles. Rév. Hémat. **9**, 364—402 (1954)

Robineaux,R.: Movements of cells involved in inflammation and immunity. In: Allen,R.D., Kamiya,N. (Eds.): Primitive Motile Systems in Cell Biology, pp. 351—364. New York: Academic Press 1964

Robineaux,R., Frédéric,J.: Contribution a l'étude des granulations des polynucléaires par la microcinématographie en contraste de phase. C.R. Soc. Biol. (Paris) **149**, 486—492 (1955)

Roseman,S.: The synthesis of complex carbohydrates by multiglycosyl transferase systems and their potential function in intercellular adhesion. Chem. Phys. Lipids **5**, 270—297 (1970)

Rühl,H., Vogt,W., Bochert,G., Schmidt,S., Moelle,R., Schaoua,H.: Effect of L-asparaginase and hydrocortisone on human lymphocyte transformation and production of a mononuclear leucocyte chemotactic factor in vitro. Immunology **26**, 989—994 (1974)

Russell,R.J., McInroy,R.J., Wilkinson,P.C., White,R.G.: Identification of a lipid chemoattractant (chemotactic) factor for macrophages from anaerobic coryneform bacteria. Behring Inst. Mitt. **57**, 103—109 (1975a)

Russell,R.J., McInroy,R.J., Wilkinson,P.C., White,R.G.: A lipid chemotactic factor from anaerobic coryneform bacteria including Corynebacterium parvum with activity for macrophages and monocytes. Immunology **30**, 935—949 (1976a)

Russell,R.J., Wilkinson,P.C., McInroy,R.J., McKay,S., McCartney,A.C., Arbuthnott,J.P.: Effects of staphylococcal products on locomotion and chemotaxis of human blood neutrophils and monocytes. J. med. Microbiol. **9**, 433—449 (1976b)

Russell,R.J., Wilkinson,P.C., Sless,F., Parrott,D.M.V.: Chemotaxis of lymphoblasts. Nature (Lond.) **256**, 646—648 (1975b)

Ryan, G. B., Borysenko, J. Z., Karnovsky, M. J.: Factors affecting the redistribution of surface bound concanavalin A on human polymorphonuclear leukocytes. J. Cell Biol. **62**, 351—365 (1974)
Ryan, G. B., Hurley, J. V.: The chemotaxis of polymorphonuclear leucocytes towards damaged tissue. Brit. J. exp. Path. **47**, 530—536 (1966)
Sandberg, A. L., Oliveira, B., Osler, A. G.: Two complement interaction sites in guinea pig immunoglobulins. J. Immunol. **106**, 282—285 (1971)
Schiffmann, E., Corcoran, B. A., Wahl, S. A.: N-formyl methionyl peptides as chemoattractants for leucocytes. Proc. Nat. Acad. Sci. (Wash.) **72**, 1059—1062 (1975a)
Schiffmann, E., Showell, H. V., Corcoran, B. A., Ward, P. A., Smith, E., Becker, E. L.: The isolation and partial characterization of neutrophil chemotactic factors from Escherichia coli. J. Immunol. **114**, 1831—1837 (1975b)
Senda, N., Tamura, H., Shibata, N., Yoshitake, J., Kondo, K., Tanaka, K.: The mechanism of the movement of leucocytes. Exp. Cell Res. **91**, 393—407 (1975)
Showell, H. J., Becker, E. L.: The effects of external K^+ and Na^+ on the chemotaxis of rabbit peritoneal neutrophils. J. Immunol. **116**, 99—105 (1976)
Showell, H. J., Freer, R. J., Zigmond, S. H., Schiffmann, E., Aswanikumar, S., Corcoran, B., Becker, E. L.: The structure-activity relations of synthetic peptides as chemotactic factors and inducers of lysosomal enzyme secretion for neutrophils. J. exp. Med. **143**, 1154—1169 (1976)
Snyderman, R., Altman, L. C., Hausman, M. S., Mergenhagen, S. E.: Human mononuclear leukocyte chemotaxis: a quantitative assay for humoral and cellular chemotactic factors. J. Immunol. **108**, 857—860 (1972a)
Snyderman, R., Phillips, J., Mergenhagen, S. E.: Polymorphonuclear leukocyte chemotactic activity in rabbit serum and guinea pig serum treated with immune complexes. Evidence for C5a as the major chemotactic factor. Infect. Immun. **1**, 521—525 (1970)
Snyderman, R., Phillips, J. K., Mergenhagen, S. E.: Biological activity of complement in vivo. Role of C5 in the accumulation of polymorphonuclear leukocytes in inflammatory exudates. J. exp. Med. **134**, 1131—1143 (1971a)
Snyderman, R., Shin, H. S., Hausman, M. S.: A chemotactic factor for mononuclear leukocytes. Proc. Soc. exp. Biol. (N.Y.) **138**, 387—390 (1971b)
Snyderman, R., Shin, H. S., Phillips, J. K., Gewurz, H., Mergenhagen, S. E.: A neutrophil chemotactic factor derived from C'5 upon interaction of guinea-pig serum with endotoxin. J. Immunol. **103**, 413—422 (1969)
Snyderman, R., Wohlenberg, C., Notkins, A. L.: Inflammation and viral infection: chemotactic activity resulting from the interaction of antiviral antibody and complement with cells infected with herpes simplex virus. J. infect Dis. **126**, 207—209 (1972b)
Sorkin, E. (Ed.): Chemotaxis: its biology and biochemistry. Basel: Karger 1974
Spitznagel, J. K., Chi, H. Y.: Cationic proteins and antibacterial properties of infected tissues and leukocytes. Amer. J. Path. **43**, 697—711 (1963)
Stecher, V. J., Sorkin, E., Ryan, G. B.: Relation between blood coagulation and chemotaxis of leucocytes. Nature (New Biol.) **233**, 95—96 (1971)
Stossel, T. P., Hartwig, J. H.: Interactions between actin, myosin and an actin-binding protein from rabbit alveolar macrophages. J. biol. Chem. **250**, 5706—5712 (1975)
Stossel, T., Pollard, T. D.: Myosin in polymorphonuclear leukocytes. J. biol. Chem. **248**, 8288—8294 (1973)
Tainer, J. A., Turner, S. R., Lynn, W. S.: New aspects of chemotaxis. Specific target-cell attraction by lipid and lipoprotein fractions of Escherichia coli chemotactic factor. Amer. J. Path. **81**, 401—410 (1975)
Tatsumi, N., Shibata, N., Okamura, Y., Takeuchi, K., Senda, N.: Actin and myosin from leucocytes. Biochim. biophys. Acta **305**, 433—444 (1973)
Thompson, P. L., Papadimitriou, J. M., Walters, M. N-I.: Suppression of leucocytic sticking and emigration by chelation of calcium. J. Path. Bact. **94**, 389—396 (1967)
Thrasher, S. G., Yoshida, T., Van Oss, C. J., Cohen, S., Rose, N. R.: Alteration of macrophage interfacial tension by supernatants of antigen-activated lymphocyte cultures. J. Immunol. **110**, 321—326 (1973)
Trinkaus, J. P.: Cells Into Organs. Englewood Cliffs N.J.: Prentice-Hall 1969
Tsan, M. F., Berlin, R. D.: Effect of phagocytosis on membrane transport of non-electrolytes. J. exp. Med. **134**, 1016—1035 (1971)

Tse,R.L., Phelps,P., Urban,D.: Polymorphonuclear leukocyte motility in vitro. VI. Effect of purine and pyrimidine analogues. Possible role of cyclic AMP. J. Lab. clin. Med. **80**, 264—274 (1972)

Turner,S.R., Campbell,J.A., Lynn,W.S.: Polymorphonuclear leukocyte chemotaxis toward oxidized lipid components of cell membranes. J. exp. Med. **141**, 1437—1441 (1975a)

Turner,S.R., Tainer,J.A., Lynn,W.S.: Biogenesis of chemotactic molecules by the arachidonate lipoxygenase system of platelets. Nature (Lond.) **257**, 680—681 (1975b)

Ukena,T.E., Berlin,R.D.: Effect of colchicine and vinblastine on the topographical separation of membrane functions. J. exp. Med. **136**, 1—7 (1972)

Van Oss,C.J., Gillman,C.F.: Phagocytosis as a surface phenomenon. I. Contact angles and phagocytosis of non-opsonized bacteria. J. reticuloendoth. Soc. **12**, 283—292 (1972a)

Van Oss,C.J., Gillman,C.F.: Phagocytosis as a surface phenomenon. II. Contact angles and phagocytosis of encapsulated bacteria before and after opsonization by specific antibody and complement. J. reticuloendoth. Soc. **12**, 497—502 (1972b)

Waddell,A.W., Robson,R.T., Edwards,J.G.: Colchicine and vinblastine inhibit fibroblast aggregation. Nature (Lond.) **248**, 239—241 (1974)

Wahl,S.M., Iverson,G.M., Oppenheim,J.J.: Induction of guinea pig B-cell lymphokine synthesis by mitogenic and non-mitogenic signals to Fc, Ig, and C3 receptors. J. exp. Med. **140**, 1631—1645 (1974)

Ward,P.A.: The chemosuppression of chemotaxis. J. exp. Med. **124**, 209—226 (1966)

Ward,P.A., Becker,E.L.: The deactivation of rabbit neutrophils by chemotactic factor and the nature of the activatable esterase. J. exp. Med. **127**, 693—709 (1968)

Ward,P.A., Cohen,S., Flanagan,T.D.: Leukotactic factors elaborated by virus-infected tissues. J. exp. Med. **135**, 1095—1103 (1972)

Ward,P.A., Lepow,I.H., Newman,L.J.: Bacterial factors chemotactic for polymorphonuclear leukocytes. Amer. J. Path. **52**, 725—736 (1968)

Ward,P.A., Remold,H.G., David,J.R.: Leukotactic factor produced by sensitized lymphocytes. Science **163**, 1079—1081 (1969)

Ward,P.A., Remold,H.G., David,J.R.: The production by antigen-stimulated lymphocytes of a leukotactic factor distinct from migration inhibitory factor. Cell. Immunol. **1**, 162—174 (1970)

Weiss,L.: Studies on cellular adhesion in tissue culture. XII. Some effects of cytochalasins and colchicine. Exp. Cell Res. **74**, 21—26 (1972)

Wilkinson,P.C.: Characterization of the chemotactic activity of casein for neutrophil leucocytes and macrophages. Experientia (Basel) **28**, 1051—1052 (1972)

Wilkinson,P.C.: Recognition of protein structure in leukocyte chemotaxis. Nature (Lond.) **244**, 512—513 (1973)

Wilkinson,P.C.: Surface and cell membrane activities of leukocyte chemotactic factors. Nature (Lond.) **251**, 58—60 (1974a)

Wilkinson,P.C.: Recognition in leucocyte chemotaxis: some observations on the nature of chemotactic proteins. In: Veld,G.P., Willoughby,D.A., Giroud,J.P. (Eds.): Future Trends in Inflammation, pp. 125—134. Padua: Piccin 1974b

Wilkinson,P.C.: Chemotaxis and Inflammation. Edinburgh: Churchill-Livingstone 1974c

Wilkinson,P.C.: Inhibition of leukocyte locomotion and chemotaxis by lipid-specific bacterial toxins. Nature (Lond.) **255**, 485—487 (1975a)

Wilkinson,P.C.: Leucocyte locomotion and chemotaxis. The influence of divalent cations and cation ionophores. Exp. Cell Res. **93**, 420—426 (1975b)

Wilkinson,P.C.: Chemotaxis of leucocytes. In: Carlile,M.J. (Ed.): Primitive Sensory and Communication Systems. The Taxes and Tropisms of Microorganisms and Cells, pp. 205—243. New York: Academic Press 1975c

Wilkinson,P.C.: Cellular and molecular aspects of chemotaxis of macrophages and monocytes. In: Nelson,D.S. (Ed.): Immunobiology of the Macrophages, pp. 349—365. New York: Academic Press 1976

Wilkinson,P.C.: A requirement for albumin as carrier for low-molecular weight leucocyte chemotactic factors. Exp. Cell Res. **103**, 415—418 (1976)

Wilkinson,P.C., McKay,I.C.: The chemotactic activity of native and denatured serum albumin. Int. Arch. Allergy **41**, 237—247 (1971)

Wilkinson, P.C., McKay, I.C.: The molecular requirements for chemotactic attraction of leucocytes by proteins. Studies of proteins with synthetic side groups. Europ. J. Immunol. **2**, 570—577 (1972)
Wilkinson, P.C., McKay, I.C.: Recognition in leucocyte chemotaxis. Studies with structurally modified proteins. Antibiot. Chemother. **19**, 421—441 (1974)
Wilkinson, P.C., O'Neill, G.J., McInroy, R.J., Cater, J.C., Roberts, J.A.: Chemotaxis of macrophages: the role of a macrophage specific cytotaxin from anaerobic corynebacteria and its relation to immunopotentiation in vivo. In: Wolstenholme, G.E.W., Knight, J. (Eds.): Immunopotentiation. Ciba Foundation Symposium 18, pp. 121—135. Amsterdam: ASP 1973a
Wilkinson, P.C., Roberts, J.A., Russell, R.J., McLoughlin, M.: Chemotaxis of mitogen-activated human lymphocytes and the effects of membrane-active enzymes. Clin. exp. Immunol. **25**, 280—287 (1976)
Wilkinson, P.C., O'Neill, G.J., Wapshaw, K.G.: Role of anaerobic coryneforms in specific and non-specific immunological reactions. II. Production of a chemotactic factor specific for macrophages. Immunology **24**, 997—1006 (1973b)
Wissler, J.H., Stecher, V.J., Sorkin, E.: Biochemistry and biology of a leucotactic binary peptide system related to anaphylatoxin. Int. Arch. Allergy **42**, 722—747 (1972)
Wissler, J.H., Stecher, V.J., Sorkin, E.: Cyclic AMP and chemotaxis of leukocytes. In: Braun, W., Lichtenstein, L.M., Parker, C.W. (Eds.): Cyclic AMP, Cell Growth and the Immune Response, pp. 270—283. Berlin-Heidelberg-New York: Springer 1974
Woodin, A.M.: Staphylococcal leucocidin. In: Cohen, J.O. (Ed.): The Staphylococci, pp. 281—299. New York: Wiley 1972
Woodin, A.M., Wieneke, A.A.: Action of DFP on the leucocyte and the axon. Nature (Lond.) **227**, 460—463 (1970a)
Woodin, A.M., Wieneke, A.A.: Leukocidin: tetraethylammonium ions and the membrane acyl phosphatases in relation to the leukocyte potassium pump. J. gen. Physiol. **56**, 16—32 (1970b)
Woodruff, J., Gesner, B.M.: Lymphocytes: circulation altered by trypsin. Science **161**, 176—178 (1968)
Zigmond, S.H.: Mechanisms of sensing chemical gradients by polymorphonuclear leukocytes. Nature (Lond.) **249**, 450—452 (1974)
Zigmond, S.H., Hirsch, J.G.: Effects of cytochalasin B on polymorphonuclear leucocyte locomotion, phagocytosis and glycolysis. Exp. Cell Res. **73**, 383—393 (1972)
Zigmond, S.H., Hirsch, J.G.: Leukocyte locomotion and chemotaxis. New methods for evaluation and demonstration of cell-derived chemotactic factor. J. exp. Med. **137**, 387—410 (1973)

Addendum

Since this review was completed, a considerable volume of new and interesting work has appeared. Readers are referred to a multiauthor text "Leukocyte Chemotaxis; Methodology, Physiology, Clinical Implications," ed. Gallin, J.I. and Quie, P.G., Raven, New York 1978, for many studies it was not possible to include here. A proposal by an international group of workers for a nomenclature to be used for locomotor reactions in leucocytes and other cells, based on the distinction between *chemokinesis* and *chemotaxis*, mentioned earlier in this review, has appeared (Keller et al., Clin. Exp. Immunol. **27**, 377—380, 1977). The importance of this distinction is emphasized by the fact that serum albumin behaves as a chemokinetic medium for all types of leucocyte since it enhances their rate of locomotion without influencing its direction. Chemokinesis appears to play a major role in the locomotor reactions of lymphocytes, judged by the locomotor responses of primed lymphocytes to antigen. Wilkinson, Parrott, Russell and Sless (J. Exp. Med. **145**, 1158—1168 1977) suggest that antigen mediates both chemokinetic and chemotactic reactions in antigen-primed lymphocytes. The eosinophil chemotactic factors of anaphylaxis have been identified as tetrapeptides, Val-Gly-Ser-Glu and Ala-Gly-Ser-Glu (GOETZL and AUSTEN, Proc. nat. Acad. Sci. U.S. **72**, 4123, 1975). Formyl methionyl tripeptides are not only chemotactic for leucocytes at very low doses but induce degranulation and enzyme release at similar doses (SHOWELL et al., op. cit. 1976). Some interesting work on inhibitors which bind to the cell surface and prevent responses to chemotactic factors is appearing. For example, polymeric IgA binds to neutrophils to act in this way (VAN EPPS and WILLIAMS. J. Exp. Med. **144**, 1227—1242, 1976).

CHAPTER 5

Platelet Aggregation Mechanisms and Their Implications in Haemostasis and Inflammatory Disease

A. L. WILLIS

A. Introduction

The platelet is arguably the most widely studied of all human cells. It has lent itself well to biochemical investigations, because it is so readily available and can be isolated free from other cell types. Biochemical studies of the platelet have taught us a great deal about amine uptake, storage, and release, lysosomal enzymes, contractile proteins, and the biological significance of cyclic nucleotides. Furthermore, study of the factors involved in platelet adhesion promises to teach us a great deal about the events involved in cell-to-cell and cell-to-substrate contact.

The recent work on platelet prostaglandins (PGs), endoperoxides and arachidonate lipoxygenase, has also given us new insight into mechanisms and means of treatment for haemostatic defects, arterial thrombosis and inflammatory diseases.

It has not been possible to deal here in detail with all of these topics. However, I have described mechanisms and biochemical mediators of platelet aggregation with particular emphasis on the prostaglandin area.

The implications of such mechanisms in thrombosis are beyond the scope of this chapter. Instead I have attempted to analyse their role in the related processes of haemostasis and inflammation.

B. Relationship of Morphology to Physiological Function in the Blood Platelet

In all animals except the most primitive, aggregation of free single cells is utilised for the rapid blocking of wounds which would otherwise allow fatal loss of essential body fluids. In man and other mammals, platelets ("thrombocytes") are the cells that circulate in the blood, adhere to damaged vessel constituents and aggregate to produce haemostatic plugs.

Platelets are different from other mammalian cells in that they are anucleated and derived by fragmentation of the cytoplasm of single large polyploid cells (megakaryocytes) located in the bone marrow. Each megakaryocyte can produce 3000–4000 platelets by coalescence of the cytoplasmic membranes following invagination of the cell surface (BEHNKE, 1970; BORN, 1972). The usual platelet count in man is in the range of 200000–400000 cells per cubic millimetre of blood. In other species it may be different (nearly 1000000 cells/mm^3 in the rat). Life span of the human platelet in the circulation is usually 7–10 days (WEISS, 1975b; VAINER, 1972).

Platelets recently liberated from the bone marrow ("young platelets") are larger, have a higher specific gravity and may be more efficient in haemostatic function compared with "old platelets" that have remained in the circulation for several days. Young and old populations of platelets can be separated from each other by sucrose gradient centrifugation (VAINER, 1972). Overall, the average diameter of a human platelet is about 2 μM (WEISS, 1975b).

Uniquely characteristic biological properties of the platelet include *adherence* to various constituents of blood vessel walls, perivascular tissue or to artificial surfaces; only the blood vessel endothelium appears to be completely inert to platelets. Platelets can, of course also adhere to each other by the process of "*aggregation*." This can be produced in response to pro-aggregatory substances released from platelet granules during the "platelet *release reaction*," or to aggregation-stimulating substances present in the plasma and released from cells other than the platelet (e.g. adrenaline or bacterial endotoxin). These concepts are dealt with in some detail by MUSTARD and PACKHAM (1970) and in Section C of this chapter.

How is the morphology of platelets suited to performance of the above functions? Basic morphological features of the human blood platelet are outlined in Figure 1A and they are as follows:

I. The Amorphous Coat

The amorphous coat (about 20 nm/thick) that covers the platelet surface is undoubtedly of considerable importance, since it contains substances considered necessary for platelet aggregation and blood coagulation (see MUSTARD and PACKHAM, 1970; WEISS, 1975b). This coat consists partly of protein and partly of sulphated mucopolysaccharide (WHITE and KRIVIT, 1967; HOVIG, 1974). Present in this periplatelet atmosphere are coagulation factors I (fibrinogen), V and XI (HOROWITZ and FUJIMOTO, 1965; NACHMAN, 1968). Other coagulation factors (II, VII, VIII, IX, X, and XII) have also been detected but are to a varying degree washed from the platelets by platelet isolation procedures (BOUNAMEAUX, 1957; HOROWITZ and FUJIMOTO, 1965; NACHMAN, 1968; KARPATKIN and KARPATKIN, 1969; JENKINS et al., 1976).

In addition, "platelet factor 3" (PF3) consisting of lipoprotein or phospholipid is made available at the platelet surface when platelets are stimulated to aggregate in response to adenosine diphosphate (ADP) or other agents (CASTALDI et al., 1965; MARCUS, 1966; HARDISTY and HUTTON, 1966; MUSTARD et al., 1967).

II. The Trilaminar Plasma Membrane

Like other plasma membranes, the platelet membrane consists of a phospholipid bilayer with various integral and peripheral proteins.

An actomyosin-like contractile protein ("thrombasthenin") is apparently present near the platelet surface (BOOYSE and RAFELSON, 1971; NACHMAN and FERRIS, 1972) and other sulphydryl-containing proteins (NACHMAN and FERRIS, 1972; STEINER, 1974). One of these proteins may be associated with Na^+/K^+-activated ATPase which is sensitive to modification by E-type PGs (JOHNSON and RAMWELL, 1973). This may account for the modulatory effects of E-type PGs on platelet aggregation and its blockade by sulphydryl-blocking agents (JOHNSON et al., 1974). Adenylate cyclase (BRODIE et al., 1972) which regulates platelet cAMP levels and consequently aggregability of the platelets (SALZMAN, 1972), is also associated with the platelet membrane as are various glycosyl transferases (BOSMANN, 1971); these may be involved in the interaction of platelets with collagen.

III. The Surface-Connecting ("Open Channel" or "Cannicular") System

This is a sponge-like system of channels which open through the platelet membrane probably accounting for the appearance of "vacuoles" in most sections of platelets (BEHNKE, 1970).

The surface-connecting system enormously increases the surface area of the platelet and would therefore serve to amplify uptake of plasma-born substances into the platelet or the discharge of substances from the platelet during the release reaction (WEISS, 1975b). Platelets phygocytose particles such as polystyrene particles or antigen/antibody complexes (see MUSTARD and PACKHAM, 1968, 1970). Such uptake of particles may involve the surface-connecting system (BEHNKE, 1970; WHITE, 1968).

IV. The Dense-Tubular System

This runs close to canals of the surface-connecting system. Like the sarcoplasmic reticulum of skeletal muscle it may be involved in transport of calcium ions (WHITE, 1972a) and membranes of the dense tubular system appear to be a site where arachidonate is converted to PG endoperoxides (GERRARD et al., 1976).

V. Microtubules

Platelets contain microtubules which are similar to those described in other cells. The microtubules are apparently hollow tubes, consisting of protofilaments of about 3–5 nm diameter. These disappear when platelets are cooled (MUSTARD and PACKHAM, 1970) or exposed to colchicine (WHITE, 1971; HOLMSEN, 1972). Platelets also contain a protein ("tubulin") which binds colchicine (PUSZKIN et al., 1971) or colcemid (UKENA and BERLIN, 1972) and may thus be the protein component of the microtubules. The role of platelet microtubules is probably to maintain the discoid shape of the "resting" platelet since the tubule bundles are located circumferentially just under the platelet surface (BEHNKE, 1965) and could thus be capable of acting as an endoskeleton. The discoid shape of the platelet is otherwise thermodynamically improbable (WEISS, 1975b).

The microtubules may be involved in the shape change of platelets that precedes aggregation (Section C). Microtubules appear also to be involved in the "spreading" of platelets on non-endothelial surfaces (BOYLE-KAY and FUDENBERG, 1973).

VI. Microfilaments

These are present in the pseudopodia which appear during the shape change phenomenon (ZUCKER-FRANKLIN and BLOOMBERG, 1969; WESSELLS et al., 1971). Treatment of platelets with cytocholasin B, a drug that disrupts microfilaments (ZUCKER-FRANKLIN and BLOOMBERG, 1969) shows that formation of elongated pseudopodia, spreading, and aggregation are all inhibited. Such results indicate that microfilaments are important in these processes (BOYLE-KAY and FUDENBERG, 1973).

VII. Granules

These are of two main types. The most common "α-granules" are similar to lysosomes in that they contain cathepsins and acid hydrolases (GORDON, 1975; DAY et al., 1969). Other important platelet granules are electron dense and consequently called "dense bodies". Dense bodies contain calcium, 5-hydroxytryptamine (5-HT), adenosine triphosphate (ATP), and ADP, probably complexed as high molecular weight aggregates (DAVIS and WHITE, 1968; HOLMSEN et al., 1969a, 1969b; PLETSCHER et al., 1971; SKAER et al., 1974). The 5-HT probably is not synthesised in the platelet but is taken up from the plasma. Platelets can actively take up 5-HT from plasma into dense granules against a concentration gradient of 1000:1 (BORN and GILLSON, 1959) although uptake is lacking in platelets that have been degranulated by exposure to thrombin (REIMERS et al., 1975a). The uptake and metabolism of 5-HT by platelets has been extensively studied by PLETSCHER and others (PLETSCHER et al., 1966a, 1966b, 1967; PLETSCHER, 1968).

The ADP stored in the dense granules is of obvious importance because ADP induces platelet aggregation and accounts for about 60% of the total platelet ADP content. However, this "storage pool" of adenine nucleotides does not participate (at least to any significant extent) in processes involving the "metabolic pool" of ADP and ATP utilised in energy producing reactions. Hence, radio-labelled adenine or adenosine are incorporated only very slowly into dense granules, although the metabolic pool is rapidly filled with labelled adenine nucleotides (DA PRADA and PLETSCHER, 1970; HOLMSEN, 1972; HOLMSEN et al., 1969a, 1969b; REIMERS et al., 1975b, 1975c) and they probably play their usual role as sources of stored energy.

The α-granules and dense bodies are involved in the platelet release reaction and the accompanying aggregation response. It is also possible that enzymes and amines from both types of granule participate in inflammatory reactions (see Section E). Enzymes from the α-granules are released when platelets are exposed to thrombin or to "high" (supra-aggregatory) concentrations of collagen ("release II" of DAY and HOLMSEN, 1971).

In both cases, when release II is produced, aspirin-type drugs are not able to block either the release of granular contents or the accompanying aggregation response (although there may be some reduction in release of dense body contents) (ZUCKER and PETERSON, 1970; WEISS, 1975b). This implies involvement of a non-PG mechanism (WILLIS et al., 1974a; WEISS, 1975b).

In contrast, when only contents of the dense bodies are released ("release I" of DAY and HOLMSEN, 1971), as during the "second phase" aggregation response to ADP or adrenaline, then both the release reaction and the accompanying aggregation component can be completely suppressed by aspirin-type drugs (WEISS et al., 1968; ZUCKER and PETERSON, 1968, 1970; O'BRIEN, 1968; EVANS et al., 1968) or TYA[1], another inhibitor of arachidonate oxygenation (WILLIS et al., 1974b). This aspect of platelet aggregation will be discussed further in later sections.

[1] TYA [5,8,11,14-eicosatetraynoic acid;] an acetylenic analogue of arachidonate that blocks arachidonate utilisation by PG synthetase (AHERN and DOWNING, 1970;) or lipoxygenases (DOWNING, 1972; HAMBERG and SAMUELSSON, 1974).

VIII. Organelles Concerned With Carbohydrate, Protein and Lipid Metabolism

Although present in small numbers (1–6 per section, as observed by electron microscopy) and poorly developed morphologically, the mitochondria of the platelet seem to be important in the generation of metabolic energy. Thus, most platelet functions, including aggregation and clot retraction, are completely inhibited when both the glycolytic and oxidative phosphorylation pathways are blocked (MUSTARD and PACKHAM, 1970; WEISS, 1975b).

Protein synthesis has been demonstrated in platelets and a small amount of RNA is present, although there are no nuclei and no DNA. Ribosomes have been seen only rarely (BOOYSE and RAFELSON, 1971; TS'AO, 1971) although there is difficulty in distinguishing histologically between ribosomes and the glycogen granules (MUSTARD and PACKHAM, 1970).

Platelets are able to synthesise phospholipids from glycerol (MAJERUS et al., 1971; DEYKIN and DESSER, 1968), and can synthesise fatty acids de novo or by chain elongation and desaturation of linoleate (MAJERUS et al., 1971; MARCUS, 1972). Platelet lipid metabolism is important as a substrate source (arachidonate of membrane phospholipids) for the prostaglandin endoperoxides (see "Section C.VI.3").

C. Mechanisms of Platelet Aggregation (see Fig. 1B)

When platelets adhere to vascular subendothelium or foreign surfaces, they spread out on the surface and release their granular contents. This induces other platelets to adhere to those already attached to the surface (aggregation). When aggregation is induced directly by a soluble aggregating agent, then a prior shape change is seen which may be related to the spreading phenomenon.

I. Adhesion and Spreading

A unique property of platelets is the ease with which they adhere to any particle or surface, with the sole exception of normal undamaged vascular endothelium. This unique property of vascular endothelium may be partly due to its ability to generate PGI_2 ("prostacyclin"; PGX) from the arachidonate-derived endoperoxides. PGI_2 is a short-lived, but extremely potent inhibitor of platelet adhesion and aggregation, which also has vasodilator properties (GRYGLEWSKI et al., 1976; JOHNSON et al., 1976). There are obviously varying degrees of thrombogenicity for different surfaces. Vascular *sub*endothelium is probably the most thrombogenic natural substance and studies by BAUMGARTNER and associates have shown that fibrillar collagen in the subendothelium is probably the most important stimulus to adherence (and subsequent aggregation) of the platelets. Possibly platelet glucosyl transferases are involved in this reaction with collagen (see BAUMGARTNER, 1974b; WEISS, 1975b). One of the most sticky artifical surfaces upon which platelets adhere is non-siliconised glass, while teflon (now used in many prosthetic devices such as artifical heart valves) is probably the least thrombogenic. Early materials used in such prosthetic devices and the membranes of artifical kidney machines are, however, sufficiently thrombogenic to platelets to pose a problem in their use and have, incidentally, provided a test

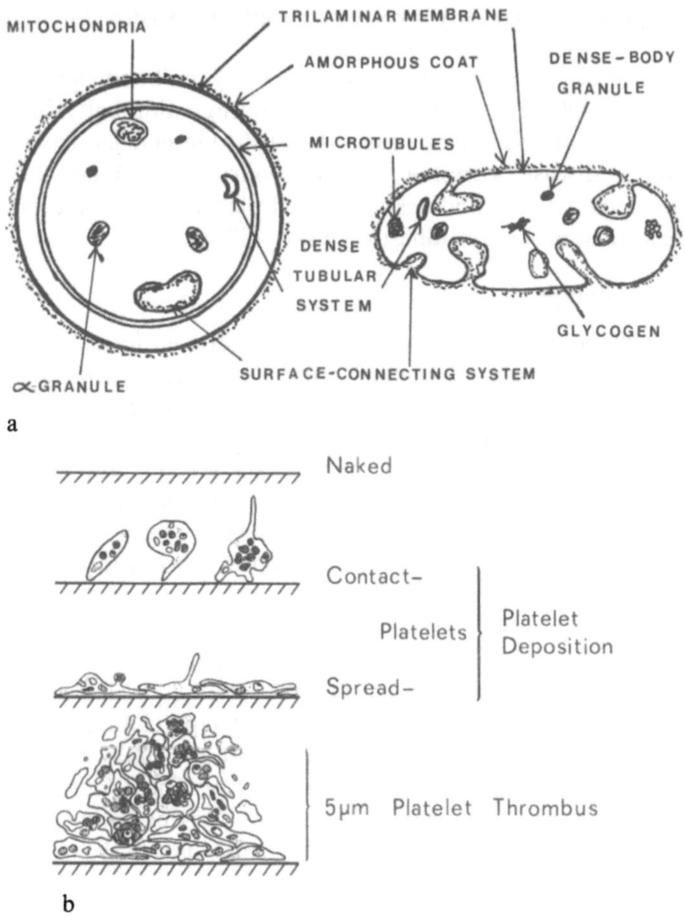

Fig. 1a and b. (a) Diagrammatic representation of main morphological features in the "resting" human platelet. Modified from WEISS (1975b). (b) Diagrammatic representation of the events occurring when platelets in flowing blood come into contact with naked vascular subendothelium. From electron microscopic studies using the perfusion chamber method. From BAUMGARTNER et al. (1976). Reprinted by permission

bed for the experimental evaluation of anti-thrombotic drugs in man (McNICOL et al., 1976).

When platelets come into contact with thrombogenic surfaces under the right rheological conditions (BAUMGARTNER, 1974a, 1974b; BAUMGARTNER et al., 1976), they first form elongated pseudopodia which adhere to the substrate. After adhesion, the pseudopodia thicken as cytoplasm flows into them and so this process continues until the spaces between the pseudopodia are obliterated and the platelet appears as a central elevation surrounded by a skirt of membrane. This latter process is called spreading (BORN, 1970, 1972; BARNARDT et al., 1972). Studies with inhibitors of microtubule function (colcemid) and microfilament formation (cytochalasin B) have confirmed that integrity of microtubules is necessary for the resting discoid shape of the platelets and is thus functionally involved in the formation of pseudopodia, while the spreading process apparently involves microfilaments (BOYLE-KAY and FUDENBERG, 1973).

The processes of adhesion and spreading are not inhibited significantly by normal concentrations of the usual anti-aggregatory drugs, although adhesion of platelets to vascular subendothelium or glass is diminished in platelets from patients with Von Willebrand's disease or Bernard Soulier syndrome (see WEISS, 1975b and Section D of this chapter); such findings imply that plasma factors and platelet surface glyco-proteins are important in adhesion (WEISS, 1975b).

II. The Shape Change

The change in shape of platelets, from the normal discoid form to that with spiky pseudopodia and small blebs, is similar to the events seen when platelets begin to adhere to thrombogenic surfaces; some common mechanisms may be involved. This similarity is exemplified by the shape change of platelets during adhesion of platelets to collagen, present in the form of a microfibrilar suspension, rather than as part of a surface. The shape change produced can readily be detected on the light transmission tracing of an "aggregometer;" it appears to be obligatory to the subsequent aggregation of platelets, at least in so far as "physiological" aggregation stimuli are concerned[2].

The shape change can also occur without subsequent platelet aggregation. Thus when platelets are pre-incubated with the calcium chelator, ethylene diamine tetra acetic acid (EDTA), or with low concentrations of PGE_1, the shape change response to ADP occurs without subsequent aggregation. Shape change in the absence of aggregation is also seen with platelets from patients with thrombasthenia, a congenital haemostatic defect (WEISS, 1975b; MILLS, 1973, 1974). These findings indicate that (unlike aggregation) the shape change of platelets does not require plasma Ca^{++} and does not principally involve cAMP mechanisms (since PGE_1 stimulates platelet adenylate cyclase).

However, with prolonged exposure of platelets to high concentrations of EDTA (which chelates cell-bound Ca^{++} in addition to plasma Ca^{++}), the shape change is reduced (BORN, 1974). Similarly, high concentrations of PGE_1 can reduce the shape change (see MUSTARD and PACKHAM, 1975) as well as adhesion (TSCHOPP, personal communication). The shape change induced by ADP or 5-HT (but not adrenaline) may be causally related to the rapid fall in "energy change" observed (MILLS, 1973, 1974; see Section C.VI.2.a of this chapter).

The shape change phenomenon has sometimes been termed "platelet swelling". However, scanning electron microscopy shows that there is probably no change in net platelet volume. Furthermore, although the packed cell volume of platelets may increase, this is attributable to an increase in the volume of plasma trapped in the spaces between them (see BORN, 1972, 1974).

III. Aggregation

The aggregation response of platelets induced by "physiological" aggregating agents (ADP, collagen, etc.) has an absolute requirement for two co-factors, viz calcium and

[2] The question of whether or not platelets change shape in response to adrenaline is discussed later (Section C.VI.2.c).

fibrinogen[3] (see MUSTARD and PACKHAM, 1970; BORN, 1974; WEISS, 1975b). Sialic acid attached to fibrinogen may be essential for its aggregation co-factor activity. Platelet aggregation could thus depend on the formation of calcium bridges between sialic acid residues of fibrinogen and the same or other acid groups on the platelet surface (AHTEE and MICHAL, 1972). Since these co-factors are always present in normal circulating blood, the question arises, "Why do platelets not always spontaneously aggregate?" An explanation that has been put forward is that the platelets also have to become activated in some way to make them "sticky."

This activation of the platelets by aggregating agents could involve the platelet shape change. Normally there is a strong mutual repulsion between resting platelets because of the negative surface charge, resulting from the excess of anionic over cationic groups in the surface layer of platelets. Sialic acid residues apparently account for most of this electronegativity (BORN, 1974). However, the platelet shape change means that the long, thin pseudopodia can adhere together and overcome the normally strong mutual repulsion of the platelets, allowing them to become "zippered" together into loose aggregates (BOYLE-KAY and FUDENBERG, 1973; BORN, 1974). Such events may take place during the "first phase" of aggregation induced by ADP, explaining why disaggregation takes place so readily.

Given appropriate conditions, the platelet aggregates become consolidated and fuse into a few large masses in which individual platelets can only be distinguished from each other by thin section electron microscopy (BORN, 1972, 1974). This process, once termed "viscous metamorphosis" is, under normal conditions, irreversible[4], and is causally related to the release of pro-aggregatory substances from the platelets themselves. This latter process has been termed the "platelet release reaction" (GRETTE, 1962).

IV. The Platelet Release Reaction

This occurs simultaneously with and is apparently obligatory for the irreversible-type of platelet aggregation described above, and is thus seen during aggregation induced by collagen or during "second phase" aggregation produced by ADP or adrenaline (see Section C.VI.1). Substances released from the platelet during the platelet release reaction come either from dense granules (ADP, Ca^{++}, 5-HT), or from α-granules (lysosomal enzymes) (see Section B). The release of the contents of dense granules has been termed release I and those of α-granules as release II (DAY and HOLMSEN, 1971). Among the other substances released from platelets are PGE_2 and $PGF_{2\alpha}$ together with the labile aggregation stimulating substances (LASS) enzymically derived from arachidonate (consisting of endoperoxides and thromboxanes). Unlike the other substances released, these derivatives of arachidonate are synthesised de novo in the platelets immediately prior to release. Their role in

---

[3] Other plasma proteins, including factor XII (Hageman factor), γ-globulins, and possibly factor V, also promote aggregation, (SOLUM, 1966), although aggregation can still take place in their absence (BORN, 1974).

[4] Such "irreversible" aggregation *can* be reversed by agents that increase platelet cAMP, viz PGE_1 (CHANDRA-SEKHAR, 1970) or dihomo-γ-linolenic acid (FARROW and WILLIS, 1975).

inducing release reaction I explains why this process can be largely or completely inhibited by drugs (e.g. aspirin) that inhibit platelet PG synthesis.

Although the 15-hydroxy endoperoxide, PGH_2 (PGR_2) can directly activate the aggregation machinery of the platelet independently of the release reaction (WILLIS et al., 1974a), endoperoxides are clearly implicated in production of release reaction I. Higher concentrations of PGH_2, produce an aggregation response that is partially attributable to the release of dense granule ADP, especially when the platelets are sensitised by prior exposure to PGE_2 (WILLIS et al., 1974a). This finding explains why PGE_2 can enhance the collagen-induced release reaction (WILLIS, unpublished observations).

More recently, MALMSTEN et al. (1975) have shown that aggregation produced by the endoperoxide PGG_2 (15-hydroperoxy PGR_2) is largely mediated through the release of ADP. Although it has been suggested that PGG_2 acts through release of platelet ADP (MALMSTEN et al., 1975), it has also been postulated that it acts through conversion to "thromboxane A_2" (HAMBERG et al., 1975), although the latter substance appears to be able to induce aggregation independent of ADP release. This discrepancy will have to be resolved; perhaps additional substances formed from arachidonate are also involved in the pro-aggregatory effects of arachidonate. Certainly, arachidonate added exogenously produces much of its platelet aggregation response through release of platelet ADP (VARGAFTIG and ZIRINIS, 1973; SILVER et al., 1973).

Release reaction I seen during the "second phase" of aggregation induced by ADP or adrenaline, is probably mediated by a PG endoperoxide mechanism since this process is blocked by aspirin, regardless of the concentrations of ADP or adrenaline used to induce the release reaction (see WILLIS et al., 1974a and Fig. 2). However, release I induced by thrombin or by high concentrations of collagen, is only reduced to a minor extent by aspirin and therefore some unknown mechanism ("X") must be involved, also accounting for the failure of aspirin to inhibit the resulting aggregation response (see later). Release I induced by low concentrations of collagen, however, is almost completely attributable to prostaglandin endoperoxide formation (WILLIS et al., 1974a and Fig. 2).

Release II (of α-granule enzymes) is not extensively activated during normal second phase aggregation as produced by adrenaline or ADP, but is induced by collagen or thrombin (MILLS et al., 1968). The exact mechanisms involved in release II are not known, although the release reaction as a whole shows similarities with glandular secretion, and there is a considerable consumption of energy derived from metabolic pools of ATP (see HOLMSEN, 1972).

The burst in oxygen consumption that occurs during the platelet release reaction (see HOLMSEN et al., 1969b) could, in part, reflect the rapid cyclo-oxygenation of arachidonate that takes place. It has been shown, for instance, that PGH_2 production from arachidonate by sheep vesicular gland microsomes occurs during a period when oxygen uptake is near maximal and that endoperoxide (PGH_2) is not synthesised under anaerobic conditions (HAMBERG and SAMUELSSON, 1973; WILLIS, 1974b). Of course, in such experiments, both oxygen uptake and PGH_2 production is suppressed by aspirin and one might therefore expect that aspirin would reduce the "oxygen burst" during the platelet release reaction in platelets. Unfortunately, this crucial experiment does not seem to have been done.

V. An Outline of Methods for Studying Platelet Aggregation and Related Processes

Over the years several methods have been devised which provide some quantitative measure of platelet adhesiveness and/or aggregation. The earlier methods, measured adhesion of platelets to the sides of a rotating glass bulb (WRIGHT, 1942) or their retention from platelet rich plasma (PRP) or blood on glass bead columns; no anti-coagulant is required if the blood is drawn over the glass beads directly from a vein (HELLEM, 1960; SALZMAN, 1963).

An interesting method devised by BREDDIN (BREDDIN et al., 1974) measures "spontaneous" platelet aggregation (determined histologically or photometrically) in citrated PRP rotated in a siliconised glass bulb at 37° C. The aggregation is apparently initiated through activation of some endogenous factor (thrombin, perhaps). This test has the advantage of not only measuring "aggregability" of the platelets, but also the propensity of the plasma to generate pro-aggregatory activity. A more common method that may involve similar mechanisms is the rotating plastic loop method of CHANDLER (1958). It has been used with anti-coagulated PRP, or whole blood. Aggregation (or thrombus formation) can be induced spontaneously or by injection of ADP.

It has recently been realised that studies with PRP cannot take into account the rheological role of erythrocytes in thrombus formation (they act as miniature stirring bars). Such considerations arise from studies with the elegant perfusion chamber technique of BAUMGARTNER in which platelet adhesion, spreading and aggregation ("mural thrombus formation") can be quantified by electron microscopy under various flow conditions, after drug ingestion, in congenital bleeding disorders, etc. This technique has revealed a great deal about the physiology of thrombus formation but, in its present form, it is not suitable as a rapid screening procedure. GORDON (1973) has introduced a method by which platelet aggregation can be routinely measured in small samples of citrated whole blood by determination of the reduction in platelet count following sedimentation of the erythrocytes and aggregates.

Ideally, platelet aggregation should be measured in vivo (i.e. quantification of arterial thrombus formation). However, such methods are time-consuming and difficult to quantify. HORNSTRA and GIELEN (1972) introduced an elegant technique by which formation of intravascular platelet aggregates can be detected by monitoring the pressure gradient across a 20-μm filter interposed in the flow of anti-coagulated blood through an extracorporeal bypass in anaesthetised animals. This technique allows the anti-aggregatory effects of drug administration to be determined in the blood of the animal while it is still alive. A modification of this technique has also been employed in man to demonstrate the anti-aggregatory effects of linoleate administration. A disadvantage of this method is that it does not take platelet adhesiveness into account.

A method with many of the drawbacks discussed above, has nevertheless found a favoured place in platelet research. This method introduced by BORN (1962) and by O'BRIEN (1962) simply gives a measure of platelet aggregation in citrated or heparinised PRP by photometric recording of the light transmission through it. The PRP has to be rapidly stirred (the stirring rate of 1000 rpm is fairly critical) and warmed to 37° C. Aggregation, following addition of ADP, collagen, etc., is indicated by an increase in light transmission and large, irregular excursions on the tracing, give some estimate of the size of the aggregates (Fig. 2). Initially, under resting conditions there are rapid oscillations in the base line as the PRP is stirred, attributable to rotation of the platelets around their horizontal axes. When the platelets undergo the shape change (see Section C.II), then periodic oscillations are no longer produced by the spiky platelets and there is a transient decrease in light transmission (due to an increase in scattered light from the spiky projections). Obviously, the full extent and time curve of the shape change is usually eclipsed by the much greater decrease in turbidity (and increase in light transmission) resulting from the onset of platelet aggregation. Light scattering is best measured by recording the amount of light emerging at 90° to the incident, since interference by changes in light transmission are then minimised. Such a light-scattering attachment has been used on an aggregometer to measure shape change simultaneously with aggregation (MICHAL, 1972).

VI. Mechanisms of Platelet Aggregation (Fig. 2)

1. Semantics—First and Second Phase Aggregation

Some confusion exists concerning the terms first and second phase aggregation. In human citrated PRP, when adrenaline or critical concentrations of ADP are used as stimuli, the aggregation response produced consists of two phases, which represent, respectively, the loose aggregates first formed (as described above), and their subsequent transformation into the fused masses of irreversibly aggregated platelets seen during the platelet release reaction. The first phase of aggregation produced by ADP (Fig. 2) is spontaneously reversible. It is produced by small concentrations of ADP, or any concentration of ADP provided that the platelets have first been exposed to aspirin (which blocks the second phase of aggregation). In contrast, the first phase aggregation response to adrenaline or noradrenaline (exposed by treatment of the platelets by aspirin) is not normally reversible (Fig. 2). This is probably because different mechanisms are involved in aggregation directly produced by these agents.

When the terminology of first and second phase aggregation is restricted to discussion of the response to ADP or adrenaline [5], no confusion can ensue. However, confusion may arise when these terms are used with reference to other aggregating agents particularly when directly induced aggregation is equated with first phase and indirectly induced aggregation with second phase. For instance, PGH_2 is produced during the second phase of aggregation response to adrenaline. In turn, PGH_2 is a mediator of second-phase aggregation, producing much of its effects on platelets by a direct action (which some may regard as first phase). Does PGH_2 produce second-phase or first-phase aggregation? The answer is a paradox. A similar question could arise if one considers ADP which, again, is produced during the release reaction occurring during second phase aggregation, but which produces much of its effects on platelets directly.

Clearly, if the terms first and second phase are to be used unambiguously, they should refer to a biphasic *shape* of the aggregation curve, and should ideally be restricted to discussion of ADP and adrenaline only.

[5] Use of this terminology has been stretched to describe biphasic aggregation patterns seen with agents such as Zymosan (CHRISTIAN and GORDON, 1975).

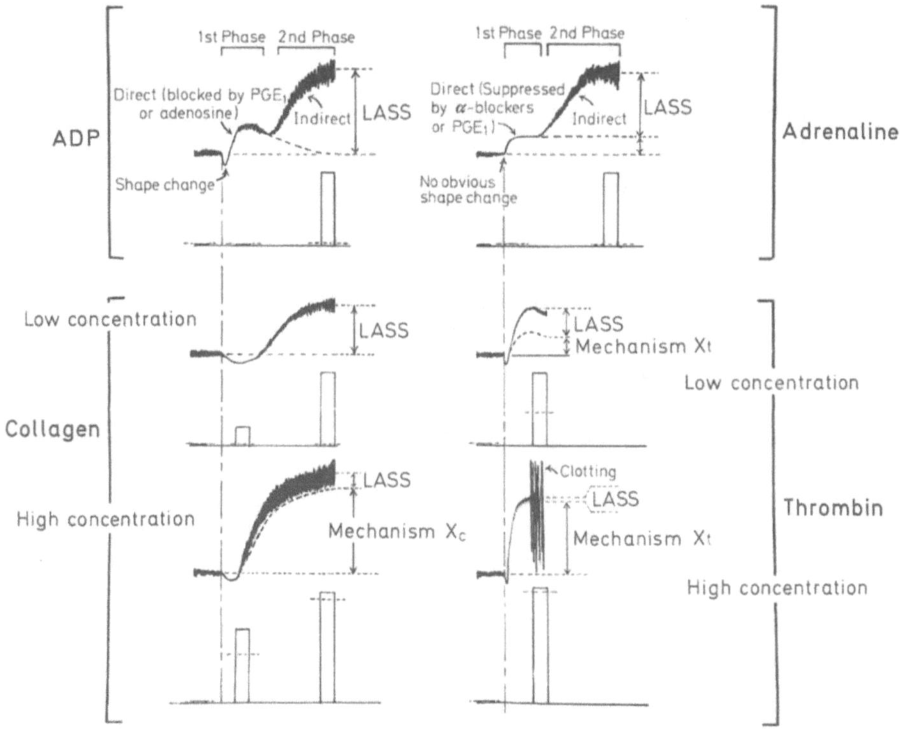

Fig. 2. Platelet aggregation mechanisms. Diagrams represent aggregometer tracings in stirred citrated human PRP at 37° C after addition of various aggregating agents. Histograms represent ADP release from the platelets. Dotted lines on the histogram bars indicate level of ADP release after exposure of platelets to aspirin. Dotted lines on aggregation tracings represent the base line aggregation response in the presence of aspirin. *ADP* produces an initial shape change followed by two phases of aggregation. The first phase is induced directly and is not associated with endogenous ADP release. It is not reduced by aspirin but is blocked by adenosine and other ADP antagonists. The second phase of ADP aggregation is produced indirectly through biosynthesis of endoperoxides and thromboxane A_2 (≡LASS), and is thus abolished by aspirin, exposing the first phase of aggregation which is spontaneously reversible. LASS-mediated aggregation is produced in part through release of platelet stores of ADP and so this too is blocked by aspirin. *Adrenaline* produces no obvious shape change and two distinct phases of aggregation. In this case the first phase is not spontaneously reversible and is blocked by α-adrenoceptor blocking agents. Second phase response is again mediated through synthesis of LASS and release of platelet ADP. *Collagen* produces its effects indirectly through release of pro-aggregatory material from the platelets. Low concentrations of collagen produce effects that are entirely attributable to production of LASS and so are completely blocked by aspirin. With high concentrations of collagen, an additional mechanism (X_c) becomes predominant, so that both aggregation and ADP release are not significantly reduced by aspirin, even though it can be shown (WILLIS and WEISS, 1973) that PG synthesis is blocked. *Thrombin* also produces much of its aggregation response and ADP release through some unknown mechanism (X_t); clotting may also be seen. PGE_1 is capable of completely suppressing aggregation induced by ADP, adrenaline collagen or thrombin

To avoid confusion, I shall generally refer to the ability of various stimuli to produce aggregation by a *direct* effect on the aggregation machinery of platelets or by an *indirect* effect through the release and mediation of active substances from the platelets, rather than use the terms first and second phase aggregation.

2. Mechanisms of Directly Induced Platelet Aggregation

As one might expect, the mechanisms through which different agents activate the platelet aggregation machinery differ somewhat. In some cases a type of receptor (as in smooth muscle) is apparently involved while in other cases enzymic mechanisms have been proposed.

a) ADP

This is undoubtedly one of the most important aggregating agents physiologically. Various theories have been put forward to explain its action on platelets. It has been suggested, for instance, that ADP and Ca^{++} together form a physical bridge between platelets (GAARDER and LALAND, 1964), or that ADP acts by inhibition of an ATPase on the platelet surface (SALZMANN et al., 1966). Alternatively, a nucleoside diphosphate kinase on the platelet surface acts as the receptor for ADP and phosphorylation of ADP by this enzyme stimulates aggregation (GUCCIONE et al., 1971). Another theory has involved the ability of aggregating agents to decrease platelet-cAMP levels. Validity of this theory rests upon the assumption that basal levels of platelet cAMP suppress the tendency of the platelet to change shape and aggregate (perhaps by maintaining the integrity of microtubules). This assumption is an extrapolation of the data suggesting that PGE_1 and the phosphodiesterase inhibitors exert their anti-aggregatory effects (which are synergistic) through increasing platelet levels of cAMP. PGE_1 activates the adenylate cyclase while phosphodiesterase inhibits the enzymic destruction of cAMP.

One reservation about this proposed mechanism of action for ADP lies in the design of some of the experiments by which evidence for the theory was obtained. In order to show that platelet cAMP was decreased by ADP, platelet levels of cAMP had first to be raised by addition of PGE_1 and a phosphodiesterase inhibitor. (SALZMANN, 1972; MILLS and SMITH, 1972), which is hardly physiological. Stimulation of platelet cGMP (which often has the opposite effect to cAMP) might be an additional or alternative explanation (HASLAM and MCCLENAGHAN, 1974).

Objections can be raised to most of the above hypotheses (MILLS, 1974) especially when considered in isolation. MILLS (1973, 1974) has recently shown that the first event following addition of ADP to platelets is probably a rapid and profound change in platelet energy metabolism, expressed as a decrease in energy charge[6]. It was suggested by MILLS that this metabolic event is causally related to the shape change phenomenon (considered to be a prerequisite for aggregation). To support this assumption, it was shown that both metabolic events and the shape change induced by ADP were related temporally and that both events could be seen in the presence of EDTA (which blocks aggregation and not the shape change) or in thrombasthenic platelets which are naturally deficient in ability to aggregate but still

[6] Energy change (EC) = $(ATP + 1^1/_2ADP)/(ATP + ADP + AMP)$

undergo the shape change (see Section D). MILLS attributed this early metabolic change to an increase in cellular ATP utilisation and suggested that this process could be involved in the inhibition of platelet adenylate cyclase by ADP, since this latter process is apparently indirect, involving a sulphydryl enzyme which may be selectively inhibited by critical concentrations of N-ethyl maleimide (NEM) (see MILLS, 1974). However, the exact nature of any such biochemical link has yet to be ascertained.

The ADP aggregation response does appear to involve some type of receptor, explaining, for instance, why it is blocked by prior exposure to high concentrations of ADP under conditions which do not allow aggregation to take place (NUNN, 1973), i.e. "tachyphylaxis" or "receptor paralysis" may take place.

The direct aggregation response to ADP is also inhibited in a fairly selective way by adenosine, dichloro-adenosine and other adenosine analogues (BORN, 1962, 1964; MICHAL, 1974) as well as by ATP (MCFARLANE, 1974), or by high concentrations of furosamide (ROSSI, 1974). Such inhibitors can thus be used to indicate whether a given aggregation stimulus exerts its effects indirectly through liberation of platelet ADP. Another way of providing such evidence is to add to the platelet suspension an enzyme system which can destroy the ADP before it acts. Such enzymes can be derived from snake venom or potatoes (HASLAM, 1967; ARDLIE et al., 1971). Alternatively, pure creatinine phosphate-creatinine phosphokinase (CP-CPK) can be used (TSCHOPP and BAUMGARTNER, 1976; PACKHAM et al., 1977).

b) 5-HT

Platelet dense bodies contain much 5-HT, and its release (in ^{14}C form after uptake into the granules from plasma) is usually taken as a marker for release I (DAY and HOLMSEN, 1971). However, 5-HT is apparently of limited importance as a direct aggregating agent. In citrated PRP of man, 5-HT induces a shape change, followed by a reversible aggregation response (MITCHELL and SHARP, 1964). This effect seems to be mediated by 5-HT D receptors (as in guinea pig ileum), since it can be blocked by agents such as methysergide, or LSD-25 (MUSTARD and PACKHAM, 1970). It was concluded by BAUMGARTNER (1969) and BAUMGARTNER and BORN (1968, 1969) that 5-HT produced platelet aggregation following its uptake into the platelets through release of ADP. Aggregation can also be produced by 5-HT in PRP of the rabbit or cat, although spontaneous aggregation is a problem with cat platelets (TSCHOPP, 1970).

Prior exposure of platelets to 5-HT can render platelets insensitive to the aggregatory effects of ADP, adrenaline or 5-HT itself (MUSTARD and PACKHAM, 1970). Adrenaline in concentrations too small to induce aggregation alone can markedly enhance aggregation induced by 5-HT (BAUMGARTNER and BORN, 1969).

c) Adrenaline

Adrenaline induces an aggregation of human platelets which has two characteristic phases (O'BRIEN, 1963), regardless of how much adrenaline is added. In this respect it differs from ADP which only produces clear first and second phases of aggregation with critical concentrations. In very low concentrations, adrenaline sensitises platelets to aggregation induced by other aggregating agents (MUSTARD and PACKHAM, 1970) including the endoperoxide PGH_2 (WILLIS, unpublished results).

The first phase aggregation response to adrenaline is attributable to a direct effect on the aggregation machinery (it is not inhibited by aspirin and ADP is not released). This effect apparently involves α-adrenoceptors, since the aggregation response is blocked by α-adrenoceptor blocking drugs. Nevertheless, these α-receptors appear to differ from those in smooth muscle. Blockade occurs with phentolamine and dihydroergotamine, but not with normal concentrations of phenoxybenzamine or dibenzylene, two other commonly used α-adrenoceptor antagonists (MILLS and ROBERTS, 1967a; MUSTARD and PACKHAM, 1970).

It is interesting to speculate that the PG synthesis that mediates the second phase of adrenaline-induced aggregation (see Section C.VI.4.a) may involve α-adrenoceptors, since these are involved in PG production by spleen (GILMORE et al., 1968).

Involvement of β-adrenoceptors does not appear to be significant. High concentrations of β-blockers do inhibit the aggregation response (MUSTARD and PACKHAM, 1970), although this effect seems to be due to a non-specific membrane stabilising effect (SMITH, 1971) as reported for other anti-adrenergic compounds (MILLS and ROBERTS, 1967b). β-adrenoceptors could be involved in platelet disaggregation, since reversal of aggregation is reduced by β-adrenoceptor blocking drugs (SMITH, 1971).

The aggregating properties of adrenaline might also involve inhibition of platelet adenylate cyclase (thereby combating the antiaggregatory effects of basal cAMP synthesis). Unlike the effects of ADP (which also lowers previously elevated cAMP levels) those of adrenaline are more direct; it inhibits adenylcyclase in broken cell preparations from platelets (MILLS, 1974). This brings us to the question of whether or not adrenaline induces a platelet shape change. MILLS (1973, 1974) did not obtain a fall in adenylate energy charge after addition of adrenaline to platelets and attributed this result to the inability of adrenaline to induce a platelet shape change, since the fall in energy charge is apparently related to this phenomenon. It is true that no apparent shape change is seen in the usual aggregometer tracings. However, MICHAL (1972), using a light-scattering technique to measure shape change in the presence of aggregation, did obtain evidence for a shape change; micrographs have also been published that indicate this possibility (MUSTARD and PACKHAM, 1970). Perhaps adrenaline produces a biochemically different (and slower?) type of shape change than that seen with ADP.

d) Thrombin

Aggregation of platelets in response to thrombin undoubtedly involves the platelet release reaction (see Section C.VI.4) but thrombin may also induce aggregation directly. Unlike those of most other aggregating agents, the effects of thrombin on platelets are produced regardless of the presence or absence of plasma factors and in the absence of external Ca^{++} ions (chelated by EDTA). The aggregation produced by thrombin involves a shape change effect and is (like thrombin-induced clotting) blocked by heparin. For the various active forms of thrombin now known to exist, clotting activity runs parallel to ability to produce platelet aggregation (MOHAMMED et al., 1976).

These findings suggest that thrombin produces aggregation through an action on platelet surface fibrinogen, but current evidence (WEISS, 1975b) is against this possibility. Other mechanisms may be involved. PHILLIPS and AGIN (1973) showed that thrombin appears to attack a membrane glycoprotein with a molecular weight of

118000 daltons. This finding has been confirmed by some workers but not by others. Other platelet proteins that are altered by thrombin include thrombasthenin M (platelet myosin) but the mechanism of action of thrombin on platelets still remains to be definitively established (WEISS, 1975b).

Like ADP and adrenaline (see Sections C.VI.2.a and c above), thrombin appears also to decrease the activity of adenylate cyclase (BRODIE et al., 1972; SALZMAN, 1972); the fact that all three of these aggregating agents produce this effect favours its relationship to a mode of action.

3. The Labile Aggregation-Stimulating Substances (LASS) Derived From Arachidonic Acid

a) Background Information

SMITH and WILLIS (1971) discovered that platelet PG biosynthesis in response to thrombin was suppressed after oral ingestion of aspirin or indomethacin, but not by codeine; paracetamol (acetaminophen) and sodium salicylate are also ineffective (WILLIS and SMITH, unpublished; KOCSIS et al., 1973). This finding correlated well with the ability of aspirin or indomethacin (but not the other three drugs) to inhibit second phase aggregation and aggregation to low concentrations of collagen, as first discovered by WEISS and ALEDORT (1967), O'BRIEN (1968) and others (WEISS, 1972b). There is clearly a difference between PG synthetase in human platelets and that at other sites. Thus paracetamol does block PG synthesis in brain, but not in inflammatory exudate or dog spleen (WILLIS et al., 1972; FLOWER and VANE, 1972; FLOWER et al., 1972).

At that time we were unable to provide an explanation for the coincidence between these two effects of aspirin since PGE_2 and $PGF_{2\alpha}$ do not induce aggregation of human platelets[7].

The reports that arachidonic acid, the precursor of PGE_2 and $PGF_{2\alpha}$ could antagonise the effects of aspirin and itself induce aggregation that was blocked by aspirin (LEONARDI et al., 1972; VARGAFTIG and ZIRINIS, 1973; SILVER et al., 1973) cast new light on the problem. These findings led me to test the hypothesis that one or more LASS were responsible for mediating the type of aggregation response (and ADP release) that is inhibited by aspirin.

Direct evidence was produced in 1973, when we showed that microsomal preparations of human platelets or sheep vesicular gland converted arachidonate (but not related fatty acids) into a short-lived material detectable by platelet aggregation and whose generation was blocked by aspirin or indomethacin (WILLIS, 1973a, 1973b; WILLIS and KUHN, 1973; WILLIS, 1974a). This was the first demonstration of an enzymic basis for the antihaemostatic and antithrombotic properties of aspirin (WILLIS, 1974a; FLOWER, 1975; DE GAETANO, 1975). We then examined the temporal relationships between the appearance of LASS, rabbit aorta-contracting substances (RCS), PGE_2 and oxygen uptake. We also devised extraction and isolation procedures (WILLIS, 1974b).

---

[7] MACINTYRE and GORDON (1975) have now shown that PGE_2 produces aggregation in heparinised pig PRP.

By this time, NUGTEREN and HAZELHOF (1973) and HAMBERG and SAMUELSSON (1973) had reported the isolation and chemical characterisation of an endoperoxide (15, α-hydroxy, 9α, 11α-peroxidoprosta-5,13-dienoic acid; PGH_2; PGR_2) intermediate in PGE_2 biosynthesis. Application of some of their techniques to our own isolated material (inactivation by stannous chloride and non-enzymic conversion to PGs) supported an identification of the LASS from sheep vesicular gland as PGH_2 (WILLIS, 1974b). Subsequently we were also able to confirm this identification regorously on material purified by high resolution high pressure liquid chromatography, using gas chromatography/mass spectrometry to assay the non-enzymically derived PGs. We were thus able to prepare the pure endoperoxide for use in biological testing procedures using radioactivity derived from the ^{14}C-arachidonate precursor for its quantitation. Using identical techniques, we isolated and identified the corresponding endoperoxide of PGE_1 synthesis, derived from dihomo-γ-linolenic acid; interestingly, this substance was completely devoid of effects on platelets (WILLIS et al., 1974a).

HAMBERG et al. (1974b) found that their preparations of PGH_2 and PGG_2 (15-hydroperoxy PGR_2) produced aggregation of washed human platelets and they provided some indirect evidence (increased $PGF_{2\alpha}$ production in the presence of stannous chloride) that one or both of these endoperoxides had been formed in washed platelets stimulated with thrombin. SMITH et al. (1974a) also reported that some labile material reducable to $PGF_{2\alpha}$ was formed in human PRP during aggregation induced by collagen, arachidonate and the second phase of adrenaline induced aggregation. Using washed platelets stimulated with thrombin, collagen, or arachidonate, we isolated a semi-purified LASS, detected by its ability to aggregate platelets [8]; its production was blocked by aspirin (WILLIS et al., 1974a).

One of the puzzles in considering the role that endoperoxides play in aggregation was that the amounts produced in platelets were about 10–100 times higher than the amounts of platelet PGE_2 and $F_{2\alpha}$ usually detected (e.g. SMITH et al., 1973a; WILLIS and WEISS, 1973; WILLIS et al., 1974a, 1974b). This is particularly evident when ADP is used to stimulate aggregation. Amounts of ADP about 20-fold greater than those needed to produce second-phase aggregation can induce production of only a few nanograms of PGE_2 (SMITH et al., 1973a). The discovery by HAMBERG and SAMUELSSON (1974) that platelets (unlike many other tissues) convert much of their endoperoxides to non-prostanoate substances, provides an explanation. These latter substances have been termed "thromboxanes" (HAMBERG et al., 1975) and it has been postulated that a labile thromboxane (thromboxane A_2) produces platelet aggregation and that conversion of PGG_2 and PGH_2 to this substance (Fig. 7) may account for much of the pro-aggregatory properties of the endoperoxides. In addition, NEEDLEMAN et al. (1976a) reported the generation of a thromboxane A_2-like material from PGG_2 and PGH_2 in platelets by a microsomal enzyme (NEEDLEMAN et al., 1976a). This "thromboxane synthetase" is specifically inhibited by several compounds including imidazole (MONCADA et al., 1977; NEEDLEMAN et al., 1977).

[8] Interestingly, this material could not be detected in PRP whether or not isolation was attempted. This may also be the reason why HAMBERG et al. (1975) used washed platelets to detect thromboxanes. PRP from rabbits can be used to generate LASS, however (CHIGNARD and VARGAFTIG, 1976).

Thromboxane A_2 is extracted into cold diethyl ether at neutral pH, and distinguished from the endoperoxide PGG_2 and PGH_2 by ability to produce contractions (not relaxations) of isolated strips of rabbit mesenteric and coeliac artery of rabbits (BUNTING et al., 1976b). The rapidity with which findings in this area are now being published suggests that soon the thromboxanes, like the endoperoxides, will become available in pure form as research tools. In the meantime, it is possible to generate platelet-aggregating material from arachidonate in crude incubates, without the necessity for extraction and chromatographic separation. There are successful examples of this approach. GERRARD et al. (1975) showed that LASS can act as an intercellular messenger in restoring the aggregation defect in aspirin-treated platelets. Also BUNTING et al. (1976a) have described a simple procedure for enzymically generating thromboxane-like biological activity from arachidonate, by an enzyme cascade of sheep vesicular gland microsomes (which produce mainly endoperoxides) followed by platelet microsomes (which convert the endoperoxides into thromboxanes). VARGAFTIG and CHIGNARD (1975) showed that agents which increased platelet cAMP could inhibit the release of thromboxane A_2/endoperoxide-like material (RCS) following stimulation by arachidonic acid.

b) Aggregation Produced by PGH_2 (PGR_2; Pure LASS Generated From Arachidonate by Phenol-Activated Sheep Vesicular Gland Microsomes)

WILLIS et al. (1974a) extensively studied the effects of PGH_2 on platelets. In a concentration range of 0.02–2 µg/ml, PGH_2 produces aggregation in PRP of man, rat, and rabbit. The finding with rabbit PRP was confirmed by CHIGNARD and VARGAFTIG (1976) who also reported that dog platelets are insensitive to PGH_2, unpurified LASS or their arachidonate precursor.

Aggregation induced by PGH_2 is preceded by a shape change and is dependent upon plasma Ca^{++} ions. Washed platelets tend to be more sensitive to PGH_2, suggesting that, like arachidonate (SILVER et al., 1973), PGH_2 is partially inactivated by binding to plasma constituents. However, when platelets are isolated by gel filtration, so that plasma constituents are removed more completely, the aggregation response to PGH_2 is diminished, although it can be restored by addition of a small amount of platelet-free plasma; this may indicate that fibrinogen is necessary as a cofactor, as it is for other aggregating agents (WILLIS et al., 1974a). Low concentrations of PGH_2 induce aggregation that tends to be reversible, is not accompanied by 5-HT release or blocked by adenosine and therefore almost certainly is due to a direct aggregating effect of the endoperoxides[9]. When higher concentrations of PGH_2 are used, the aggregation response and size of aggregates are greater and 5-HT release is seen. Since the aggregation response is partially inhibited by adenosine (an ADP antagonist) it is partly attributable to induction of release reaction I (WILLIS et al., 1974a).

Endoperoxide-induced aggregation is finely modulated by E-type PGs. Thus, aggregation induced by PGH_2 is strongly inhibited by PGE_1 in concentrations

---

[9] PACKHAM et al. (1977) showed that platelets previously degranulated by a special treatment with thrombin can still be aggregated by arachidonate: this supports the concept (WILLIS et al., 1974a) that endoperoxides can produce part of their effect by direct activation of the aggregation machinery.

which do not similarly reduce the first phase aggregation response to ADP[10]. In contrast, PGE_2 markedly potentiates aggregation produced by pure PGH_2 (or crude LASS); a potentiation of several hundred percent can sometimes be observed. This potentiation effect seems to be principally concerned with sensitisation of the platelets to the platelet release reaction induced by PGH_2. In a related manner, PGE_2 antagonised the inhibitory effects of adenosine on PGH_2-induced aggregation (WILLIS et al., 1974a). This potentiation of endoperoxide-induced aggregation explains a rather old finding that low concentrations of PGE_2 potentiated the aggregation response induced by ADP, adrenaline and collagen (KLOEZE, 1967; CHANDRA-SEKHAR, 1970; SHIO and RAMWELL, 1972; AMER and MARQUIS, 1972), and that this effect was prevented by aspirin (SHIO and RAMWELL, 1972). Presumably, PGE_2 had sensitised the platelets to PGH_2 produced in the platelets and its endogenous production could, of course, be blocked by aspirin.

MACINTYRE and GORDON (1975) reported that the ability of PGE_2 to enhance second phase aggregation is highly Ca^{++} dependent. This is not surprising, since PGE_2 acts by potentiating the effects of PGH_2, the ability of which to produce platelet aggregation is itself Ca^{++} dependent.

Aspirin acts by inhibiting the generation, but not the actions of the endoperoxides. In the absence of exogenous PGE_2, aspirin does cause a slight decrease in aggregation response to PGH_2 in human PRP; this is possibly due to a reduction in basal synthesis of PGE_2 which might exert some "tonal" potentiation of the PGH_2 response (WILLIS et al., 1974a). In PRP to which PGE_2 had been added (WILLIS et al., 1974a), or in saline-suspended platelets (HAMBERG et al., 1974b; WEISS et al., 1976)[11] aspirin produces a slight potentiation of the aggregation response to PGH_2. In rabbit PRP, indomethacin failed to inhibit the aggregation response to PGH_2 as did catalase, a free radical scavenger that inhibits the pro-aggregatory effects of arachidonate by preventing its conversion to endoperoxides (VARGAFTIG et al., 1975; CHIGNARD and VARGAFTIG, 1976).

Finally, the concept that endoperoxides were a "chemical trigger" for thrombosis was supported by the demonstration that crude or pure PGH_2 produced thrombocytopenia when injected in rats or mice and sufficient amounts of endoperoxide could be injected into mice to produce sudden death. Histology showed that intravascular platelet aggregation had taken place in the circulation of heart and lungs. No lethal effects were seen with material enzymically derived from other unsaturated fatty acids (including dihomo-γ-linolenic acid). The lethal effects of crude or pure endoperoxide were not blocked by treatment of the animals with aspirin (WILLIS, 1974b; WILLIS et al., 1974a).

c) PGG_2 (15-hydroperoxy-PGR_2)

The properties of this substance on platelets have not been so extensively investigated. HAMBERG et al. (1974b) reported that PGG_2 in nanogram concentrations

[10] Aggregation induced by collagen is more sensitive to inhibition by PGE_1 than is ADP-induced aggregation (GORDON, personal communication). The reason could well be that collagen induces aggregation through generation of PGH_2 (the action of which, as described here, is highly sensitive to inhibition by PGE_1).

[11] Processes involved in resuspending platelets in saline, induce platelet production of PGs (SALZMAN, 1974).

could produce aggregation of washed human platelets and MALMSTEN et al. (1975) reported that it produced aggregation in citrated human PRP, apparently through inducing release of ADP (which was measured directly). The modulatory effects of E-type PGs on PGG_2-induced aggregation have not been reported although NISHIZAWA et al. (1975) showed that PGD_2 was a potent inhibitor of aggregation induced in human PRP by various agents, including PGG_2.

Thus, PGG_2 may differ from PGH_2 in producing more of its effect through the release reaction and less of its effects through a direct action on the platelet aggregation machinery.

d) Thromboxane A_2

It was reported by HAMBERG et al. (1975) that when PGG_2 was added to a platelet suspension, the aggregation response reached maximal levels when most of the added endoperoxide (estimated chemically) had disappeared. These workers had earlier shown that in washed platelets, endoperoxides were largely metabolised to non-prostanoate substances and that a major metabolite was PHD (8-(1-hydroxy-3-oxopropyl)-9,-12S-dihydroxy-5 *cis*, 10 *cis*, heptadecadienoic acid), (now called thromboxane B_2, Fig. 7[12]). Thromboxane B_2 did not induce aggregation but it was postulated that a labile intermediate with platelet aggregating properties is formed between the endoperoxides (PGG_2 and PGH_2) and thromboxane B_2. To support this assumption it was shown that there was a formation of aggregating activity (distinguishable from ADP) upon addition of PGG_2 to platelets and that this activity increased as the PGG_2 (estimated chemically) disappeared. This activity was apparently attributable to a very unstable substance with a half-life of only about 30 s. A structure (thromboxane A_2; Fig. 7) was attributed to this activity and supporting evidence for the postulated structure was obtained when it was "trapped" (as an inactive but chemically identifiable derivative) by ethanol or sodium azide.

The RCS from lung described earlier by PIPER and VANE (1969) seems to consist mainly of thromboxane A_2 (SVENSSEN et al., 1975; NEEDLEMAN et al., 1976a, 1976b) although many lipoperoxides are capable of producing contractions of this tissue (GRYGLEWSKI and VANE, 1972; VARGAFTIG and ZIRINIS, 1973; WILLIS and KUHN, 1973; WILLIS, 1974b). The biological properties of pure thromboxane A_2 have not yet been delineated. However, according to HAMBERG et al. (1975) the actions of thromboxane A_2 on platelets differ from those of PGG_2 in that it produces aggregation in the virtual absence of ADP release. This finding is not consistent with the results of SMITH et al. (1977) which indicate that thromboxane generation is a prerequisite for the platelet release reaction. It is also not consistent with an opinion that conversion of endoperoxides (PGG_2 and PGH_2) is largely responsible for their pro-aggregatory properties, since PGG_2 seems to produce its effects mainly through release of platelet ADP (MALMSTEN et al., 1975), while PGH_2 does not (WILLIS et al., 1974a); both PGG_2 and PGH_2 are converted to thromboxane A_2 by washed platelets (HAMBERG et al., 1975).

Studies with inhibitors of thromboxane synthetase in washed human platelets (NEEDLEMAN et al., 1977) or PRP (FITZPATRICK and GORMAN, 1977) have provided conflicting evidence for an obligatory role of thromboxane A_2 in arachidonate-

[12] See WILLIS and STONE (1976) for alternative systematic nomenclature.

mediated aggregation. Furthermore, stable endoperoxide analogues (U44069 and U46619) cannot be converted into thromboxanes and still produce aggregation that is not blocked by aspirin (SMITH et al., 1976). Taken together, the available evidence suggests that endoperoxides may, to some extent, mediate aggregation independent of thromboxane A_2 generation.

According to NUGTEREN (1976) and NEEDLEMAN et al. (1976b) little of the monoenoic thromboxanes (A and B) are formed from the endoperoxides (PGG_1 and PGH_1) derived from dihomo-γ-linolenic acid. In addition, it is possible that they are devoid of the ability to produce platelet aggregation since neither incubates of platelet microsomal enzymes + dihomo-γ-linolenate, nor pure PGH_1 (PGR_1) are capable of producing platelet aggregation (WILLIS, 1974a, 1974b; WILLIS et al., 1974a).

The surplus endoperoxides (PGG_2 and PGH_2) that are not converted to thromboxane A_2 within the platelets escape into the extra-platelet milieu. They may then be converted into PGE_2 and PGD_2 in plasma (SMITH et al., 1977) or into PGI_2 upon contact with the blood vessel wall (GRYGLEWSKI et al., 1976). The latter two substances have actions that are the antithesis of those for thromboxane A_2. Thus thromboxane synthetase could play a central modulatory role in haemostasis and thrombosis.

e) Other Substances

Because many substances are produced enzymically from arachidonate, it would not be surprising if yet more constituents of platelet LASS exist besides the endoperoxides and thromboxane A_2. For instance, some of the free radicals that have been postulated as intermediates might produce aggregation (but would probably defy isolation).

A platelet lipoxygenase also converts arachidonate to 12-hydroperoxy and 12-hydroxy fatty acids (HAMBERG and SAMUELSSON, 1974; NUGTEREN, 1975, 1977). This enzyme is unlikely to be of importance in platelet aggregation, however, since its action is blocked by TYA but not by aspirin (both drugs inhibit endoperoxide formation by the cyclo-oxygenase) and we were unable to distinguish between the effects of TYA and aspirin on platelet aggregation (WILLIS et al., 1974b). Finally, it is as well to add that in at least one species (the pig) PGE_2 itself can produce platelet aggregation in heparinised PRP (MACINTYRE and GORDON, 1975).

4. Mechanisms of Aggregation Induced Indirectly (i.e. Mediated Through Pro-Aggregatory Platelet Substances)

a) Second Phase Aggregation Induced by ADP or Adrenaline

The secondary aggregation response to ADP and adrenaline is irreversible and is always accompanied by release (release I) of ADP and 5-HT although release II of lysosomal enzymes is not similarly activated (MILLS et al., 1968; MUSTARD and PACKHAM, 1970).

This second phase aggregation response is suppressed by aspirin-type drugs (see MUSTARD and PACKHAM, 1970, 1975; WEISS, 1975b) that selectively block the cyclo-oxygenation of arachidonate to PG endoperoxides (HAMBERG et al., 1974a, 1974b; WILLIS et al., 1974a). An identical effect is seen with TYA which blocks both the cyclo-oxygenase and the lipoxygenase of platelets (WILLIS et al., 1974b; HAMBERG and SAMUELSSON, 1974; HAMBERG et al., 1974a).

From recent work on endoperoxides and thromboxanes, it seems that second phase aggregation to ADP or adrenaline is mediated entirely through endoperoxides (PGH_2 and PGG_2) and perhaps thromboxane A_2 and other pro-aggregatory substances i.e. a LASS mechanism is involved (Fig. 2). There is indirect evidence that an endoperoxide-like substance is formed during the second phase of aggregation produced by adrenaline (SMITH et al., 1974a).

Endoperoxides (and PGE_2) are generated from arachidonate which is liberated from platelet phosphatidylcholine and phosphatidylinositol by phospholipases whose activity is known to be induced by the common aggregating agents including adrenaline (SHOENE and IACONO, 1976), or thrombin (BILLS and SILVER, 1975; BILLS et al., 1977; BLACKWELL et al., 1977). This hypothesis explains several findings, such as a lack of second phase aggregation in children with essential fatty acid (EFA) deficiency; this abnormal aggregation response can be reversed by correction of the EFA deficiency (FRIEDMAN et al., 1976).

Similarly, in EFA-deficient rats (in rats the first and second phase aggregation to ADP coalesce into one), platelet PG production is low and the ability of aspirin or indomethacin to reduce the aggregation response and release I (of 5-HT) is mostly lacking (VINCENT et al., 1976).

Platelets from diabetics produce abnormally high amounts of prostaglandin in response to adrenaline (or collagen) and the second phase (and interestingly enough, also the first phase) of aggregation is produced by much lower than normal concentrations of ADP or adrenaline. The resulting aggregation response is abnormally sensitive to inhibition by aspirin-type drugs or TYA (HALUSHKA et al., 1976; KWAAN et al., 1972; COLWELL et al., 1973).

b) Aggregation Induced by Collagen

Collagen cannot directly produce platelet aggregation, but adhesion of platelets to collagen microfibrils indirectly produces aggregation by initiating events (including endoperoxide synthesis) leading to platelet aggregation and to release of platelet ADP which also produces aggregation. Aggregation produced by collagen is greatly dependent upon its size, form and dispersion (MUGGLI and BAUMGARTNER, 1973). When low to moderate concentrations of collagen are used to induce platelet aggregation, the aggregation response may be considered to be identical to that occurring during the second phase aggregation response to ADP or adrenaline (there is no direct effect of collagen on platelets and, therefore, no first phase of aggregation).

The aggregation response is, therefore, produced entirely through conversion of platelet arachidonate to the prostaglandin endoperoxides and thromboxane A_2 (see Section C.VI.4.a). Thus, the aggregation response to these low concentrations of collagen can be almost completely suppressed by aspirin-type drugs or by TYA (Fig. 2), with a parallel reduction in platelet PG production (MUSTARD and PACKHAM, 1970, 1975; WEISS, 1972b, 1975b; WILLIS et al., 1974a, 1974b). Similarly, aggregation to low collagen concentrations is diminished or absent in storage pool deficient (SPD) platelets which are relatively unresponsive to aggregation produced by PGH_2 and lack releasable ("storage") pools of ADP (WILLIS and WEISS, 1973; WEISS,

1975b). However, when high concentrations of collagen are used, an additional mechanism, defined here as mechanism X_c (for collagen), comes further into prominance with increasing collagen concentration so that the endoperoxide-mediated mechanism eventually becomes completely eclipsed. Aspirin now fails significantly to inhibit platelet aggregation; collagen-induced aggregation in SPD platelets is then also no different from normal.

Whether there are one or more components to mechanism X_c remains to be established, but it is apparently involved in both aggregation and release I, since ZUCKER and PETERSON (1970) showed that platelet 5-HT release, like the aggregation response, could not be greatly reduced by aspirin, when high concentrations of collagen were used (Fig. 2).

Nevertheless, mechanism X_c probably is not significantly mediated through ADP release. Hence, NUNN (1973) showed that the aggregation response to high concentrations of collagen was undiminished in platelets made insensitive to ADP aggregation (by tachyphylaxis). High concentrations of collagen can also produce a normal aggregation response in SPD platelets which (by definition) have a lack of releasable ADP (WILLIS and WEISS, 1973; WEISS, 1975b). Mechanism X_c could, however, be causally related to the release of lysosomal enzymes from α granules (release II), that is seen with high concentrations of collagen and which is not inhibited by aspirin (see MUSTARD and PACKHAM, 1970; HOLMSEN et al., 1969b; DAY and HOLMSEN, 1971).

The elevation in platelet cGMP that is induced by exposure to collagen (HASLAM and MCCLENAGHAN, 1974) is attributable to liberation of arachidonate and its conversion to endoperoxides, since similar increases in cGMP are produced by arachidonic acid (GLASS et al., 1975) and both collagen-induced and arachidonate-induced cGMP accumulation are blocked by aspirin, a known inhibitor of arachidonate cyclo-oxygenation (HASLAM and MCCLENAGHAN, 1974; GLASS et al., 1975).

c) Aggregation Induced by Thrombin

The ability of thrombin to produce aggregation by a direct effect on the platelets has already been discussed (Section C.VI.2.d). However, thrombin probably exerts much of its platelet aggregatory effects indirectly. Consistent with this assumption, thrombin is known to be a potent inducer of platelet PGE_2 and $PGF_{2\alpha}$ production (SMITH and WILLIS, 1970; SILVER et al., 1972) and there is ample indirect evidence that it induces platelet endoperoxide synthesis (HAMBERG et al., 1974b; HAMBERG and SAMUELSSON, 1974). Thrombin also induces platelet production of LASS, detected by platelet aggregation following its rapid isolation (WILLIS et al., 1974a). Thrombin is also very potent in initiating release reaction I (of ADP and 5-HT) and release II (of lysosomal enzymes) (HOLMSEN et al., 1969a, 1969b).

However, aspirin-sensitive mechanisms appear to play a minor role in the aggregation response to thrombin. Only if small concentrations of thrombin are used, can aspirin-type drugs (EVANS et al., 1968) or TYA (WILLIS et al., 1974b) inhibit aggregation and release of 5-HT and even then the inhibition is not complete. With higher concentrations of thrombin, inhibitors of endoperoxide production are virtually without effect on aggregation or release (Fig. 2).

Thus, as already postulated in the case of collagen, one (or more) additional mechanism(s) (mechanism X_t) must be involved in the aggregation and release reaction induced by thrombin (Fig. 2).

It is felt by this author that in vivo the mechanism(s) *X* involved in aggregation to both collagen and thrombin could eclipse the contribution of mechanisms involving PG endoperoxides and ADP release.

Thus, in situations where platelet function is impaired by a congenital lack of releasable ADP (storage pool disease) or endoperoxide biosynthesis is blocked (by ingestion of aspirin), then haemostasis is only partially impaired and a serious bleeding disorder does not usually occur unless some other mechanism is also inhibited, for instance, by ingestion of oral anticoagulants (see Section D.II). Similarly, chronic ingestion of aspirin may produce only a limited protection against stroke and heart attack (GENTON et al., 1975).

5. "Special Cases" (e.g. Zymosan and Ristocetin)

The events occurring and possible mechanisms involved in aggregation produced by the "physiological" aggregating agents (collagen, thrombin, ADP, and adrenaline and endoperoxides) have already been discussed. There are certain factors in common to each case. Thus, the aggregation response usually requires plasma Ca^{++} ions and fibrinogen, is preceded by a shape change (in which the platelets become spiky) and can be completely suppressed by PGE_1 or other agents that increase platelet cAMP. In cases where part of the aggregation response is induced indirectly, then release of ADP and 5-HT is seen and (if endoperoxides are involved) prostaglandins, and other endoperoxide metabolites, are produced by the platelets and both aggregation and PG production is blocked by aspirin.

There are, however, some stimuli that apparently induce platelet aggregation through other mechanisms (see MUSTARD and PACKHAM, 1975; PACKHAM et al., 1977). Two important examples of such stimuli are zymosan and ristocetin.

a) Zymosan

In PRP of rabbit or man, zymosan produces a biphasic aggregation response following an initial lag period, during which no evidence of a shape change has yet been produced (ZUCKER and GRANT, 1974; CHRISTIAN and GORDON, 1975). Experiments with washed platelets show that in order to produce any aggregation, the zymosan has to be activated by combination with a plasma factor (possibly IgG) which is present in both normal and C_6 complement deficient plasma. However, in order to produce the release reaction (and hence the second phase of aggregation), the later components of complement are apparently necessary. Thus, only addition of normal plasma (not that from C_6-deficient rabbits) can support both phases of aggregation. Similar results are obtained in rabbit PRP. Only the initial aggregation response is seen in PRP from C_6 deficient rabbits but both phases in normal rabbit PRP (CHRISTIAN and GORDON, 1975). Except for its dependancy on complement, the second phase of zymosan aggregation (probably attributable to release of ADP) appears to involve normal aggregation mechanisms, since it can be suppressed by PGE_1. However, the initial aggregation response does involve an abnormal mechanism since it is not affected by PGE_1 (MACINTYRE and GORDON, personal communication). The mechanisms of this initial aggregation at present remain unknown.

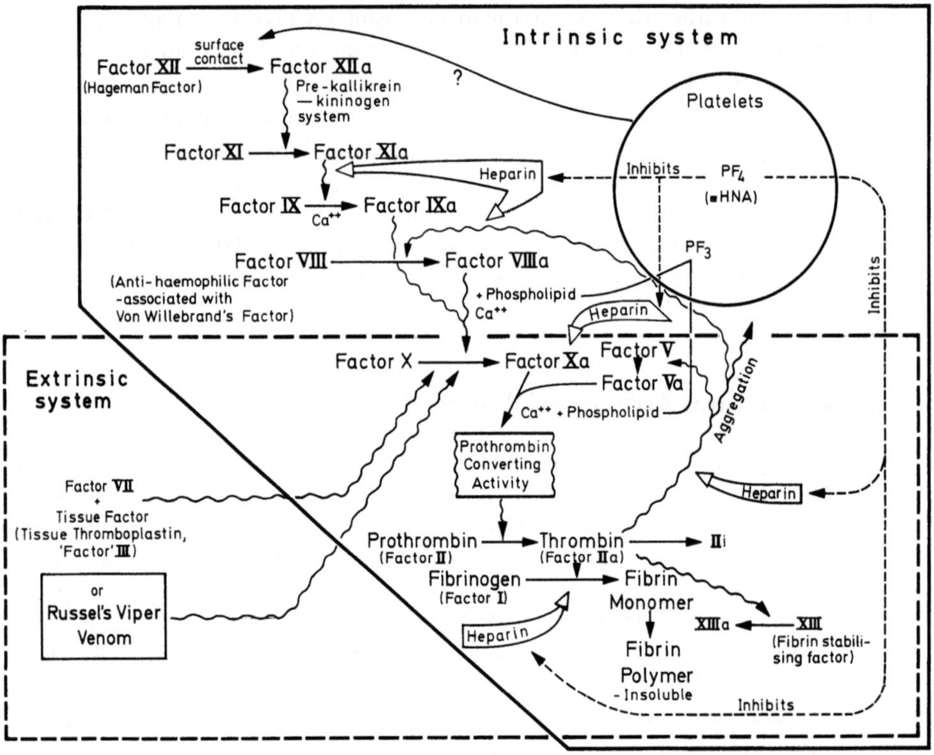

Fig. 3. Blood clotting mechanisms and the role of platelets (modified from WILLIAMS, 1968; BIGGS, 1969; STORMORKEN and OWREN, 1971; WEISS, 1975b). Nearly all the plasma coagulation factors circulate in blood as pro-enzymes and are converted to enzymes during process of clotting. In general, the function of each enzyme appears to be activation of the pro-enzyme which succeeds it in the coagulation sequence. Internationally agreed Roman nomenclature is used for each clotting factor, except where common usage is otherwise (e.g. prothrombin is used instead of factor II, Ca^{++} instead of factor IV). It should be noted that the numerals were assigned on the basis of chronological discovery, that there is no factor VI, and that Arabic numerals are used for clotting factors of platelet origin. The suffix "a" denotes the "activated" form of the clotting factor and "i" the inactive form. Platelets are a source of the phospholipid (PF_3) necessary for activation of several factors and generation of prothrombin-converting activity. PF_3 is made available at the platelet surface during the release reaction induced by collagen or by thrombin which is itself generated during the coagulation process (MARCUS and ZUCKER, 1965; HARDISTY and HUTTON, 1966). Platelets may also be involved in the "contact activation" which initiates coagulation through activation of factor XII (WEISS, 1975b). Thus, whole blood contains all the constituents necessary for activation of coagulation through the so-called *intrinsic clotting system*. Damage of vascular or extravascular tissue may also induce clotting and platelet aggregation by release of tissue factor (alternatively named tissue thromboplastin or factor III). This is composed of phospholipid and protein (NEMERSON, 1968) and it activates the coagulation cascade by activation of factor X. This so-called *extrinsic clotting system* can also be activated by Russel's Viper venom, commonly used in laboratory clotting tests (WILLIAMS, 1968). Decalcification inhibits clotting by interfering with several key enzyme steps requiring Ca^{++} ions. Similarly, heparin inhibits other stages in the clotting process (as indicated) in addition to its widely known ability to block the action of thrombin in producing clotting (fibrinogen→fibrin) and platelet aggregation. The actions of heparin are attenuated by heparin-neutralising activity (HNA). This is produced during blood clotting and is attributable, at least in part, to PF_4 released from platelets during the release reaction induced by thrombin or collagen (WALSH, 1972; DONATI et al., 1972). Heparin exerts its anti-coagulant action by acting as a co-factor for an inhibitor in plasma known as antithrombin III (AT III) or antifactor Xa (Anti Xa). Anti-thrombin

b) Ristocetin

Ristocetin is an antibiotic that produces aggregation in citrated PRP from normal human individuals or from patients with congenital haemostatic defects, in which aggregation to physiological aggregating agents is diminished (storage pool disease) or even absent (thrombasthenia). Clearly then, the aggregation response to ristocetin involves an unusual mechanism. Possibly, some type of adhesion process is involved in the formation of platelet/ristocetin complexes. Support for this idea is present in the findings that ristocetin aggregation is diminished or absent in the congenital haemostatic defects known as Bernard Soulier syndrome and von Willebrand's disease, or in normal platelets which are washed sufficiently to remove factor VIII from the platelet surface (JENKINS et al., 1974).

It has been shown that factor VIII is composed of at least three separable components and that ristocetin aggregation co-factor activity requires two or more of these components (BAUGH et al., 1974). Platelet membrane glycoproteins have also been implicated in the mechanism of ristocetin-induced aggregation (JENKINS et al., 1976). In both von Willebrand's disease and Bernard Soulier syndrome, aggregation to physiological aggregating agents is normal, although *adhesion* (retention on glass or vascular sub-endothelium) is abnormally low (details are given in Sections D.3 and D.4 of this chapter and in WEISS, 1975b).

Superimposed upon this direct aggregation effect of unknown mechanism, there appears to be some degree of indirect aggregation which (as one might expect) is not seen in aspirin-treated, SPD, or thrombasthenic platelets and it might, therefore, involve an endoperoxide/ADP mechanism (see WEISS, 1975b; and JENKINS et al., 1974 for representative aggregation tracings.) This indirect component of aggregation, is also inhibited by PGE_1, although the direct aggregating effect of ristocetin is more resistant (MACINTYRE and GORDON, personal communication).

D. The Role of Platelets in Haemostasis and Haemostatic Defects

Haemostasis is the means by which blood loss from a wound surface is staunched. Even in the nineteenth century, the role of platelets in haemostasis was recognised (ARDLIE, 1973) and this involvement is now well documented (MARCUS and ZUCKER, 1965; RODMAN and MASON, 1967; MUSTARD and PACKHAM, 1970; ARDLIE, 1973; WEISS, 1975b and references therein). A scenario along the lines below is generally accepted:

I. Events Occurring in Haemostasis

Platelets play an initiating role in haemostasis by adhering to the subendothelial constituents, exposed in severed blood vessels. They then release substances which produce aggregation and formation of a platelet plug. Among the substances released are ADP, PG endoperoxides and thromboxanes. These induce platelet aggre-

III inactivates coagulation factors such as thrombin and factor Xa (see WEISS, 1975b; SUTTIE and JACKSON, 1977). Coumarin-type oral anti-coagulant drugs act in the liver to antagonise the actions of vitamin K in promoting the synthesis of clotting factors IX, X, VII and prothrombin (SUTTIE and JACKSON, 1977). Dextran precipitates clotting factors (ALEXANDER et al., 1975) including factor VIII and fibrinogen, which are also co-factors for platelet adhesion and the platelet release reaction (see Sections C.III.2 and C.VI.5.b)

gation (and further release of ADP) (WILLIS et al., 1974a; HAMBERG et al., 1974a, 1974b; 1975; SMITH et al., 1974a; Section C.V.3 of this chapter).

These latter substances are also potent vasoconstrictors, thus constricting lumen of the severed vessel which further tends to reduce blood loss.

Availability of coagulation factors (including PF 3 and PF 4) coupled with local sluggish blood flow (due to the platelet plug) help to initiate the clotting process through activation of thrombin (Fig. 3). The relative contribution of platelet aggregation per se and coagulation is dependent upon blood flow conditions (Fig. 6).

Thrombin further promotes haemostasis in two ways. It induces irreversible aggregation of platelets with accompanying production of PG endoperoxides (HAMBERG et al., 1974a, 1974b; WILLIS et al., 1974a) and release of pro-aggregatory contents from both dense bodies *and* α granules (DAY and HOLMSEN, 1971; HOLMSEN et al., 1969a, 1969b). The net result is extension and consolidation of the area of aggregated platelets.

Thrombin also plays its more widely known role in converting fibrinogen to fibrin. The network of fibrin polymer stabilises the platelet plug and traps red cells and other blood constituents in a gelatinous mass formed immediately behind it. At this stage, platelets play an additional role in consolidating the clot and perhaps pulling severed edges of the blood vessel together. Platelets do this by the process of *clot retraction* in which contractile protein of the platelets (thrombasthenin) shortens, pulling the fibrin strands (to which platelets have adhered) closer together. Thus, platelets play an essential role both early and late in the haemostatic process.

II. Haemostatic Defects

The mechanisms through which platelets exert their actions in haemostasis are now understood to a considerable degree, because platelets are easily available for study and because various congenital or drug-induced platelet defects in haemostasis are known. These are usually detectable by a prolonged bleeding time[13], difficulty in producing haemostasis during surgery and (often) easy bruising. These defects can also be detected in the laboratory by examination of platelet function. Main examples of such haemostatic defects are discussed below; a more detailed account has been recently published by WEISS (1975b).

1. **Thrombocytopenia** (Decreased Level of Circulating Platelets)

Since platelets are necessary for normal haemostasis (see above) one would expect haemostasis to be impaired in thrombocytopenia. However, there is a large safety margin in the number of circulating platelets required to support normal haemostasis. Platelet count can be reduced to levels of only 10–20% of normal and haemostasis may not be greatly impaired (MUSTARD and PACKHAM, 1970) although HARKER and SCHLICHTER (1972) have reported that bleeding time is prolonged. This excess of platelets is probably necessary to meet the eventualities of major trauma.

In spite of these considerations, it has been shown by several groups that severe thrombocytopenia is associated with impaired haemostasis (see MUSTARD and

[13] Bleeding time is the average time taken for arrest of bleeding in a superficial cut in the skin (see PRAGA et al., 1972 for details of methodology).

PACKHAM, 1970). There is also some evidence that platelets may be necessary to repair small defects in the vascular endothelium (MARCUS and ZUCKER, 1965).

Thrombocytopenia may result from auto-immunity as in idiopathic thrombocytopenic purpura in which there appears to be accelerated destruction of platelets (ASTER, 1966; DAVEY, 1966; NAJEAN et al., 1967; EBBE, 1968). In other cases, thrombocytopenia may result from abnormally low production of platelets in the bone marrow, as during aplastic anaemia (SCOTT et al., 1959). Congenitally low platelet counts have also been described (MUSTARD and PACKHAM, 1970).

2. Afibrinogenemia

Fibrinogen is necessary, not only for the clotting process but also as a co-factor in platelet aggregation (see Section C.III. of this chapter). Thus, in individuals with a congenital lack of fibrinogen (afibrinogenemia), there is deficient haemostasis attributable to both impaired platelet function and impaired fibrin formation. Such patients usually have a prolonged bleeding time and an impaired platelet aggregation response to ADP (GUGLER and LÜSCHER, 1965; INCEMAN et al., 1966; CRONBERG, 1968) and adrenaline (WEISS, personal communication).

Retention of the platelets in glass bead columns is also low in afibrinogenemia (GUGLER and LÜSCHER, 1965; INCEMAN et al., 1966). This is to be expected since the mechanisms involved in glass bead tests involve aggregation of the platelets in response to released ADP (O'BRIEN, 1972). The aggregation defect in vitro can be corrected by addition of a small amount of fibrinogen or plasma from a normal individual (see MUSTARD and PACKHAM, 1970; GUGLER and LÜSCHER, 1965). Aggregation induced by PGH_2 may also require fibrinogen (WILLIS et al., 1974a) as does aggregation induced by the PG analogue WY-17186 (SMITH et al., 1976).

3. Von Willebrand's Disease

This is another congenital defect in haemostasis in which there is absence of a plasma protein (VON WILLEBRAND'S factor) which seems necessary for adhesion of platelets to vascular subendothelium. This factor is associated with clotting factor VIII (see WEISS, 1975b) and thus transfusion of normal human plasma, cryoprecipitate or purified factor VIII can reverse the haemostatic defect in von Willebrand's disease (WEISS, 1975a, 1975b).

In view of such findings, it is surprising that the defect in haemostasis in this disease principally involves not the clotting process but formation of the haemostatic platelet plug (JØRGENSEN and BORCHGREVINK, 1964). Using the in vitro perfusion chamber technique of BAUMGARTNER, it was shown that adhesion of platelets to vascular subendothelium is diminished in blood from patients with the disease, but the platelets that do adhere aggregate normally (TSCHOPP et al., 1974; WEISS et al., 1975). In spite of this clear implication of defective platelet function in vivo, aggregation to the usual physiological aggregating agents (collagen, ADP, adrenaline and thrombin) is normal (CRONBERG, 1968; WEISS, 1968).

There is a reduced retention of the platelets by glass beads in von Willebrand's disease (SALZMAN, 1963), although critical experimental conditions have resulted in a degree of non-reproducibility (MUSTARD and PACKHAM, 1970). The relative lack of easy laboratory tests for this disease was previously a drawback to diagnosis and research in the area. This situation has recently been remedied by the findings that ristocetin produces aggregation in stirred PRP of normal individuals, but that such aggregation is absent in von Willebrand's disease. The aggregation defect can be eliminated by addition of factor VIII or normal plasma (HOWARD and FIRKIN, 1971; WEISS et al., 1973; MEYER et al., 1974). Precipitating antibodies against factor VIII and von Willebrand's factor have recently been implicated in the aetiology of the disease (MANNUCCI et al., 1976). The ristocetin test now forms a basis for routine diagnosis (WEISS, 1975a).

4. Bernard Soulier (Giant Platelet) Syndrome

In this rather rare syndrome, the platelets are abnormally large and the haemostatic defect has some similarities to that in von Willebrand's disease. Adhesion (but not aggregation) is reduced when platelets are exposed to vascular subendothelium (WEISS et al., 1974a). Similarly, retention on glass beads is low and ristocetin aggregation is absent, although that to ADP, collagen etc. is not (WEISS, 1975b). Unlike the situation with von Willebrand's disease, however, the defect is not reversed by normal plasma and so resides in the platelets themselves.

This platelet defect may involve decreased binding of clotting factors on the platelet surface and an abnormality in surface glycoproteins that is distinct from that observed in thrombasthenia (WEISS, 1975b; NURDEN and CAEN, 1974; JENKINS et al., 1976). It bears comparison with the loss in ristocetin aggregation seen when normal platelets are thoroughly washed to remove factor VIII (and von Willebrand's factor) as reported by JENKINS et al. (1974).

5. Thrombasthenia

In the haemostatic defect known as Glanzmann's thrombasthenia, it is the aggregation machinery of the platelets that appears to be defective. The platelets do not aggregate, even to high concentrations of ADP, collagen, thrombin, adrenaline (WEISS, 1975b) or to arachidonate and PG endoperoxides (WEISS et al., 1976). Adhesion of thrombasthenic platelets to collagen is thus normal (ZUCKER et al., 1966; CAEN, 1972), as well as adhesion to vascular subendothelium as a whole (TSCHOPP et al., 1975).

In agreement with a role of PG endoperoxides in inducing release reaction I, which normally produces second phase aggregation (WILLIS et al., 1974a; MALMSTEN et al., 1975), the platelet release reaction (liberation of ADP, 5-HT etc.) in response to collagen, thrombin or vascular subendothelium, is normal in thrombasthenia (WEISS, 1975b; TSCHOPP et al., 1975), as is production of PGE_2 and $PGF_{2\alpha}$ which are formed from endoperoxides produced in the platelets (WILLIS and WEISS, 1973); the platelets are, of course, incapable of aggregation in response to these released substances.

Interestingly, and in contrast to findings in von Willebrand's disease or Bernard Soulier syndrome, thrombasthenic platelets are induced to aggregate in response to ristocetin (WEISS, 1975b). In this way, thrombasthenic platelets behave similarly to normal platelets exposed to PGE_1. In both cases, aggregation is produced by ristocetin but not by ADP, collagen or any of the usual aggregating agents, although the shape change is usually present (MILLS, 1973).

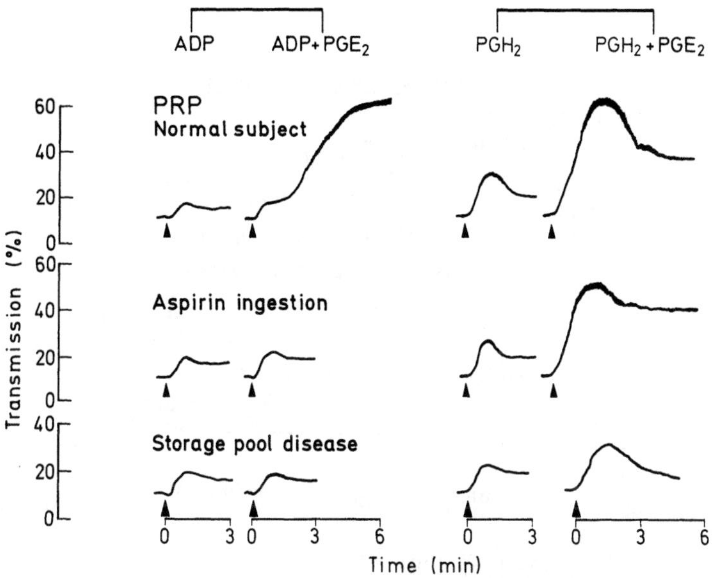

Fig. 4. Use of endoperoxide-induced aggregation to diagnose storage pool disease using the Born aggregometer. With PRP from normal individuals, PGE_2 potentiates ADP (second phase) aggregation as well as that induced by pure PGH_2. After aspirin ingestion PGH_2-induced aggregation is still potentiated by PGE_2, although no potentiation of ADP aggregation is seen (because the platelets are no longer able to produce PGH_2 endogenously). SPD deficient platelets show a diminished or absent second-phase aggregation response to ADP, whether or not they are preincubated with PGE_2. Similarly PGH_2-induced aggregation is not significantly altered by exposure to PGE_2. This is probably because PGE_2 acts principally to sensitise platelets to release of ADP (release I) induced by endoperoxide. PGE_2: 1 µg/ml: PGH_2 (800 ng/ml). Platelet count: 250000 cells mm^3. From WEISS et al. (1976) reprinted by permission

The exact cause of thrombasthenia is not yet known, although there are several abnormal biochemical findings in thrombasthenic platelets (see WEISS, 1975a). For instance, BOOYSE et al. (1972) found that platelet levels of actomyosin-like protein ("thrombasthenin") were lower in thrombasthenic platelets (the similar terminology is coincidental!). More recently, NURDEN and CAEN (1975) have reported an absence of one of the three membrane-specific platelet glycoproteins Either or both of the above findings could be a primary cause for the aggregation defect.

6. Storage Pool Disease

WEISS (1967) and HARDISTY and HUTTON (1967) independently discovered two groups of patients who lacked a second phase aggregation response, but who had not ingested aspirin or any other drug known to induce an abnormality in aggregation.

a) General Features

This defect could apparently be explained by the finding that platelet ADP release was low (as it is after aspirin treatment). However, release per se of the ADP was not the primary defect. Instead, there was a diminished dense granule content of Ca^{++},

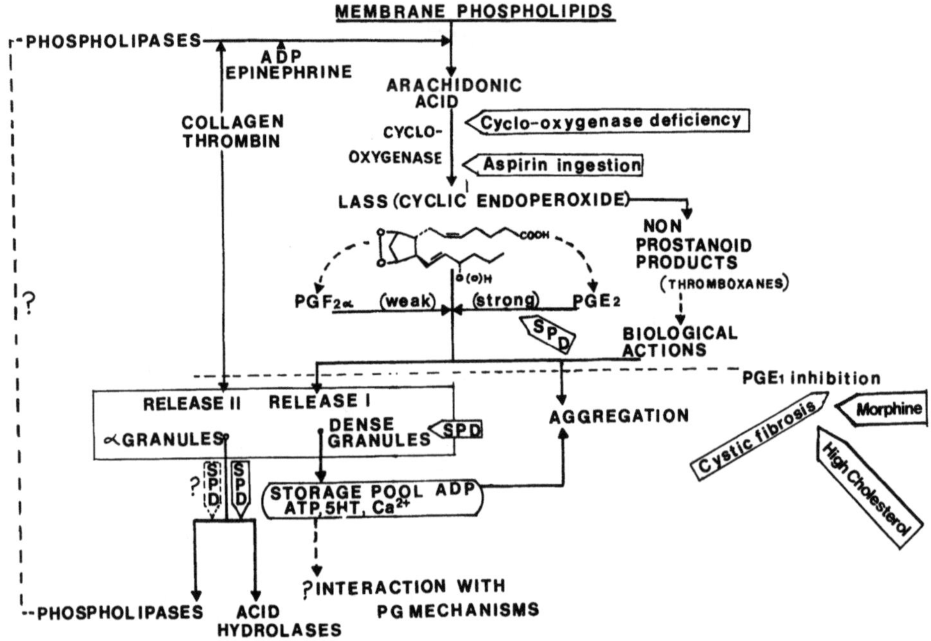

Fig. 5. PG-related defects in platelet aggregation. Activation of phospholipases (mechanism unknown) results in cleavage of arachidonate from membrane phospholipids. Then cyclo-oxygenase converts arachidonate into the endoperoxides PGG_2 and PGH_2, some of which is converted to PGE_2 and $PGF_{2\alpha}$ which are also available from sources outside the platelet. The endoperoxides produce aggregation both directly and through the release of storage pool contents (release I of DAY and HOLMSEN, 1971). Some of the pro-aggregatory effects of endoperoxide may be exerted through conversion to thromboxane A_2 (HAMBERG et al., 1975). The release reaction (I) and consequent aggregation is strongly potentiated by PGE_2. Abnormalities are indicated by large open arrows: (a) *Cyclo-oxygenase defects:* Aspirin ingestion inhibits platelet aggregation through blockade of the cyclo-oxygenase (WILLIS, 1974a; WILLIS et al., 1974a; HAMBERG et al., 1974b; HAMBERG and SAMUELSSON, 1974). Among individuals with aspirin-like defect (WEISS, 1972a), cyclo-oxygenase activity has been reported to be absent in at least one (MALMSTEN et al., 1975). (b) *Storage pool deficiency:* In storage pool disease, PGE_2 is unable to potentiate endoperoxide-induced aggregation (WEISS et al., 1976), partly because of lack of storage pool ADP (PGE_2 potentiates mainly endoperoxide-induced release I). Thus aggregation mediated through ADP release is diminished. (c) *Deficient release of α-granule contents:* SPD platelets also exhibit an impaired release of acid hydrolases (release II), among which is phospholipase A_1 (WILLIS et al., 1972). This may explain why platelet PG production in response to thrombin or high collagen concentrations (which stimulate release II) is abnormally low in storage pool disease (WILLIS and WEISS, 1973). (d) *Cystic fibrosis and EFA deficiency:* Cystic fibrosis patients often have a form of EFA deficiency. In both cystic fibrosis (SAMUELS et al., 1975) and EFA deficiency in rats or man (VINCENT et al., 1974; PRESS et al., 1974), PGE_1 fails to produce its usual inhibition of the platelet aggregation machinery. (e) *High blood cholestrol* can also block the anti-aggregatory effects of PGE_1 (COLMAN et al., 1975). (f) *Morphine-type drugs:* Morphine blocks the anti-aggregatory effect of PGE_1, probably by interfering with the ability of PGE_1 to activate adenylate cyclase (GRYGLEWSKI et al., 1975b)

ATP, ADP, and 5-HT with an increase in ATP/ADP ratio, fewer dense granules but undiminished adhesion to vascular subendothelium (WEISS et al., 1969; HOLMSEN and WEISS, 1970, 1972; WEISS et al., 1974b, 1975, 1976; WEISS, 1975b). A similar SPD defect in haemostasis (Hermansky-Pudlak syndrome) is seen in some albino patients (see WEISS, 1975b) and in fawn hooded rats (TSCHOPP and ZUCKER, 1972; TSCHOPP and WEISS, 1974).

b) PG Mechanisms (Fig. 5)

Recently, additional data has been forthcoming to explain the aggregation defect in storage pool disease and its differentiation from that seen after ingestion of aspirin by normal individuals. SPD platelets, either in PRP or isolated by a gel-filtration technique, are insensitive to the aggregation-inducing effects of arachidonate, although the accompanying production of PGE_2 is not similarly diminished (WEISS et al., 1976). These findings differ markedly from those seen with normal platelets that have been exposed to aspirin and which do not aggregate to arachidonate. In this instance, conversion of arachidonate to PGE_2 is inhibited (SMITH and WILLIS, 1971), through blockade of the cyclo-oxygenase that produces the PG endoperoxide intermediates (WILLIS, 1974a; HAMBERG et al., 1974a, 1974b; WILLIS et al., 1974a; HAMBERG et al., 1975). A logical possibility, therefore, was that responsiveness to endoperoxides is abnormally low in storage pool disease. This hypothesis was confirmed using either crude incubates containing endoperoxides or using highly purified PGH_2. Aggregation induced by PGH_2 was significantly lower in gel-filtered SPD platelets, compared with those from normal individuals, regardless of whether or not they had been taken from patients who had ingested aspirin. Similar results were obtained in PRP. However, the most striking result was seen when the effects of PGH_2 were examined in the presence of PGE_2 (WEISS et al., 1976).

It had earlier been reported (WILLIS, 1974a; WILLIS et al., 1974a) that aggregation produced by small amounts of LASS could be potentiated several fold by pre-incubation of the platelets with PGE_2 (0.01–1 μg/ml), regardless of whether or not aspirin was present. The potentiating effect of PGE_2 was largely or completely lacking when SPD platelets were examined (Fig. 4). This finding can be explained by the ability of PGE_2 to sensitise platelets to release I (of ADP and 5-HT) induced by PGH_2 as previously reported by WILLIS et al. (1974a), i.e. aggregation induced by $PGH_2 + PGE_2$ is mediated largely through release of ADP.

This explains why a potentiation of PGH_2 aggregation by PGE_2 is virtually absent in storage pool disease since (by definition) the dense granule ADP and 5-HT content is low. The fact that PGH_2 alone causes some aggregation of SPD platelets is consistent with the reported ability of PGH_2 to activate platelet aggregation machinery, independent of effects on the release reaction (WILLIS et al., 1974a); the aggregation machinery of SPD platelets is not abnormal (WEISS, 1975b).

To summarise: aspirin-treated platelets respond by aggregation (largely mediated through ADP release) to $PGH_2 + PGE_2$, but cannot themselves produce these pro-aggregatory substances because aspirin has blocked activity of the cyclo-oxygenase (see Fig. 5). The opposite occurs in storage pool disease: the patelets synthesise PGH_2 and PGE_2, but (because of lack of releasable ADP) are rather insensitive to endoperoxide-induced aggregation. Further, fairly conclusive evidence for this hypothesis has emerged from the work of WHITE and WITKOP (1972). They showed that in mixtures of aspirin-treated and SPD (Hermansky-Pudlak syndrome) platelets the second-phase aggregation response was restored to that seen with normal platelets, although, of course, it was absent in SPD or aspirin-treated platelets examined separately. We have confirmed this result in a different group of patients, using adrenaline, collagen or arachidonate as the aggregation stimuli (WEISS et al., 1976). Finally, GERRARD et al. (1975) showed directly that this mutual correction is due to formation of LASS in SPD platelets which acts as an intercellular messenger to produce aggregation of the aspirin-treated platelets.

c) Phospholipase Defects?

To add further interest to the basic picture in storage pool disease, the release II (of α-granule acid hydrolases) which is produced in response to thrombin or "high" concentrations of collagen (DAY and HOLMSEN, 1971) is also abnormally low (HOLMSEN et al., 1975).

A deficient release II might also result in a low output of the lysosomal phospholipase A described by SMITH et al. (1973) the release of which is always closely associated with thrombin-induced PGE_2 and $PGF_{2\alpha}$ formation (WILLIS et al., 1972). These considerations raise the possibility that SPD platelets produce much less PGE_2 and $PGE_{2\alpha}$ than normal platelets when stimulated by thrombin or by high concentrations of collagen[14]. Such findings have been reported by WILLIS and WEISS (1973). In agreement with a phospholipase-(not cyclo-oxygenase) related defect, it was shown that PG production in response to arachidonate (i.e. by-passing the phospholipase stage) was not abnormally low in comparison to that in normal platelets (WEISS et al., 1976).

Consistent with the above hypothesis it was also shown that platelet PG production in SPD platelets was not abnormally low during aggregation stimulated by low concentrations of collagen, although the aggregation response was diminished (WILLIS and WEISS, 1973 and unpublished data). Under these conditions, release II does not occur (and so lysosomal phospholipase would not be released). Instead, another phospholipase A_2 (SCHOENE and IACONO, 1976) which may not reside in lysosomes[15] must be responsible for liberation of the arachidonate precursor for LASS.

The aggregation response is, of course, diminished in storage pool disease because the platelets are insensitive to the pro-aggregatory effects of LASS (through lack of releasable ADP).

d) Phospholipid Defect

In experiments in which mutual correction of the second phase aggregation defect was attempted in mixtures of SPD and aspirin-treated platelets one anomalous finding was obtained. No mutual correction of the aggregation response was ob-

[14] When thrombin or high concentrations of collagen are used to produce aggregation, the response in normal, aspirin-treated or SPD platelets is virtually the same (i.e. maximal). This is because any participation of endoperoxides is swamped by some other aggregation mechanism (mechanism X: see Section C.VI.4).

[15] This enzyme (probably not of lysosomal origin) can even be activated by agents such as adrenaline which can induce release reaction I but not release reaction II.

served when platelets from two members of one particular family were used, though in the same experiments restoration of the aggregation response was seen with SPD platelets from all the other patients examined (WEISS et al., 1976). Earlier, SAFRIT et al. (1972) had reported that the platelet ratio of phosphatidylcholine to phosphaditylethanoline was abnormally high in members of this family, but not in other storage pool disease patients (some of whom were also used in our mutual correction studies). It is, therefore, possible that the aggregation and platelet phospholipid abnormalities in this family are causally related.

e) Significance of Biochemical Findings

Clearly the biochemical and morphological studies of storage pool disease have cast much light on the mechanisms of platelet aggregation. They have, for instance, shown that endoperoxides and/or thromboxane A_2 (LASS) have a role as an intercellular messenger for inducing platelet aggregation (GERRARD et al., 1975). This could explain why transfusion of platelets from donors who have ingested aspirin does not adversely effect haemostasis in the recipient (O'BRIEN, personal communication); presumably the normal platelets already present in the circulation can generate sufficient endoperoxide to cause aggregation of the aspirin-treated platelets.

Perhaps the most important application of basic biochemical investigations of storage pool disease, however, is the development of a rapid and specific platelet aggregation test, i.e. the characteristic lack of PGE_2 potentiation of aggregation induced by PGH_2 (WEISS et al., 1976). Although the pure endoperoxide used in our studies is at present available in only a handful of laboratories, similar results can be obtained using crude enzyme incubates (as described by WILLIS, 1974a). Moreover, past experience suggests that endoperoxides or their stable analogues may soon be commercially available. For instance, a stable analogue of PGH_2 with identical platelet-aggregating properties has recently been described by COREY et al. (1975).

7. **Congenital Aspirin-Like Defects in Aggregation** (see Fig. 5)

There are several individuals with idiopathic haemostatic defects in which there is a characteristic absence of second phase aggregation and a diminished release of ADP (and other dense granule contents) even though the storage pools of these materials are adequate. This platelet defect (or group of defects) is identical to that seen in normal individuals after ingestion of aspirin. For this reason, such patients have been defined as having "aspirin-like defect" (WEISS, 1972a). This similarity with the effects of aspirin-ingestion appears to have an identical biochemical basis to that induced by aspirin, in at least one patient with aspirin-like defect. MALMSTEN et al. (1975) showed that in this individual, the platelet cyclo-oxygenase that converts arachidonate to endoperoxides and thromboxanes was apparently absent, although responsiveness to aggregation induced by pure endoperoxide (PGG_2) was normal. The patient was thus defined as having platelet "cyclo-oxygenase deficiency."

In normal individuals who take aspirin, of course, platelet cyclo-oxygenase is also inhibited. Perhaps the rather more severe haemostatic defect described in cyclo-oxygenase deficiency (compared to that produced by aspirin) is due to the described complete inactivity of the enzyme (MALMSTEN et al., 1975). Aspirin treatment produces a large but still incomplete inhibition of the enzyme (SMITH and WILLIS, 1971;

HAMBERG and SAMUELSSON, 1974; HAMBERG et al., 1974a). In the view of this author, it is unlikely that cyclo-oxygenases throughout the body could be similarly absent in the patient studied by MALMSTEN et al. (1975). If so, one would expect to see symptoms of EFA deficiency, since prostaglandins have many important modulatory roles in most physiological systems (WILLIS and STONE, 1976).

8. Other Platelet Abnormalities

Various additional platelet defects have been described, some of which are associated with altered haemostasis. Such defects may be congenital (as in May-Hegglin anomaly) or in patients who lack PF_3. Other abnormalities may be acquired (as during uremia). A detailed account of these many abnormalities is given by WEISS (1975b).

A recent discovery of interest to prostaglandin workers is the inability of PGE_1 to inhibit platelet aggregation in PRP from patients with cystic fibrosis (SAMUELS et al., 1975) (Fig. 5). Some of these individuals have a form of essential fatty acid deficiency (RIVERS and HASSAM, 1975) and interestingly, a similarly reduced ability of PGE_1 to inhibit aggregation is seen during EFA deficiency in rats (VINCENT et al., 1974) or man (PRESS et al., 1974). High plasma cholesterol levels can also interfere with the antiaggregating effects of PGE_1 (but not of dibutyryl cAMP); interference with PG/platelet membrane interactions is suggested (COLMAN et al., 1975). Morphine can similarly inhibit the ability of PGE_1 to elevate cAMP (GRYGLEWSKI et al., 1975b), although the effects of morphine on haemostosis do not seem to have been studied.

E. The Role of Platelets in Inflammatory Processes

As ZUCKER (1974) pointed out, "platelets play a pivotal role when blood or blood vessels are injured." While it is probably true to say that in general, platelets do not often play the central role in inflammatory processes, they probably do influence the course of many inflammatory reactions by acting as a source for release of pharmacologically active substances. This release can be reduced in part by non-steroid anti-inflammatory agents. In addition, the extraordinary rapidity with which platelets adhere to damaged tissue, aggregate and release potent biologically active materials, suggests that the platelet (like the mast cell) is ideally suited as a cellular trigger for the inflammatory process. Other reviews of the participation of platelets in inflammatory processes have been published (PACKHAM et al., 1968; MUSTARD et al., 1969; RATNOFF, 1969; MUSTARD and PACKHAM, 1971; DE PREZ and MARNEY, 1971; NACHMAN and WEKSLER, 1972; MCFARLANE, 1973; ZUCKER, 1974; SILVER et al., 1974). The role of patelet lysosomes has been reviewed by GORDON (1975), and the lysosomal field in general by HIRSCHHORN (1974).

I. The Platelet as a Source of Pro-Inflammatory Materials

For platelets to play a significant role, they should be able to release pro-inflammatory and injurious substances in response to biological events which initiate inflammation.

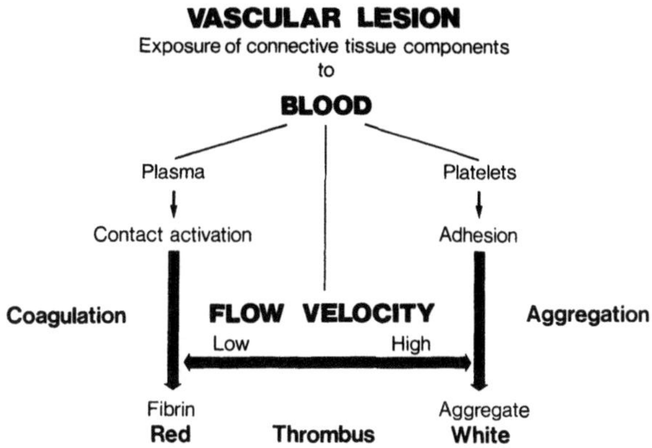

Fig. 6. Whether platelet aggregation or coagulation predominates may depend upon blood flow conditions. Thus, "white thrombi", composed of aggregated platelets are formed most readily in the rapid flow conditions of the arterial circulation. "Red thrombi" (composed of blood cells and serum trapped in a fibrin network) are formed most readily in the sluggish flow conditions of the venous circulation. From BAUMGARTNER (1974b). Reprinted by permission

1. Mediators of Acute Inflammation Released From Platelets

During the release I (DAY and HOLMSEN, 1971) of platelets in response to adhesion or other stimuli (see below), contents of the dense granules are discharged. Among the substances thus released are histamine (in the case of rabbit but not man) and 5-HT. Both amines are potent in inducing increased vascular permeability.

PGE_2, one of the most important mediators of inflammation, is also synthesised and released during the platelet release reaction (SMITH and WILLIS, 1970; SMITH et al., 1973a; WILLIS and WEISS, 1973; WILLIS et al., 1974b). PGE_2 not only increases vascular permeability and releases histamine from mast cells (CRUNKHORN and WILLIS, 1969, 1971a), but also potentiates the pro-inflammatory effects of other mediators (WILLIAMS and MORLEY, 1973; MONCADA et al., 1973). Furthermore, PGE_2 (or its metabolites?) induces a prolonged painfulness of any area in which its concentration has been locally elevated (FERREIRA, 1972; WILLIS and CORNELSEN, 1973; KUHN and WILLIS, 1973). PGD_2 (see Fig. 7) is also produced in platelets (OELZ et al., 1977). It is a potent inducer of increased vascular permeability in rat and man and can potentiate some pro-inflammatory effects of histamine, although not those of bradykinin (FLOWER et al., 1976).

The possible importance of platelet prostaglandin synthesis in inflammation was first suggested by the discovery that ingestion of aspirin or similar non-steroid anti-inflammatory drugs suppresses the biosynthesis of PGE_2 in human platelets (SMITH and WILLIS, 1971). This effect persists for some days (KOCSIS et al., 1973). Interestingly, aspirin also decreases release of dense granule contents and second phase aggregation (see MUSTARD and PACKHAM, 1970).

2. Chemotactic Factors From Platelets

Although there is some evidence to suggest that E-type PGs may be involved in chemotaxis of leucocytes (KALEY and WEINER, 1971a, 1971b; MCCALL and YOULTEN, 1974) or platelets (VALONE et al., 1974, 1975) it is the opinion of this author that

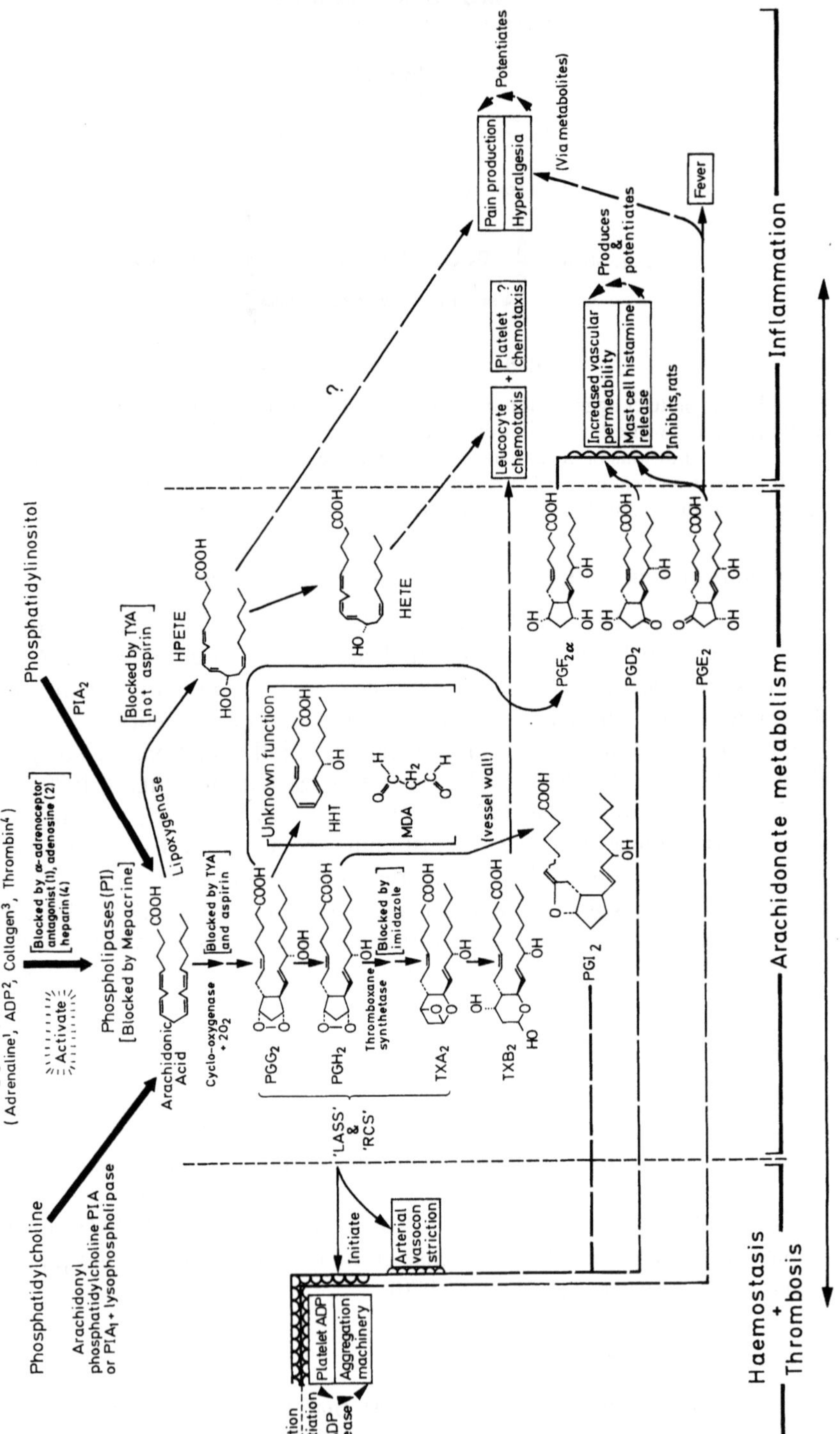
Platelet
Aggregation stimuli
(Adrenaline[1], ADP[2], Collagen[3], Thrombin[4])
Activate
Blocked by α-adrenoceptor antagonist (1), adenosine (2) heparin (4)
Phospholipases (PI)
[Blocked by Mepacrine]
Phosphatidylcholine
Arachidonyl phosphatidylcholine PIA or PIA1 + lysophospholipase
Phosphatidylinositol
PIA2
Arachidonic Acid
COOH
Lipoxygenase
[Blocked by TYA not aspirin]
HPETE
HETE
Cyclo-oxygenase + 2O2
[Blocked by TYA and aspirin]
PGG2
PGH2
Thromboxane synthetase
[Blocked by imidazole]
TXA2
TXB2
PGI2
(vessel wall)
Unknown function
HHT
MDA
PGF2α
PGD2
PGE2
'LASS' & 'RCS'
Initiate
Arterial vasoconstriction
Inhibition
Potentiation
ADP release
Platelet ADP
Aggregation machinery
?
Leucocyte chemotaxis
Platelet chemotaxis ?
Pain production
Hyperalgesia
Potentiates
(Via metabolites)
Fever
Increased vascular permeability
Mast cell histamine release
Inhibits, rats
Produces & potentiates
Haemostasis + Thrombosis
Arachidonate metabolism
Inflammation

PGs per se are not of clearly demonstrable importance in chemotaxis. For instance, high concentrations of PGE_1 are necessary for chemotactic activity in the rabbit and PGE_2 is inactive (KALEY and WEINER, 1971a, 1971b; KALEY et al., 1972) even though PGE_2 and *not* PGE_1 most commonly occurs in inflammatory exudate (WILLIS et al., 1972). It is possible that PGE_1 could have a chemotactic role in the rabbit, since rabbit polymorphonuclear leucocytes have been reported to produce PGE_1 during phagocytosis (HIGGS et al., 1975) and it appears in ocular inflammatory exudate in this species (EAKINS et al., 1972). In the rat, where PGE_2 is the principal PG detected (WILLIS, 1970), the chemotactic properties (if any) of PGE_2 have not yet been reported. However, in vivo experiments with PG synthetase inhibitors such as indomethacin (VANE, 1971) indicate that PG synthesis could be involved in leucocyte chemotaxis in the rat and that platelets are a source of this chemotactic activity (MCCALL and YOULTEN, 1974; SMITH et al., 1976). Perhaps generation of thromboxane B_2 could be responsible for these findings since this is chemotactic (BOOT et al., 1976) and its generation in platelets is inhibited by PG synthesis inhibitors such as indomethacin (Fig. 7). It has been suggested recently that the chemotactic properties of PGE_1 may be an artifact attributable to an easily formed breakdown product (FORD-HUTCHINSON et al., 1976), or to contamination with pyrogens. More recently, MCCLATCHNEY and SNYDERMAN (1976) reported that PGE_2 (but not PGE_1) in

---

◀ Fig. 7. Biological significance of products enzymically formed from arachidonate by platelets. Arachidonate, liberated from membrane phospholipids by platelet phospholipases (see text) is converted by cyclo-oxygenase to the labile endoperoxides PGG_2 and PGH_2. Much of the endoperoxide is then converted to thromboxane B_2 [previously termed PHD; 8-(1-hydroxy-3-oxopropyl)-9,12S-dihydroxy-5Z,10E, heptadecadienoic acid]. A labile intermediate (thromboxane A_2) in this reaction is probably responsible for some of the pro-aggregatory effects of the endoperoxides. They release platelet ADP, thus producing platelet aggregation largely through an indirect mechanism and also produce aggregation by a direct effect on the aggregation machinery of platelets. Vasoconstriction is also produced. PGE_2 and PGD_2 are both derived from the PGG_2 and PGH_2; but PGE_2 strongly potentiates endoperoxide-induced platelet aggregation (mainly through increased ADP release), while PGD_2 is a powerful inhibitor of platelet aggregation in man (WILLIS et al., 1974a; SMITH et al., 1974b; MILLS and MCFARLANE, 1974; NISHIZAWA et al., 1975). Both PGE_2 and PGD_2 produce increased vascular permeability, (in part through release of mast cell histamine) and PGE_2 can potentiate the effects of other inflammatory mediators. PGD_2 acts similarly to PGE_2 in producing increases in vascular permeability. $PGF_{2\alpha}$ can inhibit pro-inflammatory effects of PGE_2 (CRUNKHORN and WILLIS, 1969, 1971a, 1971b). Anti-inflammatory effects are also seen with PGD_1 (FLOWER and KINGSTON, 1976). Similarly, PGE_2 produces hyperalgaesia by potentiating the pain-producing effects of other mediators, among which may be HPETE (12S-hydroperoxy-5,8Z, 10E, 14Z—eicosatetraenoic acid) formed from arachidonate by platelet lipoxygenase; fatty acid hydroperoxides are known to produce pain in man (FERREIRA, 1972). HETE and thromboxane B_2 are potent chemotactic agents. PGE_2 enhances the effects of chemotactic agents (MCCLATCHNEY and SNYDERMAN, 1976) and can produce fever. Also formed from the endoperoxides (PGG_2/PGH_2) are malondialdehyde (MDA) and a C_{17} fatty acid HHT (12S-hydroxy-5Z, 8Z, 10E-heptadecatrienoic acid), but biological actions have not yet been ascribed to these substances. The processes of thrombosis and inflammation are obviously interrelated. For instance, platelet thrombus formation may initiate an inflammatory process, while the formation of PGE_2 in inflammatory tissue could increase the tendency for platelet aggregation to occur. Also shown is the newly discovered unstable PGI_2 (prostacyclin). This is formed by an enzyme in blood vessel walls from PGG_2 or PGH_2 that is generated locally or donated by platelets. (GRYGLEWSKI et al., 1976; JOHNSON et al., 1976). This potently inhibits platelet aggregation or adhesion and it dilates blood vessels However, the exact role of PGI_2 in inflammation has not yet been established.

concentrations of 100 ng/ml or more can sensitize monocytes to the chemotactic activity of complement-activated serum.

In spite of this conflicting evidence concerning the PGs, platelets are undoubtedly a source of potent chemotactic activity. Thus, formation of intravascular platelet thrombi in vivo or accumulation of platelets in subcutaneously implanted sponges is quickly followed by accumulation of leucocytes, which are attracted to the site (see ZUCKER, 1974; SMITH et al., 1976). The release of such chemotactic activity is closely associated with the release reaction (particularly release II) induced by thrombin, as during clotting (STECHER et al., 1971; WEKSLER and COUPAL, 1973). At least part of this activity has recently been attributed by TURNER et al. (1975) to a hydroxy derivative of arachidonate (12S-hydroxy-5,8,10,14-eicosatetraenoic acid; HETE). This is generated from arachidonate by a soluble lipoxygenase in platelets (HAMBERG and SAMUELSSON, 1974; NUGTEREN, 1975, 1977). However, it has also been shown that cationic protein from platelet α-granules is responsible for production of chemotactic activity from the C_5 component of complement (WEKSLER and COUPAL, 1973). This observation extends that of WILKINSON et al. (1969) and STECHER et al. (1971) who showed that two chemotactic proteins were produced in rabbit blood during clotting.

Finally, it must be added that platelets themselves may migrate and that a PG-related mechanism seems to be involved. Thus, indomethacin and TYA inhibit random platelet migration which, in turn, is stimulated by PGE_2, PGE_1 and their respective biosynthetic precursors arachidonate and dihomo-γ-linolenate. An interesting aspect of this work is that the PG synthetase inhibitors block migration stimulated by PGE_2 (the end product of PG synthesis) as well as that of its precursor arachidonic acid (VALONE et al., 1974, 1975).

3. Cationic Proteins and Peptides Which Induce Increased Vascular Permeability

It is interesting to compare the above findings with earlier work of PACKHAM et al. (1968). They observed that a permeability factor from pig platelets produced a delayed effect in association with leucocyte accumulation, while its acute effect was attributable to mast cell amine release. It also induced contractions of guinea pig isolated ileum. This material is probably a cationic protein from platelet α-granules. It is heat stable and has an apparent molecular weight of 39000 daltons (see MUSTARD et al., 1965; PACKHAM et al., 1968; NACHMAN et al., 1970; NACHMAN and WEKSLER, 1972; WEKSLER and COUPAL, 1973).

Bradykinin is an extremely potent pro-inflammatory agent (see Chapters 1 and 14 of this book) and the formation of plasma kinins could well result from release of platelet α-granule contents. These are implicated in initiation of the clotting process and clotting is accompanied by activation of the plasma kinin-forming system (SUZUKI et al., 1970). One of these α-granule pro-coagulation factors (platelet factor 4[PF_4]) acts by blocking the anticoagulant effects of heparin. Although some part of PF_4 activity appears to be associated with the "dense bodies" (DAY et al., 1973), a cationic protein from α-granules may also account for much of this activity (NACHMAN et al., 1972); indeed, the anti-heparin activity of platelets has been shown to consist of a protein of 25000–30000 daltons molecular weight. After release, it may polymerise or complex with macromolecules to form higher molecular weight material (SEAR and POLLER, 1973). SMITH (1974) has suggested that one of the platelet cationic proteins could be a phospholipase, therefore producing its effects indirectly through metabolites of arachidonate.

The other coagulation-promoting material from platelets is PF_3, a phospholipid which helps initiate clotting by acting at various stages in the enzymic cascade, including activation of clotting factor VIII (see Fig. 3). The α-granules may be a source of PF_3, released in association with a lipoprotein that binds acid phosphatase, one of the α-granule acid hydrolases (POLASEK and KUBISZ, 1968; KUBISZ and CAEN, 1972). Both factors (acid phosphatase and PF_3) have a high degree of latency, i.e. they are not released to a significant extent in active form into fluid surrounding the platelets; rather, they become available at the platelet surface.

4. Pro-Inflammatory and Autolytic Enzymes From Platelets

Enzymes from platelet α-granules are also well suited for participation in the pathogenesis of inflammation and tissue injury. They may, for instance, be involved in liberation of arachidonate.

a) Phospholipases

Availability of arachidonate for conversion to prostaglandins and to HETE is almost certainly controlled by activity of the phospholipases A which liberate arachidonate from phospholipids. Arachidonate is the most plentiful single fatty acid in platelet phospholipids, where it accounts for about 20% of the total fatty acid content (MARCUS et al., 1969) and like other unsaturated fatty acids is located mainly at the "2" position of the glyceryl backbone. Saturated fatty acids mainly occupy the "1" position (see BOLDINGH, 1975).

ANDERSON et al. (1971) first suggested that lysosomes were a likely source of phospholipases for production of PGs during inflammation. This suggestion was based upon the clear association between appearance of lysosomal marker enzymes and PGE_2 during carrageenin inflammation in the rat (ANDERSON et al., 1971) and the reported presence of phospholipases A in lysosomes of polymorphonuclear leucocytes and macrophages (ELSBACH and RIZACK, 1963; ELSBACH, 1966) and other tissues (e.g. SMITH and WINKLER, 1968). The discovery that PGs are synthesised by thrombin-treated platelets (SMITH and WILLIS, 1970), a homogenous population of isolated cells, allowed a more meaningful examination of the concept that activity of lysosomal phospholipases is a controlling factor in PG production. Platelet α-granules apparently did contain a phospholipase A (A_1) with an acid pH optimum (SILVER et al., 1971; SMITH et al., 1973b). We observed that there was a parallelism between release of acid hydrolases, phospholipase A_1 (both presumably from α-granules) and PGE_2 and $PGF_{2\alpha}$. This similarity was not seen for platelet 5-HT release and was apparent when either ascending concentrations of thrombin were used to stimulate the platelets or when temporal relationships were examined (WILLIS et al., 1972; WILLIS and SMITH, unpublished results).

Although phospholipase A_1 preferentially attacks the "1" position of phospholipids (which would not contain a great deal of arachidonate), activity of this enzyme could still be the rate-limiting step in formation of PGs, because lysophospholipase

("phospholipase B") can cleave arachidonate from the "2" position, but after the "1" position substituent has first been removed (WILLIS and STONE, 1976). It is also possible that platelet lysosomes contain phospholipase A_2, but that the conditions used for its detection were not optimised. More recently phospholipase A_2 has been detected in platelets (SCHOENE and IACONO, 1976). This is sensitive to activation by various aggregating agents, including adrenaline which does not induce release II but only release I (MILLS et al., 1968). Phosphatidylinositol appears to be the principal source of arachidonate liberated by this platelet phospholipase A_2 (SCHOENE and IACONO, 1976).

This conclusion differs from that of BILLS and SILVER (1975) and BILLS et al. (1977), who used thrombin as the stimulus and determined that phosphatidylcholine was the principal source of arachidonate. Such discrepancies may be reconciled when one considers that the platelet phospholipase A_2 (SCHOENE and IACONO, 1976) is associated with release of platelet amines and ADP (release I) and that the lysosomal phospholipase A of SILVER et al. (1971) and SMITH et al. (1973b) is associated with thrombin-induced release of lysosomal enzymes from α-granules (release II). It would, therefore, not be surprising if substrate specificity of these two enzymes is different. In confirmation of the above findings, BLACKWELL et al. (1977) showed that phosphatidylcholine was a major source of arachidonate release in rabbit platelets stimulated by thrombin or collagen. This release was blocked by mepacrine, which apparently acts through inhibition of platelet phospholipases.

A new aspect of this problem is that the phospholipase that releases arachidonate from phosphatidylcholine cannot release similar fatty acids, including dihomo-γ-linolenate (precursor for PGE_1), although release of both arachidonate and dihomo-γ-linolenate can occur from platelet phosphatidylinositol (BILLS et al., 1977).

One final point to consider in discussion of platelet phospholipases is that the lysosomal phospholipase liberated from platelets during release II could be involved in liberation of arachidonate (and hence PGs or related products) at sites adjacent to platelet aggregates, thus propagating the inflammatory response. Although this possibility might appear remote, it would explain, for instance, why thrombin-like mechanisms may be involved in inflammation (WISEMAN and CHANG, 1968). However, corticosteroids cannot act to inhibit platelet PG production and release (SMITH and WILLIS, 1971) as they have been reported to do in rabbit adipose tissue, perfused guinea pig lungs and cultures of rheumatoid synovia and mouse fibrosarcoma (LEWIS and PIPER, 1975; GRYGLEWSKI et al., 1975a; KANTROWITZ et al., 1975; TASHJIAN et al., 1975).

Since this particular anti-inflammatory effect has been attributed to inhibition of arachidonate release by phospholipases (HONG and LEVINE, 1976), there is further reason to suggest that platelet phospholipases differ from those in several other tissues [16].

b) PG Synthetases

It goes almost without saying that platelets contain the necessary enzymes to convert arachidonate (liberated by phospholipases) into PG endoperoxides (see WILLIS et al.,

---

[16] Hydrocortisone also does not inhibit prostaglandin release in perfused dog spleen (FERREIRA et al., 1971) or superfused rabbit spleen (WILLIS, unpublished data 1970).

1974a). A recent advance in this area has been the apparent isolation of the PG synthetase (cyclo-oxygenase) of platelets. It has long been known that aspirin irreversibly acetylates platelet protein (AL-MONDHIRY et al., 1970), thus explaining why aspirin ingestion induces a prolonged and parallel inhibition of second phase platelet aggregation and platelet production of PGs (KOCSIS et al., 1973); presumably a new population of aspirin-free platelets has to be produced (WEISS, 1975b). ROTH and MAJERUS (1975) used [acetyl ^{3}H] aspirin and isolated a labelled protein (approximate molecular weight of 85000 daltons) from the particulate fraction of platelets, which was identical to or associated with the cyclo-oxygenase enzyme. A similar protein present in sheep vesicular gland has also been shown to be labelled with [acetyl ^{3}H aspirin] and to have a molecular weight that is virtually the same as the platelet protein (ROTH et al., 1975). It has yet to be shown that the isolated cyclo-oxygenase capable of acetylation by aspirin is indeed capable of converting arachidonate into PG endoperoxides. However, acetylation of the 85000 daltons molecular weight protein does parallel inhibition of PG synthesis (ROTH et al., 1975). According to GERRARD et al. (1976) membranes of the dense tubular system (Fig. 1A) are the main site of arachidonate cyclo-oxygenation.

c) Proteases

Other enzymes (Table 1) in platelet α-granules (lysosomes) are well suited to play a role in chronic inflammation and tissue damage. For instance, cathepsins can cause loss of proteoglycan ground substance in cartilage (MORRISON et al., 1973). Furthermore, the acid cathepsin activity of human platelets is similar to the cathepsin found in carrageenin granuloma (LEGRAND et al., 1973). Elastase and collagenase from platelet α-granules could also attack the fibrous support of connective tissue, cartilage, and vascular subendothelium. The implication of elastase in pulmonary emphysema (MITTMAN, 1972) is of interest when it is considered how readily platelet aggregates accumulate in the lungs and adhere to damaged tissue (ZUCKER, 1974). Finally, the possibility cannot be ruled out that proteases and other substances from platelets could be involved in the pathogenesis of rheumatoid arthritis. It has, for instance, already been suggested that the PGs present in the synovial fluid of inflamed joints may be of platelet origin (GLATT et al., 1974; SWINSON et al., 1976).

The collagenase of human platelets (CHESNEY et al., 1974) is of special interest, since it is readily activated (and simultaneously released) by exposure of the platelets to ADP, even in concentrations too low to induce release of 5-HT or β-glucuronidase. Indeed, this activation/release of platelet collagenase appears to be associated with the ADP-induced shape change rather than release reaction I or II. This platelet collagenase destroys the platelet-aggregating properties of collagen and its activity is suppressed by EDTA and by factors (including α_1-antitrypsin) from normal human plasma (CHESNEY et al., 1974). This activity of platelet collagenase could be an important regulatory factor in the pathogenesis of haemostasis, thrombosis and inflammatory processes involving platelets.

d) Other Platelet Lysosomal Enzymes

Other lysosomal enzymes present in the α-granules include glycosidases (e.g. β-glucuronidase), phosphatases and aryl sulphatase (GORDON, 1975), although no clear pathophysiological function has yet been ascribed to them.

Table 1. Lysosomal enzymes from platelets

a) Proteolytic enzymes in lysosomes of human platelets

Enzyme	Substrate	Optimum pH
Cathepsin A	Bovine haemoglobin Carbobenzoxy-α-L-Glu-L-Tyr	3.5
Cathepsin C(?)	Bovine haemoglobin	3.5–5.0
Cathepsin D	Bovine haemoglobin	3.3
Collagenase	[^{14}C]glycine-labelled collagen	Not reported
Elastase	^{125}I-labelled elastin $AcAla_3OMe$	8.0

b) Glycosidases in lysosomes of human platelets

Enzyme	Substrate	pH
β-glucuronidase	phenolphthaleinmono-β-glucuronide	5.0
β-N-acetyl-glucosaminidase	p-nitrophenyl-N-acetyl-glucosaminidase	4.5
D-galactosidase	p-nitrophenyl-β-D-galactoside	3.6
α-mannosidase	p-nitrophenyl-α-D-mannoside	4.8

c) Characteristics of platelet enzymes liberating 4-methyl-umbelliferone from glycoside conjugates

Enzyme	Substrate	Optimum pH	Substrate conc (mM)
β-glucuronidase	4MU-β-D-glucuronide trihydrate	4.5	1.5
β-N-acetyl-glucosaminidase	4MU-2-acetamido-2-deoxy-β-D-glucopyranoside	4.9	3.0
β-galactosidase	4MU-β-D-galactopyranoside monohydrate	4.3	1.5
α-galactosidase	4MU-α-D-galactopyranoside	4.5	1.5
β-glucosidase	4MU-β-D-glucopyranoside	5.3	3.0
α-glucosidase	4MU-α-D-glucopyranoside	5.5	3.0
α-mannosidase	4MU-α-D-mannopyranoside	4.7	3.0
α-arabinosidase	4MU-α-L-arabinopyranoside	4.8	3.0
β-xylosidase	4MU-β-D-xylopyranoside	5.6	3.0

d) Aryl sulphatase activity in platelets

Animal species	Sulphatase activity (μmol 4MU-phosphate/10^{11} platelets/h)
Man	4.6
Rat	2.0
Rabbit	2.6

Data compiled by GORDON (1975), reprinted by permission.

II. Evidence for Participation of Platelets in Various Inflammatory Diseases

From the information reviewed above (Section E.I), platelets may be involved in various inflammatory conditions. Let us now examine the available evidence for this possibility.

1. Acute Inflammatory Responses Induced in the Rat by Non-Immunological Mechanisms

Evidence for involvement of platelets in non-immunological types of inflammation is rather scant.

a) Carrageenin Inflammation

Prior to 1975, some circumstantial evidence existed to implicate platelets in inflammation induced by carrageenin. In vitro, carrageenin potentiates second phase aggregation of human platelets (SHIO and RAMWELL, 1972) and releases PGs from rat platelets (GLENN et al., 1972). Also, WISEMAN and CHANG (1968) showed that a thrombin-like mechanism appeared to be involved in carrageenin-induced paw oedema in the rat, while accumulation of lysosomal enzymes in the inflamed paws (COPPI and BONARDI, 1968) could possibly be related to platelet accumulation.

UBATUBA et al. (1975) used anti-rat platelet serum (produced by immunisation of rabbits with rat platelets) to examine the role of platelets in acute inflammation in rat hind paws. They found that anti-platelet serum reduced the blood platelet count to <2% of that in untreated rats. However, in such thrombocytopenic rats the paw oedema response to carrageenin was unaltered, as was the ability of indomethacin to reduce the carrageenin response. Thus, neither platelets nor platelet PGs may be involved in carrageenin oedema. This evidence should not, however, be regarded as immutable; it is possible that in normal animals, platelets release a non-prostanoate pro-inflammatory material the release of which is not inhibited by indomethacin and of which the effects are usually eclipsed by the presence of other mediators.

b) In vivo Bronchoconstriction

Bronchoconstriction in the guinea pig is a model of inflammation (VANE, 1973) in which accumulation of platelet clumps in the pulmonary circulation could be partially responsible for the bronchoconstrictor response. Bronchoconstrictor agents (including PG endoperoxides) are released from aggregating platelets (HAMBERG et al., 1974a, 1974b; WILLIS et al., 1974a) while lung tissue itself releases PGs and RCS when the pulmonary circulation is disrupted by emboli (PIPER and VANE, 1971).

In line with such possibilities, LEFORT and VARGAFTIG (1975) used anti-platelet serum to show that the bronchoconstrictor response to intravenous ADP or ATP (which is converted to ADP in vivo) or arachidonate did involve formation of pulmonary platelet emboli. Bronchoconstriction induced by bradykinin did not appear to be secondary to platelet aggregation and indeed bradykinin was devoid of platelet-aggregating activity in vitro, even allowing for its rapid inactivation by kininases (LEFORT and VARGAFTIG, 1975). The bronchoconstriction produced by intravenous injection of anti-platelet serum clearly involves platelets since it can be prevented by previous treatment of the animals with anti-platelet serum (LEFORT and VARGAFTIG, 1975).

c) Inflammation Engendered by Local Injection of Arachidonate

Possibly another situation in which platelets may be involved is the inflammation engendered by injection of arachidonate in the rat hind paw. It is now well known, for instance, that injection of arachidonate into the blood vessels of various species can induce intravascular platelet aggregation (see SPECTOR et al., 1975).

If platelets are involved in this response, then pro-inflammatory material released from them cannot be attributable completely to prostaglandins since indomethacin (10 mg/kg intraperitoneally) only partially reduces the pro-inflammatory effects of arachidonate in the rat paw (WILLIS and BARUTH, unpublished results; COTTNEY et al., 1976); perhaps a non-specific detergent effect of the sodium arachidonate (SPECTOR et al., 1975) could be involved.

2. Inflammation Produced by Immunological Mechanisms

a) The Reaction to Anti-Platelet Serum

Platelets would be expected to be involved in the inflammatory response produced by injection of anti-platelet serum, since this produces aggregation and lysis of platelets in vitro and release of vasoactive substances from platelets in vivo (UBATUBA et al., 1975). The bronchoconstrictor or hypotensive response to anti-platelet serum clearly involves platelets (LEFORT and VARGAFTIG, 1975). In the rat hind paw, however, the inflammatory response following sub-plantar injection of anti-platelet serum is not reduced by prior depletion of circulating platelet levels (by intravenous injection of anti-platelet serum). Interestingly, the pharmacological mechanisms involved in this inflammatory response are obscure since the paw oedema is not reduced by indomethacin, or by anti-5-HT or anti-histamine agents alone or in combination (UBATUBA et al., 1975).

b) Passive Cutaneous Anaphylaxis (PCA)

This is the cutaneous inflammation produced at localised sites previously injected with antibody (sensitisation) when the animal is intravenously injected with antigen (challenge). When this test is carried out 24 h or more after sensitisation, the response involves a "homocytotropic" ("mast-cell sensitising" or "reagenic") type of antibody which is heat labile and has a high affinity for binding to tissue at the injection site. Reactions involving homocytotropic antibody usually involve release of histamine and 5-HT from the sensitised mast cells and are independent of complement. In contrast, when the animal is challenged only a few hours after sensitisation, precipitating-type antibodies are involved (and antigen/antibody complexes may be formed); both blood cells and complement may be involved. This topic is further dealt with by STECHSHULTE and AUSTEN (1974).

In the rabbit, HENSON and COCHRANE (1969a) showed that the PCA reaction involving homocytotropic antibody did not appear to require platelets (depleted by injection with anti-platelet serum) or complement (depleted with cobra venom). The pharmacological mediators involved were not examined. However, in skin sensitised by the precipitating type of antibody, the inflammatory reaction appeared to involve platelets, neutrophils, complement and release of histamine (which in the rabbit is mainly contained in the platelets). It was suggested that antigen/antibody complexes reacted with complement and aggregated platelets by an immune adherence mechanism which also induced them to release histamine (HENSON and COCHRANE, 1969a).

In the rat hind paw, the PCA system involving only homocytotropic antibody has been examined for involvement of platelets (UBATUBA et al., 1975). It was shown that the PCA reaction involved (as previously shown in many laboratories) release of mast cell amines. Treatment with anti-platelet serum or indomethacin did not reduce that PCA reaction, thus eliminating involvement of both PGs and platelets. Rat PCA reactions involving non-homocytotropic antibody do not yet seem to have been similarly examined.

c) Anaphylactic Shock

This is a sudden, usually fatal reaction following intravenous injection of antigen into highly sensitised animals (LEAK and BURKE, 1974). The principal signs of anaphylaxis in various species depend upon the main "shock organ" (in dog, the liver; in guinea pig, the lungs). In the rabbit, the main feature of anaphylaxis is pulmonary embolism and circulatory collapse, following intravascular aggregation of platelets and the release from them of vasoactive material (see BECKER and AUSTEN, 1968; MOVAT et al., 1968) including histamine and 5-HT (WAALKES et al., 1957a, 1957b), although release of these amines does not appear to be the principal cause of death (which is not prevented by anti-5-HT or anti-histamine agents) (FISCHER and LECOMTE, 1956; REUSE, 1956). High doses of heparin, however, do exert a protective effect with an associated reduction in platelet consumption (JOHANSSON, 1960). The pharmacological mediation of anaphylaxis in rabbits is incompletely understood but the role of platelets is certainly known to be important. Post-mortem examination of rabbits killed by anaphylactic shock shows that the lungs are congested with platelet aggregates and antigen/antibody complexes, and so it is likely that the mechanism observed by HENSON and COCHRANE (1969b) (i.e. basophil release of pro-aggregatory substances) might be involved (see Section E.II.2.d). To support this assumption, intravenous injection of antigen/antibody complexes into rabbits produces a similar fatal congestion of the lungs by platelet aggregates and this effect is prevented by pretreatment of the rabbits with non-steroid anti-inflammatory drugs which prevent platelet aggregation (MUSTARD et al., 1969). Unfortunately, no one seems to have similarly examined whether anti-aggregatory drugs can protect rabbits against anaphylactic shock!

d) The Arthus Reaction and Serum Sickness

The Arthus reaction is the localised inflammatory and necrotic reaction produced when antigen is injected into the skin of highly sensitised animals (see COCHRANE and JANOFF, 1974). Serum sickness of the acute type follows a single injection (for therapeutic purposes) of a foreign serum (usually horse serum) for its content of antibody. Some 8–12 days after the injection, urticaria, fever, oedema, neutropenia and lymph-node enlargement are seen; but this reaction is non-fatal and reversible.

Chronic serum sickness after repeated injection of foreign serum is more serious, producing glomerular lesions in the kidney and arteritis. This topic is dealt with in depth by LEBER and MCCLUSKY (1974).

In both the Arthus reaction and serum sickness, tissue damage is produced by localisation of antigen/antibody complexes in the tissues. Some of the inflammation and most of the tissue damage is produced by the release of injurious substances from accumulating neutrophils (HENSON, 1971). Thus, such reactions are diminished in neutropenic animals (see HIRSCH, 1974) and in the Arthus reaction, neutrophils have been demonstrated by electron microscopy (DAEMS and OORT, 1962). Substances from the neutrophils probably include autolytic enzymes and cationic proteins (JANOFF and ZWEIFACH, 1964; ZEYA and SPITZNAGEL, 1971; see WEISSMAN, 1967). However, there is ample evidence to show that these events do not take place unless vascular permeability is increased sufficiently for tissue deposition of the antigen/antibody complexes to occur. This has clearly been shown for serum sickness in rabbits (KNIKER and COCHRANE, 1968; COCHRANE and DIXON, 1968). In mice and guinea pigs, mast cells are apparently the source of the amines which produce this increased vascular permeability. However, in rabbits, these amines are released mainly from platelets undergoing the release reaction (there are few tissue mast cells). Thus, prior depletion of platelets, or pretreatment with antagonists of histamine and 5-HT, inhibit the tissue changes in serum sickness (COCHRANE, 1971) or the Arthus reaction (MARGARETTEN and MCKAY, 1971). HENSON and COCHRANE (1969b, 1970) have provided in vitro evidence that the clumping of platelets in serum sickness and the Arthus reaction probably involve a reaction between the antigen and sensitised basophils, which then release agents inducing aggregation and release reaction in the platelets. This mechanism is apparently independent of the complement system.

Additional evidence that platelet aggregation is involved in the Arthus reaction has been provided by the ability of sulphinpyrazone to inhibit the Arthus reaction and accompanying thrombocytopenia (BUTLER and WHITE, 1975): sulphinpyrazone is an anti-aggregating drug with reported clinical efficacy against thrombosis (see MUSTARD and PACKHAM, 1975).

e) Reaction to Endotoxin and the Shwartzman Reaction

Endotoxin is the lipopolysaccharide(s) from the wall of gram-negative bacteria (E. Coli, for instance). Addition of endotoxin in vitro to platelets of rabbit or dog can induce them to aggregate and release their content of amines; PF_3 is also "made available" (MCKAY et al., 1958; DES PREZ et al., 1961; HINSHAW et al., 1961; HOROWITZ et al., 1962). Platelet PGs may also be released, since in vivo work shows a protective effect of PG synthetase inhibitors (see below). Only slight effects of endotoxin are seen on human platelets (MEULLER-ECKHARDT and LÜSCHER, 1968; REAM et al., 1965; NAGAYAMA et al., 1971).

The reaction of platelets with endotoxin requires Ca^{++} ions and a plasma protein which is heat labile and inactivated by zymosan. Although this is not the C_3 component of complement, it could be properdin (DES PREZ et al., 1961; DES PREZ and BRYANT, 1966; DES PREZ, 1967; DES PREZ and MARNEY, 1971). In contrast to these findings, ZIMMERMAN and MÜLLER-EBERHARD (1971) observed that the C_6 component of complement was necessary for endotoxin-induced prothrombin consumption (with enhanced coagulation) in rabbit blood. Platelet phagocytosis of endotoxin with accompanying degranulation (DAVIS, 1966; SPIELVOGEL, 1967) may also be involved in the reaction to endotoxin. The possibility of an immunological basis of the endotoxin reaction involving a naturally present antibody has still not been resolved.

SHWARTZMAN (1928) originally described two reactons to endotoxin injection in the rabbit. The final event consists of a local inflammatory response in the skin upon intradermal injection of bacterial endotoxin (a localised in vivo endotoxin reaction). The second reaction follows an intravenous injection of endotoxin in the same animals and characteristically produces haemhorragic necrosis of the previously injected skin site (the local Schwartzman reaction).

When injected intravenously, endotoxin produces marked cardiovascular symptoms, which in the cat, for instance, consist of an acute phase of arterial hypotension and decrease in myocardial contractility. This is followed by a delayed response (shock) with systemic hypotension (probably involving increased vascular permeability), reduced cardiac output and metabolic acidosis (PARRAT, 1973). In animals which have been previously sensitised (18–24 h earlier) with intravenous endotoxin, the injection of endotoxin results in a generalised Shwartzman reaction. This may be regarded as a model of disseminated intravascular coagulation (see RODMAN, 1973).

Sensitisation by the endotoxin may involve the intervention of polymorphonuclear leucocytes (COCHRANE and JANOFF, 1974) which are a rich source of pro-inflammatory and injury producing substances (JANOFF, 1972). However, an immunological basis for the Shwartzman reactions has not been established. It is interesting that sensitisation to endotoxin can be produced in vitro, since platelets are rendered more sensitive to aggregation by endotoxin when the plasma had previously been exposed to endotoxin (DES PREZ et al., 1961; SPIELVOGEL, 1967).

As expected from the in vitro data discussed already, platelets are essential for the reaction to endotoxin in vivo (MARGARETTEN and MCKAY, 1969) and it is probable that they are responsible for initiation of coagulation through increased availability of PF_3 and other pro-coagulation factors from the aggregating platelets. Thus, when injected intravenously in dog or rabbit, endotoxin rapidly accumulates in platelets rather than other blood cells [17] (BRAUDE et al., 1955; HERRING et al., 1963) and there is an elevation in plasma levels of 5-HT and PF_3 activity (DAVIS et al., 1960; DES PREZ et al., 1961; HOROWITZ et al., 1962).

Furthermore, as would be expected if platelets were involved, the cardiovascular platelet response to endotoxin in dogs can be inhibited by drugs which inhibit aggregation, such as BL 3459 (FLEMING et al., 1975) and non-steroid anti-inflammatory drugs such as indomethacin (NORTHOVER and SUBRAMANIAN, 1962; ERDÖS, 1968; SOLOMON and HINSHAW, 1968; HALL et al., 1972). A similar protective effect of indomethacin has also been observed in the cat (PARRAT and STURGESS, 1973), while VAN ARMAN (1970) showed that indomethacin could suppress the local Shwartzman reaction in rabbit skin.

Heparin also provides protection against the in vivo effects of endotoxin by preventing activation of coagulation (GOOD and THOMAS, 1953; CLUFF and BER-

[17] In primates, endotoxin adheres to erythrocytes rather than platelets. The opposite occurs in rabbits, rats, dogs, and guinea pigs (SPIELVOGEL, 1967).

THRONG, 1953). This would also mean that thrombin-induced platelet PG output would be reduced (WILLIS and SMITH, unpublished) and that formation of plasma kinins by clotting would be suppressed.

Supporting histological evidence for the above pharmacological studies is available. Thus, platelet aggregates have been detected in the microvasculature following the provocative injection of endotoxin in rabbits or hamsters. The platelet aggregates are found in association with leucocytes and fibrin (SILVER and STEHBENS, 1965; TAICHMAN et al., 1965).

Recent work has shown that PG endoperoxides are involved in the irreversible platelet aggregation response, in turn suggesting that PG mechanisms are involved in the pathophysiological changes induced by endotoxin. Such involvement has been shown directly in the dog knee-joint; HERMAN and MONCADA (1975) and HERMAN (1975), showed that the painful and incapacitating inflammation of the knee produced by local injection of endotoxin (with or without a prior sensitising injection) was accompanied by an output of PGs (probably PGE_2 and $PGF_{2\alpha}$) into the synovial space. Furthermore, indomethacin prevented the incapacitation and concomitantly suppressed PG production. It had earlier been shown that intra-articular injection of E- and F-type PGs in the dog results in a prolonged incapacitation (ROSENTHALE et al., 1972). Clearly, the use of endotoxin may continue to provide us with models for the study of thrombotic and inflammatory conditions involving platelets, prostaglandins and clotting.

f) Reaction to Bacteria and Viruses

CLAWSON and WHITE (1971) showed that staphylococci and other bacteria could induce aggregation of human platelets in citrated PRP, provided that there was a 1:1 ratio of bacteria to platelets. Rabbit platelets have been reported to be more sensitive to aggregation by bacteria (see ZUCKER, 1974). Washed human platelets in the presence of γ-globulin also aggregate when exposed to bacteria and release their granular substituents (PACKHAM et al., 1968), although phagocytosis of the bacteria does not seem to take place (MUSTARD and PACKHAM, 1970). In PRP, neither human nor rabbit platelets killed the bacteria within 2 h of aggregation induced by them (CLAWSON and WHITE, 1971). In contrast, WEKSLER and NACHMAN (1971) showed that endotoxin (from gram-negative bacteria) did release an anti-bacterial cationic protein from platelet granules, the activity of which was inhibited by heparin.

These discrepancies may be explained if in the studies of CLAWSON and WHITE, (1971), and other similar investigations, only release I (of dense body constituents) was produced. Thus, anti-bacterial protein was not liberated, since this is presumably located in the α-granules and would only be released during release II produced by endotoxin. (There is evidence that α-granule constituents are released during endotoxin shock—see Section E.II.2.e.) This idea could explain why antibacterial material including that from platelets, is released into serum during clotting (ZUCKER, 1974). It would also explain why platelets fail to kill bacteria which do not produce endotoxin (i.e. gram-positive strains).

The reaction of platelets with viruses could be of greater significance. There are several reports that both live and dead influenza viruses are: a) absorbed by human platelets (TERADA et al., 1966); b) in vivo produce prolonged thrombocytopenia, possibly attributable to platelet aggregation, as seen in vitro (MOTULSKY, 1953; LU, 1958; JERUSHALMY et al., 1961; BROUN and BROUN, 1962), and c) induce the platelet release reaction (PACKHAM et al., 1968). The reaction of viruses with human platelets appears to involve absorption onto the platelet surface, followed by phagocytosis (SCHULZ and LANDGRÄBER, 1966). This may involve interaction with platelet surface glycoproteins (PEPPER and JAMEISON, 1968). The uptake of viruses into platelets may, as in the case of Chitungunya virus, lead to protection of the viruses against heat inactivation (LARKE and WHEELOCK, 1969).

From the facts above it is difficult to assess whether or not the formation of platelet aggregates around bacteria or viruses has any biological significance. A possible exception is the case of the anti-bacterial protein released by the endotoxin of some bacteria (WEKSLER and NACHMAN, 1971). It has, however, been shown that phagocytosis of particles by platelets, with resulting thrombocytopenia, may result in increased uptake of the platelets (+particles) into the reticuloendothelial system (VAN AKEN et al., 1968). In this way, perhaps, uptake of viruses into platelets aids defensive mechanisms of the body.

g) Graft Rejection

The rejection and deterioration of function in allografts is a good example of a situation where aggregation and the release reaction of platelets is centrally involved. This is particularly well documented in the case of kidney transplants. Organisation of thrombi leads to intinal thickening and chronic obliterative vascular lesions with progressive ischaemic atrophy of the renal parenchyma distal to the narrowed vessels. Graft failure coincides with these histological changes. These events have been shown experimentally in dogs (LOWENHAUPT and NATHAN, 1969) and in human patients (PORTER, 1967; KINCAID-SMITH, 1967). Biopsies in man have shown the appearance of platelet thrombi within 24 h of rejection, but the earliest histological change is adherence of cells (mainly polymorphs) to the endothelium (KINCAID-SMITH, 1967).

It is probable that antigen/antibody complexes are involved in the rejection phenomenon, because γ-globulin is found in association with the endothelium and basement membrane of vessels in renal allografts undergoing rejection (PORTER, 1967; LOWENHAUPT and NATHAN, 1968). The sequence of such events has been followed by transplanting a small piece of kidney into transparent ear chambers and carrying out time-lapse photo-microscopy, and the results compared with those of electron microscopy (HOBBS, 1973). In this study, the initial cellular response at 2 days was adherence of single platelets, and leucocytes to the vascular endothelium of the graft. Electron micrographs revealed that the platelets released contents of their granules (particularly the electron-dense amine-storage granules). These results suggest that release of substances from platelets (and leucocytes) produces or accelerates the blood vessel injury and other tissue changes leading to rejection of the transplant. The substances thus released from the platelets would include the PG endoperoxides and thromboxanes (see Section E.I) which are potent platelet-aggregating and vasoconstrictor agents.

Also, it should be remembered that kidney lipid droplets can be a source of free arachidonic acid (COMAI et al., 1975) which could (through endoperoxide mechanisms) produce many of the platelet aggregation changes described. Chemotactic substances from the platelets could be involved in attraction of leucocytes (see Section E.I.2).

Pharmacological evidence for the above ideas is available from the clinical work of MOWBRAY (1966) who showed that ^{51}Cr-labelled platelets accumulated in rejecting kidney transplants, but that in cases where the threatened rejection was successfully treated with drugs, the platelets escaped from the kidney back into the circulation. The drugs used were hydrocortisone (an immunosuppressive anti-inflammatory agent) and phenylbutazone, which is known to inhibit the irreversible type of platelet aggregation and the release (release I) of vasoactive and pro-aggregatory amines and nucleotides from the platelets. MATTHEW et al. (1971) reported that similar protective effects were produced in dogs by aspirin and prednisolone, although dipyridamole was without effect. The mechanism of action of phenylbutazone or aspirin in these studies was almost certainly through blockade of PG endoperoxide biosynthesis (see WILLIS et al., 1974a; WEISS, 1975b; Section E.I). The corticosteroids probably acted through their immunosuppressive and anti-inflammatory properties.

There is also some evidence that rejection of skin allografts involves platelets. Thus, BALLANTYNE et al. (1972) showed that there was a profound fall in circulating platelet levels during rejection of skin allografts in rats. A similar drop in platelet count did not occur in rats receiving autografts. In contrast to the findings with kidney allografts, platelets did not appear to accumulate in the skin. One possibility put forward involved formation of antigen/antibody complexes which activate complement (circulating complement levels fall). This would produce platelet aggregates with their elimination via the reticuloendothelial system.

F. Concluding Remarks

The following is a summary of the most important points covered in this chapter.

I. Haemostasis

Platelets as morphologically and biochemically equipped to act as "patrolling prison wardens" in the blood circulation. When the vascular wall is breached, the platelets adhere together over the exposed subendothelium and form a platelet plug which staunches the leakage of blood. They also release substances (PF_3 and PF_4) that help in formation of the network of fibrin laid down over the damaged area; this more effectively prevents leakage.

II. Platelet Aggregation Mechanisms

In haemostasis and thrombosis, collagen and thrombin may be the most important stimuli to platelet aggregation. The principal biochemical mechanism (defined here as mechanism X) is still not understood. Platelet production of pro-aggregatory endoperoxides and thromboxanes (LASS+RCS) is important but probably plays a secondary role to mechanism X in thrombosis and haemostasis. Thus, drugs such as aspirin that inhibit synthesis of endoperoxides usually have only a slight effect in prolonging bleeding and preventing thrombosis.

Involvement of endoperoxides in haemostasis is, however, indicated by the existence of congenital platelet disorders in which there is prolonged bleeding. In such cases platelet synthesis of endoperoxides may be absent (cyclo-oxygenase deficiency), or the platelets may be insensitive to endoperoxide-induced aggregation (storage pool disease).

III. Inflammation

Release of inflammatory mediators (histamine, 5-HT, PGE_2, HETE, and cationic proteins) from platelets may play an initiating role in some types of inflammatory disease, including the Arthus reaction, the Shwartzman reaction, endotoxin shock and tissue graft rejection.

In addition, release of chemotactic agents and lysosomal enzymes from the platelet may be involved in some types of chronic inflammation.

Acknowledgments. Thanks are due to Dr. L. O. RANDALL, Dept. of Pharmacology, Hoffmann-La Roche Inc. for his hospitality to me during my tenure as Visiting Scientist, 1972–1974; to Ms. DIANE TURNER for preparation of the typescript and to Mr. P. MARPLES and Mr. N. MEEN for help with the bibliography. Most of all I thank my wife Tina for her help and support.

References

Ahern, D. G., Downing, D. T.: Inhibition of prostaglandin biosynthesis in sheep vesicular tissue by eicosa-5,8,11,14-tetraynoic acid. Biochim. biophys. Acta (Amst.) **210**, 456—461 (1970)

Ahtee, L., Michal, F.: Effects of sympathomimetic amines on rabbit platelet aggregation in vitro. Brit. J. Pharmacol. **44**, 363 P—364 P (1972)

Alexander, B., Odake, K., Lawlor, D., Swangler, M.: Coagulation, haemostasis and plasma expanders; a quarter century enigma. Fed. Proc. **34**, 1429—1440 (1975)

Al-Mondhiry, H., Marcus, A. J., Spaet, T. H.: On the mechanism of platelet function inhibition by acetylsalicyclic acid. Proc. Soc. exp. Biol. (N.Y.) **133**, 632—636 (1970)

Amer, M. S., Marquis, N. R.: The effect of prostaglandins, epinephrine and aspirin on cyclic AMP phosphodiesterase activity of human blood platelets and their aggregation. In: Ramwell, P. W., Pharriss, B. B. (Eds.): Prostaglandins in Cellular Biology, pp. 93—110. New York-London: Plenum Press 1972

Anderson, A. J., Brocklehurst, W. E., Willis, A. L.: Evidence for the role of lysosomes in the formation of prostaglandins during carrageenin-induced inflammation in the rat. Pharmacol. Res. Commun. **3**, 13—19 (1971)

Ardlie, N. G.: Mechanism of platelet aggregation and disease. Their possible role in vascular injury. Perspect. Nephrol. Hypertens. **1**, 891—905 (1973)

Ardlie, N. G., Perry, D. W., Packham, M. A., Mustard, J. F.: Stability of suspensions of washed rabbit platelets. Proc. Soc. exp. Biol. (N.Y.) **136**, 1021—1023 (1971)

Aster, R. H.: Observations on survival time, sites of sequestration and production rate of platelets in idiopathic thrombocytopenic purpura. Blood **28**, 1014—1015 (1966)

Ballantyne, D. L., Jr., Coburn, R. J., Hawthorne, G. A., Nathan, P.: Platelet levels during rat skin allograft rejection. Transplantation **13**, 531—533 (1972)

Barnhardt, M. I., Walsh, R. T., Robinson, J. A.: Three dimensional view of platelet responses to chemical stimuli. Ann. N.Y. Acad. Sci. **201**, 360—390 (1972)

Baugh, R., Brown, J., Sargeant, R., Hougie, C.: Separation of human factor VIII activity from the von Willebrand's antigen and ristocetin platelet aggregating activity. Biochim. biophys. Acta **371**, 360—367 (1974)

Baumgartner, H. R.: 5-hydroxytryptamine uptake and release in relation to aggregation of rabbit platelets. J. Physiol. (Lond.) **201**, 409—423 (1969)

Baumgartner, H. R.: Morphometric quantitation of adherence of platelets to an artificial surface and components of connective tissue. Thrombos. Diathes. haemorrh. (Stuttg.) Suppl. **60**, 39—49 (1974a)

Baumgartner, H. R.: New aspects in thrombogenesis. J. Vascular Diseases (VASA) **3**, 60—64 (1974b)

Baumgartner, H. R., Born, G. V. R.: Effects of 5-hydroxytryptamine on platelet aggregation. Nature (Lond.) **218**, 137—141 (1968)

Baumgartner, H. R., Born, G. V. R.: The relation between the 5-hydroxytryptamine content and aggregation of rabbit platelets. J. Physiol. (Lond.) **201**, 397—408 (1969)

Baumgartner, H. R., Muggli, R., Tschopp, T. B., Turitto, U. T.: Platelet adhesion, release and aggregation in flowing blood; effects of surface properties and platelet function. Thrombos. Diathes. Haemorrh. (Stuttg.) **35**, 125—138 (1976)

Becker, E. L., Austen, K. F.: Anaphylaxis. In: Miescher, P. A., Müller-Eberhard, H. J. (Eds.): Textbook of Immunopathology, Vol. 1, pp. 76—93. New York: Grune and Stratton 1968

Behnke, O.: Further studies on microtubules. A marginal bundle in human and rat thrombocytes. J. Ultrastruct. Res. **13**, 469—477 (1965)

Behnke, O.: The morphology of blood platelet membrane systems. Ser. Haematol. **3**, 3—16 (1970)

Biggs, R.: The observations on which the theory of blood coagulation is based. Proc. roy. Soc. B **173**, 277—284 (1969)

Bills, T. K., Silver, M. J.: Phosphatidylcholine is the primary source of arachidonic acid utilised by platelet prostaglandin synthetase. Fed. Proc. **34**, 790 (1975)

Bills, T. K., Smith, J. B., Silver, K. J.: Platelet uptake, release and oxidation of 14C-arachidonic acid—specificity of metabolic pathways. In: Prostaglandins in Haematology, pp. 27—55. New York: Spectrum Publications 1977b

Blackwell, G. J., Duncombe, W. G., Flower, R. J., Parsons, M. F., Vane, J. R.: The distribution and metabolism of arachidonic acid in rabbit platelets during aggregation and its modification by drugs. Brit. J. Pharmacol. **59**, 353—366 (1977)

Boldingh, J.: Lipid metabolism in relation to human health. Chem. Ind. **23**, 984—993 (1975)

Boot, J. R., Dawson, W., Kitchen, E. A.: The chemotactic activity of thromboxane B_2: a possible role in inflammation. J. Physiol. (Lond.) **257**, 47P—49P (1976)

Booyse, F., Kisieleski, D. I., Seeler, R.: Possible thrombasthenin defect in Glanzmann's thrombasthenia. Blood **39**, 377—381 (1972)

Booyse, F. M., Rafelson, M. E.: Human platelet contractile proteins: location, properties and function. Ser. Haematol. **4**, 152—174 (1971)

Born, G. V. R.: Aggregation of blood platelets by adenosine diphosphate and its reversal. Nature (Lond.) **194**, 927—929 (1962)

Born, G. V. R.: Strong inhibition by 2-chloroadenosine of the aggregation of blood platelets by adenosine diphosphate. Nature (Lond.) **202**, 95—96 (1964)

Born, G. V. R.: Observations in the change in shape of blood platelets brought about by adenosine diphosphate. J. Physiol. (Lond.) **209**, 487—511 (1970)

Born, G. V. R.: The functional physiology of blood platelets. In: Mannucci, P. M., Gorini, S. (Eds.): Platelet Function and Thrombosis. A Review of Methods, pp. 3—21. New York-London: Plenum Press 1972

Born, G. V. R.: Aggregation of haemostatic cells as an example of specialised cell function. In: Caprino, L., Rossi, E. C. (Eds.): Platelet Aggregation and Drugs, pp. 1—19. London-New York-San Fransisco: Academic Press 1974

Born, G. V. R., Gillson, R. E.: Studies on the uptake of 5-hydroxytryptamine by blood platelets. J. Physiol. (Lond.) **146**, 472—491 (1959)

Bosmann, H. B.: Platelet adhesiveness and aggregation: the collagen glycosyl, polypeptide; N-acetylgalactosominyl and glycoprotein galactosyl transferase of human platelets. Biochem. biophys. Res. Commun. **43**, 1118—1124 (1971)

Bounameaux, Y.: Dosage de facteurs coagulation contenus dans l'atmosphere plasmatique de plaquettes humaines. Rev. Franç. Et. clin. biol. **2**, 52—63 (1957)

Boyle-Kay, M. M., Fudenberg, H. H.: Inhibition and reversal of platelet activation by cytochalasin B or colcemid. Nature (Lond.) **244**, 288—289 (1973)

Braude, A. I., Carey, F. J., Zalesky, M.: Studies with radioactive endotoxin II. Correlation of physiological effects with distribution of radioactivity in rabbits injected with lethal doses of *E. coli* endotoxin labelled with radioactive sodium chromate. J. clin. Invest. **34**, 858—866 (1955)

Breddin, K., Krzywanek, H. J., Bald, M., Kutschera, J.: Is enhanced platelet aggregation a risk factor for thrombo-embolic complications in atherosclerosis? In: Caprino, L., Rossi, E. C. (Eds.): Platelet Aggregation and Drugs, pp. 197—212. London-New York-San Fransisco: Academic Press 1974

Brodie, G. N., Baenziger, N. L., Chase, L. R., Majurus, P. W.: The effects of thrombin on adenyl cyclase activity and membrane protein from human platelets. J. clin. Invest. **51**, 81—88 (1972)

Broun, G. O., Jr., Broun, G. O., Snr.: Reactions between platelets and viruses. In: Proceedings of VIII International Congress for Hematology, Tokyo, 1960, Vol. 3, p. 1756. Tokyo: Pan Pacific Press 1962

Bunting, S., Moncada, S., Needleman, P., Vane, J. R.: Formation of prostaglandin endoperoxides and rabbit aorta contracting substance (RCS) by coupling two enzyme systems. Brit. J. Pharmacol. **56**, 344 P (1976 a)

Bunting, S., Moncada, S., Vane, J. R.: The effects of prostaglandin endoperoxides and thromboxane A_2 on strips of rabbit coeliac artery and certain other smooth muscle preparations. Brit. J. Pharmacol. **57**, 462 P—463 P (1976 b)

Butler, K. D., White, A. M.: The effect of sulphinpyrazone on the thrombocytopenia occurring in the Arthus reaction. Brit. J. Pharmacol. **55**, 256—257 P (1975)

Caen, J. P.: Glanzmann thrombasthenia. In: O'Brien, J. R. (Ed.): Clinics in Haematology, Vol. 1, pp. 383—392. Philadelphia: W. B. Sanders. Co. 1972

Castaldi, P. A., Larrieu, M. J., Caen, J.: Availability of platelet factor 3 and activation of factor XII in thrombasthenia. Nature (Lond.) **207**, 422—424 (1965)

Chandler, A. B.: In vitro thrombotic coagulation of the blood. A method for producing a thrombus. Lab. Invest. **7**, 110—114 (1958)

Chandra-Sekhar, N. C.: Effect of eight prostaglandins on platelet aggregation. J. med. Chem. **13**, 34—44 (1970)

Chesney, C. M., Harper, E., Colman, R. W.: Human platelet collagenase. J. clin. Invest. **53**, 1647—1654 (1974)

Chignard, M., Vargaftig, B. B.: Dog platelets fail to aggregate when they form aggregating substances upon stimulation with arachidonic acid. Europ. J. Pharmacol. **38**, 7—18 (1976)

Christian, F. A., Gordon, J. L.: Platelet function in C_6-deficient rabbits. Aggregation and secretion induced by collagen and zymosan. Immunology **29**, 131—141 (1975)

Clawson, C. C., White, J. G.: Platelet interaction with bacteria. I. Reaction phases and effects of inhibitors. Amer. J. Path. **65**, 367—381 (1971)

Cluff, L. E., Berthrong, M.: The inhibition of the local Schwartzman reaction by aspirin. Bull. Johns Hopk. Hosp. **92**, 353—363 (1953)

Cochrane, C. G.: Mechanisms involved in the deposition of immune complexes in tissues. J. exp. Med. **134**, 755 (1971)

Cochrane, C. G., Dixon, F. J.: Cell and tissue damage through antigen-antibody complexes. In: Miescher, P. A., Müller-Eberhardt, H. J. (Eds.): Textbook of Immunopathology, Vol. 1, pp. 94—110. New York: Grune and Stratton 1968

Cochrane, S. G., Janoff, A.: The Arthus reaction: a model of neutrophil and complement—mediated injury. In: Zweifach, B. W., Grant, L., McCluskey, R. T. (Eds.): The Inflammatory Process, 2nd Edit., Vol. III, pp. 85—102. London-New York: Academic Press 1974

Colman, R. W., Shattil, S. J., Bennett, J. S.: Cholesterol-rich platelets are resistant to inhibition by prostaglandin E_1. Blood **46**, 1033 (1975)

Colwell, J. P., Sagel, J., Pennington, R., Meeks, M., Scarpatia, R., Laminus, M.: Effect of therapy on platelet aggregation in diabetes. Clin. Res. **21**, 884 (1973)

Comai, K., Farber, S. J., Paulsrud, J. R.: Analyses of renal medullary lipid droplets from normal, hydronephrotic and indomethacin-treated rabbits. Lipids **10**, 555—581 (1975)

Coppi, G., Bonardi, G.: Effect of two non-steroidal anti-inflammatory agents on alkaline and acid phosphatases of inflamed tissue. J. Pharm. (Lond.) **20**, 661—662 (1968)

Corey, E. J., Nicolaou, K. C., Machida, Y., Malmsten, C. L., Samuelsson, B.: Synthesis and biological properties of a 9,11-azo-prostanoid: highly active biochemical mimic of prostaglandin endoperoxides. Proc. nat. Acad. Sci. (Wash.) **72**, 3355—3358 (1975)

Cottney, J., Lewis, A. J., Nelson, D. J.: Arachidonic acid-induced paw oedema in the rat. Brit. J. Pharmacol. **58**, 311 P (1976)

Cronberg, S.: Investigations in haemorrhogic disorders with prolonged bleeding time but normal number of platelets. With special reference to platelet adhesiveness. Acta med. scand. **486**, Suppl. 1—54 (1968)

Crunkhorn, P., Willis, A. L.: Actions and interactions of prostaglandins administered intradermally. Brit. J. Pharmacol. **36**, 216 P—217 P (1969)

Crunkhorn, P., Willis, A. L.: Cutaneous reactions to intradermal prostaglandins. Brit. J. Pharmacol. **41**, 49—56 (1971 a)

Crunkhorn, P., Willis, A. L.: Interaction between prostaglandin E and F given intradermally in the rat. Brit. J. Pharmacol. **41**, 507—512 (1971 b)

Daems, W. T., Oort, J.: Electron microscopic and histochemical observations on polymorphonuclear leucocytes in the reversed Arthus reaction. Exp. Cell Res. **28**, 11—20 (1962)

Da Prada, M., Pletscher, A.: Synthesis and storage of nucleotides in blood platelets. Life Sci. **9**, 1271—1282 (1970)

Davey, M. G.: The survival and destruction of human platelets. Basel-New York: S. Karger 1966

Davis, R. B., White, J. G.: Localisation of 5-hydroxytryptamine in blood platelets: an autoradiographic and ultrastructural study. Brit. J. Haemat. **15**, 93—99 (1968)

Davis, R. B.: Electron microscopic changes in blood platelets induced by bacterial lipopolysaccharide. Exp. molec. Path. **5**, 559—574 (1966)

Davis, R. B., Meeker, W. R., McQuarrie, D. G.: Immediate effects of intravenous endotoxin on serotonin concentrations and blood platelets. Circulat. Res. **8**, 234—239 (1960)

Day, H. J., Holmsen, H.: Concepts of the blood platelet release reaction. Ser. Haematol. **4**, 3—27 (1971)

Day, H. J., Holmsen, H., Hovig, T.: Subcellular particles of human platelets. Scand. J. Haemat. **7** Suppl., 1—35 (1969)

Day, H. J., Stormorken, H., Holmsen, H.: Subcellular localization of platelet factor 3 and platelet factor 4. Scand. J. Haemat. **10**, 254—260 (1973)

Des Prez, R. M.: The effects of bacterial endotoxin on rabbit platelets. V. Heat labile plasma factor requirements of endotoxin-induced platelet injury. J. Immunol. **99**, 966—973 (1967)

Des Prez, R. M., Bryant, R. E.: Effects of bacterial endotoxin on rabbit platelets. IV. The divalent ion requirements of endotoxin-induced and immunologically-induced platelet injury. J. exp. Med. **124**, 971—982 (1966)

Des Prez, R. M., Horowitz, H. I., Hook, E. W., Jr.: Effects of bacterial endotoxin on rabbit platelets. I. Platelet aggregation and release of platelet factors in vitro. J. exp. Med. **114**, 857—874 (1961)

Des Prez, R. M., Marney, S. R., Jr.: Immunological reactions involving platelets. In: Johnson, S. A. (Ed.): The Circulating Platelet, pp. 415—471. New York: Academic Press 1971

Deykin, D., Desser, R. K.: The incorporation of acetate and palmitate into lipids by human platelets. J. clin. Invest. **47**, 1590—1602 (1968)

Donati, M. B., Palester-Chlebowczyk, M., de Gaetano, G., Vermylen, J.: Platelet factor 4—methods of study. In: Platelet Function and Thrombosis. Advances in Experimental Medicine and Biology, Vol. 34, pp. 295—308. New York: Pharm. Rec. 1972

Downing, D. T.: Differential inhibition of prostaglandin synthetase and soyabean lipoxygenase. Prostaglandins **1**, 437—441 (1972)

Eakins, K. E., Whitelocke, R. A. F., Perkins, E. S., Bennett, A., Unger, W. G.: Release of prostaglandins in ocular inflammation in the rabbit. Nature (New Biol.) **239**, 248—249 (1972)

Ebbe, S.: Megakaryocytopoiesis and platelet turnover. Ser. Haematol. **2**, 65—68 (1968)

Elsbach, P.: Phospholipid metabolism by phagocytic cells. I. A comparison of conversion of lysolecithin-^{32}P to lecithin and glycerylphosphorylcholine by homogenates of rabbit polymorphonuclear leucocytes and alveolar macrophages. Biochim. biophys. Acta **125**, 510—524 (1966)

Elsbach, P., Rizack, M. A.: Acid lipase and phospholipase activity in homogenates of rabbit polymorphonuclear leukocytes. Amer. J. Physiol. **205**, 1154—1158 (1963)

Erdös, E. G.: Effect of non-steroidal anti-inflammatory drugs in endotoxin shock. Biochem. Pharmacol. Suppl., 283—291 (1968)

Evans, G., Packham, M. A., Nishizawa, E. E., Mustard, J. F., Murphy, E. A.: The effect of acetylsalicyclic acid on platelet function. J. exp. Med. **128**, 877—894 (1968)

Farrow, J. F., Willis, A. L.: Thrombolytic and anti-thrombotic properties of dihomo-γ-linolenate in vitro. Brit. J. Pharmacol. **55**, 316 P—317 P (1975)

Ferreira, S. H.: Prostaglandins, aspirin-like drugs and analgesia. Nature (New Biol.) **240**, 200—203 (1972)

Ferreira, S. H., Moncada, S., Vane, J. R.: Indomethacin and aspirin abolish prostaglandin release from the spleen. Nature (New Biol.) **231**, 237—239 (1971)

Fischer, P., Lecomte, J.: Anaphylactic shock in the rabbit treated with reserpine. C.R. Soc. Biol. (Paris) **150**, 1026—1028 (1956)

Fitzpatrick, F. A. and Gorman, R. R.: Platelet rich plasma transforms exogenous endoperoxide H_2 into thromboxane A_2.: Prostaglandins **14**, 881—889 (1977)

Fleming, J. S., Buyniski, J. P., Cavanagh, R. L., Bierwagen, M. E.: Pharmacology of a potent new anti-thrombotic agent, 6-methyl-1,2,3,5-tetrahydroimidazo[2,1-b]quinazolin-2-one hydrochloride monohydrate (BL-3459). J. Pharmacol. exp. Ther. **194**, 435—449 (1975)

Flower, R. J.: Aspirin, prostaglandins, endoperoxides and platelets. Nature (Lond.) **253**, 88—90 (1975)

Flower, R. J., Gryglewski, R., Herbaczynska-Cedro, K., Vane, J. R.: Effects of anti-inflammatory drugs on prostaglandin biosynthesis. Nature (New Biol.) **238**, 104—106 (1972)

Flower, R. J., Harvey, E. A., Kingston, W. P.: Inflammatory effects of prostaglandin D_2 in rat and human skin. Brit. J. Pharmacol. **56**, 229—233 (1976)

Flower, R. J., Kingston, W. P.: Prostaglandin D_1 inhibits the increase in vascular permeability produced by prostaglandin E_1, E_2, and D_2. Brit. J. Pharmacol. **55**, 230 P—240 P (1975)

Flower, R. J., Vane, J. R.: Inhibition of prostaglandin synthetase in brain explains the anti-pyretic activity of paracetamol (4-acetamidophenol). Nature (Lond.) **240**, 410—411 (1972)

Ford-Hutchinson, A. W., Smith, M. J. H., Walker, J. R.: Chemotactic activity of solutions of prostaglandin E_1. Brit. J. Pharmacol. **56**, 345 P (1976)

Friedman, Z., Lamberth, E. L., Stahlman, M. T., Oates, J. A.: Platelet aggregation in infants with essential fatty acid deficiency. In: Samuelsson, B., Paoletti, R. (Eds.): Advances in Prostaglandin and Thromboxane Research, Vol. 2, pp. 852—855. New York: Raven Press 1976

Gaarder, A., Laland, S.: Hypothesis for the aggregation of platelets by nucleotides. Nature (Lond.) **202**, 909—910 (1964)

Gaetano, G., de: Pharmacology of platelet aggregation. Pharmacol. Res. Commun. **7**, 301—309 (1975)

Genton, E., Gent, M., Hirsh, J., Harper, L. A.: Platelet inhibiting drugs in the prevention of clinical thrombotic disease. New Engl. J. Med. **293**, 1174—1178, 1236—1240, 1296—1300 (1975)

Gerrard, J. M., White, J. G., Rao, G. N. R.: Labile aggregation stimulating substances (LASS): the factor from storage pool deficient platelets correcting defective aggregation release in normal platelets. Brit. J. Haemat. **29**, 657—665 (1975)

Gerrard, J. M., White, J. G., Rao, G. N. R., Townsend, D.: Localization of platelet prostaglandin production in the platelet dense tubular system. Amer. J. Path. **83**, 283—298 (1976)

Gilmore, N., Vane, J. R., Wyllie, J. H.: Prostaglandin released by the spleen. Nature (Lond.) **218**, 1135—1140 (1968)

Glass, D. B., Gerrard, J. M., White, J. G., Goldberg, W. D.: Cyclic GMP formation in human platelets aggregated by arachidonic acid. Blood **46**, 1033 (1975)

Glatt, M., Peskar, B., Brune, K.: Leucocytes and prostaglandins in acute inflammation. Experientia (Basel) **30**, 1257—1259 (1974)

Glenn, E. M., Wilks, J., Bowman, B.: Platelets, prostaglandins, red cells, sedimentation rates, serum and tissue proteins and non-steroidal anti-inflammatory drugs. Proc. Soc. exp. Biol. (N.Y.) **141**, 879—886 (1972)

Good, R. A., Thomas, L.: The generalised Schwartzman reaction. IV. Prevention of the local and generalised Schwartzman reaction with heparin. J. exp. Med. **97**, 871—888 (1953)

Gordon, J. L.: Evaluation of a semi-micro method for measuring platelet aggregation in whole blood samples. Thrombos. Diathes. haemorrh. (Stuttg.) **30**, 160—172 (1973)
Gordon, J. L.: Blood platelet lysosomes and their contribution to the pathophysiological role of platelets. In: Dingle, J. T., Dean, R. T. (Eds.): Lysosomes in Biology and Pathology, pp. 2—31. Amsterdam-Oxford: North-Holland Publishing Co. 1975
Grette, K.: Studies on the mechanism of thrombin-catalysed haemostatic reactions in blood platelets. Acta physiol. scand. **56**, Suppl. 195, 5—93 (1962)
Gryglewski, R. J., Bunting, S., Moncada, S., Flower, R. J., Vane, J. R.: Arterial walls are protected against deposition of platelet thrombi by a substance (prostaglandin X) which they make from prostaglandin endoperoxide. Prostaglandins **12**, 685—713 (1976)
Gryglewski, R. J., Panczenko, B., Korbut, R., Grodzinska, L., Ocetkiewicz, A.: Corticosteroids inhibit prostaglandin release from perfused mesenteric blood vessels of rabbit and from perfused lungs of sensitized guinea pig. Prostaglandins **10**, 343—355 (1975a)
Gryglewski, R. J., Szczeklik, A., Bieron, K.: Morphine antagonises prostaglandin E_1-mediated inhibition of human platelet aggregation. Nature (Lond.) **236**, 56—57 1975b)
Gryglewsky, R., Vane, J. R.: The generation from arachidonic acid of rabbit aorta contacting substance (RCS) by a microsomal enzyme preparation which also generates prostaglandins. Brit. J. Pharmacol. **46**, 449—457 (1972)
Guccione, M. A., Packham, M. A., Kinlough-Rathbone, R. L., Mustard, J. F.: Reactions of [^{14}C]-ADP and [^{14}C]-ATP with washed platelets from rabbits. Blood **37**, 542—555 (1971)
Gugler, E., Lüscher, E. F.: Platelet function in congenital afibinogenemia. Thrombos. Diathes. haemorrh. (Stuttg.) **14**, 361—373 (1965)
Hall, R. C., Hodge, R. L., Irvine, R., Katic, F., Middleton, J. M.: The effect of aspirin on the response to endotoxin. Aust. J. exp. Med. **50**, 589—601 (1972)
Halushka, P. V., Weiser, C., Chambers, A., Colwell, J.: Synthesis of prostaglandin E-like material (PGE) in diabetic and normal platelets. In: Samuelsson, B., Paoletti, R. (Eds.): Advances in Prostaglandin and Thromboxane Research, Vol. 2, p. 853. New York: Raven Press 1976
Hamberg, M., Samuelsson, B.: Detection and isolation of an endoperoxide intermediate in prostaglandin biosynthesis. Proc. nat. Acad. Sci. (Wash.) **70**, 899—903 (1973)
Hamberg, M., Samuelsson, B.: Prostaglandin endoperoxides. Novel transformations of arachidonic acid in human platelets. Proc. nat. Acad. Sci. (Wash.) **71**, 3400—3404 (1974)
Hamberg, M., Svensson, J., Samuelsson, B.: Prostaglandin endoperoxides. A new concept concerning the mode of action and release of prostaglandins. Proc. nat. Acad. Sci. (Wash.) **71**, 3824—3828 (1974a)
Hamberg, M., Svensson, J., Samuelsson, B.: Thromboxanes: A new group of biologically active compounds derived from prostaglandin endoperoxides. Proc. nat. Acad. Sci. (Wash.) **72**, 2994—2998 (1975)
Hamberg, M., Svensson, J., Wakabayashi, T., Samuelsson, B.: Isolation and structures of two prostaglandin endoperoxides that cause platelet aggregation. Proc. nat. Acad. Sci. (Wash.) **71**, 345—349 (1974b)
Hardisty, R. M., Hutton, R. A.: Platelet aggregation and availability of platelet factor 3. Brit. J. Haemat. **12**, 764—776 (1966)
Hardisty, R. M., Hutton, R. A.: Bleeding tendency associated with "new" abnormality of platelet behaviour. Lancet **1**, 983—985 (1967)
Harker, L. A., Slichter, S. J.: The bleeding time as a screening test for evaluation of platelet function. New Engl. J. Med. **287**, 155—159 (1972)
Haslam, R. J.: Mechanisms of blood platelet aggregation. In: Johnson, S. A., Segers, W. H. (Eds.): Physiology of Hemostasis and Thrombosis, pp. 88—112. Springfield, Ill.: Charles C. Thomas 1967
Haslam, R. J., McClenaghan, M. D.: Effects of collagen and of aspirin on the concentration of guanosine 3′5-cyclic monophosphate in human blood platelets. Measurement by a permeability technique. Biochem. J. **138**, 317—320 (1974)
Hellem, A. J.: The adhesiveness of human blood platelets in vitro. Scand. J. clin. Lab. Invest. **12**, Suppl. 51, 1—117 (1960)
Henson, P. M.: Interaction of cells with immune complexes. Adherence, release of constituents and tissue injury. J. exp. Med. **134**, 114s—115s (1971)

Henson, P. M., Cochrane, C. G.: Immunological induction of increased vascular permeability. I. A rabbit passive cutaneous anaphylactic reaction requiring complement, platelets and neutrophils. J. exp. Med. **129**, 153—165 (1969 a)
Henson, P. M., Cochrane, C. G.: Antigen-antibody complexes, platelets and increased vascular permeability. In: Movat, H. Z. (Ed.): Cellular and Humoral Mechanisms of Anaphylaxis Allergy, Proceedings 3rd International Symposium Canadian Society Immunology, 1968, pp. 129—143. Basel: Karger 1969 b
Henson, P. M., Cochrane, C. G.: Cellular mediators of immunological tissue injury. J. reticuloendoth. Soc. **8**, 124—138 (1970)
Herman, A. G.: Release of prostaglandins in the knee joint of the dog during local Shwartzmann-like reaction. Brit. J. Pharmacol. **55**, 241 P—242 P (1975)
Herman, A. G., Moncada, S.: Release of prostaglandins and incapacitation after injection of endotoxin in the knee joint of the dog. Brit. J. Pharmacol. **53**, 405 P (1975)
Herring, W. B., Herion, J. C., Walker, R. I., Palmer, J. G.: Distribution and clearance of circulating endotoxin. J. clin. Invest. **42**, 79—87 (1963)
Higgs, G. A., McCall, E., Youlten, L. J. F.: A chemotactic role for prostaglandins released from polymorphonuclear leucocytes during phagocytosis. Brit. J. Pharmacol. **53**, 539—546 (1975)
Hinshaw, L. B., Jordon, M. M., Vick, J. A.: Mechanism of histamine release in endotoxin shock. Amer. J. Physiol. **200**, 987—989 (1961)
Hirsch, J. G.: Neutrophil leukocytes. In: Zweifach, B. W., Grant, L., McCluskey, R. T. (Eds.): The Inflammatory Process, 2nd Edit., Vol. II, pp. 411—447. New York-London: Academic Press 1974
Hirschhorn, R.: Lysosomal mechanisms in the inflammatory process. In: Zweifach, B. W., Grant, L., McCluskey, R. T. (Eds.): The Inflammatory Process, 2nd Edit., Vol. II, pp. 259—285. New York-London: Academic Press 1974
Hobbs, J. B.: Platelets and the renal vascular endothelium. Perspect. Nephrol. Hypertens. **1**, 907—914 (1973)
Holmsen, H.: The platelet: its membrane, physiology and biochemistry. Clin. Haematol. **1**, 235—266 (1972)
Holmsen, H., Day, H. J., Storm, E.: Adenine nucleotide metabolism of blood platelets. VI. Subcellular localisation of nucleotide pools with different functions in the platelet release reaction. Biochim. biophys. Acta **186**, 254—266 (1969 a)
Holmsen, H., Day, H. J., Stormorken, H.: The blood platelet release reaction. Scand. J. Haemat. **8**, Suppl. 1—26 (1969 b)
Holmsen, H., Setowsky, C. A., Lages, B.: Content and thrombin induced release of acid hydrolases in gel-filtered platelets from patients with storage pool disease. Blood **46**, 131—142 (1975)
Holmsen, M., Weiss, H. J.: Hereditary defect in the platelet release reaction caused by a deficiency in the storage pool of platelet adenine nucleotides. Brit. J. Haemat. **19**, 643—649 (1970)
Holmsen, H., Weiss, H. J.: Further evidence for a deficient storage pool of adenine nucleotides in platelets from some patients with thrombocytopathia "storage pool disease". Blood **39**, 197—209 (1972)
Hong, S. L., Levine, L.: Inhibition of arachidonic acid release from cells as the biochemical action of anti-inflammatory corticosteroids. Proc. nat. Acad. Sci. (Wash.) **73**, 1730—1734 (1976)
Hornstra, G., Gielen, S. Y.: Measurement of platelet aggregation and thrombus formation in circulating blood. In: Manucci, P. M., Gorini, S. (Eds.): Platelet Function and Thrombosis: A Review of Methods. Advances in Experimental Medicine and Biology, Vol. 34, pp. 321—333. New York-London: Plenum Press 1972
Horowitz, H. I., Des Prez, R. M., Hook, E. W.: Effects of bacterial endotoxin on rabbit platelets. II. Enhancement of platelet factor 3 activity in vitro and in vivo. J. exp. Med. **116**, 619—633 (1962)
Horowitz, H. I., Fujimoto, M. M.: Association of factors XI and XII with blood platelets. Proc. Soc. exp. Biol. (N.Y.) **119**, 487—492 (1965)
Hovig, T.: The ultrastructure basis of platelet function. In: Baldini, M. G., Ebbe, E. (Eds.): Platelets, Production, Function, Transfusion, and Storage, pp. 221—233. New York: Grune and Stratton 1974
Howard, M. A., Firkin, B. G.: Ristocetin—a new tool in the investigation of platelet aggregation. Thrombos. Diathes. Haemorrh. (Stuttg.) **26**, 362—369 (1971)

Inceman, S., Caen, J., Bernard, J.: Aggregation, adhesion, and viscous metamorphosis of platelets in congenital fibrinogen deficiencies. J. Lab. clin. Med. **68**, 21—32 (1966)
Janoff, A.: Neutrophil proteases in inflammation. Ann. rev. Med. **23**, 177—190 (1972)
Janoff, A., Zweifach, B. W.: Adhesion and emigration of leukocytes produced by cationic proteins of lysosomes. Science **144**, 1456—1458 (1964)
Jenkins, C. S. P., Meyer, D., Dreyfus, M. D., Larrieu, M. J.: Willebrand factor and ristocetin. I. Mechanism of ristocetin-induced platelet aggregation. Brit. J. Haemat. **28**, 561—578 (1974)
Jenkins, C. S. P., Phillips, D. R., Clemetson, K. J., Meyer, D., Larrieu, M. J., Luscher, E. E.: Platelet membrane glycoproteins implicated in ristocetin-induced aggregation. J. clin. Invest. **57**, 112—124 (1976)
Jerushalmy, Z., Kohn, A., De Vries, A.: Interaction of myxoviruses with human blood platelets in vitro. Proc. Soc. exp. Biol. (N.Y.) **106**, 462—466 (1961)
Johansson, S. A.: Inhibition of thrombocytopenia and 5-hydroxytryptamine release in anaphylactic shock by heparin. Acta physiol. scand. **50**, 95—104 (1960)
Johnson, M., Jessup, R., Ramwell, P. W.: The significance of protein disulphide and sulphydryl groups in prostaglandin action. Prostaglandins **5**, 125—136 (1974)
Johnson, M., Ramwell, P. W.: Prostaglandin modification of membrane-bound enzyme activity. Advanc. Biosci. **9**, 205—212 (1973)
Johnson, R. A., Morton, D. R., Kinner, J. H., Gorman, R. R., McGuire, G. C., Sun, F. F., Whittaker, N., Bunting, S., Salmon, J., Moncada, S., Vane, J. R.: Prostaglandins **12**, 915—928 (1976)
Jørgensen, L., Borchgrevink, C. F.: The haemostatic mechanism in patients with haemostatic diseases. A histological study of wounds made for primary and secondary bleeding time tests. Acta path. microbiol. scand. **60**, 55—82 (1964)
Kaley, G., Messina, E. J., Weiner, R.: The role of prostaglandins in microcirculatory regulation and inflammation. In: Ramwell, P. W., Phariss, B. B. (Eds.): Prostaglandins in Cellular Biology, pp. 309—327. New York-London: Plenum Press 1972
Kaley, G., Weiner, R.: Prostaglandin E_1: a potential mediator of the inflammatory response. Ann. N.Y. Acad. Sci. **180**, 338—350 (1971 a)
Kaley, G., Weiner, R.: Effect of prostaglandin E_1 on leukocyte migration. Nature (New Biol.) **234**, 114—115 (1971 b)
Kantrowitz, F., Robinson, D. R., McGuire, M. B., Levine, L.: Corticosteroids inhibit prostaglandin production by rheumatoid synovia. Nature (Lond.) **258**, 737—739 (1975)
Karpatkin, M. H., Karpatkin, S.: In vivo and in vitro binding of factor VIII to human platelets. Thrombos. Diathes. Haemorrh. (Stuttg.) **21**, 129—133 (1969)
Kincaid-Smith, P.: Histological diagnosis of rejection of renal homografts in man. Lancet **2**, 849—852 (1967)
Kloeze, J.: Influence of prostaglandins on platelet adhesiveness and platelet aggregation. In: Bergstrom, S., Samuelsson, B. (Eds.): Nobel Symposium, 2. Prostaglandins, pp. 241—252. Stockholm: Almquist and Wiksell 1967
Kniker, W. T., Cochrane, C. G.: The localisation of circulating immune complexes in experimental serum sickness—the role of vasoactive amines and hydrodynamic forces. J. exp. Med. **127**, 119—135 (1968)
Kocsis, J. J., Hernandovich, J., Silver, M. J., Smith, J. B., Ingerman, C.: Duration of inhibition of platelet prostaglandin formation and aggregation by ingested aspirin on indomethacin. Prostaglandins **3**, 141—144 (1973)
Kubisz, P., Caen, J.: Interaction of alpha and beta receptor blocking agents with platelet release and availability reaction induced by ADP, adrenaline and collagen. Path. Biol. **20**, Suppl., 34—40 (1972)
Kuhn, D. C., Willis, A. L.: Prostaglandin E_2, inflammation and pain threshold in rat paws. Brit. J. Pharmacol. **49**, 183 P—184 P (1973)
Kwaan, A. C., Colwell, J. A., Cruz, S., Suwanwela, N., Dobbie, J.: Increased platelet aggregation in diabetes mellitus. J. Lab. clin. Med. **80**, 236—246 (1972)
Larke, R. P. B., Wheelock, E. F.: Stabilisation of Chikungunya virus infectivity by human blood platelets. Bact. Proc. 184 (1969)
Leak, L. V., Burke, J. F.: Early events of tissue injury and the role of the lymphatic system in early inflammation. In: Zweifach, B. W., Grant, B. W., McCluskey, R. T. (Eds.): The Inflammatory Process, 2nd Edit., Vol. III, pp. 163—199. New York-London: Academic Press 1974

Leber, P. D., McCluskey, R. T.: Immune complex diseases. In: Zweifach, B. W., Grant, B. W., McCluskey, R. T. (Eds.): The Inflammatory Process, 2nd Edit., Vol. III, pp. 401—441. London-New York: Academic Press 1974

Lefort, J., Vargaftig, B. B.: Role of platelet aggregation in bronchoconstriction in guinea-pigs. Brit. J. Pharmacol. **55**, 254 P—255 P (1975)

Legrand, Y. J., Caen, F. M., Booyse, M. E., Rafelson, B., Rafelson, L.: Human blood platelet protease with elastolytic activity. Biochim. biophys. Acta **309**, 406—413 (1973)

Leonardi, R. G., Alexander, B., White, F.: Prevention of the inhibitory effect of aspirin on platelet aggregation. Fed. Proc. **31**, Abs. 202 (1972)

Lewis, G. P., Piper, P. J.: Inhibition of release of prostaglandins as an explanation of some of the actions of anti-inflammatory corticosteroids. Nature (Lond.) **254**, 308—311 (1975)

Lowenhaupt, R., Nathan, P.: Platelet accumulation observed by electron microscopy in the early phase of renal allo-transplant rejection. Nature (Lond.) **220**, 822—825 (1968)

Lowenhaupt, R., Nathan, P.: The participation of platelets in the rejection of dog kidney allo-transplants; hematologic and electron microscopic studies. Transplant. Proc. **1**, 305—310 (1969)

Lu, W. C.: Agglutination of human platelets by influenza (PR 8 strain) virus and mumps virus. Fed. Proc. **17**, 446 (1958)

McCall, E., Youlten, L. J. F.: The effects of indomethacin and depletion of complement on cell migration and prostaglandin levels in carrageenin-induced air bleb inflammation. Brit. J. Pharmacol. **52**, 452 P (1974)

McClatchley, W. and Snyderman, R.: Prostaglandins and inflammation: enhancement of monocyte chemotactic responsiveness by prostaglandin E_2. Prostaglandins **12**, 415—426 (1976)

McFarlane, D. E.: ATP specifically inhibits ADP effects on blood platelets. Fed. Proc. **33**, 269 (1974)

McFarlane, R. G.: Hemostatic mechanisms in tissue injury. In: Zweifach, B. W., Grant, L., McCluskey, R. T. (Eds.): The Inflammatory Process, 2nd Edit., Vol. II, pp. 335—362. New York-London: Academic Press 1973

MacIntyre, D. E., Gordon, J. L.: Calcium-dependent stimulation of platelet aggregation by PGE_2. Nature (Lond.) **258**, 337—338 (1975)

McKay, D. G.: Disseminated intravascular coagulation. An intermediary mechanism of disease. New York: Hoeber Med. Division, Harper and Row

McKay, D. G., Shapiro, S. S., Shanberge, J. N.: Alterations in the blood coagulation system induced by bacterial endotoxins. II. In vitro. J. exp. Med. **107**, 369—376 (1965)

McNicol, G. P., Mitchell, J. R. A., Reuter, H., Van de Loo, J.: Platelets in thrombosis, their clinical significance and the evaluation of potential drugs. Thrombos. Diathes. haemorrh. (Stuttg.) **31**, 381—394 (1974)

Majerus, P. Q., Baenziger, N. L., Brodie, G. N.: Lipid metabolism in human platelets. Ser. Haematol. **4**, 59—74 (1971)

Malmsten, C., Hamberg, M., Svensson, J.: Physiological role of an endoperoxide in human platelets: haemostatic defect due to platelet cyclo-oxygenase deficiency. Proc. nat. Acad. Sci. (Wash.) **72**, 1440—1450 (1975)

Mannucci, P. M., Meyer, D., Ruggeri, Z. M., Koutts, J., Lavergne, J. M.: Precipitating antibodies in von Willebrand's disease. Nature (Lond.) **262**, 141—142 (1976)

Marcus, A. J.: The role of lipids in blood coagulation. In: Paoletti, R., Krutshevsky, D. (Eds.): Advances in Lipid Research, pp. 1—37. New York: Academic Press 1966

Marcus, A. J.: Recent advances in platelet lipid metabolism research. Ann. N.Y. Acad. Sci. **201**, 102—108 (1972)

Marcus, A. J., Ullman, M. L., Safier, L. B.: Lipid composition of subcellular particles of human blood platelets. J. Lipid Res. **10**, 108—114 (1969)

Marcus, A. J., Zucker, M. B.: The physiology of blood platelets. New York: Grune and Stratton 1965

Margaretten, W., McKay, D. G.: The role of the platelet in the generalised Shwartzman reaction. J. exp. Med. **129**, 585—590 (1969)

Margaretten, W., McKay, D. G.: The requirement for platelets in the active Arthus reaction. Amer. J. Path. **64**, 257—263 (1971)

Matthew, T. H., Hogan, G. P., Lewers, D. T., Bauer, H., Maher, J. F., Schreiner, G. E.: Controlled, double-blind trial of antiplatelet aggregating agents in vascular allograft rejection. Transplant. Proc. **3**, 901—904 (1971)

Meuller-Eckhardt, C., Lüscher, E. F.: Immune reactions of human blood platelets. I. A comparative study on the antigen-antibody complexes, aggregated γ-globulin and thrombin. Thrombos. Diathes. haemorrh. (Stuttg.) **20**, 155—167 (1968)

Meyer, D., Jenkins, C. S. P., Dreyfus, D.: Willebrand factor and ristocetin-II. Relationship between Willebrand factor, Willebrand antigen and factor VIII activity. Brit. J. Haemat. **28**, 579—599 (1974)

Michal, F.: Measurement of platelet aggregation and shape change. In: Mannucci, P. M., Gorini, S. (Eds.): Platelet Function and Thrombosis. A Review of Methods, pp. 257—262. New York-London: Plenum Press 1972

Michal, F.: Pharmacology of platelet aggregation and its therapeutic implications. In: Caprino, L., Rossi, E. C. (Eds.): Platelet Aggregation and Drugs, pp. 185—195. London-New York-San Francisco: Academic Press 1974

Mills, D. C. B.: Changes in the adenylate energy charge in human blood platelets induced by adenosine diphosphate. Nature (New Biol.) **243**, 220—222 (1973)

Mills, D. C. B.: Early metabolic effects of ADP on platelets. In: Caprino, L., Rossi, E. C. (Eds.): Platelet Aggregation and Drugs, pp. 159—168. London: Academic Press 1974

Mills, D. C. B., McFarlane, D. E.: Stimulation of human platelet adenylate cyclase by prostaglandin D_2. Thrombos. Res. **5**, 401—412 (1974)

Mills, D. C. B., Robb, I. A., Roberts, G. C. K.: The release of nucleotides, 5-hydroxytryptamine and enzymes from blood platelets during aggregation. J. Physiol. (Lond.) **195**, 715—729 (1968)

Mills, D. C. B., Roberts, G. C. K.: Effects of adrenaline on human blood platelets. J. Physiol. (Lond.) **193**, 443—453 (1967a)

Mills, D. C. B., Roberts, G. C. K.: Membrane active drugs and the aggregation of human blood platelets. Nature (Lond.) **213**, 35—38 (1967b)

Mills, D. C. B., Smith, J. B.: Control of platelet responsiveness by agents that influence cyclic AMP metabolism. Ann. N.Y. Acad. Sci. **201**, 391—399 (1972)

Mitchell, J. R. A., Sharp, A. A.: Platelet clumping in vitro. Brit. J. Haemat. **10**, 78—93 (1964)

Mittman, C., Ed.: Pulmonary emphysema and proteolysis. London-New York: Academic Press 1972

Mohammed, S. F., Whitworth, C., Chuang, H. Y. K., Lundblad, R. L., Mason, R. G.: Multiple active forms of thrombin binding to platelets and effects on platelet function. Proc. nat. Acad. Sci. (Wash.) **73**, 1660—1663 (1976)

Moncada, S., Bunting, S., Mullane, K., Thorogood, P., Vane, J. R., Raz, A., Needleman, P.: Imidazole: a selective inhibitor of thromboxane synthetase. Prostaglandins **13**, 611—618 (1977)

Moncada, S., Ferreira, S. H., Vane, J. R.: Prostaglandins, aspirin-like drugs and the oedema of inflammation. Nature (Lond.) **246**, 217—219 (1973)

Morrison, R. I. G., Barrett, A. J., Dingle, J. T., Prior, D.: Cathepsins B1 and D. Action on human cartilage proteoglycans. Biochim. biophys. Acta **302**, 411—419 (1973)

Motulsky, A. G.: Platelet agglutination by influenza virus. Clin. Res. Proc. **1**, 100 (1953)

Movat, H. Z., Uriuhara, T., Taichman, N. S., Rowsell, H. C., Mustard, J. F.: The role of PMN-leukocyte lysosomes in tissue injury, inflammation and hypersensitivity. Immunology **14**, 637—648 (1968)

Mowbray, J. F.: Methods of suppression of immune responses. In: Dunning, A. J., Burrows, E. H., Compston, N. D., Hamilton, S. W., Kerr, D. N. S., Thompson, M. (Eds.): Proceedings of IX International Congress for Internal Medicine, Excerpta Medica Int. Congr. Ser. No. 137, pp. 106—110. Amsterdam: Excerpta Medica 1966

Muggli, R., Baumgartner, H. R.: Collagen-induced platelet aggregation requirement for tropocollagen. Thrombos. Res. **3**, 713—728 (1973)

Mustard, J. F., Evans, G., Packham, M. A., Nishizawa, E. E.: The platelet in intravascular immunological reactions. In: Movat, H. Z. (Ed.): Cellular and humoral mechanisms in anaphylaxis allergy. Proceedings 3rd International Symposium Canadian Society Immunology, 1968, pp. 151—163. Basel: Karger 1969

Mustard, J. F., Glynn, M. F., Nishizawa, E. E., Packham, M. A.: Platelet surface interactions; relationship to thrombosis and haemostasis. Fed. Proc. **20**, 106—114 (1967)

Mustard, J. F., Movat, H. Z., McMorine, D. R. L., Senyi, A.: Release of permeability factors from the blood platelet. Proc. Soc. exp. Biol. (N.Y.) **119**, 988—991 (1965)
Mustard, J. F., Packham, M. A.: Platelet phagocytosis. Ser. Haematol. **2**, 168—184 (1968)
Mustard, J. F., Packham, M. A.: Factors influencing platelet function: adhesion, release and aggregation. Pharmacol. Rev. **22**, 97—187 (1970)
Mustard, J. F., Packham, M. A.: Role of platelets and thrombosis in atherosclerosis. In: The Platelet—International Academy of Pathology. Monograph No. 11, pp. 215—232. Baltimore: Williams and Wilkins 1971
Mustard, J. F., Packham, M. A.: Platelets, thrombosis and drugs. Drugs **9**, 19—76 (1975)
Nachman, R. L.: Platelet proteins. Semin. Hematol. **5**, 18—31 (1968)
Nachman, R. L., Ferris, B.: Studies on the proteins of human platelet membranes. J. biol. Chem. **247**, 4468—4475 (1972)
Nachman, R. L., Weksler, B.: Platelet as an inflammatory cell. Ann. N.Y. Acad. Sci. **201**, 131—137 (1972)
Nachman, R. L., Weksler, B. B., Ferris, B.: Increased vascular permeability produced by human platelet granule cationic extract. J. clin. Invest. **49**, 274—281 (1970)
Nachman, R. L., Weksler, B. B., Ferris, B.: Characterisation of human platelet vascular permeability-enhancing activity. J. clin. Invest. **51**, 549—556 (1972)
Nagayama, M., Zucker, M. B., Beller, F. K.: Effects of a variety of endotoxins on human and rabbit platelet function. Thrombos. Diathes. haemorrh. (Stuttg.) **26**, 467—473 (1971)
Najean, Y., Ardaillou, N., Dresch, C., Bernard, J.: The platelet destruction site in thrombocytopenic purpuras. Brit. J. Haemat. **13**, 409—426 (1967)
Needleman, P., Bryan, B., Wyche, A., Bronson, S. D., Eakins, Ferrendelli, J. A., Minkes, M.: Thromboxane synthetase inhibitors as pharmacological tools: differential biochemical and biological effects on platelet suspensions. Prostaglandins **14**, 897—907 (1977)
Needleman, P., Minkes, M., Raz, A.: Thromboxanes: selective biosynthesis and distinct biological properties. Science **193**, 163—165 (1976b)
Needleman, P., Moncada, S., Bunting, S., Vane, J. R., Hamberg, M., Samuelsson, B.: Identification of an enzyme in platelet microsomes which generates thromboxanes A_2 from prostaglandin endoperoxides. Nature (Lond.) **261**, 558—560 (1976a)
Nemerson, Y.: The phospholipid requirement of tissue factor in blood coagulation. J. clin. Invest. **47**, 72—80 (1968)
Nishizawa, E. E., Miller, W. L., Gorman, R. R., Bundy, G. L., Svensson, J., Hamberg, M.: Prostaglandin D_2 as a potential anti-thrombotic agent. Prostaglandins **9**, 109—121 (1975)
Northover, B. J., Subramanian, G.: Analgesic-antipyretic drugs as antagonists of endotoxin shock in dogs. J. Path. Bact. **83**, 463—468 (1962)
Nugteren, D. H.: Arachidonate lipoxygenase in blood platelets. Biochim. biophys. Acta **380**, 299—307 (1975)
Nugteren, D. H.: Arachidonate lipoxygenase. In: Silver, M. J., Smith, J. B., Kocsis, J. J. (Eds.): Prostaglandins in Haematology, pp. 11—23. Holliswood, New York: Spectrum Publications 1977
Nugteren, D. H., Hazelhof, E.: Isolation and properties of intermediates in prostaglandin biosynthesis. Biochim. biophys. Acta **326**, 448—461 (1973)
Nunn, B.: Role of ADP in collagen induced platelet aggregation. Brit. J. Pharmacol. **46**, 579P—580P (1973)
Nurden, A. T., Caen, J. P.: Specific roles for platelet surface glycoproteins in platelet function. Nature (Lond.) **255**, 720—722 (1975)
Nurden, A. T., Caen, J. P.: An abnormal platelet glycoprotein problem in three cases of Glanzmann's thrombasthenia. Brit. J. Haemat. **28**, 253—260 (1974)
O'Brien, J. R.: Platelet aggregation II. Some results from a new method of study. J. clin. Path. **15**, 452—455 (1962)
O'Brien, J. R.: Some effects of adrenaline and anti-adrenaline compounds on platelets in vitro and in vivo. Nature (Lond.) **200**, 763—764 (1963)
O'Brien, J. R.: Effect of anti-inflammatory agents on platelets. Lancet **1**, 894—895 (1968)
O'Brien, J. R.: Platelet function tests and thrombosis. In: Mannucci, P. M., Gorini, S. (Eds.): Platelet Function and Thrombosis. A Review of Methods, pp. 43—54. New York-London: Plenum Press 1972

Oelz, O., Oelz, R., Knapp, H. R., Jr., Sweetman, B. J., Oates, J. A.: Biosynthesis of prostaglandin D_2. Formation of prostaglandin D_2 by human platelets. Prostaglandins **13**, 225—234 (1977)

Packham, M. A., Kinlough-Rathbone, R. L., Reimers, H. J., Scott, S., Mustard, J. F.: Mechanisms of platelet aggregation independant of adenosine diphosphate. In: Silver, M. J., Smith, J. B., Kocsis, J. J. (Eds.): Prostaglandins in Haematology, pp. 247—276. Holliswood, New York: Spectrum Publications 1977

Packham, M. A., Nishizawa, E. E., Mustard, J. F.: Response of platelets to tissue injury. Biochem. Pharmacol. Suppl., 171—184 (1968)

Parratt, J. R.: Myocardial and circulatory effects of *E. coli* endotoxin: modification of responses to catecholamines. Brit. J. Pharmacol. **47**, 12—25 (1973)

Parratt, J. R., Sturgess, R.: The effect of indomethacin on the cardiovascular responses of cats to E. coli endotoxin. Brit. J. Pharmacol. **49**, 163P—164P (1973)

Pepper, D. S., Jamieson, G. A.: Isolation of a glycoprotein fraction from human platelet membranes which inhibit viral haemagglutination. Nature (Lond.) **219**, 1252—1253 (1968)

Piper, P. J., Vane, J. R.: Release of additional factors in anaphylaxis and its antagonism by anti-inflammatory drugs. Nature (Lond.) **223**, 29—35 (1969)

Piper, R., Vane, J. R.: The release of prostaglandin from lung and other tissues. Ann. N.Y. Acad. Sci. **180**, 363—385 (1971)

Phillips, D. R., Agin, P. P.: Thrombin-induced alterations in the plasma membrane. Ser. Haematol. **6**, 292—310 (1973)

Pletscher, A.: Metabolism, transfer and storage of 5-hydroxytryptamine in blood platelets. Brit. J. Pharmacol. **32**, 1—16 (1968)

Pletscher, A., Bartholini, G., Da Prada, M.: Metabolism of monoamines by blood platelets and relation to 5-hydroxytryptamine liberation. In: von Euler, U. S., Rosell, S., Uvnas, B. (Eds.): Mechanisms of Release of Biogenic Amines, pp. 165—175. Oxford-London: Pergamon Press 1966a

Pletscher, A., Burkard, W. P., Tranzer, J. P., Gey, K. F.: Two sites of 5-hydroxytryptamine uptake in blood platelets. Life Sci. **6**, 273—280 (1967)

Pletscher, A., Da Prada, M., Bartholini, G.: Temperature dependance of the passive in and outflow of 5-hydroxytryptamine in blood platelets. Biochem. Pharmacol. **15**, 419—424 (1966b)

Pletscher, A., Da Prada, M., Berneis, K. H.: New aspects on the storage of 5-hydroxytryptamine in blood platelets. Experientia (Basel) **27**, 993—1002 (1971)

Polasek, J., Kubisz, P.: Acid phosphatases and platelet factor 3. Scand. J. Haemat. **5**, 390—400 (1968)

Porter, K. A.: Rejection in treated allografts. J. clin. Path. **20**, Suppl. 518—523 (1967)

Praga, C., Valentine, L., Maiorano, M., Cortellaro, M.: A new automatic device for the standardised. Ivy Bleeding Time. In: Mannucci, P. M., Gorini, S. (Eds.): Platelet Function and Thrombosis. A Review of Methods, pp. 271—279. New York-London: Plenum Press 1972

Press, M., Hartop, P. J., Hawkey, C.: Correction of essential fatty acid deficiency and "sticky" platelets in man by the cutaneous administration of sunflower seed oil. Clin. Sci. molec. Med. **46**, 138 (1974)

Puszkin, E., Puszkin, S., Aledort, L. M.: Colchicine-binding protein from human platelets and its effect on muscle myosin and platelet myosin-like thrombasthenin-M. J. biol. Chem. **246**, 271—276 (1971)

Ratnoff, O. D.: Relation among hemostasis, fibrinolytic phenomena, immunity, and the inflammatory response. Advanc. Immunol. **10**, 145—227 (1969)

Ream, V. J., Deykin, D., Gurewich, V., Wessler, S.: The aggregation of human platelets by bacterial endotoxin. J. Lab. clin. Med. **66**, 245—252 (1965)

Reimers, H. J., Allen, D. J., Feurstein, A., Mustard, J. F.: Transport and storage of serotonin by thrombin-treated platelets. J. Cell Biol. **65**, 359—372 (1975a)

Reimers, H. J., Mustard, J. F., Packham, M. A.: Transfer of adenine nucleotides between the releasable and non-releasable compartements of rabbit blood platelets. J. Cell Biol. **67**, 61—67 (1975b)

Reimers, H. J., Packham, M. A., Mustard, J. F.: Labelling of the releasable adenine nucleotide pool of human platelets. Fed. Proc. **34**, Abs. 3595 (1975c)

Reuse, J. J.: Antihistamine drugs and histamine release, especially in anaphylaxis. In: Wostenholme, G. W., O'Connor, C. M. (Eds.): Histamine, Ciba Foundation Symposium, pp. 150—154. London: Churchill 1956
Rivers, J. P. W., Hassam, A. G.: Defective essential fatty acid metabolism in cystic fibrosis. Lancet **1975 I**, 642
Rodman, N. F.: Thrombosis. In: Zweifach, B. W., Grant, L., McCluskey, R. T. (Eds.): The Inflammatory Process, 2nd Edit., Vol. II, pp. 363—392. New York-London: Academic Press 1973
Rodman, N. F., Mason, R. G.: Platelet-platelet interaction: relationship to haemostasis and thrombosis. Fed. Proc. **26**, 95—105 (1967)
Rosenthale, M. E., Dervinis, A., Kassarich, J.: Prostaglandins and anti-inflammatory drugs in the dog knee joint. J. Pharm. (Lond.) **24**, 149—150 (1972)
Rossi, E. C.: The search for a clinically useful inhibitor of primary ADP-induced platelet aggregation. In: Caprino, L., Rossi, E. C. (Eds.): Platelet Aggregation and Drugs, pp. 221—233. London-New York-San Fransisco: Academic Press 1974
Roth, G. J., Majerus, P. W.: The mechanism of the effect of aspirin on human platelets. I. Acetylation of a particulate fraction protein. J. clin. Invest. **56**, 624—632 (1975)
Roth, G. J., Stanford, D., Majerus, P. W.: Acetylation of prostaglandin synthetase by aspirin. Proc. nat. Acad. Sci. (Wash.) **72**, 3073—3076 (1975)
Safrit, H., Weiss, H. J., Phillips, G.: Platelet phospholipids and fatty acids in patients with primary defects of platelet function. Lipids **7**, 60—67 (1972)
Salzman, E. W.: Measurement of platelet adhesiveness: a simple in vitro technique demonstrating an abnormality in von Willebrand's disease. J. Lab. clin. Med. **62**, 724—735 (1963)
Salzman, E. W.: Cyclic AMP and platelet function. New. Engl. J. Med. **286**, 358—363 (1972)
Salzman, E. W.: Prostaglandins, cyclic AMP and platelet function. Thrombos. Diathes. haemorrh. (Stuttg.) **60** Suppl., 311—319 (1974)
Salzman, E. W., Chambers, D. A., Neri, L. L.: Possible mechanism of aggregation of blood platelets with ADP. Nature (Lond.) **210**, 167—169 (1966)
Samuels, C. E., Robinson, P. G., Elliot, R. B.: Decreased inhibition of platelet aggregation by PGE_1 in children with cystic fibrosis and their parents. Prostaglandins **10**, 617—621 (1975)
Shoene, N. W., Iacono, J. M.: The influence of phospholipase A_2 on prostaglandin production in platelets. In: Samuelsson, B., Paoletti, R. (Eds.): Advances in Prostaglandin and Thromboxane Research, Vol. 2, pp. 763—766. New York: Raven Press 1976
Schulz, H., Landgräber, E.: Elektronenmikroskopische Untersuchungen über die Adsorption und Phagocytose von Influenza-Viren durch Thrombocyten. Klin. Wschr. **44**, 998—1006 (1966)
Scott, J. L., Cartwright, G. E., Wintrobe, M. M.: Acquired aplastic anaemia: an analysis of thirty nine cases and review of the pertinant literature. Medicine (Baltimore) **38**, 119—172 (1959)
Sear, C. H. J., Poller, L.: Antiheparin activity of human serum and platelet factor 4. Thrombos. Diathes. haemorrh. (Stuttg.) **30**, 93—105 (1973)
Shio, H., Ramwell, P. W.: Effect of prostaglandin E_2 and aspirin on the secondary aggregation of human platelets. Nature (New Biol.) **236**, 45—46 (1972)
Shwartzman, G.: A new phenomenon of local skin reactivity to B. Typhosus culture filtrate. Proc. Soc. exp. Biol. (N.Y.) **25**, 560—561 (1928)
Silver, M. D., Stehbens, W. E.: The behaviour of platelets in vivo. Quart. J. exp. Physiol. **1**, 241—248 (1965)
Silver, M. J., Smith, J. B., Ingerman, C. M.: Blood platelets and the inflammatory process. Agents Actions **4**, 233—240 (1974)
Silver, M. J., Smith, J. B., Ingerman, C., Kocsis, J. J.: Human blood prostaglandins: formation during clotting. Prostaglandins **1**, 429—436 (1972)
Silver, M. J., Smith, J. B., Ingerman, C., Kocsis, J. J.: Arachidonic acid-induced human platelet aggregation and prostaglandin formation. Prostaglandins **4**, 863—875 (1973)
Silver, M. J., Smith, J. B., Webster, G. R.: Phospholipase activity in human platelets. Pharmacologist **13**, 474 (1971)
Skaer, R. J., Peters, P. D., Emmines, J. P.: The localisation of calcium and phosphorus in human platelets. J. Cell Sci. **15**, 679—692 (1974)
Smith, A. D., Winkler, H.: Lysosomal phospholipases A_1 and A_2 of bovine adrenal medulla. Biochem. J. **108**, 867—874 (1968)

Smith, G. M.: The influence of β-adrenergic blocking drugs on platelet aggregation. In: Ditzel, J., Lewis, D. H. (Eds.): 6th European Conference on Microcirculation, Aalborg 1970, pp. 335—338. Basel: Karger 1971

Smith, J. B.: Platelets and permeability factors. In: Van Arman, C. G. (Ed.): White Cells in Inflammation, pp. 3—14. Springfield, Ill.: Charles C. Thomas 1974

Smith, J. B., Ingerman, C., Kocsis, J. J., Silver, M. J.: Formation of prostaglandins during the aggregation of human blood platelets. J. clin. Invest. **52**, 965—969 (1973a)

Smith, J. B., Ingerman, C., Kocsis, J. J., Silver, M. J.: Formation of an intermediate in prostaglandin biosynthesis and its association with the platelet release reaction. J. clin. Invest. **53**, 1468—1472 (1974a)

Smith, J. B., Ingerman, C. M., Silver, M. J.: Platelet prostaglandin production and its implications. In: Samuelsson, B. and Paoletti, R. (Eds.): Advances in Prostaglandin and Thromboxane Research, Vol. 2, pp. 747—753. New York: Raven Press 1976

Smith, J. B., Ingerman, E. M., Silver, M. J.: Effects of prostaglandin precursors on platelets. In: Silver, M. J., Smith, J. B., Kocsis, J. J. (Eds.): Prostaglandins in Haematology, pp. 277—292. Holliswood, New York: Spectrum Publications 1977

Smith, J. B., Silver, M. J., Ingerman, C., Kocsis, J. J.: Prostaglandin D_2 inhibits the aggregation of human platelets. Thrombos. Res. **5**, 291—299 (1974b)

Smith, J. B., Silver, M. J., Webster, G. R.: Phospholipase A_1 of human blood platelets. Biochem. J. **131**, 615—618 (1973b)

Smith, J. B., Willis, A. L.: Formation and release of prostaglandins by platelets in response to thrombin. Brit. J. Pharmacol. **40**, 545P—546P (1970)

Smith, J. B., Willis, A. L.: Aspirin selectively inhibits prostaglandin production in human platelets. Nature (New Biol.) **231**, 235—237 (1971)

Smith, M. J. H., Walker, J. R., Ford-Hutchinson, A. W., Pennington, D. G.: Platelets, prostaglandins and inflammation. Agents Actions **6**, 701—704 (1976)

Solomon, L. A., Hinshaw, L. B.: Effect of acetyl salicylic acid on the liver response to endotoxin. Proc. Soc. exp. Biol. (N.Y.) **127**, 225—332 (1968)

Solum, N. O.: Platelet aggregation during fibrin polymerization. Scand. J. clin. Invest. **18**, 577—587 (1966)

Spector, A. A., Hoak, J. C., Furlow, T. W., Bass, N. H., Silver, M. J., Hoch, W. S., Kocsis, J. J., Ingerman, C. M., Smith, J. B.: Fatty acids, platelets and microcirculatory obstruction. Science **190**, 490—492 (1975)

Spielvogel, A. R.: An ultrastructural study of the mechanisms of platelet-endotoxin interaction. J. exp. Med. **126**, 235—249 (1967)

Stecher, V. J., Sorkin, E., Ryan, G. B.: Relation between blood coagulation and chemotaxis of leukocytes. Nature (New Biol.) **233**, 95—96 (1971)

Stechschulte, D. J., Austen, K. F.: Anaphylaxis. In: Zweifach, B. W., Grant, L., McCluskey, R. T. (Eds.): The Inflammatory Process, 2nd Edit., Vol. III, pp. 237—276. London-New York: Academic Press 1974

Steiner, M.: The role of membrane proteins in platelet aggregation. In: Baldini, M. G., Ebbe, E. (Eds.): Platelets, Production, Function, Transfusion, and Storage, pp. 197—206. New York: Grune and Stratton 1974

Stormorken, H., Owren, P. A.: Physiopathology of haemostasis. Semin. Haematol. **8**, 3—29 (1971)

Suttie, J. W., Jackson, C. M.: Prothrombin structure, activation and biosynthesis. Physiol. Rev. **57**, 1—70 (1977)

Suzuki, T., Nagasawa, M. Y., Takahashi, H., Kato, H.: Liberation mechanisms of kinins in bovine plasma. In: Sicuteri, F., Rocha e Silva, M., Back, N. (Eds.): Bradykinin and Related Kinins. Cardiovascular, Biochemical and Neural Actions, pp. 15—22. New York: Plenum Press 1970

Svensson, J., Hamberg, M., Samuelsson, B.: Prostaglandin endoperoxides. IX. Characterisation of rabbit aorta contracting substance (RCS) from guinea pig lung and human platelets. Acta. physiol. scand. **94**, 222—228 (1975)

Swinson, D. R., Bennet, A., Hamilton, E. B. D.: Synovial prostaglandins in joint disease. In: Lewis, G. P. (Ed.): The role of prostaglandins in Inflammation, pp. 41—46. Stuttgart-Vienna: Hans Huber 1976

Taichmann, N. S., Uriuhara, T., Movat, H. Z.: Ultrastructural alterations in the local Shwartzman reaction. Lab. Invest. **14**, 2160—2176 (1965)

Tashjian, A. H. J., Voelkel, E. F., McDonough, J., Levine, L.: Hydrocortisone inhibits prostaglandin production by mouse fibrosarcoma cells. Nature (Lond.) **258**, 739—741 (1975)

Terada, H., Baldini, M., Ebbe, S., Madoff, M. A.: Interaction of influenza virus with blood platelets. Blood **28**, 213—228 (1966)

Tomlinson, R. V., Ringold, H. J., Qureshi, M. C., Forchielli, E.: Relationship between inhibition of prostaglandin synthesis and drug efficacy. Support for the current theory on mode of action of aspirin-like drugs. Biochem. biophys. Res. Commun. **46**, 552—559 (1972)

Ts'ao, C. H.: Rough endoplasmic reticulum and ribosomes in blood platelets. Scand. J. Haemat. **8**, 134—140 (1971)

Tschopp, T. B.: Aggregation of cat platelets in vitro. Thrombos. Diathes. haemorrh. (Stuttg.) **23**, 601—620 (1970)

Tschopp, T. B., Baumgartner, H. R.: Enzymatic removal of ADP from plasma. Unaltered platelet adhesion but reduced aggregation on sub-endothelium and collagen fibrils. Thrombos. diathes. haemorrh. (Stuttg.) **35**, 334—341 (1976)

Tschopp, T. B., Weiss, H. J.: Decreased ATP, ADP, and serotonin in young platelets of fawn-hooded rats with storage pool disease. Thrombos. Diathes. haemorrh. (Stuttg.) **32**, 670—677 (1974)

Tschopp, T. B., Weiss, H. J., Baumgartner, H. R.: Decreased adhesion of platelets to sub-endothelium in von Willebrand's disease. J. Lab. clin. Med. **83**, 296—300 (1974b)

Tschopp, T. B., Weiss, H. J., Baumgartner, H. R.: Interaction of platelets with sub-endothelium in thrombasthenia: normal adhesion, impaired aggregation. Experientia (Basel) **31**, 113—116 (1975)

Tschopp, T. B., Zucker, M. B.: Hereditary defect in platelet function in rats. Blood **40**, 217—226 (1972)

Turner, S. R., Tainer, S. A., Lynn, W. J.: Biogenesis of chemotactic molecules by the arachidonate lipoxygenase system of platelets. Nature (Lond.) **257**, 680—681 (1975)

Ubatuba, F. B., Harvey, E. A., Ferreira, S. H.: Are platelets important in inflammation? Agents Actions **5**, 31—34 (1975)

Ukena, T. E., Berlin, R. D.: Effect of colchicine and vinblastine on the topographical separation of membrane functions. J. exp. Med. **136**, 1—7 (1972)

Vainer, H.: Platelet populations. Advanc. exp. Med. Biol. **34**, 191—217 (1972)

Valone, F. H., Austen, K. F., Goetzl, E. J.: Modulation of the random migration of human platelets. J. clin. Invest. **54**, 1100—1106 (1974)

Valone, F. H., Austen, K. F., Goetzl, E. J.: Inhibition by aspirin of the enhanced migration of human platelets in response to prostaglandin precursors. Immunol. Commun. **4**, 139—148 (1975)

Van Aken, W. G., Croote, T. M., Vreeken, J.: Platelet aggregation: an intermediary mechanism in carbon clearance. Scand. J. Haemat. **5**, 333—338 (1968)

Van Arman, C. G., Carlson, R. P., Brown, W. R., Itkin, A.: Indomethacin inhibits the local Shwartzman reaction. Proc. Soc. exp. Biol. (N.Y.) **134**, 163—168 (1970)

Vane, J. R.: Inhibition of prostaglandin synthesis as a mechanism of action for aspirin-like drugs. Nature (New Biol.) **231**, 232—235 (1971)

Vane, J. R.: Inhibition of prostaglandin biosynthesis as the mechanism of action of aspirin-like drugs. Advanc. Biosci. **9**, 395—411 (1973)

Vargaftig, B. B., Chignard, M.: Substances that increase the cyclic AMP content prevent platelet aggregation and the concurrent release of pharmacologically active substances evoked by arachidonic acid. Agents. Actions **5**, 137—144 (1975)

Vargaftig, B. B., Trainier, Y., Chignard, M.: Blockade by metal complexing agents and by catalase of the effects of arachidonic acid on platelets; relevance to the study of antiinflammatory mechanisms. Europ. J. Pharmacol. **33**, 19—29 (1975)

Vargaftig, B. B., Zirinis, P.: Platelet aggregation induced by arachidonic acid is accompanied by release of potential inflammatory mediators distinct from PGE_2 and $PGF_{2\alpha}$. Nature (New Biol.) **244**, 114—116 (1973)

Vincent, J. E., Melai, A., Bonta, I. L.: Comparison of the effects of prostaglandin E_1 on platelet aggregation in normal and essential fatty acid deficient rats. Prostaglandins **5**, 369—373 (1974)

Vincent, J. E., Zijlstra, F. J., Bonta, I. L.: The effects of non-steroid anti-inflammatory drugs (NSAID), dibutyryl cyclic 3′5′adenosine monophoshate and phosphodiesterase inhibitors on platelet aggregation and platelet serotonin release in normal and essential fatty acid deficient (EFAD) rats. In: Samuelsson, B., Paoletti, R. (Eds.): Advances in Prostaglandin and Thromboxane Research, Vol. 2, p. 854. New York: Raven Press 1976

Waalkes,T.P., Weissbach,H., Bozicevich,J., Udenfriend,S.: Serotonin and histamine release during anaphylaxis in the rabbit. J. clin. Invest. **36**, 1115—1120 (1957a)
Waalkes,T.P., Weissbach,H., Bozicevich,J., Udenfriend,S.: Further studies on release of serotonin and histamine during anaphylaxis in the rabbit. Proc. Soc. exp. Biol. (N.Y.) **95**, 479—482 (1957b)
Walsh,P.N.: Platelet coagulant activities in thrombasthenia. Brit. J. Haemat. **23**, 553—569 (1972)
Weiss,H.J.: Platelet aggregation, adhesion and adenosine diphosphate release in thrombopathia (platelet factor 3 deficiency); a comparison with Glanzmann's thrombasthenia and von Willebrand's disease. Amer. J. Med. **43**, 470—578 (1967)
Weiss,H.J.: Von Willebrand's disease—diagnostic criterion. Blood **32**, 668—679 (1968)
Weiss,H.J.: Abnormalities in platelet function due to defects in the release reaction. Ann. N.Y. Acad. Sci. **201**, 161—173 (1972a)
Weiss,H.J.: The pharmacology of platelet inhibition. Prog. Haemostasis Thromb. **1**, 199—231 (1972b)
Weiss,H.J.: Abnormalities of factor VIII and platelet aggregation—use of ristocetin in diagnosing the von Willebrand's syndrome. Blood **45**, 403—412 (1975a)
Weiss,H.J.: Platelet physiology and abnormalities of platelet function. New Engl. J. Med. **293**, 531—541, 580—588 (1975b)
Weiss,H.J., Aledort,L.M.: Impaired platelet connective-tissue reaction in man after aspirin ingestion. Lancet **2**, 495—497 (1967)
Weiss,H.J., Aledort,L.M., Kochwa,S.: The effect of salicylates on the haemostasis properties of platelets in man. J. clin. Invest. **47**, 2169—2180 (1968)
Weiss,H.J., Chervinick,P.A., Zulusky,R., Factor,A.: A familiar defect in platelet function associated with impaired release of adenosine diphosphate. New Engl. J. Med. **28**, 1264—1270 (1969)
Weiss,H.J., Rogers,J., Brand,H.: Defective ristocetin-induced platelet aggregation in von Willebrand's disease and its correction by factor VIII. J. clin. Invest. **52**, 2697—2707 (1973)
Weiss,H.J., Tschopp,T.B., Baumgartner,H.R.: Decreased adhesion of giant (Bernard-Soulier) platelets to sub-endothelium: further implications on the role of the von Willebrand's factor in haemostasis. Amer. J. Med. **57**, 920—925 (1974a)
Weiss,H.J., Tschopp,T.B., Baumgartnèr,H.R.: Impaired interaction (adhesion-aggregation) of platelets with the sub-endothelium in storage-pool disease and after aspirin ingestion: a comparison with von Willebrand's disease. New Engl. J. Med. **293**, 619—623 (1975)
Weiss,H.J., Tschopp,T., Rogers,J., Brand,H.: Studies of platelet 5-hydroxytryptamine (serotonin) in patients with storage pool disease and albinism. J. clin. Invest. **54**, 421—432 (1974b)
Weiss,H.J., Willis,A.L., Kuhn,D.C., Brand,H.: Prostaglandin E_2 potentiation of platelet aggregation induced by LASS endoperoxide; absent in storage pool disease, normal after aspirin ingestion. Brit. J. Haemat. **32**, 257—272 (1976)
Weissman,G.: Role of lysosomes in inflammation and disease. Ann. Rev. Med. **18**, 97—112 (1967)
Weksler,B.B., Coupal,C.E.: Platelet-dependent generation of chemotactic activity in serum. J. exp. Med. **137**, 1419—1430 (1973)
Weksler,B.B., Nachman,R.L.: Rabbit platelet bactericidal protein. J. exp. Med. **134**, 1114—1130 (1971)
Wessells,N.K., Spooner,B.S., Ash,J.F., Bradley,M.O., Luduena,M.A., Taylor,E.L., Wrenn,J.T., Yamada,K.M.: Microfilaments in cellular and development processes. Science **171**, 135—143 (1971)
White,J.G.: The transfer of thorium particles from plasma to platelets and platelet granules. Amer. J. Path. **53**, 567—575 (1968)
White,J.G.: Platelet morphology. In: Johnson,S.A. (Ed.): The circulating platelet, pp. 46—122. New York: Academic Press 1971
White,J.G.: Interaction of membrane systems in blood platelets. Amer. J. Path. **66**, 295—312 (1972)
White,J.G., Krivit,W.: An ultrastructure basis for the shape change induced in platelets by chilling. Blood **30**, 625—635 (1967)
White,J.G., Witkop,J.G.: Effects of normal and aspirin-treated platelets on defective secondary aggregation in the Hermansky-Pudlak syndrome. Amer. J. Path. **68**, 57—66 (1972)

Wilkinson, P. C., Basel, J. F., Stecher-Levin, V. J., Sarkin, E.: Macrophage and neutrophil specific chemotactic factors in serum. Nature (Lond.) **222**, 244—247 (1969)

Williams, T. J.: Recent concepts of the clotting mechanism. Semin. Haematol. **5**, 32—44 (1968)

Williams, T. J., Morley, J.: Prostaglandins as potentiators of increased vascular permeability in inflammation. Nature (Lond.) **246**, 215—217 (1973)

Willis, A. L.: Identification of prostaglandin E_2 in rat inflammatory exudate. Pharmacol. Res. Commun. **2**, 297—304 (1970)

Willis, A. L.: Biosynthesis of prostaglandins E_2 and $F_{2\alpha}$ generates labile material which induces platelet aggregation. Abstracts 4th International Congress Thrombosis Haemostasis, Vienna, p. 79, 1973a

Willis, A. L.: Platelet synthesis of aggregatory material from arachidonate and its blockade by aspirin. Circulation Suppl., IV **8**, 10—25 (1973b)

Willis, A. L.: An enzymatic mechanism for the anti-thrombotic and anti-haemostatic actions of aspirin. Science **183**, 325—327 (1974a)

Willis, A. L.: Isolation of a chemical trigger for thrombosis. Prostaglandins **5**, 1—25 (1974b)

Willis, A. L., Cornelsen, M.: Repeated injection of prostaglandin E_2 in rat paws induces chronic swelling and a marked decrease in pain threshold. Prostaglandins **3**, 353—357 (1973)

Willis, A. L., Davison, P., Ramwell, P. W., Brocklehurst, W. E., Smith, B.: Release and actions of prostaglandins in inflammation and fever: Inhibition by anti-inflammatory and antipyretic drugs. In: Ramwell, P. W., Phariss, B. B. (Eds.): Prostaglandins in Cellular Biology, pp. 227—268. New York-London: Plenum Press 1972

Willis, A. L., Kuhn, D. C.: A new potential mediator of arterial thrombosis whose biosynthesis is inhibited by aspirin. Prostaglandins **4**, 127—130 (1973)

Willis, A. L., Kuhn, D. C., Weiss, H. J.: Acetylenic analogue of arachidonate that acts like aspirin on platelets. Science **183**, 327—330 (1974b)

Willis, A. L., Stone, K. J.: Prostaglandins, thromboxanes, their precursors, intermediates, metabolites and analogs—a compendium. In: Fasman, G. D. (Ed.): Handbook of Biochemistry and Molecular Biology, 3rd Ed., Vol. II, pp. 312—423. Cleveland, Ohio: CRC Press 1976

Willis, A. L., Vane, F. M., Kuhn, D. C., Scott, C. G., Petrin, M.: An endoperoxide aggregator (LASS) formed in platelets in response to thrombotic stimuli, purification, identification and unique biological significance. Prostaglandins **8**, 453—507 (1974a)

Willis, A. L., Weiss, H. J.: A congenital defect in platelet prostaglandin production associated with impaired haemostasis in storage pool disease. Prostaglandins **4**, 783—794 (1973)

Wiseman, E. H., Chang, Y.: The role of fibrin in the inflammatory response to carrageenin. J. Pharmacol. exp. Ther. **159**, 206—210 (1968)

Wright, H. P.: The adhesiveness of blood platelets following parturition and surgical operations. J. Path. Bact. **54**, 461—468 (1942)

Zeya, H. I., Spitznagel, J. K.: Characterisation of cationic protein-bearing granules of polymorphonuclear leukocytes. Lab. Invest. **24**, 229—236 (1971)

Zimmerman, T. S., Müller-Eberhard, H. J.: Blood coagulation initiation by a complement-mediated pathway. J. exp. Med. **134**, 1601—1607 (1971)

Zucker, M. B.: Platelets. In: Zweifach, B. W., Grant, L., McCluskey, R. T. (Eds.): The Inflammatory Process, 2nd Edit., Vol. 1, pp. 511—543. New York-San Francisco-London: Academic Press 1974

Zucker, M. B., Grant, R. A.: Aggregation and release reaction induced in human blood platelets by zymosan. J. Immunol. **112**, 1219—1230 (1974)

Zucker, M. B., Pert, J., Hilgartner, M. W.: Platelet function in a patient with thrombasthenia. Blood **28**, 524—534 (1966)

Zucker, M. B., Peterson, J.: Inhibition of adenosine diphosphate-induced secondary aggregation and other platelet functions by acetylsalicylic acid ingestion. Proc. Soc. exp. Biol. (N.Y.) **127**, 547—551 (1968)

Zucker, M. B., Peterson, J.: Effect of acetylsalicylic acid, other non-steroidal anti-inflammatory agents and dipyridamole on human blood platelets. J. Lab. clin. Med. **76**, 66—75 (1970)

Zucker-Franklin, D., Bloomberg, N.: Microfibrils of blood platelets: their relationship to microtubules and the contractile protein. J. clin. Invest. **48**, 167—175 (1969)

CHAPTER 6

Regeneration and Repair

L. E. GLYNN

A. The Replacement of Lost Tissue

Except in the most trivial examples of inflammation, tissue is lost during the inflammatory process. This can result from the direct action of the injurious agent itself upon the living cells in its vicinity, e.g. the dermo-necrotic factor of staphylococci, or indirectly from ischaemia as a consequence of local vascular stasis or thrombosis. The replacement of the necrotic tissue by a living tissue requires two preconditions: the removal of the necrotic material by a combination of phagocytosis and enzymic digestion, both intra- and extra-cellular, and the presence of viable cells able to reproduce. Moreover, the reproduction of such viable cells and the formation of their corresponding extra-cellular secretions are dependent upon local and systemic factors, such as the persistence or otherwise of the original irritant, the ability of the local blood supply to adapt itself readily to the increased demands resulting from the metabolic activity of the proliferating cells, and the nutritional status of the organism.

The replacement of lost tissue may be of two kinds:

I. Tissues Capable of Regeneration

These include the liver, the skin and most epithelia, but regeneration is inadequate in striated and cardiac muscle and is probably entirely absent in the CNS, at least as far as the nerve cells themselves are concerned. What determines whether a particular cell type in its mature state is still capable of proliferation is not understood. It is not merely a question of specialisation, since cells of the parenchymal organs are hardly less specialised than a smooth muscle fibre or a cell of the adipose tissue. To some extent at least, it appears to be a question of metabolic demand. For example, after a partial hepatectomy there must inevitably be an increased functional demand upon the remaining liver cells. It is difficult, however, to translate this to the situation of epithelial cells when the surface they cover has been breached; and metabolic demand, as for example in muscular exercise, may lead to cell enlargement (hypertrophy) but not to proliferation. There can be little doubt that the stimuli for cell proliferation must vary enormously between cell types and possibly even for similar cells under different conditions. In view of the readiness with which most cells can be induced to proliferate in tissue culture, it seems probable that the inherent tendency of cell proliferation thus revealed is held in check in vivo by mechanisms still mostly obscure. Contact between adjacent cells undoubtedly plays a role in some instances, e.g. fibroblasts (ABERCROMBIE, 1970) but there is also evidence for the existence of specific antimitotic agents termed chalones (HOUCK, 1973), which may operate in certain areas, e.g. the epidermis and the thymus. They are polypeptides of less than 30000 molecular weight, and although organ specific they are not species specific. To what extent substances of this kind are responsible for the control of cell proliferation in regeneration or repair is, however, unknown. They may perhaps be regarded as the counterpart of the trophic hormones whose presence stimulates the proliferation of the specific cells of their target organs and whose absence is followed by atrophy.

Although metabolic demand would appear to constitute an adequate stimulus for the increase in quantity of any tissue involved, there are probably several intermediate steps in the chemical sequence, most of which still remain to be discovered. Even as easily demonstrable an effect as anoxia upon the proliferation of the red cell precursors in the bone marrow is mediated by another substance namely erythropoietin (KRANTZ and JACOBSON, 1970) synthesised in the kidney. This is a mucoprotein of molecular weight 46000 and containing about 30% polysaccharide made up of approximately equal parts of hexosamine and nucleic acid.

Its mode of action in turn is also obscure but its study does illustrate the complexity of the events between what appears to be an adequate stimulus and the cell proliferation expected to result from it.

II. Tissues Incapable of Adequate Regeneration

Here it is important to recognise that even in organs capable of a high degree of regeneration such as the liver, situations can arise which interfere with parenchymal cell replacement, and the cell loss is in consequence made good by other tissue, presumably more adapted to the new environmental state. Thus, in organs like the liver, kidneys and glands, both exocrine and endocrine, the regenerative capacity of the specific epithelial cells is closely dependent upon the persistence of the original connective tissue framework, in order to supply an adequate scaffolding for the support of the newly formed cells. Even extensive loss of parenchymal cells, as in carbon tetrachloride-induced hepatic necrosis or in the average case of viral hepatitis, is usually rapidly and entirely replaced by the centripetal spread of cells from the proliferating survivors in the periportal zones (CAMERON and KARUNARATNE, 1936). If, however, the initial necrosis is so extensive that the fibrous framework of the lobules collapses before regeneration is completed, the end result is a scarred liver in which the bulk of the scar tissue is not newly formed but represents the collapsed remains of the original fibrous framework. Similarly in the kidney, the renal tubule cells are capable of proliferating and relining long stretches of a damaged nephron but if the extent of the damage is too great, or if other factors impede cell proliferation, collapse of the denuded nephron ensues with a characteristic linear scarring of the affected organ.

When large blocks of tissue are destroyed, as for example in areas of infarction as a consequence of acute vascular insufficiency, the result, even in organs capable of considerable parenchymal cell proliferation, is a permanent scar, which marks the site of initial damage. Here the situation is the converse of framework collapse and arises from the inability to clear the site of damaged tissue to make room for the ingrowth of newly formed parenchymal cells. This is an excellent example of the importance of site clearance as a necessary prerequisite for parenchymal regeneration. Interference with site clearance can arise in many ways, such as persistence of the initial injurious agent, the presence of protease inhibitors, or the sheer mass of necrotic tissue to be removed. Indispensable for adequate clearance is a vascular supply capable of providing the macrophages and removing the digestive products. For any or all of these reasons, site clearance may be impaired: the consequence is encapsulation with the necrotic mass regarded as a foreign body. Such necrotic lesions, if less than a few millimetres in diameter, undergo a slow but progressive invasion by fibroblasts; larger lesions are invaded with difficulty and frequently become calcified structures surrounded by a fibrous capsule.

B. The Nature of the Stimulus Leading to Formation of Scar Tissue

Scar tissue is a form of connective tissue rich in collagen fibres and, in its mature form, relatively poor in blood vessels. This presumably correlates with the low metabolic demand of a tissue composed mainly of extra-cellular material with few living cells. These cells are the survivors of those which produced the collagen fibres and other inter-cellular components of which scar tissue is largely composed. The origin of these cells is still not fully established but there is general agreement that they are derived from the fixed cells of connective tissue and not from the white cells of the circulation. Controversy is mainly concerned with the nature of these fixed connective tissue cells: are they already committed fibroblasts or are they derived from more primitive connective tissue cells with a wider potential for differentiation? The probability is that both types of cell can be involved depending upon the intensity of the stimulus. Since the precise nature of this stimulus is unknown, the measurement of its strength can only be assessed by the results. There is in fact very little evidence for a connective tissue stem cell. LASH (1972) states that "as far back in the embryo as one can go one finds that the tissues are making the normal constituents of extra cellular matrix—chondromucoprotein and (presumably) collagen fibrils. In fact it has been found in amphibians that unfertilised eggs can synthesise chondromucoprotein and collagen (KLOSE and FLICKINGER, 1971)."

It seems, therefore, that the fixed connective tissue cells, even in their resting state, can synthesise an inter-cellular matrix and probably do so at an extremely low level of activity. The appropriate stimulus, therefore, is not an instruction to perform a new activity but to increase the rate of one already in progress. What is this stimulus? Mention has already been made of inhibitory chalones, and the readiness with which connective tissue grows and forms a matrix in tissue culture seems to imply that release from inhibition is more important than direct stimulation. The phenomenon of contact inhibition, first shown with fibroblasts in culture (ABERCROMBIE, 1970) also emphasises the importance of inhibitory agents. Evidence from cells separated by cell-impermeable membranes excludes the participation of diffusible agents (BURGER, 1972), whereas the effect of proteases in releasing the cells from inhibition suggests the participation of a surface protein in the phenomenon. Transformed cells, in contrast to normal fibroblasts, do not exhibit contact inhibition but can be induced to show it by the introduction of protease inhibitors. The conclusion, therefore, is that transformed cells do not show contact inhibition because they, unlike normal cells, produce their own protease which, it is inferred, removes the inhibitory surface material.

The connective tissue cells in normal tissue, however, are not in contact with each other and their non-proliferating state must therefore be the result of other restraints. Does the inter-cellular maxtrix itself, or some particular constituent of it, inhibit cell proliferation, and is this eluted or destroyed in tissue culture? That matrix materials can influence the behaviour of associated cells has been claimed by KANG et al. (1966), who found in the amputated salamander forelimb that hyaluronic acid inhibits the production of chondroitin sulphate and collagen. It may well be, therefore, that the stimulus to cell proliferation and matrix formation in injured connective tissue is the change in the matrix itself consequent upon the enzyme release associated with the injury inflicted. Further evidence for the participation of hyaluronic acid in the control of connective tissue cell activity, is provided by the work of MUIR and her associates on the inhibition of proteoglycan biosynthesis by isolated cartilage cells of adult tissues (WIEBKIN and MUIR, 1973; HARDINGHAM and MUIR, 1974; WIEBKIN and MUIR, 1975).

Of all the known constituents of cartilage, only hyaluronic acid and its relatively large fragments (i.e. down to oligmers of not less than ten repeating units) inhibited the production of proteoglycans by the cartilage cells in tissue culture. This depended upon the interaction of the hyaluronic acid with some surface component of the cells, probably itself a proteoglycan, since neutralisation of the inhibitory effect resulted from enzyme treatment of the cells designed to remove either protein or chondroitin sulphate.

There is no reason to suppose that all types of connective tissue cell are subject to control by the same chemical entities. It would indeed be functionally more appropriate if the inhibitory agents bore some relationship to the normal matrix products of the cells in question. Thus hyaluronic acid, which plays a key role in aggregate formation of the proteoglycans in cartilage, is well suited by this function to exert some control over the cells synthesising these substances.

In other connective tissue sites e.g. the dermis, the matrix differs both qualitatively and quantitatively from that of cartilage, and it is therefore not surprising that hyaluronic acid has no effect on cells from non-cartilage connective tissue (WIEBKIN ct al., 1974). The possible existence and identification of the compounds in the various connective tissues with a role comparable to that of hyaluronic acid in cartilage, holds promising possibilities for the control of unwanted or excessive connective tissue proliferation and its associated matrix formation.

C. The Generation of Scar Tissue

The formation of scar tissue is seen in two contrasting situations: in the first, the presence of an acute inflammatory exudate results in the formation of considerable quantities of fibrin; in the second, inflammation is non-exudative and fibrin is virtually absent. Since fibrin itself seems to exert a potent stimulating effect upon fibroblastic activity, as well as providing a scaffold for the support of invading cells, the details of scar formation are strikingly different in the two situations.

I. Generation of Scar Tissue in the Presence of Fibrin

This is seen in its most characteristic and least complicated form when the exudate occurs on the surface of a body cavity, e.g. the pericardial sac. In such a situation, the process is unobscured by other components of the connective tissue. Within the first 24 h of the development of such an exudate, the natural gloss of the surface is lost owing to a combination of desquamation of the lining cells with the formation of a loosely adherent layer of interlacing fibrin filaments. At this stage, there is a modest to severe infiltration with polymorphonuclear cells, partly in response to the inflammatory agent but also partly in response to the fibrin itself, as can be shown by the subcutaneous implantation of a fragment of autochthonous fibrin in an experimental subject (BANERJEE and GLYNN, 1960; GLYNN and DUMONDE, 1965).

The invasion by polymorphonuclear cells is short-lived unless a pyrogenic agent is present, and is soon followed by an invasion of fibroblasts and endothelial cells derived from the underlying connective tissue. The stimulus for this invasion and the associated changes in the adjacent tissues is at least in part derived from the fibrin meshwork, since similar changes are seen in association with experimental fibrin implants, as already mentioned. The chemical nature of the stimulus is unknown, but it is most probably an enzymic breakdown product of fibrin or of fibrinogen. Several proteolytic enzymes are usually available: the tissue proteases, plasmin derived from plasminogen which is almost invariably present within any fibrin clot or exudate, and the lysosomal enzymes released from the polymorphonuclear cells of the early invasion. Of the various enzymes available, the latter appear to be the most important because in their absence fibrin can be seen to persist for abnormally long periods, e.g. in lobar pneumonia if for any reason the granulocyte response is impaired.

Little is known of the mechanisms involved in the formation of new vessels and their invasion of the fibrin mesh. New capillaries form by solid cellular outgrowths from the endothelial cells of pre-existing capillaries, with subsequent canalization and anastamosis with other similarly formed outgrowths. The immediate stimulus to the formation of these outgrowths seems to be a persistent increase in blood flow through the parent capillary and this in turn is consequent upon the metabolic demand of the tissues supplied by that vessel. Which metabolites are responsible is another question which can be only incompletely answered, but carbon dioxide, lack of oxygen and various intermediates of the glycolytic cycle, probably all contribute to the overall effect. That the fibrin mesh exerts a directional influence over the growth of the new vessels is evident even within the first two days, by which time sufficient ingrowth has occurred to bind the fibrin to the underlying surface. Its forcible detachment then reveals a series of minute bleeding points on the deep surface.

The ingrowth of capillaries is accompanied by migrating fibroblasts which are evidently capable of a gliding motion over the fibrillar elements of the fibrin network. The presence of contractile filaments within such fibroblasts has been especially studied by MAJNO and his colleagues (for review see GABBIANI et al., 1973) who have distinguished these cells from the classical resting fibroblast or fibrocyte by the name myo-fibroblast. There are several distinguishing features: (a) a rich fibrillar system within the cytoplasm consisting of bundles of fibrils 40–80 Å in diameter running parallel to the cell's long axis. Scattered electron-dense areas amongst these fibrils are reminiscent of similar bodies in smooth muscle cells. (b) As in smooth muscle cells, the nuclear membranes are highly indented. (c) Surface features suggestive in places of a basement membrane, and between adjacent cells maculae adhaerentes (desmosomes). (d) Chemically identifiable actomyosin in extracts of granulation tissue (4 mg/g of wet tissue). The contractile nature of these cells was confirmed by exposing strips of similar tissue to pharmacological agents known to excite smooth muscle contraction. These included 5-hydroxytryptamine (5-HT), bradykinin, and prostaglandins. (e) Specific immunofluorescence revealed that the filaments in question reacted specifically with sera containing anti-smooth muscle antibodies whereas only negative reactions were obtained with ordinary fibroblasts.

The invasion of the fibrin mesh by the myofibroblasts is rapidly followed by the appearance of collagen fibrils in the intercellular areas in intimate contact with the cells. The manner in which such a large structure as a collagen fibril is able to be assembled within a cell and then passed to the exterior has long puzzled biologists, and the puzzle has only recently approached resolution. Its complete resolution will require not only an understanding of the structure of the collagen molecule and its mode of assembly into a histological fibril, but also the steps of its intracellular synthesis, the changes undergone by the molecules after their assembly on the ribosomes and the various pathways open to them from the ribosome to the outer surface of the cell membrane. These will be considered in section D3 (p. 216).

The progressive increase in the amount of collagen is accompanied by a corresponding disappearance of the associated fibrin. The parallelism of these two events is sufficiently striking to have suggested to some of the early histopathologists that collagen was merely a physicochemically altered form of fibrin, a suggestion which is entirely ruled out by present knowledge of the strikingly different amino acid composition of these two proteins (DAVIE and RATNOFF, 1965; EASTOE, 1967).

II. Generation of Scar Tissue in the Absence of Fibrin

By no means all fibrotic processes involve the organisation of a pre-existing fibrinous exudate. In fact, the majority of progressive fibrotic processes occur independently of fibrin, e.g. nephrosclerosis, Dupuytren's contracture, cirrhosis of the liver and retroperitoneal fibrosis. Several of these conditions appear to arise by replacement of lost parenchymal cells by fibrous tissue, but whether the primary lesion is parenchymal cell loss or some pathological stimulus to the connective tissue framework is still unresolved, even in so well studied a situation as idiopathic hepatic cirrhosis. It is not even clear whether the increase in collagen in these conditions is produced by connective tissue cells or by the parenchymal cells themselves. In many situations, scirrhous mammary carcinoma for example, proline hydroxylase (GRANT and PROCKOP, 1972), an enzyme exclusively required for collagen synthesis, can be demonstrated within the neoplastic epithelial cells (KIRRANE, personal communication). It is doubtful, however, whether in non-neoplastic situations collagen is produced by epithelial cells, but it has been clearly established that smooth muscle in blood vessel walls can synthesise collagen during development and in tissue culture (ROSS and KLEBANOFF, 1971). Basement membranes, which are also rich in a collagen protein (KEFALIDES, 1973), are synthesised by epithelial cells and endothelial cells so that the absence of active fibroblasts in an area of increasing fibrosis need not be too surprising.

Not all fibrosis occurring in non-fibrinous areas need, however, be attributed to epithelial or endothelial collagen synthesis. In most situations, e.g. pulmonary silicosis, as well as other examples of progressive pulmonary fibrosis, the collagen synthesis is largely fibroblastic in origin and the stimulus is apparently derived from activated macrophages (Allison, 1973). This is highly probable in the fibrosis associated with granulomata, e.g. tuberculosis (Velo and Spector, 1973), and appears probable in other inflammatory situations even when the macrophages are less conspicuous.

The chemical nature of the stimulus provided by the macrophages has not yet been identified but could be one or more of the lysosomal enzymes, or some other secretory product within the repertoire of the macrophage at some phase of its activation.

In summary, the stimulus to collagen formation can be derived either from fibrin or macrophages, and the newly formed collagen from fibroblasts or other cells. Although in most instances fibroblasts are the principal source of the collagen, there are situations where other cells may contribute significantly or even predominantly. The recent recognition of different types of collagen in different anatomical or developmental situations (see p. 217) has drawn attention to the unique features of the collagen in basement membranes. If any forms of pathological fibrosis are indeed epithelial in origin, this may well be revealed by a study of the collagen type involved.

D. Stages in Scar Tissue Formation

I. Formation of Capillaries

When scar tissue is developing by the organisation of a fibrinous exudate, the invasion of the fibrin by fibroblasts is invariably accompanied by a parallel ingrowth of newly formed capillaries, as already described. Where the invading tissue is open to direct inspection, as in a healing ulcer, the looped ends of the capillaries impart a granular surface to the material filling the ulcer; hence the term granulation tissue. At this stage, it is bright red in colour and bleeds readily to the touch. When the defect has become filled with such tissue and its surface covered by an ingrowth of epithelial cells from the periphery, there is a progressive change in the appearance of the lesion. With the removal of the fibrin and its replacement by collagen and intercollagenous matrix, there is a progressive decrease in the synthetic activity and hence metabolism of the associated fibroblasts. This decrease is paralleled by a progressive reduction in size and then number of the fibroblasts present and a diminution in blood flow through the newly formed capillaries. This reduction in blood flow, as shown by Thoma (1896) many years ago, leads to collapse and ultimate disappearance of the majority of the vessels. The originally bright red scar progressively fades until it becomes even paler than the normal tissue around it. This pallor is partly attributable to the opacity of the collagenous tissue and partly to the low metabolic rate since the scar is now almost acellular without even the usual appendages of the normal tissue.

The change in vascularity as fibrin is organised, is presumably determined by the metabolic demand of the tissues in the immediate vicinity. The precise chemical agent or agents involved are not known but may be comparable to those responsible for the reactive hyperaemia, which occurs after periods of ischaemia that are too brief to cause cell death. Since similar changes occur in the vicinity of a fibrin implant it may be assumed that either products of fibrinolysis or the metabolic products of the activated fibroblasts can act in a similar fashion to increase the local blood flow and in consequence the formation of new capillaries. The studies of SILVER (1973) on healing wounds in rats and in rabbit ear chambers have shown that oxygen tension varies from almost zero in the wound space to between 60 and 90 mmHg in the nearest perfusing capillaries. Fibroblasts not only survive but could produce immunologically detectable collagen in the 10–30 mmHg zone, but cell proliferation was predominantly in the richer oxygen zone, namely 30–60 mmHg. In the zone of oxygen tension below 10 mmHg, the cells were incapable of synthesising an extracellular product.

The greater dependence of the proliferating cells than the synthesising cells upon the blood supply, was well demonstrated in SILVER's experiments in which the circulation was progressively impaired by the withdrawal of blood. In the growing zone, the oxygen tension fell to zero and when this was maintained for more than a few minutes, the cells in this zone showed evidence of serious damage with a fall in intracellular pH and impairment of the sodium pump. Complete arrest of the circulation in the experimental area in consequence of induced haemorragic shock resulted in much less dramatic changes in the more peripheral zones of the wound where synthesis prodominates over proliferation.

II. The Formation of Connective Tissue

All connective tissues, despite their considerable variation in macroscopic appearance, are composed of the same constituents: fibres, interstitial material amorphous by light microscopy and cells. Where the fibres predominate, the tissue is tough and resists stretching as in tendons and ligaments. Where the interstitial material predominates, the tissue is soft and gelatinous as in the umbilical cord, or firm with resistance to compression as in cartilage. Mineralisation can occur in any type of connective tissue under pathological conditions but is particularly favoured by the organisation and metabolism of the constituent elements of osteoid, the normal precursor of bone.

1. The Cells Involved

The major cell of connective tissue is the fibroblast and its quiescent counterpart the fibrocyte. Although earlier workers strongly favoured a haematogenous cell as the precursor of the fibroblast in healing wounds, kinetic studies with nuclear labelling have now clearly shown that the precursor cell is the fibrocyte which becomes activated, proliferates, and acquires the characteristic features of a fibroblast (ROSS, 1968). These features are essentially those of any cell actively sythesising protein for secretion. Thus, the nucleus is large and vesicular, with conspicuous nucleoli required for the elaboration of RNA for both messenger and other purposes. The cytoplasm is crowded with the elongated vesicles of rough endoplasmic reticulum and the Golgi vesicles are also well developed and occur in several areas not restricted to the vicinity of the nucleus. In addition, there are several small vesicles in the periphery, which observations on living cells have indicated are not pinocytotic but probably secretory in nature. Mitochondria are always present in moderate numbers and characterised by irregular cristae and pale staining matrix. Finally, and probably of importance in relation to the contractile properties of these cells (see p. 223), large numbers of fine filaments 80 Å in diameter are present, as well as contacts resembling tight junctions with adjacent cells.

Other cells do not normally contribute to the synthesis of collagen in connective tissue although there is much evidence that cells other than fibroblasts can occasionally do so. For example, epithelial basement membranes, which are largely if not exclusively secreted by the epithelial cells, contain collagen molecules although these are not aligned into fibres with the EM characteristics of collagen. Arterial smooth muscle is also a potential secretor of collagen as shown by ROSS and KLEBANOFF (1971), whilst there is also evidence that in some epithelial neoplasms, especially scirrhous carcinoma of breast, the interstitial collagen is produced by the neoplastic cells themselves. In support of this view is the presence in these cells of the enzyme prolyl hydroxylase which is apparently exclusively required for the hydroxylation of proline to hydroxyproline in the newly synthesised collagen chain (see below).

Although in addition to collagen fibres, connective tissues also contain elastic fibres, no criteria have been established for the recognition of the cells responsible for their synthesis. All the evidence available points to the fibroblast as the cell responsible, but the stimuli determining which fibre it should produce are completely unknown.

Of the cells indigenous to the connective tissues, in contrast to the migrant cells derived from the circulating blood, two remain for consideration—the histiocyte and the tissue mast cell. The histiocyte is the non-circulating counterpart of the blood monocyte and its derived form, the macrophage. Like the latter it is an actively phagocytic cell and lacks the organelles required for the synthesis of protein for extra cellular release. It presumably plays a role in removal of necrotic and effete cells and disorganised tissue. The tissue mast cell may similarly be regarded as the counterpart of the blood basophil and, like the basophil, it is characterised by granules containing heparin, histamine and sometimes 5-HT. The metachromasia of these granules gives them a superficial resemblance to the acid polysaccharides found in connective tissue ground substance and led to the erroneous view that some of these were actually derived from the granules (ASBOE-HANSON, 1954).

The role of these cells is still far from clearly understood but their usual proximity to blood vessels supports the view that their pharmacologically active ingredients play an important part in normal vascular physiology. The remarkable affinity shown by IgE immunoglobulin for the surface of these cells (ISHIZAKA et al., 1969) is responsible for allergic hypersensitivity to those substances that elicit an IgE response, e.g. ragweed pollen. There is no evidence, however, that mast cells play any direct part in the events leading to fibrosis or cell regeneration.

Finally, any of the circulating cells can on occasion be found in the connective tissues. The polymorphonuclear cells are rarely present in the absence of some irritant, but lymphocytes can always be found, although in small numbers. The occasional plasma cells are presumably derived from a precursor B-type lymphocyte, but when present in conspicuous numbers are indicative of a local immunogenic stimulus.

2. The Non-Fibrous Components of Connective Tissue

The non-fibrous components of connective tissue differ considerably between different types of tissue, but the differences are predominantly quantitative. The fundamental ingredient is the proteoglycan. This consists of a protein core in the form of a single polypeptide chain to which are attached at fairly regular intervals a series of polysaccharide side chains (ROSENBERG et al., 1970). These chains can be composed of chondroitin 4-sulphate or chondroitin 6-sulphate, dermatan sulphate or keratan sulphate. The attachment to the protein is usually via a glycosidic linkage to the hydroxyl group of either serine or threonine. The actual linkage itself is via a galactosyl-galactosylxylose (RODEN and SMITH, 1966). Because of the carboxyl and sulphate groups present, these macromonolecules carry a net negative change which is responsible for many of the physicochemical properties possessed by them, and which they impart to the connective tissue itself. These include such gel properties as swelling, entanglement of other macromolecules, excluded volume and ion exchange. It is the extended form of these molecules, by virtue of the mutual repulsion of the negative charges, that underlies these important attributes of the connective tissue.

The synthesis of the various proteoglycans is the function of the connective tissue cells i.e. the fibroblasts. The synthetic steps and the associated enzymes have been clearly identified in recent years. The hexoses to be incorporated into the polysaccharide chains are made chemically reactive by combination with a base phosphate; e.g. glucose-1-phosphate is linked by a glyosidic linkage with the terminal phosphate of uridine diphosphate (UDP) to form UDP-glucose, the enzyme responsible being known as UDP-glucose pyrophosphorylase because during the reaction pyrophosphate is liberated (NEUFELD and HASSID, 1963). In its activated form as UDP-glucose, the sugar can undergo a variety of changes involving oxidation, reduction or epimerisation so as to give rise to the other hexoses found in the polysaccharides as well as the uronic acids and the amino sugars. In addition to these modifications, the hexose in its activated form i.e. linked to UDP, can be transferred serially to another hexose so as to build up a polymer, e.g. glycogen. The enzymes responsible for these various stages have now been largely identified, although in many instances sources richer than fibroblasts have been found. Finally, since many of the sugars in the connective tissue polysaccharides are sulphated, an active form of the sulphate radical is required. This too has now been identified as phosphoadenosine phosphosulphate which is adenosine with a phosphate on the third carbon and phosphosulphate on the fifth carbon of the constituent ribose.

Factors controlling the synthesis of the various polysaccharides in connective tissue are obviously of profound importance in determining the final physical form of the tissue. Of equal importance are those factors responsible for determining the ratio of collagen to proteoglycan synthesised by individual cells, since these must dramatically influence, for example, the final appearance and efficacy of any scar tissue. The use of specific inhibitors e.g. α, α' dipyridyl for collagen and 6-diazo-5-oxo-L-norleucine for polysaccharide has clearly shown that these two functions follow independent pathways (BHATNAGAR and PROCKOP, 1966), and can therefore be independently influenced. The innumerable enzymes involved in the complex reactions of synthesis of the connective tissue polysaccharides are an obvious target for hormonal control, which is particularly well exemplified in the response to sex hormones of such secondary sex characters as the comb of the cock (BOAS, 1949; BOAS and LUDWIG, 1950) and the sex skin of the baboon (RIENITS, 1960). A brief but excellent review of the effect of hormones on the connective tissue is given by SCHUBERT and HAMERMAN (1968).

The intra-cellular sites at which the polysaccharides and sulphate radicals are added to the polypeptide chains to form the complete proteoglycan, have now been identified. Apparently, the additions do not take place, as was once supposed, whilst the peptide chain is being elaborated on the polyribosome, but after the peptide has moved into the Golgi vesicles. Here are found the various enzymes needed for the synthesis and coupling of the polysaccharides and from here the complete molecules are subsequently transported to the cell surface (DORFMAN, 1972).

3. The Fibrous Components of Connective Tissue

a) Collagen

Of the three principal components (collagen, reticulin, and elastin), collagen is with few exceptions the predominant fibre. Each collagen fibre is composed of fibrils and these in turn are built up of individual molecules, so called tropocollagen, which are rigid rods about 3000 Å long and 15 Å in diameter. The molecular weight is about 320000. Although mature collagen is highly insoluble in water or weak acid, a significant amount can be solubilised from young connective tissue by neutral salt solutions or acid at pH 3.8. From such solutions, the material may be regained in fibrous form, but this is lost if the solution is first heated to 40° C. Chromatography of such a heated solution on a carboxy methyl cellulose column allows separation of the individual chains of which the native molecules are composed (PIEZ et al., 1963). Analysis of these chains from ordinary connective tissue, e.g. that obtained from skin, tendon or fascia, has shown that each molecule consists of three chains, two of which are identical. The single chains are referred to as α chains and the brief formula for this type of collagen is therefore $(\alpha 1)_2\alpha 2$ (PIEZ et al., 1961). Each of these chains has a molecular weight of about 100000 and contains about 1000 amino acid residues. X-ray diffraction analysis has revealed that in the native state, each chain exists as a helix with a left handed turn and the three chains are then coiled together in the opposite sense forming a coiled coil structure (RAMACHANDRAN, 1967). Estimation of the individual amino acids has revealed the unique composition of collagen which underlies its specific coiled structure. Thus, one-third of all the residues is glycine and the two amino acids, proline and hydroxyproline, together contribute about one fifth (EASTOE, 1967). It is the high proportion of glycine and the two prolines that permits the peptide chains to adopt the specific coiled form characteristic of collagen, but the maintenance of this form depends initially upon the formation of hydrogen bonds between the adjacent chains. It is their disruption by heat which permits the separation of the chains by column chromatography, and as a result the chains assume a random configuration. In addition to hydroxy proline, collagen also contains one other unique amino acid, namely hydroxylysine, which together with lysine plays a fundamental part in the covalent cross linking of the chains (see below).

Although the greater part of each chain is in helical formation, and its amino acid sequence is a repetition of the tripeptide glycine-proline-X where X is any other amino acid, sequence studies have shown that a non-helical segment of entirely different composition is present both at the amino and carboxyl ends of each chain (KANG et al., 1967; FIETZEK and KUHN, 1975). These are known as telopeptides and are approximately 16 residues in length at the amino end and 25 residues at the carboxyl end. Whereas considerable homology exists between the helical portions of the collagen molecules of different species, there is much greater species variation between the telopeptides.

In addition to its constituent amino acids, all varieties of collagen contain covalently bound sugars either as single hexoses, mainly galactose, or the dipeptide glucosyl-galactose. These are joined by a glycosidal linkage to the hydroxyl groups of some of the hydroxylysyl residues present in the helical portions (BUTLER, 1970).

The mechanical properties of collagen, particularly its tensile strength, are due to the development of cross links between the peptide chains, i.e. intra-molecular cross linking as well as the formation of similar links between adjacent molecules. The most important of these are provided by lysine and hydroxylysine, which are first oxidised to their corresponding aldehydes by means of a copper-containing enzyme, lysyl oxidase. Two lysine derived aldehydes may then condense together to form the corresponding aldol or an aldehyde can react with the unoxidised lysine or hydroxylysine to form the corresponding aldimine. These cross linkages are labile when first formed in so far as they can be disrupted by reduction, but as the collagen matures they undergo a further change, not yet identified, which renders them resistant (BAILEY and ROBINS, 1973).

Although other forms of covalent cross linking probably exist in collagen, the major importance of those based on the aldehydes derived from lysine and hydroxylysine can be assessed by the effects of agents known to interfere with their formation. Thus lathyrogenic agents such as β-amino-propionitrile, which block the action of lysyl oxidase, induce a striking loss in the mechanical strength of the newly formed collagen and a corresponding increase in its solubility in neutral salt solutions (TRAUB and PIEZ, 1971). Similar effects may also be induced by agents such as D-penicillamine, which bind to aldehydes (DESHMUKH and NIMNI, 1969).

Until recently, all collagen was regarded as built on the same plan by which each tropocollagen molecule comprised two identical chains designated $\alpha 1$ and one unique chain designated $\alpha 2$. Recent studies, however, have identified at least four different types of collagen, designated types I–IV, of which type I is the classic form found predominantly in skin, fascia, and tendon. Type II is the form characteristically found in cartilage and has the composition $[\alpha 1\ (\mathrm{II})]_3$ indicating that all three constituent chains are identical, but differ from both chains of type I collagen (MILLER, 1971). Type III collagen described by the formula $[\alpha 1\ (\mathrm{III})]_3$ also possesses three identical chains and is found predominantly in human placenta, infant skin and blood vessel walls. It is also the predominant type in newly formed repair tissue (CHUNG and MILLER, 1974). Type IV collagen, described by the formula $[\alpha 1\ (\mathrm{IV})]_3$, is found exclusively in basement membrane from which it can be obtained by limited pepsin digestion (KEFALIDES, 1973).

Important differences exist in the primary structure of the four collagen types although all have in common the presence of glycine as at least one-third of the total amino acid residues and a high content of the two imino acids. The glycine contents of types III and IV are somewhat greater than one-third and both types are also richer in hydroxyproline than types I and II. Type II collagen is similar to type IV in having higher levels of glutamic acid, hydroxylysine and hydroxylysine-linked carbohydrate than types I and III, but differs from all the other types in its high threonine to serine ratio. Of special note is the presence of cysteine in types III and IV and its absence from Types I and II, and the exceptionally high proportion of 3-hydroxyproline in type IV (KEFALIDES and DENDUCHIS, 1969). How these variations modify the functional attributes of the collagen types to suit their specific requirements is virtually unknown, but they are of inestimable value in enabling the different types to be identified and quantified in the various tissues.

Of particular importance are the small variations in number as well as distribution of the methionine residues since these are the sites at which cyanogen bromide disrupts the chains into fragments (BORNSTEIN and PIEZ, 1966). These are so characteristic that each type can be recognised by its resulting peptide chromatogram.

In most collagenous tissues, the tropocollagen molecules are arranged in fibrils which are then built up into the macroscopic fibrous structure. The arrangements of the molecules in the fibrils is responsible for the characteristic banded appearance with a periodicity of 680 Å which is so typical of collagen when seen with the electron microscope. This banding is thought to arise from the regular overlapping of the molecules by one quarter of their length (HODGE and SCHMITT, 1960) and the dark band in the unstained fibril corresponds to the hole left by the overlap (Fig. 1). This is confirmed by the periodicity four times as large when soluble collagen is precipitated by ATP (HODGE et al., 1965). In this so called segment long-spacing variety, the tropocollagen molecules are regarded as arranged head to tail with adjacent columns in exact alignment with no overlap. The periodicity shown by this form of collagen is, as expected, approximately 3000 Å.

The individual peptide chains as synthesised on the ribosomes of the rough endoplasmic reticulum are quite different from the chains as they are found in the extra cellular collagen fibrils. Firstly, the newly formed chains are far longer than those found in mature collagen and the extensions are non-helical, that is they are part of the telopeptides at the amino and carboxyl ends. The triple helix formed by these extended chains is termed procollagen (DEHM and PROCKOP, 1973) and the constituent chains are pro α-chains. The amino acid composition of the polypeptide extensions differs markedly from that of tropocollagen, having both cysteine and tryptophan as well as higher levels of tyrosine, glutamic acid, aspartic acid and serine, and lower levels of proline and glycine (SCHOFIELD and PROCKOP, 1973). The C terminal extension is richer in cysteine than that of the amino terminus, which supports the suggestion that disulphide bonds are located at the C terminus.

The function of the extensions on the procollagen chains is far from clear. Amongst those suggested are: (1) facilitation of transport or secretion of the molecule; (2) initiation of triple helix formation; (3) inhibition of intracellular fibrillogenesis; (4) alignment of the peptide chains in extra-cellular fibril formation (LAYMAN et al., 1971). None of these has been experimentally demonstrated and in vitro formation of fibrils when precipitated from solution is more rapid for collagen than for

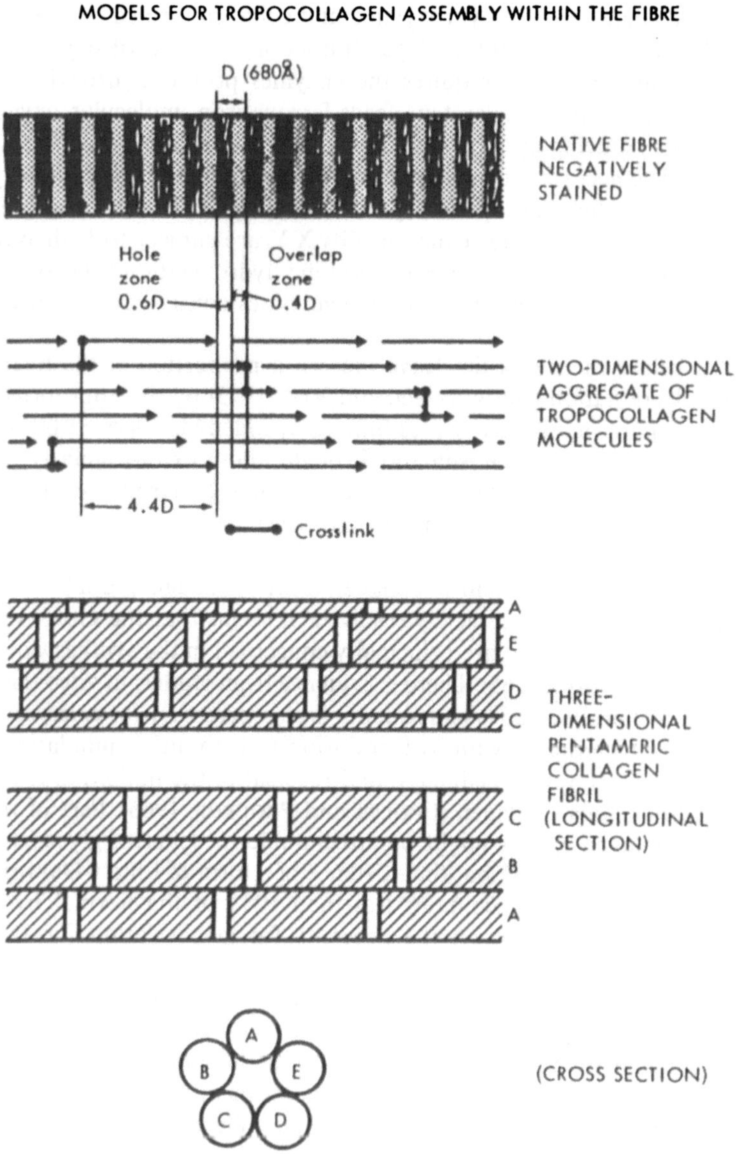

Fig. 1. Arrangement of collagen molecules within the fibrils

procollagen (MÜLLER et al., 1973). The probability therefore, is that the extensions facilitate transport and secretion, but that optimal fibril formation requires the removal of the extensions by the appropriate extra-cellular enzymes. This view is corroborated by the grossly impaired mechanical strength of the collagen in situations where these enzymes are deficient, for example in the skin of dermatosparactic calves (LENAERS et al., 1971).

The second feature which distinguishes the mature chain from the newly synthesised chain is the hydroxylation of a proportion of the proline and lysine residues. The newly formed chains are not hydroxylated and collagen formed from such chains is distinguished by the term protocollagen (PROCKOP, 1970). Hydroxylation normally occurs after translation and requires the enzymes proline hydroxylase and lysine hydroxylase. In addition, the system needs ferrous iron, molecular oxygen, α-ketoglutarate and a reducing agent, which in vivo is most probably ascorbic acid (BORNSTEIN, 1974). The necessity for iron presumably accounts for the inhibitory effect on hydroxylation of chelating agents e.g. α–α dipyridyl (HUTTON et al., 1966). Only residues in position Y of the sequences Gly X Y are subject to hydroxylation and although the proportion of prolines undergoing hydroxylation is fairly constant the proportion of lysines undergoing this change varies considerably between different tissues.

Finally, before the molecules leave the cell a proportion of the hydroxylysines undergoes glycosylation (BROWNWELL and VEIS, 1975) by the appropriate transferases, which require manganese. Cross linking by aldehydes derived by oxidation of lysine and hydroxylysine is presumably brought about extra-cellularly, since newly formed collagen extractable by neutral salt solution is free from such linkage, as can be shown by its ready dissociation into the three constituent α-chains on thermal denaturation.

The intra-cellular movement of collagen from the rough endoplasmic reticulum to the surface is still not completely resolved. It seems that the Golgi vesicles play only a minor part in this but are principally concerned in the synthesis of proteoglycans (ROSS and BENDITT, 1965). There is evidence from studies in vitro that adequate hydroxylation of proline and lysine residues is also necessary for extra-cellular delivery since factors interfering with hydroxylation lead to an accumulation of under-hydroxylated collagen intra-cellularly, and reversal of the inhibition is followed by increased extra-cellular collagen (COOPER and PROCKOP, 1966). Part of this impairment of the collagen export might be attributable to deficient glycosylation when lysine is under-hydroxylated, but the existence of a form of Ehlers-Danlos syndrome in which the skin collagen contains less than 10% of the normal hydroxylysine content throws some doubt on the necessity for glycosylation for this purpose (KRANE et al., 1972).

The actual passage of collagen into the extra-cellular space requires the participation of some of the cell's organelles. Thus, agents such as colchicine, which interfere with microtubular function, cause retardation in the conversion of procollagen to collagen (EHRLICH et al., 1974), although none of them is inhibitory of procollagen peptidase or interferes with the synthesis of non-collagen proteins. Cytochalasin B, however, which interferes with microfilament function, has no effect upon the procollagen/collagen ratio, although it does reduce the total collagen synthesised (EHRLICH and BORNSTEIN, 1972).

BORNSTEIN and EHRLICH (1973) sum up the conclusion from this work on the influence of antimitotic and other agents on collagen formation as follows: procollagen, after hydroxylation and glycosylation, is transported in vesicles through the microtubular system to the cell surface. This step is inhibited by colchicine, vinblastine and other antimitotic agents. At the cell surface, the procollagen meets the peptidase, the action of which converts the procollagen to collagen which is then delivered by exocytosis into the extra-cellular space. This stage of exocytosis probably requires the activity of the microfilaments. Interference of their function by cytochalasin B then leads to impaired collagen synthesis by negative feed-back from the retained intra-cellular collagen.

It must be stressed that this scheme is based on BORNSTEIN'S (LAYMAN et al., 1971) work on cultures of cranial bones and that the evidence from other sources shows that procollagen can be secreted as such without previous subjection to the action of procollagen peptidase (JIMENEZ et al., 1971). CLARK and VEIS (1972) have published results which suggest that the conversion of procollagen to collagen occurs in several steps, and extractable collagen from newly formed tissue contains molecules of different molecular weight depending upon how much of the extension peptide has been removed.

b) Reticulin

The relationship between collagen and reticulin has long intrigued histologists of connective tissue. Reticulin is known, both chemically and histologically, to contain collagen, but the fibrils are more delicate and arranged to form networks rather than fibres. The most striking difference, however, is in the reaction of these two fibrillar materials with ammoniacal silver, reticulin being referred to as argyrophilic because the silver is reduced and precipitated; collagen is non-argyrophilic and acquires a pinkish to brown colour, depending upon the precise technique employed, but is easily distinguished from the jet black of reticulin. The difference is probably attributable to the presence of aldehyde groups in reticulin or their formation during the mild oxidation carried out as part of the staining procedure (CULLING, 1963).

There is some evidence that the argyrophilia of reticulin might not be an attribute of its collagenous component but of the non-collagenous material, which constitutes a high proportion of the total material present. Thus PRAS and GLYNN (1973) have shown that this non-collagen component can be readily extracted with distilled water, and when precipitated displays similar argyrophilia to the tissue of origin. KEFALIDES (1973), however, has established that the collagen of reticulin is of type IV which not only differs from type I collagen in its primary amino acid structure but is much richer in sugars, 10–12% compared with about 1%. It is, therefore, conceivable that part at least of the argyrophilia of reticulin is attributable to its high sugar content.

Newly formed collagen fibres, such as occur in healing wounds, differ from mature collagen in that they stain like reticulin with silver reagents. It is claimed, however, that in contrast with reticulin, the argyrophilia is lost after a short-term extraction with neutral salt solution (JACKSON and WILLIAMS, 1956). This suggests that the argyrophilia is a function of the newly formed non-cross linked tropocollagen which presumably still retains its lysine residues in non-oxidised form and is, therefore, potentially able to yield aldehydes when exposed to appropriate oxidation. With progressive maturation of the collagen, such as accompanies wound healing and scar formation, the argyrophilia is progressively lost.

c) Elastin

Fibres readily distinguishable from both collagen and reticulin are normally present in variable proportion in all collagenous structures, even including tendon. These fibres tend to be yellowish in colour when seen in bulk, are branched and their elastic property revealed by their contraction when cut. Histologically, they are stained specifically with orcein. The fibres are apparently formed by cells indistinguishable from fibroblasts, but little is known about the conditions that determine which fibrous protein should be synthesised by a particular cell. Elastic fibres are, however, conspicuously absent from scar tissue, an absence which might well contribute to the known propensity for this tissue to yield under sustained pressure.

In chemical structure elastin, the constituent protein of elastic fibres, bears no relation to collagen even in its primary structure. Thus, its amino acid residues are predominantly non-polar: 904 out of 1000 compared with only 640 per 1000 residues in collagen (PARTRIDGE et al., 1963). Only about 1% of its residues are hydroxyproline compared with 8–10% in collagen, and hydroxylysine is entirely absent. Of major importance is the presence of two residues, desmosine and isodesmosine, which occur exclusively in elastin. Each consists of a pyridine nucleus with four α amino acid side chains so that each of these novel residues can act as a link for four peptide chains. This imparts a complex net-like structure which is now accepted as the basis of the rubber-like elasticity which characterises elastic tissue.

As would be expected from such a highly cross-linked structure composed predominantly of non-polar amino acids, elastin is resistant to the majority of animal proteases. Enzymes capable of attacking elastin, however, do exist, in pancreatic extracts for example, although such elastases are by no means specific for elastin.

E. The Maturation of Scar Tissue: Contraction

In all areas where defects of tissue are made good by infilling with granulation tissue followed by local synthesis of collagen, the newly formed tissue undergoes a well-recognised sequence of changes which may be referred to as maturation. To the naked eye, this reveals itself as progressive pallor of the newly formed tissue, accompanied by progressive shrinkage in a direction parallel to that of the constituent fibres. The direction of these fibres is itself determined by the orientation of their cells of origin and this in turn is determined by mechanical stresses to which the cells are subjected during the healing process (WEISS, 1929).

The loss of colour in the maturing scar is due to diminishing blood flow which is determined by metabolic demand. This demand is presumably dependent upon the synthetic activities of the local fibroblasts, which decreases as the need for collagen and ground substance synthesis is satisfied. What precisely switches off the synthesis is unknown, but it is most probably based on negative feedback from one or more of the products of synthesis. With the fall in metabolic demand and consequent decrease in blood flow, capillaries and related small vessels collapse and disappear resulting eventually in an opaque, white, almost avascular fibrous scar.

The well-known tendency for scars to shrink has long been difficult to explain, especially in the face of the equally well-known tendency for scars to stretch, e.g. in incisional hernias. Collagen itself, which constitutes the bulk of any mature scar, has a remarkably high tensile strength with little elasticity, tearing when it has elongated only 1%. It is evident, therefore, that the stretching of a mature scar cannot be due to either stretching or rupture of individual collagen fibres (the forces being inadequate) but to the remoulding of the whole scar structure to adapt it to its new situation, namely increased tension. Neither is shrinkage of scar tissue a manifestation of a corresponding change in individual collagen fibrils. It is probably attributable to the contractile ability of the microfibrils of the fibroblasts. These cells are now known to be rich in actin and perhaps other proteins of the actomyosin complex and to be capable of contraction resembling that of smooth muscle (GABBIANI and MAJNO, 1972). They also contain junctions capable of transferring the contraction force through the whole tissue. Whereas in many situations, as in a healing wound, contraction of the maturing scar would be beneficial, in many other situations, e.g. in the wall of a hollow viscus, such contraction could be highly detrimental. Little is known of the factors that determine contraction, but it is evident that the more prolonged the inflammatory process and the greater the amount of granulation and scar tissue that is formed, the greater the tendency to contraction.

F. Abnormalities of Scar Tissue

There are several situations where scar tissue forms in excess of what is apparently required, and others in which there is no known adequate stimulus for its formation. Included amongst the latter are several examples in which the formation of scar tissue can be correlated with the use of certain drugs and which even necessitates their withdrawal.

I. Keloids and Hypertrophic Scars

A scar may be said to be hypertrophic or keloidal when it fails to show the signs of maturation that we have just discussed. The scar in consequence remains pink, raised above the surrounding surface and shows little tendency to contract. Such scars are unsightly when in the skin and may lead to serious obstructive consequences when in a hollow organ such as the oesophagus.

Little is known of the aetiology of such scars other than an increased tendency to occur in vertical incisions, i.e. those parallel to the long axis of the body, and in subjects with active tuberculosis. They were particularly common, therefore, in individuals subjected to surgical removal of tuberculous glands in the neck. Some influence of genetic factors is also suggested by their increased frequency in the negroid races, some of whom have taken advantage of this phenomenon by using keloidal scars as a form of body decoration.

The histology of hypertrophic scars is much as would be expected from their gross appearance and history—they differ from normal scars of comparable age in their evident cellularity and vascularity, in the greater argyrophilia of their fibrous component and stronger histochemical reactions for acid glycosominoglycans (LEVER, 1967).

A study by workers at the Institute Pasteur (BAZIN et al., 1973) revealed the following: the amount of collagen and its degree of cross linking are not significantly different in hypertrophic scars from the corresponding values in normal scars; the glycosominoglycan content is much higher; the sialoglycoproteins of hypertrophic scars are mainly soluble in neutral phosphate buffers whilst the converse is true in normal scar tissue; the increased glycosominoglycans in hypertrophic scars, unlike those in normal scars, are mainly of the acidic type.

In addition to the above findings, which are mainly confirmatory, BAZIN et al. (1973) found that, of the acid glycosominoglycans, the increase is in chondroitin sulphate-dermatan sulphate but not in hyaluronate. It is, of course, not known whether these changes are primary or secondary, but in view of the known inhibitory effect of hyaluronic acid on the synthetic activities of chondrocytes, these findings suggest the possibility of some interference with the mechanisms that normally control the anabolic activities of the connective tissue cells.

II. Dupuytren's Contracture

A second and even more puzzling example of abnormal scar formation is the condition known as Dupuytren's contracture. Although this is mainly an affection of the skin and deep fascia of the palms, the feet may also occasionally be involved. Increasing fibrosis and associated contraction of the affected areas lead to considerable deformity and limitation of movement. Histologically, the lesions reveal a striking proliferation of fibroblasts with associated formation of collagen in various stages of maturation. Although there is no sharp line of demarcation between affected and unaffected tissue, there is no tendency for the condition to develop neoplastically, even when it recurs as it often does after surgical removal. GABBIANI and MAJNO (1972) have shown that the cells participating are particularly rich in actomyosin-like fibrils characteristic of so called myofibroblasts.

The aetiology of Dupuytren's contracture is unknown. There is little evidence of any association with repeated trauma and the suggestion that auto-immunity is important is based entirely on a mathematical analysis of age-specific incidence (BURCH, 1966). There are neither histological nor immunological grounds to support this suggestion.

Peyronies disease, a progressive fibrosis affecting the cavernous tissue of the penis, is related to Dupuytren's contracture in so far as it shows similar histological features and occurs in conjunction with Dupuytren's contracture with significant frequency. Other equally obscure conditions involving the fasciae but without showing any pronounced tendency to contracture are also known, but tend to affect a younger age group and to show greater evidence of inflammatory cell participation (ENZINGER et al., 1970).

III. Scleroderma: Systemic Sclerosis

Scleroderma, a condition of progressive thickening of the skin with loss of elasticity, was first regarded as a purely skin condition. It is now known to affect the connective tissues throughout the body, hence the term systemic sclerosis. Principally involved, apart from the skin, are the gastro-intestinal tract resulting in dysphagia, and the kidneys resulting in uraemia, but impairment of cardiac and pulmonary function may also occur from fibrosis of the organs involved.

The aetiology, as with almost all these fibrotic states, is unknown although associated immunological features, such as the presence of antinuclear factors, are suggestive of an immunologically associated pathogenesis. Skin lesions resembling those of scleroderma which occur in rats suffering from a graft-vs.-host reaction (STASTNY et al., 1965) afford some support for this suggestion.

IV. Drug-Induced Fibrosis

This is only a recently observed but extremely disquieting phenomenon, since a number of otherwise invaluable drugs are having to be withdrawn or their use seriously restricted. The first observation of a drug-induced fibrosis was, surprisingly, endogenous in nature. Sclerosis of the pulmonary valve was detected in several patients suffering from malignant carcinoid tumours and this was finally attributed to the effect of 5-HT secreted by the tumour cells (ROBERTS and SJOERDSMA, 1964). Whether 5-HT is to be regarded as a drug or a hormone is a moot point, but the demonstration that it induces fibrosis indicated the potential danger of an undesirable fibrotic reaction to relatively simple non-irritant drugs.

Of the non-natural (i.e. artificially synthesised) drugs, phenytoin was apparently the first to be associated with an undesirable effect on connective tissue resulting in gingival hypertrophy in a small proportion of patients (GOODMAN and GILMAN, 1965). On rare occasions, the hypertrophy may be sufficient to lead to complete submersion of the teeth. More recently, methysergide has been incriminated as a cause of retroperitoneal fibrosis manifesting itself as obstruction of one or both ureters (GRAHAM et al., 1966) and the β-adrenoceptor blocking agent practolol (EDITORIAL, 1975) has been reported as causing an unusual form of sclerosing peritonitis. Unfortunately, in none of these drug-induced fibroses is there any indication of the pathogenesis of the lesions, nor are there any known clues for identifying susceptible subjects. It is, of course, quite conceivable that the active agent is not the drug itself but a metabolite.

G. Healing of Specialised Tissues

Although the basic principles of repair are the same for all tissues and organs, the details may be much modified by the detailed nature of the tissue concerned. Healing of fractured bone, for example, differs in several respects from that of an incision in soft tissue, for two main reasons: the damaged and necrotic tissue in bone is much more difficult to dispose of, and the newly formed tissue necessary for complete restitution is a highly specialised connective tissue. The cells invading the fibrin mass between the fractured bone ends must form not only collagen but also a combination of collagen and ground substance susceptible to calcification of the kind which characterises bone itself. The adaptation of bone structure to the forces to which it is exposed is even more remarkable than the adaptation of the newly formed collagen in a healing wound. The importance of purely mechanical factors in bone healing is perhaps nowhere more emphasised than in a comparison of healing fractures in rib and skull. Healing of a rib fracture is invariably rapid and satisfactory; healing of a virtually immobile fracture as in the skull is slow and unsatisfactory.

Cartilage, like bone, is a highly specialised form of connective tissue, presenting its own healing problems. Although the mature cartilage cell may be regarded as a special form of fibroblast, since it synthesises both the collagenous and the non-collagenous components, its capacity to form new cartilage matrix is seriously restricted. In consequence, replacement of cartilage defects resulting from either traumatic or infectious causes is notoriously inadequate, and anything but the smallest lesion is repaired by fibrous and not by cartilaginous tissue. This is surprising, because cartilage cells can proliferate, as in osteoarthrosis, and connective tissue cells can synthesise cartilaginous tissue, as in a healing bone fracture. Why do they not do so in healing cartilage itself?

Healing in parenchymal organs, such as the liver and kidney is more frequently associated with natural disease than with physical trauma. In such situations, exudation of fibrin and its subsequent organisation is inconspicuous or entirely absent. It is not even clear whether the fibrous tissue formed in these situations is to be regarded as part of a repair process consequent upon preceding damage to the parenchymal cell or is itself the result of some insult to the connective tissue whose resulting overgrowth then leads to secondary damage to the parenchymal cells, possibly by interference with blood flow and the exchange of metabolites. This question has been largely resolved for the liver, for which most observers now accept that parenchymal injury is primary. In the kidney, however, although the primary lesion most frequently involves the glomeruli, subsequent loss of tubules is attributable to ischaemia secondary to obliteration of the glomerular capillaries by the intra-glomerular healing process.

The CNS is unique in that its connective tissue, apart from that surrounding the larger vessels, is ectodermal in origin and its fibrous component is entirely intracellular. The supporting tissue is provided by the complex network formed by the processes of the astrocytes, which are richly provided with fibrils. Repair in the CNS is achieved mainly by proliferation of these so-called fibrous astrocytes resulting in areas of gliosis, essentially comparable to areas of fibrosis in other tissues. When lesions in the nervous system exceed a few millimetres in diameter, part of the healing process is provided by fibroblasts derived from connective tissue surrounding the arteries and veins in the vicinity. Macroscopic scars in the brain frequently act as epileptic foci, and it is possible that the collagenous component of such scars may be responsible.

Summary

1. Replacement of lost tissue is mainly achieved by the formation of a new tissue composed at first of capillaries and fibroblasts, so called granulation tissue.

2. This matures by the formation of collagen fibres, followed by progressive loss of the newly formed blood vessels and progressive reduction in size and number of the fibroblasts.

3. The end result is a densely fibrous, poorly vascular, poorly cellular structure characteristic of scar tissue.

4. The nature of the stimulus to the formation of scar tissue is still unknown, but at least in some instances is probably provided by fibrin degradation products, activated macrophages and probably by lymphocytes.

5. In many situations the formation of scar tissue occurs without any obvious preceding loss of other tissue, e.g. hepatic cirrhosis, or scleroderma. The nature of the stimulus is here even more obscure, and the controversy as to whether the initial injury is to the parenchyma or the connective tissue itself is still unresolved.

6. The higher forms of animal life may perhaps each be regarded as a microcosm where the individual cells compete for space and nutriments, and in any area those cells survive which are best adapted to the prevailing environmental conditions. The

replacement of specialised parenchymal cells by scar tissue may be the expression of the greater suitability of the micro-environment for fibroblasts than for parenchymal cells.

References

Abercrombie, M.: Contact inhibition in tissue culture. In vitro **6**, 128—142 (1970)

Allison, A. C.: On the role of macrophages in some pathological processes. In: Van Furth, R. (Ed.): Mononuclear Phagocytes, pp. 422—440. Oxford: Blackwell Scientific Publications 1973

Asboe-Hanson, G.: The mast cell. Int. Rev. Cytol. **3**, 399—435 (1954)

Bailey, A. J., Robins, S. P.: Development and maturation of the crosslinks in the collagen fibres of skin. Front. Matrix Biol. **1**, 130—136 (1973)

Banerjee, S., Glynn, L. E.: Reactions to homologous and heterologous fibrin implants in experimental animals. Ann. N.Y. Acad. Sci. (Wash.) **86**, 1064—1075 (1960)

Bazin, S., Nicoletis, C., Delaunay, A.: Intercellular matrix of hypertrophic scars and keloids. In: Kulonen, E., Pikkarainen, J. (Eds.): Biology of the Fibroblast, pp. 571—578. London: Academic Press 1973

Bhatnagar, R. S., Prockop, D. J.: Dissociation of the synthesis of sulphated nucopolysaccharides and the synthesis of collagen in embryonic cartilage. Biochim. biophys. Acta. (Amst.) **130**, 383—392 (1966)

Boas, N. F.: Isolation of hyaluronic acid from the cock's comb. J. biol. Chem. **181**, 573—575 (1949)

Boas, N. F., Ludwig, A. W.: The mechanism of estrogen inhibition of comb growth in the cockerel, with histologic observations. Endocrinology **46**, 299—306 (1950)

Bornstein, P.: The biosynthesis of collagen. Ann. Rev. Biochem. **43**, 567—603 (1974)

Bornstein, P., Ehrlich, H. P.: The intracellular translocation and secretion of collagen. In: Kulonen, E., Pikkarainen, J. (Eds.): Biology of the Fibroblast, pp. 321—338. London: Academic Press 1973

Bornstein, P., Piez, K. A.: The nature of the intra-molecular cross-links in collagen. The separation and characterisation of peptides from the cross-link region of rat skin collagen. Biochemistry **5**, 3460—3473 (1966)

Brownwell, A. G., Veis, A.: The intracellular location of the glycosylation of hydroxylysine of collagen. Biochem. biophys. Res. Commun. **63**, 371—377 (1975)

Burch, P. R. J.: Dupuytren's contracture: an auto-immune disease? J. Bone Jt. Surg. **48B**, 312—319 (1966)

Burger, M. M.: Cell surfaces: cell interactions. In: Slavkin, H. C. (Ed.): The Comparative Molecular Biology of Extracellular Matrices, pp. 118—124. New York-London: Academic Press 1972

Butler, W. T.: Chemical studies on the cyanogen bromide peptides of rat skin collagen. The covalent structure of α1-CB 5, the major hexose-containing cyanogen bromide peptide of α1. Biochemistry **9**, 44—50 (1970)

Cameron, G. R., Karunaratne, W. A. E.: Carbon tetrachloride cirrhosis in relation to liver regeneration. J. Path. Bact. **42**, 1—21 (1936)

Chung, E., Miller, E. J.: Collagen polymorphism: characterisation of molecules with the chain composition $[\alpha 1\ (III)]_3$ in human tissues. Science **183**, 1200—1201 (1974)

Clark, C. C., Veis, A.: High molecular weight chains in acid-soluble collagen and their role in fibrillogenesis. Biochemistry **11**, 494—502 (1972)

Cooper, G. W., Prockop, D. J.: Intracellular accumulation of protocollagen and extrusion of collagen by embryonic cartilage cells. J. Cell Biol. **38**, 523—537 (1966)

Culling, C. F. A.: Tissues requiring special treatment or techniques. Reticulin fibres. In: Handbook of Histopathological Techniques, 2nd Ed., pp. 345—348. London: Butterworth 1963

Davie, E. W., Ratnoff, O. D.: The proteins of blood coagulation. In: Neurath, H. (Ed.): The Proteins, 2nd Ed., Vol. II, pp. 359—443. New York-London: Academic Press 1965

Dehm, P., Prockop, D.J.: Biosynthesis of cartilage procollagen. Europ. J. Biochem. **35**, 159—166 (1973)

Deschmukh, A.D., Nimni, M.E.: In vitro formation of intramolecular crosslinks in tropocollagen. Biochem. biophys. Res. Commun. **35**, 845—853 (1969)

Dorfman, A.: The developmental aspects of extracellular matrices. In: Slavkin, H.C. (Ed.): The Comparative Molecular Biology of Extracellular Matrices, pp. 27—33. New York-London: Academic Press 1972

Eastoe, J.E.: Composition of collagen and allied proteins. In: Ramachadran, G.N. (Ed.): Treatise on Collagen, Vol. I, pp. 1—72. New York-London: Academic Press 1967

Editorial: Side effects of practolol. Brit. med. J. **2**, 577—578 (1975)

Ehrlich, H.P., Bornstein, P.: Microtubultes in transcellular movement of procollagen. Nature (New Biol.) **238**, 257—260 (1972)

Ehrlich, H.P., Ross, R., Bornstein, P.: Effects of antimicrotubular agents on the secretion of collagen. J. Cell Biol. **62**, 390—405 (1974)

Enzinger, F.M., Lattes, R., Torloni, H.: Histological typing of soft tissue tumour. In: International Histological Classification of Tumours, No. 3. Geneva: World Health Organisation 1970

Fietzek, P.P., Kuhn, K.: Information contained in the amino acid sequence of the α1 (1)-chain of collagen and its consequences upon the formation of the triple helix, of fibrils and crosslinks. Molec. Cell Biochem. **8**, 141—157 (1975)

Gabbiani, G., Majno, G.: Dupuytren's contracture: fibroblast contraction? Amer. J. Path. **66**, 131—146 (1972)

Gabbiani, G., Majno, G., Ryan, G.B.: The fibroblast as a contractile cell: the myo-fibroblast. In: Kulonen, E., Pakkarainen, J. (Eds.): Biology of the Fibroblast, pp. 139—154. New York-London: Academic Press 1973

Glynn, L.E., Dumonde, D.C.: The reaction of guinea-pigs to autologous and heterologous fibrin implants. J. Path. Bact. **90**, 649—657 (1965)

Goodman, L.S., Gilman, A.: The Pharmacological Basis of Therapeutics, 3rd Ed. London: Macmillan 1965

Graham, J.R., Suby, H.I., Le Compte, P.R., Sadowsky, N.L.: Fibrotic disorders associated with methysergide therapy for headache. New Engl. J. Med. **274**, 359—368 (1966)

Grant, M.E., Prockop, D.J.: The biosynthesis of collagen. New Engl. J. Med. **286**, 194—199, 242—249, 291—300 (1972)

Hardingham, T.E., Muir, H.: Hyaluronic acid in cartilage and proteoglycan aggregation. Biochem. J. **139**, 565—581 (1974)

Hodge, A.J., Petruska, J., Bailey, A.J.: The subunit structure of the tropocollagen macromolecule and its relation to various ordered aggregation states. In: Fitton Jackson, S., Harkness, R.D., Partridge, S.M., Tristram, G.R. (Eds.): Structure and Function of Connective and Skeletal Tissues, pp. 31—41. London: Butterworth 1965

Hodge, A.G., Schmitt, F.O.: The charge profile of the tropocollagen macromolecule and the packing arrangement in native-type collagen fibrils. Proc. nat. Acad. Sci. (Wash.) **46**, 186—197 (1960)

Houck, J.C.: General introduction to chalone concept. Nat. Canad. Inst. Monog. **38**, 1—9 (1973)

Hutton, J.J., Jr., Tappel, A.L., Udenfriend, S.: Requirements for α-ketoglutarate, ferrous ion and ascorbate by collagen proline hydroxylase. Biochem. biophys. Res. Commun. **24**, 179—184 (1966)

Ishizaka, T., Ishizaka, K., Johansson, G.O., Bennich, H.: Histamine release from human leukocytes by anti-γ E antibodies. J. Immunol. **102**, 884—892 (1969)

Jackson, D.S., Williams, G.: Nature of reticulin. Nature (Lond.) **178**, 915—916 (1956)

Jimenez, S.A., Dehm, P., Prockop, D.J.: Further evidence for a transport form of collagen, its extrusion and extracellular conversion to tropocollagen in embryonic tendon. FEBS Lett. **17**, 245—248 (1971)

Kang, A.H., Nagai, Y., Piez, K.A., Gross, J.: Studies on the structure of collagen utilizing a collagenolytic enzyme from tapole. Biochemistry **5**, 509—521 (1966)

Kang, A.H., Bornstein, P., Piez, K.A.: The amino acid sequence of peptides from the cross-linking region of rat skin collagen. Biochemistry **6**, 788—795 (1967)

Kefalides, N. A.: Structure and biosynthesis of basement membranes. Int. Rev. Conn. Tiss. Res. **6**, 63—104 (1973)
Kefalides, N. A., Denduchis, B.: Structural components of epithelial and endothelial basement membranes. Biochemistry **8**, 4613—4621 (1969)
Klose, J., Flickinger, R. A.: Collagen synthesis in frog embryo endoderm cells. Biochim. biophys. Acta **232**, 207—211 (1971)
Krane, S. M., Pinnell, S. R., Erbe, R. W.: Lysyl-protocollagen hydroxylysine-deficient collagen. Proc. nat. Acad. Sci. (Wash.) **69**, 2899—2903 (1972)
Krantz, S. B., Jacobson, L. O.: Erythropoietin and the Regulation of Erythropoiesis. Chicago: University of Chicago Press 1970
Lash, J.: The developmental aspects of extracellular matrices. In: Slavkin, H. C. (Ed.): The Comparative Molecular Biology of Extracellular Matrices, p. 19. New York-London: Academic Press 1972
Layman, D. L., McGoodwin, E. B., Martin, G. R.: The nature of the collagen synthesized by cultured human fibroblasts. Proc. nat. Acad. Sci. (Wash.) **68**, 454—458 (1971)
Lenaers, A., Ansay, M., Nusgens, B. V., Lapiere, C. M.: Collagen made of extended chains, procollagen, in genetically defective dermatosparaxic calves. Europ. J. Biochem. **23**, 533—543 (1971)
Lever, W. F.: Nerves and nerve end-organs: keloid. In: Histopathology of the Skin, 4th Ed., pp. 30—33 and 622—623. London-Philadelphia: Pitman Medical Publishing Co. 1967
Miller, E. J.: Isolation and characterisation of a collagen from chick cartilage containing three identical α chains. Biochemistry **10**, 1652—1659 (1971)
Müller, P. K., McGoodwin, E. B., Martin, G. R.: Intracellular forms of collagen—underhydroxylated collagen. In: Kulonen, E., Pikkarainen, J. (Eds.): Biology of the Fibroblast, pp. 349—364. London: Academic Press 1973
Neufeld, E. F., Hassid, W. Z.: Biosynthesis of saccharides from glycopyranosyl esters of nucleotides (sugar nucleotides). Advanc. Carbohyd. Chem. **18**, 309—356 (1963)
Partridge, S. M., Elsden, D. F., Thomas, J.: Constitution of the cross-linkages in elastin. Nature (Lond.) **197**, 1297—1298 (1963)
Piez, K., Lewis, M. S., Martin, G. R., Gross, J.: Subunits of the collagen molecule. Biochim. biophys. Acta **53**, 596—598 (1961)
Piez, K. A., Eigner, E. A., Lewis, M. S.: The chromatographic separation and amino acid composition of the subunits of several collagens. Biochemistry **2**, 58—66 (1963)
Pras, M., Glynn, L. E.: Isolation of a non-collagenous reticulin component and its primary characterisation. Brit. J. exp. Path. **54**, 449—456 (1973)
Prockop, D. J.: Intracellular biosynthesis of collagen and interactions of protocollagen proline hydroxylase with large polypeptides. In: Balazs, E. A. (Ed.): The Chemistry and Molecular Biology of the Intercellular Matrix, pp. 335—370. New York: Academic Press 1970
Ramachandran, G. N.: Structure of collagen at the molecular level. In: Ramachandran, G. N. (Ed.): Treatise on Collagen, Vol. I, pp. 103—183. New York-London: Academic Press 1967
Rienits, K. G.: The acid mucopolysaccharides of the sexual skin of apes and monkeys. Biochem. J. **74**, 27—38 (1950)
Roberts, W. C., Sjoerdsma, A.: The cardiac disease associated with the carcinoid syndrome (carcinoid heart disease). Amer. J. Med. **36**, 5—34 (1964)
Roden, L., Smith, R.: Structure of the neutral trisaccharide of the chondroitin 4-sulfate-protein linkage region. J. biol. Chem. **241**, 5949—5954 (1966)
Rosenberg, L., Hellman, W., Kleineschmidt, A. K.: Macromolecular models of proteinpolysaccharides from bovine nasal cartilage based on electron microscopic studies. J. biol. Chem. **245**, 4123—4130 (1970)
Ross, R.: The connective tissue fibre forming cell. In: Gould, B. S. (Ed.): Treatise on Collagen, Vol. 2, Part A, pp. 48—51. New York-London: Academic Press 1968
Ross, R., Benditt, E. P.: Wound healing and collagen formation. V. Quantitative electron microscope radioautographic observations of proline—H^3 utilization by fibroblasts. J. Cell Biol. **27**, 83—106 (1965)
Ross, R., Klebanoff, S. J.: The smooth muscle cell. 1. In vivo synthesis of connective tissue proteins. J. Cell Biol. **50**, 159—171 (1971)

Schofield,J.D., Prockop,D.J.: A precursor form of collagen procollagen. Clin. Orthop. **97**, 175—195 (1973)

Schubert,M., Hamerman,D.: A Primer on Connective Tissue Biochemistry. Philadelphia: Lea and Febiger 1968

Silver,I.A.: Local and systemic factors which affect the proliferation of fibroblasts. In: Kulonen,E., Pikkarainen,J. (Eds.): Biology of the Fibroblast, pp. 507—519. New York-London: Academic Press 1973

Stastny,P., Stembridge,V.A., Vischer,T., Ziff,M.: Homologous disease in the adult rat, a model for autoimmune disease. II. Findings in the joints, heart, and other tissues. J. exp. Med. **122**, 681—692 (1965)

Thoma,R.: Textbook of General Pathology and Pathological Anatomy. (Tr. Bruce,A.). Vol. I. London: Adam and Charles Black 1896

Traub,W., Piez,K.A.: The chemistry and structure of collagen. Advanc. Protein Chem. **25**, 243—352 (1971)

Velo,G.P., Spector,W.G.: The origin and turnover of alveolar macrophages in experimental pneumonia. J. Path. **109**, 7—19 (1973)

Weiss,P.: Erzwingung elementarer Strukturverschiedenheiten am in vitro wachsenden Gewebe (die Wirkung mechanischer Spannung auf Richtung und Intensität des Gewebewachstums und ihre Analyse). Arch. Entwickl. Mech. Org. **116**, 438—554 (1929)

Wiebkin,O.W., Hardingham,T.E., Muir,H.: The interaction of proteoglycans and hyaluronic acid and the effect of hyaluronic acid on proteoglycan synthesis by chondrocytes of adult cartilage. In: Burleigh,P.M.C., Poole,A.R. (Eds.): Dynamics of Connective Tissue Macromolecules, p. 81. Amsterdam: North-Holland 1974

Wiebkin,O.W., Muir,H.: The inhibition of sulphate incorporation in isolated adult chondrocytes by hyaluronic acid. FEBS Lett. **37**, 42—46 (1973)

Wiebkin,O.W., Muir,H.: Influence of the cells on the pericellular environment. Phil. Trans. roy. Soc. B **271**, 283—291 (1975)

CHAPTER 7

Immunological and Para-Immunological Aspects of Inflammation

J. L. TURK and D. A. WILLOUGHBY

A. Introduction

Investigations into the causes of inflammatory processes in the body stem from the recognition by JOHN HUNTER that inflammation is not a disease process in its own right, and that every inflammatory process has a cause (HUNTER, 1812). There is no doubt that at the present time we know more about the immunological causes of inflammation than about the mechanisms underlying the processes that, for want of a better term, are described as "non-specific" inflammatory processes. It is therefore logical to divide inflammatory mechanisms into two broad groups (1) immunological (2) non-immunological. This chapter is concerned with a review of the immunological causes of inflammation and, in addition, with those phenomena which may lack the specificity normally associated with the "specific adaptive immune response" but which use some of the pathways normally associated with immunological reactions, such as the alternative pathway of complement activation.

The earliest association of inflammatory changes in the skin with immunological phenomena was made in studies of two groups of phenomena, the "Koch phenomenon" and those originally collected together under the broad title of "cutaneous anaphylaxis." The Koch phenomenon (KOCH, 1890) and the reaction of immunity to vaccinia virus (JENNER, 1798) are both examples of the group of phenomena known later as bacterial allergies, and now as delayed hypersensitivity reactions. In an investigation of the reaction to vaccinia, VON PIRQUET (1906) suggested the term allergy to describe the increased reactivity that occurs in an individual on second exposure to a foreign substance such as a bacterium, virus or heterologous protein. In two classic papers *Bacterial allergy and tissue reaction* (ZINSSER, 1925) and *On the nature of bacterial allergies* (ZINSSER and MUELLER, 1925), ZINSSER formally separated bacterial allergies to tuberculin, mallein, and abortin from anaphylactic reactions. VON PIRQUET and SCHICK (1903) had believed earlier that the tuberculin reaction was another manifestation of cutaneous anaphylaxis similar to that described by ARTHUS (1903) following the daily subcutaneous injection of horse serum in rabbits. Anaphylactic reactions and Arthus reactivity can be passively transferred with serum, whereas tuberculin reactivity cannot.

One may now subdivide strictly immunological reactions in the skin into those mediated by humoral antibody and those mediated by cell-mediated immune processes through specifically sensitized T-lymphocytes (Fig. 1). The former group include (1) anaphylactic reactions mediated by IgE antibody through, amongst other processes, mast cell activation, and (2) immune complex reactions of the Arthus type mediated by IgG or IgM antibody through the classical pathway of complement

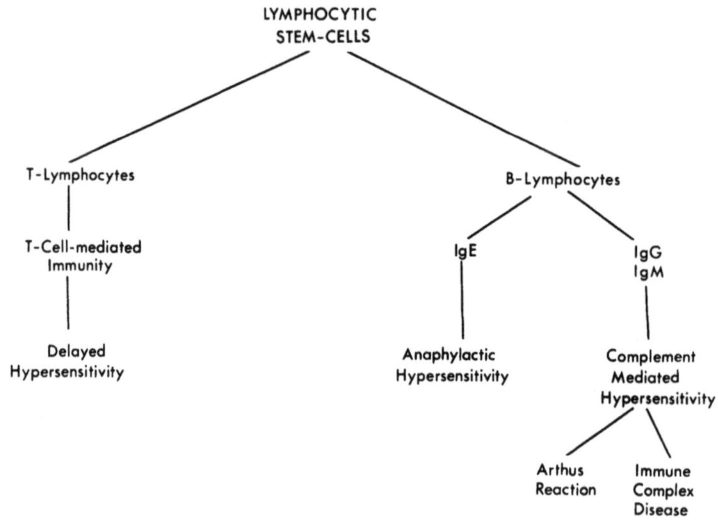

Fig. 1. Classification of Hypersensitivity Reactions

activation. Anaphylactic reactions take between 5 and 20 min to reach maximum intensity, whereas Arthus reactions reach maximum intensity between 2 and 8 h. These reactions are known as "immediate hypersensitivity reactions." In contrast, cell-mediated immune processes result in "delayed hypersensitivity" reactions which reach their maximum intensity between 24 and 48 h after contact with antigen.

A further type of inflammatory reaction with some immunological features, is that which occurs in the skin of an animal prepared with an endotoxin or related polysaccharide followed by the i.v. injection of the same or another endotoxin or polysaccharide. This type of reaction is now known as the local Shwartzman reaction (SHWARTZMAN, 1928) and has a number of features that suggest that it might be mediated through the alternative pathway of complement activation. Morphologically, this reaction may resemble the Arthus phenomenon and have the same time course of development in experimental animals. Chronic inflammatory reactions of the epithelioid granuloma type can also be induced by the deposition of immune complexes in antibody excess (SPECTOR and HEESOM, 1969) or by a chronic delayed hypersensitivity reaction. Other immunological models of inflammation that will be described include allergic arthritis and the inflammatory response in the pleural cavity following the instillation of antigen into the pleural cavity of the appropriately sensitized animal. As with granuloma formation, both these models of inflammation may be produced by either humoral antibody action or cell-mediated immunity, or as will become more apparent, may depend on a contribution from both mechanisms.

B. Mechanisms of Reactions in the Skin, Joints, and Body Cavities

I. Complement-Dependent

1. Classical Pathway of Complement Activation

Complement is recognised as a system of factors that occur in normal serum, that are activated characteristically by antigen-antibody interaction and that subsequently mediate a number of biologically significant consequences (WHO, 1968). Complement is normally studied in its role in immune haemolysis, which is a process associated with the development of certain lesions in the erythrocyte membrane (HUMPHREY and DOURMASHKIN, 1969). These circular lesions (100 Å diameter) develop as the end result of a sequence of events involving nine components of complement reacting in five stages.

Homeostasis of complement reaction is controlled by a series of inhibitors or inactivators. The classical pathway of complement is generally considered to be activated by IgG or IgM antibody interacting with antigen. There is little evidence for a role in IgE mediated anaphylactic reactions or for its activation by IgA antibodies.

Activation of the classical pathway of complement plays a central role in the development of Arthus and similar immune complex reactions. Apart from the membrane lytic effect of C9, the main direct biological effect of complement is through C3 and C5, C6 and C7. C3 plays a major role through the immune adherence phenomenon by which antigens adhere to membrane receptors and which is important in phagocytosis by macrophages and polymorphs as well as in platelet agglutination in certain species. A small fragment of C3, produced by the action of C3 convertase and known as C3a, has a series of biological actions which have been grouped together under the title of anaphylatoxins. C5a produced during the activation of C5 by C3 convertase, is also an anaphylatoxin as well as being chemotactic for polymorphonuclear leucocytes. The trimolecular complex $C\overline{567}$ (WARD et al., 1966) is also chemotactic for polymorphs but it has no action as an anaphylatoxin.

a) Immune-Adherence

Immune-adherence was described by NELSON in 1953, although the phenomenon had been known and studied for the previous 40 years. It may be defined as the propensity of immune complexes that have reacted with complement to bind to the platelets of certain non-primate species (rabbit, guinea pig, mouse, rat, cat, dog, horse) or the erythrocytes of others (primates, including man, pig, ox, sheep, and goat) (HENSON, 1969). Immune-adherence occurs only after C3 has been bound to the immune complex (GIGLI and NELSON, 1968). It is thought that a configurational change in the C3 molecule takes place after the fixation that allows it to combine with C3 receptors on the surface of some cells (NELSON, 1965). It is also believed that the mechanism involved in immune-adherence is the same as that which underlies the opsonization of C3 coated complexes or particles in vivo (GIGLI and NELSON, 1968). The promotion of phagocytosis by immune complexes may have further relevance at an inflammatory site, since it has been estimated that polymorphonuclear leucocytes stimulated to phagocytose in vitro, release 10% of the enzyme content of their granules into the surrounding medium (COHN and HIRSCH, 1960). Moreover, release of polymorph granules into the medium can be induced by immune complexes in the presence of complement components up to C3. In non-primates, the immune-adherence phenomenon may play an important role in inflammation by causing intravascular platelet aggregation.

b) Anaphylatoxins

Anaphylatoxins C3a and C5a are two peptides of 7500 and 17000 M.W. that are derived from C3 and C5 respectively. In vitro, these substances can be demonstrated by their ability to contract guinea pig ileum and they will be discussed in more detail in a later section (AUSTEN et al., Chapter 13). The intradermal injection of human C3a into human skin causes pruritus, wheal and erythema associated with mast cell degranulation and polymorphonuclear leucocyte accumulation (WUEPPER et al., 1972). Both in vitro and in vivo effects were associated with a release of histamine and 5-hydroxytryptamine (5-HT); the effects of anaphylatoxin can be partially reversed by antihistamine drugs. Anaphylatoxin activity has also been demonstrated in porcine and guinea pig serum. It is now established that both C3a and C5a are pharmacologically distinct (DIAS DA SILVA and LEPOW, 1965, 1967; DIAS DA SILVA et al., 1967; COCHRANE and MÜLLER-EBERHARD, 1967; JENSEN, 1967; BOKISCH et al., 1969; BUDZKO et al., 1971).

c) Neutrophil Chemotaxis

Initially it was thought that complement-dependent chemotaxis was mediated through a trimolecular complex $C\overline{567}$ (WARD et al., 1966). More recently, C5a has been shown to be a potent chemotactic factor (SNYDERMAN and MERGENHAGEN, 1972). It appears that the chemotactic action of C5a is independent of the anaphylatoxin activity and is due to another peptide fragment present in the preparation (WISSLER, 1972); a chemotactic action has also been attributed to peptide fragments derived from C3 (WARD, 1967). The role of the trimolecular complex $C\overline{567}$ has recently been questioned. Although chemotactic activity can be found in the serum of C6 deficient rabbits (STECHER and SORKIN, 1969), it cannot be detected in the serum of C5 deficient mice (SNYDERMAN et al., 1968). So far the evidence suggests that the major complement chemotactic factor is C5a, especially as C5 related chemotactic factors can be isolated in vivo from reversed passive Arthus reactions (WARD and HILL, 1970).

2. The Arthus Reaction

The Arthus reaction or phenomenon was first described by ARTHUS in 1903. In these experiments he noted that repeated injections of horse serum into the skin of rabbits resulted in a severe inflammatory reaction characterized by erythema, oedema, and haemorrhage. The reaction became so intense that there was thrombosis of the local blood vessels and the skin became necrotic and ulcerated. As will be discussed later, these reactions belong to the group of immediate-type hypersensitivities, as they occur with maximum intensity within the first 4 h after skin testing. The immunological basis of the Arthus reaction was demonstrated by OPIE (1924), who injected large amounts of precipitating rabbit anti-horse serum intravenously into normal rabbits and demonstrated that they had developed Arthus-type sensitivity. Quantitative data are available that indicate that approximately 0.1 mg of precipitating antibody per ml is required in the serum of a rabbit for it to show Arthus reactivity (CULBERTSON, 1935). Moreover, minimal Arthus reactivity can be induced by the local injection of 25 μg antibody nitrogen into the skin. This indicates that a large amount of antibody is necessary for an Arthus reaction to develop; between 1000 and 3000 times as much antibody is necessary to produce a local Arthus reaction as compared with that necessary to produce passive cutaneous anaphylaxis in the guinea pig (KABAT and MAYER, 1961). The demonstration of a class of antibody that would produce Arthus reactions different from which would induce cutaneous anaphylaxis was made by BLOCH et al. (1963) who showed that in the guinea pig severe passive Arthus reactions could be induced by an electrophoretically slow γ_2 (IgG) antibody, whereas passive cutaneous anaphylaxis reactions were induced by an electrophoretically fast γ_1 antibody. The association of complement with Arthus reactions was derived from these studies, as it was shown that the γ_2 antibody was also that involved in complement fixation and haemolysis. This suggestion was followed up by WARD and COCHRANE (1965) who inhibited Arthus reactions in rats and guinea pigs by depleting complement by treatment with, among others, heat aggregated γ globulin and anti-β_{1C} globulin. Moreover, they confirmed that only those antibodies that reacted with complement would induce an immunological vasculitis of the Arthus type.

3. The Alternative Pathway of Complement Activation

Evidence for an alternative pathway of complement action comes from early studies showing that complement could be inactivated by yeast or by zymosan, an insoluble carbohydrate derived from yeast. This is due to inactivation of the factor known now as C3. Moreover, the removal of C3 occurs in a two-stage reaction in which firstly the zymosan combines non-specifically with a protein called properdin (PILLEMER et al., 1954) and then the resulting complex inactivates the C3. This inactivation of C3 is independent of the classical pathway through C1, C4, and C2 that is activated by immune complexes. C3 can also be inactivated by a wide range of bacterial and other polysaccharides, including bacterial endotoxins and carrageenin. Inactivation of C3 by the alternative pathway is also associated with the production of anaphylatoxin in the serum and activation of the rest of the stages of complement activation down to C9 (LACHMANN and THOMPSON, 1970).

C3 can also be inactivated by a factor present in cobra venom (CVF). However, it is not clear how this differs from the alternative pathway of complement activation. CVF reacts with a serum factor called C3 proactivator (C3PA) to form a stable complex that reacts with C3 (MÜLLER-EBERHARD et al., 1966). This could be equivalent to the substance known as Factor B that is necessary for C3 inactivation through the zymosan-properdin pathway (BRADE et al., 1974)

The alternative pathway of complement activation can also interact with the blood coagulation system. So far, this association has been shown in rabbits where activation was in vivo following the intravenous injection of endotoxin (BROWN and LACHMANN, 1973). It has been suggested that endotoxin causes platelets to release platelet factor 3 (PF 3) through the immune-adherence phenomenon. It is only seen in species in which immune-adherence to platelets occurs, and not in C6-deficient rabbits, although it can occur in C4-deficient guinea pigs. It appears that platelets are disrupted in large numbers, releasing PF 3, which accelerates coagulation once it has already begun. This is associated with basophil and mast cell degranulation induced by anaphylatoxin, which results in increased vascular permeability leading to haemoconcentration and stasis. Together, those two processes will then result in widespread small vessel vasculitis and diffuse intravascular coagulation (BROWN, 1974).

4. Non-Specific Reactions to Endotoxin and the Local Shwartzman Phenomenon

The local Shwartzman phenomenon is an inflammatory reaction in the skin associated with haemorrhage that has many of the morphological and histological features of an Arthus reaction. First described by SHWARTZMAN (1928), it is produced typically by a series of two injections of bacterial endotoxin. The first (preparatory injection) is administered intradermally, while the second (challenging injection) is given intravenously 18–24 h later. The local Shwartzman reaction is elicited with endotoxin from Gram-negative bacteria; other polysaccharides from plant and animal tissues, tuberculin and vaccinia virus can be shown to prepare the skin test site, whilst provoking agents also include kaolin, glycogen, starch, agar, and dextran. The haemorrhagic reaction begins within 1 to 2 h after the intravenous injection, reaching its maximum intensity within 4 h. It develops in an area of inflammation induced by the preparatory injection of the endotoxin 24 h previously. Histologically, the reaction is associated with a marked polymorphonuclear infiltration. In addition there is increased vascular permeability (THOMAS and STETSON, 1948). Distinction has to be made between the effect of the initial preparatory dose of endotoxin and the changes that occur at the site subsequent to the second (intravenous) dose of endotoxin. In addition to the inflammatory changes of a polymorphonuclear leucocyte infiltration with a marked perivascular distribution induced by the intradermal injection of endotoxin, the intravenous injection results in intravascular changes. These occur within 1 h of the injection, and include occlusion of the lumen of cutaneous blood vessels by thrombi consisting of masses of platelets and leucocytes. The blood vessels most affected are the venules, while the arteries and arterioles are usually patent. The changes then result in local infarction of the skin and necrosis. These changes may be averted by treatment with an anticoagulant such as dicoumarol (SPANOUDIS et al., 1955).

The role of the alternative pathway of complement activation in the local Shwartzman reaction was originally suggested by the similarity of the agents that prepare and provoke the Shwartzman reaction with those that activate the properdin pathway and stimulate the formation of anaphylatoxin. This impression has been partially confirmed by studies in which the haemorrhagic component of the Shwartzman reaction was suppressed by treatment of guinea pigs with antiserum prepared against C3 administered before the provoking injection (POLAK and TURK, 1969). In another study, FONG and GOOD (1971) decomplemented rabbits with CVF before the preparatory injection of endotoxin, and although there were no changes found in the direct endotoxin reaction, haemorrhage was prevented at the site following the intravenous provoking injection. These findings suggest that depletion of C3 might suppress the local Shwartzman phenomenon by preventing the intravascular coagulation that would follow the local immune-adherence of platelets by endotoxin activating the alternative pathway of complement action.

II. Cell-Mediated Immunity

Inflammatory reactions due to cell-mediated immune processes are mainly delayed type hypersensitivities, although there is increasing evidence for the role of cell-mediated immune processes in the formation of certain chronic granulomas. Cell-mediated immunity was originally defined in relation to its role in the tuberculin reaction. The criteria for classifying an inflammatory reaction as cell-mediated has always been with respect to its similarity to the tuberculin reaction as it is found in the guinea pig or man. Thus, such reactions generally reach their maximum intensity between 24 and 48 h after skin testing and are characterized by erythema and thickening of the skin, described as induration. This would appear to be mainly swelling of collagen rather than the extracellular oedema typical of the Arthus reaction. The cellular infiltrate, although described typically as mononuclear, may vary considerably from species to species. In the early stages of development of the reaction there may be a large infiltration of polymorphonuclear leucocytes. However, by 24 h 50% or more of the cells may be mononuclear, with a marked perivascular distribution; there are usually equal numbers of small lymphocytes and macrophages. By 48 h, the infiltrate is almost exclusively mononuclear.

Tuberculin reactivity, as with all cell-mediated delayed hypersensitivities, cannot be transferred by serum containing specific antibody. Transfer is possible, however, with cell suspensions containing lymphocytes from specifically sensitized donors. Active suspensions may be obtained from peripheral blood, peritoneal exudates induced by mineral oil 24–48 h previously, thoracic duct, lymph nodes, spleen and under certain circumstances, bone marrow. Thymus lymphocytes are not capable of such transfers. The specifically sensitized cell in these suspensions is a T-lymphocyte, as opposed to a B-lymphocyte, and in the mouse and rat can be shown to be dependent on thymus integrity in late foetal or neonatal life. Passive transfer may be by systemic injection, either intravenously or intraperitoneally. Local passive transfer may be performed by injecting cell suspensions intradermally, together with antigen, or by injecting the cells alone intradermally and giving antigen 24–48 h later systemically.

Antigen recognition in cell-mediated immunity is by a specifically sensitized T-lymphocyte, presumably with a membrane-bound recognition unit. The nature of the recognition has not been chemically defined. However, from the specificity of its action, it has a number of features in common with the F(ab) unit of the immunoglobulin molecule. It is reasonable, therefore, to speculate that it consists of a polypeptide chain or chains with variable amino acid domains, which might account for specificity for antigen in the same way as for antibody. The main difference between antigen recognition in delayed hypersensitivity and that in antibody production is related to carrier specificity in response to hapten-protein conjugates. Specificity for carrier as well as hapten indicates that the antigen recognition site in cell-mediated immunity may be considerably broader than that on the antibody molecule.

The role of the carrier in immunization was first demonstrated in experiments on the induction of delayed hypersensitivity to dinitrophenylated (DNP-) and trinitrophenylated (TNP-) protein conjugates. In experiments of this type, the carrier protein is more than just a means of increasing the molecular weight of the complex to that which will induce an immune response; it also contributes significantly to the overall antigenicity of the molecule (BENACERRAF and GELL, 1959).

Such carrier specificity may occur in antibody formation but is frequently more apparent in delayed hypersensitivity. An example of this is found in guinea pigs immunized with TNP-coupled to bovine γ globulin (BGG). Antibody reactions can be detected towards TNP-conjugated to a wide range of carrier proteins. However, delayed hypersensitivity may only be detected to the specific carrier used in immunization. Another example of this occurs when the hapten is coupled to one of the body's own proteins (BENACERRAF and LEVINE, 1962). When guinea pigs are sensitized with TNP-guinea pig albumin, specificity in delayed hypersensitivity may be directed to the immunizing antigen only. Antibody may, however, react with a wide range of TNP-conjugates including TNP-rabbit albumin and TNP-ovalbumin. The specificity of the carrier in cell-mediated immune reactions of this type is further emphasised by experiments in which guinea pigs sensitized with DNP-linked to a copolymer of L-glutamic acid and L-lysine (DNP-GL), react only with the immunizing antigen and not to challenge with DNP-conjugates of D-glutamic acid. Furthermore, conjugates with D-lysine (DNP-D-L) react only to the immunizing antigen and not to challenge with DNP conjugates of D-glutamic acid and D-lysine (DNP-D-GL) (BENACERRAF et al., 1970).

The minimum size of the carrier for cell-mediated immunity to develop was demonstrated by SCHLOSSMANN et al. (1966) in studies on the immunogenicity of oligo L-lysines. Immunization was only possible with a molecule equal to or larger than a heptamer. Delayed hypersensitivity, however, can only be elicited with the octamer or nonamer. In contrast, antibody-induced Arthus reactions can be elicited with the hapten substituted tetramer, pentamer, and hexamer. This could indicate that carrier specificity needs a chain length equivalent to that of the octamer, whereas hapten-specific reactions can be induced by the hapten-substituted tetramer.

A state of delayed hypersensitivity is related to specific proliferation of T-lymphocytes in the paracortical areas of lymph nodes draining the site of antigen deposition during sensitization. Proliferating T-lymphocytes may be recognized as "large pyroninophilic cells" and the proportion of these cells in the paracortical area at any period of time can be counted. In addition, an estimate can be made of the increase in paracortical area size in relation to the increase in lymph node weight. In the guinea pig, large pyroninophilic cells may reach a maximum of 20% of all cells in the paracortical area 4 days after the beginning of sensitization. This is frequently the day before the first signs of sensitivity can be detected. After this, the proportion of these cells begins to decline. The increased proliferation of T-lymphocytes is paralled by an increase in lymph node weight and an increase in the size of the paracortical area.

At the time that animals become sensitive, there are lymphocytes capable of transferring delayed hypersensitivity in the circulation. In addition, there are lymphocytes in lymphoid tissues and in the circulation that respond to antigen by transformation and incorporation of radioactive nucleic acid precursors, such as ^{3}H-thymidine. Similar cells can produce lymphokines (see Chapter 10) in vitro in the presence of specific antigen. Using histocompatible animals it is possible to transfer a state of "adoptive immunity", with lymphocytes from sensitized donors, which is different from the "passive" immune state transferred among outbred animals and which is a temporary state like the serum transfer of humoral immunity. In adoptive immunity the donor cells continue in a state of active immunity while colonising the reticuloendothelial system of the recipient.

It is considered by many workers that the inflammatory reaction that occurs as part of a delayed hypersensitivity reaction is the direct result of the interaction between antigen and sensitized lymphocytes, causing the local release of lymphokines into the tissues. Lymphokines have been demonstrated both by migration inhibitory activity and mitogenic activity in the lymph draining the site of delayed hypersensitivity in sheep (TRNKA et al., 1973). However, lymphocytes from guinea pigs showing delayed hypersensitivity induced by antigen in Freund's incomplete adjuvant (FIA) (JONES-MOTE reactivity), do not seem capable of producing lymphokines in vitro (KATZ et al., 1975). There is no doubt that the local injection of lymphokines into the skin produces inflammatory reactions with increased vascular permeability (PICK et al., 1969; MAILLARD et al., 1972). These reactions differ from delayed hypersensitivity particularly in their time course; the time of onset and maximum intensity is more like that of the Arthus reaction with a peak at 3 h. This is shown not only by the intensity of erythema and induration, but also by the increased vascular permeability. Moreover, the reactions are sometimes oedematous and may also have a central haemorrhage as early as 3 h after injection. There is also more of a polymorphonuclear leucocyte reaction at the peak than there is in the tuberculin reaction at its peak. The similarity between these reactions and the Arthus reaction needs some thought, but could be explained by the rapid release of a large dose of mediators at one time, whereas in delayed hypersensitivity there would normally be a much slower release of mediators, associated with the slower recruitment of sensitized cells into the area.

As well as being involved in delayed hypersensitivity reactions to the intradermal injection of antigens, cell-mediated immune processes are involved in tissue and organ allograft rejection and chemical contact sensitivity. Other allergic reactions in which cell-mediated immunity plays a part are granuloma formation and certain autoimmune inflammatory processes including autoimmune allergic arthritis. Some of these will be considered in more detail later in this chapter.

C. Complement-Dependent Inflammation—Classical Pathway

I. Arthus Reaction

1. Experimental

In this section it is intended to discuss the different forms of Arthus reaction and how they may differ from model to model. The Arthus reaction was initially studied mainly in the rabbit. Most of these models involve the intradermal injection of about 100 µg of antigen, normally a purified bovine or human serum protein (albumin or γ-globulin) or ovalbumin, into rabbits with at least 1 mg/ml circulating precipitating antibody. The amount of antibody present is generally estimated by quantitative precipitation and expressed as μg antibody nitrogen/ml serum (COCHRANE et al., 1959). This is an expression generally of the amount of complement activating antibody present, and takes little account of non-precipitating or homocytotropic antibodies that are also present. In some cases, animals are immunized by repeated injections with saline solutions of antigens either subcutaneously or intravenously. In some they are primed with antigen in Freund's complete adjuvant (FCA) or FIA; in others they may be primed with a subcutaneous injection of alum-precipitated antigen. Similar forms of immunization have the same effect in the guinea pig. It is usual to continue immunization until reactions in the animals show central haemorrhage as well as oedema and erythema. Reversed passive Arthus reactions can be induced in rabbits by intravenous injection of 20–30 mg of protein antigen or 2–3 mg pneumococcal polysaccharide. After 30–60 min, 0.5 ml of serum containing 3–5 mg precipitating antibody/ml is injected intradermally. Oedema develops rapidly at the site of injection and reaches maximum intensity 10 h after the injection (HUMPHREY, 1955a). A similar reversed passive transfer of Arthus reactivity can be achieved in guinea pigs using the same rabbit antiserum (HUMPHREY, 1955b). Reversed passive Arthus reactions can be induced using guinea pig antiserum. Guinea pigs may be injected intravenously with 1 ml of a 2 mg/ml of protein antigen and the antibody solutions injected immediately afterwards intradermally in an 0.1 ml volume. Reactions may then be observed 2 h later (BLOCH et al., 1963). Frequently these passively induced reactions are not associated with any evidence of central haemorrhage.

The time course of Arthus-type reactivity may vary considerably in the rabbit and guinea pig. In the rabbit, reactions begin to appear about 4 h after the challenge and reach maximum intensity at about 10 h, after which the intensity of reaction begins to decrease. However, in neurotic haemorrhagic reactions there will be considerable residual inflammation at the reaction site at 24 h. In the guinea pig, the reaction may begin as early as 1 h after challenge and reach maximum intensity between 2 and 4 h. In many cases, especially in animals actively sensitized with antigen in FCA, an Arthus reaction may be associated with an intense inflammatory reaction persisting for 24 h or longer. It is important to assess whether these animals are showing delayed hypersensitivity as well as Arthus type sensitivity. This is only possible by taking frequent readings of the intensity of skin swelling at 2 h, 4 h, 8 h, 24 h, 48 h, 72 h, and 96 h; then it can be easily determined whether the intense inflammation at 24 h is the tail end of the Arthus reaction or the result of a superimposed delayed hypersensitivity reaction.

In guinea pigs sensitized with a single injection of protein antigen in FIA, the animals may show Jones-Mote type delayed hypersensitivity 7 days after immunization, but at 14 days there may be an intense Arthus reaction without any delayed component. Similar immunization in FCA will result in a delayed hypersensitivity reaction at 7 days. However, at 14 days there will be both Arthus reactivity and delayed hypersensitivity superimposed. Delayed hypersensitivity reactions may be induced on challenge 5–7 days after sensitization; Arthus-type reactivity does not develop until about 14 days. Arthus reactivity developing 14 days after immunization with 1–10 μg ovalbumin in FCA or FIA, may be present without any evidence of precipitating antibody in the serum. Antibody may be detected either by haemagglutination of coated erythrocytes or by passive cutaneous anaphylaxis. The most readily detectable antibody is a γ_1 homocytotropic antibody that classically is not complement activating. In fractionation of hyperimmune guinea pig antibody, it is the 7S γ_2 antibody that is the most efficient in provoking haemorrhagic reverse passive Arthus reactions. Animals sensitized with 1 µg ovalbumin in FIA 14 days earlier, have passive cutaneous anaphylaxis (PCA) titres of 1:128–1:512 and γ_1 haemagglutinating antibody titre of 1:48, and a titre in the γ_2 fraction of 1:192. Neither of these antibodies were found to be lytic with complement. Reverse passive Arthus reactivity was present in both fractions. In these experiments, treatment of the animals with CVF had no effect on the active Arthus reaction as compared with a group of similarly sensitized animals not treated with CVF. The total haemolytic complement levels in the CVF-treated animals were reduced to less than 5% of the pre-CVF levels. CVF treatment also reduced the complement levels to less than 5% in animals used for reversed passive Arthus, but this had no effect on the intensity or induration of these reactions as compared to non-CVF controls. Complement reduction to 50% by treatment with zymosan or anti β_{1C}/β_{1A} globulin, markedly reduced reverse passive Arthus reactivity (KATZ, 1974). The role of complement and the type of antibody that can induce Arthus reactions is not as clear-cut as a superficial view of the literature indicates. The role of γ_1 antibody in the induction of Arthus reactions has been further emphasised by MAILLARD and VOISIN (1970) using direct passive Arthus reactions rather than reverse passive Arthus reactions. In these studies, γ_1 antibody was found to bring about a strong exudative non-haemorrhagic reaction. γ_2 antibody by itself was ineffective. The reactions induced by the γ_1 antibody were observed microscopically between 20 min and 48 h; they showed a similar emigration of polymorphonuclear leucocytes from the venules to that seen in the active Arthus reaction despite being non-complement fixing. In these studies γ_2 antibody, although ineffective alone, when added to the γ_1 antibody was capable of inducing haemorrhage in these reactions.

The role of complement in the Arthus reaction was studied by WARD and COCHRANE (1965), who demonstrated inhibition of Arthus reactions in rats and guinea pigs depleted of complement by heat aggregated γ-globulin, zymosan, anti-β_{1C} globulin and carrageenin. The role of the CVF in the Arthus reaction has been studied in guinea pigs by MAILLARD and ZARCO (1968) and in rabbits and rats by COCHRANE et al. (1970). Despite massive depletion of complement by CVF, the Arthus reaction was not inhibited in the guinea pig (MAILLARD and ZARCO, 1968). In rats and rabbits, however, there was prevention of haemorrhage and reduction in oedema. Reduction in the polymorphonuclear leucocyte infiltrate in the lesion was variable. The effect of anti-β_{1C}/β_{1A} globulin (anti-C3) and zymosan was compared with the effect of CVF on direct Arthus and reversed passive Arthus reactions in the guinea pig (LEWIS and TURK, 1975). The anti-complement sera and zymosan caused a 50–60% reduction in serum complement and an equivalent reduction in the Arthus reactions. CVF reduced the complement level by 80–90% but did not affect active or passive Arthus reactions. There was complete inhibition of polymorphonuclear leucocyte infiltration in the anti-C3 and zymosan treated animals, but this was normal in the CVF-treated animals. The main difference, however, was that both anti-C3 serum and zymosan dropped the circulating platelet levels to about 100000/cu mm, probably by immune-adherence. The oedema component of the Arthus reaction was not dependent on complement but rather on the level of circulating platelets. The haemorrhagic component did, however, show some delay in CVF treated animals, indicating some degree of complement dependence.

The time course of immune complex and complement deposition in relation to the polymorphonuclear leucocyte infiltrate has been studied in the rabbit (COCHRANE et al., 1959) and in the guinea pig (CREAM et al., 1971). Deposition of immune complexes, as indicated by the presence of complement and immunoglobulin, starts 20 min after challenge and by 4 h there is a granular deposition some distance from the vessel. Between 8 and 18 h there is evidence of removal of complexes, since they cannot be demonstrated by the fluorescent antibody technique after this time. Histologically, the disappearance of immune complexes and complement from the lesion is associated with the disappearance of polymorphonuclear leucocytes, leaving a patchy mononuclear cell infiltrate at the site and a reduction of inflammation as detected macroscopically.

2. Clinical

The direct analogy between the Arthus reaction in experimental models and a similar state in man is difficult to find. However, KOHN et al. (1938) described a massive haemorrhagic necrotic lesion following the injection of horse serum into a sensitive child. Arthus-like reactions have also been observed after skin testing with *Aspergillus fumigatus*, *Candida albicans* and avian extracts (PEPYS, 1969), when precipitating antibodies were present in the serum. Lesions with many of the characteristics of the Arthus phenomenon may be found in erythema nodosum leprosum. This complication of lepromatous leprosy occurs mainly in the first 6 months after initiation of sulphone therapy. It is characterized by red painful oedematous nodules which occasionally have a haemorrhagic centre and are necrotic. Histologically, the lesions are characterized by severe vascular damage and a marked polymorphonuclear leucocyte infiltrate. These lesions develop when the bacteria are becoming degenerate as a result of treatment (providing a source of soluble antigen), and there are high levels of precipiting antimycobacterial antibody in the circulation. Fluorescent antibody studies have demonstrated the presence of granular deposits of immunoglobulin and β_{1C}/β_{1A} globulin (C3) both outside vessels and within the vessel walls (WEMAMBU et al., 1969). Other lesions, due possibly to circulating immune complexes, such as arthritis, iridocyclitis and nephritis, can occur in parallel.

The role of immune complex formation in the lesions of allergic vasculitis and polyarteritis nodosa, is far less clear, although immunoglobulin and complement may be detected in these lesions. Streptococcal and candidal antigens have been found in the lesions of several patients. However, doubt has been expressed as to the significance of these findings, since the immunoglobulin in the lesion has only rarely been found to be directed against the antigen found in the lesion. Moreover, it has been suggested that these findings might be due to the fortuitous deposition of these substances in tissue damaged by other means (PARISH, 1971). The demonstration of immune complexes of hepatitis B antigen, IgM and complement in the vessel walls of certain patients with polyarteritis nodosa (GOCKE et al., 1970), would appear to have a more solid basis related to the aetiology of the condition.

II. Circulating Immune Complexes

1. Experimental

Serum sickness is produced in rabbits by a single injection of a large dose of horse serum (10 ml/kg) or an equivalent amount (250 mg/kg) of a more purified preparation such as BGG (bovine γ globulin). The lesions that develop include a vasculitis resembling polyarteritis nodosa, myocarditis, endocarditis, and glomerulonephritis.

Lesions develop about one week after injection, at a time when the circulating antibody begins to form and the soluble antigen begins to be eliminated because of its complexing with the antibody. Chronic serum sickness produced by daily injections over a long period will result in the development of a membranous or membrano-proliferative nephritis. The development of acute or chronic serum sickness is associated with the deposition of immunoglobulin and complement, with the typical "lumpy bumpy" distribution along the basement membrane of the glomeruli. When serum sickness was induced by the injection of preformed immune complexes, it was found that these have to be of a sedimentation rate of 19S (equivalent to 900000 mol wt) before being able to localize in blood vessel walls (COCHRANE and HAWKINS, 1968). In addition, optimal localization was obtained with complexes in which the antigen to antibody ratio was in antigen excess and 20 times equivalence. The localization and deposition of immune complexes in blood vessels is associated with an increase in vascular permeability (COCHRANE and HAWKINS, 1968) and can be prevented by administration of antagonists of histamine and 5-HT or by depletion of circulating platelets (KNIKER and COCHRANE, 1965).

As with the Arthus phenomenon, the role of complement in the development of serum sickness lesions is controversial. In many of these lesions, C3 can be detected by the fluorescent antibody technique, particularly in the lesions of glomerulonephritis. Treatment of animals with CVF in amounts sufficient to drop the complement (C3) level to below 15%, did not prevent the normal appearance of serum sickness nephritis. This was despite the maintenance of low levels over the period of the 6th to 8th day after antigen administration, the time during which proteinuria normally develops (HENSON and COCHRANE, 1971). In addition to the demonstration that complement does not play a critical role in these lesions, there was a strong correlation between a leucocyte-dependent release of vasoactive amines from platelets by antigen and the development of glomerular injury, as determined by the onset of proteinuria.

A wide range of other models of glomerulonephritis exist in which the nature of the immune complex is less well-defined than in the classic serum sickness model using purified protein antigens. These include (DIXON et al., 1970):

1. Those due to induced or natural viral infections—lymphocytic choriomeningitis, Aleutian disease of mink, lactic dehydrogenase infection of mice.

2. Those associated with antinuclear antibodies—NZB/W mice.

3. Other chronic viral infections—murine leukaemia virus, Coxsackie B virus, polyoma virus, equine infectious anaemia.

4. Those following experimental manipulation of the immune response—neonatal X-irradiation of mice, neonatal thymectomy, chronic allogeneic disease.

In many of these conditions, renal disease may develop associated with the deposition of immunoglobulin and complement on the glomerular basement membrane.

2. Clinical

Serum sickness in man may be associated with the development of nephritis and arthritis. Apart from serum sickness, the most widely studied immune complex disease has been systemic lupus erythematosus (SLE). In this condition, using fluorescein-labelled anti-DNA antibodies, the antigen (DNA) was detected in the glomerulus with a distribution similar to that of immunoglobulin and complement (KOFFLER et al., 1967). This condition is usually associated with a depression of circulating complement. It is now recognized that many infectious diseases may be complicated by immune complex nephritis or arthritis. The association between immune complex nephritis and streptococcal infection is well known, but more recently the immune complex aetiology of malarial nephrosis has been investigated (ALLISON et al., 1969). In this condition, there is a proliferative glomerulonephritis in which immunoglobulin and complement is deposited on the glomerular basement membrane. In a few cases, *P. malariae* antigen was also found in the deposits. A similar nephrotic syndrome develops in patients infected with *Schistosoma mansoni.* These are also associated with granular deposits of immunoglobulin and complement on the basement membrane, suggesting an immune complex aetiology (WHO, 1974). Other infective conditions in which there is evidence suggestive of immune complex nephritis include syphilis and leprosy.

The association between infection and arthritis is also well known. Arthritis has been described, for instance, as a complication of erythema nodosum leprosum (KARAT et al., 1967). Immune complex disease associated with meningococcal infection has been investigated by WHITTLE et al. (1973) and GREENWOOD et al. (1973). Out of 717 subjects with meningococcal disease, 53 showed one or more of three allergic complications, 47 (6.6%) developed arthritis, 12 (1.7%) developed cutaneous vasculitis and 6 developed episcleritis. Immunological investigation of four of the patients with arthritis or cutaneous lesions showed circulating meningococcal antigen at the time of presentation; two showed a marked fall in the serum C3 level. Deposits of meningococcal antigen, immunoglobulin and C3 were detected in the synovial fluid leucocytes in two of the patients studied and in the skin biopsy in one case. Other infectious states where there is a similar association with arthritis include Shigella dysentery, gonococcal infection, and the viral infections mumps and measles.

An interesting condition that may have an immune complex aetiology is dengue haemorrhagic fever. This has been the subject of a recent combined international study (WHO, 1973) and occurs in patients with secondary dengue infection. During the condition, there was convincing evidence of in vivo complement consumption, and marked depression of serum levels of complement components was correlated with the severity of the disease. The reduction in complement was associated with a reduction of platelets and fibrinogen in plasma and the presence of split products of fibrin and fibrinogen. Thus, as a result of dengue virus infection in a patient with pre-existing antibody, there may be massive activation of complement. This is accompanied by the liberation of anaphylatoxins and the initiation of intravascular blood coagulation, followed by severe depletion of complement and activation of the kinin system leading to increased vascular permeability and shock.

D. Complement-Dependent Inflammation—Alternative Pathway

The group of non-specific inflammatory reactions induced by bacterial endotoxins and related polysaccharides might be mediated through the alternative pathway of complement activation. This allows deeper insight into the mechanism behind these reactions. Four reactions can be recognized in experimental models:

1. Local skin inflammation induced by the intradermal injection of endotoxin.
2. Endotoxin shock.
3. Local Shwartzman reaction.
4. Generalised Shwartzman reaction.

These reactions have in common that the particular inflammatory reaction can occur in a normal animal that has not been previous sensitized and in which there is no evidence of humoral antibody or cell-mediated immunity directed against the provoking antigen.

1. Local Skin Inflammation—Local Shwartzman Reaction

It is impossible to understand the mechanism of the local Shwartzman reaction without first understanding the local inflammatory response that develops following the intradermal injection of endotoxin. This erythematous induration reaction, of maximal intensity between 4 and 24 h, can be induced by a wide range of polysaccharides and other related substances (including carrageenin) capable of activating the alternate pathway of complement activation. In the rabbit, Shwartzman reactions can be induced by the intradermal injection of 10 µg endotoxin followed by an intravenous injection of an equivalent dose. In the guinea pig, it is necessary to use a dose of 1 mg endotoxin for both the preparatory and eliciting dose.

There is a lack of specificity in the reaction in that, for instance, *Serratia marcescens* endotoxin can induce a haemorrhagic reaction at an *E. coli* prepared site. However, KOVATS and VEGH (1967) demonstrate an unexpected specificity in the reaction by the use of endotoxin resistance. Animals in which specific endotoxin resistance had been induced by intravenous injection on five consecutive days of *Serratia* endotoxins, still showed Shwartzman reactions at the skin test site that had been prepared with *E. coli*, but not at skin sites prepared with *Serratia* endotoxin. *Serratia* endotoxin, however, could still be used to provoke the reaction at the *E. coli* site. The effect of endotoxin resistance would be particularly to reduce the intensity of inflammation at the preparatory site. Thus, the intensity of the hypersensitivity reaction at the preparatory site is important in the production of the final haemorrhagic reaction. The production of endotoxin resistance, by blocking the development of the preparatory reaction, specifically blocks the haemorrhagic component as well. No such specificity exists for the second part of the Shwartzman reaction (the intravenous provocation), as it can be induced not only by endotoxin, but also by agar, glycogen and kaolin (STETSON, 1951). The importance of the preparatory injection is also shown in the study of Fong and Good (1971), who gave CVF to rabbits 24 h before the preparatory injection of endotoxin. These animals failed to develop a haemorrhagic reaction at the endotoxin prepared site following intravenous injection of endotoxin. Curiously, there was no difference in the histological appearance of the biopsy of the preparatory intradermal site in normal and CVF treated animals, and the area of inflammation was reduced rather than abolished. Despite this, haemorrhagic necrosis failed to develop in the CVF treated animals.

The role of complement in the haemorrhagic reaction following the intravenous provocation, was studied more fully in guinea pigs by Polak and Turk (1969) and Lewis and Turk (1975). In these experiments, the various procedures were undertaken 2–4 h before the i.v. provocation injection. The haemorrhagic component of the reaction was reduced in intensity by anti-C3 sera but decomplementation with CVF, zymosan or immune complexes failed to affect the reaction, even though the circulating complement level had been reduced to 10% of the normal level. The effect of anti-C3 serum could also be reproduced by antiserum prepared against properdin and against zymosan. From these experiments, the mechanism of the haemorrhagic reaction remains obscure. Thus, in addition to the reaction occurring in the presence of low levels of complement, agents which reduce circulating platelets, such as antiserum against guinea pig immunoglobulin, injection of immune complexes and injection of zymosan, failed to alter the intensity of haemorrhage. Association of a block in the haemorrhagic component of the Shwartzman reaction with a reduction in platelets or clotting factors would anyhow be paradoxical, as thrombocytopenia is usually associated with increased fragility of the vasculature and an increased tendency to haemorrhage, rather than the reverse. Despite this, it is clear that the reaction depends on a normal clotting system with adequate fibrinogen concentrations and platelets (Good and Thomas, 1953; Bell et al., 1972; Margaretten and McKay, 1969).

The role of polymorphonuclear leucocytes in the Shwartzman reaction is as important as in the Arthus reaction. Thus, rabbits made leucopenic by treatment with nitrogen mustard, but which normal platelet count, fail to develop haemorrhagic reactions (Stetson and Good, 1951) and the skin test site can be prepared by the local injection of lysosomes from polymorphonuclear leucocytes alone (Thomas, 1965).

2. The Effect of Intravenous Injection of Endotoxin— The Generalised Shwartzman Reaction

The intravenous injection of endotoxin in the normal guinea pig leads to a 95% fall in the level of circulating platelets within 15 min, as well as a fall in circulating polymorphonuclear leucocytes. This appears to be dependent on the classical pathway of complement activation, as it does not occur in C4-deficient guinea pigs (Kane et al., 1973). Thrombocytopenia and neutropenia similarly cannot be induced in CVF treated guinea pigs. Endotoxin also causes a shortening of the clotting time in guinea pigs, and this does not occur in the C4-deficient strain or those treated with CVF. The intravenous injection of endotoxin will produce a local Shwartzman reaction in C4-deficient animals in the same way as in animals treated with CVF.

Despite these reports, there is evidence that CVF treatment will block the development of a generalised Shwartzman reaction in the rabbit (FONG and GOOD, 1971). This is associated in this species with a block in the development of thrombocytopenia following the two doses of endotoxin, and in the appearance of fibrinogen and fibrin degradation products in the circulation. There are, therefore, differences in the role of the two pathways of complement activation in the rabbit and guinea pig, particularly in their response to endotoxin.

In the generalised Shwartzman reaction, a single injection of endotoxin is not enough to produce the generalised pattern of the phenomenon. This only occurs following the second injection 24 h later, which in the rabbit is correlated in time with development of the thrombocytopenia and a hypercoagulable state of the blood. This is then associated with aggregation of platelets in the lungs liver, spleen, and kidneys, with haemorrhagic necrosis and with fibrin deposition. When animals are made leucopenic with nitrogen mustard, they fail to show fibrin deposition, and haemorrhagic lesions fail to develop in the kidneys, lungs, liver, and spleen (WOLFF and KOVATS, 1974).

The role of the Shwartzman reaction in human disease is poorly understood. Patients with infections by Gram-negative organisms, such as *Enterobacteriaceae*, develop high levels of fibrinogen and fibrin degradation products in the circulation. This may be accompanied by a thrombocytopenia at the height of the bacteraemia (WOLFF and KOVATS, 1974). However, the relationship between these findings and intravascular clotting in man needs to be elucidated. Until this has been undertaken, the role of the Shwartzman reaction in human disease must remain at the most conjectural, and the phenomena, both local and generalised, no more than laboratory-induced artefacts.

E. Delayed Hypersensitivity

1. "Jones-Mote" vs. "Tuberculin-Type" Reactivity— Normal Homeostasis by Suppressor Cells

The most frequently used species in delayed hypersensitivity research is the guinea pig. Much of our knowledge of the mechanism of cell-mediated immunity is derived from research into the mechanism behind delayed hypersensitivity to defined proteins in the guinea pig. The other experimental model is that of chemical contact sensitivity to a defined hapten, such as 2,4-dinitrochlorobenzene (DNCB). Two types of delayed hypersensitivity reaction are recognized to defined antigens (TURK, 1975). Most delayed hypersensitivity reactions are characterized by their similarity to the tuberculin reaction in guinea pig skin tested with protein-purified derivative of tuberculin (PPD), in animals sensitized with Bacille Calmette-Guerin (BCG) vaccine, or heat-killed *Mycobacterium tuberculosis* suspended in a water in oil emulsion (FCA). Animals show the earliest evidence of sensitivity 4–5 days after immunization, and reactions may be read either by the diameter of the area of skin erythema and induration, or by the increase in skin thickness as recorded by calipers such as the "Schnelltäster" (Kröplin AO2T). In order to obtain a suitable profile of the kinetics of a delayed hypersensitivity reaction, it is important to make multiple recordings of

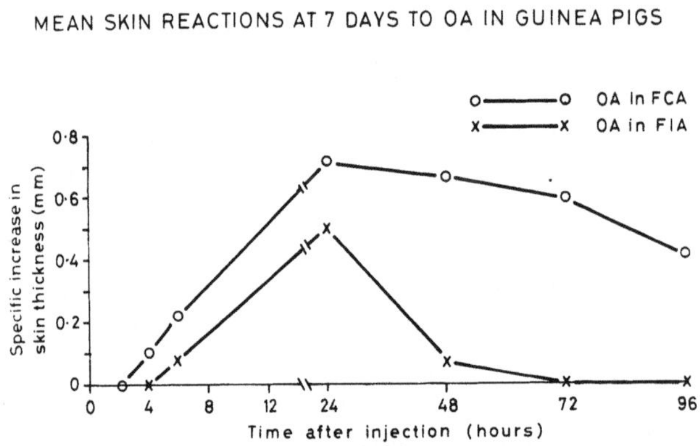

Fig. 2. Comparison of time course of tuberculin type and Jones-Mote-type of delayed hypersensitivity reactions. Animals sensitized with ovalbumin *(OA)* in Freund's complete adjuvant *(FCA)* showing tuberculin-type time course. Animals sensitized with ovalbumin *(OA)* in Freund's incomplete adjuvant *(FIA)* showing Jones-Mote-type time course

the increase in skin thickness at 4, 8, 24, 48, 72, and 96 h. The earlier times are necessary to determine whether one is dealing with a pure delayed hypersensitivity reaction or whether there is a mixed delayed and Arthus (immediate) reaction, as so frequently occurs. The later readings at 48, 72, and 96 h, are to distinguish the tuberculin type of delayed hypersensitivity from the Jones-Mote form of the reaction (Fig. 2). Tuberculin types of delayed hypersensitivity develop when animals are sensitized with soluble proteins such as ovalbumin emulsified in FCA (containing *M. tuberculosis*), and have the same profile as tuberculin reactions. In these reactions the erythema and induration appear after 6 h, reach their maximum intensity after about 24–30 h and are still fairly marked after 48–72 h, persisting up to 96 h.

Jones-Mote reactions are found classically in animals sensitized 7 days previously with a soluble antigen such as ovalbumin in a water in oil emulsion without added micro-organisms (FIA). These reactions are characterized by a slight thickening of the skin accompanied by erythema, often covering quite a large area. The onset of these reactions is delayed 12–30 h, but they do not persist and begin to disappear by 48 h. Reactivity of this type is transient; by 14 days after sensitization animals sensitized in this way fail to show delayed type hypersensitivity and are only capable of showing humoral antibody-mediated Arthus type sensitivity. This is in marked contrast to the reactivity of animals sensitized with antigen in FCA, in which the delayed hypersensitivity reactions get stronger as the time interval between sensitization and skin test increases. The nature of Jones-Mote reactivity has been a matter of controversy for a number of years. Recently, the association of this type of reaction with a strong infiltration of basophilic leucocytes has been pointed out by RICHERSON et al. (1970), and is sometimes referred to as "cutaneous basophilic hypersensitivity." The time course of the delayed hypersensitivity reactions in the guinea pig that can be elicited by skin contact with a simple chemical sensitizer, such as DNFB or 4-ethoxymethylene-2-phenyl oxazolone, is similar to that of a Jones-Mote reaction, being markedly reduced by 48 h. However, it differs from Jones-Mote sensitivity in that delayed reactivity can be elicited beyond 14 days. One of the main features that has always distinguished delayed hypersensitivity and contact sensitivity from antibody-mediated reactions, is that the former reactions cannot be transferred passively with serum, but can be with cells derived from lymphoid tissues. In a similar manner, Jones-Mote hypersensitivity cannot be transferred with serum, but can be transferred passively with cells of lymphoid origin.

It has been possible to analyse the relationship between Jones-Mote and contact reactivity to tuberculin type delayed hypersensitivity by methods of selectively depleting animals of B-lymphocytes, leaving the T-lymphocyte population of effector cells unaffected. In studies on the histological appearance of lymphoid tissues following treatment with different antimitotic agents, a single intraperitoneal injection of cyclophosphamide (CY) of 300 mg/kg selectively depleted of lymphocytes from the B cell areas of lymph nodes and spleen, without affecting the T cell areas. Maximum depletion occurred at 3 days and repopulation began 4 days later (TURK and POULTER, 1972). A protocol was therefore devised in which guinea pigs were treated with CY (300 mg/kg i.p.) 3 days prior to contact sensitization with DNFB or oxazolone. When skin tested 7 days later, the animals showed markedly increased skin reactivity. Furthermore, these contact reactions, in CY-pretreated animals, were prolonged in that they could still be detected 8 days after skin testing. This increased reactivity could be partially reversed by the i.p. transplant of spleen fragments from normally sensitized animals (TURK et al., 1972).

CY pretreatment did not increase delayed hypersensitivity to tuberculin in BCG immunized animals, nor did it increase delayed hypersensitivity to ovalbumin in animals sensitized with ovalbumin in FCA. In contrast, the effect of CY pretreatment on guinea pigs immunized with ovalbumin in FIA, was to increase the skin reactions elicited at 7 days. These Jones-Mote skin reactions had been converted, by the CY pretreatment, into skin reactions with the intensity and time course found in normal animals sensitized with ovalbumin in FCA (TURK and PARKER, 1973).

On the basis of these findings, it is postulated that CY pretreatment removes a population of cells that normally modulate the expression of delayed hypersensitivity, since strongly enhanced skin reactions result without this cell population. It also seems that the cells which are depleted by CY are B-lymphocytes. To demonstrate the presence of suppressor cells in normally sensitized animals, lymphoid cell population from normally sensitized donors were transferred to animals in which suppressor cells had been depleted by treatment with CY before sensitization. Cells which reduced the intensity of skin reactions in these recipients were found in the spleen and peritoneal exudates of normal guinea pigs immunized with ovalbumin in FIA 8 days and 14 days previously. This suppression was found to be antigen specific and to need live cells (KATZ et al., 1974a). These suppressor cells could be removed by passage through a column that had been coated with specifically purified anti-guinea pig gamma globulin; this process also removed 95% of B-lymphocytes from the suspension (KATZ et al., 1974b). A similar demonstration of suppressor cells in guinea pigs immunized with ovalbumin or diphtheria toxoid has been reported by NETA and SALVIN (1973) in transfers of mixed spleen and peritoneal exudate cells. These suspensions suppressed the expression of delayed hypersensitivity in already sensitized animals.

The role of the basophil in delayed hypersensitivity has also been studied in CY pretreated animals. Delayed hypersensitivity and contact sensitivity reactions occured in the absence of basophils in animals sensitized with ovalbumin in FIA or with DNFB (KATZ et al., 1974c). It may be, however, that the accumulation of basophils is related more to the interaction between antigen and suppressor cells or their products, than to the direct action of effector lymphocytes in producing the delayed hypersensitivity reaction.

A similar effect to that described in the guinea pig occurs in the mouse. A single intraperitoneal injection of CY (300 mg/kg) 8 h prior to immunization with sheep red cells results in an increase in delayed hypersensitivity (KERCKHAERT et al., 1974). Transfusion of syngeneic bone marrow or spleen cells at the same time as immunization will reverse the effect of CY. As in the guinea pig, experiments removing one population of cells (in this case T cells), indicate that the effect is mediated by the B cell population. This phenomenon of homeostasis by suppressor B cells appears to be different from the state of specific immunological unresponsiveness induced in mice in contact sensitivity experiments. In these experiments, mice are made specifically unresponsive to picryl chloride by systemic injection of picryl sulphonic acid before sensitization. This state of unresponsiveness has been demonstrated as being mediated by suppressor T cells rather than suppressor B cells (ZEMBALA and ASHERSON, 1973).

The demonstration that CY pretreatment could increase certain forms of delayed hypersensitivity by elimination of the precursors of a population of specifically sensitized suppressor cells, led to a study of its action on a state of immunological unresponsiveness similar to that described above. Guinea pigs were be made specifically unresponsive by intravenous injection of dinitrobenzene sulphonic acid ($DNBSO_3$) 500 mg/kg on two separate before attempted sensitization with DNCB. A similar state of unresponsiveness can be induced by oral administration of DNCB. Both these states were reversible when the animals had been injected with CY (300 mg/kg) strategically 3 days before attempted sensitization (POLAK and TURK, 1974; POLAK et al., 1975).

The ability to manifest a delayed hypersensitivity reaction is, therefore, dependent on the balance between effector and suppressor cells. Elimination of suppressor cells by a strategically given dose of CY, restores the ability of the animal to show a delayed hypersensitivity reaction 14 days after immunization with ovalbumin in FIA, or after being made specifically unresponsive with $DNBSO_3$. In other situations, such as 7 days after immunization with ovalbumin in FIA or contact sensitization with DNFB, reactivity is normally dampened by suppressor cells and can be increased to its full potential by similar treatment. The demonstration of such a homeostatic mechanism as part of a normal immune response, has enabled considerable clarification of the waxing and waning of peripheral reactivity in the hypersensitive state.

2. Humoral Antibody Reactions Resembling Delayed Hypersensitivity

It is immunological dogma that delayed hypersensitivity reactions are mediated by specifically sensitized lymphocytes and not by humoral antibody. There are, however, a number of well-documented demonstrations of "delayed-in-onset" hypersensitivity reactions that can be transferred from animal to animal by serum and which are mediated by humoral antibody. One such system is that described by PICK and

FELDMAN (1968). In these experiments, guinea pigs immunized with tubercle bacilli were given an intracardiac injection of old tuberculin. The serum from these animals taken 4 h later was found to contain a γG_2 immunoglobulin, which, when injected systemically into normal recipients, sensitized them so that they would produce an erythematous skin reaction to old tuberculin, which was at maximum intensity between 12 and 18 h.

A further system is that described by HULLIGER et al. (1968) using cytophilic antibody. Intradermal injection into guinea pigs of macrophages coated with cytophilic antibody against sheep red cells together with an extract of sheep red cells, produces a delayed hypersensitivity reaction maximum at 24 h. Another system in which a delayed hypersensitivity reaction is mediated by cytophilic antibody, is that of ZEMBALA and ASHERSON (1970) in chemical contact sensitivity to oxazolone in the mouse. Skin reactivity with a delayed time course as indicated by an increase in skin (ear) thickness, can be transferred systemically by intravenous injection of immune serum, or normal peritoneal exudate macrophages incubated with immune serum, into recipients irradiated the day before transfer.

3. Granuloma Formation

A granuloma may be defined as a chronic inflammatory reaction containing a predominance of cells of the mononuclear-phagocyte series. Depending on the agent that excites the granuloma, there is varying participation by other inflammatory cell types. Granulomas can be:

1. *Non toxic*—due to a reaction against a chemically and biologically inert substance such as carbon particles.

2. *Toxic*—due to the direct toxic action of certain chemicals, such as colloidal silica or asbestos, on tissue macrophages. These substances act particularly by causing increased permeability of the lysosomal membrane.

3. *Immunological*—these may be mediated by humoral antibody, cell-mediated immunity or a mixture of both mechanisms.

Whereas the injection of antigen-antibody complexes in antigen excess induces a transient acute inflammatory reaction of the Arthus type, characterized by a marked polymorphonuclear leucocyte reaction (COCHRANE and WEIGLE, 1958), the injection of similar immune complexes at equivalence will give rise to local granuloma formation (SPECTOR and HEESOM, 1969). The immunological basis of granuloma formation in chronic infection has been defined in a series of experiments on the development of schistosome granulomas in mice (WARREN et al., 1967; DOMINGO and WARREN, 1967). The transformation of undifferentiated macrophages into "epithelioid cells" in these granulomas appears to be related to the development of delayed hypersensitivity, as the reaction is reduced in neonatally thymectomized animals. The non-specific reaction to plastic beads, however, is the same in thymectomized as in normal mice. The immunological basis for epithelioid cell formation is further emphasized by in vitro studies on macrophage cultures. In these cultures, macrophages will transform into cells resembling epithelioid cells in the presence of a cell-mediated immune reaction (BLANDEN, 1968; GODAL et al., 1971). Macrophages activated in this way have an increased capacity to phagocytose and eliminate ingested micro-organisms, including mycobacteria. Macrophage activation in cell-mediated immunity is produced in the non-specific mediators or "lymphokines" that are secreted by sensitized T-lymphocytes reacting with antigen. The changes observed in these cells include increases in activity of enzymes of the hexose monophosphate shunt, Krebs cycle and also lysosomal enzymes (NATHAN et al., 1971; NATH et al., 1973). Activated macrophages have enzyme activity two to four times that of normal cells.

Granulomas generally occur at the site of immunological reaction in which there is delayed elimination of the irritating complex. Such granulomas are associated with marked lymphocytic infiltration as well as epithelioid changes in the macrophages. The infiltrating lymphocytes in a granuloma are frequently organized into typical T cell areas round postcapillary venules, or, B cells, may form lymph follicles and germinal centres, or be transformed into plasma cells making immunoglobulins. Granulomas of this type are found especially in infection with mycobacteria and similar obligate or facultative intracellular parasites. They also occur round the ova of helminths such as schistosomes, and are the basis of nodule formation in autoimmune conditions such as rheumatoid arthritis. Granulomas are also the site of fibrosis due to the presence of fibroblasts laying down collagen, and can lead to fibrotic changes in organs such as lungs and liver. Granulomas due to the deposition of inorganic substances may also be immunologically derived, as in the case of zirconium, which only form in people who have been previously sensitized to the metal. However, although beryllium is a powerful sensitizing agent, there is no evidence that granulomas formed by this substance in the lung are due to immunological mechanisms. They are probably due to a direct toxic action similar to that which occurs in silicosis.

F. Endogenous Antigen and Autoimmune Phenomena in Acute and Chronic Inflammation

There is little doubt that following severe tissue damage, e.g. thermal injury, circulating antibodies are detected in the circulation against modified DNA. Obviously, under these conditions, such antibodies are not participating in the inflammatory reaction. On the other hand, it might be of interest to know whether people in the type of occupation which exposes them to constant burns and scalds, develop a cutaneous hypersensitivity associated with such a non-immunological form of trauma. The situation must not be confused, however, with that in which antibodies arise as a consequence of the inflammatory stimulus and do not persist.

The most convincing evidence for an endogenous antigen participating in inflammation came from the experiments of DUMONDE and GLYNN (1962). These authors showed that by sensitizing rabbits to products of an inflammatory response and then repeating the inflammatory insult, a greatly enhanced reaction followed. This hypothesis gained further support from the experiments of WILLOUGHBY and RYAN (1970), who found that animals not only could be sensitized to give a greater inflammatory response, but could also be made unresponsive by injecting the products of the inflammatory response neonatally. It is interesting that this particular model of inflammation was apparently non-immunological; it was merely the implantation of cotton pellets.

A similar role for endogenous antigen, namely modified protein, was ascribed to adjuvant arthritis in the rat (BERRY et al., 1974). It was found in this model that, following the development of hypersensitivity, there was a better correlation of hypersensitivity measured in vitro to modified tissue proteins than to tuberculin.

Recently, much interest has been aroused in the use of immunostimulants in rheumatoid arthritis, a disease which also responds to immunosuppressive agents. This apparent anomaly may be explained on the basis of the formation of super macrophages which remove antigen completely or sequester antigen after immunostimulant therapy.

There is abundant evidence for an immune process underlying rheumatoid disease. A possible explanation could be a primary antigen e.g. an infectious agent, whether it be microbial, viral or mycoplasmal. Such an agent could lead to the formation of a secondary antigen, i.e. the modified tissue proteins. These would then act as the antigenic stimulus for the perpetuation of the arthropathy.

The role of endogenous antigen, most probably the product of an inflammatory response, is likely to be more important in chronic than in acute inflammatory phenomena.

G. Allergic Arthritis

1. Experimental Models

It should be stressed from the outset that no perfect model exists for the study of arthritis in animals. There have been many attempts to produce an allergic arthritis but each model has its own shortcomings, as will be described.

a) Rats

The standard method for the production of an experimental arthritis in rats is the so-called adjuvant-arthritis or, as should be better termed, adjuvant-disease (PEARSON, 1956). In this model, a small quantity of FCA is injected into the hind paw of rats, resulting in a swelling in the paw—the primary lesion. After a period of 14–21 days, according to the strain of the rat, secondary lesions appear, manifesting themselves as a swelling of the contralateral paw. The front paws also show involvement and lesions appear along the length of the tail. It is generally accepted that this reaction wanes after onset; in other words, it fails to resemble human arthritis in that it lacks chronicity.

There is a wide variability in the response of different strains of rats to adjuvant in their ability to respond with secondary lesions. This has recently been subjected to an interesting mathematical analysis by KAHAN and co-workers (1975).

It is often not recognized that animals injected with FCA develop lesions in the liver, kidneys and in the gut, i.e. these animals are not normal in their metabolic behaviour. This is a most important factor when considering the effect of potentially new anti-rheumatic compounds in these animals.

That the reaction is an allergic one has been clearly established by a number of workers. It has been demonstrated that hypersensitivity develops to BCG during the course of the reaction (BERRY et al., 1974), although a better correlation exists to endogenous antigen than to BCG or wax fraction D of tuberculin (see above). NEW-

BOULD (1963) found that when the draining lymph nodes are removed within the first 5 days after injection of the adjuvant, the appearance of secondary lesions is prevented. Treatment with immunosuppressive agents also prevents the onset of secondary lesions (see WHITEHOUSE and JASANI later in this volume).

In our hands, we have found the passive transfer of the adjuvant disease into sensitized lymphocytes to be an unsatisfactory procedure.

It is of interest that ZURIER and WEISSMANN (1972) and GLENN and co-workers (1972) have found that adjuvant disease may be suppressed by treatment with prostaglandins of the E type. Thus the E-type prostaglandins, usually regarded as anti-inflammatory, may suppress this reaction. Attempts were made to correlate the anti-inflammatory activity with their effects on lysosomal enzyme release; no correlation was found.

This model has many uses provided that one regards its limitations. It is simple to perform, requires rats which are cheap, and may be quantified by relatively unskilled staff. Of great value is the differential effect that may be observed with a new anti-inflammatory agent acting first on the primary (non-specific) lesion, or on the secondary lesion. Should such a compound be discovered, it is necessary to confirm that one is not merely observing a slow-acting anti-inflammatory agent such as gold, or penicillamine.

b) Guinea Pigs

Allergic arthritis is rarely used as a model in guinea pigs, although various toxic agents have been injected into the joints. The disadvantages of guinea pigs are their seasonal variation in response to these agents, and the fact that they are more expensive than rats. On the other hand, they are a good test species to use for cell-mediated immunity. Usually these are cutaneous reactions which are difficult to quantify.

c) Rabbits

The model of allergic arthritis used in rabbits is commonly referred to as the Glynn arthritis model, which was described by GLYNN and co-workers (DUMONDE and GLYNN, 1962; see GLYNN, 1968). This group have successfully utilised this method over a number of years. It consists of a sensitizing injection of an antigen, usually ovalbumin, in FCA; hypersensitivity cannot be induced in the absence of FCA. After an appropriate period of sensitization, the rabbits are challenged with an intra-articular injection of the antigen. A mono-articular arthritis develops which closely resembles the lesion seen in human arthritis, with pannus formation, infiltration with plasma cells and lymphocytes. The most important feature of this lesion is the chronicity, so that it not only resembles human arthritis in appearance but also in duration, with concomitant destruction of cartilage and bone. However, it differs from human arthritis in that it remains mono-articular, only affecting the injected joint.

Using rabbits has many advantages; it is possible to follow the intensity of the lesion by using methods of measurement similar to those used in man, namely size of joint, or by application of thermography (see Chapter 40).

The exact reason for persistence of the lesion in the rabbit is not clearly understood. It has been suggested that it may be persistence of the injected challenging dose of antigen. Alternatively, it may be the response to endogenous antigen; once again the response to modified tissue components which behave as non-self and subsequently act as antigens.

FOX and GLYNN (1975) have recently shown that antigen persists at the injected site for long periods of time following intra-articular challenge. The fascinating aspect of this recent work was that antigen persisted, whether the animals were sensitized with the antigen in FCA or FIA. The animals immunized with antigen in FIA do not develop the mono-articular arthritis. Yet antigen (IgG and C3) persisted for long periods of time in this group, in the absence of inflammation. Therefore mere persistence of antigen cannot itself explain the chronicity of the lesion. The antibody produced following injection of FIA plus antigen, does initiate an Arthus-type reaction. Thus, immune complexes remaining at the site do not seem to explain the chronicity of the lesion when rabbits are immunized with antigen plus FCA. STASTNY et al., (1973) have shown the continued production of macrophage inhibition factor (MIF). Experiments using the presence of MIF should be treated with caution, as YAMAMOTO et al. (1976) have shown that different forms of MIF activity may be present in Arthus exudate and serum from animals responding to a reverse passive Arthus reaction.

Nevertheless, in view of the ability of tuberculin to produce lymphocyte transformation from animals with experimental arthritis (BERRY et al., 1974), it seems likely that cell-mediated immunity is involved. DOBLE and GLYNN (quoted by FOX and GLYNN, 1975) favour the third possibility that during the acute phase, macrophages may carry to the joint breakdown products of tubercle bacilli, where they may then act as an adjuvant per se, or be chemotactic for more macrophages. In support of this hypothesis they quote the findings of COOK et al. (1969), who showed that dead streptococcal L-forms injected intra-articularly may cause a long-lasting inflammation.

Similarly WHITE and PULS (1969) showed that cell free extracts of *Erysipelothrix insidosa* also produce an arthritis. Probably the best evidence in favour of the transport of material by macrophages is that from GINSBURG and TROST (1971), who showed that macrophages carrying fluorescinated group A streptococci pass to joints made arthritic by injection of streptolysin S.

The certain advantages of this model of allergic arthritis are as follows:

1. With such a long lasting lesion, drugs may be tested on an *established lesion* rather than using a prophylactic treatment.
2. For the same reason, drugs which have a slow onset in action may be tested on this model, for long periods of time.
3. Measurement is not difficult, but remains crude.
4. There is close resemblance to the histology of human arthritis.

Among the disadvantages must be listed:

1. Principally the cost of rabbits; this cannot be envisaged as a primary screen for anti-rheumatic drugs even by its most ardent supporters.
2. Whereas measurement is simple and parallels those parameters used in man, it is very crude in explaining the mode of action.
3. The mono-articular nature of the disease makes one question the parallelism between this and human rheumatoid arthritis.

2. Arthritis in Swine

The role of mycoplasmas (PPLO) in arthritis and in other diseases has been extensively reviewed by SHARP and RIGGS (1967)—notably *M. hyorhinis* (ROBERTS et al., 1963) and later *M. granularum*. The latter strain induced arthritis within 8–10 days and, unlike *M. hyorhinis*, the animals did not develop fever or polyserositis. It is believed that this experimental form of arthritis is at times either chronic or recurrent.

The histology of the lesions produced by these PPLO resemble those seen in man with rheumatoid arthritis, the dominant features being the chronic non-suppurative character of the inflammation, the development of lymphoid follicles and the appearance of the cells in the synovial fluid.

Swine erysipelas is a naturally occurring disease in swine; the agent responsible is *E. rhusiopathiae*. If affected animals survive the acute phase of the disease, they develop a chronic arthritis at about 2–3 weeks after exposure. In view of the failure to isolate the organisms from the affected joints (SIKES, 1959), it has been suggested that the erysipelothrix arthritis may be the result of hypersensitivity rather than direct infection (STASTNY and ZIFF, 1967; NEHAR and SWENSON, 1959; FREEMAN, 1964). Certainly this disease is chronic in nature and is characterized by large numbers of mononuclear cells both in synovial fluid and in the synovium.

At this point in time, it would seem almost certain that this form of arthritis represents a model of hypersensitivity. Once again, although this is a fascinating model of an experimental arthropathy, the cost of pigs probably makes it prohibitive to utilise them as a model. Further, the precise mechanism remains to be resolved.

In this section we have discussed allergic arthritis: there is a host of other models of autoimmune disease (see STASTNY and ZIFF, 1967; GLYNN and HOLBOROW, 1965).

H. The Inflammatory Response in the Pleural Cavity

1. As an Experimental Model for Inflammation of Serosal Surface Including the Synovia

One of the gravest hazards in the quantitation of immunological models is the inability to quantitate the sequence of events. Thus, many of the tests are cutaneous and depend upon measurement of skin thickness (induration), and erythema (subjective, but made to appear quantitative by measuring diameter). In closer studies of the cutaneous reactions, at best only estimates may be made of the number and types of cells involved.

It is virtually impossible to perform assays on the extracellular enzymes participating in the reaction or on the pharmacologically active mediators. Attempts have been made to assay mediators and enzymes, but these have inevitably involved elaborate perfusion methods, which may themselves introduce a source of artefact. Thus when perfusing skin, having grossly dilated vessels as a consequence of an inflammatory response, various factors may become activated. It is not a control to perfuse non-inflamed skin; this does not permit the flow of perfusate past the engorged vessels or even through tissues containing possible pharmacological precursors, which may become activated by this procedure.

The obvious answer to this problem was to seek a body cavity in which immunological reactions could be performed. The cavity should preferably be such that it permitted easy collection of exudate and quantitation of cell types and numbers. The pleural cavity would seem to be best suited. This cavity has previously been used extensively by a number of workers for the study of non-specific inflammatory responses, and it has been shown that the collection of cells from the pleural cavity is a simple procedure which gives highly reproducible results (VELO et al., 1973; CAPASSO et al., 1975).

2. The Arthus Reaction

The first workers to use the pleural cavity for the study of the Arthus reaction were APICELLA and ALLEN (1969), who used an intrapleural method of sensitization followed by a challenge by the same route.

More recently, YAMAMOTO et al. (1975a) have used the reverse passive Arthus reaction (RPA) in rats. Rabbits were immunized with bovine serum albumin (BSA) and the resultant antibody was carefully purified. It is most important to purify the γ-globulin fraction of the anti-BSA. Injections of whole rabbit serum intrapleurally into rats produces an exudate which is rich in polymorphs.

To produce the RPA, rats are injected intravenously with BSA; 20 min later they are injected intrapleurally with 0.2 ml of anti-BSA. The resultant exudate is maximal at approximately 6 h and consists of up to 2 ml protein-rich fluid with large numbers of polymorphs. After this time, the reaction rapidly wanes. It is highly reproducible as a method, and intracellular and extracellular mediators, enzymes and cyclic nucleotides can all be assayed. The reaction is almost completely suppressed following depletion of peripheral haemolytic complement with CVF.

Assay of mediators has shown that the predominant pharmacologically active substance is histamine, which reaches a peak at 1–3 h after challenge, rising up to 70 $\mu g/10^8$ cells; by 12 h the histamine content of the cells has fallen to sub-microgram levels/10^8 cells. Simultaneously, there is a rise in the intracellular levels of 5-HT which peak between 1 and 3 h. At the height of the vascular response prostaglandin E (PGE) becomes maximal; as the vascular reaction wanes, the $PGF_{2\alpha}$ levels rise. This is consistent with the hypothesis of the PG's activity as a modulating system for the inflammatory reaction, i.e. PGE promoting increased vascular permeability, and PGF subsequently inhibiting this phase of the reaction. Intracellular cAMP levels fall by up to 40% (DUNN et al., unpublished).

This would seem to be an ideal model for the study of RPA reactions in the rat. It is cheap, reproducible, and permits absolute quantification of a variety of parameters.

It is of interest that macrophage inhibition activity has been found in the blood and exudates of animals undergoing RPA reactions (YAMAMOTO et al., 1976).

3. Cell-Mediated Immunity

a) Tuberculin Reaction

Attempts to produce a consistent response to the intrapleural injection of tuberculin in rats, have to date been unsuccessful. On the other hand, this has been successfully achieved in guinea pigs, following sensitization with FCA. The animals are subsequently challenged between $2^1/_2$ and 4 weeks later with an intrapleural injection of PPD (ALLEN and APICELLA, 1968; APICELLA and ALLEN, 1969; LEIBOWITZ et al., 1973; YAMAMOTO et al., 1975b). This method has proved reliable, once the technique of intrapleural injection has been mastered and exudates are produced free of blood.

As has been described for the RPA reaction, absolute quantitation of cell numbers and types, enzymes, cyclic nucleotides and pharmacological mediators, may be performed. It is also easy to study ultrastructural changes in the cells migrating into the pleural cavity. For electron microscopy it is best to harvest the cells from the pleural cavity using the appropriate EM fixative. This method avoids distortion of ultrastructure, which is otherwise often incurred when the cells are collected in Medium 199, centrifuged, and then fixed. The reaction is slow in onset, becoming maximal at 18–24 h after challenge. A typical reaction produces an exudate of 0.5 ml at 6 h after challenge, rising to 5.0 ml at 18 h and then slowly returning to normal by 48–72 h. The exudate is rich in cells, mainly of the mononuclear type.

Assay of both intracellular, and extracellular cAMP, shows a prolonged fall between 6 and 24 h, returning to normal by 48–72 h. Once again, during the peak of the response (as with the Arthus reaction), there is the maximum fall in cAMP. It is of interest that during this period of reduced cAMP levels, there is a rise in PGs. This is contrary to the hypothesis that the PGs should provoke a rise in cAMP, based on in vitro findings (WEISSMANN et al., 1971).

In contrast to the Arthus reaction, the tuberculin reaction leads to almost no release of histamine into the pleural cavity and only a modest quantity of 5-HT. The prostaglandins become maximal at about 12 h, which is close to the peak of the inflammatory response. Almost total depletion of the peripheral complement titres failed to affect the development of the reaction, either cellular or vascular. Thus, this tuberculin model in the pleural cavity of guinea pigs was in complete contrast to the RPA reaction in rats.

b) Pertussis Vaccine Pleurisy

DIEPPE et al. (1976b) have described a model of cell-mediated immunity produced in the pleural cavity of rats. In this model, rats are sensitized with pertussis vaccine in FIA. Twelve days after sensitization, the animals were challenged with an intrapleural injection of pertussis vaccine. This led to an exudate which became maximal 48 h later and was dominated by mononuclear cells.

The work on this model has not yet been extended to such detailed studies as those performed on the tuberculin reaction in the guinea pig. It is, however, one of the few models which show suppression of inflammation with D-penicillamine, indomethacin or levamisole. Dosing prior to sensitization and continuing throughout that period caused suppression with each of the three agents. On the other hand, dosing just at the time of challenge showed a marked enhancement of the reaction with levamisole and D-penicillamine, whereas indomethacin caused a suppression. Thus, the problem remains of finding a model capable of showing positive results with the immuno-stimulant drugs and D-penicillamine. Both of these drugs have already shown activity in human rheumatoid arthritis.

I. New Experimental Models for the Assay of Anti-Inflammatory Drugs

Mention has been made already of the use of the pleural cavity for the assay of anti-inflammatory drugs. Thus, cell-mediated immunity and RPA reactions have been described which include two important possible pathways in the maintenance of chronicity in human rheumatoid arthritis.

Recently, DIEPPE et al. (1976a) have described a new crystal deposition disease, namely "apatite deposition disease." Crystals of apatite have been identified in human synovial fluid and subjected to intensive analysis, using X-ray diffraction patterns, electron probe analysis and infrared spectometry. Once identification is absolute, identical crystals have been injected into the pleural cavity of rats. Similarly, calcium pyrophosphate crystals have been identified and injected into the pleural cavity of rats. The ensuing inflammatory responses are once again easy to quantify. Indeed, using a calcium pyrophosphate—induced pleurisy, there was, during the time course of the reaction, a clear-cut yin yang effect of cAMP and cGMP. This is an example of the advantage of this system, in that it permits for the first time an in vivo assay of intracellular cAMP vs. cGMP in inflammation. Hitherto, one was dependent upon in vitro systems.

GIROUD et al. (1973) showed the usefulness of implantation of coverslips into the subcutaneous tissues of rats and mice, to quantify the migration of a glass adherent cell population. This method showed the effect of slow-acting anti-inflammatory agents by prior dosing. It is relatively simple. Sterile glass cover slips are implanted into the subcutaneous tissues; these are then removed at different times, stained heavily and projected onto a piece of paper. This enables a calculation of the percent age of area of the cover slip covered with cells. Treatment with a potential anti-inflammatory agent may reduce the number of adherent cells. The method has the advantage of allowing the numbers of binucleated or giant cells on the cover slip to be counted. Additional evidence regarding kinetics may be obtained by a small injection of tritiated thymidine into the pocket containing the cover slip. This immediately provides information on how the new drug will be affecting cell turnover.

VERNON-ROBERTS et al. (1973), utilised a modified skin window technique (REBUCK and CROWLEY, 1955), in which they abraded the skin and then placed on the skin a glass slide coated in carbon. The "skin windows" were removed 24 h later and showed numbers of phagocytic cells adherent to the glass cover slip. Using such methods, they demonstrated the anti-inflammatory effect of prednisolone and gold salts.

JASANI and his colleagues (JASANI, 1973; JASANI et al., 1974) advocate the usefulness of skin homografts as a method for the assessment of potential anti-rheumatic drugs (see Chapter 37).

ANDREIS et al. (1974) produced a chronic synovitis in the rabbit following the injection of lymphokines obtained from keyhole limpex haemocyanin-sensitized lymphocytes. Repeated injections of these mediators of cell-mediated immunity were required to produce the arthritis. This was proposed not so much as a model, but as a method for the study of the mechanism of arthritis.

There seems little doubt that the main body of opinion is in favour of moving away from models which depend upon "swelling." Today, the research worker is more concerned with the effects of drugs upon the intracellular nucleotides (DE-

PORTER et al., 1976). Certainly there is agreement upon the central role of the macrophage (see review by ALLISON and DAVIES, 1974). To this end, the reader is referred to the volume *Future Trends in Inflammation II* (GIROUD et al., 1975). In this volume the mitogenic factors capable of causing proliferation of macrophages or monocytes present in exudates are discussed. Such models may prove to be invaluable in the future for the control of proliferative arthritic lesions.

Later chapters will be dealing specifically with assessment of anti-inflammatory drugs, and it would be repetitious to outline present in vitro and in vivo methods for their assessment.

References

Allen, J. C., Apicella, M. A.: Experimental pleural effusion as a manifestation of delayed hypersensitivity to tuberculin PPD. J. Immunol. **101**, 481—487 (1968)

Allison, A. C., Davies, P.: Mechanisms underlying chronic inflammation. In: Velo, G. P., Willoughby, D. A., Giroud, J. P. (Eds.): Future Trends in Inflammation, pp. 449—480. Padua-London: Piccin Medical Books 1974

Allison, A. C., Houba, V., Hendrickse, R. G., de Petris, S., Edington, G. M., Adeniyi, A.: Immune complexes in the nephrotic syndrome of African children. Lancet **1969 I**, 1232—1237

Andreis, M., Stastny, P., Ziff, M.: Experimental arthritis produced by injection of mediators of delayed hypersensitivity. Arthr. Rheum. **17**, 537—551 (1974)

Apicella, M. A., Allen, J. C.: A physiologic differentiation between delayed and immediate hypersensitivity. J. clin. Invest. **48**, 250—259 (1969)

Arthus, M.: Injections répetées de sérum de cheval chez le lapin. C.R. Soc. Biol. (Paris) **55**, 817—820 (1903)

Bell, W. R., Miller, R. E., Levin, R. J.: Inhibition of the generalised Shwartzman reaction by hypofibrinogenaemia. Blood **40**, 697—708 (1972)

Benacerraf, B., Gell, P. G. H.: Studies on hypersensitivity. III. The relation between delayed reactivity to the picryl group. Immunology **2**, 219—229 (1959)

Benacerraf, B., Levine, B. B.: Immunological specificity of delayed and immediate hypersensitivity reactions. J. exp. Med. **115**, 1023—1035 (1962)

Benacerraf, B., Paul, W. E., Green, I.: Hapten carrier relationships. Ann. N.Y. Acad. Sci. **169**, 93—104 (1970)

Berry, H., Giroud, J. P., Willoughby, D. A.: Evidence for an endogenous antigen in the adjuvant arthritic rat. In: Velo, G. P., Willoughby, D. A., Giroud, J. P. (Eds.): Future Trends in Inflammation, pp. 285—286. London-Padua: Piccin Medical Books 1974

Blanden, R. V.: Modification of macrophage function. J. reticuloendoth. Soc. **5**, 179—202 (1968)

Bloch, K. J., Kourilsky, F. M., Ovary, Z., Benacerraf, B.: Properties of guinea pig 7S antibodies. III. Identification of antibodies involved in complement fixation and hemolysis. J. exp. Med. **117**, 965—981 (1963)

Bokisch, V. A., Müller-Eberhard, H. J., Cochrane, C. G.: Isolation of a fragment (C3a) of the third component of human complement containing anaphylatoxin and chemotactic activity and description of an anaphylatoxin inactivator of human serum. J. exp. Med. **129**, 1109—1130 (1969)

Brade, V., Nicholson, A., Lee, G. D., Mayer, M. M.: The reaction of zymosan with the properdin system: Isolation of purified Factor D from guinea pig serum and study of its reaction chracteristics. J. Immunol. **112**, 1845—1854 (1974)

Brown, D. L.: Complement and coagulation. In: Brent, L., Holborow, J. (Eds.): Progress in Immunology II. Immunological Aspects, Vol. I, p. 191. Amsterdam: North Holland 1974

Brown, D. L., Lachmann, P. J.: The behaviour of complement and platelets in lethal endotoxin shock in rabbits. Int. Arch. Allergy **45**, 193—205 (1973)

Budzko, D. B., Bokisch, V. A., Müller-Eberhard, H. J.: A fragment of the third component of human complement with anaphylatoxin activity. Biochemistry **10**, 1166—1172 (1971)

Capasso, F., Dunn, C. J., Yamamoto, S., Deporter, D. A., Giroud, J. P., Willoughby, D. A.: Pharmacological mediators of various immunological and non-immunological inflammatory reactions produced in the pleural cavity. Agents Actions **5**, 528—533 (1975)
Cochrane, C. G., Hawkins, D.: Studies on circulating immune complexes. III. Factors governing the ability of circulating complexes to localize in blood vessels. J. exp. Med. **127**, 137—154 (1968)
Cochrane, C. G., Müller-Eberhard, H. J.: The derivation of two distinct anaphylatoxin activities from the third and fifth components of human complement. J. exp. Med. **127**, 371—386 (1967)
Cochrane, C. G., Müller-Eberhard, H. J., Aiken, B. S.: Depletion of plasma complement in vivo by a protein of cobra venom: its effect on various immunologic reactions. J. Immunol. **105**, 55—67 (1970)
Cochrane, C. G., Weigle, W. O.: The cutaneous reaction to soluble antigen antibody complexes. J. exp. Med. **108**, 591—604 (1958)
Cochrane, C. G., Weigle, W. O., Dixon, F. J.: The role of polymorphonuclear leucocytes in the initiation and cessation of Arthus vasculitis. J. exp. Med. **110**, 481—494 (1959)
Cohn, Z. A., Hirsch, J. G.: The influence of phagocytosis on intracellular distribution of granule associated components of polymorphonuclear leucocytes. J. exp. Med. **112**, 1015—1022 (1960)
Cook, J., Fincham, W. J., Lack, C. H.: Chronic arthritis induced by streptococcal L forms. J. Path. **19**, 283—299 (1969)
Cream, J. J., Bryceson, A. D. M., Ryder, G.: Disappearance of immunoglobulin and complement from the Arthus reaction and its relevance to studies of vasculitis in man. Brit. J. Derm. **84**, 106—109 (1971)
Culbertson, J. T.: Relationship of circulating antibody to the Arthus phenomenon. J. Immunol. **29**, 29—39 (1935)
Deporter, D. A., Capasso, F., Willoughby, D. A.: The effects of modifying intracellular cyclic nucleotides on the inflammatory response. J. Path. (1976) (in press)
Dias da Silva, W., Eisele, J. W., Lepow, I. H.: Complement as a mediator of inflammation. III. Purification of the activity with anaphylatoxin properties generated by interaction of the first four components of complement and its identification as a cleavage product of C'3. J. exp. Med. **126**, 1027—1048 (1967)
Dias da Silva, W., Lepow, I. H.: Anaphylatoxin formation by purified human C'1 esterase. J. Immunol. **95**, 1080—1089 (1965)
Dias da Silva, W., Lepow, I. H.: Complement as a mediator of inflammation. II. Biological properties of anaphylatoxin prepared with purified components of human complement. J. exp. Med. **125**, 921—946 (1967)
Dieppe, P. A., Huskisson, E. C., Crocker, P., Willoughby, D. A., Balme, H. W.: A new form of crystal deposition disease: apatite arthropathy. Lancet **1976a** (in press)
Dieppe, P. A., Willoughby, D. A., Huskisson, E. C., Anigoni-Martelli, E.: Pertussis vaccine pleurisy a model of delayed hypersensitivity. Agents Actions (1976 b) (in press)
Dixon, F. J., Oldstone, M. B. A., Tonietti, G.: The etiologies of immune complex type glomerulonphritis. In: Bonoma, L., Turk, J. L. (Eds.): Proceedings of the International Symposium on Immune Complex Diseases, pp. 15—18. Milan: Carlo Erba 1970
Domingo, E. C., Warren, K. S.: The inhibition of granuloma formation around *Schistomsoma mansoni* eggs. II. Thymectomy. Amer. J. Path. **51**, 757—767 (1967)
Dumonde, D. C., Glynn, L. E.: The production of arthritis in rabbits by an immunological reaction to fibrin. Brit. J. exp. Path. **43**, 373—383 (1962)
Fong, J. S. C., Good, R. A.: Prevention of the localised and generalised Shwartzman reaction by an anti-complementary agent—cobra venom factor. J. exp. Med. **134**, 642—655 (1971)
Fox, A., Glynn, L. E.: Persistence of antigen in nonarthritic joints. Ann. rheum. Dis. **34**, 431—437 (1975)
Freeman, J. J.: Effects of vaccination on the development of arthritis in swine with erysipelas: clinical, haematologic, and gross pathologic observations. Amer. J. vet. Res. **25**, 589—608 (1964)
Gigli, I., Nelson, R. A., Jr.: Complement dependent immune phagocytosis. I. Requirements for C'1, C'4, C'2, C'3. Exp. Cell Res. **51**, 45—67 (1968)

Ginsburg, I., Trost, R.: Localization of group A streptococci and particles of titanium dioxide in arthritic lesions in the rabbit. J. infect. Dis. **123**, 292—296 (1971)

Giroud, J. P., Timsit, J., Spector, W. G., Willoughby, D. A.: The pharmaco-cellular assessment of slow acting anti-inflammatory drugs. Agents Action **314**, 205—209 (1973)

Giroud, J. P., Willoughby, D. A., Velo, G. P. (Eds.): Future Trends in Inflammation. II. Basel: Birkhauser Verlag 1975

Glenn, E. M., Rohloff, N.: Anti-arthritic and anti-inflammatory effects of certain prostaglandins. Proc. Soc. exp. Biol. (N.Y.) **139**, 290—294 (1972)

Glynn, L. E.: The chronicity of inflammation and its significance in rheumatoid arthritis (Heberden Oration). Ann. rheum. Dis. **27**, 105—121 (1968)

Glynn, L. E., Holborow, E. J.: Autoimmunity and disease. Oxford: Blackwell 1965

Gocke, D. J., Hsu, K., Morgan, C., Bombardieri, S., Lockshin, M., Christian, C. L.: Association between polyarteritis and Australia antigen. Lancet **1970 II**, 1149—1153

Godal, T., Rees, R. J. W., Lamvik, J. O.: Lymphocyte mediated modification of blood derived macrophage function in vitro: inhibition of growth of intracellular mycobacteria with lymphokines. Clin. exp. Immunol. **8**, 625—637 (1971)

Good, R. A., Thomas, L.: Studies on the generalised Shwartzman reaction. IV. Prevention of the local and generalised Shwartzman reactions with heparin. J. exp. Med. **97**, 871—888 (1953)

Greenwood, B. M., Whittle, H. C., Bryceson, A. D. M.: Allergic complications of meningococcal disease. II. Immunological investigations. Brit. med. J. **1973 II**, 737—740

Henson, P. M.: The adherence of leucocytes and platelets induced by fixed IgG antibody or complement. Immunology **16**, 107—121 (1969)

Henson, P. M., Cochrane, C. G.: Acute immune complex disease in rabbits. The role of complement and of a leukocyte dependent release of vasoactive amines from platelets. J. exp. Med. **133**, 554—571 (1971)

Hulliger, L., Blazkovec, A. A., Sorkin, E.: A study of the passive cellular transfer of local cutaneous hypersensitivity. IV. Transfer of hypersensitivity to sheep erythrocytes with peritoneal exudate cells coated with antibody. Int. Arch. Allergy **33**, 281—291 (1968)

Humphrey, J. H.: The mechanism of Arthus reaction. I. The role of polymorphonuclear leucocytes and the factors in reversed passive reactions in rabbits. Brit. J. exp. Path. **36**, 268—282 (1955a)

Humphrey, J. H.: The mechanism of Arthus reactions. II. The role of polymorphonuclear leucocytes and platelets in reversal passive reactions in the guinea pig. Brit. J. exp. Path. **36**, 283—289 (1955b)

Humphrey, J. H., Dourmashkin, R. R.: The lesions in cell membranes caused by complement. Advanc. Immunol. **11**, 75—115 (1969)

Hunter, J.: A Treatise on the Blood Inflammation and Gunshot Wounds, Vol. I, p. 438. London 1812

Jasani, M. K.: A new approach for studying the influence of cyclophosphamide upon the rejection of rabbit skin homografts. Brit. J. Pharmacol. **48**, 334 P—334 P (1973)

Jasani, M. K., Parsons, R. R., Roberts, J. M., Tweed, M. F.: The usefuness of homologous pairs of rabbit skin grafts for studying the pharmacology of anti-rheumatic drugs. Proc. Brit. pharm. Soc. 152 P (1974)

Jenner, E.: An enquiry into the cause and effects of variolae-vaccinae. London: 1798

Jensen, J.: Anaphylatoxin in its relation to the complement system. Science **155**, 1122—1123 (1967)

Kabat, E. A., Mayer, M. M.: Experimental Immunochemistry, 2nd Ed., p. 278. Illinois: Charles C. Thomas 1961

Kahan, A., Perlik, F., Le Go, A., Delbarre, F.: In: Giroud, J. P., Willoughby, D. A., Velo, G. P. (Eds.): Future Trends in Inflammation II. Basel: Birkhauser Verlag 1975

Kane, M. A., May, J. E., Frank, M. M.: Interactions of the classical and alternate complement pathway with endotoxin lipopolysaccharide. J. clin. Invest. **52**, 370—376 (1973)

Karat, A. B. A., Karat, S., Job, C. K., Furness, M. A.: Acute exudative arthritis in leprosy. Rheumatoid-arthritis-like syndrome in association with erythema nodosum leprosum. Brit. med. J. **1967 III**, 770—772

Katz, S. I.: Mechanisms involved in the express of Jones-Mote hypersensitivity. Ph.D. Thesis, University of London 1974

Katz, S. I., Heather, C. J., Parker, D., Turk, J. L.: Basophilic leucocytes in delayed hypersensitivity reactions. J. Immunol. **113**, 1073—1078 (1974c)
Katz, S. I., Parker, D., Sommer, G., Turk, J. L.: Suppressor cells in normal immunisation as a basic homeostatic mechanism. Nature (Lond.) **248**, 612—614 (1974a)
Katz, S. I., Parker, D., Turk, J. L.: B-cell suppression of delayed hypersensitivity reactions. Nature (Lond.) **251**, 550—551 (1974b)
Katz, S. I., Parker, D., Turk, J. L.: Mechanisms involved in the expression of Jones-Mote hypersensitivity. II. Lymph node morphology and in vitro correlates. Cell. Immunol. **16**, 404—412 (1975)
Kerckhaert, J. A. M., Van den Berg, G. J., Willers, J. M. N.: Influence of cyclophosphamide on the delayed hypersensitivity of the mouse. Ann. Immunol. **125c**, 415—425 (1974)
Kniker, W. J., Cochrane, C. G.: Pathogenic factors in vascular lesions of experimental serum sickness. J. exp. Med. **122**, 83—97 (1965)
Koch, R.: Weitere Mitteilungen über ein Heilmittel gegen Tuberculose. Dtsch. med. Wschr. **16**, 1029—1032 (1890)
Koffler, D., Schur, P. H., Kunkel, H. G.: Immunological studies concerning the nephritis of systemic lupus erythematosus. J. exp. Med. **126**, 607—623 (1967)
Kohn, J. L., McCabe, E. J., Brem, J.: Anaphylactic gangrene following administration of horse serum. Arthus or Shwartzman phenomenon? Amer. J. Dis. Child. **55**, 1018—1030 (1938)
Kovats, T. G., Vegh, P.: Shwartzman reaction in endotoxin resistant rabbits induced by heterologous endotoxin. Immunology **12**, 445—453 (1967)
Lachmann, P. J., Thompson, R. A.: Reactive lysis: the complement mediated lysis of unsensitized cells. II. The characterization of the activated reactor as $C\overline{56}$ and the participation of C8 and C9. J. exp. Med. **131**, 643—657 (1970)
Leibowitz, S., Kennedy, L., Lessof, M. H.: The tuberculin reaction in the pleural cavity and its suppression by antilymphocyte serum. Brit. J. exp. Path. **54**, 152—162 (1973)
Lewis, E., Turk, J. L.: Comparison of the effect of various antisera and cobra venom factor on inflammatory reactions in guinea pig skin. II. The Arthus reaction and local Shwartzman reaction. J. Path. **115**, 111—125 (1975)
Maillard, J. L., Pick, E., Turk, J. L.: Interaction between "sensitized lymphocytes" and antigen in vitro. V. Vascular permeability induced by a skin reactive factor. Int. Arch. Allergy **42**, 50—68 (1972)
Maillard, J. L., Voisin, G. A.: Elicitation of Arthus reactions in guinea pigs by homologous γ_1 and γ_2 immunoglobulin. Proc. Soc. exp. Biol. (N.Y.) **133**, 1188—1194 (1970)
Maillard, J. L., Zarco, R. M.: Décomplementation par un factour extrait du venin de cobra. Effet sur plusieurs reactions immunes du cobaye et du rat. Ann. Inst. Pasteur **114**, 756—774 (1968)
Margaretten, W., McKay, D. G.: The role of the platelet in the generalised Shwartzman reaction. J. exp. Med. **129**, 585—590 (1969)
Müller-Eberhard, H. J., Dalmasso, A. P., Calcott, M. A.: The reaction mechanism of β_{1C}-globulin (C'3) in immune hemolysis. J. exp. Med. **123**, 33—54 (1966)
Nath, I., Poulter, L. W., Turk, J. L.: Effect of lymphocyte mediators on macrophages in vitro. A correlation of morphological and cytochemical changes. Clin. exp. Immunol. **13**, 455—466 (1973)
Nathan, C. F., Karnovsky, M. L., David, J. R.: Alteration of macrophage function by mediators from lymphocytes. J. exp. Med. **133**, 1356—1376 (1971)
Neher, G. M., Swenson, C. B.: Does vaccination against swine erysipelas afford protection against arthritis? Lab. Invest. **8**, 1419—1426 (1959)
Nelson, D. S.: Immune adherence. In: Wolstenholm, G. E. W., Knight, J. (Eds.): Ciba Foundation Symposium on Complement, p. 22. London: Churchill 1965
Nelson, R. A., Jr.: The immune adherence phenomenon. An immunologically specific reaction between microorganisms and erythrocytes leading to enhanced phagocytosis. Science **118**, 733—737 (1953)
Neta, R., Salvin, S. B.: Specific depression of delayed hypersensitivity to purified proteins, with relation to production of circulating antibody. Cell. Immunol. **9**, 242—250 (1973)
Newbould, B. B.: Studies on adjuvant arthritis in rats. Brit. J. Pharmacol. **21**, 127—134 (1963)
Opie, E. L.: Inflammatory reaction of the immune animal to antigen (Arthus phenomenon) and its relation to antibodies. J. Immunol. **9**, 231—245 (1924)

Parish, W. E.: Studies on vasculitis. I. Immunoglobulin β_{1C}, C reactive protein and bacterial antigens in cutaneous vasculitis lesions. Clin. Allergy **1**, 97—110 (1971)

Pearson, C. M.: Experimental production of arthritis in rats. Ann. rheum. Dis. **15**, 379—385 (1956)

Pepys, J.: Hypersensitivity diseases of the lung due to fungi and organic diseases. Monogr. Allergy **4**. Basel: Karger 1969

Pick, E., Feldman, T. J.: Transfer of cutaneous hypersensitivity to tuberculin in the guinea pig by γ_2 from immunised donors. J. Immunol. **100**, 858—862 (1968)

Pick, E., Krejci, J., Cech, K., Turk, J. L.: Interaction between "sensitized lymphocytes" and antigen in vitro. I. The release of a skin-reactive factor. Immunology **17**, 741—767 (1969)

Pillemer, L., Blum, L., Lepow, I., Ross, O., Todd, E., Wardlaw, A.: The properdin system and immunity. I. Demonstration and isolation of a new serum protein, properdin, and its role in immune phenomena. Science **120**, 279—285 (1954)

Pirquet, C. von: Allergie. Münch. med. Wschr. **53**, 1457—1459 (1906)

Pirquet, C. von, Schlick, B.: Zur Theorie der Inkubationszeit. Wien. klin. Wschr. **16**, 758—759 (1903)

Polak, L., Geleick, H., Turk, J. L.: Reversal of tolerance in contact sensitization by cyclophosphamide: tolerance induced by prior feeding with DNCB. Immunology **28**, 939—942 (1975)

Polak, L., Turk, J. L.: Suppression of the haemorrhagic component of the Shwartzman reaction with anti-complement serum. Nature (Lond.) **223**, 738—739 (1969)

Polak, L., Turk, J. L.: Reversal of immunological tolerance by cyclophosphamide through inhibition of suppressor cell activity. Nature (Lond.) **249**, 654—656 (1974)

Rebuck, J. W., Crowley, J. H.: A method of studying leukocytic functions in vivo. Ann. N.Y. Acad. Sci. **59**, 757—760 (1955)

Richerson, H. B., Dvorak, H. F., Leskowitz, S.: Cutaneous basophil hypersensitivity. I. A new look at the Jones-Mote reaction. General characteristics. J. exp. Med. **132**, 546—557 (1970)

Roberts, E. D., Switzer, W. P., Ramsey, F. R.: The pathology of *M. hyorhinis* arthritis produced experimentally in swine. Amer. J. vet. Res. **24**, 19—31 (1963)

Schlossman, S. F., Ben-Efraim, S., Yaron, A., Sober, H. A.: Immunochemical studies n the antigenic determinants required to elicit delayed and immediate hypersensitivity reactions. J. exp. Med. **123**, 1083—1095 (1966)

Sharp, J. T., Riggs, S.: Mycoplasmas and rheumatic disease. In: Rotstein, J. (Ed.): Rheumatology, Vol. I, pp. 51—84. Basel: S. Karger 1967

Sikes, D.: A rheumatoid-like arthritis in swine. Lab. Invest. **8**, 1406—1415 (1959)

Shwartzman, G.: A new phenomenon of local skin reactivity to *B. typhosus* culture filtrate. Proc. Soc. exp. Biol. (N.Y.) **25**, 560—561 (1928)

Snyderman, R., Gewurz, H., Mergenhagen, S. E.: Interations of the complement system with endotoxic lipopolysaccharide. Generation of a factor chemotactic for polymorphonuclear leukocytes. J. exp. Med. **128**, 259—275 (1968)

Snyderman, R., Mergenhagen, S. E.: Characterization of polymorphonuclear chemotactic activity in serums activated by various inflammatory agents. In: Ingram, D. G. (Ed.): Biological Activities of Complement, p. 117. Basel: Karger 1972

Spanoudis, S., Eichbaum, F., Rosenfeld, G.: Inhibition of the local Shwartzman reaction by dicumarol. J. Immunol. **75**, 167—170 (1955)

Spector, W. G., Heesom, N.: The production of granulomata by antigen-antibody complexes. J. Path. **98**, 31—39 (1969)

Stastny, P., Cooke, T. D., Ziff, M.: Production of a macrophage migration inhibitory factor in rabbits with experimental arthritis. Clin. exp. Immunol. **14**, 141—147 (1973)

Stastny, P., Ziff, M.: Immunologically induced experimental models of human connective tissue diseases. In: Rotstein, J. (Ed.): Rheumatology, Vol. I, pp. 189—230. Basel: S. Karger 1967

Stecher, V. J., Sorkin, E.: Studies on chemotaxis. XII. Generation of chemotactic activity for polymorphonuclear leucocytes in sera with complement deficiencies. Immunology **16**, 231—239 (1969)

Stetson, C. A. Jr.: Similarities in the mechanisms determining the Arthus and Shwartzman phenomena. J. exp. Med. **94**, 347—357 (1951)

Stetson, C. A. Jr., Good, R. A.: Studies on the mechanism of the Shwartzman phenomenon. Evidence for the participation of polymorphonuclear leucocytes in the phenomenon. J. exp. Med. **93**, 49—63 (1951)

Thomas, L.: The role of lysosomes in tissue injury. In: Zweifach, B. W., Grant, L., McCluskey, R. T. (Eds.): The Inflammatory Process, p. 449. New York: Academic Press 1965
Thomas, L., Stetson, C. Jr.: Inhibition of the Shwartzman phenomenon by local application of bromobenzene and other solvents. Proc. Soc. exp. Biol. (N.Y.) **69**, 409—413 (1948)
Trnka, Z., Hay, J. B., Lachmann, P. J.: Production of MIF and mitogenic factor in vivo. Int. Arch. Allergy **45**, 292—294 (1973)
Turk, J. L.: Delayed Hypersensitivity, 2nd Ed. Amsterdam: North-Holland Elsevier 1975
Turk, J. L., Parker, D.: Further studies on B-lymphocyte suppression in delayed hypersensitivity, indicating a possible mechanism for Jones-Mote hypersensitivity. Immunology **24**, 751—758 (1973)
Turk, J. L., Parker, D., Poulter, L. W.: Functional aspects of the selective depletion of lymphoid tissue by cyclophosphamide. Immunology **23**, 493—501 (1972)
Turk, J. L., Poulter, L. W.: Selective depletion of lymphoid tissue by cyclophosphamide. Clin. exp. Immunol. **10**, 285—296 (1972)
Velo, G. P., Dunn, C. J., Giroud, J. P., Timsit, J., Willoughby, D. A.: Distribution of prostaglandin in inflammatory exudate. J. Path. **111**, 149—158 (1973)
Vernon-Roberts, B., Jessop, J. D., Dore, J.: Effects of gold salts and prednisolone on inflammatory cells. Ann. rheum. Dis. **32**, 301—307 (1973)
Ward, P. A.: A plasmin-split fragment of C'3 as a new chemotactic factor. J. exp. Med. **126**, 189—206 (1967)
Ward, P. A., Cochrane, C. G.: Bound complement and immunologic injury of blood vessels. J. exp. Med. **121**, 215—234 (1965)
Ward, P. A., Cochrane, C. G., Müller-Eberhard, H. J.: Further studies on the chemotactic factor of complement and its formation in vivo. Immunology **11**, 141—154 (1966)
Ward, P. A., Hill, J. H.: C5 Chemotactic Fragments produced by an enzyme in lysosomal granules of neutrophils. J. Immunol. **104**, 535—543 (1970)
Warren, K. S., Domingo, E. C., Cowan, R. B. T.: Granuloma formation around schistosome eggs as a manifestation of delayed hypersensitivity. Amer. J. Path. **51**, 755—756 (1967)
Weissmann, G., Dukor, P., Zurier, R. B.: Effect of cyclic AMP on release of lysosomal enzymes from phagocytes. Nature (New Biol.) **231**, 131—135 (1971)
Wemambu, S. N. C., Turk, J. L., Waters, M. F. R., Rees, R. J. W.: Erythema nodosum leprosum: a clinical manifestation of the Arthus reaction phenomenon. Lancet **1969 II**, 933—935
White, T. G., Puls, J. L.: Induction of experimental chronic arthritis in rabbits by cell free fragments of erysipelothrix. J. Bact. **98**, 403—406 (1969)
Whittle, H. C., Abdullahi, M. J., Fakunle, F. A., Greenwood, B. M., Bryceson, A. D. M., Parry, E. H. C., Turk, J. L.: Allergic complications of meningococcal disease. I. Clinical aspects. Brit. med. J. **1973 II**, 733—737
Willoughby, D. A., Ryan, G. B.: Evidence for a possible endogenous antigen in chronic inflammation. J. Path. **101**, 233—239 (1970)
Wissler, J. H.: Chemistry and biology of the anaphylatoxin related serum peptide system. I. Purification, crystallisation and properties of classical anaphylatoxin from rat serum. Europ. J. Immunol. **2**, 73—83 (1972)
WHO Memorandum: Nomenclature of complement. Bull. Wld Hlth Org. **39**, 935—938 (1968)
WHO Memorandum: Immunology of schistosomiasis. Bull. Wld Hlth Org. **51**, 553—595 (1974)
WHO Report: Pathogenetic mechanisms in dengue haemorrhagic fever: Report of an international collaborative study. Bull. Wld Hlth Org. **48**, 117—133 (1973)
Wolff, S. M., Kovats, T. G.: The Shwartzman reaction. In: Brent, L., Holborow, J. (Eds.): Progress in Immunology II, Vol. 4, pp. 359—362. Amsterdam: North Holland 1974
Wuepper, K. D., Bokisch, V. A., Müller-Eberhard, H. J., Stoughton, R. B.: Cutaneous responses to human C3 anaphylatoxin in man. Clin. exp. Immunol. **11**, 13—20 (1972)
Yamamoto, S., Dunn, C. J., Capasso, F., Deporter, D. A., Willoughby, D. A.: Quantitative studies on cell-mediated immunity in the pleural cavity of guinea-pigs. J. Path. **117**, 65—73 (1975b)
Yamamoto, S., Dunn, C. J., Deporter, D. A., Capasso, F., Willoughby, D. A., Huskisson, E. C.: A model for the quantitative study of Arthus hypersensitivity in rats. Agents Actions **5/4**, 374—377 (1975a)
Yamamoto, S., Dunn, C. J., Willoughby, D. A.: Studies on delayed hypersensitivity pleural exudates in guinea pigs II. The interrelationship of monocytic and lymphocytic cells with respect to migration. Immunology **30**, 513—519 (1976)

Zembala, M., Asherson, G. L.: Contact sensitivity in the mouse. V. The role of macrophage cytophilic antibody in passive transfer and the effect of trypsin and anti-gamma globulin serum. Cell. Immunol. **1**, 276—289 (1970)
Zembala, M., Asherson, G. L.: Depression of the T cell phenomenon of contact sensitivity by T cells from unresponsive mice. Nature (Lond.) **244**, 227—228 (1973)
Zinsser, H.: Bacterial allergy and tissue reactions. Proc. Soc. exp. Biol. (N.Y.) **22**, 35—39 (1925)
Zinsser, H., Mueller, J. H.: On the nature of bacterial allergies. J. exp. Med. **41**, 159—177 (1925)
Zurier, R. B., Weissmann, G.: Effect of prostaglandin upon enzyme release from lysosome in experimental arthritis. In: Ramwell, P. W., Pharris, B. B. (Eds.): Proceedings Alza Conference on Prostaglandins in Cellular Biology and the Inflammatory Process, pp. 151—172. New York: Plenum Press 1972

CHAPTER 8

The Release of Hydrolytic Enzymes From Phagocytic and Other Cells Participating in Acute and Chronic Inflammation

P. DAVIES and A. C. ALLISON

Introduction

The release of hydrolytic enzymes by cells present at sites of inflammation is now well recognized. These enzymes are released following either the death of cells after interaction with cytotoxic agents or in a selective manner, where hydrolase release occurs by secretion from viable cells. The latter process has attracted much attention in recent years since it constitutes a mechanism by which hydrolytic enzymes can be released in a directed manner towards an extracellular stimulus. Also viable cells under certain conditions, can be induced to release newly synthesized hydrolases over a long period of time, illustrating a possible mechanism by which tissue damage, degradation and remodelling seen during chronic inflammatory processes can occur.

In this chapter we first discuss the mechanisms by which enzymes can be released from cells. Secondly, we give a concise account of the way in which different stimuli can induce the release of hydrolytic enzymes from various cell types involved in inflammation, and thirdly, we consider some of the ways in which hydrolytic enzymes can contribute to the initiation and evolution of inflammatory responses.

A. Mechanism of Release of Hydrolytic Enzymes From Cells

I. Lysis of Membranes

There are at least two ways by which agents can cause non-selective enzyme release by breaking down integrity of membranes. A cytotoxic agent can rupture the plasma membrane causing release of cytoplasmic enzymes, such as those of the glycolytic pathway, as well as enzymes associated with mitochondria, lysosomes, the endoplasmic reticulum and nucleus. In addition, cytotoxic agents may break down the membrane of lysosomes after interiorization into the cell by pinocytosis or phagocytosis. In many instances such materials do not exert a cytotoxic effect at the plasma membrane because of their association with non-toxic substances. For example, the cytotoxic effect of silica particles phagocytosed by macrophages is not seen until adsorbed proteins on the surface of the particles are digested by the hydrolytic enzymes of lysosomes. Similarly, if a toxic agent is coupled to a digestible carrier its effects will be seen only after catabolism of the carrier within lysosomes (BARBANTI-BRODANO and FIUME, 1973).

A toxic agent may also exert a cytolytic effect after being formed from a non-toxic precursor by the activity of the enzymes of the smooth endoplasmic reticulum in certain cell types.

II. Selective Release of Hydrolytic Enzymes Following Membrane Fusion

The selective release of hydrolytic enzymes by the fusion of subcellular organelles containing these enzymes with the plasma membrane, can occur in several ways. In phagocytic cells, the selective release of acid hydrolases contained within lysosomes during the phagocytosis of particulate substances is well established. Polymorphonuclear leucocytes show selective release of acid hydrolases when exposed to any kind of phagocytic stimulus while macrophages release a large proportion of their lysosomal acid hydrolases in response to inflammatory stimuli only.

Release may occur by incomplete closure of phagocytic vacuoles before their fusion with lysosomes, allowing free passage of lysosomal enzymes into the extracellular environment. In other instances, perturbation of the plasma membranes of non-phagocytic cells or of phagocytic cells when their phagocytic capacity has been inhibited, leads to the selective release of acid hydrolases. The former is illustrated by complement-sufficient antiserum-induced release of enzymes from organ cultures of embryonic limb bones, while the latter is demonstrated by the selective release of acid hydrolases from polymorphonuclear leucocytes and macrophages exposed to a phagocytic stimulus in the presence of cytochalasin B.

In other instances, neutral proteinases (which may not reside within lysosomes) can be secreted from cells such as macrophages and synovial fibroblast-like cells over a long period of time. The secretion of neutral proteinases is not totally dependent on stimulation of the plasma membrane, although the secretion of these enzymes can be greatly enhanced by phagocytosis.

B. The Selective Release of Acid Hydrolases by Polymorphonuclear Leucocytes

I. Factors Influencing Enzyme Release

The hydrolytic enzymes of polymorphonuclear leucocytes are contained within more than one population of granules (BAGGIOLINI et al., 1969; BRETZ and BAGGIOLINI, 1974). The azurophilic granules contain the bulk of acid hydrolases and neutral proteinases (BAGGIOLINI et al., 1969; DAVIES et al., 1971; FOLDS et al., 1972; SPITZNAGEL et al., 1974; DEWALD et al., 1975) while specific granules contain lysozyme and alkaline phosphatase (BAGGIOLINI et al., 1969; BRETZ and BAGGIOLINI, 1973).

The release of acid hydrolases from viable polymorphonuclear leucocytes during phagocytosis was described by CROWDER et al. (1969) and later studies confirmed that this was selective (HAWKINS and PEETERS, 1971; HENSON, 1971a; WEISSMANN et al., 1971).

More recently, conditions and stimuli have been defined in response to which there is a differential secretion of the contents of specific and azurophilic granules. ESTENSEN et al. (1974) and WHITE and ESTENSEN (1974) have shown that human polymorphonuclear leucocytes exposed to phorbol myristate acetate (PMA) release lysozyme and alkaline phosphatase but not acid hydrolases. This finding has been confirmed by GOLDSTEIN et al. (1974) who have further shown that PMA also enhances the release of acid hydrolases from cytochalasin B-treated polymorphonuclear leucocytes exposed to C5a (GOLDSTEIN et al., 1975a). These authors have also shown that lysozyme could be released selectively from human polymorphonuclear leucocytes suspended in HEPES-buffered sodium chloride containing increasing amounts of calcium ions. Detectable lysozyme release was seen with as little as 0.01 mM calcium with maximal release being obtained with 1.0 mM calcium ion. The effect of calcium was temperature-dependent, lysozyme release being greatly reduced at 20° C and absent at 0° C in the presence of 2.5 mM calcium. Manganese, strontium and zinc ions were found to mimic the effects of calcium ions to varying extents, but magnesium and barium inhibited the effect of calcium ions. The effects of calcium ions were also potentiated by the ionophore A23187. There was no detectable release of lysosomal enzymes under these conditions where cells were suspended in an extracellular medium containing only HEPES-buffered sodium chloride with increasing amounts of calcium ions.

Calcium ions also play a role in the release of lysosomal enzymes from polymorphonuclear leucocytes induced by stimuli such as immune complexes and zymosan-treated serum (IGNARRO and GEORGE, 1974; GOLDSTEIN et al., 1975b).

II. Mechanism of Selective Release of Acid Hydrolases From Polymorphonuclear Leucocytes

The pharmacological modulation of the selective release of hydrolytic enzymes from polymorphonuclear leucocytes will be discussed in detail in chapter 9 by ZURIER and KRAKAUER. It is becoming clear that contractile proteins showing the properties of actin and myosin and found within polymorphonuclear leucocytes (SHIBATA et al., 1972; STOSSEL and POLLARD, 1973), macrophages (ALLISON et al., 1971; AXLINE and REAVEN, 1974) and other cell types (ISHIKAWA et al., 1969; YANG and PERDUE, 1972), play a role in the retention of acid hydrolases within cells. Speculation regarding the function of contractile proteins in cells has been stimulated by studies with cytochalasin B, which is a natural product derived from *Helminthosporium dematoideum*. The effects of this substance on cells were first described by CARTER in 1967 when he found that it inhibited cell movement, ruffled membrane activity and cytokinesis after cell division without any apparent toxic effects.

Subsequently, WESSELS et al. (1971) suggested that all the effects of cytochalasin B could be explained on the basis of inhibition of the function of the contractile microfilament system. In 1972, SPUDICH and LIN showed that cytochalasin B interacted directly with isolated contractile elements, but it has also been found that cytochalasin B in low doses inhibits specific membrane transport of glucose and glucosamine (KLETZIEN et al., 1972; MIZEL and WILSON, 1972; ESTENSEN and PLAGEMAN, 1972; ZIGMOND and HIRSCH, 1972). LIN et al. (1974) have shown that blood platelets, HeLa cells and SV40-transformed fibroblasts all have two classes of receptors for cytochalasin B. One has a high affinity for cytochalasin B with a dissociation constant of about 10^{-7} M and the other has a lower affinity with a dissociation constant of about 10^{-5} M. LIN et al. (1974) have suggested that these two classes of receptors represent hexose transport sites (high affinity) and cell components being responsible for cell movement and maintaining cell shape (low affinity), respectively.

Cytochalasin B is a potent inhibitor of phagocytosis by both polymorphonuclear leucocytes and macrophages (ALLISON et al., 1971; DAVIS et al., 1971; MALAWISTA et al., 1971). However, such prevention of phagocytosis is not accompanied by an inhibition of selective release of lysosomal hydrolases. In contrast, there is an enhancement of acid hydrolase release compared with that seen with cells exposed to the phagocytic stimulus in the absence of cytochalasin B (DAVIES et al., 1973; HAWKINS, 1973; ZURIER et al., 1973a; TEMPLE et al., 1973). This release is selective since the cells remain viable as indicated by morphological observations and retention of a cytoplasmic enzyme marker, lactate dehydrogenase. A similar phenomenon is seen when polymorphonuclear leucocytes are exposed to stimuli rendered nonphagocytozable by attachment to immobile surfaces (HENSON and OADES, 1973). Electron microscopic studies showed that the selective release of acid hydrolases occurred by fusion of lysosomes with the plasma membrane of the cell close to the site of attachment of the phagocytic stimulus (DAVIES et al., 1973; HENSON and OADES, 1973; ZURIER et al., 1973a). A suggested mechanism for this phenomenon is that cytochalasin B inhibits the function of a peripheral band of microfilaments which normally confine the subcellular organelles within the inner cytoplasm or endoplasm of the cell (DAVIES et al., 1973). In the absence of this controlling influence, lysosomes and other subcellular organelles are free to move towards and come into contact with the plasma membrane. Cytochalasin B has no effect on the attachment step of phagocytosis (DAVIES et al., 1973) and it is likely that the local membrane changes which normally trigger endocytosis still occur. Since lysosomes have easier access to plasma membranes, acid hydrolases which are normally discharged into phagocytic vacuoles are released extracellularly at the plasma membrane in a selective manner. The reader is referred to chapter 9 for further discussion of the factors controlling the selective release of acid hydrolases from polymorphonuclear leucocytes.

III. Selective Release of Lysosomal Enzymes From Polymorphonuclear Leucocytes by Factors Generated During Inflammatory Responses

A number of factors generated during immune-based inflammatory responses may, under certain conditions, induce the selective release of acid hydrolases from polymorphonuclear leucocytes.

1. Immune Complexes

BURKE et al. (1964) described the release of a vascular permeability-inducing factor from polymorphonuclear leucocytes exposed to immune complexes. This factor is almost certainly one of the neutral proteinases now shown to be localized within azurophilic granules (DEWALD et al., 1975). Subsequently, the selective release of lysosomal enzymes from polymorphonuclear leucocytes has been extensively studied (HAWKINS and PEETERS, 1971; HAWKINS, 1971; HENSON, 1971a, b, c; WEISSMANN et al., 1971; HENSON et al., 1972). Rabbit (HAWKINS and PEETERS, 1971; HENSON, 1971a, b, c) or human polymorphonuclear leucocytes (WEISSMANN et al., 1971) exposed to particulate immune complexes of various kinds, release lysosomal acid hydrolases selectively in a time- and dose-dependent manner. This release does not require the presence of complement, but complexes which have been allowed to prefix complement cause an enhanced release of lysosomal enzymes (HENSON, 1971b). This increase occurred with serum deficient in C6 but was prevented by depletion of C3 with cobra venom factor (CVF), indicating a role for C3 or C5. That phagocytosis of immune complexes was not essential for inducing selective release of lysosomal hydrolases was established by studies in which immune complexes were presented to polymorphonuclear leucocytes in an immobilized form on an extracellular matrix (HENSON, 1971a, b, c; HAWKINS, 1971). HENSON applied immune complex to Millipore filters, while HAWKINS embedded antigen in membranes prepared from acid-soluble calf skin collagen. HENSON (1971b) demonstrated that immobilized immune complexes induced selective release of acid hydrolases at lower doses than seen with complexes in a free suspension. On the other hand, HAWKINS (1971) demonstrated lysosomal enzyme release only when cell death, as manifested by release of cellular lactate dehydrogenase, was detected. HAWKINS and PEETERS (1971) found that maximal enzyme release was induced by complexes precipitated at close to antigen-antibody equivalence, whereas soluble complexes made in excess antigen were ineffective in causing enzyme release.

The relative effectiveness of immunoglobulins of different subclasses in causing enzyme release has been examined by HENSON et al. (1972). Aggregated human myeloma immunoglobulins of classes IgG_1 to IgG_4, IgA_1 and IgA_2 caused selective release of lysosomal hydrolases but IgD, IgE, and IgM did not. Soluble aggregates of IgG or IgA were not effective when in solution but did cause enzyme release when adsorbed onto Millipore filters.

The in vitro selective release of lysosomal hydrolases from polymorphonuclear leucocytes exposed to immune complexes immobilized in an extracellular matrix, provides a useful model for the events occurring during a number of acute inflammatory processes involving the deposition of immune complexes (HENSON, 1972). These include the arteritis induced by the deposition of immune complexes in arterial walls (HENSON, 1972) or the nephrotoxic nephritis induced by antibodies to glomerular basement membrane (COCHRANE et al., 1965).

2. Components of the Complement System

Activation of the complement pathway results in the formation of a number of cleavage products with a variety of biological activities (for review see RUDDY et al., 1972). Recent studies have shown that these include the promotion of the fusion of phagosomes with lysosomes in polymorphonuclear leucocytes and, under certain circumstances, the selective release of lysosomal enzymes into the extracellular environment.

GOLDSTEIN et al. (1973a) showed that serum containing complement activated by the alternate pathway, by treatment with either zymosan or CVF, causes the selective release of lysosomal enzymes from cytochalasin B-treated human polymorphonuclear leucocytes in the absence of any particulate stimulus. Further studies showed that the fragment active in inducing enzyme release was C5a (GOLDSTEIN et al., 1973b). More recently, BECKER et al. (1974) have shown that selective release of acid hydrolases can be induced by C3a, C5a, and C567 immobilized on Millipore filters. The release is not as great as that reported by GOLDSTEIN et al. (1973a) but does occur in the absence of cytochalasin B.

IV. Lysis of Polymorphonuclear Leucocytes by Toxic Particles

It has been suggested that the deposition of crystals of monosodium urate is responsible for initiation of the inflammatory episodes seen in acute gout. Polymorphonuclear leucocytes exposed to monosodium urate phagocytose the crystals; this is accompanied by the burst of glucose oxidation which normally accompanies phagocytosis. Subsequently, large amounts of cytoplasmic and lysosomal enzymes are released at the same time (ZURIER et al., 1973b). Ultrastructural studies show that cell death occurs by lysis of the membranes of phagosomes (HOFFSTEIN and WEISSMANN, 1975). This is similar to the well-known effects of silica particles on macrophages (ALLISON et al., 1966).

C. Blood Platelets

Blood platelets can be induced to aggregate and release a variety of mediators by a large number of stimuli (BECKER and HENSON, 1973). Lysosomes were first identified in platelets as corresponding to α-granules by MARCUS et al. (1966). The selective release of these lysosomal enzymes by stimuli such as thrombin (SIEGEL and LUSCHER, 1967; HOLMSEN and DAY, 1968) and collagen (MILLS et al., 1968) has also been described.

NACHMAN and FERRIS (1968) found proteinase activity in platelets over a wide range of pH values, as well as cathepsin A. Fibrinogen was one of the natural substrates for these enzymes, suggesting that they have a physiological role. More recently, LEGRAND et al. (1973) have identified and purified (LEGRAND and PIGNAUD, 1975) both elastase and a trypsin-sensitive pro-elastase from human platelets. If these proteinases reside within granules corresponding to lysosomes as seen in polymorphonuclear leucocytes, their release with other lysosomal enzymes at sites of platelet aggregation and thrombus formation may contribute considerably to the tissue damage occurring at these sites.

D. Macrophages

Macrophages are present at sites of chronic inflammation regardless of whether the inciting stimulus is of immunological or non-immunological origin. We have reviewed in detail elsewhere how macrophages participate in chronic inflammatory responses (ALLISON and DAVIES, 1974) with particular reference to their function as secretory cells (DAVIES and ALLISON, 1976a, b). Since macrophages persist at sites of chronic inflammation for long periods of time, a stimulus eliciting the release of hydrolytic enzymes from these cells would be expected to induce inflammation. This has indeed been shown to be the case with lysosomal hydrolases. Many substances provoking chronic inflammatory responses also induce selective release of acid hydrolases from macrophages maintained in culture (DAVIES and ALLISON, 1976a). On the other hand, a number of inert or readily digestible substances do not cause such release (AXLINE and COHN, 1970; DAVIES et al., 1974a).

Recently, macrophages have been shown to secrete neutral proteinases in response to a number of stimuli, including some of those causing release of acid hydrolases (REICH, 1975). However, some stimuli considered not to be inflammatory also enhance the release of neutral proteinases from macrophages (GORDON et al., 1974a; WERB and GORDON, 1975a, 1975b). The timing and extent of release of acid hydrolase and of neutral proteinase differ markedly, the former being released in large amounts shortly after contact with an appropriate stimulus whilst the latter is usually released after a latent period of at least 24 h but then continues over a very long time.

I. Selective Release of Acid Hydrolases by Macrophages

Macrophages are present in chronic inflammatory lesions of both immunological and non-immunological origin, and it is now clear that non-immunogenic substances provoking chronic inflammatory responses and also certain products of stimulated T- and B-lymphocytes induce the selective release of acid hydrolases from macrophages in vitro (DAVIES and ALLISON, 1976a). This information has been determined in studies with macrophages obtained by peritoneal lavage of mice. These cells can be maintained in tissue culture over long periods as a stable population of non-dividing, surface-adherent cells.

1. The Direct Interaction With Macrophages of Substances Which Cause Chronic Inflammation of a Non-Immunological Nature

a) Group A Streptococcal Cell Walls

The association of Group A streptococci with a number of diseases, including rheumatic fever, is well established (WANNAMAKER and MATSEN, 1972; GINSBURG, 1972). A type-specific C-mucopolysaccharide-peptidoglycan complex (PPG) from Group A streptococcal cell walls causes chronic inflammatory lesions, in which macrophages are the predominant cells, after single injections at various sites (SCHWAB et al., 1959; GINSBURG, 1972; PAGE et al., 1974a). The cell-wall material is extremely resistant to the action of lysosomal enzymes (AYOUB and MCCARTY, 1968) and persists for many months at sites of chronic inflammation. The granulomatous lesion does not appear to have an immunopathological basis but is due to direct effects of PPG on macrophages, as shown with cultures of these cells (DAVIES et al., 1974a; PAGE et al., 1974a). After exposure to PPG, macrophages undergo rapid and marked morphological changes which persist for many days. These include 2- to 4-fold increase in cell size and an increase in the number of lyosomes, as shown by vital staining with acridine orange, and an increase in ruffled membrane activity. These changes are brought about by concentrations of PPG ranging from 1 to 15 µg/ml. Macrophages cultured in the presence of 15–50 µg/ml of PPG show comparable increases in size, but they tend to become more rounded and the cytoplasm exhibits more prominent but fewer vacuoles. These cells show no loss of viability, as determined biochemically by estimations of lactate dehydrogenase levels or morphologically by the capacity to hydrolyse fluorescein dibutyrate (DAVIES et al., 1974a).

The cells showed 2–3-fold increases in protein levels (Fig. 1). There are also considerable changes in the levels and distribution of various cellular enzymes. Exposure to doses of PPG in the range of 1–15 µg/ml for 72 h resulted in marked increases in the cellular levels of non-lysosomal enzymes such as lactate dehydroge-

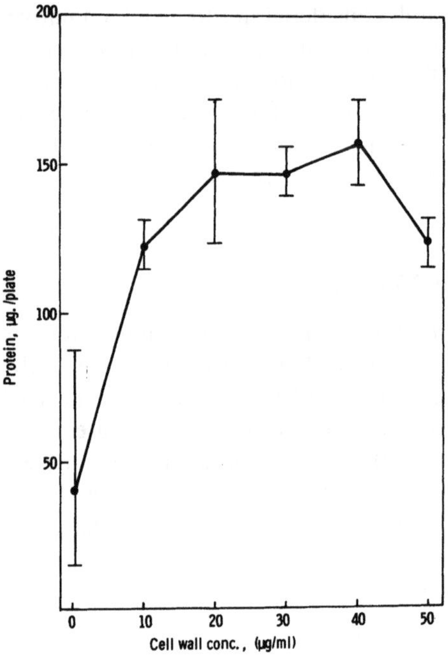

Fig. 1

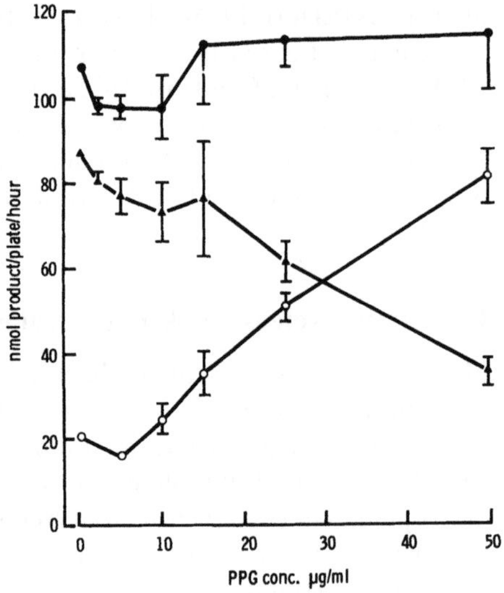

Fig. 2

Fig. 1. Dose-dependent increase in cellular protein levels in cultures of mouse peritoneal macrophages exposed to increasing concentrations of group A streptococcal cell wall for 72 h. (Reprinted with permission from J. exp. Med. **139**, 1262–1282, 1974)

Fig. 2. Dose-dependent selective release of β-glucuronidase from mouse peritoneal macrophages exposed to increasing doses of PPG (2–50 µg/ml) for 24 h. (●—●) shows total activity in culture, (▲—▲) the cellular levels of β-glucuronidase and (○—○) the amount of enzyme released into culture medium. (Reproduced with permission from J. exp. Med. **139**, 1262–1282, 1974)

nase and leucine-2-naphthylamidase. There are also smaller increases in cellular levels of lysosomal enzymes such as β-glucuronidase. At these relatively low concentrations of PPG there is no detectable release of enzymes from the cells into the culture medium. However, addition of PPG to cultures in amounts ranging from 15 to 50 µg/ml induces the release of lysosomal enzymes from viable macrophages in a dose- and time-dependent manner. Figure 2 illustrates the dose-dependent release of β-glucuronidase from macrophages exposed to increasing amounts of PPG for 24 h. The release proceeds rapidly, with much of the enzyme being redistributed within 6 h of exposure to PPG (DAVIES et al., 1974a).

b) Homogenates of Dental Plaque

Dental plaque is a mixed bacterial growth on the sheltered areas of the teeth of humans and experimental animals. It contains numerous micro-organisms of various types. There is substantial evidence that plaque is the primary aetiological agent involved in the pathogenesis of chronic periodontitis. Plaque sterilized by irradiation causes morphological changes very similar to those seen with PPG when added to cultures of macrophages (PAGE et al., 1973). Plaque in doses of 5–50 µg/ml causes a

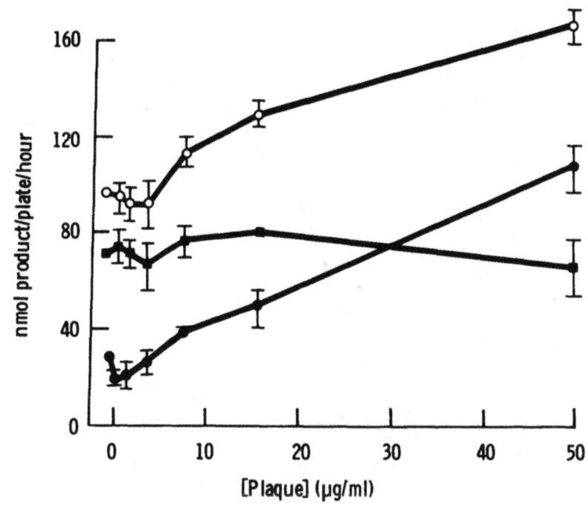

Fig. 3. Levels of β-glucuronidase in the culture medium (●—●) cells (■—■) and in total culture of mouse peritoneal macrophages after 72 h incubation in the presence of various concentrations of dental plaque

rapid and massive redistribution of acid hydrolases from the cells into the culture medium. Although no net increase in acid hydrolase levels is detected in cultures exposed to plaque for 24 h, there are significant increases in the levels of β-glucuronidase in cultures exposed to concentrations of plaque greater than 10 μg/ml for 72 h (PAGE et al., 1973) (Fig. 3). This suggests that the continuous depletion of intracellular lysosomal enzyme serves as a stimulus for the replacement of enzyme released into the culture medium. These changes also occur in the absence of any detectable cell death. The plaque constituents responsible for this effect are not known, although subsequent studies (PAGE et al., 1974b) have shown that sterile homogenates of *Actinomyces viscosus* have a similar effect to that of plaque. *A. viscosus* is a Gram-positive anaerobic filamentous micro-organism which can induce severe chronic inflammatory periodontal disease in mono-infected germ-free rodents. It is also found in high concentrations in human periodontal pockets.

c) Carrageenin

Carrageenin, a mixture of sulphated D-galactose and 3,6-dehydro-D-galactose, induces chronic inflammation in experimental animals such as guinea pigs (ROBERTSON and SCHWARTZ, 1953) and rats (BENITZ and HALL, 1959). Recent experiments in our laboratory indicate that certain preparations of carrageenin also induce intense chronic inflammatory lesions after intramuscular injection in mice (DAVIES et al., 1975). It is also clear that the same preparations of carrageenin induce selective release of acid hydrolases from macrophages in a dose- and time-dependent manner (ALLISON and DAVIES, 1975). Enzyme release is delayed in comparison with the particulate stimuli discussed above, approximately 10 h elapsing before significant amounts of acid hydrolases above control levels are detected in the culture medium. This may be accounted for by the solubility of carrageenin which means that it enters cells by pinocytosis, a process less rapid than phagocytosis.

We have compared three commercially available preparations of carrageenin for their ability to induce chronic inflammation in vivo and selective release of lysoso-

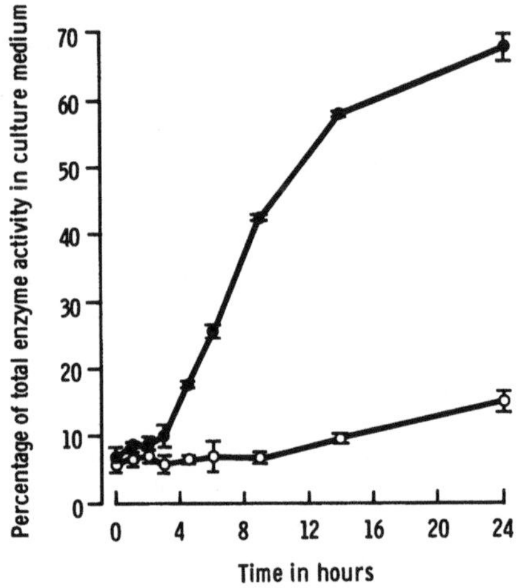

Fig. 4. Time-dependent release of β-galactosidase from mouse peritoneal macrophages exposed to chrysotyle asbestos (50 µg/ml). (●—●) represents percentage of total enzyme activity in medium of asbestos-treated cultures and (○—○) represents enzyme in medium of control cultures not exposed to asbestos. (Reproduced with permission from Nature (Lond.) **251**, 423–425, 1974)

mal enzymes in vitro. Native undegraded carrageenin (Gelcarin HMR, Marine Colloids) produces an intense chronic inflammatory reaction after intramuscular injection as well as inducing the greatest increase in selective release of acid hydrolases. In contrast, the calcium salt of carrageenin (Sigma Chemical Company) has negligible inflammatory activity and lacks the ability to induce selective release of acid hydrolases, while the potassium salt of carrageenin shows intermediate activity in both tests. Structure-activity relationships show that lambda carrageenin, a linear polymer of D-galactose with α-1,3 linkages and sulphated on carbon-4, has the greatest activity. Kappa-carrageenin, containing alternate units of 4-sulphated D-galactose and 3,6-anhydro-D-galactose with α-1,3 and β-1,4 linkages, possesses lower inflammatory activity. The correlation of the inflammatory activity of purified preparations of the various forms of carrageenin with their activity on macrophages should give further information on the relevance of selective release of lysosomal enzymes in chronic inflammation.

d) Inhaled Cytotoxic Particles

The most common route of entry into the body of cytotoxic particles is by inhalation into the lungs. The toxic effects of such particles result in a number of lung diseases known collectively as the pneumoconioses (SPENCER, 1968). Many of the pneumoconioses are characterized by a chronic inflammatory lesion which has an immunological or non-immunological basis depending on the nature of the inhaled material.

It is accepted that the initial event after inhalation of toxic particles is their phagocytosis by macrophages in the pulmonary alveoli (ALLISON, 1968). Failure of the macrophages to digest or remove the particles from the lungs results in a chronic inflammatory process leading to irreversible damage. In vitro studies of the interaction of toxic particles, such as silica and asbestos, with mononuclear phagocytes has demonstrated the cytotoxic effects of these substances (ALLISON et al., 1966; ALLISON, 1971). Although asbestos is less cytotoxic than silica, recent work has shown that small amounts of chrysotile asbestos fibres induce the selective release of lysosomal enzymes from cultured macrophages (DAVIES et al., 1974 b).

As little asbestos as 2 μg/ml causes a significant increase in the selective release of lysosomal enzymes. This release increases in a dose-dependent manner until 80% of the enzyme is found in the culture medium. The enzyme release is also time-dependent, the majority occurring within 12 h (DAVIES et al., 1974 b) (Fig. 4). The release of lysosomal enzymes is accompanied by marked increases in cellular levels of the cytoplasmic enzyme lactate dehydrogenase. Extracellular levels of lactate dehydrogenase do not increase significantly, indicating that the cultures have remained viable. Morphological observations show that the mononuclear phagocytes have phagocytosed most of the asbestos fibres and contain an increased number of vacuoles, which are probably secondary lysosomes. At higher doses of asbestos (25–100 μg/ml) the cells tend to form clusters, but the majority retain the cytoplasmic extensions characteristic of normal mononuclear phagocytes.

Investigations with another type of asbestos, the amphibole crocidolite, shows it to be a less potent stimulus of lysosomal enzyme release than chrysotile asbestos. Two other amphiboles, namely amosite and anthophyllite, show potencies intermediate between that of chrysotile and crocidolite for releasing acid hydrolases from macrophages.

2. The Release of Macrophage Lysosomal Enzymes by Products of Immune Reactions

The products of both T- and B-lymphocytes have many effects on macrophages. Tissue macrophages (BERKEN and BENACERRAFF, 1966) and also human peripheral blood monocytes (HUBER et al., 1968) have Fc receptors for immune complexes containing either IgG or IgM antibodies (for review see SHEVACH et al., 1973). The binding site for immune complexes on human mononuclear phagocytes displays a specificity for the γ_1 and γ_3 subclasses of human IgG (HUBER and WAGNER, 1974). The endocytosis of immune complexes by macrophages has been studied by STEINMAN and COHN (1972) who reported that aggregates of horseradish peroxidase and the corresponding antibody were taken up into and degraded within secondary lysosomes of mouse peritoneal macrophages.

a) The Release of Acid Hydrolases From Macrophages Exposed to Immune Complexes

Immune complexes are deposited at sites of chronic inflammation in several common diseases, including rheumatoid arthritis and certain types of glomerulonephritis. The intradermal injection into rats of immune complexes formed at equivalence results in a chronic inflammatory lesion characterized by many macrophages containing residual immune complexes (SPECTOR and HEESOM, 1969). As we have already discussed, there is considerable evidence showing that immune complexes interact with polymorphonuclear leucocytes in vitro to cause selective release of acid hydrolases. However, until recently there has been no information concerning this process in macrophages exposed to immune complexes. We have studied the interaction of immune complexes with mouse peritoneal macrophages and found that small

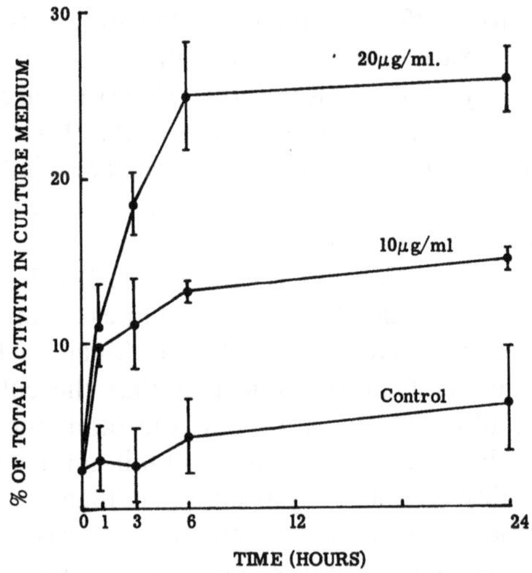

Fig. 5. Time- and dose-dependent release of β-glucuronidase from mouse peritoneal macrophages exposed to increasing concentrations of rabbit antibovine serum albumin antigen-antibody complexes over a 24 h time period. (Reproduced with permission from Nature (Lond.) **247**, 46–48, 1974

amounts of complexes formed at equivalence induce selective release of various acid hydrolases (CARDELLA et al., 1974). The release increases with time of exposure to complexes over a period of at least 24 h and is dependent upon the dose of immune complex (Fig. 5). Selective release of lysosomal hydrolases is not seen in cells exposed to antigen or antiserum. Cultures exposed to immune complexes for 24 h show elevated levels of acid hydrolases compared with control values. This may be due to a cellular response to a digestible substrate (see AXLINE and COHN, 1970) or result from the depletion of the cellular pool of lysosomal enzymes.

b) The Selective Release of Acid Hydrolases From Macrophages Exposed to the Products of Stimulated T-Lymphocytes

The exposure of T-lymphocytes to specific antigens or non-specific mitogens results in the release of several biologically active macromolecules (DAVID and DAVID, 1972), a number of which influence macrophage function (see ALLISON and DAVIES, 1974). PANTALONE and PAGE (1975) have incubated mouse peritoneal macrophages with culture media from human peripheral blood leucocytes incubated with phytohaemagglutinin for 72 h. The macrophages show elevated levels of both lysosomal and non-lysosomal enzymes, and selective release of acid hydrolases was observed without any detectable loss of cell viability. Macrophages incubated with supernatants from unstimulated cells or with phytohaemagglutinin alone for a 48-h time period showed no significant changes in their levels of lysosomal hydrolases, nor in the release of these enzymes into the culture medium compared with control cultures. Maximal stimulation of enzyme release, amounting to between 70 and 80% of the total in the culture for β-glucuronidase (Fig. 6) and N-acetyl-β-D-glucosaminidase, occurred with the supernatant obtained from approximately 0.5×10^6 lymphoid cells added to between 2 and 4×10^6 macrophages. It is not clear whether the

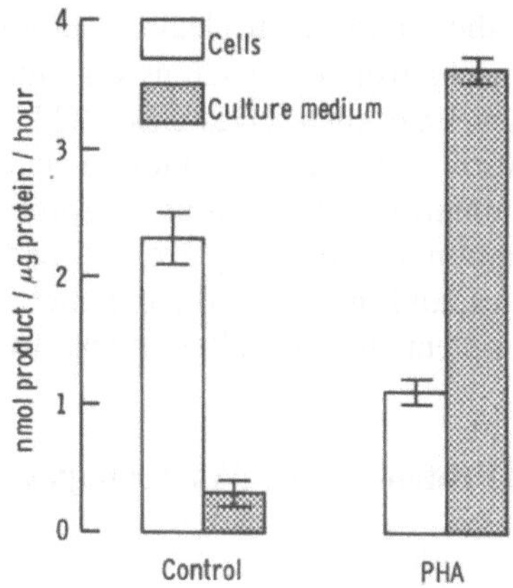

Fig. 6. Selective release of β-glucuronidase from mouse peritoneal macrophages exposed for 48 h to supernatants from human peripheral blood lymphocytes cultured in the presence and absence of phytohaemagglutinin (*PHA*) for 72 h. (Reproduced with permission from Pantalone, R. M., Page, R. C., Proc. nat. Acad. Sci. (Wash.) **72**, 2091—2094, 1975)

selective release of lysosomal enzyme described above is caused by factors of the type described by RUDDLE and WAKSMAN (1968), GRANGER and WILLIAMS (1968) and DAVID and DAVID (1972), or by previously undescribed factors. Macrophages are resistant to the cytotoxic effects of lymphotoxin (DAVID and DAVID, 1972) although this does not exclude the possibility that lymphotoxins may cause selective release of lysosomal enzymes. This in vitro phenomenon may form the basis of tissue damage seen in delayed hypersensitivity, where factors released from T-lymphocytes lead to the recruitment of macrophages into the site of inflammation and their immobilization there, with subsequent release of acid hydrolases.

c) Role of Complement in the Release of Lysosomal Enzymes by Macrophages

In looking for a common factor in the variety of agents that induce chronic inflammation in vivo and hydrolase secretion from macrophages in culture, our attention has been drawn to the fact that they all activate complement by the alternative pathway. This is true of carrageenins and dextran sulphates (BURGER et al., 1975), zymosan and mouldy hay dust containing *Micropolysporum faeni* (EDWARDS, personal communication) and streptococcal cell walls (BITTER-SUERMAN, personal communication).

An early event in such activation is the cleavage of the complement component C3 to a smaller fragment C3a and a larger fragment C3b. The highly purified C3a component, when incubated with mouse peritoneal macrophages in culture, was found to release both lysosomal hydrolases and lactate dehydrogenase, thus indicating cell death (SCHORLEMMER et al., 1976). In contrast, when highly purified C3b was incubated with the macrophages, selective, dose- and time-dependent release of several glycosidases, but not of lactate dehydrogenase, was observed. Similar results have been obtained with guinea pig peritoneal macrophages using highly purified guinea pig C3a and C3b (SCHORLEMMER and ALLISON, 1976). Supernatants from macrophages stimulated by asbestos, but not unstimulated macrophages, are also able to cleave C3. Thus, the complement cleavage product C3b appears to be a common and important mechanism for switching on hydrolase secretion by macrophages. The secreted enzymes can themselves cleave C3, thereby generating further C3b, so that an amplification system is set in motion. This may well play an important role in chronic inflammation. The various substances that induce chronic inflammation have two common features: they are not readily biodegradable, so that they persist in macrophages; and they have the polymeric acidic structural requirements for activation of complement by the alternate pathway.

II. Secretion of Neutral Proteinases by Macrophages

1. Collagenase

The presence of this enzyme at sites of both acute and chronic inflammation has been reported. It is likely that collagenase found at sites of acute inflammation is derived from polymorphonuclear leucocytes, which have been shown to contain the enzyme (LAZARUS, 1973). However, collagen breakdown is most evident during chronic inflammation, when relatively few polymorphonuclear leucocytes are present. Although these lesions usually contain many macrophages, it was not until very recently that the presence of collagenase within these cells was demonstrated. Reports by SENIOR et al. (1972) and ROBERTSON et al. (1973) demonstrated the presence of this enzyme in alveolar macrophages. WAHL et al. (1974) showed the production and secretion of significant amounts of collagenase by macrophages maintained in tissue culture. These workers have shown that guinea pig peritoneal exudate macrophages exposed to bacterial lipopolysaccharide in culture, produce considerable amounts of collagenase over a period of several days. It is clear that the enzyme was newly synthesized by the macrophages, since its appearance in the culture medium was inhibited by cycloheximide. It is also notable that no collagenase activity was detected in freshly isolated cells after detergent lysis or freeze thawing. The appearance of the collagenase was delayed for at least 24 h after the addition of the lipopolysaccharide. Control cultures not exposed to lipopolysaccharide did not show any detectable collagenase activity during 5 days of culture. It was found that the lipid A fraction was the most active of the lipopolysaccharide components in inducing synthesis and release of collagenase.

The glycolipid portion was less active than the lipid A, while the lipid-free polysaccharide fraction induced only low levels of collagenase production and secretion. The macrophage collagenase resembles other collagenases in many respects. It is inhibited by serum and EDTA and was found to cleave native collagen molecules into $^3/_4$ and $^1/_4$ portions. It is not known whether stimulated macrophages synthesize collagenase as such or in the form of pro-enzyme, as reported in other tissues. WAHL et al. (1975) found that sensitized lymphocytes treated with specific antigen or with concanavallin A release a factor or factors that stimulate macrophages to produce collagenase. Maximal collagenase secretion was detected after exposure of macrophages to supernatants of stimulated lymphocytes for 48 h and continued for at least 3 days afterwards.

WERB and GORDON (1975a) have reported that peritoneal macrophages obtained from mice, to which an intraperitoneal injection of thioglycollate broth had been administered 4 days previously, secrete considerable amounts of collagenase over a period of at least 7 days. On the other hand, macrophages from unstimulated mice secreted only barely detectable amounts of enzyme. These cells did, however, secrete some collagenase after the ingestion of latex particles or dextran sulphate, although in considerably smaller amounts than were obtained from cells taken from thioglycollate stimulated animals. The failure of unstimulated macrophages to secrete the enzyme was not due to the simultaneous production of inhibitors of collagenase by these cells.

The enzyme was identical to other collagenases in terms of its specific cleavage products and sensitivity to inhibitors, including α_2-macroglobulin. Collagenase production was abolished by treatment of the macrophages with cycloheximide.

Collagenase production by macrophages did not, however, approach the amount shown to be secreted by fibroblast-like cells obtained from rabbit synovial tissue (Werb and Reynolds, 1974). Macrophages from thioglycollate stimulated mice produced 0.11 unit collagenase/day/mg cell protein while rabbit synovial cells produced 1.8 units enzyme/day/mg cell protein. Harris et al. (1975) have reported that the secretion of collagenase by rabbit synovial fibroblasts can be increased as much as 100-fold by treatment with cytochalasin B.

2. Elastase

Werb and Gordon (1975b) have described the secretion of elastase by peritoneal macrophages stimulated by thioglycollate. Janoff et al. (1971) had previously described such an enzyme in lysates of alveolar macrophages. Werb and Gordon (1975b) showed elastase secretion by macrophages to be time-dependent, continuing for at least 12 days, and to be sensitive to inhibitors of protein synthesis. As with collagenase, macrophages from unstimulated mice secreted very little elastase; such cells did, however, secrete some enzyme after phagocytosis of latex beads. The enzyme secreted by macrophages was found to differ significantly from enzymes with elastinolytic activity purified from pancreas and polymorphonuclear leucocytes. The macrophage elastase is more restricted in its substrate specificity, not showing any activity towards synthetic substrates such as N-acetyl-L-alanyl-L-alanyl-L-alanine-*p*-nitroanilide or benzyloxycarbonyl-L-alanine-2-naphthol ester. It is also resistant to inhibitors of other elastases, such as the active site-directed alanyl chloromethyl ketones and turkey ovomucoid. The enzyme shows marked affinity for elastin complexed to sodium dodecyl sulphate; the cationic nature of the enzyme makes such a complex a suitable substrate.

3. Plasminogen Activator

Unkeless et al. (1974) and Gordon et al. (1974a) have shown that macrophages which have been stimulated in certain ways will secrete large amounts of plasminogen activator. It was found that mouse macrophages obtained after intraperitoneal injection of thioglycollate broth secrete large amounts of plasminogen activator when cultured. In contrast, macrophages from unstimulated mice do not synthesize or secrete this enzyme. In vivo stimulation with agents such as endotoxin, calf serum, BCG or mineral oil, induces the in vitro secretion of much smaller amounts of plasminogen activator than does thioglycollate. However, if cells stimulated in vivo by these agents are exposed to phagocytic stimuli in vitro, such as latex beads, their secretion of plasminogen activator is greatly enhanced. Other phagocytic stimuli besides latex beads induce secretion of plasminogen activator from stimulated macrophages in vitro, although non-digestible materials are more efficient in this respect than digestible substrates such as *Micrococcus lysodeikticus*, heat aggregated gammaglobulin or peroxidase-antiperoxidase immune complexes. The production and secretion of plasminogen activator by stimulated macrophages continues for periods of up to 9 days, as was observed when latex particles were added to cultures obtained from mice injected intraperitoneally with endotoxin.

III. Secretion of Lysozyme by Macrophages

Lysozyme is a low molecular weight cationic protein, which hydrolyses N-acetyl muramic β-1,4 N-acetyl glucosamine linkages in bacterial cell walls. High concentrations of lysozyme are found in both polymorphonuclear leucocytes and in rabbit alveolar macrophages. In the polymorphonuclear leucocyte the enzyme is largely particulate, being found in both azurophilic and specific granules of this cell. The early studies of COHN and WIENER (1963) showed that BGC-induced rabbit alveolar macrophages released a large fraction of their intracellular lysozyme during phagocytosis. Large amounts of this enzyme accumulate in both the serum and urine of humans and experimental animals suffering from monocytic leukemia. Recent studies by GORDON et al. (1974b) have shown that mouse peritoneal macrophages and also human peripheral blood monocytes synthesize and secrete substantial amounts of lysozyme in vitro. This enzyme is a major secretory product of both macrophages and monocytes since its daily production represents 0.5–2.5% of the total cell protein (GORDON et al., 1974b). The enzyme is secreted under a wide variety of conditions, is not drastically changed by the presence or absence of serum in the culture medium, and is not stimulated either by phagocytosis or the introduction of its substrate *M. lysodeikticus*. Secretion in vitro begins after a latent period but then continues for up to 17 days. Macrophages secrete the equivalent of their cellular pool of lysozyme within a period of between 5 and 8 h, and this secretion can be almost completely abolished in the presence of an inhibitor of protein synthesis such as cycloheximide. The secretion of lysozyme seems to be restricted to macrophages since other cell types, such as epithelioid cell lines, fibroblasts and lymphocytes, do not secrete lysozyme. Although polymorphonuclear leucocytes release their intracellular store of lysozyme when cultured, there is no evidence of synthesis of new enzyme by these cells.

E. Secretion of Lysosomal Enzymes by Cells of Soft Connective Tissue

Under certain conditions, the exposure of differentiated connective tissues to complement-sufficient antiserum results in the degradation of the extracellular matrix accompanied by proliferation of cells and secretion of large quantities of lysosomal hydrolases. Such responses correspond to type II allergic reactions in the classification of COOMBS and GELL (1968), where antibody and complement react with antigenic components of basement membranes or cells. They are exceptional, however, in that cells are stimulated rather than lysed by the action of complement.

COOMBS and FELL (1969) have summarized studies showing extensive loss of metachromatic material from the matrix of limb bone explants leading to their disintegration on exposure to complement-sufficient antisera. Cell death was detectable only in areas in immediate contact with antiserum; osteoclasts and chondrocytes remained viable but had lost their characteristic morphology, becoming transformed into fibroblast-like cells which showed active mitosis. Removal of the antiserum led to the reversal of these changes.

Biochemical assessment of these cultures showed a depression of growth, as measured by dry weight and DNA content. However, after addition of complement-sufficient antiserum, more lysosomal enzyme was released into the culture medium in treated cultures, and total enzyme activity in the limb and culture medium was increased. The release of lysosomal acid proteinase was selective since the total level and release of a non-lysosomal enzyme, lactate dehydrogenase, was unchanged compared with control cultures.

The use of specific antisera has provided strong supporting evidence for the role of secreted lysosomal enzymes in the degradation of cartilage. POOLE et al. (1974) have demonstrated extracellular cathepsin D by immuno-histochemical methods in chicken and rabbit cell cultures. Enzyme was detectable in normal tissue and to a much greater extent in tissues exposed to supraphysiological doses of retinol. That enzyme released in this way causes tissue degradation, is suggested by observations that both pepstatin (DINGLE et al., 1972) and a specific inhibitor of cathepsin D (DINGLE et al., 1971) inhibit the autolytic degradation of cartilage.

LACHMANN et al. (1969) provided further evidence that the changes were induced by antibody and complement by fractionating antisera. Both IgG and IgM were effective in inducing the morphological changes described above. The possibility that the heat-labile factor in the antisera was complement was supported by several lines of evidence. Complement-depleting agents such as antigen-antibody aggregates, zymosan and CVF reduced the effectiveness of the antisera. The addition of purified IgG or IgM fractions of antisera to cultures in the presence of fresh serum from rabbits deficient in C6, failed to induce the morphological changes seen in cultures exposed to immunoglobulins and fresh rabbit serum.

This activity of the complement system can be added to its well-recognized functions of causing membrane lysis and opsonisation of foreign particles or damaged cells. Its target in the limb bone rudiment was not identified, but immunofluorescence studies showed that in unaffected rudiments, complement and antibody were restricted to the perichondrium while in moderately affected rudiments only limited penetration was seen. In severely affected rudiments, penetration throughout the rudiments was demonstrable but chondrocytes were not lysed. The possibility that the action of the complement-sufficient antiserum on the peripheral areas of the explant leads to the release of humoral factors—possibly lysosomal enzymes—which diffused into and damaged the cartilage, was considered unlikely but not discounted. There was no evidence that a product of the complement system activated by zymosan was able to reproduce the damage caused by complement-sufficient antiserum.

Recently, further information on the nature of the cells involved in the reaction of cartilaginous tissue to complement-sufficient antiserum, has been provided by Dame Honor Fell and her colleagues. They examined the reaction of four types of cartilage explants from the distal ends of the 3rd and 4th metacarpals of bacon pigs to complement-sufficient mixed rabbit antiserum against washed pig erythrocytes of groups A and O (FELL and BARRATT, 1973). The explants, all cut parallel to the articular surface, were (a) slices cut above the invasion zone of bone marrow into the cartilage, (b) slices including portions of the invasion zone, (c) slices containing the fibrous cartilage located at the junction of the cartilage with the periosteum, (d) explants of cartilage without invasion zone grown in close contact with pieces of joint capsule (affronted explants). At the same time, the penetration of the immunoglobulin of the rabbit antiserum into the explant was studied by the use of fluorescein-labelled pig anti-rabbit IgG (POOLE et al., 1973).

Cartilage slices of type (a) lacking any invasion zone were found to be unreactive to antiserum and complement for periods of up to 10 days, and immunoglobulin was only detected in a very narrow zone of flattened cells at the articular surface of the cartilage. However, cartilage explants of type (b), (c), or (d) showed dramatic changes on exposure to complement-sufficient antiserum. In explants containing marrow invasion channels, exposure to media containing control (sera consisting of heat-inactivated normal rabbit serum, antiserum without complement or heat-inactivated normal rabbit serum + complement) resulted in some loss of metachromasia from a narrow zone of cartilage matrix bordering the invading marrow; similar explants exposed to complement-sufficient antiserum showed much more extensive loss of cartilage metachromasia, which was most pronounced in explants containing large amounts of invading marrow. In addition, the antiserum killed most of the cells in the marrow channels, but the chondrocytes remained alive and were seen to proliferate except in the immediate vicinity of the invasion zones. In these explants, rabbit immunoglobulin also penetrated into the depleted matrix and reacted with the surface of the chondrocytes and also with extracellular material.

In explants of fibrous cartilage of type (c), complement-sufficient antiserum caused only slight loss of metachromasia in the cartilage, the remainder of the cartilage in the explant remaining strongly metachromatic. It was notable in those explants were fibrous cartilage covered only part of the articular surface, that loss of metachromasia was confined to these zones. Once again, immunoglobulin was readily detectable in those areas where metachromasia had been lost.

When explants of either condylar or fibrous cartilage were cultured in close contact with joint capsule (type d), extensive loss of metachromasia occurred in the areas of contact of the cartilage with the joint capsule in the presence of complement-sufficient antiserum. There was some necrosis of the cartilage but the surviving chondrocytes were actively dividing. The capsular tissue showed no significant change in appearance. The binding of IgG antibody by the cells of the joint capsule was found to vary. In the synovial intima the more deeply lying cells stained more intensely than those at the surface and the authors suggest that they may represent the B-type synovial cell described originally by BARLAND et al. (1962). Another cell type, scattered in the tissue near the edges of the villi, stained more brilliantly for the fluorescein-labelled IgG antibody than any other kind of cell. These findings are analogous to those of BARRATT (1972) who showed a similar requirement for soft connective tissue for the degradation of cartilage induced by retinol.

The nature of the cell or cells in the soft connective tissues associated with the pig metacarpal cartilage, which reacted with the complement-sufficient antiserum to cause cartilage degradation, remains unknown. POOLE et al. (1973) conclude that the most likely mechanism of cartilage degradation is enzymic; possibly acid hydrolytic enzymes are released from target cells in soft connective tissue by interaction with immune complexes formed in the presence of complement-sufficient antiserum. In view of the findings of CARDELLA et al. (1974) that immune complexes induce selective release of acid hydrolases from mouse peritoneal mononuclear phagocytes, a similar response by phagocytic cells in soft connective tissue to complement-sufficient antiserum would lead to degradation of associated cartilage. If this were the case, osteoclasts of the invading marrow and tissue macrophages or phagocytic A cells of the capsular tissue would be possible sources of acid hydrolases released after exposure to complement-sufficient antiserum. A possible contribution of cartilage degradation by chondrocytes cannot be excluded, but POOLE et al. (1973) found that in cartilage explants devoid of soft connective tissue, the chondrocytes of the articular surface reacted quite strongly with IgG antibody without being able to deplete the underlying metachromatic matrix. MILLROY and POOLE (1974) have provided further evidence that chondrocytes are not the targets for the action of complement-sufficient antiserum for the release of cartilage-degrading mediators. Matrix depletion by trypsin treatment of slices of pig articular cartilage allowed the penetration of IgG during subsequent incubation in complement-sufficient antiserum. Although IgG was shown to react with chondrocytes, many of these cells underwent mitosis and formed pericellular capsules of new matrix which excluded antibody. There was no evidence that the chondrocytes produced mediators which caused matrix breakdown similar to that seen when soft connective tissue was exposed to complement-sufficient antiserum.

The deposition of immune complexes in cartilage may have relevance to the pathology of rheumatoid arthritis since a similar deposition of immune complexes has been observed in both experimental antigen-induced arthritis (COOKE et al., 1972) and in articular cartilage of patients with rheumatoid arthritis, but not in normal cartilage (ISHIKAWA et al., 1975). The interaction of such complexes with chondrocytes, or more likely with mononuclear phagocytes from invading pannus, could result in the release of hydrolytic enzymes with the subsequent damage and destruction of cartilage that is characteristic of this disease.

F. Effect of Released Enzymes on Macromolecular Natural Substrates

I. Degradation of Connective Tissue Components

The capacity of lysosomal enzymes to degrade natural substrates has been amply documented (BARRETT, 1969; ARONSON and DEDUVE, 1968; COFFEY and DEDUVE, 1968; FOWLER and DEDUVE, 1969). Studies with specific antisera to cathepsin D have demonstrated the activity of secreted enzyme (DINGLE et al., 1971) in organ culture and of intralysosomal cathepsin D (DINGLE et al., 1973) in cultured macrophages. ORONSKY et al. (1973) have shown that the release of polymorphonuclear leucocyte neutral proteinase induced by aggregated gammaglobulin entrapped in cartilage, leads to the degradation of the proteoglycan matrix as indicated by release of a preincorporated $^{35}SO_4$ label.

The activities of collagenase, elastase and plasminogen activator on their respective natural substrates has been extensively discussed elsewhere (LAZARUS, 1973; JANOFF et al., 1975; REICH, 1975) and the reader is referred to these reviews for further information. Elastase is active against a wide range of connective tissue substrates besides elastin, including cartilage proteoglycan (JANOFF, 1972). Similarly, plasmin generated by the activity of plasminogen activator is active against a variety of natural substrates.

II. Generation of Inflammatory Mediators by Hydrolytic Enzymes

The activation of the clotting, kinin, complement and fibrinolytic systems are all features of the inflammatory process. In each case, proteinases play an important part in the activation process (DAVIES et al., 1975; GREENBAUM, 1975; MÜLLER-EBERHARD, 1975; REICH, 1975). Consequently, proteinases secreted by phagocytic cells at sites of inflammation may initiate the activity of one or more of the cascade systems mentioned above.

CHANG et al. (1972) have shown that an acid proteinase from polymorphonuclear leucocytes or macrophages, probably cathepsin D, can generate polypeptides with kinin activity from plasma leucokininogen.

The cleavage of C3 and C5 by plasmin or lysosomal enzymes (SNYDERMAN et al., 1972; GOLDSTEIN and WEISSMANN, 1974; WARD and HILL, 1970) results in the formation of cleavage products with chemotactic, anaphylotoxic and lysosomal enzyme mobilizing activity.

It is also notable that lysosomal enzymes are able to degrade certain inflammatory mediators. For example, aryl sulphatase from eosinophils degrades SRS-A released by mast cells at sites of inflammation (WASSERMAN et al., 1975).

G. The Effects of Drugs on the Release of Hydrolytic Enzymes at Sites of Inflammation

Many studies have shown that anti-inflammatory drugs affect the stability of isolated lysosomes (WEISSMANN, 1969; IGNARRO, 1971), but their relevance to the secretion of hydrolytic enzymes by intact cells is not clear.

I. Steroid Anti-Inflammatory Drugs

Steroid anti-inflammatory drugs interfere with the secretion of hydrolytic enzymes in several situations. DINGLE et al. (1967) showed that hydrocortisone (0.1 μg/ml) inhibited the secretion of lysosomal enzymes induced by complement-sufficient antiserum from embryonic limb bones maintained in organ culture.

Recently, RINGROSE et al. (1975) have shown that steroid anti-inflammatory drugs, such as dexamethasone, prednisolone and hydrocortisone, inhibit the selective release of acid hydrolases from macrophages caused by the phagocytosis of zymosan particles. The response showed a biphasic concentration-dependence, the maximum inhibitory effect being seen at between 3×10^{-6} M and 3×10^{-7} M.

It is clear that glucocorticoids can interfere with the interaction of lymphocyte activation products with macrophages (LOCKSHIN, 1972; WESTON et al., 1972; BALOW and ROSENTHAL, 1973). It will be of interest to determine whether glucocorticoids also inhibit the secretion of lysosomal enzymes (PANTALONE and PAGE, 1975) and collagenase (WAHL et al., 1975) induced by these products.

KOOB et al. (1974) have shown that low doses of hydrocortisone and dexamethasone (maximal effects seen at doses of 10^{-7} M and 10^{-8} M, respectively) prevent the secretion of collagenase in cultures of normal human skin, rheumatoid synovium and rat uterus. This inhibition is not accompanied by a detectable decrease in protein synthesis, although cessation of tissue collagen degradation is seen. It will be of great interest to determine whether steroids inhibit the secretion of collagenase by other cells such as macrophages. REICH (1975) and his colleagues have shown that small amounts of dexamethasone, prednisolone and hydrocortisone inhibit the secretion of plasminogen activator by macrophages at doses of 10^{-7} M to 10^{-9} M; this inhibition is reversible on withdrawal of the drug.

II. Nonsteroid Anti-Inflammatory Drugs

There are conflicting reports on the effects of nonsteroid anti-inflammatory drugs on the release of acid hydrolases by polymorphonuclear leucocytes exposed to phagocytic stimuli or to a surface containing an immobilized phagocytic stimulus. WRIGHT and MALAWISTA (1973) have reported that colchicine, but not acetylsalicylic acid and sodium salicylate, inhibits the release of lysosomal enzymes from human polymorphonuclear leucocytes induced by the phagocytosis of heat-killed staphylococci. PERPER and ORONSKY (1974) found that a number of anti-inflammatory drugs, including acetylsalicylic acid, phenylbutazone, indomethacin and hydrocortisone, inhibit the release of a cartilage-degrading neutral proteinase and β-glucuronidase from human polymorphonuclear leucocytes exposed to cartilage discs opsonised with heat-aggregated IgG.

RINGROSE et al. (1975) have reported that indomethacin has a slight inhibitory effect on the release of acid hydrolases from macrophages which had phagocytozed zymosan. Studies in our laboratories (FINLAY et al., 1975) have shown that indomethacin inhibits the release of lysosomal enzymes from macrophages exposed to PPG from Group A streptococcal cell walls. Indomethacin also increases the cellular levels of several lysosomal enzymes at doses as low as 5×10^{-8} M, maximal effects being seen at 1×10^{-6} M to 1×10^{-5} M. Despite the elevations in their cellular levels of acid hydrolases, macrophage cultures pretreated with 1×10^{-5} M indomethacin release lower amounts of these enzymes than do control cultures when exposed to PPG.

It is now clear that cells participating in both acute and chronic inflammatory responses release hydrolytic enzymes when confronted with a wide variety of inflammatory stimuli. In many instances, these enzymes are released by a secretory process indicating a specific response of the lysosomal or other intracellular vacuolar systems such as those releasing neutral proteinases or lysozyme. There are indications that these secretory processes can be interfered with by pharmacologial agents with well-established anti-inflammatory properties. Future studies with such agents should assist in the determination of the cellular mechanisms which mediate the release of the various classes of hydrolytic enzymes from cells at sites of inflammation.

References

Allison, A. C.: Lysosomes and the response of cells to toxic materials. Sci. Basis Med. 18—30 (1968)

Allison, A. C.: Lysosomes and the toxicity of particulate pollutants. Arch. intern. Med. **128**, 131—139 (1971)

Allison, A. C., Davies, P.: Mechanisms underlying chronic inflammation. In: Velo, G. P., Willoughby, D. A., Giroud, J. P. (Eds.): Future Trends in Inflammation, pp. 449—480. Padua-London: Piccin Medical Books 1974

Allison, A. C., Davies, P.: Increased biochemical and biological activities of mononuclear phagocytes exposed to various stimuli with special reference to lysosomal enzymes. In: Furth, R. (Ed.): Mononuclear Phagocytes in Immunity, Infection and Pathology, pp. 487—506. Oxford: Blackwell 1975

Allison, A. C., Davies, P., De Petris, S.: Role of contractile microfilaments in macrophage movement and endocytosis. Nature (New Biol.) **232**, 153—155 (1971)

Allison, A. C., Harington, J. C., Birbeck, M.: An examination of the cytotoxic effects of silica on macrophages. J. exp. Med. **124**, 141—153 (1966)

Aronson, Jr. N. N., De Duve, C.: Digestive activity of lysosomes. II. The digestion of macromolecular carbohydrates by extracts of rat liver lysosomes. J. biol. Chem. **243**, 4564—4573 (1968)

Axline, S. G., Cohn, Z. A.: In vitro induction of lysosomal enzymes by phagocytosis. J. exp. Med. **131**, 1239—1260 (1970)

Axline, S. G., Reaven, E. P.: Inhibition of phagocytosis and plasma membrane. Mobility of the cultivated macrophage by cytochalasin B. Role of subplasmalemmal microfilaments. J. Cell Biol. **64**, 647—659 (1974)

Ayoub, E. M., McCarty, M.: Intraphagocytic β-N-acetyl glucosaminidase: properties of the enzyme and its activity on Group A streptococcal carbohydrate in comparison with a soil bacillus enzyme. J. exp. Med. **127**, 833—851 (1968)

Baggiolini, M., Hirsch, J. G., De Duve, C.: Resolution of granules from rabbit heterophil leucocytes into distinct population by zonal sedimentation. J. Cell Biol. **40**, 529—549 (1969)

Balow, J. E., Rosenthal, A. S.: Glucocorticoid suppression of macrophage migration inhibition factor. J. exp. Med. **137**, 1031—1041 (1973)

Barbanti-Brodano, G., Fiume, L.: Selective killing of macrophages by amanitin-albumin conjugates. Nature (New Biol.) **243**, 281—283 (1973)

Barland, P., Novikoff, A. B., Hameran, D.: Electron microscopy of the human synovial membrane. J. Cell Biol. **14**, 207—220 (1962)

Barratt, M. E. J.: The role of soft connective tissue in the response of pig articular cartilage in organ culture to excess of retinol. J. Cell Sci. **13**, 205—219 (1972)

Barrett, A. J.: Properties of lysosomal enzymes. In: Dingle, J. T., Fell, H. B. (Eds.): Lysosomes in Biology and Pathology, Vol. 2, pp. 245—312. London-Amsterdam: North Holland 1969

Becker, E. L., Henson, P. M.: In vitro studies of immunologically induced secretion of mediators from cells and related phenomena. Advanc. Immunol. **17**, 93—193 (1973)

Becker, E. L., Showell, H. J., Henson, P. M., Hsu, L. S.: The ability of chemotactic factors to induce lysosomal enzyme release. I. The characteristics of release, the importance of surfaces and the relation of enzyme release to chemotactic responsiveness. J. Immunol. **112**, 2047—2054 (1974)

Benitz, K. F., Hall, L. M.: Local morphological response following a single subcutaneous injection of carrageenan in the rat. Proc. Soc. exp. Biol. (N.Y.) **102**, 442—445 (1959)

Berken, B., Benaceraff, B.: Properties of antibodies cytophilic for macrophages macrophages. J. exp. Med. **123**, 119—144 (1966)

Bretz,U., Baggiolini,M.: Association of the alkaline phosphatase of rabbit polymorphonuclear leucocytes with the membrane of the specific granules. J. Cell Biol. **59**, 696—707 (1973)

Bretz,U., Baggiolini,M.: Biochemical and morphological characterization of azurophil and specific granules of human neutrophilic polymorphonuclear leucocytes. J. Cell Biol. **63**, 251—269 (1974)

Burger,R., Hadding,U., Schorlemmer,H.U., Brade,V., Bitter-Suerman,D.: Dextran sulphate: a synthetic activator of C3 via the alternative pathway. I. Influence of molecular size and degree of sulphation on the activation potency. Immunology **29**, 549—554 (1975)

Burke,J.S., Urihara,T.S., Macmorine,D.R.L., Movat,H.Z.: A permeability factor released from phagocytosing PMN leucocytes and its inhibition by protease inhibitors. Life Sci. **3**, 1505—1512 (1964)

Cardella,C.J., Davies,P., Allison,A.C.: Immune complexes induce selective release of lysosomal hydrolases from macrophages in vitro. Nature (Lond.) **247**, 46—48 (1974)

Carter,S.D.: Effects of cytochalasins on mammalian cells. Nature (Lond.) **213**, 261—264 (1967)

Chang,J., Freer,R., Stella,R., Greenbaum,L.M.: Studies on leucokinins. II. Studies on the formation, partial amino acid sequence and chemical properties of leucokinins M and PMN. Biochem. Pharmacol. **21**, 3095—3106 (1972)

Cochrane,C.G., Unanue,E.R., Dixon,F.J.: A role of polymorphonuclear leucocytes and complement in nephrotoxic nephritis. J. exp. Med. **122**, 99—116 (1965)

Coffey,J.W., DeDuve,C.: Digestive activity of lysosomes. I. The digestion of proteins by extracts of rat liver lysosomes. J. biol. Chem. **243**, 3255—3263 (1968)

Cohn,Z.A., Wiener,E.: The particulate hydrolases of macrophages. II. Biochemical and morphological response to particulate ingestion. J. exp. Med. **118**, 1009—1018 (1963)

Cooke,T.D., Hurd,E.R., Ziff,M., Jasin,H.E.: The pathogenesis of chronic inflammation in experimental antigen-induced arthritis. II. Preferential localization of antigen-antibody complexes to collagenous tissues. J. exp. Med. **135**, 323—338 (1972)

Coombs,R.R.A., Fell,H.B.: Lysosomes in tissue damage mediated by allergic reactions. In: Dingle,J.T., Fell,H.B. (Eds.): Lysosomes in Biology and Pathology, pp. 3—18. London-Amsterdam: North Holland 1969

Coombs,R.R.A., Gell,P.G.H.: Clinical aspects of immunology, 2nd Ed., pp. 575—596. Oxford: Blackwell 1968

Crowder,J.C., Martin,R.R., White,A.: Release of histamine and lysosomal enzymes by human leucocytes during phagocytosis of staphylococci. J. Lab. clin. Med. **74**, 436—444 (1969)

Davey,M.G., Lüscher,E.F.: Release reactions of human platelets induced by thrombin and other agents. Biochim. biophys. Acta **165**, 490—506 (1968)

David,J., David,R.A.: Cell hypersensitivity and immunity. Progr. Allergy **16**, 300—449 (1972)

Davies,P., Allison,A.C.: Secretion of macrophage enzymes in relation to pathogenesis of chronic inflammation. In: Nelson,D.S. (Ed.): Immunobiology of the Macrophage, pp. 428—463. London-New York: Academic Press 1976a

Davies,P., Allison,A.C.: The macrophage as a secretory cell in chronic inflammation. Agents Actions **6**, 60—74 (1976b)

Davies,P., Allison,A.C., Ackerman,J., Butterfield,A., Williams,S.: Asbestos induces selective release of lysosomal enzymes from mononuclear phagocytes. Nature (Lond.) **251**, 423—425 (1974b)

Davies,P., Allison,A.C., Dym,M., Cardella,C.J.: The selective release of lysosomal enzymes from mononuclear phagocytes by immune complexes and other materials causing chronic inflammation. In: Dumond,D.C. (Ed.): Infection and Immunology in the Rheumatic Diseases, pp. 365—373. New York: Blackwell 1975

Davies,P., Fox,R., Polyzonis,M., Allison,A.C., Haswell,A.D.: The inhibition of phagocytosis and facilitation of exocytosis in rabbit polymorphonuclear leucocytes by cytochalasin B. Lab. Invest. **28**, 16—23 (1973)

Davies,P., Page,R.C., Allison,A.C.: Changes in cellular enzyme levels and extracellular release of lysosomal acid hydrolases in macrophages exposed to Group A streptococcal cell wall substance. J. exp. Med. **139**, 1262—1282 (1974a)

Davies,P., Rita,G.A., Krakauer,K., Weissmann,G.: Characterization of a neutral protease from lysosomes of rabbit polymorphonuclear leucocytes. Biochem. J. **123**, 559—569 (1971)

Davis, A. T., Estensen, R., Quie, P. G.: Cytochalasin B. III. Inhibition of human polymorphonuclear leucocyte phagocytosis. Proc. Soc. exp. Biol. (N.Y.) **137**, 161—165 (1971)

Dewald, B., Rindler-Ludwig, R., Bretz, U., Baggiolini, M.: Subcellular localization and heterogeneity of neutral proteases in neutrophilic polymorphonuclear leucocytes. J. exp. Med. **141**, 709—723 (1975)

Dingle, J. T., Barrett, A. J., Poole, A. R., Stovin, P.: Inhibition by pepstatin of human cartilage degradation. Biochem. J. **127**, 443—444 (1972)

Dingle, J. T., Barrett, A. J., Weston, P. D.: Cathepsin D. Characteristics of immuno-inhibition and the confirmation of a role in cartilage breakdown. Biochem. J. **123**, 1—13 (1971)

Dingle, J. T., Fell, H. B., Coombs, R. R. A.: The breakdown of embryonic cartilage and bone cultivated in the presence of complement sufficient antiserum. II. Biochemical changes and the role of the lysosomal system. Int. Arch. Allergy **31**, 283—303 (1967)

Dingle, J. T., Poole, A. R., Lazarus, G., Barrett, A. J.: Immunoinhibition of intracellular protein digestion in macrophages. J. exp. Med. **137**, 1124—1141 (1973)

Estensen, R. D., Plageman, P. G. W.: Cytochalasin B inhibition of glucose and glucosamine transport. Proc. nat. Acad. Sci. (Wash.) **69**, 1430—1434 (1972)

Estensen, R. D., White, J. G., Holmes, B.: Specific degranulation of human polymorphonuclear leucocytes. Nature (Lond.) **248**, 347—348 (1974)

Fell, H. B., Barratt, M. E. J.: The role of soft connective tissue in the breakdown of pig articular cartilage cultivated in the presence of complement-sufficient antiserum to pig erythrocytes. I. Histological changes. Int. Arch. Allergy **44**, 441—468 (1973)

Finlay, C., Davies, P., Allison, A. C.: Changes in cellular enzyme levels and the inhibition of selective release of lysosomal hydrolases from macrophages by indomethacin. Agents Actions **5**, 345—353 (1975)

Folds, J. D., Welsh, I. R. H., Spitznagel, J. K.: Neutral protease confined to one class of lysosomes of human polymorphonuclear leucocytes. Proc. Soc. exp. Biol. (N.Y.) **139**, 461—463 (1972)

Fowler, S., DeDuve, C.: Digestive activity of lysosomes. III. The digestion of lipids by extracts of rat liver lysosomes. J. biol. Chem. **244**, 471—481 (1969)

Ginsburg, I.: Mechanisms of cell and tissue injury induced by Group A streptococci: relation of poststreptococcal sequelae. J. infect. Dis. **126**, 294—340, 419—456 (1972)

Goldstein, I. M., Brai, M., Osler, A. G., Weissmann, G.: Lysosomal enzyme release from human leucocytes: mediation by the alternate pathway of complement activation. J. Immunol. **111**, 33—37 (1973a)

Goldstein, I. M., Hoffstein, S., Gallin, J., Weissmann, G.: Mechanism of lysosomal enzyme release from human leucocytes: microtubule assembly and membrane fusion induced by a component of complement. Proc. nat. Acad. Sci. (Wash.) **70**, 2916—2920 (1973b)

Goldstein, I. M., Hoffstein, S., Weissmann, G.: Mechanisms of lysosomal enzyme release from human polymorphonuclear leucocytes. Effects of phorbol myristate acetate. J. Cell Biol. **66**, 647—652 (1975a)

Goldstein, I. M., Hoffstein, S., Weissman, G.: Influence of divalent cations upon complement-mediated enzyme release from human polymorphonuclear leucocytes. J. Immunol. **115**, 665—670 (1975b)

Goldstein, I. M., Horn, J. K., Kaplan, H. B., Weissmann, G.: Calcium-induced lysozyme secretion from human polymorphonuclear leucocytes. Biochem. biophys. Res. Commun. **60**, 807—812 (1974)

Goldstein, I. M., Weissmann, G.: Generation of C5-derived lysosomal enzyme-releasing activity (C5a) by lysates of leucocytes lysosomes. J. Immunol. **113**, 1583—1588 (1974)

Gordon, S., Todd, J., Cohn, Z. A.: In vitro synthesis and secretion of lysozyme by mononuclear phagocytes. J. exp. Med. **139**, 1228—1248 (1974b)

Gordon, S., Unkeless, J. C., Cohn, Z. A.: Induction of macrophage plasminogen activator by endotoxin stimulation and phagocytosis. Evidence for a two stage process. J. exp. Med. **140**, 995—1010 (1974a)

Granger, G. A., Williams, T.: Lymphocyte cytotoxicity in vitro: activation and release of a cytotoxic factor. Nature (Lond.) **218**, 1253—1254 (1968)

Greenbaum, L. M.: Cathepsin D-generated, pharmacologically active peptides (leucokinins) and their role in ascites fluid accumulation. In: Reich, E., Rifkin, D. B., Shaw, E. (Eds.): Proteases and Biological Control, pp. 223—228. Cold Spring Harbor Laboratory 1975

Harris, Jr., E. D., Reynolds, J. J., Werb, Z.: Cytochalasin B increases collagenase production by cells in vitro. Nature (Lond.) **257**, 243—244 (1975)

Hawkins, D.: Biopolymer membrane: a model system for the study of the neutrophilic leucocyte response to immune complexes. J. Immunol. **107**, 344—352 (1971)

Hawkins, D.: Neutrophilic leucocytes in immunologic reactions in vitro: effect of cytochalasin B. J. Immunol. **110**, 294—296 (1973)

Hawkins, D., Peeters, S.: The response of polymorphonuclear leucocytes to immune complexes in vitro. Lab. Invest. **24**, 483—491 (1971)

Henson, P. M.: Interaction of cells with immune complexes: adherence, release of constituents and tissue injury. J. exp. Med. **134**, 114S—135S (1971a)

Henson, P. M.: The immunologic release of constituents from neutrophil leucocytes. I. The role of antibody and complement on nonphagocytosable surfaces or phagocytosable particles. J. Immunol. **107**, 1535—1546 (1971b)

Henson, P. M.: The immunologic release of constituents from neutrophil leucocytes. II. Mechanisms of release during phagocytosis and adherence to nonphagocytosable surfaces. J. Immunol. **107**, 1547—1557 (1971c)

Henson, P. M.: Pathologic mechanisms in neutrophil-mediated injury. Amer. J. Path. **68**, 593—612 (1972)

Henson, P. M., Johnson, H. B., Spiegelberg, H. L.: The release of granule enzymes from human neutrophils stimulated by aggregated immunoglobulins of different classes and subclasses. J. Immunol. **109**, 1182—1192 (1972)

Henson, P. M., Oades, Z. G.: Enhanced of immunologically induced granule exocytosis from neutrophils by cytochalasin B. J. Immunol. **110**, 290—293 (1973)

Hoffstein, S., Weissmann, G.: Mechanism of lysosomal enzyme release from leucocytes. IV. Interaction of monosodium urate crystals with dogfish and human leucocytes. Arthr. Rheum. **18**, 153—165 (1975)

Holmsen, H., Day, H. J.: Thrombin-induced platelet release reaction and platelet lysosomes. Nature (Lond.) **219**, 760—761 (1968)

Huber, H., Polley, M. J., Linscott, W. D., Fudenberg, H. M., Müller-Eberhard, H. J.: Human monocytes: distinct receptor sites for the third component of complement and for immunoglobulin G. Science **162**, 1281—1283 (1968)

Huber, H., Wagner, M.: Binding of immune complexes to human macrophages: the role of membrane receptor sites. In: Wagner, W. H., Hahn, H. (Eds.): Activation of Macrophages Workshop Conferences Hoescht, Vol. 2, pp. 54—62. Amsterdam: Excerpta Medica Foundation 1974

Ignarro, L. J.: Dissimilar effects of antiinflammatory drugs on stability of lysosomes from peritoneal and circulating leucocytes and liver. Biochem. Pharmacol. **20**, 2861—2870 (1971)

Ignarro, L. J., George, W. J.: Mediation of immunological discharge of lysosomal enzymes from human neutrophils by guanosine 3'5'-monophosphate. Requirement of calcium and inhibition by adenosine 3',5'-monophosphate. J. exp. Med. **140**, 225—238 (1974)

Ishikawa, H., Bischoff, R., Holtzer, H.: Formation of arrowhead complexes with heavy meromyosin in a variety of cells. J. Cell Biol. **43**, 312—328 (1969)

Ishikawa, H., Smiley, J. D., Ziff, M.: Electron microscopic demonstration of immunoglobulin deposition in rheumatoid cartilage. Arthr. Rheum. **18**, 563—576 (1975)

Janoff, A.: Human granulocyte elastase. Further delineation of its role in connective tissue damage. Amer. J. Path. **68**, 579—591 (1972)

Janoff, A., Blondin, J., Sandhaus, R. A., Mosser, A., Malemud, C.: Human neutrophil elastase: in vitro effects on natural substrates suggest important physiological and pathological actions. In: Reich, E., Rifkin, D. B., Shaw, E. (Eds.): Proteases and Biological Control, pp. 603—620. Cold Spring Harbor Laboratory 1975

Janoff, A., Rosenberg, R., Galdston, M.: Elastase-like esteroprotease activity in human and rabbit alveolar macrophage granules. Proc. Soc. exp. Biol. (N.Y.) **136**, 1054—1058 (1971)

Kletzien, R. F., Perdue, J. F., Springer, A.: Cytochalasin A and B. Inhibition of sugar uptake in cultured cells. J. biol. Chem. **247**, 2964—2966 (1972)

Koob, T. J., Jeffrey, J. J., Eisen, A. Z.: Regulation of human skin collagenase activity by hydrocortisone and dexamethasone in organ culture. Biochem. biophys. Res. Commun. **61**, 1083—1088 (1974)

Lachmann, P. J., Coombs, R. R. A., Fell, H. B., Dingle, J. T.: The breakdown of embryonic (chick) cartilage and bone cultivated in the presence of complement-sufficient antiserum. III. Immunological analysis. Int. Arch. Allergy **36**, 469—485 (1969)
Lazarus, G. S.: Studies on the degradation of collagen by collagenases. In: Dingle, J. T. (Ed.): Lysosomes in Biology and Pathology, pp. 338—364. Amsterdam-London: North Holland 1973
Legrande, Y., Caen, J. P., Booyse, F. M., Rafelson, M. E., Robert, B., Robert, L.: Studies on a human blood platelet protease with elastolytic activity. Biochim. biophys. Acta **309**, 406—413 (1973)
Legrande, Y., Pignaud, G.: Human blood platelet elastase and proelastase. Path. et Biol. **23**, 546—549 (1975)
Lin, S., Santi, D. V., Spudich, J. A.: Biochemical studies on the mode of action of cytochalasin B. Preparation of [^{3}H] cytochalasin B and studies on its binding to cells. J. biol. Chem. **249**, 2268—2274 (1974)
Lockshin, M. D.: Normal macrophage migration inhibition in dexamethasone-treated guinea-pigs. Experientia (Basel) **28**, 571—572 (1972)
Malawista, S. E., Gee, J. B. L., Bensch, K. G.: Cytochalasin B reversibly inhibits phagocytosis; functional, metabolic and ultrastructural effects in human blood leucocytes and rabbit alveolar macrophages. Yale J. Biol. Med. **44**, 286—300 (1971)
Marcus, A. J., Zucker-Franklin, D., Safier, L. B., Ullman, H. L.: Studies on human platelets and granules. J. clin. Invest. **45**, 14—28 (1966)
Millroy, S. J., Poole, A. R.: Pig articular cartilage in organ culture. Effect of enzymatic depletion of the matrix on the response of chondrocytes to complement-sufficient antiserum against pig erythrocytes. Ann. rheum. Dis. **33**, 500—508 (1974)
Mills, D. C. B., Robb, I. A., Roberts, G. C. K.: The release of nucleotides, 5-hydroxytryptamine and enzymes from human blood platelets during aggregation. J. Physiol. (Lond.) **195**, 715—729 (1968)
Mizel, S. B., Wilson, L.: Inhibition of the transport of several hexoses in mammalian cells by cytochalasin B. J. biol. Chem. **247**, 4102—4105 (1972)
Müller-Eberhard, H. J.: Initiation of membrane attack by complement: assembly and control of C3 and C5. In: Reich, E., Rifkin, D. B., Shaw, E. (Eds.): Proteases and Biological Control, pp. 229—241. Cold Spr. Harb. Lab. 1975
Nachman, R. L., Ferris, B.: Studies on human platelet protease activity. J. clin. Invest. **47**, 2530—2540 (1968)
Oronsky, A., Ignarro, L., Perper, R.: Release of cartilage mucopolysaccharide-degrading neutral protease from human leucocytes. J. exp. Med. **138**, 461—472 (1973)
Page, R. C., Davies, P., Allison, A. C.: Effects of dental plaque on the production and release of lysosomal hydrolases by macrophages in culture. Arch. oral Biol. **18**, 1481—1495 (1973)
Page, R. C., Davies, P., Allison, A. C.: Pathogenesis of the chronic inflammatory lesion induced by Group A streptococcal cell walls. Lab. Invest. **30**, 568—581 (1974a)
Page, R. C., Davies, P., Allison, A. C.: Participation of mononuclear phagocytes in chronic inflammatory diseases. J. reticuloendoth. Soc. **15**, 413—438 (1974b)
Pantalone, R. M., Page, R. C.: Lymphokine-induced production and release of lysosomal enzymes by macrophages. Proc. nat. Acad. Sci. (Wash.) **72**, 2091—2094 (1975)
Perper, R. J., Oronsky, A. L.: Enzyme release from human leucocytes and degradation of cartilage matrix. Effects of antirheumatic drugs. Arthr. Rheum. **17**, 47—55 (1974)
Poole, A. R., Barratt, M. E. J., Fell, H. B.: The role of soft connective tissue in the breakdown of pig articular cartilage cultivated in the presence of complement sufficient antiserum to pig erythrocytes. II. Distribution of immunoglobulin G (IgG). Int. Arch. Allergy **44**, 469—488 (1973)
Poole, A. R., Hembry, R. M., Dingle, J. T.: Cathepsin D in cartilage: the immunohistochemical demonstration of extracellular enzyme in normal and pathological conditions. J. Cell Sci. **14**, 139—161 (1974)
Reich, E.: Plasminogen activator—secretion by neoplastic cells and macrophages. In: Reich, E., Rifkin, D. B., Shaw, E. (Eds.): Proteases and Biological Control, pp. 333—341. Cold Spr. Harb. Lab. 1975
Ringrose, P. S., Parr, M. A., McLaren, M.: Effects of anti-inflammatory and other compounds on the release of lysosomal enzymes from macrophages. Biochem. Pharmacol. **24**, 607—614 (1975)

Robertson, P.B., Shru, K.W., Vail, M.S., Taylor, R.E., Fullmer, H.M.: Collagenase: demonstration in rabbit macrophages. J. dent. Res. **52**, 189 (1973)
Robertson, W., Van, Schwartz, B.: Ascorbic acid and the formation of collagen. J. biol. Chem. **201**, 689—696 (1953)
Ruddle, N.H., Waksman, B.H.: Cytotoxicity mediated by soluble antigen and lymphocytes in delayed hypersensitivity. II. Correlation of the in vitro response with skin reactivity. J. exp. Med. **128**, 1255—1265 (1968)
Ruddy, S., Gigli, I., Austen, K.F.: The complement system of man. New Engl. J. Med. **287**, 489—495, 545—549, 592—596, 642—646 (1972)
Schorlemmer, H.U., Allison, A.C.: Effects of activated complement components on enzyme secretion by macrophages. Immunology **31**, 181—188 (1976)
Schorlemmer, H.U., Davies, P., Allison, A.C.: Ability of achivated complement components to induce lysosomal enzyme release from macrophages. Nature (Lond.) **261**, 48—49 (1976)
Schwab, J.H., Cromartie, W.J., Robertson, B.S.: Identification of a toxic cellular component of Group A streptococci as a complex of group specific C-polysaccharide and A protein. J. exp. Med. **109**, 43—54 (1959)
Senior, R.M., Bielefeld, D.R., Jeffrey, J.J.: Collagenolytic activity in alveolar macrophages. Clin. Res. **20**, 88 (1972)
Shevach, E.M., Jaffe, E.S., Green, I.: Receptors for complement and immunoglobulin on human and animal lymphoid cells. Transplant. Rev. **16**, 3—28 (1973)
Shibata, N., Tatsumi, N., Tanaka, K., Okamura, Y., Senda, N.: A contractile protein possessing Ca sensitivity (natural actomyosin) from leucocytes. Its extraction and some of its properties. Biochim. biophys. Acta **256**, 565—576 (1972)
Siegel, A., Lüscher, E.F.: Non-identity of the α-granules of human blood platelets with typical lysosomes. Nature (Lond.) **215**, 745—747 (1967)
Snyderman, R., Shin, H.S., Dannenberg, A.M.: Macrophage proteinase and inflammation: the production of chemotactic activity from the fifth component of complement by macrophage proteinase. J. Immunol. **109**, 896—898 (1972)
Spector, W.G., Heesom, N.: The production of granulomata by antigen-antibody complexes. J. Path. **98**, 31—39 (1969)
Spencer, H.: Pathology of the Lung, 2nd Ed., pp. 434—471. London: Pergamon Press 1968
Spitznagel, J.K., Dalldorf, F.G., Leffell, M.S., Folds, J.D., Welsh, I.R.H., Cooney, M.H., Martin, L.E.: Character of azurophil and specific granules purified from human polymorphonuclear leucocytes. Lab. Invest. **30**, 774—785 (1974)
Spudich, J.A., Lin, S.: Cytochalasin B. Its interaction with actin and actomyosin from muscle. Proc. nat. Acad. Sci. (Wash.) **69**, 442—446 (1972)
Steinman, R.M., Cohn, Z.A.: The interaction of particulate horseradish peroxidase (HRP)-anti HRP immune complexes with mouse peritoneal macrophages in vitro. J. Cell Biol. **55**, 616—634 (1972)
Stossel, T.P., Pollard, T.D.: Myosin in polymorphonuclear leucocytes. J. biol. Chem. **248**, 8288—8294 (1973)
Temple, A., Loewi, G., Davies, P., Howard, A.: Cytotoxicity of immune guinea pig cells. II. The mechanism of macrophage cytotoxicity. Immunology **248**, 655—670 (1973)
Unkeless, J.C., Gordon, S., Reich, E.: Secretion of plasminogen activator by stimulated macrophages. J. exp. Med. **139**, 834—850 (1974)
Wahl, L.M., Wahl, S.M., Mergenhagen, S.E., Martin, G.R.: Collagenase production by endotoxin-activated macrophages. Proc. nat. Acad. Sci. (Wash.) **71**, 3598—3601 (1974)
Wahl, L.M., Wahl, S.M., Mergenhagen, S.E., Martin, G.R.: Collagenase production by lymphokine-activated macrophages. Science **187**, 261—263 (1975)
Wannamaker, L.W., Matsen, J.M.: Streptococci and streptococcal diseases. New York: Academic Press 1972
Ward, P.A., Hill, J.H.: C5 chemotactic fragments produced by an enzyme in lysosomal granules of neutrophils. J. Immunol. **104**, 535—543 (1970)
Wasserman, S.I., Goetzl, E.J., Austen, K.F.: Inactivation of slow reacting substance of anaphylaxis by eosinophil arylsulfatase. J. Immunol. **114**, 645—649 (1975)

Weissmann, G.: The effects of steroids and drugs on lysosomes. In: Dingle, J. T., Fell, H. B. (Eds.): Lysosomes in Biology and Pathology, Vol. 1, pp. 276—298. London-Amsterdam: North Holland 1969
Weissmann, G., Zurier, R. B., Spieler, P. T., Goldstein, I. M.: Mechanism of lysosomal enzyme release from leucocytes exposed to immune complexes and other particles. J. exp. Med. **134**, 149 S—165 S (1971)
Werb, Z., Gordon, S.: Secretion of a specific collagenase by stimulated macrophages. J. exp. Med. **142**, 346—360 (1975 a)
Werb, Z., Gordon, S.: Elastase secretion by stimulated macrophages. Characterization and regulation. J. exp. Med. **142**, 361—377 (1975 b)
Werb, Z., Reynolds, J. J.: Stimulation by endocytosis of the secretion of collagenase and neutral proteinase from rabbit synovial fibroblasts. J. exp. Med. **140**, 1482—1497 (1974)
Wessels, N. K., Spooner, B. G., Ash, J. F., Bradley, M. D., Luduena, M. A., Taylor, E. L., Wrenn, J. T., Yamada, K. M.: Microfilaments in cellular and developmental processes. Science **171**, 135—143 (1971)
Weston, W. L., Mandel, M. J., Krueger, G. G., Claman, H. N.: Differential suppressive effect of hydrocortisone on lymphocytes and mononuclear macrophages in delayed hypersensitivity of guinea pigs. J. invest. Derm. **59**, 345—348 (1972)
White, R. G., Estensen, R. D.: Selective labilization of specific granules in polymorphonuclear leucocytes by phorbol myristate acetate. Amer. J. Path. **75**, 45—54 (1974)
Wright, D. G., Malawista, S. E.: Mobilization and extracellular release of granular enzymes from human leucocytes during phagocytosis: inhibition by colchicine and cortisol but not by salicylate. Arthr. Rheum. **16**, 749—758 (1973)
Yang, Y. Z., Perdue, J. F.: Contractile proteins of cultured cells. I. The isolation and characterization of an actin-like protein from cultured chick embryo fiborblasts. J. biol. Chem. **247**, 4503—4509 (1972)
Zigmond, S. H., Hirsch, J. G.: Cytochalasin B: inhibition of D-2-deoxyglucose transport into leucocytes and fibroblasts. Science **176**, 1432—1434 (1972)
Zurier, R. B., Hoffstein, S., Weissmann, G.: Cytochalasin B: effect on lysosomal enzyme release from human leucocytes. Proc. nat. Acad. Sci. (Wash.) **70**, 844—848 (1973 a)
Zurier, R. B., Hoffstein, S., Weissmann, G.: Mechanisms of enzyme release from human leucocytes. I. Effect of cyclic nucleotides and colchicine. J. Cell Biol. **58**, 27—41 (1973 b)

CHAPTER 9

Lysosomal Enzymes

R. B. ZURIER and K. KRAKAUER

A. Lysosomes as Organelles

The study of cellular organelles, while a collaborative effort, usually begins with the morphological observations of the cell anatomist followed by the biochemist's analysis of the isolated organelles and their molecular components. The pattern was reversed for lysosomes, the nature and function of which were not recognized until they had been characterized chemically. The discovery of lysosomes began in 1949 by Dr. CHRISTIAN DE DUVE and his colleagues, with an investigation of rat liver enzymes involved in carbohydrate metabolism. Using the then newly developed technique of centrifugal fractionation of cells, a class of subcellular particles having centrifugal properties intermediate between those of mitochondria and microsomes was isolated. These were found to have a high content of acid phosphatase and other hydrolytic enzymes. By centrifugation, it was calculated that the size of the particles was 0.2–0.8 μ. It was also determined that these enzymes were inactive towards their potential substrates if the fraction was carefully prepared to avoid disruption of the organelles. However, preparation of the fraction without regard to cellular organization, or exposure of the fraction to decreased osmotic pressure or surface active agents, resulted in a considerable increase in enzyme activity (DE DUVE et al., 1949; DE DUVE, 1959, 1965). This special relationship between particle and enzymes whereby disruption of the organelle is required for maximum enzyme activity is termed "structure-linked latency" and its establishment led to the hypothesis that the acid hydrolases were packaged together in a previously undescribed, membrane-bounded organelle.

Because of its cargo of hydrolytic enzymes, the particle was called a lysosome (Greek: lysis = dissolution; soma = body). An interesting question concerning the enzymes of lysosomes is whether they are free in the interior of the particles or bound to the enclosing membrane. Initially, it appeared that lysosomal enzymes were simply retained within the granules by a membranous barrier. However, studies on the availability of lysosomal enzymes at acid, alkaline and neutral pH indicate that at least some lysosomal enzymes are bound to differing, perhaps polar sites, of the membrane. There is also evidence for the possibility of salt-like linkages between the enzymes and non-enzymatic charged constituents, such as basic proteins. Some problems, such as the failure of intralysosomal cathepsin to attack the other hydrolytic enzymes, might be explained by the fact that some enzymes are bound to other constituents which preserve it from attack, or that they are associated with discrete

Supported by National Institutes of Health Grants AM 17309 and AI 12225.

portions of the surface membrane, thus accessible only to substrates that are freely diffusible within the organelle.

NOVIKOFF (1961) obtained the first electron micrographs of DE DUVE'S cell fractions containing partially purified lysosomes. Particles morphologically distinct from mitochondria were seen which gave a positive staining reaction for acid phosphatase. The cytochemical definition, then, of lysosomes as particles which are bounded by a single unit membrane and yield a positive staining reaction for acid phosphatase, has been considered as equivalent to the biochemical definition. It may be time, however, to expand the definition to similar organelles which do not contain acid phosphatase.

B. Polymorphonuclear Leucocyte Lysosomes

I. Granule Type

The phagocytic cells of blood and exudates—polymorphonuclear (PMN) leucocytes and macrophages—have provided good sources of material for studies of lysosomes. PMN granules are lysosomes and at least three (and perhaps four) types have been characterized in humans (BRETZ and BAGGIOLINI, 1974), by use of both sucrose density zonal and isopycnic centrifugation. Granules with the highest modal density (1.23 g/ml sucrose) are *azurophils* or true lysosomes. These contain 100% of the peroxidase, 60–90% of the total lysosomal acid hydrolase activities and 50% of the lysozyme activity. Acid β-glycerophosphatase activity but not acid 4-nitrophenyl phosphatase activity is also present in this fraction. *Specific* granules are of medium density (1.19 g/ml sucrose) and contain lysozyme but not hydrolase, peroxidase or alkaline phosphatase activities. LEFELL and SPITZNAGEL (1972) and SPITZNAGEL et al. (1973) have demonstrated that human specific granules also contain lactoferrin. At the same modal density as the specific granules, some acid hydrolase-containing organelles were found which, though difficult to separate from the specific granules, were considered to be a distinct granule species. They therefore represent a second population of lysosomes which contain both acid β-glycerophosphatase and acid 4-nitrophenyl phosphatase activities. Finally, a light fraction (1.16 g/ml sucrose) composed of membrane fragments contains all of the alkaline phosphatase activity along with some acid 4-nitrophenyl phosphatase. Similar data which indicate three to four different organelle populations in human PMN have been reported by other investigators (SCHULTZ et al., 1965; JOHN et al., 1967; OLSSON, 1969; WELSH et al., 1971; WEST and KIMBALL, 1971). Species differences do exist. Thus, for example, rabbit specific granules contain an alkaline phosphatase not present in their human counterpart (BAGGIOLINI et al., 1970).

II. Vacuolar Apparatus and Types of Lysosomes

While the characteristic structure of the mitochondrion makes it readily distinguishable in any type of cell, lysosomes come in a bewildering assortment of shapes and sizes, even in a single cell type. This polymorphism varies with the state of the cell in which the lysosomes are found. It is now recognized, therefore, that the term lysosome rather than referring to a particular "soma", encompasses all the various forms of vesicles, granules and pockets of the vacuolar system or apparatus, the role of which involves the intracellular digestion of endogenous and exogenous substrates. The vacuolar apparatus is a dynamic system which enables materials to move into, through and out of the cell while remaining at all times screened from the cytoplasm. Materials enter the cell by "endocytosis" a word which represents all the cell's engulfing properties including phagocytosis, pinocytosis and micropinocytosis. A portion of the cell membrane first attaches itself to the material to be ingested and then appears to be sucked inwards to form an internal pocket containing the material. The pocket pinches free from the cell membrane and is now a phagosome (endocytic vacuole).

There are four principal varieties of lysosome: the storage granule, the heterophagic vacuole, the autophagic vacuole and the residual body. The first is a primary or pure lysosome, the other three are secondary lysosomes. As described above, the primary lysosome is a membrane limited structure containing newly synthesized acid hydrolases which have not as yet participated in acts of digestion. Electron microscopic observations (NOVIKOFF et al., 1964; BRANDES, 1965; COHN et al., 1966; FRIEND and FARQUHAR, 1967; HELMINEN and ERICSSON, 1970) lead to the conclusion that lysosomal enzymes are synthesized by ribosomes, accumulate in the rough surfaced endoplasmic reticulum (ER), enter the cisternae of these ER and are then transported to the smooth ER. Packaging is usually accomplished by elements of the Golgi apparatus. Azurophil granules of rabbit and human PMN in the early progranulocyte stage have been demonstrated (BAINTON and FARQUHAR, 1966, 1968a, 1968b; BAINTON et al., 1971) to arise from the proximal or concave face of the Golgi by budding and subsequent coalescence of vesicles. Later, in the myelocyte stage, specific granules are formed from the distal convex face of the Golgi. The Golgi also serve to concentrate lysosomal contents by removal of water and low molecular weight constituents. Addition of monosaccharides to protein and lipid moieties of the new organelles also occurs at the Golgi (COOK, 1973).

The initial phagosome, an enclave of external milieu separated from the cytoplasm by a bit of plasma membrane, rapidly leaves the periphery where it was formed and moves toward the centre of the cell. During this migration it may become fragmented by budding or may merge with other phagosomes. Its journey ends when it comes in contact and fuses with the membrane of a primary lysosome. The lysosomal enzymes are discharged in an explosive fashion into the phagosome, there to degrade the ingested material. The new vacuole is a phagolysosome or heterophagic vacuole. The presence of acid lipids (BARRETT and DINGLE, 1967) and acidic lipoproteins (GOLDSTONE et al., 1970) in lysosomes may be an essential part of the buffering system within heterophagic vacuoles which allows digestion to proceed at an acid pH.

The merger of phagosome with primary lysosome is generally assumed to occur by fusion of the phagosomal membrane with that of the lysosome. It is not yet clear why lysosomal membranes fuse only with those of phagosomes or with plasma membrane, but not with mitochondrial or nuclear membranes. Different populations of granules react differently to a variety of stimuli. This specificity is discussed more fully by DAVIES and ALLISON (Chapter 8) and is mentioned here only to emphasize further the differences in types of lysosomes. BAINTON (1970) has shown histochemically that fusion of specific granules with phagocytic vacuoles in rabbit PMN occurs approximately three minutes before the fusion of azurophils with these same vacuoles. Concurrent, time-dependent pH changes within secondary lysosomes were noted in rat peritoneal PMN and mononuclear phagocytes following uptake of dye-stained yeast (JENSEN and BAINTON, 1973). Approximately 10 min after yeast ingestion, the pH of a majority of phagocytic vacuoles had dropped from neutrality to pH 5.0; by 20–25 min pH 3.5 had been reached and was maintained for at least 18 h. These experiments indicate that neutral-acting enzymes of specific granules were the first to attack the vacuolar contents. Following this initial onslaught, neutral proteinases, acid proteinases and acid hydrolases of the azurophils degraded the substrates to diffusible, harmless and possibly re-usable metabolites.

It is possible to differentiate granule populations similarly by monitoring their fusion with plasma membrane. Thus, ESTENSEN et al. (1974) and WHITE and ESTENSEN (1974) have shown that treatment of human PMN with phorbol myristate acetate (PMA) caused release of enzymes from specific granules, but not those from azurophils. GOLDSTEIN et al. (1974) observed that low concentrations of calcium, manganese, strontium or zinc induced the selective release of lysozyme, but not β-glucuronidase, from human PMN. These results indicate that a particular population of enzymes may mediate a digestive process because of the specific reactivity of its organelles.

C. Lysosomes, Polymorphonuclear Leucocytes, and Inflammation

Questions of lysosomal permeability are not restricted to the passage of substances into lysosomes but also concern the outward movement of end products of digestion, since smaller molecules such as amino acids, nucleotides and monosaccharides presumably cross the membrane subsequent to degradation by hydrolytic enzymes of the engulfed material from which they derive. Perhaps of prime consideration is the outward movement of the lysosomal enzymes themselves. An important property of lysosomes is their stability in living cells. Among the first suggestions relating the lysosomal concept to pathology was the possibility that lysosomal membranes might rupture and that an excessive or inappropriate release of enzymes into the cell sap or surrounding medium would cause cell and tissue damage. It is now clear that although lysosomes are suitably equipped for this role, the circumstances under which they act as "suicide sacs" are rare. The major macromolecules of cells and extracellular materials such as collagen, protein, polysaccharides, nucleic acids, etc. can be broken down by lysosomal enzymes. Furthermore, mixtures of enzymes can degrade whole tissues. Neutral and acid proteases, ordinarily contained within lysosomes, can split molecules whose biological function is to initiate and propagate inflammation. They can cleave complement components to subfractions which are chemotactic for PMN. They can disrupt mast cells with resultant release of vasoactive amines. They can cause increased vascular permeability.

Considerable experimental evidence has been accumulated to support the concept that PMN and their contents are critical to the production in vivo of inflammation and tissue injury. Thus, removal of PMN by treatment with nitrogen mustard or heterologous antineutrophil antisera inhibits the vasculitis of the Arthus phenomenon (STETSON, 1951; HUMPHREY, 1955; COCHRANE et al., 1959; PARISH, 1969; DESHAZO et al., 1972). Similarly, the necrotizing arteritis of experimental serum sickness in rabbits (KNIKER and COCHRANE, 1965) and the proteinuria associated with acute nephrotoxic nephritis in rats and rabbits (COCHRANE et al., 1965) is prevented by depletion of PMN in these animals. HENSON (1972) has produced glomerular injury in PMN depleted rabbits by i.v. injection of sheep anti-basement membrane antiserum and homologous leucocytes; degree of injury varied directly with the number of PMN transfused.

The presence of a substance in an inflammatory focus suggests that it may be a mediator. Increased activities of lysosomal enzymes have been reported in human rheumatoid synovial fluid and synovial membrane as well as in other inflamed tissues (SMITH and HAMERMAN, 1962; BARLAND et al., 1964; KERBY and TAYLOR, 1967; BARNHART et al., 1968; ANDERSON, 1970). Morphological evidence of degranulation has been considered to be an indication that lysosomal enzyme release from intact leucocytes occurs in vivo. HENSON (1972) used ultrastructural histochemical techniques in rabbits with nephrotoxic nephritis to demonstrate degranulation and alkaline phosphatase activity on the external surface of PMN plasma membranes at the point of contact with glomerular basement membranes. SCHUMACHER and AGUDELO (1972) examined venules in human synovial membranes from patients with inflammatory arthritis and observed that intact PMN had degranulated. It was concluded that lysosomal contents could have mediated the observed vascular damage.

The first direct evidence that lysosomes themselves were capable of initiating tissue injury was reported by THOMAS (1964) who showed in rabbits that the i.d. injection of PMN granules, followed by the intravenous injection of endotoxin, produced skin lesions (haemorrhagic necrosis) resembling those seen in the localized Schwartzman reaction. Similar treatment allowed production of the reversed passive Arthus reaction in neutropenic animals. Lysates of homologous PMN lysosomes produce acute synovitis and chronic inflammation and tissue injury after intra-articular injection in rabbits (WEISSMANN et al., 1969).

The mechanisms whereby lysosomal enzymes are released from inflammatory cells are discussed by DAVIES and ALLISON (Chapter 8). In this chapter we will consider the potential roles in the production of inflammation and tissue injury of lysosomal enzymes and non-enzymic lysosomal substances. We will also detail the means by which release of lysosomal enzymes from human PMN may be regulated.

D. Lysosomal Enzymes as Mediators of Inflammation and Tissue Injury

I. Acid Proteinases

Lysosomal acid cathepsins include both endopeptidases, cathepsin B_1, D, and E, and exopeptidases, cathepsin A, C and the carboxypeptidases A and B. These enzymes work synergistically, the endopeptidases cleaving large polypeptide chains to smaller fragments, while cathepsin A removes amino acids from the carboxyl terminus and cathepsin C attacks the amino terminus (GREENBAUM, 1971). Recently, BARRETT

(1975) described a new endopeptidase, cathepsin F, in rabbit ear and human articular cartilage. The subcellular distribution of this enzyme is unknown, but it appears to be firmly associated with some element of the cartilage, cells, or matrix.

Cathepsin D has been the most widely studied of the lysosomal proteinases and has been shown to be important in tissue remodelling, in the digestion of serum proteins, and may also have a role in initiating the action of certain hormones and enzymes. Several serum proteins are susceptible to attack by cathepsin D. These include haemoglobin, which is used as a standard substrate for cathepsin D assay, bovine serum albumin, globulins, fibrinogen, and fibrin (LEBEZ et al., 1971), immunoglobulin G (GHETIE and MIHAESCU, 1973; KEISARI and WITZ, 1973), immunoglobulin M (FERENCIK and STEFANOVIC, 1973) and α_1-antitrypsin (SANDHAUS and JANOFF, 1974). Some indication of control of these activities is reflected in the observations that a haptoglobin-haemoglobin complex has been shown to have a reduced susceptibility to digestion when compared to haemoglobin alone (SATO et al., 1973) and that macroglobulin is a potent inhibitor of many proteinases (BARRETT and STARKEY, 1973). The use of a specific antiserum to cathepsin D has allowed for the localisation and specific intra- and extracellular inhibition of the enzyme (WESTON, 1969; DINGLE et al., 1973; WESTON et al., 1969). In addition, the specific inhibitor pepstatin (UMEZAWA et al., 1970; DINGLE et al., 1972) has permitted the identification of some in vitro extracellular roles for cathepsin D. Purified cathepsin D has been shown to degrade isolated proteoglycan and cartilage (DINGLE et al., 1971). An acid autolysis of cartilage at pH 5.0 was inhibited 100% by specific antiserum (DINGLE et al., 1972; WESTON et al., 1969). At pH 6.0 only 59% of the autolytic activity was inhibited and the residual activity was attributed to cathepsin B_1. It appears, therefore, that at an appropriate stimulus, such as cell damage, cartilage lysosomal enzymes can influence the state of repair of the tissue.

There is evidence that cathepsin D of macrophages, granulocytes and granulation tissue may be active at the site of inflammation (LAZARUS, 1974). Firstly, intracellular digestion of radioactively labelled haemoglobin by macrophages is inhibited by anti-cathepsin D antiserum. Secondly, in rabbits following an intradermal injection of turpentine in peanut oil, infiltration by granulocytes at the site of inflammation within 24 h was followed by an acute inflammatory reaction during the next 4 days. By day 9, epithelial hyperplasia was visible as well as round cell proliferation and new vessel formation. Concomitantly, a biphasic increase in cathepsin D and a neutral protease was seen in this tissue. The first peak of activity was at day 2 and was coincident with the granulocyte infiltration. A peak at day 9 coincided with the granulomatous response. The elevation in proteinase activity coincided with evidence of resorption. Both granulocytes and skin were found to be the source of activity. Cathepsin D has been localized immunocytochemically to skin cells (LAZARUS and DINGLE, 1974). In agreement with these results is the observation by BAZIN and DELANEY (1972) that cathepsin D activity isolated from partially purified cell preparations derived from inflamed granulation tissue could degrade chondromucoprotein, haemoglobin, fibrinogen, serum albumin, and histone, but not collagen.

Cathepsin D and other cathepsins (E and B) have been implicated in formation of kinins (GREENBAUM, 1971). Increased vascular permeability may result from the action of this enzyme. In addition, carboxypeptidases A and B hydrolyse bradykinin and kallidin (GREENBAUM, 1971; GREENBAUM and YAMAFUJI, 1966); therefore, an inherent control mechanism seems to be present. Carboxypeptidase and cathepsin B, but not cathepsin A or D activity have been found in the oedema fluid of direct passive Arthus reaction in rat paws (FÖRSTER, 1972).

Cathepsin B_1 (for review see BARRETT, 1975) digests proteoglycan and collagen (MORRISON et al., 1973) of connective tissue and acts as a procollagenase activator (VAES and EECHOUT, 1975). The action of PMN or monocyte cathepsin B_1 may therefore be essential to tissue repair following the acute inflammatory reaction, or to the tissue damage seen in such chronic inflammatory states as rheumatoid arthritis. It is likely that cathepsin B_1 is as ubiquitous as cathepsin D and future investigations will reveal more functions of this enzyme in mediating the inflammatory response.

Cathepsin C has been localized to human PMN granules (DAVIES et al., 1974). This enzyme is similar to chymotrypsin in its substrate specificity and can attack glucagon, angiotensin II amide, gastrin, corticotrophin (GREENBAUM, 1971) and prothrombin (PURCELL and BARNHART, 1963). This enzyme may participate in the blood clotting scheme as well as in digestion of inflammation-mediating peptides.

II. Neutral Proteinases

Neutral proteinases derived from lysosomes have been implicated in the activation of complement components (TAUBMAN et al., 1970). Human peripheral blood leukocyte lysosomal enzymes have been shown to degrade the C1, C3, and C5 components of complement at neutral pH and therefore to induce the alterations usually associated with the sequential immunological activation of the complement system. One product formed from C5 cleavage (C5a) by human and rabbit PMN lysosomal enzymes has been shown to be chemotactic (TAUBMAN et al., 1970; WARD and HILL, 1970; SNYDERMAN et al., 1971; WRIGHT and GALLIN, 1974) and to induce the release of lysosomal enzymes from PMN treated with cytochalasin B (GOLDSTEIN and WEISSMANN, 1974). The action of lysosomal enzymes might mediate anaphylaxis (VALLOTA and MÜLLER-EBERHARD, 1973), chemotaxis and lysosomal enzyme release. WARD and ZVAIFLER (1971) have shown that a large percentage of rheumatoid synovial fluids contain chemotactic activity for neutrophils, an activity attributed to $C\overline{567}$ and C5a. This C5 cleaving enzyme, on the basis of substrate specificity and susceptibility to inhibitors, was similar to the enzyme extractable from lysosomes of human and rabbit granulocytes.

C3 cleaving enzyme was found in synovial fluid of patients with non-rheumatoid arthritis-derived inflammation (WARD and ZVAIFLER, 1971). These authors noted that the chemotactic activity was related to C3a, but TAUBMAN et al. (1970) have reported that incubation of C3 with lysosomal enzymes gave large and small reaction products which were without chemotactic activity. C3a has also been shown to be an anaphylatoxin (VALLOTA and MÜLLER-EBERHARD, 1973). The active form of C3 proactivator has been shown to be produced by incubation of PMN granules with fresh serum (GOLDSTEIN and WEISSMANN, 1974).

Other neutral proteinases which are present in lysosomes are: a plasminogen activator localized to rabbit kidney lysosomes (ALI and LACK, 1965; ALI and EVANS, 1968); an elastase which can degrade vascular basement membrane (JANOFF and ZELIGS, 1968); a histonase which may derepress lymphocytes (DAVIES et al., 1971); an enzyme which digests fibrin, protein of proteoglycans and extrahelical telopeptides of rat skin salt-soluble collagen (PRYCE-JONES and WOOD, 1975); an angiotensinase C (KAKIMOTO et al., 1973).

III. Other Lysosomal Enzymes

TAPPEL (1969) and BARRETT (1969) have reviewed the properties of all enzymes known to be localized within lysosomes. Most of these have not been proven to participate in the inflammatory reaction. Interestingly, arylsulphatase of human eosinophils has been shown to inactivate the slow-reacting substance of anaphylaxis (SRS – A) which is released from mast cells (WASSERMAN et al., 1975). Thus, lysosomal enzymes may also serve to *modulate* the inflammatory response.

IV. Collagenase

Thought to reside in specific granules (ROBERTSON et al., 1972), collagenases are not considered as lysosomal enzymes. They clearly have a key role in tissue injury and remodelling. Collagenases are enzymes which cleave native collagen molecules in a characteristic fashion to yield two specific products which have been termed "TC^A" and "TC^B". The TC^A fragment is the C-terminal one-quarter length product (KANG et al., 1966). A specific collagenase, active at neutral and alkaline pH, has been found in granule fractions from human PMN (LAZARUS et al., 1968a). This leucocyte collagenase was inhibited by ethylene diamine tetra acetic acid (EDTA), cysteine and reduced glutathione, but not by human serum, distinguishing it from previously described tissue collagenases and from other neutral proteases of leucocytes (LAZARUS et al., 1968b). Incubation of collagen with crude granule extracts at neutral pH results in cleavage of the collagen molecules into two specific products and in extensive lysis of fibrils. Degradative activity is lost during purification of collagenase, although cleavage of the collagen molecule into TC^A and TC^B fragments still takes place. The lost activity was identified as a non-specific protease system. The protease can be inhibited by serum, a factor found in the cytosol and soybean trypsin inhibitor. In addition to degrading TC^A and TC^B fragments, the protease may hydrolyse collagen to a limited extent. However, both specific collagenase and the protease system are required for maximal collagen degradation (LAZARUS et al., 1972).

E. Non-Enzymatic Mediators of Inflammation

A heterogeneous group of basic (cationic) proteins, devoid of enzymatic activity, have been isolated from rabbit PMN lysosomes. The proteins have diverse biological activities and are capable of either directly or indirectly producing tissue damage and inflammation. They can cause extravascular migration of leucocytes (JANOFF and ZWEIFACH, 1964), an acute dermatitis (GOLUB and SPITZNAGEL, 1966) and histamine release from mast cells (RANADIVE and COCHRANE, 1968). When peritoneal PMN of rabbits, guinea pigs and rats are incubated in vitro with antibody-antigen precipitates, they release a substance—"Pf/Phag"—which enhances vascular permeability (MOVAT et al., 1971). The substance, and another—"SRS/Phag"—were shown to be derived from lysosomes. Lysosomal cationic protein fractions from rabbit PMN also have anticoagulant (SABA et al., 1967), coagulant (HAWIGER et al., 1969), pyrogenic (HERION et al., 1966), chemotactic (WARD, 1968) and bactericidal (ZEYA and SPITZNAGEL, 1968) activities. The role of these cationic proteins in producing human disease is not clear. They have been isolated from human PMN but attempts to demonstrate pyrogenic (HERION et al., 1966) or vascular permeability enhancing activities (SCHERER and JANOFF, 1968) in these fractions have not been successful.

F. Regulation of Lysosomal Enzyme Release From Phagocytic Cells

Phagocytic cells often become the centre of inflammatory lesions (METCHNIKOFF, 1905) due in part to release of substances previously sequestered within lysosomes. A clear definition of discrete mechanisms which account for release of such materials from inflammatory cells is beginning to emerge and is discussed thoroughly in Chapter 8 by DAVIES and ALLISON. One mechanism of enzyme release—"regurgitation during feeding" (WEISSMANN et al., 1971; HENSON, 1971a; WRIGHT and MALAWISTA, 1972)—may be important to the propagation of joint inflammation in rheumatoid arthritis. When cells engage in phagocytosis (e.g. leucocytes or synovial lining cells which engulf immune complexes in the joint space of patients with rheumatoid arthritis) they release a portion of their lysosomal hydrolases to the surrounding medium. This effect appears due to extrusion of lysosomal materials from incompletely closed phagosomes open at their external border to tissue space while joined at their internal border with granules discharging enzymes into the phagolysosome. A second mechanism has been called "reverse endocytosis" (HENSON, 1971b; HENSON, 1972; WEISSMANN et al., 1972) and may be pertinent to the pathogenesis of tissue injury in immune complex nephritis, vasculitis, and rheumatoid arthritis. When leucocytes encounter immune complexes which have been dispersed along a non-phagocytosable surface there is release of lysosomal enzymes directly to the outside of the cell (HAWKINS, 1971; HENSON, 1971c). Similar enzyme release may occur when leucocytes are in apposition to immune complexes in blood vessel walls or glomerular basement membrane, or when pannus encounters articular cartilage. Under both circumstances, lysosomal enzymes are selectively released (without release of cytoplasmic enzymes) to the outside without necessarily causing cytoplasmic damage. Another mechanism for enzyme release, "perforation from within" (ALLISON, 1971; WEISSMANN and DUKOR, 1970), occurs when certain materials gain access to the vacuolar system wherein they interact with, and finally rupture, lysosomal membranes. A wave of membrane damage results with release of cytoplasmic and lysosomal enzymes and followed by cell and tissue death. The inflammatory episodes of acute gout appear due to this type of encounter between leucocytes and crystals of monosodium urate (MCCARTY and HOLLANDER, 1961).

In all of these model systems, addition of cyclic 3'5' adenosine monophosphate (cAMP), of compounds that influence the accumulation of the nucleotide or of drugs such as colchicine and vinblastine that directly affect microtubule integrity (WEISENBERG et al., 1968; BENSCH and MALAWISTA, 1968) reduce extrusion of acid hydrolase from phagocytic cells (WRIGHT and MALAWISTA, 1973; ZURIER et al., 1973a; ZURIER et al., 1974; IGNARRO, 1974; IGNARRO et al., 1974). It therefore appeared as though agents that influence intracellular levels of cyclic nucleotides might regulate the movement of lysosomes to phagocytic vacuoles and/or to the cell periphery by virtue of effects on microtubules. In such studies, however, it was not always clear that reduced enzyme release did not result simply from inhibition of phagocytosis per se. It has in fact been shown that cAMP inhibits phagocytosis (COX and KARNOVSKY, 1973).

It has been demonstrated (ZURIER et al., 1973b; HENSON and OADES, 1973; HAWKINS, 1973) that the cytochalasin B (CB)-treated leucocyte resembles a secretory cell in which the influence of various compounds on membrane fusion and enzyme extrusion may be measured directly. These cells, upon contact with a phagocytic stimulus, selectively merge lysosomes with the plasma membrane as if the latter were a phagocytic vacuole. Selective secretion of lysosomal materials after this merger occurs in the absence of cell death and despite absence of particle ingestion (particles adhere to the plasma membrane). Furthermore, the complement component C5a causes selective release of lysosomal enzymes from CB-treated PMN in the absence of particles (GOLDSTEIN et al., 1973). Thus, regulation of granule movement, merger of granule with plasma membrane and enzyme secretion may be studied independent of particle-membrane contact. In this model, too, increases in cyclic adenosine 3′5′-monophosphate (cAMP) levels are associated with reduced enzyme release and increased cGMP concentrations with enhanced enzyme release.

Intracellular movement of lysosomes, and of secretory granules in a variety of cell types, appears to be regulated by an as yet unclear interaction between cyclic nucleotides, microtubules and microfilaments (ALLISON, 1971). Although microtubules are in a dynamic state of assembly and disassembly, it is probably in their aggregated state that microtubules exert their influence on cell mechanics (WEISENBERG et al., 1968). Exogenous cAMP and colchicine both favor disassembly of microtubules (GILLESPIE, 1971) and both reduce selective enzyme release (WRIGHT and MALAWISTA, 1973; ZURIER et al., 1973a; ZURIER et al., 1974). In contrast, deuterium oxide (D_2O) favors formation of microtubules (MARSLAND et al., 1971) and augments enzyme release from leucocytes. Moreover, prior incubation of cells with colchicine reduces the potentiating effect of D_2O, suggesting that granule movement and hydrolase release both depend on intact microtubules. Similarly vinblastine, which causes the disfunction of microtubules by forming dense precipitates (BENSCH and MALAWISTA, 1968), also inhibits release of lysosomal enzymes (WEISSMANN et al., 1972). However, addition of 10^{-6} M colchicine to mouse peritoneal macrophages before their exposure to particles, eradicated morphologically identifiable microtubules but did not alter transfer of acid phosphatase to phagolysosomes (PESANTI and AXLINE, 1975). Others (HAWKINS, 1974; HENSON and OADES, 1975) have also found colchicine to inhibit degranulation of neutrophils only slightly. These studies suggest that intact microtubules may not be necessary for extrusion of lysosomal hydrolases. It appears that assembly of microtubules is not itself always sufficient. Thus, calcium-induced release of lysozyme from specific granules of PMN is associated with assembly of microtubules but not release of β-glucuronidase (GOLDSTEIN et al., 1975). Therefore, another signal appears to be required for lysosomal enzyme release. Particles or a humoral agent such as C5a (possibly acting via cyclic nucleotides) can fulfill that role. Calcium, too, may exert its influence upon exocytosis via effects on intracellular cyclic nucleotides or their interaction with structural proteins (SMITH and IGNARRO, 1975; IGNARRO and GEORGE, 1974a). It appears then that the accumulation of cAMP causes inhibition of enzyme secretion. Similarly, exogenously added cAMP inhibits the release of lymphocytotoxins (HENNEY et al., 1971) histamine and SRS-A (ORANGE et al., 1971a, 1971b). When purified (>95%) preparations of PMN rather than mixed leucocyte suspensions are studied, β-adrenoceptor stimulants, prostaglandin E_1 (PGE_1), histamine and cholera enterotoxin act to increase cAMP and to inhibit release of lysosomal enzymes in the absence of mononuclear cells (ZURIER et al., 1974). However, far greater increments of cAMP are found in mononuclear fractions (BOURNE et al., 1973; PARKER and SMITH, 1973) and reduction of enzyme release is more marked in suspensions of mixed leucocytes than in suspensions of purified PMN. This would suggest that mononuclear cells, perhaps by releasing their cAMP, may further reduce enzyme release from PMN. The nucleotide is present in most body fluids (BROADUS et al., 1971) and extracellular cAMP might therefore have a regulatory function. Addition to rat peritoneal macrophages of PGE_1 results in rapid accumulation of intracellular cAMP followed by its steady progressive release to the medium (GEMSA et al., 1975). In human diploid lung fibroblasts there is a dramatic progressive release of cAMP from cells during a 60 min incubation with PGE_1 (KELLEY and BUTCHER, 1974). The nature and extent of intercellular cAMP fluxes in the inflammatory response require greater definition.

After incubation with polystyrene latex beads (PARK et al., 1971) or zymosan, the cAMP content of human peripheral blood leucocytes is increased several-fold and the increase appears to be due to accumulation of the nucleotide mainly in mononuclear cells (MANGIANELLO et al., 1971). CB-treated human neutrophils exposed to zymosan respond with only modest increments in cAMP. However, when the cells are incubated with compounds which produce small increases in cAMP levels and are then exposed to zymosan, the cAMP burst is enhanced and sustained. The reason for this is not apparent. It is possible that adenylate cyclase stimulated by zymosan contact with the plasma membrane acts synergistically with adenylate cyclase stimulated by the test compound to produce the striking elevation in cAMP. There is evidence (PETERSON and EDELMAN, 1964; FLORES et al., 1975) for the existence of two distinct adenylate cyclases controlling sodium transport and water flow in toad bladder and for the presence of two distinct pools of cAMP within the same cell. Thus, intracellular shifts of cyclic nucleotides may help regulate cell function.

Exogenous cGMP and compounds which enhance its intracellular concentration *enhance* secretion of lysosomal hydrolases from human leucocytes (ZURIER et al., 1974; IGNARRO, 1974; IGNARRO and GEORGE, 1974b; IGNARRO et al., 1974; GOLDSTEIN et al., 1973), results which are concordant with studies in which the introduction of cGMP analogues to sensitized lung tissue was associated with enhancement of antigen-induced release of histamine and SRS-A (ORANGE et al., 1971a, 1971b). In addition, PMN are able to mediate the immunologically specific cytolysis of antibody-coated target cells—antibody-dependent cellular cytotoxicity (ADCC). Agents capable of elevating intracellular cAMP and exogenous cAMP, inhibit PMN mediated ADCC, whereas cholinergic agents which elevate cGMP concentrations enhance ADCC. This reciprocal relationship between cGMP and cAMP, whether exogenously added or endogenously accumulated after appropriate stimulation, has been observed in other biological systems. Thus, exogenous cAMP inhibits the uptake of uridine, leucine and 2-deoxyglucose by cultured mouse fibroblasts, an effect counteracted by cGMP (KRAM and TOMKINS, 1973). In addition, exogenous cAMP as well as agents that elevate intracellular concentrations of cAMP prevent the transformation of lymphocytes by phytohemagglutinin (HIRSCHHORN et al., 1970; SMITH et al., 1971), and prevent the cytotoxic actions of lymphocytes upon cells bearing alloantigens to which they are sensitized (HENNEY et al., 1971), whereas cholinergic agents enhance the cytotoxicity of lymphocytes (STROM et al., 1972). Indeed, mitogenic concentrations of PHA have been shown to produce 10–50-fold increments in the concentrations of lymphocyte cGMP whereas lymphocyte cAMP was not elevated (HADDEN et al., 1972).

A unique protein kinase, active upon histone, has been isolated from purified human PMN (TSUNG et al., 1972). This enzyme phosphorylates a number of substrates when exposed to cAMP but not when exposed to cGMP. At present no enzyme has been isolated of which the activity is uniquely susceptible to stimulation by cGMP. It has been shown (LOUIE and DIXON, 1973) that phosphorylation of histone promotes disassembly of histones; such experiments provide a precedent for disassembly of tubulin after protein kinase mediated phosphorylation. Thus, it is possible that cAMP and cGMP affect the state of assembly of microtubules in PMN, which in turn regulates the flow of lysosomes and the secretion of enzymes to the outside. In fact, it has been demonstrated (WEISSMANN et al., 1975) that the number of microtubules observed in thin sections of normal human PMN is enhanced greatly after brief exposure of cells to agents which elevate cGMP levels.

Alternatively, or additionally, cAMP may play a dual role. For example, the nucleotide could first stimulate phosphorylation of proteins and later activate a phosphatase, which in turn cleaves phosphate from the phosphorylated protein (ABELL and MONAHAN, 1973). Some evidence is available to suggest that cAMP may control phosphatase in cells (KOYAMA et al., 1972; DELORENZO et al., 1973). In the liver cell, the protein kinase system (cAMP-dependent) phosphorylates the enzyme which catalyzes both formation and breakdown of glycogen. However, the synthetase is more catalytically active in its dephosphorylated form. Thus, the cAMP-dependent protein kinase when activated simultaneously stimulates glycogen breakdown and inhibits its formation. This dual control obviates the possibility that the nucleotide effect would simply be enhanced synthesis to keep pace with accelerated breakdown. It is conceivable that a similar mechanism regulates microtubule assembly/disassembly in leucocytes.

The reciprocal relationships between cAMP and cGMP can be demonstrated not only when these agents are added exogenously, but also when compounds which influence their endogenous accumulation are used.

It is not clear, of course, whether the nucleotides influence microtubule assembly directly or via membrane effects (or both). It has been shown (IGNARRO and COLUMBO, 1973) that osmotic release of β-glucuronidase from guinea pig PMN lysosomes is inhibited by cAMP and accelerated by cGMP. In addition, an increase in cAMP in rat mast cells prevents complement mediated cytolysis and osmotic lysis, as assessed by both histamine release and vital dye exclusion (KALINER and AUSTEN, 1974). Thus, the cyclic nucleotides may alter cellular and/or granular membranes and thereby influence intracellular events.

G. Summary

The precise roles of lysosomal enzymes in initiation, perpetuation, and modulation of the inflammatory response are not well understood. Control mechanisms which determine release from inflammatory cells of lysosomal enzymes appear to be influenced in part by cyclic nucleotides. Further delineation of the biochemical events regulated by cyclic nucleotides may well dictate new approaches to the management of patients with diseases characterized by chronic inflammation and tissue injury.

References

Abell,C.W., Monahan,T.M.: The role of adenosine 3'5'-cyclic monophosphate in the regulation of mammalian cell division. J. Cell Biol. **59**, 549—558 (1973)
Ali,S.Y., Evans,L.: Purification of rabbit kidney cytokinase and a comparison of its properties with human urokinase. Biochem. J. **107**, 293—303 (1968)
Ali,S.Y., Lack,C.H.: Studies in the tissue activator of plasminogen. Distribution of activator and proteolytic activity in the subcellular fractions of rabbit kidney. Biochem. J. **96**, 63—74 (1965)
Allison,A.C.: Lysosomes and the toxicity of particulate pollutants. Arch. intern. Med. **128**, 131—139 (1971)
Anderson,A.J.: Lysosomal enzyme activity in rats with adjuvant-induced arthritis. Ann. rheum. Dis. **29**, 307—314 (1970)
Baggiolini,M., Hirsch,J., de Duve,C.: Further biochemical and morphological studies of granule fractions from rabbit heterophil leukocytes. J. Cell Biol. **45**, 586—597 (1970)
Bainton,D.F.: Sequential discharge of polymorphonuclear leukocyte granules during phagocytosis of microorganisms. J. Cell Biol. **47**, 11 a, abstract (1970)
Bainton,D.F., Farquhar,M.G.: Origin of granules in polymorphonuclear leukocytes. Two types derived from opposite faces of the Golgi complex in developing granulocytes. J. Cell Biol. **28**, 277—301 (1966)
Bainton,D.F., Farquhar,M.: Differences in enzyme content of azurophil and specific granules of polymorphonuclear leukocytes. I. Histochemical staining of bone marrow smears. J. Cell Biol. **39**, 256—298 (1968 a)
Bainton,D.F., Farquhar,M.G.: Differences in enzyme content of azurophil and specific granules of polymorphonuclear leukocytes. II. Cytochemistry and electron microscopy of bone marrow cells. J. Cell Biol. **39**, 299—371 (1968 b)
Bainton,D.F., Ullyot,J.L., Farquhar,M.G.: The development of neutrophilic polymorphonuclear leukocytes in human bone marrow. J. exp. Med. **134**, 907—934 (1971)
Barland,P., Novikoff,A.B., Hammerman,D.: Lysosomes in the synovial membrane in rheumatoid arthritis: mechanism for cartilage erosion. Trans. Ass. Amer. Phycns **77**, 239—246 (1964)
Barnhart,M.I., Quintana,C., Lenon,H.L., Bluhm,G.B., Riddle,J.M.: Proteases in inflammation. Ann. N.Y. Acad. Sci. **146**, 527—532 (1968)
Barrett,A.J.: Properties of lysosomal enzymes. In: Lysosomes in Biology and Pathology, Vol. II, pp. 245—312. Amsterdam-London: North-Holland 1969
Barrett,A.J.: The enzymic degradation of cartilage matrix. In: Dynamics of Connective Tissue Macromolecules, pp. 189—226. Amsterdam-Oxford: North-Holland 1975
Barrett,A.J., Dingle,J.T.: A lysosomal component capable of binding cations and a carcinogen. Biochem. J. **105**, 208 (1967)
Barrett,A.J., Starkey,P.M.: The interaction of α_2-macroglobulin with proteinases. Characterization and specificity of the reaction, and a hypothesis concerning the molecular mechanism. Biochem. J. **133**, 709—724 (1973)
Bazin,S., Delanay,A.: Role of cathepsins in granulation tissue. J. dent. Res. **51**, 244—250 (1962)
Bensch,K.G., Malawista,S.E.: Microtubule crystals: a new biophysical phenomenon induced by Vinca alkaloids. Nature (Lond.) **218**, 1176—1178 (1968)
Bourne,H.R., Lehrer,R.I., Lichtenstein,L.M., Weissmann,G., Zurier,R.B.: Effects of cholera enterotoxin on cyclic AMP and neutrophil function. Comparison with other compounds which stimulate leucocyte adenylcyclase. J. clin. Invest. **52**, 698—708 (1973)

Brandes, D.: Observations on the apparent mode of formation of "pure" lysosomes. J. Ultrastruct. Res. **12**, 63—80 (1965)
Bretz, U., Baggiolini, M.: Biochemical and morphological characterization of azurophil and specific granules of human neutrophilic and polymorphonuclear leukocytes. J. Cell Biol. **63**, 251—269 (1974)
Broadus, A. E., Hardman, J. G., Kaminsky, N. I., Ball, J. H., Sutherland, E. W., Liddle, G. W.: Extracellular cyclic nucleotides. Ann. N.Y. Acad. Sci. **185**, 50—62 (1971)
Cochrane, C. G., Unanue, E. R., Dixon, F. J.: A role for polymorphonuclear leukocytes and complement in nephrotoxic nephritis. J. exp. Med. **122**, 99—109 (1965)
Cohn, Z. A., Fedorko, M. E., Hirsch, J. G.: The in vitro differentiation of mononuclear phagocytes. V. The formation of macrophage lysosomes. J. exp. Med. **123**, 756—766 (1966)
Cook, G. M. W.: The Golgi apparatus: form and function. In: Lysosomes in Biology and Pathology, Vol. III, pp. 237—271. Amsterdam-London: North-Holland 1973
Cox, J. P., Karnovsky, M. L.: The depression of phagocytosis by exogenous cyclic nucleotides, prostaglandins and theophylline. J. Cell Biol. **59**, 480—490 (1973)
Davies, P., Rita, G. A., Krakauer, K., Weissmann, G.: Characterization of a neutral protease from lysosomes of rabbit polymorphonuclear leucocytes. Biochem. J. **123**, 559—569 (1971)
Davies, P., Allison, A. C., Hylotar, W. J.: The identification, properties and subcellular distribution of cathepsins B and C (dipeptidyl aminopeptidase 1) in human peripheral blood leucocytes. Biochem. Soc. Trans. **2**, 432—434 (1974)
de Duve, C., Berthet, J., Hers, H. G., Dupret, L.: Le systeme hexose phosphatique. I. Existence d'une glucose 6-phosphatase specifique dans la foie. Bull. Soc. Chem. biol. (Paris) **31**, 1242—1253 (1949)
de Duve, C.: Lysosomes. A new group of cytoplasmic particles. In: Hiyashi, T. (Ed.): Subcellular Particles, pp. 128—159. New York: Ronald Press 1959
de Duve, C.: The separation and characterization of subcellular particles. Harvey Lect. Ser. **59**, 49—88 (1965)
Delorenzo, R. J., Walton, K. G., Curran, P. F., Greengard, P.: Regulation of phosphorylation of a specific protein in toad bladder membrane by antidiuretic hormone and cyclic AMP and its possible relation to membrane permeability changes. Proc. nat. Acad. Sci. (Wash.) **70**, 880—884 (1973)
Deshazo, C. V., Mcgrade, M. T., Henson, P. M., Cochrane, C. G.: The effect of complement depletion of neutrophil migration in acute immunologic arthritis. J. Immunol. **108**, 1414—1422 (1972)
Dingle, J. T., Barrett, A. J., Weston, P. D.: Characteristics of immunoinhibition and the confirmation of a role in cartilage breakdown. Biochem. J. **123**, 1—3 (1971)
Dingle, J. T., Barrett, A. J., Poole, A. R., Stovin, P.: Inhibition by pepstatin of human cartilage degradation. Biochem. J. **127**, 443—444 (1972)
Dingle, J. T., Poole, A. R., Lazarus, G. S., Barrett, A. J.: Immunoinhibition of intracellular protein digestion in macrophages. J. exp. Med. **137**, 1124—1141 (1973)
Estensen, R. D., White, J. G., Holmes, B.: Specific degranulation of human polymorphonuclear leukocytes. Nature (Lond.) **248**, 347—348 (1974)
Ferencik, M., Stefanovic, J.: The interaction of protein substrates (antigens) during an in vitro degradation by rabbit cathepsin D. Folia microbiol. (Praha) **18**, 402—409 (1973)
Flores, J., Witkum, P. A., Beckman, B., Sharp, G. W. G.: Stimulation of osmotic water flow in toad bladder by prostaglandin E_1. Evidence for different compartments of cyclic AMP. J. clin. Invest. **56**, 256—262 (1975)
Förster, O.: Nature and origin of proteases in the immunologically induced inflammatory reaction. J. dent. Res. **51**, 257—263 (1972)
Friend, D. S., Farquhar, M. G.: Functions of coated vesicles during protein absorption in the rat vas deferens. J. Cell Biol. **35**, 357—376 (1967)
Gemsa, D., Steggemann, L., Menzel, J., Till, G.: Release of cyclic AMP from macrophages by stimulation with prostaglandins. J. Immunol. **114**, 1422—1424 (1975)
Ghetie, V., Mihaescu, S.: The hydrolysis of rabbit immunoglubulin G with purified cathepsins D and E. Immunochemistry **10**, 251—255 (1973)
Gillespie, E.: Colchicine binding in tissue slices. Decrease by calcium and biphasic effect of adenosine 3′5′-monophosphate. J. Cell Biol. **50**, 544—549 (1971)

Goldstein, I. M., Hoffstein, S., Gallin, J., Weissmann, G.: Mechanisms of lysosomal enzyme release from human leukocytes: microtubule assembly and membrane fusion induced by a component of complement. Proc. nat. Acad. Sci. (Wash.) **70**, 2916—2920 (1973)

Goldstein, I. M., Hoffstein, S., Weissmann, G.: Influence of divalent cations upon complement-mediated enzyme release from human polymorphonuclear leukocytes. J. Immunol. **115**, 665—670 (1975)

Goldstein, I. M., Horn, J. K., Kaplan, H. B., Weissmann, G.: Calcium induced lysozyme secretion from human polymorphonuclear leukocytes. Biochem. biophys. Res. Commun. **60**, 807—812 (1974)

Goldstein, I. M., Weissmann, G.: Generation of C5-derived lysosomal enzyme-releasing activity (C5a) by lysates of leukocyte lysosomes. J. Immunol. **113**, 1583—1588 (1974)

Goldstone, A., Szabo, E., Koenig, H.: Isolation and characterization of acidic lipoprotein in renal and hepatic lysosomes. Life Sci. **9**, 607—616 (1970)

Golub, E. S., Spitznagel, J. K.: The role of lysosomes in hypersensitivity reactions: tissue damage by polymorphonuclear neutrophil lysosomes. J. Immunol. **95**, 1060—1066 (1966)

Greenbaum, L. M.: Cathepsins and kinin-forming and destroying enzymes. In: The Enzymes, 3rd. Ed., Vol. III, pp. 475—483. New York: Academic Press 1971

Greenbaum, L. M., Yamafuji, K.: The in vitro inactivation and formation of plasma kinins by spleen cathepsins. Brit. J. Pharmacol. **27**, 230—238 (1966)

Greenbaum, L. M., Grebow, P., Johnston, M., Prakash, A., Semente, G.: Pepstatin, an inhibitor of leukokinin formation and ascitic fluid accumulation. Cancer Res. **35**, 706—710 (1975)

Hadden, J. W., Hadden, E. M., Haddox, M. K., Goldberg, N. D.: Guanosine 3′5′-cyclic monophosphate: a possible intracellular mediator of mitogenic influences in lymphocytes. Proc. nat. Acad. Sci. (Wash.) **69**, 3024—3027 (1972)

Hawiger, J., Collins, R. D., Horn, R. G.: Precipitation of soluble fibrin monomer complexes by lysosomal protein fraction of polymorphonuclear leukocytes. Proc. Soc. exp. Biol. (N.Y.) **131**, 349—353 (1969)

Hawkins, D.: Biopolymer membrane: a model system for the study of the neutrophilic leukocyte response to immune complexes. J. Immunol. **107**, 344—352 (1971)

Hawkins, D.: Neutrophilic leukocytes in immunologic reactions in vitro: effect of cytochalasin B. J. Immunol. **110**, 284—286 (1973)

Hawkins, D.: Neutrophilic leukocytes in immunologic reactions in vitro. III. Pharmacologic modulation of lysosomal constituent release. Clin. Immunol. Immunopath. **2**, 141—151 (1974)

Helminen, H. J., Ericsson, J. L. E.: On the mechanism of lysosomal enzyme secretion: electron microscopic and histochemical studies on the epithelial cells of the rat's ventral prostate lobe. J. Ultrastruct. Res. **33**, 528—549 (1970)

Henney, C. S., Bourne, H. R., Lehrer, R. I., Cline, M. J., Melmon, K. L.: Cyclic AMP in the human leucocyte: synthesis, degradation and effects on neutrophil candidacidal activity. J. clin. Invest. **50**, 920—930 (1971)

Henson, P. M.: The immunologic release of constituents from neutrophil leukocytes. I. The role of antibody and complement on nonphagocytosable surfaces or phagocytosable particles. J. Immunol. **107**, 1535—1546 (1971a)

Henson, P. M.: The immunologic release of constituents from neutrophil leukocytes. II. Mechanisms of release during phagocytosis and adherence to non-phagocytosable surfaces. J. Immunol. **107**, 1547—1557 (1971b)

Henson, P. M.: Interaction of cells with immune complexes: adherence, release of constituents and tissue injury. J. exp. Med. **134**, 114s—135s (1971c)

Henson, P. M.: Pathologic mechanisms in neutrophil mediated injury. Amer. J. Path. **68**, 593—612 (1972)

Henson, P. M., Oades, Z. G.: Enhancement of immunologically induced granule exocytosis from neutrophils by cytochalasin B. J. Immunol. **110**, 290—293 (1973)

Henson, P. M., Oades, Z. G.: Stimulation of human neutrophils by soluble and insoluble immunoglobulin aggregates. J. clin. Invest. **56**, 1053—1061 (1975)

Herion, J. C., Spitznagel, J. K., Walker, R. I., Zeya, H. I.: Pyrogenicity of granulocyte lysosomes. Amer. J. Physiol. **211**, 693—699 (1966)

Hirschhorn, R., Grossmann, R. J., Weissmann, G.: Effect of cyclic AMP and theophylline on lymphocyte transformation. Proc. Soc. exp. Biol. (N.Y.) **133**, 1361—1365 (1970)
Humphrey, J. H.: The mechanism of the Arthus reaction. I. The role of polymorphonuclear leukocytes and other factors in reversed passive Arthus reactions in rabbits. Brit. J. exp. Path. **36**, 268—279 (1955)
Ignarro, L. J.: Nonphagocytic release of neutral protease and B-glucuronidase from human neutrophils. Regulation by autonomic neurohormones and cyclic nucleotides. Arthr. Rheum. **17**, 25—36 (1974)
Ignarro, L. J., Columbo, C.: Enzyme release from polymorphonuclear leukocyte lysosomes: regulation by autonomic drugs and cyclic nucleotides. Science **180**, 1181—1183 (1973)
Ignarro, L. J., George, W. J.: Mediation of immunologic discharge of lysosomal enzymes from human neutrophils by guanosine 3′, 5′-monophosphate. J. exp. Med. **140**, 225—238 (1974a)
Ignarro, L. J., George, W. J.: Hormonal control of lysosomal enzyme release from human neutrophils: elevation of cyclic nucleotide levels by autonomic neurohormones. Proc. nat. Acad. Sci. (Wash.) **71**, 2027—2031 (1974b)
Ignarro, L. J., Lint, T. F., George, W. J.: Hormonal control of lysosomal enzyme release from human neutrophils. Effects of autonomic agents on enzyme release, phagocytosis and cyclic nucleotide levels. J. exp. Med. **139**, 1395—1414 (1974)
Janoff, A., Zeligs, J. D.: Vascular injury and lysis of basement membrane in vitro by neutral protease of human leukocytes. Science **161**, 702—704 (1968)
Janoff, A., Zweifach, B. W.: Adhesion and emigration of leukocytes produced by cationic proteins of lysosomes. Science **144**, 1456—1460 (1964)
Jensen, M. S., Bainton, D. F.: Temporal changes in pH within the phagocytic vacuole of the polymorphonuclear neutrophilic leukocyte. J. Cell Biol. **56**, 379—388 (1973)
John, S., Berger, N., Bonner, M. J., Schultz, J.: Localization of lactic dehydrogenase isozymes in lysosomal fraction of the neutrophil of normal human blood. Nature (Lond.) **215**, 1483—1485 (1967)
Kaliner, M., Austen, K. F.: Adenosine 3′5′-monophosphate: inhibition of complement-mediated cell lysis. Science **183**, 659—661 (1974)
Kakimoto, T., Oshima, G., Yeh, H. S. J., Erdös, E. G.: Purification of lysosomal prolylcarboxypeptidase angiotensinase C. Biochim. biophys. Acta. **302**, 178—182 (1973)
Kang, A. H., Nagai, Y., Piez, K. A., Gross, J.: Studies on the structure of collagen using collagenolytic enzyme from tadpole. Biochemistry **5**, 509—517 (1966)
Keisari, Y., Witz, J. P.: Degradation of immunoglobulins by lysosomal enzymes of tumors. I. Demonstration of the phenomenon using mouse tumor. Immunochemistry **10**, 565—570 (1973)
Kelley, L. A., Butcher, R. W.: The effects of epinephrine and prostaglandin E_1 on cyclic adenosine 3′:5′-monophosphate levels in WI-38 fibroblasts. J. biol. Chem. **249**, 3098—3102 (1974)
Kerby, G. P., Taylor, S. M.: Enzymatic activity in human synovial fluid from rheumatoid and non-rheumatoid patients. Proc. Soc. exp. Biol. (N.Y.) **126**, 865—869 (1967)
Kniker, W. T., Cochrane, C. G.: Pathogenic factors in vascular lesions of experimental serum sickness. J. exp. Med. **122**, 83—91 (1965)
Koyama, H., Kato, R., Ono, T.: Induction of alkaline phosphatase by cyclic AMP or its dibutyryl derivative in a hybrid line between mouse and chinese hamster in culture. Biochem. biophys. Res. Commun. **46**, 305—311 (1972)
Kram, R., Tomkins, G. M.: Pleiotypic control by cyclic AMP. Interaction with cyclic GMP and possible role of microtubules. Proc. nat. Acad. Sci. (Wash.) **70**, 1659—1663 (1973)
Lazarus, G. S.: The role of neutral proteinase and cathepsin D in turpentine induced inflammation. J. invest. Derm. **62**, 367—371 (1974)
Lazarus, G. S., Brown, R. S., Daniels, J. R., Fullmer, H. M.: Human granulocyte collagenase. Science **159**, 1483—1485 (1968a)
Lazarus, G. S., Daniels, J. R., Brown, R. S., Bladen, H. A., Fullmer, H. M.: Degradation of collagen by a human granulocyte collagenolytic system. J. clin. Invest. **47**, 2622—2632 (1968b)
Lazarus, G. S., Daniels, J. R., Lian, J., Burleigh, M. C.: Role of granulocyte collagenase in collagen degradation. Amer. J. Path. **68**, 565—573 (1972)
Lazarus, G. S., Dingle, J. T.: Cathepsin D of rabbit skin: an immunoenzymic study. J. invest. Derm. **62**, 61—66 (1974)

Lebez, D., Kapitar, M., Turk, V., Kregar, I.: Comparison of properties of cathepsins D and E with some new cathepsins, pp. 167—176. In: Tissue Proteinases. Amsterdam-Oxford: North-Holland 1971

Lefell, M. S., Spitznagel, J. K.: Association of lactoferrin with lysozyme in granules of human polymorphonuclear leukocytes. Infect. Immun. **6**, 761—765 (1972)

Louie, A. J., Dixon, G. H.: Kinetics of phosphorylation and dephosphorylation of testis histones and their possible role in determining chromosomal structure. Nature (New Biol.) **243**, 164—168 (1973)

McCarty, D. J., Hollander, J. L.: Identification of urate crystals in gouty synovial fluid. Ann. intern. Med. **54**, 452—460 (1961)

Mangianello, V., Evans, W. H., Stossel, T. P., Mason, R. J., Vaughan, M.: The effect of polystyrene beads on cyclic AMP concentration in leucocytes. J. clin. Invest. **50**, 2741—2744 (1971)

Marsland, D., Tilney, L. G., Hirshfield, M.: Stabilizing effects of D_2O on the microtubular components and needle-like form of heliozoan axopods—a pressure-temperature analysis. J. cell. Physiol. **77**, 187—193 (1971)

Metchnikoff, E.: Immunity in Infective Diseases, 1905. Reprinted, New York: Johnson Reprint Corp. 1968

Morrison, R. J. G., Barrett, A. J., Dingle, J. T., Prior, D.: Cathepsins B_1 and D action on human cartilage proteoglycans. Biochim. biophys. Acta **302**, 411—419 (1973)

Movat, H. Z., Poon, M. C., Takeuchi, Y.: The kinin system of human plasma. I. Isolation of a low molecular weight activator of prekallikrein. Int. Arch. Allergy **40**, 89—98 (1971)

Novikoff, A. B.: In: Brachet, J., Mirsky, A. E. (Eds.): The Cell, Vol. II, pp. 423—488. New York: Academic Press 1961

Novikoff, A. B., Essner, E., Quintana, N.: Golgi apparatus and lysosomes. Fed. Proc. **23**, 1010—1022 (1964)

Olsson, J.: Isolation of human leukocyte granules using colloidal silica-polysaccharide density gradients. Exp. Cell Res. **54**, 325—330 (1969)

Orange, R. P., Austen, W. G., Austen, K. F.: Immunological release of histamine and slow reacting substance of anaphylaxis from human lung. I. Modulation by agents influencing cellular levels of cyclic AMP. J. exp. Med. **134**, 136 s—148 s (1971 a)

Orange, R. P., Kaliner, M. A., Laraia, P. J., Austen, K. F.: Immunological release of histamine and slow reacting substance of anaphylaxis from human lung. II. Influence of cellular levels of cyclic AMP. Fed. Proc. **30**, 1725—1729 (1971 b)

Parish, W. E.: Effects of neutrophils on tissues: experiments on the Arthus reaction, the flare phenomenon, and post phagocytic release of lysosomal enzymes. Brit. J. Derm. **81**, 28—40 (1969)

Park, B. H., Good, R. A., Beck, N. P., Davis, A. B.: Concentration of cyclic AMP in human leucocyte during phagocytosis. Nature (Lond.) **229**, 27—29 (1971)

Parker, C. W., Smith, J. W.: Alterations in cyclic AMP metabolism in human bronchial asthma. I. Leukocyte responsiveness to β-adrenergic agents. J. clin. Invest. **52**, 48—59 (1973)

Pesanti, E. L., Axline, S. G.: Phagolysosomal formation in normal and colchicine-treated macrophages. J. exp. Med. **142**, 903—913 (1975)

Peterson, M. J., Edelman, I. S.: Calcium inhibition of the action of vasopressin on the urinary bladder of the toad. J. clin. Invest. **42**, 583—594 (1964)

Pryce-Jones, R. H., Wood, G. C.: Neutral proteinase activity in the cells of synovial fluids from rheumatoid patients. In: Dynamics of Connective Tissue Macromolecules, pp. 227—242. Amsterdam-Oxford: North-Holland 1975

Purcell, G. M., Barnhart, M. J.: Prothrombin activation with cathepsin C. Biochim. biophys. Acta **78**, 800—802 (1963)

Ranadive, N. S., Cochrane, C. G.: Isolation and characterization of permeability factors from rabbit neutrophils. J. exp. Med. **128**, 605—622 (1968)

Robertson, P. B., Ryel, R. B., Taylor, R. E., Shyn, K. W., Fullmer, H. M.: Collagenase: localization in polymorphonuclear neutrophils in the rabbit. Science **177**, 64—65 (1972)

Saba, H., Roberts, H. R., Herion, J. C.: The anticoagulant activity of lysosomal cationic proteins from polymorphonuclear leukocytes. J. clin. Invest. **46**, 580—588 (1967)

Sandhaus, R., Janoff, A.: Degradation of human α_1-antitrypsin by hepatocyte-acid cathepsins. Rev. resp. Dis. **110**, 263—272 (1974)

Sato, H., Sasazuki, T., Tsuno, H., Nakajima, H.: Studies on haptoglobin. IX. Effect of haptoglobin on hydrolysis of hemoglobin by some proteases. Proc. Jap. Acad. **49**, 549—554 (1973)

Scherer, J., Janoff, A.: Mediators of inflammation of leukocyte lysosomes. VII. Observations on mast cell rupturing agents in different species. Lab. Invest. **18**, 196—201 (1968)

Schultz, J., Corlin, R., Oddi, F., Kaminker, K., Jones, W.: Myeloperoxidase of leukocytes of normal human blood. III. Isolation of the peroxidase granule. Arch. Biochem. **111**, 73—79 (1965)

Schumacher, H. R., Agudelo, C. A.: Intravascular degranulation of neutrophils: an important factor in inflammation? Science **175**, 1139—1141 (1972)

Smith, C., Hamerman, D.: Acid phosphatase in human synovial fluid. Arthr. Rheum. **5**, 411—419 (1962)

Smith, J. W., Steiner, A. L., Parker, C. W.: Human lymphocyte metabolism. Effects of cyclic and noncyclic nucleotides on stimulation by phytohemagglutinin. J. clin. Invest. **50**, 442—448 (1971)

Smith, R. J., Ignarro, L. J.: Bioregulation of lysosomal enzyme secretion from human neutrophils: roles of guanosine 3′:5′-monophosphate and calcium in stimulus-secretion coupling. Proc. nat. Acad. Sci. (Wash.) **72**, 108—112 (1975)

Snyderman, R., Phillips, J. K., Mergenhagen, S. E.: Biological activity of complement in vitro. J. exp. Med. **134**, 1131—1143 (1971)

Spitznagel, J. K., Daldorf, F. G., Leffell, M. S., Folds, J. D.: Azurophil and specific granules resolved for human polymorphs (PMN); immunochemistry, biochemistry, enzyme histochemistry. J. clin. Invest. **52**, 80a (1973)

Stetson, C. A.: Similarities in the mechanisms determining the Arthus and Schwartzman phenomenon. J. exp. Med. **94**, 347—355 (1951)

Strom, T. B., Deisseroth, A., Morganroth, J., Carpenter, C. B., Merrill, J. P.: Alteration of the cytotoxic action of sensitizer lymphocytes by cholinergic agents and activators of adenylate cyclase. Proc. nat. Acad. Sci. (Wash.) **69**, 2995—2999 (1972)

Tappel, A. L.: Lysosomal enzymes and other components. In: Lysosomes in Biology and Pathology, Vol. II, pp. 207—244. Amsterdam-London: North-Holland 1969

Taubman, S. B., Goldschmidt, P. R., Lepow, I. H.: Effects of lysosomal enzymes from human leukocytes on human complement components. Fed. Proc. **29**, 434, Abstract (1970)

Thomas, L.: Possible role of leucocyte granules in the Schwartzman and Arthus Reactions. Proc. Soc. exp. Biol. **115**, 235—241 (1964)

Tsung, P.-K., Hermina, N., Weissmann, G.: Inosine 3′5′-monophosphate and adenosine 3′5′-monophosphate-dependent protein kinase from human PMN leucocytes. Biochem. biophys. Res. Commun. **49**, 1657—1662 (1972)

Umezawa, H., Aoyagi, T., Morishima, H., Matsuzaki, M., Hamada, M., Takeuchi, T.: Pepstatin, a new pepsin inhibitor produced by actinomycetes. J. Antibiot. (Tokyo) **23**, 259—269 (1970)

Vaes, G., Eechout, Y.: Procollagenase and its activation. In: Dynamics of Connective Tissue Macromolecules, pp. 129—146. Amsterdam-Oxford: North-Holland 1975

Vallota, E. H., Müller-Eberhard, H. J.: Formation of C3a and C5a anaphylatoxins in whole human serum after inhibition of the anaphylatoxin inactivator. J. exp. Med. **137**, 1109—1124 (1973)

Ward, P. A.: Chemotaxis of mononuclear cells. J. exp. Med. **128**, 1201—1211 (1968)

Ward, P. A., Hill, J. H.: C5 chemotactic fragments produced by an enzyme in lysosomal granules of neutrophils. J. Immunol. **104**, 535—543 (1970)

Ward, P. A., Zvaifler, N. J.: Complement-derived leukotactic factors in inflammatory synovial fluids of humans. J. clin. Invest. **50**, 606—616 (1971)

Wasserman, S. I., Goetzl, E. J., Austen, K. F.: Inactivation of slow reacting substance of anaphylaxis by human eosinophil anylsulfatase. J. Immunol. **114**, 645—649 (1975)

Weisenberg, R. C., Borisy, G. G., Taylor, E. W.: The colchicine-binding protein of mammalian brain and its relation to microtubules. Biochemistry **7**, 4466—4474 (1968)

Weissmann, G., Dukor, P.: The role of lysosomes in immune responses. Advanc. Immunol. **12**, 283—331 (1970)

Weissmann, G., Dukor, P., Zurier, R. B.: Effect of cyclic AMP on release of lysosomal enzymes from phagocytes. Nature (New Biol.) **231**, 131—135 (1971)

Weissmann, G., Goldstein, I. M., Hoffstein, S., Chauvet, G., Robineaux, R.: Yin/Yang modulation of lysosomal enzyme release from polymorphonuclear leukocytes by cyclic nucleotides. Ann. N.Y. Acad. Sci. **256**, 222—232 (1975)
Weissmann, G., Spilberg, I., Krakauer, K.: Arthritis induced in rabbits by lysates of granulocyte lysosomes. Arthr. Rheum. **12**, 103—112 (1969)
Weissmann, G., Zurier, R. B., Hoffstein, S.: Leukocytic proteases and the immunologic release of lysosomal enzymes. Amer. J. Path. **68**, 539—564 (1972)
Welsh, I. R. H., Zeya, H. J., Spitznagel, J. K.: Heterogeneity of lysosomes from human peripheral blood polymorphonuclear leucocytes. Fed. Proc. **30**, 599, Abstract (1971)
West, B. C., Kimball, H. R.: Separation of human polymorphonuclear leucocytes (PMN) granules. Fed. Proc. **30**, 599, Abstract (1971)
Weston, P. D.: A specific antiserum to lysosomal cathepsin D. Immunology **17**, 421—428 (1969)
Weston, P. D., Barrett, A. J., Dingle, J. T.: Specific inhibition of cartilage breakdown. Nature (Lond.) **222**, 255—256 (1969)
White, J. G., Estensen, R. D.: Selective labilization of specific granules in polymorphonuclear leukocytes by phorbol myristate acetate. Amer. J. Path. **75**, 45—60 (1974)
Wright, D. G., Gallin, J. I.: Generation of chemotactic activity from serum by a product released from human polymorphonuclear leukocytes (PMN) during phagocytosis. Fed. Proc. **33**, 631, Abstract (1974)
Wright, D. G., Malawista, S. E.: The mobilisation and extracellular release of granular enzymes from human leukocytes during phagocytosis. J. Cell Biol. **53**, 788—797 (1972)
Wright, D. G., Malawista, S. E.: Mobilization and extracellular release of granular enzymes from human leukocytes during phagocytosis: Inhibition by colchicine and cortisol but not by salicylate. Arthr. Rheum. **16**, 749—758 (1973)
Zeya, H. I., Spitznagel, J. K.: Arginine-rich proteins of polymorphonuclear leukocyte lysosomes: antimicrobial specificity and biochemical heterogeneity. J. exp. Med. **127**, 927—935 (1968)
Zurier, R. B., Hoffstein, S., Weissmann, G.: Cytochalasin B: effect on lysosomal enzyme release from human leukocytes. Proc. nat. Acad. Sci. (Wash.) **70**, 844—848 (1973a)
Zurier, R. B., Hoffstein, S., Weissmann, G.: Mechanisms of lysosomal enzyme release from human leukocytes. I. Effects of cyclic nucleotides and colchicine. J. Cell Biol. **58**, 27—41 (1973b)
Zurier, R. B., Weissmann, G., Hoffstein, S., Kammerman, S., Tai, H. H.: Mechanisms of lysosomal enzyme release from human leukocytes. II. Effects of cAMP and cGMP, autonomic agonists and agents which affect microtubule function. J. clin. Invest. **53**, 297—309 (1974)

Chapter 10

Lymphokines

J. MORLEY

A. Discovery and Definition

Allergic responses can be broadly divided into antibody-mediated and cell-mediated responses. This division was first appreciated by ZINSSER (1925) who noted the delay in onset of skin reactions evoked in animals sensitized by intracellular parasites as compared with the relatively rapid response to antigen in animals sensitized by intradermal administration of protein antigen. An experimental basis for this distinction was provided by LANDSTEINDER and CHASE (1942), who demonstrated that delayed type hypersensitivity could be transferred to unsensitized guinea pigs by injection of live lymphoid cells from sensitized donor animals, but not by serum, dead cells or cell extracts. This contrasted with the immediate type of response which could be transferred to unsensitized animals by injection of serum and which was known to be attributable to immunoglobulins present in the serum. Subsequently, similar experimental evidence was obtained for other allergic responses of delayed onset, so that by the mid-1960s, there was general agreement as to the validity of grouping responses such as contact sensitivity, bacterial allergy and homograft rejection under the common heading of delayed hypersensitivity (TURK, 1967).

Notwithstanding such general agreement, the viewpoint persisted that delayed responses were attributable either to antibody absorbed onto mononuclear cells or to the local production of antibody, and in the absence, until recent years, of chemically defined antigens for delayed hypersensitivity reactions, this hypothesis was difficult to disprove. The considerable difficulties of establishing and maintaining such a classification are illustrated by the Jones-Mote reaction. This is a mild erythematous response to intradermal injection of antigen that is delayed in onset and appears in man or animals prior to demonstrable formation of antibodies (JONES and MOTE, 1934). The Jones-Mote reaction had been widely considered as a pure delayed hypersensitivity reaction, but more recently has been shown to be quite distinct (RICHERSON et al., 1970) despite fitting the criteria for a reaction of delayed hypersensitivity (cellular immunity) (i.e. cell transfer and hapten/carrier specificity) that were deemed adequate in 1967. In establishing a response as one of delayed hypersensitivity (cellular immunity), it would therefore seem worthwhile to include additional criteria to permit distinction from the Jones-Mote reaction.

The Jones-Mote reaction has three properties not seen in other delayed reactions: (1) transfer to unsensitized animals by serum (ASKONASE, 1973), (2) a prevalence of basophils in the skin reaction at 24 h (RICHERSON et al., 1970), and (3) the production of increased vascular permeability for a brief period early in the response, vascular permeability returning to normal within 24 h (MORLEY and WILLIAMS,

1973). The concept of delayed hypersensitivity (cellular immunity) as a response classification thus remains valid; its acceptance is of particular relevance to lymphokines as these materials are generally considered in the context of mediators of delayed hypersensitivity reactions.

The first indications that the cellular immune response might be attributable to a mediator stem from the work of RICH and LEWIS (1932), who studied the in vitro reaction of guinea pig spleen explants to old tuberculin. They showed that the emigration of cells from these explants was inhibited by antigen (old tuberculin) in sensitized, but not in normal animals. The subsequent demonstration by ARONSON (1933) that this phenomenon was a feature of antigens evoking delayed reactions but not of antigens evoking Arthus type of anaphylactic reactions, established this as an in vitro test for delayed hypersensitivity.

Despite the availability of this in vitro test system, adequate for demonstration of soluble mediator participation in reactions of cellular immunity (SVEJCAR et al., 1967), a period of over 20 years elaped before a satisfactory demonstration was achieved. In part, this was probably related to RICH and LEWIS's (1932) view that the interaction of antigen with the emigrating cells resulted in cell death, when by implication the inflammatory reaction of delayed hypersensitivity would be a secondary event to cell death. In fact, the histological features of delayed hypersensitivity are not those of a non-specific response to cell death, such as that evoked by intradermal injection of toxic agents. Delayed hypersensitivity reactions exhibit characteristic mononuclear cell infiltrates, particularly in the superficial dermis with perivascular cuffing of mononuclear cells around capillaries and small venules (GELL and HINDE, 1954; DVORAK, 1974). This histological picture indicates a rather specific sequence of cellular events that seem highly unlikely to be adequately explained simply in terms of an inflammatory response to local cell death. The first suggestion that these events were due to a mediator originating in lymphoid cells came from MARKS and JAMES (1953). By analogy with the release from mast cells of stored vasoactive amines capable of mimicking the anaphylactic response, these authors suggested that the lymphocyte might release preformed material to produce the inflammatory manifestations of delayed hypersensitivity. Experimental investigation of this concept led to the demonstration that lymphocytes contain *preformed* non-dialysable material (lymph node permeability factor—LNPF) (WILLOUGHBY et al., 1962). Interest in this biologically active material has been restricted, probably because of the emphasis on vascular manifestations of the response and because of the inability of LNPF preparations to mimic the in vitro cellular correlates of delayed hypersensitivity, such as stimulation of lymphocytes and macrophages.

In 1962, GEORGE and VAUGHAN introduced a technique for studying the emigration in vitro of inflammatory cell populations packed into capillary tubes (Fig. 1). Apart from its convenience and reproducibility in comparison with the use of explants, the particular advantage of this technique was that it permitted the use of mixtures of cell populations of different origin. With this technique, it was found that the reactivity of the cell population as a whole required as few as 2.5% of the cells to have been derived from sensitized animals (DAVID et al., 1964) and that the modification of cell migration produced by antigen was suppressed by inhibition of protein synthesis (DAVID, 1965). These observations are strongly suggestive of an amplification mechanism involving a mediator, and in 1966 DAVID showed that these cell

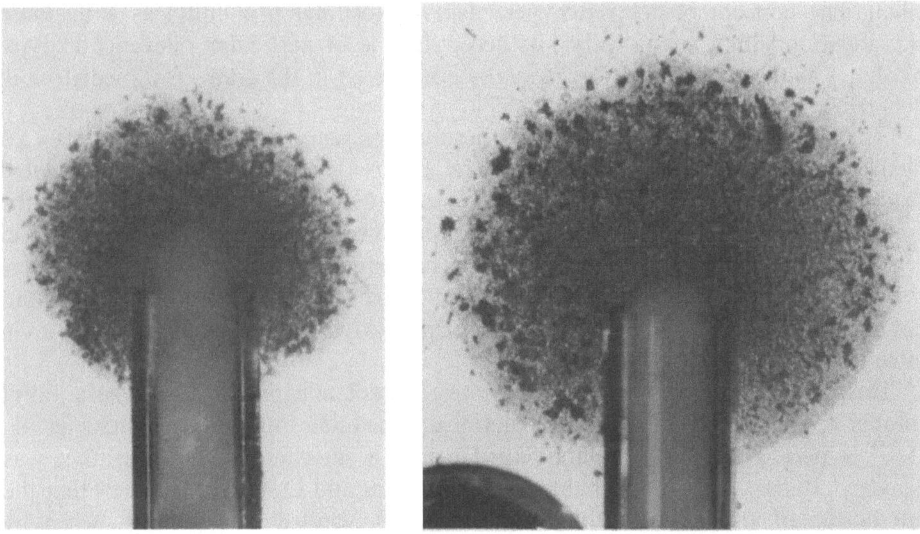

a b

Fig. 1. Inhibition of guinea pig macrophage migration by antigen. Figure 1a shows cells incubated in the presence of 5.0 (μg/ml) PPD in contrast to Figure 1b which shows cell migration in the absence of antigen (×20). (BRAY, unpublished observations)

populations released into the culture medium material capable of inhibiting the migration of both sensitized and unsensitized cell populations. At the same time, BLOOM and BENNETT (1966) demonstrated, by use of purified cell populations (macrophages >99.5% purity and lymphocytes >94% purity), that the migration of macrophages derived from sensitized animals was not inhibited by antigen whereas the migration of macrophages from non-sensitized animals was inhibited providing a small proportion (> 1%) of sensitized lymphocytes was present. This implied that the lymphocyte was the antigen responsive cell and that the macrophage serves as an effector cell responding to material released into the culture fluid, as was also confirmed by these authors (BLOOM and BENNETT, 1966). The fact that addition of antigen to extracts of sensitized cells could not reproduce the phenomenon of macrophage migration inhibition together with the effect of protein synthesis inhibitors on the production of this biological activity implied that in response to activation by specific antigen the lymphocytes generate non-specific material capable of modifying the in vitro migration of macrophages.

These observations are consistent with the proposition of MARKS and JAMES (1953) that the features of delayed hypersensitivity may be attributed to the release by sensitized lymphocytes of materials with biological properties appropriate to this type of reaction. It is clear that such materials are not preformed in the lymphocyte, as is the case for vasoactive amines in mast cells, but are generated and released following antigen activation. The active material in this test system was given the non-euphonious designation of 'migration inhibitory factor' (MIF). As there are several other in vitro tests involving the same or other cell types which could also be regarded as in vitro indicators of cellular immunity, analogous experiments were undertaken in these systems to demonstrate production of corresponding mediator material in response to antigenic stimulation (BLOOM, 1971; DAVID and DAVID, 1972; PICK and TURK, 1972; PEKÁREK and KREJČÍ, 1974). This resulted in a plethora of cumbersome terms, for in each instance the active material was described by reference to a biological action, together with its inevitable abbreviation. Examples are macrophage aggregating factor (MAF), mitogenic factor (MF) osteoclast activating factor (OAF) (see Table 1.). It was not established whether or not the active materials detected by one test were active on other test systems, and such a system for nomenclature is without limit. In 1969, it was proposed unilaterally that such products of lymphocyte activation be referred to by the generic term lymphokines (DUMONDE et al., 1969). In view of the possible involvement of kinins in the inflammatory response, the choice of this particular name is regrettable although, but for the author's veto, the term in use would have been lymphokinin. The rapidity with which the term lymphokine came into general use prompted a definition as:

> Soluble non-antibody products of lymphocyte activation by specific antigen, which produce increased vascular permeability following intradermal injection; which increase tritiated thymidine incorporation by cultured lymphocytes; and which inhibit macrophage migration in vitro. In the guinea pig, these lymphokines can be distinguished from classical immunoglobulins by their solubility in 40% saturated ammonium sulphate and by their behaviour on gel filtration chromatography. Lymphokines retain biological activity after removal of the antigen used to generate them, and, once induced, their biological activity is not dependent upon supplementation by specific antigen at the time of test. Because these substances are insufficiently characterized, it is possible that the generic term 'lymphokines' may in the future include additional biological activities (MORLEY et al., 1973).

This definition was not devised to exclude lymphokine activities other than mitogenic, inflammatory and migration inhibitory activities but merely reflected the activities that were well documented in the laboratory in which the term was coined.

A particular interest amongst immunologists has been to determine to what extent these materials depend upon the presence of antigens for the production of their biological actions, and hence to differentiate these substances from antibodies and other materials with antigenic specificity. GEORGE and VAUGHAN (1962) in their original description of the capillary test had shown that the phenomenon of macrophage migration inhibition in response to antigen was restricted to animals with cellular immunity and was not a property of cells derived from animals with strong antibody-mediated immunity but lacking cellular immunity. However, BLOOM and BENNETT, (1966) reported that following antigen activation of lymphocytes, supplementary antigen added to the culture media could enhance the inhibition of macrophage migration produced by such media. This raised the possibility that an antigen-dependent material was involved in producing macrophage migration inhibition and subsequently, by using purified protein derivative of tuberculin (PPD) or β-lactoglobulin conjugated to a polyaminopolystyrene matrix, AMOS and LACHMANN (1970) showed that in the guinea pig cell, migration inhibition had an obligatory dependence upon the presence of soluble antigen. Such antigen-dependent materials are neither immunoglobulins nor lymphokines. Additionally, it should be noted that these are not the only antigen-dependent materials capable of inhibiting macrophage migration in vitro as this is also a property of immune complexes (PICK and MANNHEIM, 1974). It is nonetheless clear that in other situations there is no evidence that supplementary antigen can affect migration inhibition (YOSHIDA et al., 1972). Fur-

Table 1. Lymphokine activities

Factor	Target cell
In vitro	
Migration inhibitory (MIF)	Macrophage
Macrophage aggregating (MAF)	Macrophage
Macrophage chemotactic (MCF)	Macrophage
Macrophage slowing	Macrophage
Macrophage arming	Macrophage
Macrophage mitogenic (MMF)	Macrophage
Factor affecting morphology	Macrophage
Macrophage activating	Macrophage
Blastogenic or mitogenic (MF)	Lymphocyte
Potentiating	Lymphocyte
Helper (cell co-operation)	Lymphocyte
Chemotactic	Lymphocyte
Immunosuppressive	Lymphocyte
Chemotactic	Eosinophil
Chemotactic	Neutrophils
Leucocyte migration inhibition (LIF)	Buffycoat cells
Osteoclast activation (OAF)	Osteoclasts
Lymphotoxin	Cultured cells (e. g. HeLa mouse cells)
Proliferation inhibition (PIF)	Cultured cells
Cloning inhibition (CIF)	Cultured cells
Interferon	Various cells
In vivo	
Macrophage disappearance (MDF)	Macrophage
Skin reactive (SRF)	Skin
Inflammatory (IF)	Skin
Lymph node activating	Lymph node (paracortex)
Lymph node activating	Lymph node (germinal centre)

thermore, although certain effects of lymphokines can be mimicked by antigen-dependent materials, lymphokines can readily be produced and detected in the absence of antigen, for example when lymphocytes are activated by plant mitogens such as concanavalin A (Con A) or Phytohaemagglutinin (PHA). Lymphokines can therefore be regarded as macromolecular products of lymphocyte activation with the capacity to act on a range of effector cells so as to mimic many of the features of a reaction of delayed hypersensitivity.

Activity	Reference
Inhibits migration	BLOOM and BENNETT (1966)
Enhances aggregation	LOLEKHA et al. (1970)
Stimulates migration through micropore filter	WARD et al. (1969)
Reduces electrophoretic mobility	CASPARY (1972)
Stimulates cytotoxicity	LOHMANN-MATTHES et al. (1973)
Stimulates proliferation	HADDEN et al. (1975)
Decreases spreading, motility, loss of pseudopodia, rounding up vacuolization	DEKARIS et al. (1971)
Increases spreading, increases metabolism	NATHAN et al. (1971)
Induces blastogenesis and increases thymidine incorporation	KASAKURA (1970)
Enhances ongoing transformation	JANIS and BACH (1970)
Enhances antibody forming cell production	MAILLARD and BLOOM (1972)
Stimulates migration through micropore filter	ALTMAN and KIRCHNER (1972)
Inhibits blast transformation	OUTTRIDGE and LEPPER (1973)
Stimulates migration through micropore filter	COHEN and WARD (1971)
Stimulates migration through micropore filter	WARD et al. (1970)
Inhibits migration	ROCKLIN (1974)
Causes decalcification of bone	HORTON et al. (1972)
Cytotoxic	KOLB and GRANGER (1970)
Inhibits proliferation	GREEN et al. (1970)
Inhibits cloning	LEBOWITZ and LAWRENCE (1971)
Protects against viral infection	GREEN et al. (1969)
Removes macrophages from peritoneal cavity	NELSON and BOYDEN (1963)
Causes inflammation of the skin	BENNETT and BLOOM (1968)
Increases vascular permeability	MORLEY and WILLIAMS (1972b)
Activates paracortex of lymph node	KELLY et al. (1972)
Causes cell proliferation in germinal centres	KELLY and WOLSTENCROFT (1974)

B. Method of Production

Lymphokines are prepared by the in vitro culture of lymphoid cells, either in the presence of antigen to which the cells will respond, or in the presence of non-specific polyclonal stimulants such as the plant mitogens. Lymphoid cells can be obtained from a variety of sources including the spleen, lymph nodes, peritoneal exudates, peripheral blood or thoracic duct. In the case of man, the most readily accessible cell population is peripheral blood. Whatever the origin of the lymphoid cell population, the yield of biological activity is low, i.e. the biological activity in the culture supernatant cannot be detected when subjected to substantial dilution. For this reason, considerable effort in both time and material must be expended to produce active lymphokine preparations in quantities sufficient to act as a reference material within a laboratory. For instance, groups of up to 40 animals were required to yield a sufficient quantity of each lymphokine preparation to obtain the data indicating the heterogeneity of these preparations summarized in Figure 6 (BRAY et al., 1976a). Not surprisingly, reference lymphokine preparations of established activity are not readily available. One possible solution would be to utilize cultured cell lines and it is therefore noteworthy that lymphoid cell lines spontaneously produce material which strongly inhibits macrophage migration (PAPAGEORGIOU et al., 1973). Such cell lines are of human origin and would seem worthy of further study, for the availability of active human lymphokine reference preparations would eliminate much inefficient laboratory effort presently directed towards their preparation. Another more recently reported source of lymphokine activity of possible relevance to standard preparations is in bacterial culture medium (YOSHIDA et al., 1975).

At present, it remains the practice of individual laboratories to produce their own lymphokine preparations. The conditions under which lymphokines are prepared vary between laboratories and have been documented by BLOOM and GLADE (1971), and MORLEY et al. (1973). Studies to determine optimal culture conditions for high yield of lymphokines are insubstantial, and evaluation of available data is hampered by the common practice in this area of research of gauging biological activity by testing at a single dose level. Furthermore, it should be noted that the selected culture conditions are often biased in favour of the preferred lymphokine test. In view of the heterogeneity of lymphokines (BRAY et al., 1976a), it is likely that optimal culture conditions for production of one activity may differ from those established for another activity. The study by FORD et al. (1976) of factors modifying the production of guinea pig lymphokines causing macrophage migration inhibition (MIF) and stimulating DNA synthesis in thymocytes (MF), illustrates this in that optimal production of the former is achieved at 10 μg antigen/ml whereas optimal production of the latter using the same cells is achieved by concentrations exceeding 2.5 mg antigen/ml.

Guinea pig lymphokine preparations that regularly exhibit mitogenic, migration inhibitory, inflammatory and chemotactic properties may be produced by the following protocol which is based upon systematic studies over several years by WOLSTENCROFT and co-workers.

Lymphoid cells are collected from animals sensitized, 10–14 days prior to sacrifice, by foot pad injection of an emulsion containing bovine gamma globulin in Freund's complete adjuvant with a total dose of 100 μg/animal. The lymphocytes used may be derived from teased lymph nodes or from the peritoneal cavity 3 days after intraperitoneal injection of 20 ml of sterile starch solution or of mineral oil, cells being collected from the peritoneal cavity by lavage with Hank's balanced salt solution. Cells are washed and counted, and their viability determined by eosin-Y or trypan blue exclusion. After centrifugation at 400 g for 10 min cells are suspended at 0.2×10^7 cells/ml in Eagle's minimal essential medium (MEM). A proportion of serum (10% heat-inactivated foetal calf serum) is included to improve cell viability in culture but this is not essential; 5% guinea pig serum may be used, although it may be preferable to achieve more constant culture conditions by using a single batch of heat-inactivated foetal calf serum for all cultures. Cells are incubated with antigen (1 mg bovine gamma globulin (BGG)/ml) or mitogen (Con A 10.0 μg/ml) at 37° C in an atmosphere of 5% CO_2 in air. After 24 h the culture is terminated and culture supernatant collected by centrifugation (700 *g*) and filtration (through an 0.45 μm membrane filter). Ammonium sulphate is added to give a final concentration of 40% saturation which precipitates the bulk of inducing antigen together with any immunoglobulin that may be present. After removal of this precipitate, further ammonium sulphate is added to give a final concentration of 90% saturation which serves to precipitate material with lymphokine activity. This material is extensively dialysed against tap water and then against volatile buffer so as to permit freeze-drying. Freeze-dried preparations stored in sealed containers retain the bulk of their biological activity after storage for 2 years.

Comparable systematic preparation of human lymphokines cannot be achieved as the most readily available cell source (human peripheral blood) contains only about 10^6 lymphocytes/ml. Detailed descriptions of the use of peripheral blood leucocytes for preparation of human lymphokines are provided by ROCKLIN (1974) and ROCKLIN et al. (1970).

C. Biological Actions and Bioassay

Lymphokines exhibit a range of biological activities and are capable of modifying the behaviour of several cell types. For this reason, lymphokine actions will be considered in terms of effector cells with, in each case, an evaluation of the use of this action for lymphokine bioassay. Although this approach is not able to include all lymphokine properties (e.g. interferon-like actions), it does cover those effects that have been extensively investigated, are widely used for lymphokine assay and of most direct relevance to their possible participation in reactions of cellular immunity.

I. Lymphocyte Transformation

The first indication that lymphokines act on lymphocytes was the observation that mixed lymphocyte cultures produce material that stimulates DNA synthesis in unstimulated lymphocytes (KASAKURA and LOWENSTEIN, 1965). The lymphokine preparations shown to produce inhibition of macrophage migration were also reported to stimulate DNA synthesis in lymphocytes (BENNETT and BLOOM, 1968; DUMONDE et al., 1968). The demonstration of a lymphokine that activated lymphocytes was less straightforward in this system than in studies utilizing macrophage migration inhibition as the in vitro indicator, since transplantation antigens, immune complexes and antigen-dependent blastogenic or mitogenic effects, can all act as strong stimulants of increased DNA synthesis in lymphocytes. It was, however, subsequently clearly established that a mitogenic lymphokine could be produced by lymphocyte stimulation in the guinea pig (WOLSTENCROFT and DUMONDE, 1970) and in man (VALENTINE and LAWRENCE, 1969). A further complication of the mitogenic test is that the response to inducing antigen may include not only mitogenic lymphokine but also material that specifically potentiates the response of sensitized lymphocytes to their inducing antigen (JANIS and BACH, 1970) or material that inhibits the capacity of lymphocytes to be stimulated by lymphokine (SMITH et al., 1970; WOLSTENCROFT and DUMONDE, 1970).

This stimulatory action of lymphokines and other agents on lymphocytes is reflected both in morphological changes (blastogenesis) and in biochemical events (mitogenesis). The morphological changes are referred to as lymphocyte transformation, whereby some of the round lymphocytes become transformed from small cells with a large nuclear/cytoplasmic ratio and few cytoplasmic organelles to much larger pyrinophyllic cells with abundant cytoplasm and abundant cytoplasmic organelles. Only a proportion of lymphocytes in a population are transformed, although increased DNA synthesis is a feature not only of this type of cell, but also of cells showing no morphological transformation. Lymphocyte transformation is not restricted to stimulation of specifically sensitized cells by antigen, and such transformation is exhibited by non-sensitized cells treated by plant mitogens (Con A, PHA). In terms of biochemical events, the response of cells to PHA has been most extensively documented, for this provides a convenient system whereby a large proportion of cells can be induced to respond, and it would seem reasonable to suggest that a similar sequence of events results from lymphokine activation of lymphocytes. Interaction with PHA results in a sequence of events in which some changes become evident within the first few seconds, whilst others require many hours before their onset (PARKER et al., 1974a). The critical nature of the early events is indicated by observations that as little as 10 min exposure to antigen is sufficient to initiate the complete sequence of events leading to stimulation of increased DNA synthesis several days later (CARON, 1967). Conversely, agents affecting lymphocyte metabolism within the first few minutes (e.g. E-type prostaglandins, external Ca^{++}, cAMP analogues) can suppress the entire sequence of events leading to increased DNA synthesis. Following interaction of lymphocytes with PHA, there are changes in transmembrane flux of K^{+}, Ca^{++} and sugar, as well as alterations in cyclic nucleotide levels (PARKER et al., 1974b). The change in cAMP levels is small and may be related to agglutinin properties of the mitogen, whilst the changes in cGMP levels are both rapid and substantial (HADDEN et al., 1972). Both exogenous cAMP (or dibutyryl cAMP) and prostaglandin E_1 (PGE_1) cause slight stimulation of DNA synthesis, which is consistent with cAMP elevation being a necessary step in the response sequence, but the more striking effect of persistent elevation of cAMP by PGE_1 is that of inhibiton of lymphocyte transformation (SMITH et al., 1971b). On the basis of present evidence it would seem likely that lymphocyte activation is accompanied by an increase in the cGMP/cAMP ratio, and that the slight elevation in cAMP may be associated with events in a restricted portion of the cell. Extracellular Ca^{++} is obligatory for stimulation of increased DNA synthesis in lymphocytes (WHITFIELD et al., 1973). The contribution of the Ca^{++} influx to the control of the biochemical events of transformation is not clear, but the sensitivity of microsomal adenyl cyclase to Ca^{++} in contrast to the insensitivity of adenyl cyclase associated with the nuclear membrane suggests that the influx of Ca^{++} may determine local changes in cAMP levels (PARKER et al., 1974a).

Subsequent events include: (1) increased turnover of phosphatidyl inositol which can be detected within 5 min (FISHER and MUELLER, 1968), (2) acetylation of histones

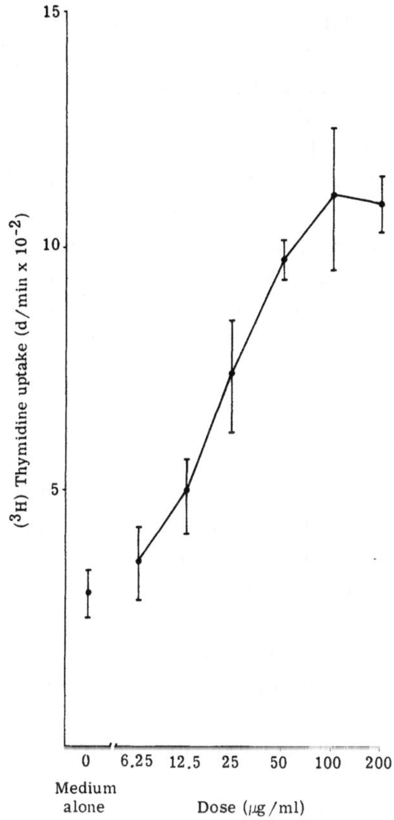

Fig. 2. Dose-response curve for a standard lymphokine preparation (LK-1) obtained by measuring stimulation of DNA synthesis in lymphocytes in vitro depicted here as ^{3}H-thymidine uptake in disintegrations/min; mean ± Standard Deviation (SD). (Data from BRAY et al., 1976)

(POGO et al., 1966), (3) increased synthesis of RNA in 30 min to 2 h (SMITH et al., 1971a) and increased incorporation of ^{3}H-thymidine into DNA after 24 h. Another rather specific change which occurs in lymphocytes following PHA stimulation is the appearance of insulin receptors on the cell surface, a phenomenon extensively studied by CUATRACASAS (1974), and whilst changes of this sort are at present difficult to relate to the transformation process, it seems unlikely that they are without significance.

Lymphokines stimulate the incorporation of ^{3}H-thymidine into DNA in cultured lymphocytes and this mitogenic action is readily assayed on the 2nd day of lymphocyte culture. Cell suspensions are prepared from regional lymph nodes, collected from animals stimulated with Freund's complete adjuvant so as to enlarge the nodes. Teased lymph nodes are pressed through a wide mesh wire filter (80 gauge) and the cells washed, counted and resuspended at a concentration of 2×10^6 viable cells/ml in Eagle's MEM supplemented with 5% heat-inactivated pooled normal guinea pig serum. The suspension is divided in 1 ml volumes into sterile containers to which a further 1 ml of medium containing test material is added. Following 24 h of incubation in 5% CO_2 in air at 38° C, 1.0 µCi of tritiated thymidine in 10 µl of 0.9% NaCl is added to each culture and incubation continued for a further 18–24 h. Incubation is terminated by cooling to 0° C and cells are washed in cold phosphate-buffered saline, lysed and the soluble protein precipitated with 5% trichloracetic acid. The precipitate, containing the incorporated ^{3}H-thymidine, is washed with methanol then solubilized using hyamine hydroxide (10% wt/vol in methanol) and washed into counting vials using 10 ml of toluene-phosphor scintillation fluid for subsequent counting in a liquid scintillation counter. Figure 2 shows a dose-response curve obtained using guinea pig lymphokine. The dose range 6.25–100 µg/ml is sufficiently linear to permit parallel line bioassay. The advantages of this method in comparison with other lymphokine bioassays are that it is more sensitive and precise and is linear over a wider dose range.

II. Macrophage Activation

The initial-observations that lymphokines exerted an action upon macrophages were those of BLOOM and BENNET (1966) who demonstrated that the material derived from incubation of sensitized lymphocytes with antigen affected the migration of purified macrophage populations. The effect of lymphokines on macrophage emigration from capillary tubes is associated with the formation of clumps of overlaid cells rather than with the more uniform layer of glass-adherent cells observed in untreated cultures. Study of events in such populations of cells have been infrequent, although DVORAK et al. (1972) in an EM study reported this clumping may be related to the loss from the surface of treated macrophages of material that could be demonstrated by electron microscopy on cells stained with ruthenium red. Other morphological studies have employed time-lapse cinematography to follow the response of individual cells. A number of changes have been observed to occur, including rounding, reduced mobility, decrease in the ruffling of the pseudopodial membrane and an increase in lysosomal inclusions (SALVIN et al., 1970). It is abundantly clear that the reduced cell migration was not a consequence of cell death.

The biochemical correlates of these alterations in cell behaviour have been less extensively documented than those in the lymphocyte. The evidence that cyclic nucleotides are involved in the reaction of macrophages to lymphokines is conflicting. REMOLD-O'DONNELL and REMOLD (1974) have reported a stimulation of adenyl cyclase and propose that the phenomenon of macrophage migration is dependent upon an elevation of intracellular cAMP. They relate their results to the report of KOOPMAN et al. (1973) that PGE_1 stimulates cell migration. Our own observations and those of PICK (1974) are at variance with this, for PGE_1 or PGE_2 up to 1 µg/ml are ineffective in modifying macrophage migration whilst these concentrations can totally inhibit lymphocyte activation (GORDON et al., 1976). The biochemical events that have been most extensively followed in lymphokine-treated macrophages are those changes associated with macrophage activation. The process of macrophage activation had been established as a feature of cells derived from animals with cellular immunity following antigen challenge. Such cells show an increased adherence to glass, increased movement of the ruffled pseudopodial membrane and increased content of mitochondria, lysosomes and lysosomal enzymes. They also exhibit a heightened bactericidal capability both for organisms to which the animal has

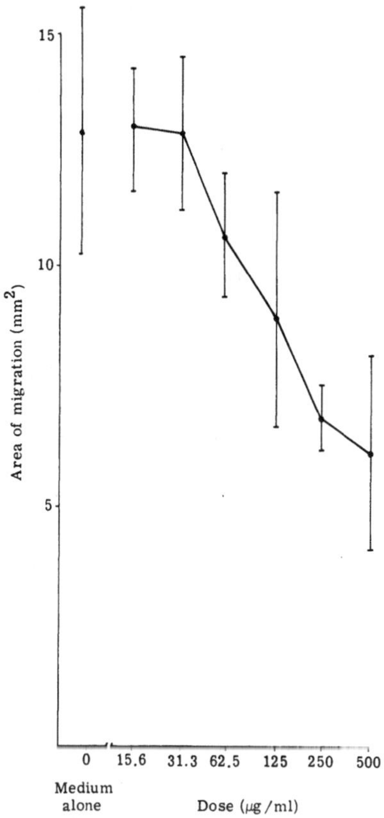

Fig. 3. Dose-response curve for a standard lymphokine preparation (LK-1) obtained by measuring inhibition of macrophage migration in vitro, migration area being measured in mm^2; mean ± SD. (Data from BRAY et al., 1976a)

been sensitized and for unrelated organisms. It is considered that these changes are associated with the protective nature of cellular immunity, i.e. the increased resistance to infection (MACKANESS and BLANDEN, 1967). Lymphokines have been shown to be capable of inducing macrophage activation in terms of increased glass adherence, spreading, motility, phagocytosis, glucose oxidation and protein synthesis, although a latent period of 2–3 days is required (NATHAN et al., 1971). More recently, it has been demonstrated that lymphokines stimulate both the release and formation of lysosomal enzymes (PANTALONE and PAGE, 1975), an observation that may account for the capacity of lymphokines to stimulate the formation of E-type prostaglandins by macrophages. These latter phenomena are of interest in pharmacology as they afford potential assay systems which rely upon the measurement of lysosomal enzymes or prostaglandins and are therefore readily available in many laboratories.

It remains uncertain whether the phenomenon of macrophage migration inhibition is directly related to macrophage activation or other actions which lymphokine preparations may exert on macrophages, such as macrophage aggregation (LOLEKHA et al., 1970), macrophage arming (LOHMANN-MATTHES et al., 1973) and changes in electrophoretic mobility (CASPARY, 1972). The measurement of inhibition of macrophage migration from capillary tubes in vitro remains the lymphokine activity most closely related to cellular immunity and is possibly the most prevalent test used for lymphokine (MORLEY, 1974). Animals receive an intraperitoneal injection of 20 ml light mineral oil or 2% soluble starch solution and are sacrificed at 3 or 4 days. Peritoneal exudate cells are collected by lavage using Hank's balanced salt solution. Cells are resuspended at approximately 4×10^7 viable cells/ml in cold (4° C) Eagle's MEM containing 10% heat-inactivated foetal calf serum. Haematocrit tubes (100 µl) are filled with the cell suspension, plugged at one end with wax and centrifuged for 5 min at 400 *g*. Tubes are cut at the cell/fluid interface and fixed by silicone grease to the floor of culture chambers (0.5 ml volume). Chambers are immediately filled with serum supplemented Eagle's MEM. For this purpose, test materials are dissolved in Eagle's MEM immediately prior to an experiment and kept at room temperature. Cultures are incubated at 37° C for up to 40 h. The border of the cell-migration fan is recorded by projection of the image of the migration fan onto paper, using either planimetry or weighing to estimate the area. Figure 3 shows a dose-response curve obtained using guinea pig lymphokine. The dose range 25–400 µg/ml has proved sufficiently linear for 3+3 parallel line assays. This method is less sensitive than the mitogenic assay, exhibits a limited response range and utilizes larger quantities of material per assay.

III. Skin Response

Cellular immunity is most conveniently detected in sensitized animals by the elicitation of reactions of delayed hypersensitivity to intradermal injection of antigen. Such delayed hypersensitivity reactions are extensively used in veterinary and medical practice, but have only infrequently been subjected to laboratory investigation. The clinical features of these lesions are erythema and induration. It is not clear to what extent the erythema represents increased blood flow, increased capacitance of superficial vessels or extravasation of erythrocytes. The induration on the other hand is clearly associated with increased vascular permeability to plasma protein that is delayed in onset (VOISIN and TOULLET, 1960; MORLEY and WILLIAMS, 1973). Attempts were made to establish that intradermal injection of lymphokine preparations were capable of evoking the cellular and vascular features of delayed hypersensitivity. BENNETT and BLOOM (1968) reported the production of extensive and persistent erythema. The analysis of vascular events by these and other authors was confined to a clinical evaluation of whether lesions displayed a similar time course to that of delayed hypersensitivity reactions as suggested by SCHWARTZ et al. (1970) or were Arthus-like (PICK et al., 1969). The vascular permeability changes produced by such materials have been studied in detail by a continuous recording technique (WILLIAMS and MORLEY, 1974) by means of which the response to lymphokines prepared in serum-free media and fractionated with ammonium sulphate were resolved into three components: The first (0–30 min) which could be totally suppressed by mepyramine (1.5 mg/µg) and two later phases which are unaffected by mepyramine, burimamide, soya bean trypsin inhibitor, bradykinin potentiating peptide (BPP 9a) or indomethacin and in this respect resemble delayed hypersensitivity reactions in their pharmacological profile (unpublished observations). These skin reac-

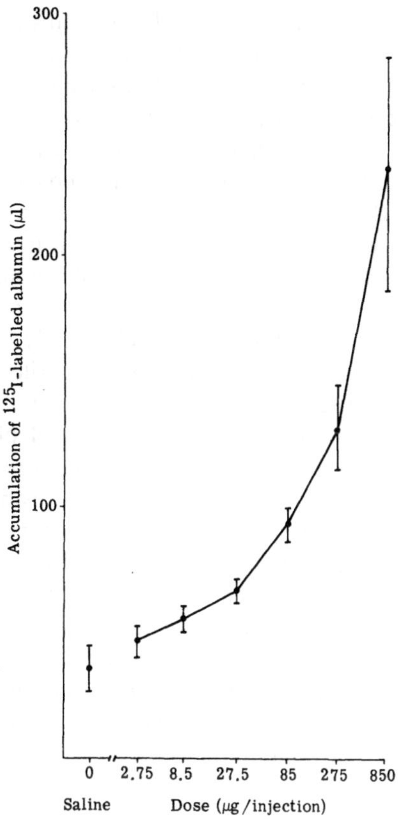

Fig. 4. Dose-response curve for a standard lymphokine preparation (LK-1) obtained by measuring increased vascular permeability, plasma protein accumulation being recorded in µl of whole blood equivalent; mean ± SD. (Data from BRAY et al., 1976a)

tions are relatively modest with little cellular infiltration despite the considerable in vitro potency of these lymphokines (FRANCO et al., 1975) and it would seem that many of the earlier reports of potent skin reactive factors stem from use of crude preparations. It is of interest to note that guinea pig LNPF produces a monophasic vascular permeability response of approximately 30 min duration, not susceptible to inhibition by mepyramine, thus differentiating this material from lymphokine. A characteristic feature of delayed hypersensitivity reactions is the involvement of superficial dermal capillaries in the response. Chemical mediators such as histamine, 5-hydroxytryptamine (5-HT), bradykinin and prostaglandins affect the venular portion of the vascular bed, and it is pertinent that the carbon labelling technique shows that in responses to intradermal injection of lymphokine, dermal capillaries show marked carbon labelling (FRANCO et al., 1975).

The production of erythema is a regular feature following intradermal injection of lymphokines. WILLIAMS (1976) has devised a technique employing local injection of ^{133}Xe for the measurement of erythema. By use of this technique it would appear that the erythema of the lesions is not related to increased blood flow (WILLIAMS, unpublished observations).

In animals pretreated with a histamine (H 1) antagonist, the intradermal injection of lymphokine produces a skin reaction exhibiting increased vascular permeability over a 3–4 h period that can readily be measured by use of isotopically labelled albumin. Groups of three animals are used for this assay. Animals are shaved and six injection sites marked on each flank in two rows of equally spaced sites. By regarding each flank as one row of a latin square, it is possible to balance the distribution of six different test injections; this permits an analysis of variance and so accomodates intersite and interanimal variation. Animals receive an intravenous injection of approximately 1 μCi of ^{125}I-labelled guinea pig serum albumin. The isotope is included in a mixture of mepyramine maleate in saline (1.5 mg/ml) and Evan's blue dye; this is injected without anaesthesia via a foot vein which usually lies between the metatarsals. Injections of test material in 0.1 ml volumes of sterile saline are given into the skin sites using a 26 or 27 gauge short bevel needle. Animals are sacrificed at 4 h by stunning followed by exsanguination, a 1 ml sample of blood being retained for counting. The skin, including the panniculus carnosus, is removed and discs of skin totally including the lesion are punched from the skin using a wad punch (usually 18 mm diameter). After counting on an automatic gamma spectrometer, plasma protein accumulation in response to lymphokine injection is estimated using the blood count to provide a unit of accumulation (μl of whole blood equivalant). Figure 4 shows a dose-response curve obtained using guinea pig lymphokine. The dose range 25–300 μg is suitable for employing parallel line bioassay. This assay is neither especially sensitive nor precise in comparison with in vitro tests. It does, however, provide a quantitative in vivo test that can be completed within a day and permits comparison with other inflammatory responses and in vivo estimation of drug actions.

IV. Chemotaxis

The phenomenon of directional migration of leucocytes in vitro has been observed in response to a range of substances (KELLER and SORKIN, 1968). Since cell accumulation, and in particular monocyte accumulation, is a characteristic feature of delayed hypersensitivity reactions, attempts have been made to demonstrate chemotactic activity of lymphokine preparations in vitro using the Boyden chamber technique whereby the cell population and the potentially chemotactic material are separated by a Millipore filter. WARD et al. (1969) reported guinea pig lymphokine to be chemotactic for mononuclear cells. In subsequent fractionation studies, it was reported that the component chemotactic for neutrophils could be separated from that chemotactic for mononuclear cells by using polyacrylamide disc electrophoresis (WARD et al., 1970). In view of a failure to observe mononuclear cell accumulation in vivo in response to intradermal injection of lymphokine preparations known to be potent in assays of mitogenicity, migration inhibition and increased vascular permeability (FRANCO et al., 1975), we decided to investigate the chemotactic properties of lymphokines. The capacity of this material to cause neutrophil accumulation in vivo was paralleled by chemotactic activity in vitro (FRANCO et al., 1975). These preparations also exhibited a marked capacity to produce mononuclear cell chemotaxis (FRANCO et al., 1977); however, examination of the cells passing through the membrane by electron microscopy shows about half of these cells to be neutrophil-like

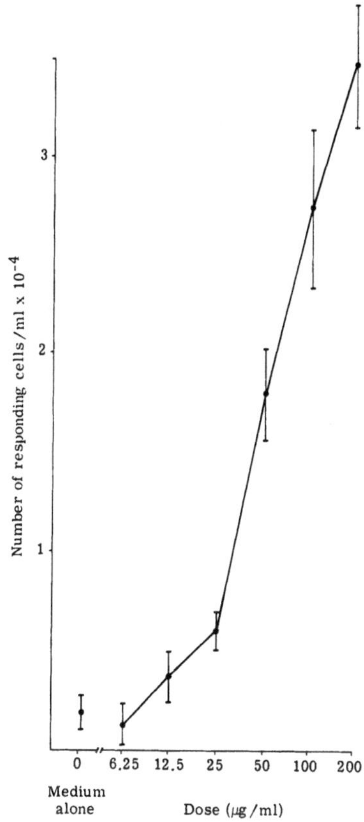

Fig. 5. Dose-response curve for a standard lymphokine preparation (KILS-14) by measuring chemotaxis of mononuclear cell populations, cell accumulation in the lower compartment being recorded by use of a Coulter counter; mean ± SD. (Data from FRANCO et al., 1976b)

despite their morphological appearance by light microscopy. Thus, although by conventional criteria the material documented in Figures 2–4 exhibits chemotaxis for mononuclear cells, our observations are that such material fails to cause chemotaxis for mononuclear cells in vivo and is of limited efficacy in vitro in comparison to its capacity to effect neutrophil chemotaxis.

Chemotaxis is the increased directional migration produced by lymphokine and is measured by counting the cells passing from a chamber in which lymphokine is absent into one in which it is present. It can be conveniently measured using a modification of the method of BOYDEN (1962). Membranes are attached to chemotactic chambers using Millipore cement (KAY, 1970). For neutrophil chemotaxis a relatively thick Millipore membrane (5 μ pore size) is used; for monocyte chemotaxis a 'Nucleopore' membrane is employed (5 μ pore size, 12 μ thick, 13 mm diameter). Cell suspensions are obtained by intraperitoneal injection of 10 ml liquid paraffin; lavage of the peritoneal cavity after 4 h gives neutrophil-rich populations, whilst after 3 or 4 days the population is predominantly mononuclear. After adjusting the cell concentration to 2×10^6 cells/ml, 1 ml aliquots are placed in the chemotaxis chambers. A few seconds are allowed to elapse to enable the filter to saturate and then 1 ml samples of Eagle's MEM containing lymphokine are added to the lower compartment (in polyethylene specimen tube, 32 × 16 mm). Chambers are incubated for 4 h at 37° C under 5% CO_2 in air. Although it is common practice to count stained cells on or in the membrane, this is both technically labourious and is subject to errors. A simpler method is to count the cells in the lower compartment either by staining the cells in a 10 µl sample or preferably by using a Coulter counter. It may be argued that the Coulter counter fails to discriminate between cell types, but in our experience, morphological criteria for identification of mononuclear cells *after* passage through these membranes are unreliable, so that this criticism would apply to all counting techniques. Figure 5 shows a dose-response curve to lymphokine using a macrophage-rich population. Parallel line bioassays can be undertaken using dose ranges from 25–100 µg/ml. This assay is comparable to that measuring macrophage migration inhibition in terms of precision, sensitivity and the manipulative procedures involved.

V. Other Lymphokine Actions

Numerous other lymphokine actions have been reported but none have been subject to systematic study to the extent accorded to mitogenic, migration inhibitory, inflammatory and chemotactic lymphokines.

Lymphotoxin (LT). Cytotoxic activity has been described in lymphokine preparations originating by antigen or mitogen stimulation or by culture of lymphoid cell lines (GRANGER, 1969). Such toxic material is active on various cell types in culture, but the mouse L cells are reported to be most susceptible (WILLIAMS and GRANGER, 1969). The effect of lymphotoxin on target cells contrasts with direct cytotoxic action of lymphocytes in requiring 24–48 h for maximal effect. The phenomenon can be simply quantified by counting viable cells using vital dye exclusion; alternatively, isotopic label may be incorporated in the cell using ^{51}Cr, ^{3}H-thymidine, ^{14}C labelled amino acids, etc. The cytopathic effects of lymphokines on such cells may result in reduced protein synthesis, but it would seem inappropriate to equate these metabolic effects with cytotoxicity especially as there is evidence of other inhibitory effects of lymphokines. Thus, LEBOWITZ and LAWRENCE (1971) observed lymphokine preparations to inhibit the cloning of HeLa cells, thus giving rise to the term *cloning inhibitory factor*; a similar type of experimental system led to the term *proliferation inhibitory activity* (GREEN et al., 1970). A possibly related phenomenon is the production of material capable of inhibiting DNA synthesis in lymphocytes by the *inhibitor of DNA synthesis* (IDS) (SMITH et al., 1970).

Interferon-like activity has also been reported in lymphokines prepared in response to PHA (FRIEDMAN and COOPER, 1967), or PPD (GREEN et al., 1969). The requirements for interferon production are serum (which is not obligatory for the other activities described above) and in PHA stimulated lymphocytes the presence of macrophages (EPSTEIN et al., 1971), although the macrophages themselves do not serve as the origin of interferon activity (MERIGAN, 1971). Participation of macrophages is also required for lymphocytes to produce OAF in response to antigen or mitogen stimulation (HORTON et al., 1972).

In view of the essentially protective nature of cellular immunity, lymphokine production is not only of interest in terms of its capacity to mimic delayed hypersensitivity reactions but may also be of relevance in promoting the host's defensive response to antigenic stimulation. Evidence supporting this view is provided by the observation that antibody production is augmented by lymphokines (MEYERS et al., 1972; KREJČÍ et al., 1973). The effect of intralymphatic injection concurs with such observations in that the action of lymphokine on lymph nodes in vivo is to produce an accelerated version of the pattern of histological events in both thymus dependent and independent areas, which normally accompanies the response to protein antigen (KELLY and WOLSTENCROFT, 1974).

D. Lymphokine Heterogeneity

Following the initial demonstration of lymphokine production by DAVID (1966) and BLOOM and BENNETT (1966), utilizing macrophage migration inhibition as a test system, similar experiments were undertaken with other test systems known to relate to cellular immunity. It quickly became evident that lymphokine preparations exhibit a wide spectrum of biological actions on several different cell types (Table 1). In the majority of instances the assumption was made that each biological activity represented a distinct substance, hence the nomenclature system (MIF, MF, MAF etc.) in which introduction of a new term did not neccesitate distinction from factors already established, in contrast to the system of nomenclature employed in pharmacology (see for example the characterisation of LNPF by SCHILD and WILLOUGHBY, 1967). Paradoxically, it was also frequently assumed that the presence of one activity was predictive of the presence of another activity.

Attempts to characterise lymphokine preparations better by purification procedures have to some extent clarified the situation. The most extensively studied activities have been the mitogenic and migration inhibitory lymphokines. It was soon established that lymphokine causing macrophage migration inhibition was not dialysable, was stable to heating at 56° C but not at 80° C for 30 min and that the active material was smaller than immunoglobulin (DAVID and DAVID, 1972). The use of sephadex, diethylaminoethyl (DEAE) and acrylamide gel electrophoresis have not achieved adequate purification on a preparative scale. The purification factors reported (DUMONDE et al., 1972; REMOLD et al., 1970) are of little value as they assume a linear dose response relationship over all doses and rely upon estimates of biological activity at one dose level (MORLEY, 1974). A fairly wide range of molecular weights has been proposed for lymphokine ranging from 12000 to 100000. It is perhaps noteworthy that a purification procedure yielding significant amounts of lymphokine beyond precipitation with ammonium sulphate (MORLEY et al., 1973) remains to be described for such activity. As a general rule, it appears that any attempted purification step results in substantial loss of total activity and only a modest increase in potency, assuming that the test permits a valid estimate of potency. Similar considerations apply to other biological activities of lymphokines and little can be said of their biochemical nature other than that they are consistent with the properties of anionic glycoproteins. Other individual facets of information have been secured, such as the sensitivity of migration inhibitory lymphokine to chymo-

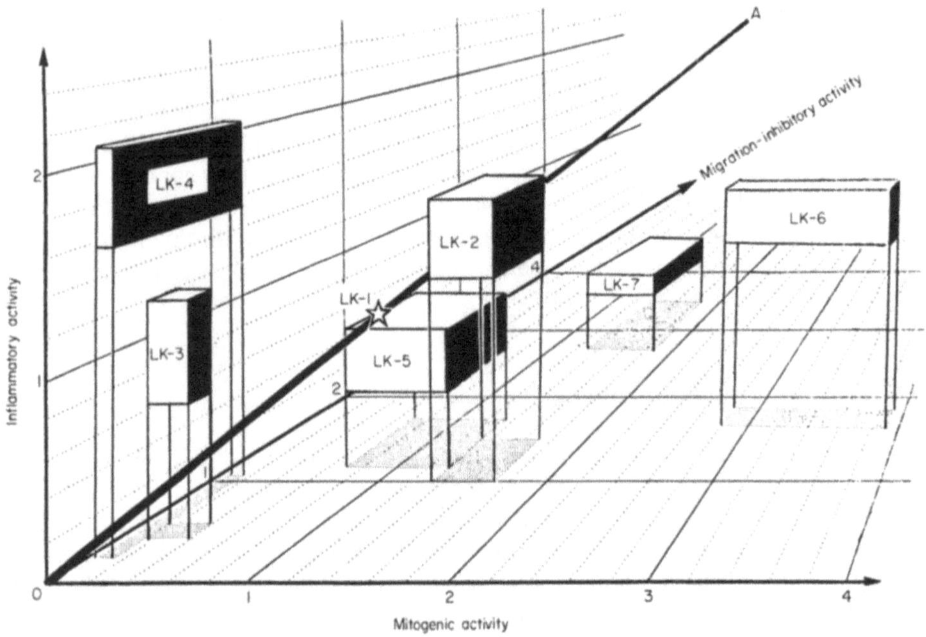

Fig. 6. Diagrammatic representation of lymphokine heterogeneity. Cuboids represent the range of potencies estimated for a series of six lymphokine preparations with reference to a standard, (from BRAY et al., 1976a)

trypsin and the suppression of its biological action by fucose, but it would seem difficult to make progress in biological characterization until some degree of purification can be achieved.

Biochemical studies of lymphokine heterogeneity have, however, permitted separation of some biological activities. Thus, the macrophage migration inhibitory lymphokine of the guinea pig has properties distinguishing it from the lymphokines that are: chemotactic for macrophages (WARD et al., 1970); cytotoxic for fibriblasts (COYNE et al., 1973) and mitogenic for lymphocytes (ASHWORTH et al., 1975). Similarly, physiochemical methods may be used to differentiate the human lymphokine identified by macrophage migration inhibition (ROCKLIN et al., 1974), PMN leucocyte migration inhibition (ROCKLIN, 1974), mononuclear cell chemotaxis (ALTMAN et al., 1973) and cytotoxicity (KOLB and GRANGER, 1970).

Other evidence of heterogeneity stems from observations that production of different lymphokines may be differentially modified. Thus, whilst guinea pigs sensitized to peptides of tobacco mosaic virus show delayed hypersensitivity reactions and inhibition of macrophage migration in response to antigenic stimulation, their lymphocytes do not transform or incorporate tritiated thymidine in vitro (SPITLER et al., 1970). Also, where both T and B cells will produce lymphokine identified by macrophage migration inhibition, only T cells appear capable of generating mitogenic lymphokine (ROCKLIN et al., 1974). In our investigation of the action of E-type prostaglandins on production of guinea pig lymphokines, we observed that whilst lymphokines produced in the presence of PGE_1 and PGE_2 showed reduced activity in terms of macrophage migration inhibition and lymphocyte mitogenicity, the increased vascular permeability produced by these same preparations was augmented. Macrophage migration inhibition, lymphocyte mitogenicity and inflammatory activities had proved particularly resistant to separation using biochemical techniques. Hence, a statistical technique utilised in the characterisation of H_1 and H_2 receptors (BLACK et al., 1972) was adapted to attempt distinction of these activites. A series of six lymphokine preparations, made under identical culture conditions, were repeatedly assayed with reference to a standard; it was clear that these three activities occured independently of one another in guinea pig lymphokines (BRAY et al., 1976a; Fig. 6).

E. Modification of Lymphokine Production and Action by Drugs

The extensive interest in lymphokines stems from their presumed role as mediators of delayed hypersensitivity, in allergic states either established to be relevant to clinical situations (e.g. graft rejection) or likely to be involved in pathogenesis of certain diseases (e.g. rheumatoid arthritis). It is therefore surprising that the action of drugs on lymphokine production has been studied rather sporadically. The established hypersensitivity response is not readily modified by drug treatment. Glucocorticosteroids have been the drugs most widely employed in such conditions. Glucocorticosteroids have long been known to affect lymphoid tissue, particularly in steroid-sensitive species (e.g. mouse, rat, rabbit), where they produce lymphopenia and atrophy of thymus, spleen and lymph nodes. Man, like the guinea pig, is a steroid-resistant species but although glucocorticosteroids are not particularly effective in causing lymphocyte lysis and cause only transitory lymphopenia, they are able to suppress the in vitro reactivity of lymphocytes to antigens and to mitogens (NOWELL, 1961; FAUCI and DALE, 1974). It might be anticipated from this that glucocorticosteroid may suppress the production of lymphokines (WAHL et al., 1975). On the other hand, experiments such as those of BALOW and ROSENTHAL (1973) suggest that steroids act not on the production of lymphokine, measured by macrophage migration inhibition, but rather by suppression of the action of lymphokines. Similar observations have been made of glucocorticosteroid suppression of the lymphokine activities of chemotaxis (KELLER and SORKIN, 1968; WAHL et al., 1975) and cytotoxicity (GRANGER, 1969). The non-steroid anti-inflammatory drugs are capable of modifying lymphocyte activation, but generally at high dose levels (HITCHENS, 1974). Aspirin may perhaps be exceptional in that therapeutic doses in normal volunteers produced a persistent impaired reactivity of their peripheral blood lymphocytes for up to 72 h (CROUT et al., 1975).

E-type prostaglandins, whilst not falling into the category of anti-inflammatory drugs, illustrate the capacity of certain agents to markedly modify lymphocyte activation (SMITH et al., 1971b). Not only are PGE_1 and PGE_2 capable at moderate dose (<1 μg/ml) of effectively suppressing lymphocyte activation, but this effect is accompanied by a corresponding decrease in mitogenic and macrophage migration inhibitory lymphokines (BRAY et al., 1976b). It would seem likely that systematic survey of the action of drugs on lymphokine production may well prove to be a productive exercise.

F. Relevance of Lymphokines to Inflammation

The production of lymphokines in response to antigenic stimulation is, in general, related to the existence of delayed hypersensitivity to that antigen in the donor from which the lymphoid cells have been collected. This relationship, taken together with the various biological actions of lymphokines which correspond to features of the delayed hypersensitivity reaction, make lymphokines putative mediators of delayed hypersensitivity (cellular immunity). Thus, the proposition has been strongly advanced that lymphokines are mediators of delayed hypersensitivity, although application of DALE's criteria (1933) indicates a paucity of evidence in comparison with other situations (MORLEY et al., 1973). Nevertheless, lymphokine preparations undoubtably possess very striking properties (e.g. lymphocyte blastogenesis, macrophage activation, activation of capillary endothelium and potent adjuvant actions on lymph nodes). Whatever their precise contribution to the process of delayed hypersensitivity and cellular immunity, lymphokine production is of considerable potential importance in those inflammatory responses where mononuclear cells predominate.

Many inflammatory responses are limited in extent and duration and can therefore be regarded as physiological events as they do not generally seriously incapacitate the host. However, reactions of excessive magnitude (i.e. hypersensitivity) or extensive duration (i.e. chronicity) may markedly impair an organism's capacity to survive and thus may be regarded as pathological processes (MORLEY, 1976b). Lymphokines exhibit a property especially pertinent to pathological inflammation, for they provide an amplification mechanism whereby following lymphocyte activation there is in turn recruitment and activation of additional lymphocytes and macrophages. This amplification step is a necessary feature of a potential mediator of delayed hypersensitivity, as it has been established that relatively few (0.1–5%) of the lymphocytes involved in a delayed hypersensitivity reaction are specifically sensitive to the eliciting antigen (NAJARIAN and FELDMAN, 1963). It is clear therefore that a mechanism resulting in persistent lymphocyte activation could readily contribute to other features of persistent inflammation as seen, for example, in an afflicted joint in rheumatoid arthritis.

The question arises as to the relative contribution of lymphokines to inflammatory responses in which there is evidence implicating other mediators. Thus, for example in the rheumatoid joint, there is evidence of lysosomal enzyme production causing cartilage and collagen degradation. It appears highly likely that prostaglandin formation also is of consequence in this disease as nonsteroid anti-inflammatory drugs used in therapy are potent inhibitors of PG-synthetase (VANE, 1971). In attempting to relate prostaglandins and lymphokines in delayed hypersensitivity, it was evident that the macrophage was capable of substantial prostaglandin production (BRAY et al., 1974). Antigen or mitogen activation of peritoneal exudate cells results in substantial prostaglandin formation and this action of antigen can be mimicked by use of preformed lymphokine (GORDON et al., 1976). Since lymphokines are also able to stimulate the production and release of lysosomal enzymes (PANTALONE and PAGE, 1975), it is evident that the lymphocyte/macrophage axis affords a medium for relating the production of these three classes of mediators (Fig. 7). This provides a convenient framework for the in vitro assessment of anti-

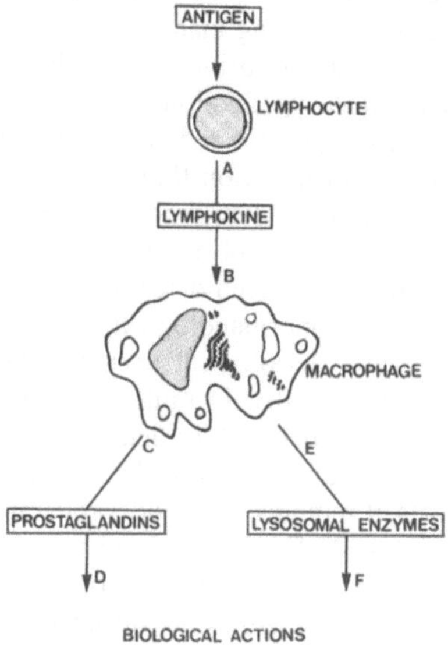

Fig. 7. The lymphocyte/macrophage axis. A–F indicates potential loci of action for anti-inflammatory drugs

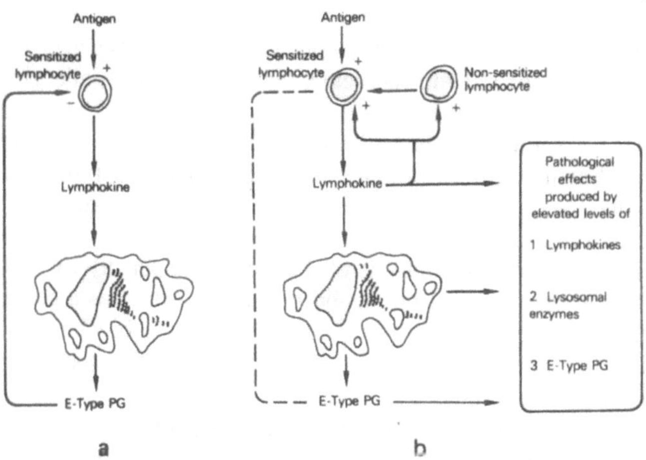

Fig. 8. (a) Physiological: Regulation of lymphokine secretion by E-type prostaglandin. (b) Pathological: Defective regulation of lymphokine secretion with consequent overproduction of lymphokines, macrophage lysosomal enzymes and E-type prostaglandins

inflammatory drug actions and has revealed a locus whereby steroids may inhibit prostaglandin formation (BRAY and GORDON, 1976). It may also explain why aspirin retains its therapeutic potential in spite of its relatively low potency as a prostaglandin synthesis inhibitor (MORLEY, 1976a).

In investigating prostaglandin/lymphokine interrelationships, it was evident that E-type prostaglandins showed considerable potency as inhibitors of lymphocyte activation and that this effect was reflected in a marked suppression of mitogenic lymphokine and lymphokines producing macrophage migration inhibition. Assuming that this reflected a reduced formation of lymphokines causing macrophage activation, it was proposed that the production of PGE by macrophages provides the basis for a negative feedback system for regulating the allergic response (Fig. 8a). This concept led in turn to the proposition that chronicity in certain inflammatory responses may result from defective lymphocyte reactivity to PGE, a condition which could result in overproduction of all three mediators under consideration (Fig. 8b). It is of especial interest that such defective reactivity can be achieved by a variety of mechanisms (genetic, pharmacological, endocrinological, bacterial and viral) thus providing for diverse aetiological agencies (MORLEY et al., 1975). This hypothesis is currently being evaluated in multiple sclerosis patients, who exhibit defective PGE_1 reactivity of peripheral blood leucocytes when compared with normal individuals (KIRBY et al., 1976). Whilst this defect may not prove to be restricted to multiple sclerosis patients, it remains of considerable interest, for, should lymphocytes show normal reactivity to PGE in diseases such as rheumatoid arthritis, rather than the proposed defective reactivity, then suppression of symptoms could be a mixed blessing, for we have shown in vitro that indomethacin enchanced the production of lymphokines in both guinea pig and man (BRAY et al., 1975).

Conclusion

An understanding of the mechanisms underlying delayed hypersensitivity reactions is of considerable importance in medicine, for in addition to allergic reactions (e.g. contact sensitivity, homograft rejection and bacterial allergy), it seems likely that a similar cellular basis underlies the pathology of many forms of chronic inflammation (e.g. rheumatoid arthritis, multiple sclerosis). The discovery and characterisation of lymphokines has been a crucial step in this process by permitting the actions of lymphokines on their target cells to be analysed in vitro—in isolation from in vivo factors which complicate the analysis of delayed hypersensitivity. Progress beyond the stage of factor characterization has been limited, largely as a consequence of the failure to achieve some degree of purification and hence biochemical characterisation of these materials, coupled with a tendency to opt for qualitative rather than quantitative studies in this field.

In spite of this, the lymphocyte/macrophage axis provides a model system for the study of anti-inflammatory drugs and by analogy with the progress achieved in Type I reactions, it is possible that this area of immunopharmacology will eventually lead to novel anti-inflammatory agents for Type IV hypersensitivity reactions.

Acknowledgements. The author wishes to acknowledge with thanks, Mr. M.A. Bray, for Figure 1, and also for helpful discussions during preparation of this manuscript; Ms. K. Howarth is also acknowledged for typing the manuscript.

References

Altman, L. C., Kirchner, H.: The production of a monocyte chemotactic factor by agammaglobulinemic chicken spleen cells. J. Immunol. **109**, 1149—1151 (1972)

Altman, L. C., Snyderman, R., Oppenheim, J. J., Mergenhagen, S. E.: A human mononuclear leucocyte chemotactic factor: characterisation, specificity and kinetics of production by homologous leucocytes. J. Immunol. **110**, 801—810 (1973)

Amos, H. E., Lachmann, P. J.: The immunological specificity of a macrophage inhibition factor. Immunology **18**, 269—278 (1970)

Aronson, J. D.: Tissue culture studies on the relation of the tuberculin reaction to anaphylaxis and the Arthus phenomenon. J. Immunol. **25**, I (1933)

Ashworth, L. A. E., Eckersley, B. J., Ford, W. H.: Comparison of the properties of two antigen-induced guinea-pig lymphokines. Int. Arch. Allergy **48**, 143—155 (1975)

Askonase, P. W.: Cutaneous basophil hypersensitivity on contact-sensitised guinea-pigs. I. Transfer with immune serum. J. exp. Med. **138**, 1144—1154 (1973)

Balow, J. E., Rosenthal, A. S.: Glucocorticoid suppression of macrophage migration inhibitory factor. J. exp. Med. **137**, 1031—1041 (1973)

Bennett, B., Bloom, B. R.: Reactions in vivo and in vitro produced by a soluble substance associated with delayed type hypersensitivity. Proc. nat. Acad. Sci. (Wash.) **59**, 756—782 (1968)

Black, J. W., Duncan, W. A. M., Durant, C. J., Ganellin, C. R., Parsons, E. M.: Definition and antagonism of histamine H_2-receptors. Nature (Lond.) **236**, 385—390 (1972)

Bloom, B. R.: In vitro approaches to the mechanism of cell-mediated immune reactions. Advanc. Immunol. **13**, 101—208 (1971)

Bloom, B. R., Bennett, B.: Mechanisms of a reaction in vitro associated with delayed type hypersensitivity. Science **153**, 80—82 (1966)

Bloom, B. R., Glade, P. R.: In vitro methods in cellular immunology. New York: Academic Press 1971

Boyden, S.: The chemotactic effect of mixtures of antibody and antigen on polymorphonuclear leucocytes. J. exp. Med. **115**, 453—466 (1962)

Bray, M. A., Dumonde, D. C., Hanson, J. M., Morley, J., Wolstencroft, R. A., Smart, J. V.: Heterogeneity of guinea-pig lymphokines revealed by parallel bioassay. Clin. exp. Immunol. **23**, 333—346 (1976a)

Bray, M. A., Gordon, D.: Effects of anti-inflammatory drugs on macrophage prostaglandin biosynthesis. Brit. J. Pharmacol. **57**, 466—467 P (1976)

Bray, M. A., Gordon, D., Morley, J.: Role of prostaglandins in reactions of cellular immunity. Brit. J. Pharmacol. **52**, 453 P (1974)

Bray, M. A., Gordon, D., Morley, J.: Regulation of lymphokine secretion by prostaglandins. In: Velo, G. P., Giroud, J. P., Willoughby, D. A. (Eds.): Future Trends in Inflammation, Vol. II. Italy: Piccin Medical Books 1975

Bray, M. A., Gordon, D., Morley, J.: Regulation of lymphokine secretion by prostaglandins. Agents Actions **6**, 171—175 (1976b)

Caron, G. A.: The effects of concentration on antigen induced lymphocyte transformation in vitro. Int. Arch. Allergy **31**, 441—448 (1967)

Caspary, E. A.: The mechanism of antigen induced electrophoretic mobility reduction of guinea-pig macrophages. Clin. exp. Immunol. **11**, 305—309 (1972)

Cohen, S., Ward, P. A.: In vitro and in vivo activity of a lymphocyte and immune complex dependent chemotactic factor for eosinophils. J. exp. Med. **133**, 133—145 (1971)

Coyne, J. A., Remold, H. G., Rosenberg, S. A., David, J. R.: Guinea-pig lymphotoxin (LT) II. Physicochemical properties of LT produced by lymphocytes stimulated with antigen or concanavallin A: its differentiation from migration inhibitory factor (MIF). J. Immunol. **110**, 1630—1637 (1973)

Crout, J. E., Hepburn, B., Ritts, R. E.: Suppression of lymphocyte transformation after aspirin injection. New Engl. J. Med. **292**, 221—223 (1975)

Cuatracasas, P.: Membrane receptors. Ann. Rev. Biochem. **43**, 169—214 (1974)

Dale, H. H.: Progress in autopharmacology: a survey of present knowledge of the chemical regulation of certain functions by natural constituents of the tissues. Bull. Johns Hopk. Hosp. **53**, 297—317 (1933)

David, J. R.: Delayed hypersensitivity in vitro: its mediation by cell-free substances formed by lymphoid cell antigen interaction. Proc. nat. Acad. Sci. (Wash.) **56**, 72—77 (1966)
David, J. R.: Suppression of delayed hypersensitivity in vitro by inhibition of protein synthesis. J. exp. Med. **122**, 1125—1134 (1965)
David, J. R., David, R. R.: Cellular hypersensitivity and immunity. Progr. Allergy **16**, 300—449 (1972)
David, J. R., Lawrence, H. S., Thomas, L.: Delayed hypersensitivity in vitro. II. Effect of sensitive cells on normal cells in the presence of antigen. J. Immunol. **93**, 274—278 (1964)
Dekaris, D., Smerdel, S., Veselić, B.: Inhibition of macrophage spreading by supernatants of antigen-stimulated sensitised lymphocytes. Europ. J. Immunol. **1**, 402—404 (1971)
Dumonde, D. C., Howson, W. T., Wolstencroft, R. A.: The role of macrophages and lymphocytes in reactions of delayed hypersensitivity. In: Miescher, P. A., Graber, P. (Eds.): Vth Annual Symposium of Immunopathology, p. 263. Basel: Schwabe 1968
Dumonde, D. C., Page, D. A., Matthew, M., Wolstencroft, R. A.: Role of lymphocyte activation products (LAP) in cell mediated immunity. I. Preparations and partial purification of guinea-pig LAP. Clin. exp. Immunol. **10**, 25—47 (1972)
Dumonde, D. C., Wolstencroft, R. A., Panayi, G. S., Matthew, M., Morley, J., Howson, W. T.: Lymphokines: non-antibody mediators of cellular immunity generated by lymphocyte activation. Nature (Lond.) **224**, 38—42 (1969)
Dvorak, A. M., Hammond, E., Dvorak, M. F., Karnovsky, M. J.: Loss of cell surface material from peritoneal exudate cells associated with lymphocyte mediated inhibition of macrophage migration from capillary tubes. Lab. Invest. **27**, 561—574 (1972)
Dvorak, H. F.: Delayed hypersensitivity. In: Zweifach, B., McClusky, R. T., Grant, L. (Eds.): The Inflammatory Process, pp. 291—345. London: Academic Press 1974
Epstein, L. B., Cline, M. J., Menigan, T. C.: The interaction of human macrophages and lymphocytes in the phytohaemagglutinin stimulated production of interferon. J. clin. Invest. **50**, 744—753 (1971)
Fauci, A. S., Dale, D. C.: The effect of in vivo hydrocortisone on sub-populations of human lymphocytes. J. clin. Invest. **53**, 240—246 (1974)
Fisher, D. B., Mueller, G. C.: An early alteration in the phospholipid metabolism of lymphocytes by phytohaemagglutinin. Proc. nat. Acad. Sci. (Wash.) **60**, 1396—1402 (1968)
Ford, W. H., Ashworth, L. A. E., Inder, S.: Effect of the concentrations of inducing agent on the output of lymphokines in the guinea-pig. Weinheim/Bergstr.: Verlag Chemie 1976. In press
Franco, M., Hanson, J. H., Morley, J., Wolstencroft, R. A.: Leucocyte chemotactic activity in the parallel bioassay of guinea-pig lymphokines. Clin. exp. Immunol. **32**, 179—190 (1977)
Franco, M., Kelly, R. H., Morley, J.: Proceedings: a comparison of the haematogenous cell infiltrate produced by intradermal injection of lymphokine with that of delayed hypersensitivity. J. med. Microbiol. **8**, Px—xi (1975)
Friedman, R. M., Cooper, H. L.: Stimulation of interferon production in human lymphocytes by mitogens. Proc. Soc. exp. Biol. (N.Y.) **125**, 901—905 (1967)
Gell, P. G. H., Hinde, I. T.: Observations on the histology of the Arthus reaction and its relation to other known types of skin hypersensitivity. Int. Arch. Allergy **5**, 23—46 (1954)
George, M., Vaughan, J. H.: In vitro cell migration as a model for delayed hypersensitivity. Proc. Soc. exp. Biol. (N.Y.) **111**, 514—521 (1962)
Gordon, D., Bray, M. A., Morley, J.: Control of lymphokine secrection by prostaglandins. Nature (Lond.) **262**, 401—402 (1976)
Granger, G. A.: In: Lawrence, H. S., Landy, M. (Eds.): Mediators of Cellular Immunity, pp. 374—388. New York: Academic Press 1969
Green, J. A., Cooperbrand, J. S., Rutstein, J. A., Kibrick, S.: Immune specific induction of interferon production in cultures of human blood lymphocytes. Science **164**, 1415—1417 (1969)
Green, J. A., Cooperbrand, S. R., Rutstein, J. A., Kibrick, S.: Inhibition of target cell proliferation by supernatants from cultures of human peripheral lymphocytes. J. Immunol. **105**, 48—54 (1970)
Hadden, J. W., Hadden, E. M., Haddox, M. K., Goldberg, N. D.: Guanosine 3′, 5′-cyclic monophosphate: a possible intracellular mediator of mitogenic influences in lymphocytes. Proc. nat. Acad. Sci. (Wash.) **69**, 3024—3027 (1972)

Hadden, J. W., Sadlik, J. R., Hadden, E. M.: Macrophage proliferation induced in vitro by a lymphocyte factor. Nature (Lond.) **257**, 483—485 (1975)
Hitchens, M.: Molecular and cellular pharmacology of the anti-inflammatory drugs: some in vitro properties related to their possible modes of action. In: Scherrer, R. A., Whitehouse, M. W. (Eds.): Anti-inflammatory Agents: Chemistry and Pharmacology, Vol. II, pp. 264—303. London: Academic Press 1974
Horton, J. E., Raisz, L. G., Simmons, H. A., Oppenheim, J. J., Mergenhagen, S. E.: Bone resorbing activity in supernatant fluid from cultured human peripheral blood leucocytes. Science **177**, 793—795 (1972)
Janis, M., Bach, F. H.: Potentiation of in vitro lymphocyte reactivity. Nature (Lond.) **225**, 238—239 (1970)
Jones, T. B., Mote, J. R.: The phases of foreign sensitisation in human beings. New Engl. J. Med. **210**, 120—123 (1934)
Kasakura, S.: Heterogeneity of blastogenic factors produced in vitro by antigenically stimulated and unstimulated leucocytes. J. Immunol. **105**, 1162—1167 (1970)
Kasakura, S., Lowenstein, L.: A factor stimulating DNA synthesis derived from the medium of leucocyte cultures. Nature (Lond.) **208**, 794—795 (1965)
Kay, A. B.: Studies on eosinophil leucocyte migration. II. Factors specifically chemotactic for eosinophils and neutrophils generated from guinea-pig serum by antigen-antibody complexes. Clin. exp. Immunol. **7**, 723—727 (1970)
Keller, H. U., Sorkin, E.: Chemotaxis of leucocytes. Experientia (Basel) **24**, 641—652 (1968)
Kelly, R. H., Wolstencroft, R. A.: Germinal centre proliferation in response to mitogenic lymphokine. Clin. exp. Immunol. **18**, 321—336 (1974)
Kelly, R. H., Wolstencroft, R. A., Dumonde, D. C., Balfour, B. H.: Role of lymphocyte activation products (LAP) in cell-mediated immunity. II. Effects of lymphocyte activation products on lymph node architecture and evidence for peripheral release of LAP following antigenic stimulation. Clin. exp. Immunol. **10**, 49—65 (1972)
Kirby, P. J., Morley, J., Ponsford, J. R., McDonald, W. I.: Defective PGE reactivity in leucocytes of multiple sclerosis patients. Prostaglandins. (1976). In press
Kolb, W. P., Granger, G. A.: Lymphocyte in vitro cytotoxicity: characterisation of mouse lymphotoxin. Cell. Immunol. **1**, 122—132 (1970)
Koopman, W. J., Gillis, M. H., David, J. R.: Prevention of MIF activity by agents known to increase cellular cylic AMP. J. Immunol. **110**, 1609—1614 (1973)
Krejčí, J., Pekarek, J., Svejcar, J., Johanovsky, J.: Role of mediators of cellular hypersensitivity in the stimulation of the antibody response to an unrelated antigen. Cell. Immunol. **7**, 323—327 (1973)
Landsteinder, K., Chase, M. W.: Experiments on transfer of cutaneous sensitivity to simple compounds. Proc. Soc. exp. Biol. (N.Y.) **49**, 688—690 (1942)
Lebowitz, A. S., Lawrence, H. S.: The technique of clonal inhibition: a quantitative assay for human lymphotoxin activity. In: Bloom, B. R., Glade, P. R. (Eds.): In vitro Methods in Cell-Mediated Immunity, pp. 375—379. New York-London: Academic Press 1971
Lohmann-Matthes, M.-L., Ziegler, F. G., Fischer, H.: Macrophage cytotoxicity factor. A product of in vitro sensitised thymus dependant cells. Europ. J. Immunol. **3**, 56—58 (1973)
Lolekha, S., Dray, S., Gotoff, S. P.: Macrophage aggregation in vitro—correlate of delayed hypersensitivity. J. Immunol. **104**, 296—304 (1970)
Mackaness, G. B., Blanden, R. V.: Cellular immunity. Progr. Allergy **11**, 89—140 (1967)
Maillard, J., Bloom, B. R.: Immunological adjuvants and the mechanism of cell co-operation. J. exp. Med. **136**, 185—190 (1972)
Marks, J., James, D. M.: The effect of tuberculin on sensitised and normal leucocytes. J. Hyg. (Lond.) **51**, 340—346 (1953)
Merigan, T. C.: In: Bloom, B. R., Glade, P. (Eds.): In vitro Methods in Cell-Mediated Immunity, pp. 81—89. New York: Academic Press 1971
Meyers, O. L., Shoji, M., Haber, E., Remold, H. G., David, J. R.: Cellular hypersensitivity: the production of antibody by cultures of lymphocytes producing migration inhibition factor. Cell. Immunol. **3**, 442—447 (1972)
Morley, J.: Cell migration inhibition: an appraisal. Acta allerg. (Kbh.) **29**, 185—208 (1974)
Morley, J.: The mode of action of aspirin. In: Dale, T. L. C. (Ed.): Proceedings of the Aspirin Symposium. London: Aspirin Foundation 1976a

Morley, J.: Prostaglandins as regulators of lymphoid cell function in allergic inflammation: a basis for chronicity in rheumatoid arthritis. In: Dumonde, D. C. (Ed.): Immunopathological Mechanisms in Relation to the Rheumatic Diseases, pp. 511—517. Oxford: Blackwell 1976b
Morley, J., Bray, M. A., Gordon, D., Paul, W.: Interaction of prostaglandins and lymphokines in arthritis. In: Silvestri, L. G. (Ed.): The Immunological Basis of Connective Tissue Disorders, pp. 129—140. Amsterdam: North Holland Publishing Company 1975
Morley, J., Dumonde, D. C. Wolstencroft, R. A.: The measurement of lymphokines. In: Weir, D. M. (Ed.): Handbook of Experimental Immunology, Chap. 28. Oxford: Blackwell 1973
Morley, J., Williams, T. J.: Increased vascular permeability in allergic inflammation. J. Physiol. (Lond.) **222**, 95 P—97 P (1972a)
Morley, J., Williams, T. J.: Inflammatory response produced by a factor released from lymphocytes. Brit. J. Pharmacol. **44**, 384 P (1972b)
Morley, J., Williams, T. J.: Characterisation of delayed hypersensitivity by measurement of some local changes in vascular permeability: the place of the Jones-Mote reaction. In: Velo, G. P., Giroud, J. P., Willoughby, D. A. (Eds.): Future Trends in Inflammation, Vol. I, pp. 227—234. Italy: Piccin Medical Books 1973
Najarian, J. S., Feldman, J. D.: Specificity of passively transferred delayed hypersensitivity. J. exp. Med. **118**, 341—352 (1963)
Nathan, C. F., Karnovsky, M. L., David, J. R.: Alterations of macrophage functions by mediators from lymphocytes. J. exp. Med. **133**, 1356—1376 (1971)
Nelson, D. S., Boyden, S. V.: The loss of macrophages from peritoneal exudates following the injection of antigens into guinea-pigs with delayed hypersensitivity. Immunology **6**, 264—275 (1963)
Nowell, P. C.: Inhibition of human leucocyte mitosis by prednisolone in vitro. Cancer Res. **21**, 1518—1521 (1961)
Outteridge, P. M., Lepper, A. W. D.: Immunosuppressive factors released by transforming lymphocytes in the delayed hypersensitivity skin response to tuberculin. Immunology **25**, 981—994 (1973)
Pantalone, R. M., Page, R. C.: Lymphokine-induced production and release of lysosomal enzymes by macrophages. Proc. nat. Acad. Sci. (Wash.) **72**, 2091—2094 (1975)
Papageorgiou, P. S., Henley, W. L., Glade, P. R.: Production and characterisation of migration inhibitory factor(s) (MIF) of established lymphoid and non-lymphoid cell lines. J. Immunol. **108**, 494—504 (1973)
Parker, C. W., Snyderman, D. E., Wedner, H. J.: The role of cyclic nucleotides in lymphocyte activation. In: Brent, L., Holborow, J. (Eds.): Progress in Immunology, Vol. II, pp. 85—94. Amsterdam: North Holland Publishing Company 1974a
Parker, C. W., Sullivan, T. J., Wedner, H. J.: In: Greengard, P., Robison, A. G. (Eds.): Advances in Cyclic Nucleotide Research, Vol. IV, p. 1. New York: Raven Press 1974b
Pekárek, J., Krejčí, J.: Survey of the methodological approaches to studying delayed hypersensitivity in vitro. J. immunol. Methods **6**, 1—22 (1974)
Pick, E.: Soluble lymphocytic mediators. I. Inhibition of macrophage migration inhibitory factor production by drugs. Immunology **26**, 649—658 (1974)
Pick, E., Krejčí, J., Cech, K., Turk, J. L.: Interaction between 'sensitised lymphocytes' and antigen in vitro. I. The release of skin reactive factor. Immunology **17**, 741—767 (1969)
Pick, E., Mannheim, S.: The mechanism of soluble lymphocytic mediators. II. Modification of macrophage migration and migration inhibitory aation by drugs, enzymes, and cationic environment. Cell. Immunol. **11**, 30—46 (1974)
Pick, E., Turk, J. L.: Biological activities of soluble lymphocyte products. Clin. exp. Immunol. **10**, 1—23 (1972)
Pogo, B. G. T., Allfrey, V. G., Mirsky, A. E.: RNA synthesis and histone acetylation during the course of gene activation in lymphocytes. Proc. nat. Acad. Sci. (Wash.) **55**, 805—812 (1966)
Remold, H. G., Katz, A. B., Haber, E., David, J. R.: Studies on migration inhibitory factor (MIF): recovery of MIF activity, purification of gel filtration and disc electrophoresis. Cell. Immunol. **1**, 133—145 (1970)
Remold, H. G., Ward, P., David, J. R.: Characterisation of migration inhibitory factor (MIF) and its separation from a chemotactic factor for monocytes. Int. Arch. Allergy **41**, 15—17 (1971)

Remold-O'Donnell, E., Remold, H. G.: The enhancement of macrophage adenyl cyclase by products of activated lymphocytes. J. biol. Chem. **249**, 3622—3627 (1974)
Rich, A. R., Lewis, M. R.: Nature of allergy in tuberculosis as revealed by tissue culture studies. Bull. Johns Hopk. Hosp. **50**, 115—128 (1932)
Richerson, B. B., Dvorak, H. F., Leskowitz, S.: Cutaneous basophil hypersensitivity. I. A new look at the Jones-Mote reaction, general characteristics. J. exp. Med. **132**, 546—557 (1970)
Rocklin, R. E.: Products of activated lymphocytes: leucocyte inhibition factor (LIF) distinct from migration inhibition factor (MIF). J. Immunol. **112**, 1461—1466 (1974)
Rocklin, R. E., MacDermott, R. P., Chess, L., Schlossman, S. E., David, J. R.: Studies on mediator production by highly purified human T and B lymphocytes. J. exp. Med. **140**, 1303—1316 (1974)
Rocklin, R. E., Meyers, O. L., David, J. R.: An in vitro assay for cellular hypersensitivity in man. J. Immunol. **104**, 95—102 (1970)
Salvin, S. B., Nishio, J., Gribik, M.: Lymphoid cells in delayed hypersensitivity. I. in vitro vs in vivo responses. Cell Immunol. **1**, 62—77 (1970)
Schild, H. O., Willoughby, D. A.: Possible pharmacological mediators of delayed hypersensitivity. Brit. med. Bull. **23**, 46—51 (1967)
Schwartz, H. J., Leon, M. A., Pelley, R. P.: Concanavallin A induced release of skin reactive factor from lymphoid cells. J. Immunol. **104**, 265—268 (1970)
Smith, J. W., Steiner, A. L., Newberry, W. M., Parker, C. W.: Cyclic adenosine 3′,5′-monophosphate in human lymphocytes. Alterations after phytohaemagglutinin stimulation. J. clin. Invest. **50**, 432—441 (1971 a)
Smith, J. W., Steiner, A. L., Parker, C. W.: Human lymphocyte metabolism. Effects of cyclic and non-cyclic nucleotides on stimulation by phytohaemagglutinin. J. clin. Invest. **50**, 442—448 (1971 b)
Smith, R. T., Bauscher, J. A. C., Adler, W. H.: Studies of an inhibitor of DNA synthesis and a non-specific mitogen elaborated by human lymphoblasts. Amer. J. Path. **60**, 495—504 (1970)
Spitler, L., Benjamini, E., Young, J. D., Kaplan, H., Fudenberg, H. H.: Studies on the immune response to a characterised antigenic determinant of the tobacco mosaic virus protein. J. exp. Med. **131**, 133—148 (1970)
Svejcar, J., Johanovsky, J., Pekárek, J.: Studies in the mechanism of delayed hypersensitivity in tissue cultures. XI. The influence of the substances released during the cultivation of lymph node cells from sensitised organism with antigen, on the migration activity of normal spleen cells. Z. Immun.-Forsch. **133**, 259—274 (1967)
Turk, J. L. (Ed.): Delayed hypersensitivity: specific cell-mediated immunity. Brit. med. Bull. **23**, 1—97 (1967)
Valentine, F. T., Lawrence, H. S.: Lymphocyte stimulation: transfer of cellular hypersensitivity to antigen in vitro. Science **165**, 1014—1016 (1969)
Vane, J. R.: Inhibition of prostaglandin synthesis as a mechanism of action for aspirin-like drugs. Nature (New Biol.) **231**, 232—235 (1971)
Voisin, G. A., Toullet, F.: Modifications of capillary permeability in immunological reactions mediated through cells. In: Wolstenholme, G. E. W., O'Connor, M. (Eds.): Ciba Foundation Symposium on Cellular Aspects of Immunity, pp. 373—408. London: Churchill 1960
Wahl, S. M., Altman, L. C., Rosenstreich, D. L.: Inhibition of in vitro lymphokine synthesis by glucocorticosteroids. J. Immunol. **115**, 476—481 (1975)
Ward, P. A., Remold, H. G., David, J. R.: Leucotactic factor produced by sensitised lymphocytes. Science **163**, 1079—1081 (1969)
Ward, P. A., Remold, H. G., David, J. R.: The production by antigen-stimulated lymphocytes of a leucotactic factor distinct from migration inhibitory factor. Cell. Immunol. **1**, 162—174 (1970)
Whitfield, J. F., Rixon, R. H., Mackmanus, J. P., Balk, S. D.: Calcium, cyclic adenosine 3′ 5′-monophosphate, and the control of cell proliferation: a review. In vitro **8**, 257—278 (1973)
Williams, T. J.: Simultaneous measurement of local plasma exudation and blood flow changes induced by intradermal injection of vaso-active substances using ^{131}I-albumin and ^{133}Xe. J. Physiol. (Lond.) **254**, 4—5 P (1976)
Williams, T. W., Granger, G. A.: Lymphocyte in vitro cytotoxicity. Mechanism of lymphotoxin-induced target cell distruction. J. Immunol. **102**, 911—918 (1969)

Williams, T. J., Morley, J.: Measurement of the rate of extravasation of plasma protein in inflammatory responses in guinea-pig skin using a continuous recording method. Brit. J. exp. Path. **55**, 1—12 (1974)

Willoughby, D. A., Boughton, B., Spector, W. G., Schild, H. O.: A vascular permeability factor extracted from normal and sensitized guinea-pig lymph node cells. Life Sci. **7**, 347—352 (1962)

Wolstencroft, R. A., Dumonde, D. C.: In vitro studies of cell mediated immunity. I. Induction of lymphocyte transformation by a soluble 'mitogenic' factor derived from interaction of sensitised guinea-pig lymphoid cells with specific antigen. Immunology **18**, 599—610 (1970)

Yoshida, T., Cohen, S., Bigazzi, P. E., Kurasuzi, T., Asmden, A.: Inflammatory mediators in culture filtrates of *Escherichia coli*. Macrophage migration inhibitory, neutrophil chemotactic, lymphocyte mitogenic and fibroblast cytotoxic activities. Amer. J. Path. **81**, 389—400 (1975)

Yoshida, T., Janeway, C. A., Paul, W. E.: Activity of migration inhibitory factor in the absence of antigen. J. Immunol. **109**, 201—206 (1972)

Zinsser, H.: Bacterial allergy and tissue reactions. Proc. Soc. exp. Biol. (N.Y.) **22**, 35—39 (1925)

Inflammatory Mediators Released From Cells

CHAPTER 11

Histamine, 5–Hydroxytryptamine, SRS–A: Discussion of Type I Hypersensitivity (Anaphylaxis)*[1]

M. PLAUT and L. M. LICHTENSTEIN

A. Immediate Hypersensitivity: General Considerations

Immunopathologic events mediating tissue injury have been divided by the scheme of COOMBS and GELL (1968) into four types: type I or anaphylactic (immediate) hypersensitivity; type II or cytotoxic; type III or immune complex-mediated; type IV or cell-mediated (delayed) hypersensitivity. Such a scheme, while useful didactically, is an oversimplification because of the complex interrelationships which actually exist between the cells and mediators involved in each 'type' of response. Thus: (1) mediator release can be triggered from mast cells by C3a and C5a (complement components usually associated with immune complex disease) (LEPOW et al., 1970; VALLOTA and MÜLLER-EBERHART, 1973), and possibly by vasoactive peptides like bradykinin (SPRAGG, 1974). On the other hand, the basophils release a kallikrein which can generate bradykinin from serum kininogen (NEWBALL et al., 1975). (2) Basophils respond to lymphocyte-derived chemotactic stimuli (presumably components of so-called type IV reactions) (WARD et al., 1975; BOETCHER and LEONARD, 1973). (3) Vasoactive amines (released during immediate hypersensitivity reactions) are important both for permitting deposition of immune complexes (KNIKER and COCHRANE, 1965), and apparently in eliciting delayed hypersensitivity reactions (GERSHON et al., 1975). (4) Immunologically activated neutrophils can produce certain mediators, such as slow-reacting substance (SRS) and eosinophil chemotactic factor (ECF) (CONROY et al., 1976; CZARNETZKI et al., 1975, 1976b; KÖNIG et al., 1976) which at least in primates were previously thought to be products only of basophils and mast cells. (5) Basophils and mast cells release both eosinophil and neutrophil chemotactic factors (KAY and AUSTEN, 1971; CZARNETZKI et al., 1976a; AUSTEN and ORANGE, 1975); neutrophils, perhaps along with the eosinophils, determine late inflammatory manifestations following immediate hypersensitivity reactions (HENSON, 1972; COCHRANE, 1968; DOLOVICH et al., 1973; SOLLEY et al., 1975; SLOTT and ZWEIMAN, 1975). (6) Mediators released from basophils (e.g., histamine and prostaglandins) can modulate the chemotactic stimuli to, and effector function of, other leukocytes which participate in inflammatory reactions (BOURNE et al., 1974, and see Section F). (7) Complex interactions occur between complement, clot-

---

* Supported by Grants Nos. AI 07290 and AI 12810 from The National Institutes of Health. From the Johns Hopkins University School of Medicine at the Good Samaritan Hospital, publication No. 299 of the O'Neill Research Laboratories, The Good Samaritan Hospital.

[1] In the 24 months following the completion of this chapter in early 1976, several important developments occured. Among them are those included in the footnotes (except 7 and 12) to this chapter.

ting and kinin-generating (and possibly also prostaglandin-generating) pathways (KAPLAN and AUSTEN, 1975; COLMAN, 1974; STONER et al., 1973; ZURIER, 1974). There are numerous other examples which might be cited but the point is clear: type I reactions cannot be considered apart from other immunopathogenetic mechanisms. The pathology following immune reactions merely begins with the reaction of antigen with antibody, and is effected by various amplication systems involving the release of mediators, interaction with serum cascade systems, etc. The time lag between antigen challenge and detectable pathological changes is primarily a function of cell (neutrophil, macrophage, etc.) recruitment. If sufficient mast cells are present locally, rapid immunological release of mediators (especially histamine) from these cells can account for such pathological changes as oedema, smooth muscle contraction, and capillary dilatation with fluid and protein extravasation—the classic manifestations of 'immediate' hypersensitivity. However, these processes blend imperceptively into 'subacute' and delayed responses to the antigen.

In this chapter, we shall discuss three mediators which have been associated classically with manifestations of anaphylaxis: histamine, 5-hydroxytryptamine (5-HT), and slow reacting substance of anaphylaxis (SRS-A). All three of these agents can effect increased vascular permeability and smooth muscle contraction. Such effector mechanisms appear to involve a direct interaction of mediator with specific receptors on end organs, and a secondary activation of biochemical mechanisms in the cells of the end organ (CUATRECASAS et al., 1975).The marked variation in sensitivity to each mediator between different species, and between different tissues in the same species, reflects both the distribution and frequency of receptors and/or the dose-response curves of tissue possessing activated receptors.

We shall discuss the mechanisms of release of these mediators, and also emphasize some multiple effects of these agents—particularly the newly described anti-inflammatory effects of histamine.

B. IgE and Other Antibodies Capable of Triggering Mast Cells and Basophils

Immediate hypersensitivity reactions are readily demonstrable by intracutaneous injection of antigen into a sensitive individual; such a stimulus results in a wheal and flare reaction at the site of injection. These reactions are elicited by 'reaginic' (skin-reactive) antibodies (ISHIZAKA and ISHIZAKA, 1975). As originally demonstrated in man by PRAUSNITZ and KÜSTNER (1921), immediate skin reactivity can be transferred by a serum factor. These antigen-induced wheal and flare reactions were later shown to be associated with 'degranulation' of tissue mast cells and release of histamine and other mediators. The serum factor was shown to be specific antibody, but its identity was established only recently, when ISHIZAKA and ISHIZAKA (1967) demonstrated that human reaginic antibodies belong to a unique class of immunoglobulin designated IgE. While IgE is present in much lower serum concentrations than other immunoglobulin classes, IgE antibodies have unique physicochemical characteristics including a (heat-labile) capacity to "fix" avidly, via the Fc portion of the molecules, to specific mast cell receptors. The interaction of antigen with appropriate mast cell-associated IgE triggers biochemical events resulting in degranulation and mediator release from the cell.

Antibodies with properties similar to those of human IgE have been described in other species (BLOCH, 1973). In several species including guinea pig, rat and mouse, some subclasses of IgG antibodies also can fix to homologous mast cells. These IgG antibodies differ from IgE by binding to mast cells less avidly, and thus for shorter times; their binding activity is not heat-labile.

In man, nearly all clinical allergy correlates with the presence of IgE antibodies (LICHTENSTEIN, 1972). While IgG fixes to human basophils (ISHIZAKA et al., 1972), and in vitro in some individuals is capable of triggering the cells for mediator release (GRANT and LICHTENSTEIN, 1972), the amounts of IgG fixed are small relative to cell-bound IgE. Several recent reports of the pathophysiological significance of IgG reagins in man (PARISH, 1974; BRYANT et al., 1975) need further confirmation.

The initial biochemical events in cell triggering occur on the basophil or mast cell surface. High affinity receptor sites for IgE have been identified on these cells, and partial purification of membrane fragments containing IgE receptors on rat mast cells and rat leukemic basophils has recently been described (KÖNIG and ISHIZAKA, 1976). There are in the order of 100000 IgE receptor sites per human basophil, and varying percentages of these sites are unoccupied.[2] (The receptor sites of allergic donors are more saturated than those of normal donors.) The receptor sites may be linked in some type of network, because anti-IgE-induced "capping" of occupied receptors also induces capping of unoccupied receptors (ISHIZAKA et al., 1974). Surprisingly, it appears that as much as 20% of IgE antibody may be directed against a single specific antigen (GLEICH and JACOB, 1975; SCHELLENBERG and ADKINSON, 1975, 1976). Mediator release triggered via IgE requires interaction of antigen with adjacent IgE molecules (ISHIZAKA and ISHIZAKA, 1975). While the distribution of IgE antibody molecules is not entirely understood, it must account for the observation that in some allergic individuals, small amounts of antigen (10^{-14} M) can in vitro induce release of 100% of intracellular histamine (LICHTENSTEIN, 1972).

C. Mast Cells, Basophils, and Platelets

Mast cells and basophils are considered to be the major cells involved in immediate hypersensitivity reactions because (1) in man, and probably other species, only these cells have IgE receptors (ISHIZAKA and ISHIZAKA, 1975), and (2) while non-mast cell-storage sites for histamine apparently exist, all blood histamine is in basophils (ISHIZAKA et al., 1972), and most tissue histamine is in mast cells (RILEY, 1963), in both cases stored in association with negatively charged (heparin-containing) metachromatic granules. Mast cells are distributed in the submucosa of the skin, gastrointestinal, respiratory, and genitourinary tracts, and especially in proximity to blood vessels (SAMTER and CZARNY, 1971). Basophils circulate—they represent 0.5% of

[2] The number of IgE receptors per basophil is now known to be approximately 500000 and to be correlated with the serum IgE level, as is the percentage of occupied receptors (MALVEAUX et al., 1978).
A linkage (network) of IgE receptor sites is controversial, since studies with rat mast cells do not reveal the linkage found with receptors on human basophils (MENDOZA und METZGER, 1976).

circulating leukocytes, or approximately 50000 per ml (LICHTENSTEIN, 1972)—and apparently also migrate into inflammatory infiltrates (DVORAK and DVORAK, 1974). In vitro they respond to chemotactic stimuli (WARD et al., 1975; BOETCHER and LEONARD, 1973). Species differences exist in distribution of these cells; guinea pigs have significant numbers of circulating basophils, while rats and mice have large numbers of peritoneal mast cells but few basophils and limited distribution of skin mast cells (LEVY, 1974). Mast cells have some features distinct from those of basophils such as site of origin, cell size and granule size (SAMTER and CZARNY, 1971; HASTIE, 1974; PARMLEY et al., 1975), and apparently activatable esterase (BECKER and HENSON, 1973), responsiveness to cholinergic agents (KALINER et al., 1972), to cromolyn (ORANGE and AUSTEN, 1971), and to C3a, and quantitative sensitivity to C5a (LEPOW et al., 1970; GRANT et al., 1975; HOOK et al., 1975). However, in this chapter we will generally make no distinction between these cells. Thus, in allergic individuals these two cell types appear to behave similarly—that is, the responses to allergen of skin and lung mast cells are quite similar to the responses to allergen of blood basophils (BRUCE et al., 1975).

The mast cells and basophils of man contain histamine but no 5-HT; in contrast, mast cells of rat and mouse contain large amounts of 5-HT. Human platelets contain 5-HT but no histamine while, in rabbits for example, histamine and 5-HT are stored in platelets.

We shall not consider platelet function in detail in this chapter. Several mechanisms of immunologically mediated secretion from platelets have been described; some of the control mechanisms of these secretory mechanisms are analogous to those involved in control of mast cell and basophil mediator secretion (HENSON, 1974; BECKER and HENSON, 1973). However, platelets to not have receptors for IgE, and thus cannot be triggered directly by antigen-IgE interaction. In rabbits, a basophil-dependent IgE-mediated release of platelet mediators involves secretion from basophils of a platelet-activating factor (PAF) (HENSON, 1970; SIRAGANIAN and OSLER, 1971; BENEVISTE, 1974). This mechanism appears to be an important means of amplifying release of vasoactive amines at the site of rabbit IgE-mediated reactions. PAF-like activity has recently been described in mast cells of several species, in human mast cells, and in a human basophilic leukemia (BENEVISTE, 1974; LEWIS et al., 1975).

While PAF could result in secondary release of 5-HT during IgE-mediated reactions in man, this reaction has not been studied extensively.

The following mediators can be released during antigen-IgE mediated reactions from human basophils and mast cells (AUSTEN and ORANGE, 1975; NEWBALL et al., 1975): histamine, SRS-A, ECF-A, PAF, the basophil kallikrein of anaphylaxis (BK-A), a neutrophil chemotactic factor (NCF), and possibly prostaglandins (from human lung mast cells). Prostaglandin release may also occur via secondary mechanisms. Secondary mediators may include prostaglandins, 5-HT (via PAF activation of platelets), and bradykinin (generated by the enzymic action of BK-A on kininogen in tissues and plasma). We have already alluded to the fact that these mediators may be released by other inflammatory cells, but in this discussion we shall consider primarily mediator release mediated by direct antigen-IgE interaction, and hence mechanisms of release from basophils and mast cells.

D. Biochemistry of Release

The mechanism of mediator release is best studied in vitro, using tissues or cell suspensions containing basophils or mast cells (LICHTENSTEIN, 1972). Basophils have been studied using washed leukocytes. Mast cells have been studied using rat peritoneal cells, lung fragments or lung cell suspensions from several species, or other tissues such as nasal polyps in man. Such cells or tissue fragments are washed, incubated in a defined medium with or without drugs, and antigen is added. After incubation, the cell-free supernatant is assayed for the presence of released mediators. Cell suspensions can be obtained either from a sensitized donor, or alternatively, cells of a nonsensitized donor may be incubated with IgE-rich sera of another donor, which then sensitizes the cells. When such cell suspensions are incubated with antigen, rapid release of histamine occurs. The reproducible and dose-dependent nature of histamine release has enabled a series of biochemical studies of the mechanisms of release.

Interaction and bridging of IgE by antigen triggers a series of steps which result in mediator secretion; only limited information on the number of steps involved is available, and the exact sequence is not certain. It has been suggested that early events include a fall in intracellular cAMP possibly followed by a cAMP-dependent aggregation of microtubules, which is an energy-requiring step, and finally increased membrane permeability to calcium (LICHTENSTEIN, 1972; KALINER and AUSTEN, 1974; SULLIVAN et al., 1975). Evidence based primarily on inhibition by agents like di-isopropylfluorophosphate suggest that many inflammatory reactions involve antigen-induced activation of serine esterase. Human lung mast cells may have an activatable esterase, but human basophils do not (BECKER and HENSON, 1973).

The release of histamine requires extracellular calcium, a temperature of 37° C, and is inhibited by microtubule-disrupting agents (colchicine), enhanced by microtubule-stabilizing agents (D_2O), and is inhibited reversibly by drugs which reversibly raise levels of intracellular cAMP (LICHTENSTEIN, 1972; FOREMAN et al., 1973). These and other observations suggest that mediator release from mast cells and basophils occurs via a non-cytotoxic secretory event analogous to 'stimulus-secretion coupling' (DOUGLAS, 1968).

It has been possible to divide histamine release in vitro into two distinct stages (LICHTENSTEIN and DEBERNARDO, 1971). In the first stage, incubation in a calcium-free medium with antigen results in 'activation' of cells but no mediator release. Activated cells are washed free of unbound antigen and the second stage initiated by the introduction of a calcium-containing medium which leads to mediator release. Drugs which raise cAMP levels act on the first stage whilst D_2O, metabolic inhibitors and agents which affect calcium flux, act on the second stage (GILLESPIE and LICHTENSTEIN, 1972; LICHTENSTEIN, 1975). The biochemical definition of activated cells is uncertain; these cells are relatively stable at 0° C, but at 37° C they rapidly become "desensitized" such that when they are rechallenged with the same or different antigens, in complete medium, they are no longer capable of releasing mediators (LICHTENSTEIN, 1971). Desensitization appears to be an important determinant of the kinetics of in vitro mediator release (BAXTER and ADAMIK, 1975).

The modulation by cyclic nucleotides of mediator release is of particular interest because cAMP has been called a 'second messenger' which regulates secretory re-

Table 1. Agents that act on specific receptors to raise cyclic AMP and inhibit histamine release

Receptor Classification	Agonist	Antagonist
β-Adrenoceptor	Isoprenaline Adrenaline	Propranolol
Histamine-2	Histamine 4-methylhistamine	Burimamide Metiamide Cimetidine
Prostaglandin	PGE_1, PGE_2, (PGA's)	—
Cholera enterotoxin	Cholera enterotoxin	Cholera toxoid

sponses of cells. BOURNE et al. (1974) have reviewed the evidence (albeit indirect) which strongly suggests that cAMP can modulate the intensity of inflammatory and immune responses. Elevation of intracellular cAMP inhibits release from basophils and mast cells of SRS-A and histamine. Three distinct mechanisms can elevate cAMP: (a) exogenous cAMP, (b) theophylline or similar compounds, which inhibit the phosphodiesterase that catabolizes cAMP, (c) β-adrenoceptor stimulants, histamine, prostaglandins, and cholera enterotoxin—which activate adenylate cyclase, the enzyme that synthesizes cAMP from ATP. The latter agents all appear to interact with specific (apparently cell-surface) receptors. Such receptors are defined pharmacologically on the basis of specific antagonists. The receptors are listed in Table 1.

The physiological significance of cholera enterotoxin receptors is unclear. There may be an endogenous cholera enterotoxin-like material which can activate these receptors, but it has not been discovered. The other three receptors are activated by endogenous agents. Histamine and prostaglandins of the E series are released during inflammatory and immune responses. Adrenaline is a hormone released under conditions of stress or other stimuli. Thus, these substances may well participate in in vivo control of inflammation. The control mechanism(s) activated by histamine are discussed in detail in Section F.

While cAMP inhibits mediator release, α-adrenoceptors and cholinoceptors when activated both enhance mediator release from lung mast cells (KALINER et al., 1972), although not from human peripheral basophils (LICHTENSTEIN et al., 1972). For example, phenylephrine (a α-receptor agonist), in the presence of propranolol to block its weak β-receptor activity, enhances release. Acetylcholine or carbamylcholine enhance histamine and especially SRS-A release, apparently through a muscarinic receptor since their effects are blocked by atropine. It is postulated that cholinoceptor agents lead to the activation of the enzyme guanylate cyclase, and to increased levels of cGMP; support for this hypothesis is provided by experiments demonstrating that 8-bromo cGMP enhances mediator release.

The biochemical events which lead to the release of other mediators appear to be similar to those leading to histamine release. However, recent experiments suggest that each mediator can be released independently (or, at least somewhat independently) of the others. Thus, ECF-A and BK-A release in vitro generally parallels that of histamine, but in dose-response and kinetic terms the ratio of absolute ECF-A/histamine or BK-A/histamine varies from individual to individual (CZARNETZKI et al., 1976a; NEWBALL et al., 1975). The kinetics of SRS-A release are quite different from that of histamine (LEWIS et al., 1974) (for further details, see Section H), presumably because SRS-A is not detectable in 'resting' cells but must be synthesized, from unknown precursors, following antigen trigger. Histamine and BK-A are preformed; ECF-A apparently is preformed in lung mast cells, but preliminary evidence suggests that it is not preformed in blood basophils (CZARNETZKI et al., 1976a).

A variety of stimuli can trigger release. Antigen, anti-IgE, and concanavalin A (Con A) all have similar mechanisms, that of bridging of adjacent IgE molecules; Con A bridges carbohydrate moieties of two adjacent IgE molecules (SIRAGANIAN and SIRAGANIAN, 1975). Some differences even among these agents exist, in that maximal anti-IgE-induced histamine release is often less than maximal antigen-induced histamine release (LICHTENSTEIN, 1972).

The classic model of 'non-specific' histamine release uses the compound 48/80, which induces histamine release from rat mast cells (GOTH, 1973). This agent does not release mediators from human mast cells except at high (possibly toxic) concentrations. A variety of 'physiological' releasers exist. Thus, aspirin-induced asthma (McDONALD et al., 1972) and exercise-induced asthma (GODFREY, 1975) may represent non-specific induction of mediator release. Several drugs (morphine, curare, radiographic contrast dye, etc.) also are releasers. Little is known of the biochemistry of these reactions.

The anaphylatoxins, C3a and C5a, are potential physiological triggers to mediator release. C3a and C5a can induce wheal and flare reactions in human skin (LEPOW et al., 1970) but, perhaps because human basophils are less sensitive to these mediators than are mast cells, histamine release in vitro can be induced only by relatively high concentrations of C5a, and not at all by C3a (GRANT et al., 1975; HOOK et al., 1975).[3] Interestingly, the mechanism of C5a-induced histamine release from human basophils (very rapid release, optimal temperature 25°–30° C, differential desensitization to C5a versus anti-IgE, lack of enhancing effect of D_2O) is distinct from that of anti-IgE, although some of the control mechanisms (comparable inhibition by some cAMP-active drugs) are similar (SIRAGANIAN, personal communication; SIRAGANIAN and HOOK, 1976; GRANT et al., 1975).

The calcium ionophore A23187 induces mediator release by a mechanism which "bypasses" the early biochemical events in antigen-induced release (LICHTENSTEIN, 1975). Thus, cAMP-active agents have no effect on release. This agent also induces synthesis and secretion of SRS (see Section H).

[3] Purified C3a has recently been shown to induce histamine release from human basophils (GLOVSKY et al., 1977). Several low molecular weight peptides, especially tripeptides with formylmethionine as N-terminal amino acid, are also potent inducers of histamine release. These peptides are thought to resemble bacterial products (HOOK et al., 1976). Several products of activated lymphocytes, including one which is identified as interferon, have been reported either to induce histamine release directly or to augment antigen-induced histamine release from human basophils (IDA et al., 1977; THUESON et al., 1977; BAMZAI et al., 1977). Phagocytic stimuli (e.g., serum-coated zymosan particles) also augment antigen-induced histamine release (THOMAS and LICHTENSTEIN, 1978).
The list of "physiologic stimuli" for mediator release may continue to grow. Many stimuli for mediator release from inflammatory cells are also chemotactic for that cell. Thus, diverse stimuli may function in many in vivo inflammatory events to attract basophils and then induce the release of histamine.

Damage to mast cells can also induce mediator release. The urticaria associated with some transfusion-associated allergic reactions (THOMPSON et al., 1971) may be related to anti-leukocyte antibody-induced histamine release from basophils and mast cells.

E. Assay of Mediators

The mediators are assayed by bioassay, chemical or radiochemical assay. Because of the marked sensitivity of guinea pig ileum to low concentrations (5–10 ng/ml) of histamine, the Schultz-Dale technique is the standard bioassay for histamine (ROCHA E SILVA, 1966). This assay is limited by changes, over multiple samples and long assay times, in the sensitivity of ileum to histamine. The identity of the contractile material as histamine can be confirmed by using an antihistamine, such as diphenhydramine or pyrilamine, to check specificity.

The fluorometric assay of histamine, described by SHORE et al. (1959) depends on quantitative interaction of histamine in aqueous medium with O-phthaldialdehyde to produce a fluorophore; a linear dose-response relationship with histamine exists over a range of 5–500 ng/ml. This assay requires multiple extractions to remove other reactive materials. Recent automation of this assay has markedly improved the convenience and sensitivity (SIRAGANIAN, 1975).

The isotopic assay described by SNYDER et al. (1966) depends on enzymic transfer by histamine-*N*-methyltransferase of the ^{14}C-CH3 of S-adenosylmethione to histamine, to form 3-methylhistamine. The assay uses a crude extract of guinea pig brain for enzyme source and one extraction to separate methylhistamine from histamine. This assay can be sensitive to 0.1 ng/ml histamine.

5-HT can be assayed by measurement of contraction of rat colon and estrus rat uterus (blocked by the 5-HT antagonist lysergic acid diethylamide), by fluorometry, and by double-isotope assay using acetylation and ^{14}C-transfer in two enzymatic steps (KAPLAN et al., 1975; SAAVADRA et al., 1973).

SRS-A is identified only by bioassay (STECHSCHULTE, 1974), typically by contraction of guinea pig ileum (made insensitive to histamine by an antihistamine). The quantity of SRS-A is defined in arbitrary units, preferably compared to aliquots of a frozen standard SRS-A preparation, or alternatively, compared to the responsiveness of the ileum to histamine.

F. Histamine

Histamine is a biologically potent low molecular weight decarboxylated amino acid possessing an imidazole ring. As discussed by BLACK (1975), the nomenclature of the imidazole ring used in this chapter designates the nitrogen adjacent to the amino-ethyl group, the '1' position. Histamine by this nomenclature is called 5-(β-amino-ethyl) imidazole.

In addition to basophil and mast cell storage sites, histamine is found in human epidermis, CNS and gastrointestinal mucosa, as a non-mast cell-associated and rapidly turned-over histamine (DOUGLAS, 1975; AUSTEN, 1971). Histamine is formed

Table 2. Histamine receptors

Receptor	Activity	Agonist	Antagonist	Mechanism
Histamine-type 1	Contract guinea pig ileum Contract guinea pig bronchi Contract human bronchi	Histamine 2-Methyl-histamine	Diphenhydramine Pyrilamine	Cyclic GMP (?) Cyclic AMP
Histamine-type 2	Stimulate gastric acid secretion Relax rat uterus Stimulate guinea pig S-A node	Histamine 4-Methyl-histamine	Burimamide Metiamide Cimetidine	Cyclic AMP

from L-histidine by the enzyme histidine decarboxylase, a pyridoxal phosphate-requiring enzyme found in mast cells and basophils. A variety of plant materials contain histamine, but exogenous intake of this material appears to be unimportant for body stores.

Histamine is metabolized by two major enzymic pathways, each of which results in biologically inactive compounds (BEAVEN, 1976; DOUGLAS, 1975; MASLINSKI, 1975): (1) histaminase (diamine oxidase), which forms imidazole acetic acid, and (2) histamine N-methyltransferase, which forms N(3)-methylhistamine. Both compounds are metabolized further. The distribution of these two distinct enzymes varies between species and between tissues; e.g., methylation is apparently the major pathway in mice, while oxidation is important in guinea pigs. In man, both pathways are active although analysis of urinary metabolites suggests that methylation is the more predominant pathway in the periphery. The two enzymes appear to have distinct distribution in leukocytes; thus, histaminase is in eosinophil and neutrophil granulocytes and histamine *N*-methyltransferase in monocytes (ZEIGER et al., 1976).

The activities of histamine are so diverse (DOUGLAS, 1975; AUSTEN, 1971; BEAVEN, 1976; LEVY, 1974) that they can be only summarized here. The classical effects of histamine are those which mimic the manifestations of acute allergic reactions—i.e., 'increased vascular permeability' and bronchial smooth muscle contraction. Histamine mediates a variety of other, and even opposing, effects. Thus, it contracts uterine smooth muscle of some species, but relaxes rat uterus. In a search for a "physiological" role, some investigators have speculated that histamine can, through its perivascular mast cell stores, regulate the microcirculation (SCHAYER, 1963), and also that through its vascular and other effects, the so-called rapidly turning-over histamine can promote tissue growth and repair (KAHLSON and ROSENGREN, 1968); thus, 'induced' histidine decarboxylase activity is found at the site of tissue repair. These speculative ideas remain controversial, and will not be discussed in detail here.

The pharmacological activity of histamine was defined by the specific inhibition of its actions by antihistamines. Thus, histamine-induced contraction of guinea pig ileum and trachea are blocked by the antihistamine agents mepyramine (also called pyrilamine) and diphenhydramine. The existence of two distinct receptors (shown in Table 2) for histamine was suggested by the work of ASH and SCHILD (1966), who showed that low concentrations of mepyramine quantitatively inhibited histamine activity on guinea pig ileum and trachea and on human bronchial muscle; receptors blocked by these antihistamines were designated histamine-type 1 receptors. The available antihistamines failed to block histamine stimulation of gastric acid secretion, nor did they block the ability of histamine to relax rat uterus or to increase guinea pig atrial rate. The existence of histamine-type 2 receptors was established by BLACK and his colleagues (1972), who synthesized the histamine-type 2 antagonist, burimamide (and more recently, metiamide and cimetidine; BLACK, 1975) and showed that this compound blocked the histamine effect on guinea pig atrial rate and on gastric acid secretion, but had no effect on the histamine-induced contraction of guinea pig ileum. Furthermore, congeners of histamine were shown to have selective agonist action; thus, 2-methylhistamine activates predominantly histamine-type 1 receptors, while 4-methylhistamine is a highly selective histamine-type 2 agonist.[4] Quantitative estimates of the dissociation constants for the antagonist-receptor complex (pA2, or K_B value) have further confirmed the distinctive nature of this histamine-type 2 receptor. It is, however, unlikely that pharmacological agents have absolutely receptor-specific actions; and it has recently been shown that the agents, tolazaline and clonidine, are not only α-adrenoceptor antagonists, but also are histamine-type 2 agonists (CSONGRADY and KOBINGER, 1974; YELLIN et al., 1975).

It has been postulated (but not proved) that the two receptors represent configurations bound by the two possible tautomers of histamine, which differ in N-N distances (MASLINKSI, 1975). The two receptors are probably structurally similar, and one series of experiments suggests that at 12° C, histamine-type 1 receptors in guinea pig ileum spontaneously convert to receptors with properties of histamine-type 2 receptors (KENATIN et al., 1974).

While the mechanism of activation of cells by histamine is not known precisely, it may be distinct for each receptor; activation of many histamine-type 2 receptors involve elevation of intracellular cAMP (BLACK, 1975). Histamine-type 1 receptor activation has been postulated to involve elevation of cGMP levels (GOLDBERG et al., 1975), but in several tissues cAMP elevation due to histamine has been blocked by histamine-type 1 antagonists (KLEIN and LEVEY, 1971; BAUDRY et al., 1975).

The physiological significance of two distinct receptors is uncertain, since to this point only one endogenous agent (histamine itself) has been shown to activate these receptors. It is possible that histamine-type 2 receptors on inflammatory cells are activated only at high concentrations of histamine, and thus provide a mechanism of feedback inhibition when large concentrations of mediator are produced. One can speculate that the pH of the stomach is in some way related to the presence of histamine-type 2 receptors, although there is very little information to this point.

Histamine can activate a variety of tissues (for review see DOUGLAS, 1975; CHAND and EYRE, 1975). We will emphasize those tissues that are apparently affected as a consequence of immediate hypersensitivity reactions; we shall also mention briefly gastric and CNS effects of histamine, although these effects are probably not directly related to anaphylactic or inflammatory responses.

Vascular system: Histamine induces wheals by 'increasing vascular permeability'—by dilatation of terminal arterioles and contraction of the endothelial cells of postcapillary venules, resulting in gaps between endothelial cells. Intravenous histamine infusion causes a generalized flush. Vascular effects of histamine are due to

[4] 2-(2-Pyridyl)ethylamine is a selective agonist for histamine-type 1 receptors (DURANT et al., 1975). The newly synthesized compound dimaprit is a highly selective agonist for histamine-type 2 receptors (PARSONS et al., 1977).

activation of both histamine-type 1 and histamine-type 2 receptors. It appears that histamine-type 2 receptors act synergistically with histamine-type 1 receptors, but that the histamine affinity for histamine-type 2 receptors may be ten times less than for histamine-type 1 receptors (BLACK, 1975).[5]

Cardiac: Direct cardiac effects of histamine may explain some manifestations of anaphylaxis, but receptors have been studied best in guinea pig hearts. In these animals, histamine-type 2 receptors mediate increased sinus node rate, and possibly increased inotropic effects, while histamine-type 1 receptors mediate decreased A-V conduction time (LEVI et al., 1975; CAPURRO and LEVI, 1975). Similar receptors have not yet been demonstrated for man.

Gastric: Histamine is found (in non-mast cell-storage sites) in the stomach and it is usually a potent stimulator of gastric acid secretion, through histamine-type 2 receptors. Recent evidence has suggested that histamine may be the final common pathway for acid secretion, although conflicting data exists. Histamine-type 2 antagonists have been used successfully in several clinical trials of treatment of peptic ulcer disease, Zollinger-Ellison syndrome and even gastric ulcer disease; trials with cimetidine are in progress (BRIMBLECOMBE et al., 1975; POUNDER et al., 1976).

Smooth muscle: The histamine-induced contraction of the uteri of several species, and of guinea pig ileum, guinea pig trachea and human bronchial smooth muscle, is mediated through histamine-type 1 receptors. In several other species, histamine-type 2 receptors on the tracheobronchial tree mediate relaxation and co-exist with the histamine-type 1 receptors mediating contraction. Thus, the net effect of histamine is the sum of its actions on these two receptors. In sheep, relaxation of bronchial smooth muscle is the predominant effect of histamine (EYRE, 1973); and in rabbits, only histamine-type 2 (relaxation) receptors exist in the upper airways (ADAMS, unpublished observation). Similarly, histamine induces relaxation of the rat uterus by stimulation of histamine-type 2 receptors. The human uterus is minimally affected by histamine.

Central nervous system: Histamine is found in specific locations in the brain; it has been postulated to be a neurotransmitter. In sympathetic ganglia, facilitation of conduction appears to be a histamine-type 1, whilst inhibition is a histamine-type 2 effect. Histamine induces cAMP elevation in guinea pig brain slices, and both histamine-type 1 and histamine-type 2 antagonists block the cAMP elevation; both antagonists together are needed to block completely the cAMP elevation (BAUDRY et al., 1975).

The effects on inflammatory cells and immune processes: Histamine can facilitate inflammation by its effects on vascular permeability; additionally, it can inhibit the effector function of many inflammatory cells. Histamine, acting through histamine-type 2 receptors, inhibits a variety of inflammatory processes (Table 3). It appears that the mechanism of action of histamine on histamine-2 receptors is through activation of adenylate cyclase, although the evidence is incomplete, and in several systems are based on cAMP measurements in heterogeneous cell populations. Also, the anti-inflammatory effects require high concentrations (usually 10^{-6} M–10^{-4} M) of

[5] Exogenous histamine preferentially activates histamine-type 1 vascular receptors. However, endogenous histamine (e.g., released from mast cells by compound 48/80) in at least some tissues may activate predominantly histamine type 2 vascular receptors (POWELL and BRODY, 1976).

Table 3. Histamine effects on inflammatory and immune responses

Activities	Receptor	Comments	References
A. "Anti-inflammatory" effects			
1. Inhibits antigen-induced histamine release from human basophils and mast cells	H2	Metiamide can enhance antigen-induced release	LICHTENSTEIN and GILLESPIE (1973; 1975) CHAKRIN et al. (1974)
2. Inhibits (in vivo) antigen-induced PCA reactions in rabbits	?		KRAVIS and ZVAIFLER (1974)
3. Inhibits (a) lysozomal enzyme release from, and (b) bacterial factor-induced chemotaxis of, human neutrophils	H2		ZURIER et al. (1974); SOSMAN and BUSSE (1976); HILL et al. (1975)
4. Causes chemotaxis of eosinophils; at higher concentrations, induces desensitization of eosinophils	Not H1, not H2	Receptor specificity unknown	CLARK et al. (1975)
5. Inhibits cytolytic activity of mouse splenic T-lymphocytes	H2	Increase of receptors during primary immune response	PLAUT et al. (1973a; 1973b; 1975a)
6. Inhibits MIF production by antigen-sensitized guinea pig lymph node cells	H2	But: no effect on responsiveness of macrophages to MIF	ROCKLIN (1976)
7. Inhibits transformation of guinea pig and mouse lymph node cells to antigen and/or mitogens	H2	Receptor specificities only partially defined	ROCKLIN (1976); ROSZKOWSKI et al. (1977a)
8. Inhibits antibody secretion by mouse B cells	?		MELMON et al. (1974)
9. Inhibits (in vivo) delayed hypersensitivity skin reactions (guinea pig)	H2 (?)		ROCKLIN (1976)
B. "Pro-inflammatory" effects			
1. Increased vascular permeability required for deposition of immune complexes in rabbits	H1	If this action is related to "increased vascular permeability," H2 receptors may also be involved	KNIKER and COCHRANE (1965)
2. Vasoactive amines are needed to elicit delayed hypersensitivity skin reactions in mice	?	5-HT is primary vasoactive amine in mice	GERSHON et al. (1975)

histamine. However, concentrations of histamine as high as 10^{-4} M are attained locally during antigen-induced histamine release.

It is of interest that several populations of leukocytes do not have measurable cAMP responses to histamine (MAKMAN, 1971; REMOLD-O'DONNELL, 1974; ROSZKOWSKI et al., 1977a). This confirms other evidence, based on functional assay, that histamine receptor-bearing cells are distinct, and histamine receptors are not uniformly distributed over all cell populations (PLAUT et al., 1973b; PLAUT et al., 1975a).

Studies which have been performed in our laboratories have shown that high concentrations (10^{-7}–10^{-6} M) of histamine inhibit histamine release from human basophils (LICHTENSTEIN and GILLESPIE, 1973, 1975). Since histamine inhibition is blocked by burimamide and metiamide but not by histamine-type 1 antagonists, histamine inhibits histamine release by interaction with histamine-type 2 receptors. The existence of this receptor has been confirmed by further studies (LICHTENSTEIN and GILLESPIE, unpublished observations) which demonstrate that the K_B values calculated for burimamide and metiamide are similar to those determined for histamine-type 2 receptors on other tissue types, and that 2-methylhistamine does not inhibit histamine release while 4-methylhistamine does. This observation suggests a potential autoregulatory feedback inhibition of histamine release, triggered by large amounts of mediator.

In assays using washed leukocytes, as described above, diffusion of antigen is as rapid as diffusion of histamine. Histamine inhibits an early biochemical step of the release mechanism. Consequently, histamine released by one basophil will not inhibit in vitro release from other basophils. However, in vivo in tissue mast cells, antigen diffusion may be rate-limiting. CHAKRIN et al. (1974) showed that histamine can inhibit antigen-induced mediator release from monkey lung tissue, and also that metiamide alone can significantly enhance histamine and SRS-A release. This suggests that histamine is released from some mast cells; diffuses rapidly in solid tissue and, unless its action is blocked by the appropriate antihistamine, inhibits mediator release from other mast cells.[6]

Histamine inhibits lysosomal enzyme release from (ZURIER et al., 1974; SOSMAN and BUSSE, 1976) and chemotaxis of (HILL et al., 1975) human neutrophils. Surprisingly, histamine can induce chemotaxis of eosinophils (CLARK et al., 1975) through a mechanism which has not been defined. Eosinophil chemotaxis by histamine is reduced in the presence of high concentrations of histamine, and this reduced chemotaxis is reversed by metiamide. The effects of histamine on modulation of the eosinophil chemotactic responsiveness to endotoxin-activated serum are complex (CLARK et al., 1977): Histamine enhances the migration of some eosinophils (this effect is blocked by histamine-type 1 antagonists), while it inhibits the chemotactic activity of other eosinophils; this inhibition is reversed by histamine-type 2 antagonists. These complex histamine effects will undoubtedly be elucidated further in the near future.

Further studies in our laboratory have demonstrated that histamine can modulate lymphocyte function (PLAUT et al., 1973a, 1973b, 1975a). Thus, the ability of cytolytically active T-lymphocytes (CTL) of alloimmune mice to kill target cells in vitro is inhibited by histamine in a dose-dependent manner (10^{-7} to 10^{-5} M); this inhibition by histamine is mediated by histamine-type 2 receptors. Further studies (PLAUT et al., 1975b) using 2-methylhistamine and 4-methylhistamine and quantitative estimation of the K_B values for burimamide and metiamide (with either histamine or 4-methylhistamine as agonist) confirm the presence of histamine-type 2

[6] Histamine also inhibits the chemotactic responsiveness (to C5a) of human basophils (LETT-BROWN and LEONARD, 1977).

receptors on killer T cells. Furthermore, the susceptibility of CTL to inhibition by histamine is not constant, but increases during the primary immune response. Thus CTL, when first detected on day 7, are not inhibited by histamine, but by day 18 cytotoxic activity is inhibited 50% by histamine, apparently reflecting the emergence of a distinct subpopulation of CTL bearing histamine receptors. The emergence of significant numbers of histamine-receptor bearing CTL is associated with a fall in cytolytic activity, suggesting a relationship between histamine and regulation of T cell numbers. Furthermore, inhibition by histamine of peritoneal exudate CTL is less than that of spleen CTL, suggesting that effector populations differ in histamine receptor display.

Several lymphocyte functions, in addition to T cell killing, can be modulated through histamine receptors. First, histamine can inhibit antigen and mitogen-induced transformation and antigen-induced production of migration inhibitory factor (Mif) (ROCKLIN, 1976; ROSZKOWSKI et al., 1977a).[7]

Histamine can also block B cell maturation into antibody-secreting cells (MELMON et al., 1974). Additionally, in a mouse model system of antigen (synthetic polypeptide)-induced immunosuppression, histamine inhibits the antigen effect (MOZES et al., 1974), although the cell-type(s) affected by histamine are not known. Histamine-type 2 antagonists were not tested, but the histamine effect was reported to be blocked by high (possibly toxic) concentrations of diphenhydramine.[8]

[7] The effects of cAMP-active agents on Mif production and action are confusing; thus, cholera enterotoxin is reported to have no effect on guinea pig Mif production (HENNEY et al., 1974), while it and other agents which raise macrophage cAMP levels, inhibit Mif action on macrophages (HENNEY et al., 1974; KOOPMAN et al., 1973). In contrast, histamine inhibits Mif production (although there is as yet no reported data on cAMP levels), but has no effect on the interaction of Mif with macrophages, and in fact, does not affect macrophage homogenate adenylate cyclase levels (ROCKLIN, 1976; REMOLD-O'DONNELL, 1974). If these differences between agents prove correct, it suggests that lymphocytes have one set of control mechanisms, and macrophages have hormone receptors distinct from those of lymphocytes.

[8] Additional evidence establishes that histamine receptors are selectively displayed on mouse lymphocyte populations. Thus, histamine receptors are present on splenic T lymphocytes but not splenic B lymphocytes. Furthermore, the maturation of T lymphocytes, from thymocytes to cortisone-resistant thymocytes to splenic T lymphocytes, is associated with complex hormone receptor changes, including reduction in number of β-adrenoceptors and development of histamine receptors (ROSZKOWSKI et al., 1977b).
While histamine receptors are not present on B lymphocytes from naive mice (ROSZKOWSKI et al., 1977a, 1977b), they may be present on maturing B lymphocytes. Histamine blocks primary in vitro antibody responses [although the target cell type(s) are not known] (FALLAH et al., 1975) and also blocks secretion of antibody (MELMON et al., 1974, as discussed in text).
Histamine inhibits lymphocyte function by several mechanisms. Its inhibition of Mif secretion and proliferation of guinea pig lymphocytes is indirect: histamine induces some cells to secrete a nondialyzable factor, "histamine-induced suppressor factor," which in turn inhibits Mif-secreting, and proliferating, cells (ROCKLIN, 1977). The inhibition of mouse cytotoxic lymphocytes appears to be direct, since no soluble factor is detectable (PLAUT, 1978).
Histamine (10^{-7} M–10^{-5} M) inhibits concanavalin A-induced proliferation of human lymphocytes (PLAUT and BERMAN, 1978; PLAUT, 1978). Several reports have suggested individual variation in sensitivity of human lymphocytes to histamine. Thus, T lymphocytes only from allergic, not nonatopic, donors are reported to possess histamine receptors, as measured by histamine-induced inhibition of E rosetting or of PHA-induced proliferation (VERHAEGEN et al., 1977; STRANNEGÅRD and STRANNEGÅRD, 1977). Our preliminary results cannot relate lymphocyte responsiveness to histamine to the presence of atopy versus nonatopy (PLAUT, 1978).

There are several other potential anti-inflammatory effects of histamine, but the evidence for these is very indirect. For example, experiments by MELMON et al. (1972) and WEINSTEIN et al. (1973) have identified putative histamine receptors by binding subpopulations of leukocytes to histamine-coated Sepharose beads. SHEARER et al. (1972, 1974), SEGAL et al. (1974), and EICHMANN (1975) have suggested that suppressor T cells possess histamine receptors, since these suppressor cells bind preferentially to histamine-coated beads. There is, however, considerable recent controversy as to whether the specificity of binding to these beads is related to the histamine moiety (MATTHYSSENS et al., 1975; PLAUT et al., 1975a). It is still possible that subpopulations of suppressor T cells, but not other cells, possess histamine receptors.

Several investigators have recently demonstrated the existence of histidine decarboxylase activity and/or histamine at the sites of immunological reactions. The role of histamine at these sites remains unknown. Thus, splenic histidine decarboxylase activity and urinary histamine excretion are increased in rats undergoing immunization to sheep red blood cells, or graft rejection; and histidine decarboxylase activity at the site of graft rejection also increases. Inhibitors of histamine decarboxylase (although not entirely specific for the enzyme) prolong graft survival (MOORE et al., 1971; SINCLAIR et al., 1973; MOORE and SCHAYER, 1969; MOORE, 1967; MOORE and LAWRENCE, 1969).

A further potential role for histamine is suggested by the work of DVORAK and DVORAK (1974), and more recently ASKENASE (1973), and KATZ et al. (1975), who have re-examined in great detail the pathology of a number of presumably cell-mediated reactions. They have shown that in so-called Jones-Mote reactivity (induced by injecting antigen in Freund's incomplete adjuvant), in contact sensitivity in guinea pigs and in poison ivy dermatitis in man, the lesions are infiltrated not only by lymphocytes and mononuclear cells, but also by large numbers of basophils. This reaction has been called cutaneous basophil hypersensitivity (CBH) and can be distinguished from classical delayed hypersensitivity (DH). However, large numbers of basophils are present (transiently) in graft rejection and in DH (tuberculin) reactions; the histamine content of guinea pig tissues parallels the basophil count.

The precise function of the basophils is unclear. While DVORAK and DVORAK (1974) have suggested that basophils infiltrating CBH reactions cannot release histamine in response to antigen, DEBERNARDO et al. (1975) have demonstrated antigen-induced mediator release at the site of CBH reactions.[9]

Since lymphocyte-derived chemotactic factors, as well as serum chemotactic factors such as C5a, are chemotactic for human and guinea pig basophils (WARD et al., 1975; BOETCHER and LEONARD, 1973), we can speculate that basophils are attracted by lymphocyte chemotactic stimuli. These basophils may then release histamine, for example, in response to triggering by antigen. The released histamine could at low concentrations facilitate an inflammatory response (see below) and at high concentrations could modulate a cell-mediated immune reaction for example, as already

[9] More recent studies strongly suggest that histamine is released during inflammatory reactions by basophils in tissue infiltrates. DVORAK et al. (1976) have established that basophils and mast cells degranulate during allergic contact dermatitis reactions in man. ASKENASE (1977) has demonstrated that augmented histamine release, induced by antigen, occurs at sites of basophil infiltrates.

discussed, by inhibiting cytotoxic T cells, Mif-producing cells, and in vivo delayed hypersensitivity skin reactions (ROCKLIN, 1976).

In contrast to these apparent anti-inflammatory effects, histamine (for example, histamine stored in the perivascular mast cells) and other mediators may be important in initiating the inflammatory process. Thus, the role of vasoactive amines (histamine and 5-HT) in delayed hypersensitivity reactions and immune complex deposition can be considered a 'pro-inflammatory' response. GERSHON et al. (1975) have shown that vasoactive amines are necessary to elicit DH skin responses in mice. Unlike guinea pigs and man, in mice it is notoriously difficult to elicit DH skin responses, and any delayed skin reactivity can be detected only in the foot pad. Basophils are apparently absent in mice, and only in the foot pad are significant numbers of skin mast cells found. Reserpine (presumed to be a 5-HT depleter) prevents antigen-induced foot pad swelling. This suggests that vasoactive amine-induced contraction of postcapillary venules allows macrophage egress into inflammatory sites. A similar role could be postulated for histamine.

A similar role for vasoactive amines (which probably occur as a consequence of immediate hypersensitivity reactions) has been postulated in the pathogenesis of immune complex disease. KNIKER and COCHRANE (1965) have shown that antihistamines can block immune complex disposition. It is presumed that histamine by increasing vascular permeability is permissive for the efflux and deposition on the basement membrane of immune complexes, which then fix complement, attract neutrophils, etc. A similar physiological role of IgE-mediated immediate hypersensitivity reactions has been postulated (by STEINBERG et al., 1974) to allow egress from the circulation to inflammatory sites of IgG and other immunoglobulin classes. Some preliminary evidence (from a prospective study during a diphtheria immunization program (KNIKER, 1972) suggests that in man prophylactic antihistamines reduce the frequency of subsequent serum sickness.

In summary, histamine may be important both in initiating the inflammatory processes via vascular changes permitting antibody efflux into tissues, and cellular infiltration of tissues; and, in high concentrations, may inhibit the action of many inflammatory cells and thus reduce the inflammatory response.

G. 5-Hydroxytryptamine

5-HT is a vasoactive amine which, like histamine, can induce smooth muscle contracting activity and increase capillary permeability (DOUGLAS, 1975; LEVY, 1974). In man, 90% of 5-HT is distributed in the mucosa of the gastrointestinal tract. Most of the remainder is present in platelets and in the CNS. The enterochromaffin cells of the gastrointestinal tract are the main storage sites in mammals. Mast cells of rats and mice, but not man, contain 5-HT (in the same granules that bind histamine). 5-HT is also present (possibly stored in mast cells) in the lung of the rat and mouse. It is synthesized by metabolic pathways involving hydroxylation and then deamination of tryptophan, and this pathway occurs in enterochromaffin cells, in neurones, and in rat mast cells. Platelets apparently have no such synthetic capacity, but can actively and passively store 5-HT. 5-HT is released from platelets during immune activation, aggregation during clotting, etc. (the vasoactive substance called "vasotonin" released during clotting is 5-HT). Such released 5-HT is either taken up again by platelets, or else metabolized by the enzyme monoamine oxidase.

A variety of effects of 5-HT appear to be mediated by multiple receptors, which can be divided into musculotropic and neurotropic, and probably can be subdivided even further (DRAKONTIDES and GERSHON, 1968; BERRIDGE, 1972; GERSCHENFELD and PAUPARDIN-TRITSCH, 1974a, 1974b). Some peripheral effects are mediated by reflex peripheral nerve stimulation. The CNS effects of 5-HT have been particularly interesting to modern pharmacologists because potent hallucinogens, like lysergic acid diethylamide, are 5-HT antagonists. [10]

The actions of 5-HT are often grouped with those of histamine, and 5-HT induces skin flushing following infusion in man. However, its original description was as a vasoconstrictor. It had been studied primarily in sensitive species (i.e., rodents). Thus, in rats it can induce bronchoconstriction, vasoconstriction, increased capillary permeability (by contraction of postcapillary venules), decreased gastric juice volume, acidity, pepsin, and increased gastric mucus (DOUGLAS, 1975).

In man, 5-HT can induce bronchoconstriction in asthmatic (but not normal) patients, and infusion of 5-HT can induce capillary dilatation (flush). The carcinoid syndrome has been thought to be due to 5-HT, but it is now believed that other mediators are involved; the diarrhoea of carcinoid syndrome is, however, blocked by 5-HT antagonists. Human smooth muscle in vitro is relatively insensitive to 5-HT.

5-HT is considered to be an inflammatory mediator, but its role has been studied only in rabbits, rats, and mice. 5-HT would appear to be the primary mediator of rat and mouse anaphylaxis (GERSHON and ROSS, 1961). Rodents are, in fact, relatively resistant to histamine. In man, since 5-HT is not found in basophils and mast cells, it has not been considered an anaphylactic mediator. Recent studies of mechanisms of platelet secretion in rabbits have demonstrated immune complex-mediated 5-HT release, as well as basophil-dependent IgE-mediated release (through the mediator PAF). The recent identification of human PAF suggests that 5-HT can be released during human immediate hypersensitivity reactions. Human PAF has not yet been demonstrated to be released under physiological conditions. KAPLAN et al. (1975) have described one patient who had elevated blood 5-HT during experimentally induced cholinergic urticaria. (However, this patient also had elevated blood histamine, and all other patients in the study had elevated histamine and not elevated 5-HT). Additionally, cyproheptadine, a drug useful in the treatment of chronic urticaria in man, has anti-5-HT as well as antihistamine properties (DOUGLAS, 1975); however, there is no evidence that the anti-5-HT activity is responsible for the effectiveness of therapy. In summary, there is no defined inflammatory role for 5-HT in man, although the fragmentary type of evidence cited above is usually adduced to support such a role.

Vasoactive amines (especially 5-HT) are permissive for delayed hypersensitivity skin reactions in mice. In rabbits, histamine and 5-HT are probably equally important in permitting immune complex deposition. To this point, no significant anti-inflammatory role for 5-HT (i.e., comparable to the previous discussion of an anti-

[10] However, in at least guinea pig brain, lysergic acid diethylamide is a histamine-type 2 antagonist (GREEN et al., 1977). Several other compounds may also be histamine-type 2 antagonists (GREEN and MAAYANI, 1977; GREEN et al., 1977).

inflammatory role of histamine) has been described; thus, in the mouse, 5-HT in vitro inhibits T cell killing modestly, but only at very high (10^{-3} M) concentrations (PLAUT, 1976).

H. SRS-A

The term "slow reacting substance" was originally introduced to describe the activity of fluid obtained from guinea pig lung perfused with cobra venom (reviewed in STECHSCHULTE, 1974). In contrast to the rapidity (within a few seconds) with which histamine induces maximal contraction of guinea pig ileum, the SRS required several minutes to produce a slow but prolonged contraction of this target tissue. Several other mechanisms for producing materials which induce 'slow' contractions have been described. For example, antigen challenge of sensitized guinea pig lung also produces a slow reacting substance; this latter material was called SRS-A (slow reacting substance of anaphylaxis) by BROCKLEHURST (1962, 1963), and is to be distinguished from SRS-C (slow reacting substance from cobra venom). SRS-C is thought to represent a mixture of several materials including prostaglandins. SRS-As from several species have been identified. It appears that SRS-A from rat, guinea pig, monkey, and human are similar (ORANGE et al., 1973).

The physicochemical uniqueness of SRS-A was demonstrated initially by BROCKLEHURST (1960), who showed that the action of SRS-A was not blocked by antihistamines and thus, that it was not histamine.

ORANGE et al. (1973, 1974) have purified SRS-A and characterized it as acidic sulfur containing lipid-soluble material, of mol w 500. Its structure has not been entirely elucidated. It is identified by its biological properties, such as contraction of guinea pig ileum, rabbit jejunum and duodenum, and human duodenal smooth muscle, but not gerbil colon or oestrus rat uterus. Furthermore, its activity is not blocked by antihistamines or anti-5-HT drugs nor by prostaglandin dehydrogenase[11]. It is inactivated by limpet arylsulfatase and human eosinophil arylsulfatase B (ORANGE et al., 1974; WASSERMAN and AUSTEN, 1976) and perhaps by other pathways.

The first evidence for in vivo production of SRS-A was provided by RAPP (1961), who showed that the interaction of heterologous antigen and antibody could induce release of SRS into the rat's peritoneal cavity. More recent investigations (ORANGE et al., 1968, 1970; STECHSCHULTE et al., 1970) have shown that two distinct rat antibodies are capable of participating in SRS-A production. IgGa antibody-induced SRS-A generation requires both an intact complement system and intact neutrophils. (This observation is strongly suggestive of the recent experiments identifying human neutrophils as a distinct source of SRS-A). A second pathway in the rat involves IgE antibody and intact mast cells.

The mechanism of SRS-A generation is difficult to study in vivo; in vitro investigation has centered primarily on SRS-A release triggered by antigen or anti-IgE in

[11] Recent evidence suggests that SRS and prostaglandins are generated from a common precursor, arachidonic acid. Thus, SRS released from rat basophilic leukemia cells appears to be derived from arachidonic acid, apparently via a newly described biochemical pathway (JAKSCHIK et al., 1977).

either human lung or human leukocytes; thus, the mediator is presumed to reside in human (and monkey) mast cells and basophils. The mechanism of formation of SRS-A is unknown. In contrast to histamine and 5-HT, no SRS-A can be detected in resting tissue. Therefore, the material must be both synthesized (from an unknown precursor) and secreted during the course of immediate hypersensitivity reactions. This process is sequential; thus, when sensitized human lung is challenged in vitro with antigen, SRS-A is detected in the pellet within 1 min; and within several additional minutes variable amounts are released into the cell-free supernatant (ORANGE, 1974; LEWIS et al., 1974).

Histamine and SRS-A release are modulated in common by several drugs; thus, calcium ions are required for release, and cAMP-active drugs inhibit in parallel release of both mediators. On the other hand, several agents have differential activity on the release of these individual mediators. Thus, the fungal metabolites, cytochalasin A and cytochalasin B, generally enhance histamine release from sensitized and antigen-challenged human lung, but they markedly inhibit SRS-A release (ORANGE, 1975). Furthermore, α-adrenoceptor or cholinoceptor stimulation may enhance release of SRS-A (from sensitized and antigen-challenged human lung) more than enhancing release of histamine (KALINER et al., 1972). Thus, the biochemical pathway following antigen challenge which leads to SRS-A synthesis and release is distinct from that leading to histamine release.

In order to study more extensively the mechanism of mediator release, rat peritoneal cells and human leukocytes were challenged with the calcium ionophore A23187, an agent which induces mediator release (e.g., histamine release from basophils) by a mechanism distinct from antigen-induced release and which apparently involves increased membrane calcium ion flux (LICHTENSTEIN, 1975). BACH and BRASHLER (1974) showed that ionophore could induce SRS-A production by rat peritoneal cells depleted of mast cells and neutrophils and speculated that many cell types could synthesize and secrete SRS. Furthermore, the ionophore was found to induce SRS release (i.e., synthesis and secretion) from human leukocytes, but in amounts far exceeding that induced by antigen or by anti-IgE, suggesting that cell(s) in addition to basophils might release SRS. Cell fractionation studies showed that (human) neutrophils represent at least one additional source of SRS. Neutrophil SRS appears physicochemically similar to SRS-A (CONROY et al., 1976).

The observation that neutrophils can synthesize a substance thought previously to be a product only of immediate hypersensitivity reactions is surprising. However, recent evidence using a more readily assayed mediator (ECF-A) has shown that not only A23187, but also activation of neutrophils by phagocytosis, induces ECF[12] synthesis and release from neutrophils (CZARNETZKI et al., 1975, 1976b). By analogy it is likely that neutrophils (and perhaps other cells) can synthesize SRS under physiologic conditions.

The defined activities of SRS are primarily on blood vessels and smooth muscle. There is only preliminary characterization of SRS-A antagonists, such as FPL 55712 (AUGSTEIN et al., 1973). (All SRS-A antagonists identified to this point also inhibit mediator release. The significance of this observation is unclear.) Thus, true receptor(s) for SRS-A are not yet defined pharmacologically.

[12] The term ECF-A is reserved for eosinophil chemotactic factor derived from anaphylactic reactions. Hence, neutrophil-derived eosinophil chemotactic factor is called ECF.

Intracutaneous injection of SRS-A can increase vascular permeability in guinea pig, rat, and monkey skin (AUSTEN and ORANGE, 1975). It can be shown to contract specific smooth muscles including guinea pig ileum and bronchi. The human bronchus in vitro is quite sensitive to SRS-A. Intravenous administration of SRS-A to unanesthetized guinea pigs results in decreased pulmonary compliance with minimal decreases in airways conductance. (In contrast, histamine decreases both compliance and conductance.) These effects are presumably not mediated via reflexes, since their effects are not blocked by atropine (DRAZEN and AUSTEN, 1974, 1975). However, some species may be insensitive to SRS-A; SRS-A has no effect on the pulmonary mechanics of anesthetized dogs (LAPIERRE et al., 1976).

Histamine and SRS may act synergistically on smooth muscle and blood vessels (BROCKLEHURST, 1962; AUSTEN and ORANGE, 1975); and they may both result in the release of secondary mediators such as prostaglandins, with diverse effects on vessels and smooth muscle depending on the type(s) of prostaglandins which are released.

I. Summary: In vivo Significance of Mediators

It is clear that the complexity which results when the in vitro observations are applied to an analysis of in vivo allergic reactions, is quite formidable. The in vivo effects will reflect synergistic, and possibly (with some agents such as prostaglandins; ZURIER, 1974), antagonistic effects of the mediators. In antigen-induced release, the relative proportion of mediators is not constant. Furthermore, distinct mechanisms for mediator release represent different biochemical sequences and thus, different control mechanisms. Conceivably, the proportions of the various mediators may differ markedly from the proportions induced following antigen-induced release.

One interesting and unsolved problem is the relative 'importance' of the various mediators in vivo. Histamine seems to be the most dominant mediator of guinea pig anaphylaxis (in that antihistamines can block anaphylaxis) and 5-HT is particularly important in rodent anaphylaxis. While histamine seems to be particularly important in human anaphylaxis, histamine-type 1 antihistamines are not clinically useful in anaphylaxis or in allergic asthma. This may be because: (1) antihistamine blood levels are inadequate to block the effects of large amounts of histamine ($\sim 10^{-4}$ M) which are released locally, (2) several histamine effects in anaphylaxis represent synergistic effects on histamine-type 1 plus histamine-type 2 receptors, and thus require combinations of two types of antihistamines to block, (3) the effects of anaphylaxis and asthma may well represent the effects of other mediators in addition to histamine, most likely SRS-A. At this point, there is evidence in favour of all these possibilities.[13]

As difficult as it is to define the role of mediators in immediate hypersensitivity reactions, attempts to define a physiological role of these mediators is even more

[13] In some recent experiments to distinguish among these possibilities, ADAMS and LICHTENSTEIN (1977) have studied the effects of mediator antagonists on in vitro antigen-induced contraction of sensitized guinea pig and human trachea. Large amounts of histamine are released within the first several minutes after antigen challenge. In the succeeding several minutes, the histamine concentration falls, and large amounts of SRS-A are secreted. These results suggest that at least the first and third possibilities are both correct.

difficult. We have already mentioned the possibility that mediators such as histamine are permissive for deposition of immune complexes and for delayed hypersensitivity reactions. This permissiveness may be important as a protective mechanism for infectious diseases, in that increased vascular permeability permits antibodies and cells to get to the appropriate site of inflammatory reactions. Furthermore, we have also shown that histamine can not only initiate inflammatory processes, but can also exert diverse anti-inflammatory activities which may limit the intensity of inflammatory processes.[14]

In searching for a physiological role, the mechanisms of mediator release must also be considered. We have emphasized mediator release following antigen-IgE interaction, but other mechanisms may occur in vivo also. For example, C3a- and C5a-induced mediator release (e.g., following immune complex activation of complement) may explain urticaria which occurs during serum sickness and immune complex disease. Since C5a is chemotactic for basophils, as are some lymphocyte products, and since SRS and ECF can be released from neutrophils and other inflammatory cells, the manifestations of immediate hypersensitivity may be triggered by pathways independent of antigen-IgE interaction. It is possible that some poorly understood phenomena, such as 'late' IgE-mediated reactions or 'late' asthma, can be explained by the delayed release by these alternate pathophysiological mechanisms of the mediators of immediate hypersensitivity reactions. If histamine plays a role in tissue growth and repair, other physiological mechanisms of histamine release must exist which have not yet been elucidated.

References

Adams, G. K., III, Lichtenstein, L. M.: Antagonism of antigen-induced contraction of guinea pig and human airways. Nature **270**, 255—257 (1977)

Adams, G. K., III: Unpublished observations (1976)

[14] The role of histamine in vivo has been evaluated by infusing histamine-releasing compounds and/or histamine receptor agonists and antagonists. The interpretation of these in vivo experiments is complicated for several reasons: 1) Apparently opposing inflammatory effects of histamine—increasing vascular permeability versus inhibiting the effector function of inflammatory cells—may both be mediated by histamine-type 2 receptors. 2) Both vascular and inflammatory cell (e.g., lymphocyte) receptors are readily desensitized in vitro and in vivo by prolonged exposure to histamine (Plaut, 1977; cf. Schwartz et al., 1977). 3) Individuals may differ in sensitivity of inflammatory cells to histamine (Verhaegen et al., 1977; Strannegård and Strannegård, 1977; Busse and Sosman, 1977). 4) Histamine receptor antagonists not only block the action of histamine on its receptors, but also a) block histamine-induced receptor desensitization and also may both b) induce histidine decarboxylase (Maudsley et al., 1973) and c) inhibit histamine metabolism. [Thus, the histamine-type 2 antagonists are relatively potent inhibitors of human neutrophil-derived histaminase (Thomas et al., 1978).] In contrast to the expected blocking action of these antihistamines, the latter three effects would tend to potentiate the activity of histamine.

In one recent study, prolonged therapy with the histamine-type 2 antagonist cimetidine appeared to enhance the delayed skin reactivity of patients with peptic ulcer disease (Avella et al., 1978). The easiest interpretation is that histamine normally is released during delayed sensitivity reactions and acts as a negative feedback control, and cimetidine inhibits this negative feedback. However, based on the considerations just described, other interpretations are possible. Further studies on in vivo inflammatory events are in progress.

Ash, A. S. F., Schild, H. O.: Receptors mediating some actions of histamine. Brit. J. Pharmacol. **27**, 427—439 (1966)
Askenase, P. W.: Cutaneous basophil hypersensitivity in contact-sensitized guinea pigs. I. Transfer with immune serum. J. exp. Med. **138**, 1144—1155 (1973)
Askenase, P. W.: Role of basophils, mast cells, and vasoamines in hypersensitivity reactions with a delayed time course. In: Kallos, P., Waksman, B. H., deWeck, A. L. (Eds.): Progress in Allergy, Vol. XXIII, pp. 199—320. Basel: Karger 1977
Augstein, J., Farmer, J. B., Lee, T. B., Sheard, P., Tattersall, M. L.: Selective inhibition of slow reacting substance of anaphylaxis. Nature (New Biol.) **245**, 215—217 (1973)
Austen, K. F.: Histamine and other mediators of allergic reactions. In: Samter, M. (Ed.): Immunologic Diseases, 2nd Ed., Vol. I, pp. 332—355. Boston: Little Brown 1971
Austen, K. F., Orange, R. P.: Bronchial asthma: the possible role of the chemical mediators of immediate hypersensitivity in the pathogenesis of subacute chronic disease. Amer. Rev. resp. Dis. **112**, 423—435 (1975)
Avella, J., Madsen, J. E., Binder, H. J., Askenase, P. W.: Effect of histamine H_2 receptor antagonists on delayed hypersensitivity. Lancet **1978I**, 624—626
Bach, M. K., Brashler, J. R.: In vivo and in vitro production of a slow reacting substance in the rat upon treatment with calcium ionophores. J. Immunol. **113**, 2040—2044 (1974)
Bamzai, A. K., Kretschmer, R. R., Gotoff, S. P.: Mononuclear cell-derived factor enhances antigen-induced leukocyte histamine release. Clinical Research **25**, 614 A (Abs.) (1977)
Baudry, M., Martres, M.-P., Schwartz, J. C.: H_1- and H_2-receptors in the histamine-induced accumulation of cyclic AMP in guinea pig brain slices. Nature (Lond.) **253**, 362—363 (1975)
Baxter, J. H., Adamik, R.: Control of histamine release: effects of various conditions on rate of release and rate of cell desensitization. J. Immunol. **114**, 1034—1041 (1975)
Beaven, M. A.: Histamine. New Engl. J. Med. **294**, 30—36 and 320—325 (1976)
Becker, E. L., Henson, P. M.: In vitro studies of immunologically induced secretion of mediators from cells and related phenomena. Advanc. Immunol. **17**, 93—193 (1973)
Benveniste, J.: Platelet activating factor, a new mediator of anaphylaxis and immune complex deposition from rabbit and human basophils. Nature (Lond.) **249**, 581—582 (1974)
Berridge, M. J.: The mode of action of 5-hydroxytryptamine. J. exp. Biol. **56**, 311—321 (1972)
Black, J. W.: Histamine receptors. In: Klinge, E. (Ed.): Proc. 6th Int. Cong. Pharmacology, Finnish Pharmacological Society, Vol. I, pp. 3—16. Helsinki 1975
Black, J. W., Duncan, W. A. M., Durant, C. J., Ganellin, C. R., Parsons, E. M.: Definition and antagonism of histamine H_2-receptors. Nature (Lond.) **236**, 385—390 (1972)
Bloch, K. J.: Reaginic and other homocytotropic antibodies: diverse immunoglobulins with common function. In: Goodfriend, L., Sehon, A. H., Orange, R. P. (Eds.): Mechanisms in Allergy. Reagin-mediated Hypersensitivity, pp. 11—32. New York: Marcel Dekker 1973
Boetcher, D. A., Leonard, E. J.: Basophil chemotaxis augmentation by a factor from stimulated lymphocyte cultures. Immunol. Commun. **2**, 421—429 (1973)
Bourne, H. R., Lichtenstein, L. M., Henney, C. S., Melmon, K. L., Weinstein, Y., Shearer, G. M.: Modulation of inflammation and immunity by cyclic AMP. Science **184**, 19—28 (1974)
Brimblecombe, R. W., Duncan, W. A. M., Durant, G. J., Ganellin, C. R., Parsons, E. M., Black, J. W.: The pharmacology of cimetidine, a new histamine H_2-receptor antagonist. Brit. J. Pharmacol. **53**, 435 P—436 P (abs.) (1975)
Brocklehurst, W. E.: The release of histamine and formation of a slow reacting substance (SRS-A) during anaphylactic shock. J. Physiol. (Lond.) **151**, 416—435 (1960)
Brocklehurst, W. E.: Slow reacting substance and related compounds. In: Waksman, B. H., Kallós, P. (Eds.): Progress in Allergy, Vol. VI, pp. 539—558. Basel: S. Karger 1962
Brocklehurst, W. E.: "SRS-A": The slow reacting substance of anaphylaxis. Biochem. Pharmacol. **12**, 431—435 (1963)
Bruce, C. A., Rosenthal, R. R., Lichtenstein, L. M., Norman, P. S.: Quantitative inhalation bronchial challenge in ragweed hay fever patients: a comparison with ragweed-allergic asthmatics. J. Allergy clin. Immunol. **56**, 331—337 (1975)
Bryant, D. H., Burns, M. W., Lazarus, L.: Identification of IgG antibody as a carrier of reaginic activity in asthmatic patients. J. Allergy clin. Immunol. **56**, 417—428 (1975)
Busse, W. W., Sosman, J.: Decreased H2 histamine response of granulocytes of asthmatic patients. J. Clin. Invest. **59**, 1080—1087 (1977)

Capurro, N., Levi, R.: The heart as a target organ in systemic allergic reactions. Comparison of cardiac anaphylaxis in vivo and in vitro. Circulat. Res. **36**, 520—528 (1975)

Chakrin, L. W., Krell, R. D., Mengel, J., Young, D., Zaher, C., Wardell, J. R.: Effect of a histamine H_2-receptor antagonist on immunologically induced mediator release in vitro. Agents Actions **4**, 297—303 (1974)

Chand, N., Eyre, P.: Classification and biological distribution of histamine receptor sub-types. Agents Actions **5**, 277—295 (1975)

Clark, R. A. F., Gallin, J. I., Kaplan, A. P.: The selective eosinophil chemotactic activity of histamine. J. exp. Med. **142**, 1462—1476 (1975)

Clark, R. A. F., Sandler, J. A., Gallin, J. I., Kaplan, A. P.: Histamine modulation of eosinophil migration. J. Immunol. **118**, 137—145 (1977)

Cochrane, C. G.: Immunologic tissue injury mediated by neutrophilic leukocytes. Advanc. Immunol. **9**, 97—162 (1968)

Colman, R. W.: Formation of human plasma kinin. New Engl. J. Med. **291**, 509—514 (1974)

Conroy, M. C., Orange, R. P., Lichtenstein, L. M.: Release of slow reacting substance of anaphylaxis (SRS-A) from human leukocytes by the calcium ionophore A23187. J. Immunol. (1976) (in press)

Coombs, R. R. A., Gell, P. G. H.: Classification of allergic reactions. In: Gell, P. G. H., Coombs, R. R. A. (Eds.): Clinical Aspects of Immunology, 2nd Ed., pp. 575—596. Oxford: Blackwell 1968

Csongrady, A., Kobinger, W.: Investigations into the positive inotropic effect of clonidine in isolated hearts. Naunyn-Schmiedebergs Arch. Pharmacol. **282**, 123—128 (1974)

Cuatrecasas, P., Hollenberg, M. D., Chang, K.-J., Bennett, V.: Hormone receptor complexes and their modulation of membrane function. In: Greep, R. O. (Ed.): Recent Progress in Hormone Research, Vol. XXXI, pp. 37—84. New York: Academic Press 1975

Czarnetzki, B. M., König, W., Lichtenstein, L. M.: Release of eosinophil chemotactic factor from human polymorphonuclear neutrophils by calcium ionophore A23187 and phagocytosis. Nature (Lond.) **258**, 725—726 (1975)

Czarnetzki, B. M., König, W., Lichtenstein, L. M.: Antigen-induced eosinophil chemotactic factor (ECF) release by human leukocytes. Inflammation **1**, 201—215 (1976a)

Czarnetzki, B. M., König, W., Lichtenstein, L. M.: Eosinophil chemotactic factor (ECF). I: Release from polymorphonuclear leukocytes by the calcium ionophore A23187. J. Immunol. **117**, 229—234 (1976b)

DeBernardo, R. M., Askenase, P., Tauben, D., Douglas, J.: Augmented anaphylaxis at sites of cutaneous basophil hypersensitivity (CBH). J. Allergy clin. Immunol. **55**, 112 (abs.) (1975)

Dolovich, J., Hargreave, F. E., Chalmers, R., Shier, K. J., Gauldie, J., Bienenstock, J.: Late cutaneous allergic responses in isolated IgE-dependent reactions. J. Allergy clin. Immunol. **52**, 38—46 (1973)

Douglas, W. W.: Stimulus-secretion coupling: The concept and clues from chromaffin and other cells. Brit. J. Pharmacol. **34**, 451—474 (1968)

Douglas, W. W.: Histamine and antihistamines: 5-hydroxytryptamine and antagonists. In: Goodman, L. S., Gilman, A. (Eds.): The Pharmacological Basis of Therapeutics, 5th Ed., pp. 590—629. New York: Macmillan 1975

Drakontides, A. B., Gershon, M. D.: 5-hydroxytryptamine receptors in the mouse duodenum. Brit. J. Pharmacol. **33**, 480—492 (1968)

Drazen, J. M., Austen, K. F.: Effects of intravenous administration of slow reacting substance of anaphylaxis, histamine, bradykinin, and prostaglandin $F_{2\alpha}$ on pulmonary mechanics in the guinea pig. J. clin. Invest. **53**, 1679—1685 (1974)

Drazen, J. M., Austen, K. F.: Atropine modification of the pulmonary effects of chemical mediators in the guinea pig. J. appl. Physiol. **38**, 834—838 (1975)

Durant, G. J., Ganellin, C. R., Parsons, M. E.: Chemical differentiation of histamine H_1- and H_2-receptor agonists. J. Med. Chem. **18**, 905—909 (1975)

Dvorak, A. M., Mihm, M. C., Jr., Dvorak, H. F.: Morphology of delayed-type hypersensitivity reactions in man. II. Ultrastructural alterations affecting the microvasculature and the tissue mast cells. Lab. Invest. **34**, 179—191 (1976)

Dvorak, H. F., Dvorak, A. M.: Cutaneous basophil hypersensitivity. In: Brent, L., Holborow, J. (Eds.): Progress in Immunology II, Vol. III, pp. 171—181. Amsterdam: North-Holland 1974

Eichmann, K.: Idiotype suppression. II. Amplification of a suppressor cell with anti-idiotype activity. Europ. J. Immunol. **5**, 511—517 (1975)

Eyre, P.: Histamine H_2-receptors in the sheep bronchus and cat trachea: the action of burimamide. Brit. J. Pharmacol. **48**, 321—323 (1973)

Fallah, H. A., Maillard, J. L., Voison, G. A.: Regulatory mast cells. I. Suppressive action of their products on an in vitro primary immune reaction. Ann. Immunol. (Inst. Pasteur) **126 C**, 669—682 (1975)

Foreman, J. D., Mongar, J. L., Gomperts, B. D.: Calcium ionophores and movement of calcium ions following the physiological stimulus to a secretory process. Nature (Lond.) **245**, 249—251 (1973)

Gerschenfeld, H. M., Paupardin-Tritsch, D.: Ionic mechanisms and receptor properties underlying the responses of molluscan neurones to 5-hydroxytryptamine. J. Physiol. (Lond.) **243**, 427—456 (1974a)

Gerschenfeld, H. M., Paupardin-Tritsch, D.: On the transmitter function of 5-hydroxytryptamine at excitatory and inhibitory monosynaptic junctions. J. Physiol. (Lond.) **243**, 457—481 (1974b)

Gershon, M. D., Ross, L. L.: Studies on the relationship of 5-hydroxytryptamine and enterochromaffin cell to anaphylactic shock in mice. J. exp. Med. **115**, 367—382 (1961)

Gershon, R. K., Askenase, P. W., Gershon, M. D.: Requirement for vasoactive amines for production of delayed-type hypersensitivity skin reactions. J. exp. Med. **142**, 732—747 (1975)

Gillespie, E., Lichtenstein, L. M.: Histamine release from human leukocytes: studies with deuterium oxide, colchicine and cytochalasin B. J. clin. Invest. **51**, 2941—2947 (1972)

Gleich, G. J., Jacob, G. L.: Immunoglobulin E antibodies to pollen allergens account for high percentages of total immunoglobulin E protein. Science **190**, 1106—1108 (1975)

Glovsky, M. M., Hugli, T. E., Ishizaka, T., Lichtenstein, L. M.: Studies on $C3a_{hu}$ on human leukocyte binding and histamine release. Fed. Proc. **36**, 1264 (abs.) (1977)

Godfrey, S.: Exercise-induced asthma—clinical, physiological, and therapeutic implications. J. Allergy clin. Immunol. **56**, 1—17 (1975)

Goldberg, N. D., Haddox, M. K., Nicol, S. E., Glass, D. B., Sanford, C. H., Kuehl, F. A., Jr., Estensen, R.: Biologic regulation through opposing influences of cyclic GMP and cyclic AMP: the Yin Yang hypothesis. In: Drummond, G. I., Greengard, P., Robison, G. A. (Eds.): Advances in Cyclic Nucleotide Research, Vol. V, pp. 307—330. New York: Raven Press 1975

Goth, A.: Histamine release by drugs and chemicals. In: Schachter, M. (Ed.): Histamine and Antihistamines, International Encyclopedia of Pharmacology and Therapeutics, Sect. 74, Vol. I, pp. 25—43. Oxford: Pergamon Press 1973

Grant, J. A., Dupree, E., Goldman, A. S., Schultz, D. K., Jackson, A. L.: Complement-induced release of histamine in human leukocytes. J. Immunol. **114**, 1101—1106 (1975)

Grant, J. A., Lichtenstein, L. M.: Reversed in vitro anaphylaxis induced by anti-IgG: specificity of the reaction and comparison with antigen-induced histamine release. J. Immunol. **109**, 20—25 (1972)

Green, J. P., Maayani, S.: Tricyclic antidepressant drugs block histamine H_2 receptor in brain. Nature **269**, 163—165 (1977)

Green, J. P., Johnson, C. L., Weinstein, H., Maayani, S.: Antagonism of histamine-activated adenylate cyclase in brain by D-lysergic acid diethylamide. Proc. nat. Acad. Sci. (Wash.) **74**, 5697—5701 (1977)

Hastie, R.: A study of the ultrastructure of human basophil leukocytes. Lab. Invest. **31**, 223—231 (1974)

Henney, C. S., Gaffney, J., Bloom, B. R.: On the relation of soluble mediators to cell-mediated cytolysis. J. exp. Med. **140**, 837—852 (1974)

Henson, P. M.: Release of vasoactive amines from rabbit platelets induced by sensitized mononuclear leukocytes and antigen. J. exp. Med. **131**, 287—306 (1970)

Henson, P. M.: Pathologic mechanisms in neutrophil mediated injury. Amer. J. Path. **68**, 593—605 (1972)

Henson, P. M.: Mechanisms of activation and secretion by platelets and neutrophils. In: Brent, L., Holborow, J. (Eds.): Progress in Immunology II, Vol. II, pp. 95—105. Amsterdam: North-Holland 1974

Hill, H. R., Estensen, R. D., Quie, P. G., Hogan, N. A., Goldberg, N. D.: Modulation of human neutrophil chemotactic responses by cyclic 3′5′-guanosine monophosphate and cyclic 3′5′-adenosine monophosphate. Metabolism **24**, 447—456 (1975)

Hook, W. A., Siraganian, R. P., Wahl, S. M.: Complement-induced histamine release from human basophils. I. Generation of activity in human serum. J. Immunol. **114**, 1185—1190 (1975)

Hook, W. A., Schiffman, E., Aswanikumar, S., Siraganian, R. P.: Histamine release by chemotactic, formyl methionine-containing peptides. J. Immunol. **117**, 594—596 (1976)

Ida, S., Hooks, J. J., Siraganian, R. P., Notkins, A. L.: Enhancement of IgE-mediated histamine release from human basophils by viruses: Role of interferon. J. exp. Med. **145**, 892—906 (1977)

Ishizaka, K., Ishizaka, T.: Identification of γE antibodies as a carrier of reaginic activity. J. Immunol. **99**, 1187—1198 (1967)

Ishizaka, K., Ishizaka, T., Kishimoto, T., Okudaira, T.: Biosynthesis of IgE antibodies and mechanisms of sensitization. In: Brent, L., Holborow, J. (Eds.): Progress in Immunology II, Vol. IV, pp. 7—17. Amsterdam: North-Holland 1974

Ishizaka, T., DeBernardo, R., Tomioka, H., Lichtenstein, L. M., Ishizaka, K.: Identification of basophil granulocytes as a site of allergic histamine release. J. Immunol. **108**, 1000—1008 (1972)

Ishizaka, T., Ishizaka, K.: Biology of immunoglobulin E. In: Kallós, P., Waksman, B. H., de Weck, A. (Eds.): Progress in Allergy, Vol. XIX, pp. 60—121. Basel: Karger 1975

Jakschik, R. A., Falkenhein, S., Parker, C. W.: Precursor role of arachidonic acid in release of slow reacting substance from rat basophilic leukemia cells. Proc. nat. Acad. Sci. (Wash.) **74**, 4577—4581 (1977)

Kahlson, G., Rosengren, E.: New approaches to the physiology of histamine. Physiol. Rev. **48**, 155—196 (1968)

Kaliner, M., Orange, R. P., Austen, K. F.: Immunological release of histamine and slow-reacting substance of anaphylaxis from human lung. IV. Enhancement by cholinergic and alpha adrenergic stimulation. J. exp. Med. **136**, 556—567 (1972)

Kaliner, M., Austen, K. F.: Cyclic AMP, ATP, and reversed anaphylactic histamine release from rat mast cells. J. Immunol. **112**, 664—674 (1974)

Kaplan, A. P., Austen, K. F.: Activation and control mechanisms of Hageman factor-dependent pathways of coagulation, fibrinolysis, and kinin generation and their contribution to the inflammatory response. J. Allergy clin. Immunol. **56**, 491—506 (1975)

Kaplan, A. P., Gray, L., Shaff, R. E., Horakowa, Z., Beaven, M. A.: In vivo studies of mediator release in cold urticaria and cholinergic urticaria. J. Allergy clin. Immunol. **55**, 394—402 (1975)

Katz, S. I., Parker, D., Turk, J. L.: Mechanisms involved in the expression of Jones-Mote hypersensitivity. I. Passive transfer studies. Cell. Immunol. **16**, 396—403 (1975)

Kay, A. B., Austen, K. F.: The IgE-mediated release of an eosinophil leukocyte chemotactic factor from human lung. J. Immunol. **107**, 899—902 (1971)

Kenatin, T. P., Krueger, C. A., Cook, D. A.: Temperature-dependent interconversion of histamine H_1 and H_2-receptors in guinea pig ileum. Nature (Lond.) **252**, 54—55 (1974)

Klein, I., Levey, G. S.: Activation of myocardial adenyl cyclase by histamine in guinea pig, cat and human heart. J. clin. Invest. **50**, 1012—1015 (1971)

Kniker, W. T.: Modulation of the inflammatory response in vivo: Prevention or amelioration of immune complex diseases. In: Lepow, I. H., Ward, P. A. (Eds.): Inflammation, Mechanisms and Control, pp. 335—363. New York: Academic Press 1972

Kniker, W. T., Cochrane, C. G.: Pathogenic factors in vascular lesions of experimental serum sickness. J. exp. Med. **122**, 83—97 (1965)

König, W., Czarnetzki, B. M., Lichtenstein, L. M.: Eosinophil chemotactic factor (ECF). II: Release during phagocytosis of human polymorphonuclear leukocytes. J. Immunol. **117**, 235—241 (1976)

König, W., Ishizaka, K.: Binding of IgE with the subcellular fragments of normal rat mast cells. Immunochemistry **13**, 345—353 (1976)

Koopman, W. M., Gillis, M. H., David, J. R.: Prevention of MIF activity by agents known to increase cellular cyclic AMP. J. Immunol. **110**, 1609—1614 (1973)

Kravis, T. C., Zvaifler, N. J.: Alteration of rabbit PCA reactions by drugs known to influence intracellular cyclic AMP. J. Immunol. **113**, 244—250 (1974)

LaPierre, J.-G., Gold, M., Levison, H., Bryan, A. C., Orange, R. P.: The effects on lung mechanics of infusion of chemical mediators through the bronchial and pulmonary arteries. Fed. Proc. **35**, 395 (abs.) (1976)

Lepow, I. H., Willms-Kretschmer, K., Patrick, R. A., Rosen, F. S.: Gross and ultrastructural observations on lesions produced by intradermal injection of human C3a in man. Amer. J. Path. **61**, 13—24 (1970)

Lett-Brown, M. A., Leonard, E. J.: Histamine-induced inhibition of normal human basophil chemotaxis to C5a. J. Immunol. **118**, 815—818 (1977)

Levi, R., Capurro, N., Lee, C.-H.: Pharmacological chracterization of cardiac histamine receptors: Sensitivity to H_1- and H_2-receptor agonists and antagonists. Europ. J. Pharmacol. **30**, 328—335 (1975)

Levy, D. A.: Histamine and serotonin. In: Weissmann, G. (Ed.): Mediators of Inflammation, pp. 85—111. New York: Plenum Press 1974

Lewis, R. A., Goetzl, E. J., Wasserman, S. I., Valone, F. H., Rubin, R. H., Austen, K. F.: The release of four mediators of immediate hypersensitivity from human leukemic basophils. J. Immunol. **114**, 87—92 (1975)

Lewis, R. A., Wasserman, S. I., Goetzl, E. J., Austen, K. F.: Formation of SRS-A in human lung tissue and cells before release. J. exp. Med. **140**, 1133—1146 (1974)

Lichtenstein, L. M.: The immediate allergic response: in vitro separation of antigen activation, decay and histamine release. J. Immunol. **107**, 1122—1130 (1971)

Lichtenstein, L. M.: Allergy. In: Bach, F., Good, R. (Eds.): Clinical Immunobiology, pp. 243—269. New York: Academic Press 1972

Lichtenstein, L. M.: The mechanism of basophil histamine release induced by antigen and by the calcium ionophore A23187. J. Immunol. **114**, 1692—1699 (1975)

Lichtenstein, L. M., DeBernardo, R.: The immediate allergic response: in vitro action of cyclic AMP-active and other drugs on the two stages of histamine release. J. Immunol. **107**, 1131—1136 (1971)

Lichtenstein, L. M., Gillespie, E.: Inhibition of histamine release by histamine is controlled by an H2 receptor. Nature (Lond.) **244**, 287—288 (1973)

Lichtenstein, L. M., Gillespie, E.: The effects of the H1 and H2 antihistamines on "allergic" histamine release and its inhibition by histamine. J. Pharmacol. exp. Ther. **192**, 441—450 (1975)

Lichtenstein, L. M., Gillespie, E., Bourne, H.: Studies on the biochemical mechanisms of IgE mediated histamine release. In: Ishizaka, K., Dayton, D. H. (Eds.): The Biological Role of the Immunoglobulin E System, pp. 165—186 National Inst. Child Hlth Human Develop. 1972

McDonald, J. R., Mathison, P. A., Stevenson, D. D.: Aspirin intolerance in asthma: detection by oral challenge. J. Allergy clin. Immunol. **50**, 198—207 (1972)

Makman, M. H.: Properties of adenyl cyclase of lymphoid cells. Proc. nat. Acad. Sci. (Wash.) **68**, 885—889 (1971)

Malveaux, F. J., Conroy, M. C., Adkinson, N. F., Jr., Lichtenstein, L. M.: IgE receptors on human basophils: Relationship to serum IgE concentration. J. clin. Invest. (1978) (in press)

Maslinski, C.: Histamine and its metabolism in mammals. Part I. Chemistry and formation of histamine. Part II. Catabolism of histamine and histamine liberation. Agents Actions **5**, 89—107 and 183—225 (1975)

Matthyssens, G. E., Hurwitz, E., Girol, D., Sela, M.: Binding of histamine- and other ligand-conjugated macromolecules to lymphocytes. Molec. cell. Biochem. **7**, 119—126 (1975)

Maudsley, D. V., Kobayashi, Y., Williamson, E., Bovaird, L.: H_2-receptor blockade and stimulation of histidine decarboxylase. Nature New Biol. **245**, 148—149 (1973)

Melmon, K. L., Bourne, H. R., Weinstein, Y., Sela, M.: Receptors for histamine can be detected on the surface of selected leukocytes. Science **177**, 707—709 (1972)

Melmon, K. L., Bourne, H. R., Weinstein, Y., Shearer, G. M., Kram, J., Bauminger, S.: Hemolytic plaque formation by leukocytes in vitro. J. clin. Invest. **53**, 13—21 (1974)

Mendoza, G., Metzger, H.: Distribution and valency of receptor for IgE on rodent mast cells and related tumor cells. Nature **264**, 548—550 (1976)

Moore, T. C.. Histidine decarboxylase inhibitors and the survival of skin homografts. Nature (Lond.) **215**, 871—872 (1967)

Moore, T. C., Lawrence, W., Jr.: Suppression of antibody formation by histidine decarboxylase inhibitors. Transplantation **8**, 224—234 (1969)

Moore, T. C., Lemmi, C. A. E., Orlando, J. C., Pinkerton, W.: Correlation of splenic histidine decarboxylase activity and antibody formation following SRBC immunization. Transplantation **11**, 346—348 (1971)

Moore, T. C., Schayer, R. W.: Histidine decarboxylase activity of autografted and allografted rat skin. Transplantation **7**, 99—104 (1969)

Mozes, E., Weinstein, Y., Bourne, H. R., Melmon, K. L., Shearer, G. M.: In vitro correction of antigen-induced immune suppression. Effects of histamine, dibutyryl cyclic AMP and cholera enterotoxin. Cell. Immunol. **11**, 57—63 (1974)

Newball, H. H., Talamo, R. C., Lichtenstein, L. M.: Release of leukocyte kallikrein mediated by IgE. Nature (Lond.) **254**, 635—636 (1975).

Orange, R. P.: The formation and release of slow reacting substance of anaphylaxis in human lung tissues. In: Brent, L., Holborow, T. (Eds.): Progress in Immunology II, Vol. IV, pp. 29—39. Amsterdam: North-Holland 1974

Orange, R. P.: Dissociation of the immunological release of histamine and slow reacting substance of anaphylaxis from human lung using cytochalasins A and B. J. Immunol. **114**, 182—186 (1975)

Orange, R. P., Austen, K. F.: The immunological release of chemical mediators of immediate type hypersensitivity from human lung. In: Amos, B. (Ed.): Progress in Immunology I, pp. 173—186. New York: Academic Press 1971

Orange, R. P., Murphy, R. C., Austen, K. F.: Inactivation of slow-reacting substance of anaphylaxis (SRS-A) by arylsulfatase. J. Immunol. **113**, 316—322 (1974)

Orange, R. P., Murphy, R. C., Karnovsky, M. D., Austen, K. F.: The physicochemical characteristics and purification of slow-reacting substance of anaphylaxis. J. Immunol. **110**, 760—770 (1973)

Orange, R. P., Stechschulte, D. J., Austen, K. F.: Immunochemical and biologic properties of rat IgE. II. Capacity to mediate the immunologic release of histamine and slow-reacting substance of anaphylaxis (SRS-A). J. Immunol. **105**, 1087—1102 (1970).

Orange, R. P., Valentine, M. D., Austen, K. F.: Antigen-induced release of slow reacting substance of anaphylaxis (SRS-A^{rat}) in rats prepared with homologous antibody. J. exp. Med. **127**, 767—782 (1968)

Parish, W. E.: Skin sensitizing non-IgE antibodies. Association between IgG S-TS and IgG4. In: Brent, L., Holborow, I., (Eds.): Progress in Immunology II, Vol. IV, pp. 19—27, Amsterdam: North-Holland 1974

Parmley, R. T., Spicer, S. S., Wright, N. J.: The ultrastructural identification of tissue basophils and mast cells in Hodgkin's disease. Lab. Invest. **32**, 469—475 (1975)

Parsons, M. E., Owen, D. A. A., Ganellin C. R., Durant, G. J.: Dimaprit-[S-[3-(N,N-dimethylamino)propyl]isothiourea]—A highly specific histamine H_2-receptor agonist. Part 1. Pharmacology. Agents and Actions **7**, 31—37 (1977)

Plaut, M.: Unpublished observations (1976)

Plaut, M., Lichtenstein, L. M., Gillespie, E., Henney, C. S.: Studies on the mechanism of lymphocyte-mediated cytolysis. IV. Specificity of the histamine receptor on effector T cells. J. Immunol. **111**, 389—394 (1973a)

Plaut, M., Lichtenstein, L. M., Henney, C. S.: Increase in histamine receptors on thymus-derived effector lymphocytes during the primary immune response to alloantigens. Nature (Lond.) **244**, 284—287 (1973b)

Plaut, M., Lichtenstein, L. M., Henney, C. S.: Properties of a subpopulation of T cells bearing histamine receptors. J. clin. Invest. **55**, 856—874 (1975a)

Plaut, M., Lichtenstein, L. M., Henney, C. S.: Activities mediated by histamine receptor-bearing T lymphocytes. Fed. Proc. **34**, 1004 (abs.) (1975b)

Plaut, M.: In vivo and in vitro desensitization of histamine receptor-bearing cytolytically active cells. Fed. Proc. **36**, 1324 (abs.) (1977)

Plaut, M.: Unpublished observations (1978)

Plaut, M., Berman, I. J.: Histamine receptors on human and mouse lymphocytes. J. Allergy clin. Immunol. **61**, 132—133 (abs.) (1978)

Pounder, R. E., Hunt, R. H., Stekelmann, R., Milton-Thompson, G. J., Misiewicz, J. J.: Healing of gastric ulcer during treatment with cimetidine. Lancet **1967 I**, 337—339

Powell, J. R., Brody, M. J.: Participation of H_1 and H_2 histamine receptors in physiological vasodilator responses. Am. J. Physiol. **231**, 1002—1009 (1976)
Prausnitz, C., Küstner, H.: Studien über die Überempfindlichkeit. Zbl. Bakt. **86**, 160—169 (1921)
Rapp, H. J.: The release of a slow-reacting substance (SRS) in the peritoneal cavity of rats by antigen-antibody interaction. J. Physiol. (Lond.) **158**, 35P (1961)
Remold-O'Donnell, E.: Stimulation and desensitization of macrophage adenylate cyclase by prostaglandins and catecholamines. J. biol. Chem. **249**, 3615—3621 (1974)
Riley, J. F.: Functional significance of histamine and heparin in tissue mast cells. Ann. N.Y. Acad. Sci. **103**, 151—163 (1963)
Rocha E Silva, M. (sub-ed.).: Histamine: Its chemistry, metabolism and physiological and pharmacological actions. In: Eichler, O., Farah, A. (Eds.): Handbook of Experimental Pharmacology, Vol. XVIII/1, New Berlin-Heidelberg-New York: Springer 1966
Rocklin, R. E.: Modulation of cellular immune responses in vivo and in vitro by histamine receptor-bearing lymphocytes. J. clin. Invest. **57**, 1051—1058 (1976)
Rocklin, R. E.: Histamine-induced suppressor factor (HSF): Effect on migration inhibitory factor (MIF) production and proliferation. J. Immunol. **118**, 1734—1738 (1977)
Roszkowski, W., Plaut, M., Lichtenstein, L. M.: Histamine receptor display on lymphocyte subpopulations. Fed. Proc. **36**, 1241 (abs.) (1977a)
Roszkowski, W., Plaut, M., Lichtenstein, L. M.: Selective display of histamine receptors on lymphocytes. Science **195**, 683—685 (1977)
Saavadra, J. M., Brownstein, M., Axelrod, J.: A specific and sensitive enzymatic isotope microassay for serotonin in tissues. J. Pharmacol. exp. ther. **186**, 509—515 (1973)
Samter, M., Czarny, P.: Secondary cells involved in the allergic reaction: eosinophils, basophils, neutrophils. In: Samter, M. (Ed.): Immunologic Diseases, Vol. I, pp. 375—399. 2nd edit. Boston: Little Brown 1971
Schayer, R. A.: Induced synthesis of histamine, microcirculatory regulation and the mechanism of action of the adrenal glucocorticoid hormones. In: Kallós, P., Waksman, B. H. (Eds.): Progress in Allergy. Vol. VII, pp. 187—212. Basel: Karger 1963
Schellenberg, R. R., Adkinson, N. F., Jr.: Measurement of absolute amounts of antigen-specific human IgE by a radioallergosorbent test (RAST) elution technique. J. Immunol. **115**, 1577—1583 (1975)
Schellenberg, R. R., Adkinson, N. F., Jr.: Absolute quantitation of serum IgE specific for two independent allergens: correlation with other allergic indices. J. Allergy clin. Immunol. **57**, 229 (abs.) (1976)
Schwartz, A., Askenase, P. W., Gershon, R. K.: The effect of locally injected vasoactive amines on the elicitation of delayed-type hypersensitivity. J. Immunol. **118**, 159—165 (1977)
Segal, S., Weinstein, Y., Melmon, K. L., McDevitt, H. O.: Termination of tolerance by removal of a suppressor cell. Fed. Proc. **33**, 723 (abs.) (1974)
Shearer, G. M., Melmon, K. L., Weinstein, Y., Sela, M.: Regulation of antobody response by cells expressing histamine receptors. J. exp. Med. **136**, 1302—1307 (1972)
Shearer, G. M., Weinstein, Y., Melmon, K. L.: Enhancement of immune response potential of mouse lymphoid cells fractionated over insolubilized conjugated histamine columns. J. Immunol. **113**, 597—607 (1974)
Shore, P. A., Burkhalter, A., Cohn, V. H., Jr.: A method for the fluorometric assay of histamine in tissues. J. Pharmol. exp. Ther. **127**, 182—186 (1959)
Sinclair, M. C., Moore, T. C., Lemmi, C. A. E., Orlando, J. C.: Increase in the urinary excretion of histamine after SRBC immunization of rats. Amer. J. Surg. **126**, 624—626 (1973)
Siraganian, R. P.: Refinements in the automated fluorometric histamine analysis system. J. immunol. Methods **7**, 283—290 (1975)
Siraganian, R. P., Hook W. A.: Complement-induced histamine release from human basophils. II. Mechanism of the histamine release reaction. J. Immunol. **116**, 639—646 (1976)
Siraganian, R. P., Osler, A. G.: Destruction of rabbit platelets in the allergic response of sensitized leukocytes. II. Evidence for basophil involvement. J. Immunol. **106**, 1252—1259 (1971)
Siraganian, R. P., Siraganian, P. A.: Mechanism of action of concanavalin A on human basophils. J. Immunol. **114**, 886—893 (1975)

Slott, R. I., Zweiman, B.: Histologic studies of human skin test responses to ragweed and compound 48/80. II. Effects of corticosteroid therapy. J. Allergy clin. Immunol. **55**, 232—240 (1975)
Snyder, S. H., Baldessarini, R. J., Axelrod, J.: A sensitive and specific enzymatic isotopic assay for tissue histamine. J. Pharmol. exp. Ther. **153**, 544—549 (1966)
Solley, G. O., Larson, J. B., Jordon, R. E., Gleich, G. J.: Late cutaneous reactions due to IgE. J. Allergy clin. Immunol. **55**, 112 (abs.) (1975)
Sosman, J., Busse, W.: Reduced H2 receptor response of granulocytes of asthmatic patients. J. Allergy clin. Immunol. **57**, 222 (abs.) (1976)
Spragg, J.: The plasma kinin-forming system. In: Weissmann, G. (Ed.): Mediators of Inflammation, pp. 85—111. New York: Plenum Press 1974
Stechschulte, D. J.: Slow-reacting substances. In: Weissmann, G. (Ed.): Mediators of Inflammation, pp. 181—197. New York: Plenum Press 1974
Stechschulte, D. J., Orange, R. P., Austen, K. F.: Immunologic and biologic properties of rat IgE. I. Immunochemical identification of rat IgE. J. Immunol. **105**, 1082—1086 (1970)
Steinberg, P., Ishizaka, K., Norman, P. S.: Possible role of IgE-mediated reaction in immunity. J. Allergy clin. Immunol. **54**, 359—366 (1974)
Stoner, J., Manganiello, V. C., Vaughan, M.: Effects of bradykinin and indomethacin on cyclic GMP and cyclic AMP in lung slices. Proc. nat. Acad. Sci. (Wash.) **70**, 3830—3833 (1973)
Strannegärd, I.-L., Strannegärd, Ö.: Increased sensitivity of lymphocytes from atopic individuals to histamine-induced suppression. Scand. J. Immunol. **6**, 1225—1231 (1977)
Sullivan, T. J., Parker, K. L., Eisen, S. A., Parker, C. W.: Modulation of cyclic AMP in purified rat mast cells. II. Studies on the relationship between intracellular cyclic AMP concentrations and histamine release. J. Immunol. **114**, 1480—1485 (1975)
Thomas, L. L., Lichtenstein, L. M.: Augmentation of IgE-mediated histamine release from human basophils by phagocytic stimuli. J. Allergy clin. Immunol. **61**, 152 (abs.) (1978)
Thomas, L. L., Bochner, B. S., Lichtenstein, L. M.: Inhibition of human PMN-derived histaminase activity by H-2 antagonists. Biochemical Pharmacol. (1978) (in press)
Thompson, J. S., Severson, C. D., Parmely, M. J., Marmorstein, B. L., Simmons, A.: Pulmonary "hypersensitivity" reactions induced by transfusion of non-HL-A leukoagglutinins. New. Engl. J. Med. **284**, 1120—1125 (1971)
Thueson, D. O., Speck, L., Grant, J. A.: Histamine releasing activity produced by human mononuclear cells. Fed. Proc. **36**, 1300 (abs.) (1977)
Vallota, E. H., Müller-Eberhard, H. J.: Formation of C3a und C5a anaphylatoxins in whole human serum after inhibition of the anaphylatoxin inactivator. J. exp. Med. **137**, 1109—1123 (1973)
Verhaegen, H., DeCock, W., DeCree, J.: Histamine receptor-bearing peripheral T lymphocytes in patients with allergies. J. Allergy clin. Immunol. **59**, 266—268 (1977)
Ward, P. A., Dvorak, H. F., Cohen, S., Yoshida, T., Data, R., Selvaggio, S. S.: Chemotaxis of basophils by lymphocyte-dependent and lymphocyte-independent mechanisms. J. Immunol. **114**, 1523—1531 (1975)
Wasserman, S. I., Austen, K. F.: Arylsulfatase of human lung. Isolation, charaterization, and interaction with slow-reacting substance of anaphylaxis. J. clin. Invest. **57**, 738—744 (1976)
Weinstein, Y., Melmon, K. L., Bourne, H. R., Sela, M.: Specific leukocyte receptors for small endogenous hormones. Detection by cell binding to insolubilized hormone preparations. J. clin. Invest. **52**, 1349—1361 (1973)
Yellin, T. O., Sperow, J. W., Buck, S. H.: Antagonism of tolazoline by histamine H_2-receptor blockers. Nature (Lond.) **253**, 561—563 (1975)
Zeiger, R. S., Yurdin, D. L., Colten, H. R.: Histamine catabolism: Localization of histaminase and histamine methyl transferase in human leukocytes. J. Allergy clin. Immunol. **57**, 244—245 (abs.) (1976)
Zurier, R. B.: Prostaglandins. In: Weissmann, G. (Ed.): Mediators of Inflammation, pp. 163—180. New York: Plenum Press 1974
Zurier, R. B., Weissmann, G., Hoffstein, S., Cameron, S., Tai, H. H.: Mechanisms of lysozomal enzyme release from human leukocytes. II. Effects of cAMP and cGMP, autonomic agonists, and agents which affect microtubule function. J. clin. Invest. **53**, 297—309 (1974)

CHAPTER 12

Prostaglandins and Related Compounds

R. J. FLOWER

A. Introduction

During the inflammatory response, cells elaborate many biologically active chemicals and the tenor of pharmacological research at any time is, not unnaturally, set by the current state of knowledge concerning these inflammatory mediators; thus, in the past, this field has been dominated by the discovery of histamine, bradykinin and 5-hydroxytryptamine (5-HT), with the subsequent invention of antihistamine and anti-5-HT drugs.

If asked a decade ago to predict which type of biological molecule would rise to a dominant position in inflammation research today, probably very few workers would have chosen the polyunsaturated fatty acids. Indeed, it was only just over 10 years ago (1964) that the transformation of these acids into the biologically active prostaglandins (PGs) was initially demonstrated (see Section G. et seq. for details); until then polyunsaturated fatty acids seem to have been regarded solely as membrane building blocks. It is now known that a whole cascade of fascinating and important molecules can be derived from these acids under the influence of specific cellular oxygenases. In the case of some of these products, such as the hydroxyacid 12 L-hydroxy-5,8,10-heptadecatrienoic acid (HHT) (see Section G.II.), their role in inflammation (if any) can only be guessed at, whereas other products such as PGs of the E series (see Section G.III. and Table 1) have been overwhelmingly implicated in inflammation, fever and pain. It seems that one of the most fertile areas in current inflammation therapy is the design of new types of drugs which interact with the metabolic pathways outlined in this chapter.

B. Reasons for Studying the Metabolism of Polyoxygenated Fatty Acid Derivatives

There are many good reasons for studying the mechanism of formation of polyoxygenated fatty acid derivatives, and in the main these are discussed in the various chapters of this book; by way of summary the reasons are:

(1) PGs are found in increased quantities in inflammatory exudates and,

(2) PGs themselves can reproduce many of the cardinal clinical signs of inflammation including the vascular events and cell chemotaxis (see FERREIRA and VANE in Chapter 31; YOULTEN, Chapter 16), the genesis of fever (see FELDBERG and MILTON, Chapter 18), as well as hyperalgesia and pain (see MONCADA et al., Chapter 17).

(3) There is a strong correlation between the anti-inflammatory action of the aspirin-like drugs and their anti-cyclo-oxygenase activity—indeed, this seems to be

Table 1. Some proinflammatory effects of arachidonic acid metabolites

Metabolite	Present in inflammatory exidates etc.	Fever	Erythema and Vasodilatation	Oedema and vascular permeability	Pain and hyperalgesia	Leucotaxis	Granuloma formation	Bronchoconstrictor	Platelet aggregation	Other effects
Arachidonic acid	+	?	?	?	?	?	?	+	++	
PGG_2 or H_2	?	?	?	+	+	?	?	+	+++	
PG F	+	Very weak	Very weak or inhibits	No effects or inhibits	+	0	?	+	$F_{1\alpha}$ Very weak inhibitor	
E	++	+++	+++	+++	+++	+	+(E_1)	Bronchodilator	E_1 Potent inhibitor E_2 Weak potentiator	
D	?	?	+($D_2>D_1$)	+(D_2)	+(D_2)	?	?	++(D_2)	D_2 Potent inhibitor	
HHT and MDA	?	?	?	?	?	?	?	?	?	General cytotoxic effects (MDA)
HPETE and HETE	+(HETE)	?	?	?	?	++ (HETE)	?	?	?	Cytotoxic actions by HPETE?
TX A_2	?	?	?	?	?	?	?	?	+++++	
B_2	?	?	?	?	?	?	?	?	No effect	

Data for this table were compiled from the following reviews or articles: FERREIRA and VANE (1974); FLOWER et al. (1973, 1976); HAMMARSTRÖM et al. (1975); MILTON and WENDLANDT (1971); SMITH and MACFARLANE (1974); TURNER et al. (1975); VANE (1976).
HETE = 12L-hydroxy-5,8,10,14-eicosatetraenoic acid.
HPETE = 12L-hydroperoxy-5,8,10,14-eicosatetraenoic acid.

their main mode of action (see GRYGLEWSKI, Chapter 19; SHEN, Chapter 30; FERREIRA and VANE, Chapter 31).

(4) Other non-prostaglandin products of the cyclo-oxygenase such as thromboxane A_2 (TXA_2) (see Section G.IV.) are responsible for irreversible platelet aggregation which may be amongst the sequelae of the inflammatory process (see WILLIS, Chapter 5).

(5) PGs are in large measure responsible for the hypotension and bronchoconstriction induced by bradykinin (see VARGAFTIG, Chapter 25; PIPER and VANE, Chapter 24).

(6) A product of the lipoxygenase has been shown to have a profound effect on white cell migration (TURNER et al., 1975).

In this chapter, the transformation of certain polyunsaturated fatty acids by the membrane bound cyclo-oxygenase and the soluble lipoxygenase will be examined in detail. The distribution of these two enzymes will be discussed, and recent evidence concerning the nature and cellular location of the substrates for the cyclo-oxygenase will also be mentioned. The metabolism of PGs will be dealt with briefly. The inhibition of the cyclo-oxygenase is dealt with by GRYGLEWSKI and SHEN in Chapters 19 and 30 respectively and will not be covered here. Inhibition of PG metabolism will however be discussed (as this could lead to an exacerbation of the inflammatory response), as will the possibility of blocking the generation of lipoxygenase and cyclo-oxygenase products by preventing substrate accumulation.

C. A Note on Nomenclature

I. Enzyme Nomenclature

Until comparatively recently, it was believed that the ubiquitously distributed, membrane-bound cyclo-oxygenase synthesised only PGs E and F from endoperoxide intermediates. Not unnaturally, therefore, this enzyme became widely known as 'prostaglandin synthetase.' It will be evident from the forthcoming pages however, that in some tissues (most notably lungs and platelets) the endoperoxide intermediates are converted almost entirely to non-prostaglandin products. In the light of these findings, it seems illogical to persist in calling the enzyme system 'prostaglandin synthetase.' Throughout this chapter therefore the more general term 'cyclo-oxygenase' will be used when referring to this enzyme.

II. Fatty Acid Nomenclature

The numbering system used for fatty acid carbon skeletons in this chapter is as follows: each carbon is numbered consecutively along the chain beginning with the carboxyl terminal (hence the carboxylic carbon is C-1), the carbon most remote from C-1 is referred to as the ω-carbon. Occasionally it is desirable to indicate a specific position relative to the ω-carbon. In this case, the ω-carbon is designated C-1, and the carbon atoms numbered consecutively in the reverse direction along the chain, the carboxyl carbon being the most distant. Thus, when referring to a 20 carbon fatty acid, C-1 (carboxyl carbon) is equivalent to ω-20, C-2 to ω-19, etc.

The following abbreviations are sometimes used when describing the nature and geometry of carbon-carbon bonds in fatty acids:

c = *cis*, t = *trans*	—c=c—	(ethylenic bonds)
a =	—c≡c—	(acetylenic bonds)

The C-20 fatty acids 8, 11, 14-eicosatrienoic acid, and 5, 8, 11, 14-eicosatetraenoic acid will be referred to by their trivial names (dihomo-γ-linolenic and arachidonic acid) throughout.

III. Prostaglandin Nomenclature

The PGs may be considered derivatives of prostanoic acid (see Fig. 1) and the nomenclature is based on that carbon skeleton. There are several groups of PGs distinguished by the nature and geometry of the substituent groups in the ring (for example E, F, D) and the number of double bonds in the side chains (for example E_1, E_2, E_3; F_1, F_2, F_3 etc.). Figure 1 shows the structures of these primary PGs (see NELSON, 1974 and HAMBERG, 1973a for more complete details of this nomenclature system).

D. Nature and Origin of Fatty Acid Substrates for the Cyclo-Oxygenase

Substrates for the cyclo-oxygenase enzyme belong to the group of so-called essential fatty acids. The substrate requirements for the sheep vesicular gland cyclo-oxygenase were tested by VAN DORP (1967) who investigated the relative reaction rates of three trienoic, five tetraenoic, and one pentaenoic acid with double bonds at the 5, 8, 11; 5, 8, 11, 14; and 5, 8, 11, 14, 17 positions (all bonds *cis*). Table 2 shows the relative reaction rates of these fatty acids during conversion into PGs. Small yields were obtained with the 19:3 and 21:4 acids whilst only very small amounts of PGs were formed from 18:4, 22:4, and 20:5. No positional isomers of these acids were tested, but 5, 8, 11, 14, 17 20:5 and 2, 5, 8, 11, 14, 17 20:6 are inhibitors of the cyclo-oxygenase (LANDS et al., 1972), as are several *trans* isomers of 20:4 and 20:3 acids (NUGTEREN, 1970). Onc may surmise therefore that the structural requirement for conversion to prostaglandins by the cyclo-oxygenase was the presence of *cis* double bonds at least at positions 8, 11, 14 and—since the methyl esters are not substrates—a free carboxyl group also. For optimal activity, however, a chain length of 20-C is required with *cis* double bonds in positions 8, 11, 14 or 5, 8, 11, 14.

PGs, and by implication other cyclo-oxygenase products, are not stored within cells (PIPER and VANE, 1971) and so biosynthesis must immediately precede release. The substrates must be in a nonesterified form (LANDS and SAMUELSSON, 1968; VONKEMAN and VAN DORP, 1968) for synthesis of the products to occur and yet the level of such substrates in cells—as free acids at least—is extremely low (KUNZE and VOGT, 1971; HAYE et al., 1973; SAMUELSSON, 1972). However, these acids are present in high concentrations in cells as esters, mainly in the form of phospholipids. In an analysis of sheep vesicular gland phospholipids for example, SAMUELSSON (1969) found high concentrations of dihomo-γ-linolenic acid in both the phosphatidyl

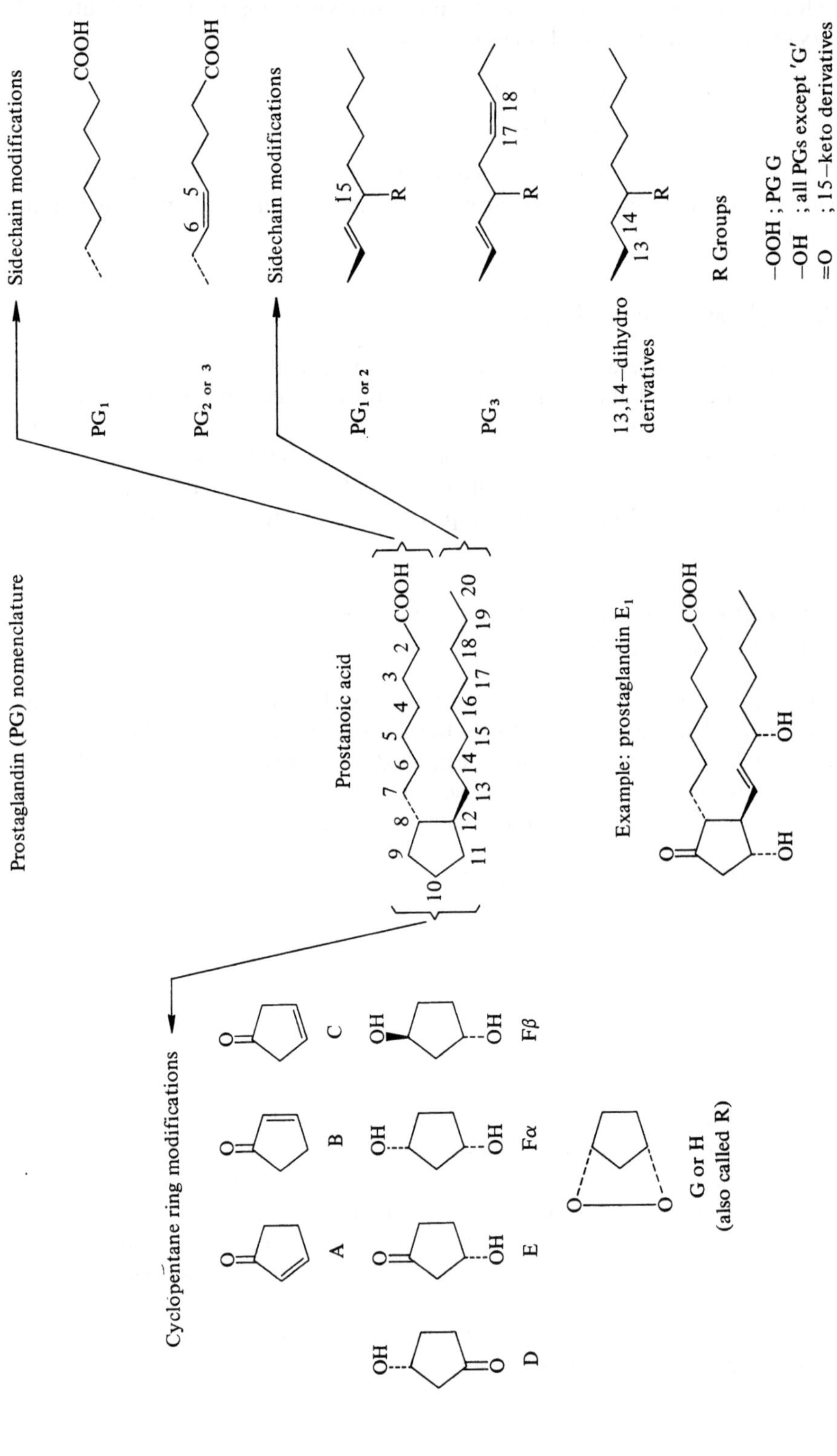

Fig. 1. Structures of prostaglandins,, prostaglandin intermediates, and major metabolites

Table 2. Substrate specificity of the cyclo-oxygenase[a]

Chain length	Double bonds (*cis*)	Position	Reaction rate (relative to arachidomic)
19C	3	8,11,14	57.1
20C[b]	3	8,11,14	91.4
21C	3	8,11,14	28.5
18C	4	5,8,11,14	7.1
19C	4	5,8,11,14	21.4
20C[c]	4	5,8,11,14	100.0
21C	4	5,8,11,14	21.4
22C	4	5,8,11,14	7.1
20C[d]	5	5,8,11,14,17	5.7

[a] Data compiled from VAN DORP (1967).
[b] Precursor of E_1 etc.
[c] Precursor of E_2 etc.
[d] Precursor of E_3 etc.

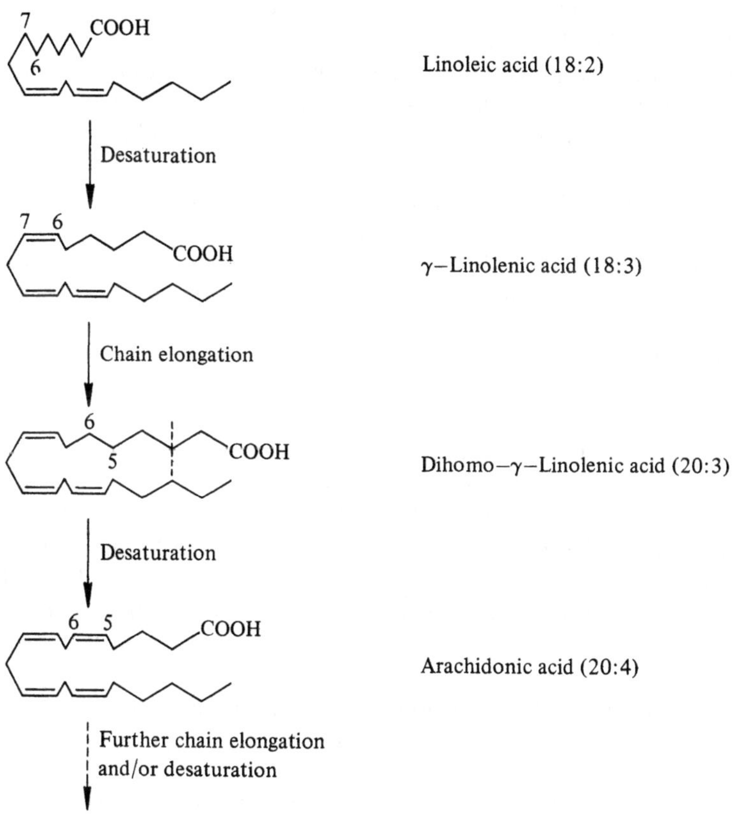

Fig. 2. Biosynthesis of dihomo-γ-linolenic acid and arachidonic acid by the rat

choline (17.5 moles %) and ethanolamine (21.8 mol %) fractions. Arachidonic acid was also present in other phosphatides but in 7–11 fold less concentration. This situation appears to be atypical and in most tissues it is arachidonic, rather than dihomo-γ-linolenic acid which appears to be the major substrate (DANON et al., 1975), even though the latter is apparently an intermediate in the preferred pathway for synthesis of arachidonic acid—at least in the rat (SPRECHER and LEE, 1975; MARCEL et al., 1968) (see Fig. 2). It seems that the presence of the precursors of dihomo-γ-linolenic (linolenic and γ-linolenic) increase the final desaturation step—perhaps explaining why dihomo-γ-linolenic acid does not accumulate in tissues to any marked degree. As a corollary to this, DANON et al. (1975) found that feeding of dihomo-γ-linolenic acid (as the ethyl ester) to rats caused a rise nor only in tissue and plasma ester levels of dihomo-γ-linolenate but that in most tissues, it also caused a rise in esterified arachidonate as well. Two interesting exceptions to this were the platelets and the renal medulla where a rise in dihomo-γ-linolenate occurred without a rise in arachidonic acid. The possible significance of these findings will be discussed later.

It seems from the foregoing discussion that the vast majority of the cyclo-oxygenase substrate is present in tissues in an esterified form. Clearly, before synthesis can occur the substrate must first be released. These precursor acids could arise from a number of intracellular lipid pools; cholesterol esters, phosphatides, mono, di, or triglycerides might all contain sufficient substrate to support biosynthesis. Thus, several enzymes are potentially capable of mobilising fatty acid substrates. The suggestion which has received most attention, however, is that the free substrate originates from the phospholipid fraction of the cell, under the influence of the hydrolytic enzyme phospholipase A_2.

The implication of this idea is that the appearance of substrate is a rate limiting step in cyclo-oxygenase activity and that phospholipase A_2 is a regulatory enzyme. The experimental evidence for this important concept may by summarised thus:

(1) Phospholipids can act as stores of precursor fatty acid (LANDS and SAMUELSSON, 1968; VONKEMAN and VAN DORP, 1968).

(2) Infusion of arachidonic acid through frog intestine (BARTELS et al., 1970) or lungs (VARGAFTIG and DAO HAI, 1972; PALMER et al., 1973), results in a release of PGs.

(3) Perfusion of guinea pig lungs or frog intestine with phospholipase A leads to a rapid release of large quantities of PGs (VOGT et al., 1969; BARTELS et al., 1970).

(4) Infusion of arachidonic acid or bradykinin through guinea pig lungs leads to an appearance of PGs in the perfusate; mepacrine, a phospholipase inhibitor, blocks the releasing action of bradykinin but not of arachidonic acid (VARGAFTIG and DAO HAI, 1972). These results are consistent with the idea that bradykinin releases PGs by stimulating phospholipase, whereas arachidonic acid is converted to PGs directly.

(5) Thyroid stimulating hormone apparently increases the synthesis of PGs in the thyroid by stimulating the activity of an endogenous phospholipase (HAYE et al., 1973).

(6) When incubated with labelled arachidonic acid, slices of guinea pig spleen incorporate the substrate into neutral lipid and phosphatide pools. The majority is incorporated into the 2′ position of a phosphatide with the chromatographic mobil-

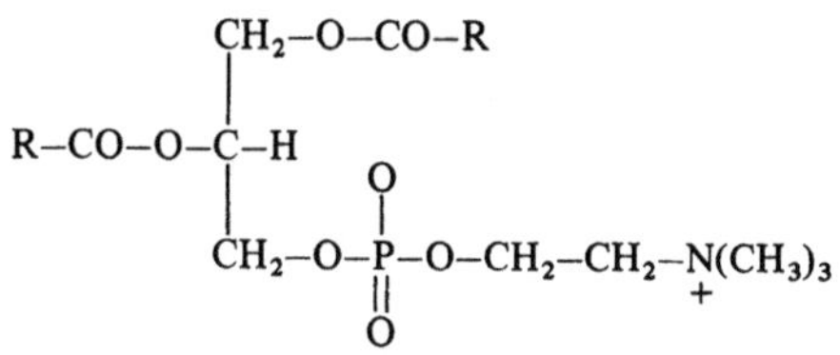

Fig. 3. The structure of lecithin. The R groups are occupied by fatty acids, generally a saturated acid in the 1′ position and an unsaturated acid in the 2′ position

Table 3. Changes in the distribution of ^{14}C-arachidonic acid following mechanical vibration

Treatment	p mol %			
	Phospholipids	Arachidonic acid	Neutral lipids	PGs
Control ($n=5$)	67.16 (±3.52)	25.36 (±3.35)	5.13 (±0.55)	2.06 (±0.13)
Vibrated ($n=5$)	41.52 (±2.67)	44.98 (±3.04)	5.34 (±1.06)	8.02 (±0.84)
P	< 0.001	< 0.01	NS	<0.001

Data taken from FLOWER and BLACKWELL (1976).

Table 4. Changes in the distribution of ^{14}C-arachidonic acid following anaphylactic shock

Treatment	p mol %			
	Phospholipids	Arachidonic acid	Neutral lipids	PGs
Control (n=5)	83.57 (±1.12)	6.38 (±1.84)	10.77 (±0.98)	0.86 (±0.26)
Anaphylaxis (n=5)	78.20 (±2.12)	8.55 (±1.35)	10.39 (±0.46)	3.25 (±0.80)
P	<0.05	NS	NS	<0.02

Data taken from FLOWER and BLACKWELL (1976).

ity of lecithin (see Fig. 3). During mechanical vibration, homogenisation or immunological stimulation, radioactive arachidonic acid is released from the lecithin fraction and converted into PGs. No release of arachidonate is observed from the neutral lipid pools at any time (see Tables 3. and 4.) (FLOWER and BLACKWELL, 1976).

(7) Experiments similar to these (6) were performed using platelets which depend upon the generation of TXA_2 for aggregation. Platelets, like spleen slices, incorporate labelled arachidonic acid into the 2′ position of phosphatides—chiefly choline and inositol phosphatides. During exposure of the platelets to aggregating agents, significant losses of arachidonic acid from the phosphatidyl choline and phosphotidylinositol and phosphatidylethanolamine fractions are observed, with the concomitant generation of cyclo-oxygenase products. The experiments have been repeated using gas chromatography to estimate the arachidonate content of platelet phosphatides. Again, a striking fall in the phosphatidylcholine and phosphatidylinositol and phosphatidylethanolamine arachidonate content is seen after the addition of collagen (BLACKWELL et al., 1976).

Although the foregoing evidence in favour of phospholipase A_2 as the regulator of cyclo-oxygenase activity is as yet incomplete, it is highly suggestive. The possibility that lipid pools other than phosphatides are important for cyclo-oxygenase activity cannot be ruled out at this stage, but nonetheless the possibility of a regulatory mechanism involving phospholipase A_2 is certainly very attractive. Because the cellular membrane system to a large extent controls the integrity of the cell (the cyclo-oxygenase is also membrane bound), its function as a storehouse of fatty acid substrates and as a regulator of permeability are intimately linked. Thus, damage to a section of membrane resulting in a turnover of phosphatides could not only release fatty acids but also result in an increased diffusion of those precursors into the cyclo-oxygenase compartment. AUDET et al. (1974) investigated the activity of phospholipase A in three different strains of *E. coli*. Very little activity was found in two of the strains which had rigid cell envelopes and were thus relatively resistant to lysis. The other strain, however, had high phospholipase activity, was easily lysed and during growth released lipid, protein and polysaccharide material into the medium. There was also production of free fatty acids. Other workers have also noticed that the activity of this enzyme is greater in cells subjected to adverse conditions (SCANDELLA and KORNBERG, 1971; BENNET et al., 1971; PATRIARCA et al., 1972). On the basis of this evidence, it is attractive to speculate that a primary lesion in cell damage is disruption of the cellular membrane system leading to a release of fatty acids and an increase in permeability which enables the liberated fatty acids to reach the cyclo-oxygenase enzyme, culminating in a release of PGs and other lipid mediators.

Of course, as one might expect, the type of PGs produced by a cell depends upon the type of fatty acid present in the phospholipid stores. Such an idea has been used as the basis of an ingenious experiment by WILLIS and his co-workers (1974a). Utilising the fact that E_1 blocks platelet aggregation, these authors fed rats with oral dihomo-γ-linolenate, a procedure which results in increased ratios of this acid to arachidonic acid in the phospholipid fraction. Platelets from these rats were much less susceptible to the aggregating activity of several agents, which normally act by generating arachidonate oxidation products such as TXA_2.

E. Nature and Location of the Cyclo-Oxygenase

The cyclo-oxygenase enzyme system which catalyses the oxidation of polyunsaturated fatty acids to endoperoxides and their subsequent transformation to PGs and other products is a multienzyme complex located in the high speed particulate fraction of cells. The actual membrane fraction to which the enzyme is bound is not entirely clear, although in careful experiments on the intracellular distribution of rabbit kidney cyclo-oxygenase, BOHMAN and LARSSON (1975) found that the bulk of the activity was associated with the endoplasmic reticulum membranes.

The membrane-bound nature of the enzyme complex has frustrated most efforts to characterize the individual enzymes. Quite recently, however, two important advances have occurred. MIYAMOTO and his colleagues (1974) succeeded in solubilising the prostaglandin synthetase system from bovine seminal vesicles using Tween 20 as a detergent (there were previous reports that prostaglandin synthetase could be solubilised with non-ionic detergents—see SIH and TAKEGUCHI, 1973). MIYAMOTO et al. (1974) found that the soluble fraction could be further separated by O-(diethylaminoethyl) cellulose chromatography into two fractions: 'fraction 1', which was eluted first from the DEAE column, catalysed the generation from dihomo-γ-linolenic acid of the PG endoperoxide PGH_1, and 'fraction 2,' which was eluted from the column with increased (200 mM) phosphate buffer concentrations, catalysed the isomerisation of the endoperoxide to PGE_1.

Another approach to characterisation was used by ROTH et al. (1975). These workers used an ingenious adaptation of the finding that aspirin (acetylsalicylic acid) and its congeners inhibit the cyclo-oxygenase (see SHEN, Chapter 30). Although the intimate mechanism of aspirin inhibition of the enzyme was unknown, the group used as a working hypothesis the known ability of the drug to acetylate proteins. After synthesising aspirin with a tritium label on the labile acetyl group, they incubated the drug with crude cyclo-oxygenase preparations derived from human platelets and sheep and ox seminal vesicles. After incubation, the insoluble enzyme was solubilised in sodium dodecyl sulphate and subjected to polyacrylamide gel electrophoresis. The bulk of the radioactivity in each of the tissue digests was found to migrate as a protein of 85000 mol wt. No incorporation of radioactivity was found when aspirin was labelled in the aromatic ring. Evidence that the cyclo-oxygenase (and not other microsomal proteins) was specifically acetylated came from comparisons of the (low) concentrations of aspirin required, and the (short) time taken to inactivate the cyclo-oxygenase and acetylate the protein. A good correlation was found in each case. The authors claim was further substantiated when it was found that protein acetylation was blocked by fatty acid substrates of the enzyme (arachidonic and dihomo-γ-linolenic acid) as well as by another potent cyclo-oxygenase inhibitor, indomethacin. Aspirin is thought to block the initial dioxygenase reaction (FLOWER, 1974a) and it would thus seem that the catalytic unit (or subunit) of the dioxygenase enzyme has a mol wt of about 85000 and that acetylation of the active site is the mechanism of aspirin inhibition—although, as the authors are careful to point out, aspirin binding at a distant 'allosteric' site could also prevent arachidonic acid binding at the true catalytic site too.

At the time of writing, no further work has been undertaken on the characterization of the enzyme at the molecular level and thus any statements are essentially speculative in nature.

F. Distribution of the Cyclo-Oxygenase

The distribution of the cyclo-oxygenase appears to be ubiquitous. 'PG synthetase' activity appears to be present in every mammalian tissue so far investigated (as well as several non-mammalian tissues); HORTON (1969) and RAMWELL and SHAW (1970) have listed tissues from which PG release has been elicited after the application of suitable stimuli. CHRIST and VAN DORP (1972, 1973) have conducted extensive investigations into the PG biosynthetic capacity of a wide range of tissues including those from vertebrates, arthropods molluscs and coelenterates. These authors measured enzyme activity in a wide variety of mammalian tissues by measuring the conversion of labelled precursor acid to PGE_1. They classified tissues into three broad categories: (1) those such as kidney medulla and lung in which 10–40% conversion occurred, (2) tissues such as gut in which only some 3% occurred and (3) other tissues such as spleen and aorta in which the conversion was 1% or less. These workers also found cyclo-oxygenase activity in the lung tissues or homologous structures of other vertebrates (i.e. frog lung and carp gills) and from members of other phyla.

PGs—and therefore PG synthesis—also occur in the coral *plexaura homamalla* (LIGHT and SAMUELSSON, 1972) as well as in some plants (MIYARES-CAO and MENENDEZ-CEPERO, 1976).

The only tissues which seem to possess very high PG biosynthetic activity (75% conversion of substrate, or more) are sheep and ox seminal vesicles. For this reason much of the experimental work on the biosynthetic mechanisms have been conducted using these organs as a source of enzyme.

The recognition that different tissues can metabolise PG endoperoxide intermediates to different products is a comparatively recent event (see succeeding sections) and we do not yet know which tissues metabolise endoperoxides mainly to PGs, and which tissues transform endoperoxides chiefly to non-PG end products. Clarification of this aspect may show that a tissue with low prostaglandin biosynthetic activity has a high level of endoperoxide synthesis.

G. Chemical Transformations Catalysed by the Cyclo-Oxygenase

The enzymic conversion of certain essential fatty acids into PGs was demonstrated in 1964 by two groups of workers, VAN DORP et al. (1964a, 1964b) in Holland, and BERGSTRÖM et al. (1964a, 1964b) in Sweden. Most of the subsequent biochemistry of PG synthesis has also been pioneered by these two groups. Although much of the original experimental work on the reaction mechanism utilised the cyclo-oxygenase from sheep seminal vesicles, there is no reason to suspect that the generation of endoperoxides catalysed by enzymes from other tissues proceeds by a radically different pathway. As pointed out in the previous section, fatty acid cyclo-oxygenase is a multienzyme complex which catalyses several reactions. Furthermore, the end products of the reaction vary from tissue to tissue. For this reason, the description of the reaction mechanism which follows is divided into different sections.

In the first experiments with sheep seminal vesicles, arachidonic acid was used as a substrate, but another set of papers by the same two groups later in 1964 (BERGSTRÖM et al., 1964a, 1964b; VAN DORP et al., 1964a, 1964b) demonstrated that dihomo-γ-linolenic acid and arachidonic acid could be converted into PGE_1 and PGE_2 and also that 5,8,11,14,17-eicosapentaenoic acid could be converted to PGE_3.

A year later, WALLACH (1965) demonstrated that arachidonic acid was converted to PGE_2 by acetone powders of bull seminal vesicles, and ÄNGGÅRD and SAMUELSSON (1965) showed that PG biosynthesis was not restricted to seminal vesicles but also occurred in guinea pig lung tissue. Figure 4 gives an overview of the known tranformations of arachidonic acid in cells by the cyclo-oxygenase and lipoxygenase.

I. Generation of the Cyclic Endoperoxides

Evidence for the formation of an endoperoxide structure as an intermediate in the cyclo-oxygenase reaction first came from $^{18}O_2$–$^{16}O_2$ experiments of SAMUELSSON (1965). However, in experiments with guinea pig lung (ÄNGGÅRD and SAMUELSSON,

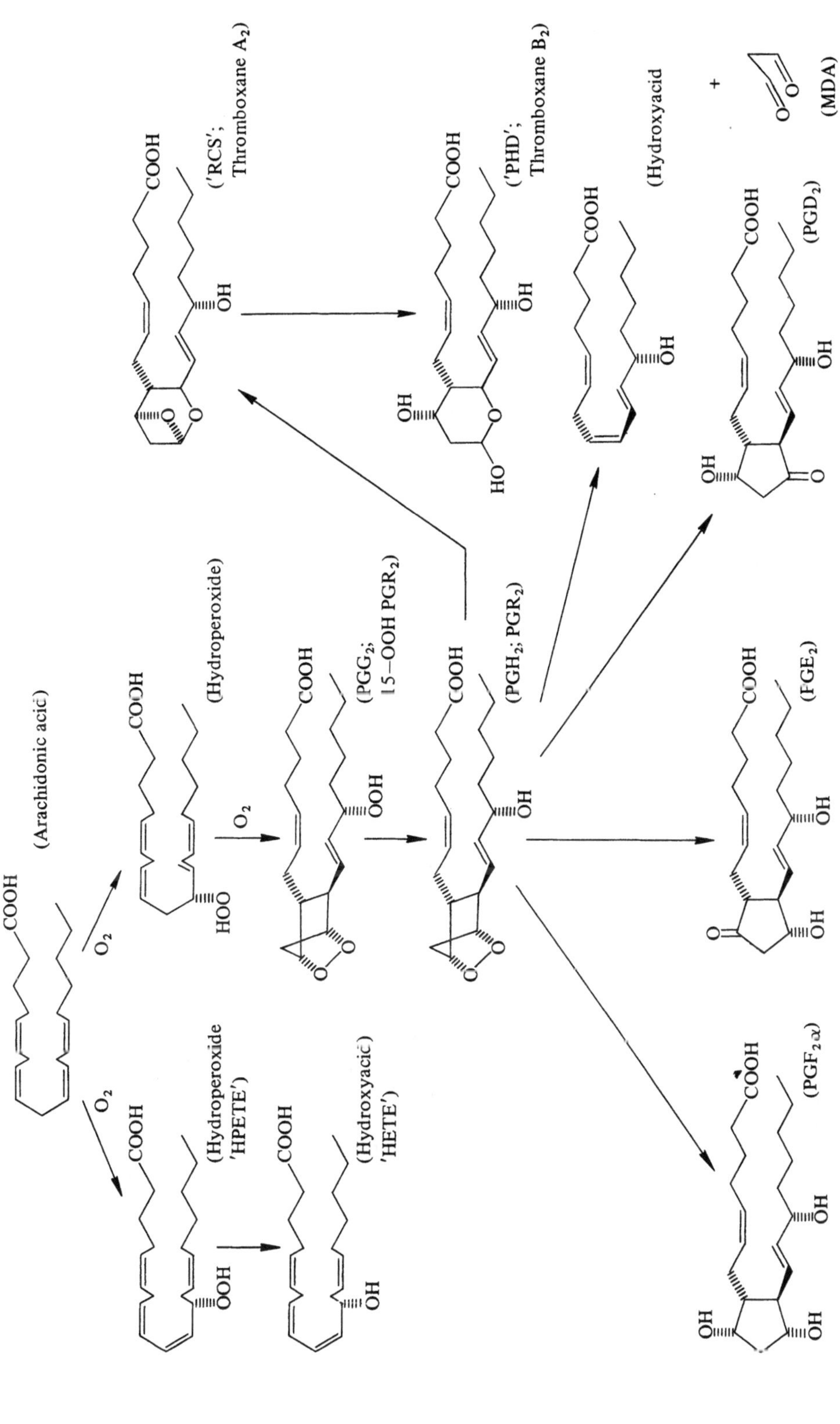

Fig. 4. An overview of arachidonic acid transformation by cells

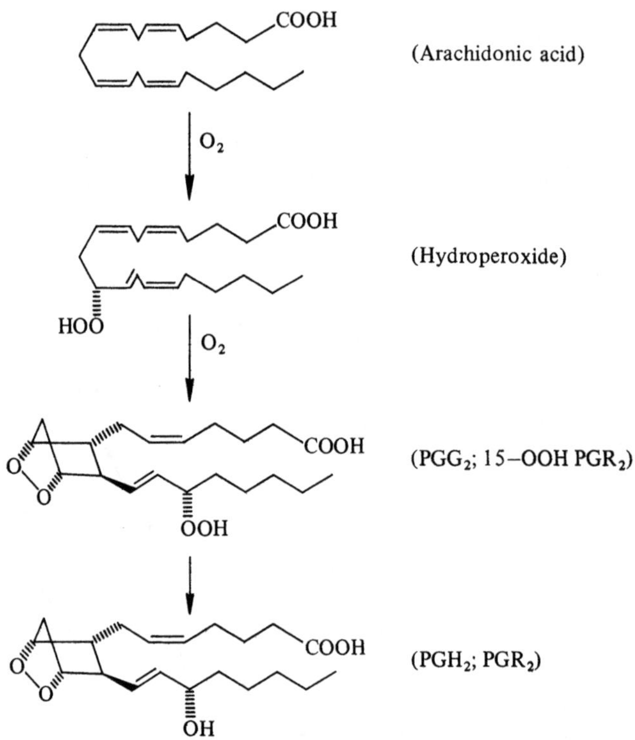

Fig. 5. Generation of cyclic endoperoxides from arachidonic acid by the cyclo-oxygenase

1965), it was found that the PGE and PGF formed could not be interconverted, thus indicating their formation from a common intermediate which was confirmed later by the studies of WLODAWER and SAMUELSSON (1973).

The initial step (HAMBERG and SAMUELSSON, 1967a; NUGTEREN et al., 1966) of this dioxygenase reaction is initiated by a stereospecific (L) removal of the ω-8 hydrogen and the conversion of the substrate to an ω–10 hydroperoxide (see Fig. 5). This step is somewhat reminiscent of the reaction catalysed by the plant enzyme soyabean lipoxidase which also removes this hydrogen stereospecifically although here, an ω-6 hydroperoxide is formed (HAMBERG and SAMUELSSON, 1967c). The next stage is a concerted reaction; the addition of oxygen at C-15 is followed by an isomerisation of the C-12 double bond, ring closure between C-8 and C-12 and an attack by an oxygen radical (of the C-11 hydroperoxide) at C-9 thus forming a 'cyclic endoperoxide'. The resulting intermediate is referred to as 'PGG' by SAMUELSSON's group (HAMBERG and SAMUELSSON, 1973; HAMBERG et al., 1974b) and as '15-hydroperoxy PG-R' by NUGTEREN and HAZELHOF (1973). The next stage involves reduction of the C-15 hydroperoxy group to the corresponding hydroxyl moiety, giving rise to a compound known as 'PGH' by SAMUELSSON's group and as 'PGR' by NUGTEREN and HAZELHOF. Both of these endoperoxide intermediates are rather unstable, spontaneously decomposing in aqueous solutions to mixtures of prostaglandins. Temperature and pH are very important in determining their half-life in aqueous solutions (NUGTEREN and HAZELHOF, 1973). Notwithstanding their insta-

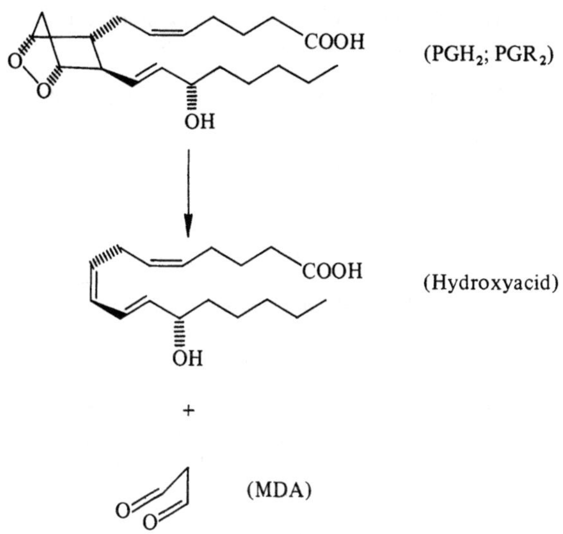

Fig. 6. Generation of the 17-C hydroxyacid (HHT) and malondialdehyde (MDA) from the cyclic endoperoxide

bility, however, the endoperoxides can be isolated in organic solvents and are stable in dry acetone at −20° C for some weeks. The 'Labile Aggregation Stimulating Substance' (LASS) of WILLIS et al. (1974b) is probably a mixture of PGG_2 and H_2 (see also WILLIS, Chapter 5).

In some systems, for example platelet aggregation, the endoperoxide intermediates have distinct pharmacological actions of their own which are different in many respects from that of their ultimate end products.

II. Transformation of the Endoperoxide to HHT

The 17-C monohydroxy fatty acid HHT had been isolated from incubation mixtures of arachidonic acid and sheep seminal vesicle homogenates by WLODAWER and SAMUELSSON (1973) and was also found to be a by-product of chemical reduction of the endoperoxides PGG_2 and PGH_2 by $SnCl_2$ (HAMBERG et al., 1974b, 1974c). Formation by sheep seminal vesicle homogenates of the analagous hydroxy fatty acid from dihomo-γ-linolenic acid had previously been demonstrated by NUGTEREN et al. (1966) and by HAMBERG and SAMUELSSON (1966, 1967a, 1967b), who postulated that it was derived from the endoperoxide intermediate after the expulsion of malondialdehyde (MDA) from PGG_2 in platelets (HAMBERG and SAMUELSSON, 1974a). Later the same year, HAMBERG, and his co-workers (HAMBERG et al., 1974c) performed quantitative measurements of the hydroxy acid (now known as HHT) released from aggregating human platelets and demonstrated that it represented a very considerable proportion (about 30%) of total endoperoxide metabolism (Fig. 6). In a further paper, HAMBERG and SAMUELSSON (1974b) demonstrated that the transformation of PGG_2 to HHT also occurs in guinea pig lungs once again, it represents a major metabolic pathway (see Table 5). As a product of fatty acid cyclo-oxygenase, the formation of this compound is blocked by aspirin-like drugs.

Table 5. Products formed from arachidonic acid by guinea pig isolated perfused lungs

Product	% Conversion of arachidonic acid[a]
PHD	2.18–7.68
HHT	0.64–1.29
F_{2a}	0.31–0.57
HETE	0.22–0.37
E_2	0.05–0.31

[a] Data calculated from HAMBERG and SAMUELSSON (1974b). Arachidonic acid (30 µg) was injected into guinea pig lungs perfused through the pulmonary artery with Krebs-Henseleit solution. The effluent was collected and the amounts of products determined by multiple-ion analysis using deuterated internal standards.

The formation of HHT is accompanied by the generation of MDA this compound may be readily measured by a simple colorimetric method using thiobarbituric acid (TBA), and this assay has been used successfully as an index of cyclo-oxygenase activity (FLOWER et al., 1973; HAMBERG et al., 1974c). The TBA reaction has also been used for many years as an index of 'lipid peroxidation' (DAHLE et al., 1962; SCHULTZ, 1962) and a question which must be asked is whether much of the MDA measured in the early literature actually originated from the cyclo-oxygenase pathway. According to NIEHAUS and SAMUELSSON (1968), the formation of MDA which occurs during lipid peroxidation, whilst derived mainly from phospholipid arachidonate, is generated by a different mechanism.

III. Transformation of the Endoperoxide to PGs

Opinion seems to be divided as to which of the endoperoxide intermediates is the precursor of PGE. NUGTEREN and HAZELHOF (1973) propose that PGH is the precursor of PGE, (as well as PGF and PGD), whereas SAMUELSSON and HAMBERG (1974) believe that the reaction proceeds via the intermediate 15-hydroperoxy PGE. However, as NUGTEREN and HAZELHOF point out, when 15-hydroperoxy PGE decomposes in the absence of a reducing factor it gives rise to significant quantities of 15-keto PGE, explaining perhaps why this compound is sometimes found as a product of prostaglandin biosynthesis (see Figs. 7 and 8).

Using labelled PGH_1 and PGH_2 as a precursor, NUGTEREN and HAZELHOF (1973) investigated the formation of labelled prostaglandins in different tissues. In the lung, stomach and intestine, PGD was the predominant product formed from the endoperoxide, whereas in the liver and sheep vesicular gland, PGE was the major product. The enzyme responsible for the formation of PGE ('endoperoxide—PGE isomerase') was found by these authors to be particulate in nature and to require glutathione for maximal activity; it could perhaps be identical to glutathione peroxidase. The enzyme catalysing the formation of PGD ('endoperoxide—PGD isomerase') was apparently a soluble protein of mol wt $36–42 \times 10^3$ daltons, which also required GSH for activity. NUGTEREN and HAZELHOF concluded that the formation

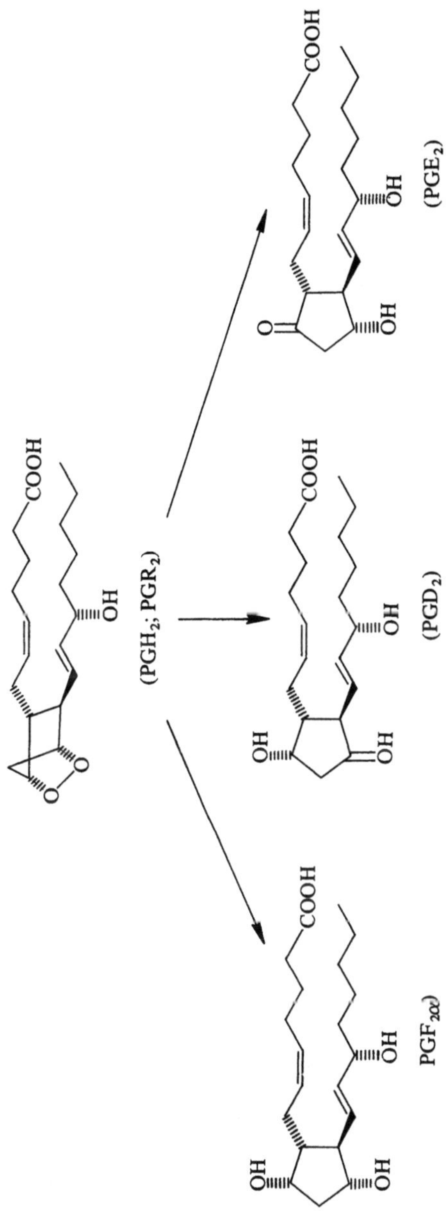

Fig. 7. Generation of PGs F, E and D from the cyclic endoperoxide

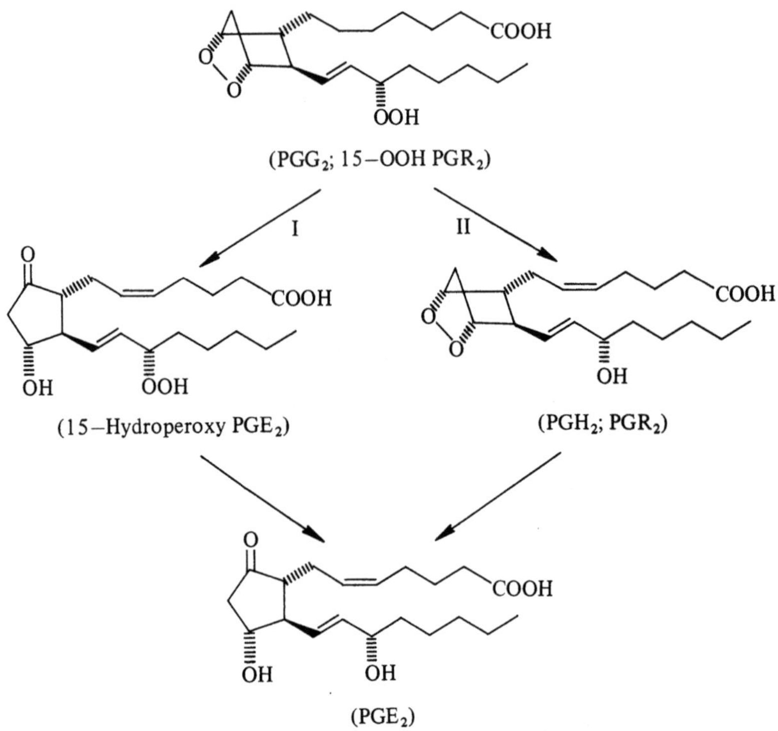

Fig. 8. Alternative routes for the synthesis of PGE_2 from the cyclic endoperoxide

of PGF (by an 'endoperoxide reductase') could simply be a non-enzymic phenomenon since reduction of endoperoxide to PGF occurs when tissue homogenates contain reducing agents (i.e. SH-compounds, ferrihaem compounds, etc.), and an appreciable conversion of endoperoxide to PGF could be seen even when such homogenates were boiled, thus ruling out an enzymic conversion. Possibly, then, there is no 'endoperoxide reductase' enzyme at all, and PGF occurs in tissues having a relative deficiency of 'E' or 'D' isomerase enzymes and a sufficient level of reducing factors. This conclusion is also supported by the experiments of Chan et al. (1975) who demonstrated that chemical reducing agents promote PGF biosynthesis by bovine seminal vesicle microsomes.

IV. Transformation of the Endoperoxide to Thromboxane 'A' and 'B' (PHD)

The recent discovery by Hamberg, Samuelsson and their colleagues (Hamberg and Samuelsson 1974a, 1974b; Hamberg et al., 1974c) that in certain tissues, such as lungs and platelets, PGG_2 is transformed mainly into non-prostaglandin end products has proved to be critical to our understanding of the mechanism of platelet aggregation (see Willis, Chapter 5). Furthermore, it is now possible to state with virtual certainty that the mysterious substance 'rabbit aorta contracting substance (RCS)' first described by Piper and Vane in 1969, is in fact a mixture of endoperoxides and TXA_2.

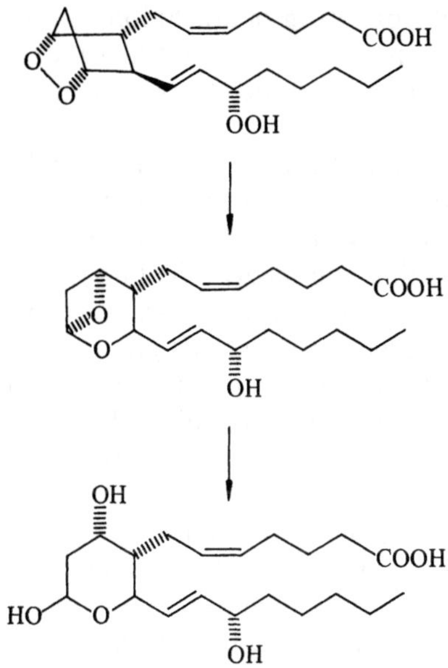

(PGG_2; 15–OOH PGR_2)

('RCS'; Thromboxane A_2)

('PHD'; Thromboxane B_2)

Fig. 9. Generation of TXA_2 and B_2 from the cyclic endoperoxide

The first demonstration that PGG_2 could be transformed to 'thromboxanes' was reported in September 1974 (HAMBERG and SAMUELSSON, 1974a) although at that time this term had not yet been coined (see Fig. 9). In the September paper, HAMBERG and SAMUELSSON described the transformation of PGG_2 in human platelets; the two major compounds formed from the endoperoxide were a 17-C hydroxy fatty acid (HHT) (see previous section for details) and a very polar compound not previously described—the hemi-acetal derivative of 8-(1-hydroxy-3-oxopropyl)-9, 12 L-dihydroxy-5, 10-heptadecadienoic acid. Experiments with $^{18}O_2$ demonstrated that both the endoperoxide oxygens were incorporated into the six-membered ring of this polar compound, although the exact mechanism of its formation was not elucidated at that time. In October of the same year, a further paper by SAMUELSSON's group appeared (HAMBERG et al., 1974c) in which quantitative measurements of the formation of this very polar product (provisionally called PHD), HHT, and PGs were performed, using multiple-ion analysis with deuterated internal standards for the HHT and PHD estimations. When washed human platelets were aggregated by thrombin, large quantities of arachidonate oxidation products were released, approximately one-third of which was PHD. The remainder comprised equal quantities of HHT and the lipoxygenase product HETE (see Section J.) The amounts of PGs (E_2 and $F_{2\alpha}$) formed were some two orders of magnitude less than the total amounts of PGG_2 biosynthesised, thus clearly indicating that PGs as such were formed in insignificant amounts compared with other endoperoxide products. The formation of PHD (as well as HHT, but not HETE) was blocked by aspirin-like drugs, as might be anticipated. A further paper by HAMBERG and SAMUELSSON (1974b) reported that guinea pig lung homogenates or perfused intact lungs could generate PHD as well as platelets (although the possibility that platelets in the lung were responsible for the transformation cannot be ruled out). When quantitative measurements of the products formed from 30 μg of arachidonic acid injected into perfused guinea pig isolated lungs were made, it was found that the major product formed was again PHD (see Table 5), which accounted for approximately 2—8% of the injected substrate.

The mechanism of the transformation of PGG_2 to its major metabolite in lungs and platelets, PHD, was not understood until HAMBERG et al. published in August 1975 an account of the enzymic reaction by which PGG_2 is converted to PHD via a highly unstable intermediate. Because this intermediate had an oxane ring, was a potent platelet aggregating substance and in this case was derived from arachidonic acid (and therefore had two double bonds), SAMUELSSON'S group named it 'thromboxane A_2'. The metabolite of TXA_2 which had been provisionally named PHD was then renamed 'thromboxane B_2' (TXB_2). As with the initial work on transformations of PGG_2, this first demonstration of the generation of TXA_2 was made using human platelets.

In their experiments, the authors noted that a very unstable compound (half-life in aqueous media at 37° C about 32 s) could be detected during the conversion of PGG_2 to TXB_2. Various nucleophilic reagents such as ethanol, methanol and sodium azide when added to the platelet incubation medium, resulted in the formation of derivatives from which the structure of the intermediate was deduced.

In another series of experiments, incubation of washed platelets with arachidonic acid or PGG_2 was found to give rise to a highly unstable factor which could induce irreversible platelet aggregation and cause the release of ^{14}C-5-HT from platelets. The properties and mode of formation of this product strongly suggested that it was TXA_2.

One interesting spin-off from these experiments was that the question of identity of the RCS of PIPER and VANE (1969) (and also in the experiments of GRYGLEWSKI and VANE, 1972a, 1972b) could be finally solved. Initially, when the endoperoxide G_2 was described and found to posses rabbit aorta contracting activity, it was thought that RCS may have been PGG_2 or PGH_2. However, comparison of their half-lives in aqueous solution (endoperoxide about 8 min, RCS 1–2 min) made this unlikely. The half-life of RCS, its mode of formation and the existence of the thromboxane pathway in lung, makes it seem certain that the activity of RCS is caused mainly by TXA_2 with a small amount of PGG_2 or PGH_2 or both.

V. Other Products Formed by the Cyclo-Oxygenase

In addition to the pathways already detailed in this section, there are reports in the literature of several other derivatives of polyunsaturated fatty acids, some of which are as yet uncharacterised, such as the 'activating factor' which is reported by COOK and LANDS (1975) to be generated during the oxygenation of arachidonic acid by acetone powders of sheep vesicular glands. These authors found that a 'lag' phase in the oxygenase reaction occurred when inhibitory concentrations of NaCN were present in the incubation medium. The lag phase was greatly reduced when fresh enzyme, or an ether extract of an uninhibited reaction mixture, was added to the inhibited samples. These experiments suggest that an activating factor formed during the oxygenation reaction is necessary for optimal activity of the enzyme. The nature of this factor is unknown but it could be a hydroperoxide. Another uncharacterized

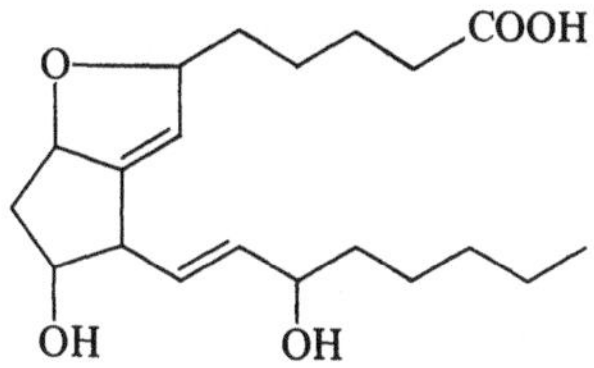

Fig. 10

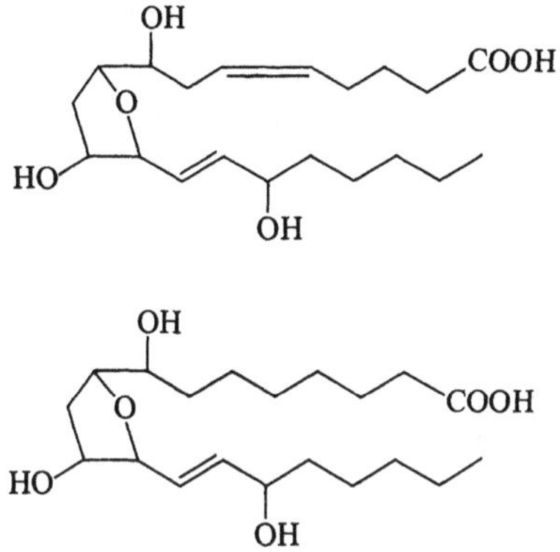

Fig. 11

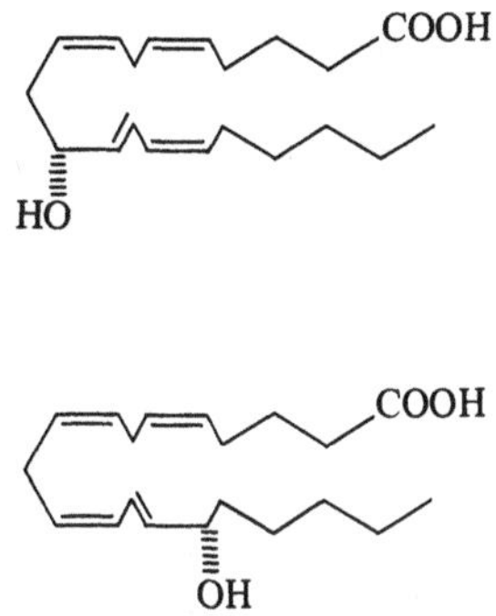

Fig. 12

Fig. 10. Proposed structure of product formed by rat fundus homogenates from arachidonic acid. It is also formed to a small extent by sheep seminal vesicles

Fig. 11. Proposed structure of a minor product formed from arachidonic acid by sheep seminal vesicles. An analogous compound lacking a 5,6 double bond is formed from dihomo-γ-linolenic acid

Fig. 12. Two hydroxy fatty acids formed in small quantities from arachidonate by the cyclo-oxygenase

product 'prostaglandin MI,' described by PARKES and ELING (1974) as being the major product of guinea pig lung cyclo-oxygenase, would now seem to be identical to TXB_2. The chromatographic mobility and other properties of 'MI' fit well with those described by HAMBERG and SAMUELSSON (1974a, 1974b) for this compound. PACE-ASCIAK and WOLFE (1971) described the formation by rat stomach homogenates of a novel prostanoic acid derivative together with a smaller amount of an isomeric form—6(9)-oxy-11,15-dehydroxy prosta—7,13-dienoic acid (see Fig. 10) which was formed in addition to E_2 and $F_{2\alpha}$. Two possible pathways of generation from endoperoxide intermediates are suggested by the authors. It is not known whether these derivatives are released from stimulated intact stomachs as are E_2 and $F_{2\alpha}$ (BENNETT et al., 1967; COCEANI et al., 1967). Although formed in excess of E_2 and $F_{2\alpha}$, the derivative has much less biological activity than these compounds. PACE-ASCIAK (1971) also reported that homogenates of sheep seminal vesicles incubated with arachidonic acid produce this derivative along with another novel compound (see Fig. 11). However, the amount of these products was only some 2% of the PGE_2 formed, so that in this case they constitute only a very minor pathway.

Apart from 15-keto E_1 which has already been referred to as a by-product of PG biosynthesis, NUGTEREN et al. (1966) and DANIELS et al. (1968) found that 8-iso-PGE_1 was formed as a minor product (<2%) when bovine seminal vesicles were incubated with dihomo-γ-linolenic acid.

Finally, HAMBERG and SAMUELSSON (1974b) reported the formation in guinea pig lung homogenates of two C-20 hydroxy fatty acids (in addition to HETE). These were 15-hydroxy-5,8,11,13-eicosatetraenoic, and 11-hydroxy-5,8,12,14-eicosatetraenoic acid (see Fig. 12). These acids were present in small yields (<2% of recovered radioactivity), and were probably formed by reduction of the parent fatty acid hydroperoxides thought to be intermediates in endoperoxides formation. Analogous compounds have been isolated from sheep seminal vesicle homogenates incubated with dihomo-γ-linolenic acid (HAMBERG and SAMUELSSON, 1967a, 1967b; WLODAWER and SAMUELSSON, 1973).

The role in inflammation (if any) of the compounds referred to in this section has not been delineated, and they will not be referred to again.

H. Enzymology of the Cyclo-Oxygenase

In this section it is proposed to compare data on those (regrettably few) preparations of the cyclo-oxygenase enzyme which have been carefully examined, and to extend and amplify those remarks made in Section G concerning the nature of the enzyme.

I. Purification of the Enzyme

Apart from the experiments of MIYAMOTO et al. (1974) already referred to in Section G, there have been several other attempts to purify the cyclo-oxygenase. Since it is membrane-bound, the first stages of any such purification inevitably involve a solubilisation step. The first workers to solubilise the microsomal biosynthetic system were SAMUELSSON et al. in 1967 and GRANSTRÖM in 1968. Although deoxycholate and sodium lauryl sulphate failed to produce soluble preparations which retained activity, these workers found that the non-ionic detergent cutscum worked quite well. When solubilised, the material was precipiated with ammonium sulphate (40–60% saturation) and the detergent-free material further purified by DEAE cellulose chromatography. The final material was purified some tenfold by these procedures and was obtained in yields of about 20%. The catalytic activity was stimulated by hydroquinone and reduced glutathione. Amongst others who have worked with partially purified preparations of the cyclo-oxygenase are CHAN et al. (1975) who obtained again about a tenfold purification and a 40% yield, using cutscum as a detergent and a purification scheme similar to that of SAMUELSSON et al. (1967). RAZ et al. (1975) found that Lubrol Px, Lubrol Wx and Tween 20 yielded active soluble synthetase preparations from sheep vesicular glands, rabbit kidney medulla and rat papilla. The soluble enzyme preparations retained their activity for several weeks when stored at −18° C at pH 5 but deteriorated rapidly at pH 8. Interestingly, the soluble enzymes were less sensitive to the inhibitory activity of aspirin-like drugs.

II. Co-Factor Requirements

Few data are available on the co-factor requirements (if any) for HETE, HHT, TXA_2 or TXB_2 formation, but considerable data have been published on the co-factor requirements for PG biosynthesis per se. PG biosynthesis by sheep vesicular gland fractions is greatly stimulated by the addition of boiled supernatant, reduced glutathione, or by tetrahydrofolate, but not by NADH[1] or NADPH[2] (see SAMUELSSON, 1969). The differential effects of co-factors on the cyclo-oxygenase products have

[1] Nicotinamide-adenine dinucleotide (reduced) [NADH].
[2] Nicotinamide-adenine dinucleotide phosphate (reduced) [NADPH].

been investigated by GRANSTRÖM (1968). Tetrahydrofolate, glutathione, ascorbic acid and supernatant (but not NADH or NADPH) stimulated the production of E_1, $F_{1\alpha}$ as well as monohydroxy acids. A very interesting observation was that the addition of *fresh* supernatant stimulated the production of PGD_1 in excess of other products, suggesting perhaps that in intact cells this is the major product formed. VAN DORP (1967) followed up the original observation of NUGTEREN et al. (1966) that GSH exerted a stimulating influence on synthesis and tested several other thiol compounds—cysteine, homocysteine, Co A-SH, thioglycolic acid and thiophenol. None of these compounds could substitute for GSH in the reaction; the most active, thiophenol and cysteine were only about one-third as active as GSH. TAKEGUCHI et al. (1971) confirmed that GSH was unique amongst thiol compounds in this respect. VAN DORP (1967) also reported that low concentrations of phenolic antioxidants such as hydroquinone should be present for optimal enzyme activity. Other authors have also found that a wide range of aromatic compounds can substitute for hydroquinone (but not for GSH) as a co-factor in PG biosynthesis: TAKEGUCHI et al. (1971) found that p-aminophenol, L-noradrenaline, L-adrenaline, 5-HT and 5-hydroxyindolacetic acid were also suitable co-factors (providing GSH were present). These authors further found that the pH optimum of the synthetic reaction depended to some extent on the co-factor utilized, as did the ratio PGD:PGE:PGF (SIH and TAKEGUCHI, 1973). PACE-ASCIAK (1972) found stimulation of PG biosynthesis in rat stomach homogenates by a number of amines. L-noradrenaline was the most potent followed by dopamine and L-adrenaline. Tyramine, DL-normetanephrine DL-Dopa and β-phenyl ethylamine were only weakly active whilst L-ephedrine and L-tyrosine produced a slight inhibition. The stimulant effect of noradrenaline was blocked by propanalol. An important feature of the stimulation by hydroquinone and other related co-factors is that in excess (in the case of hydroquinone $>5 \times 10^{-4}$ M) they cause inhibition of the reaction (NUGTEREN et al., 1966).

YOSHIMOTO et al. (1970) found that prostaglandin production by bovine seminal vesicles was markedly stimulated by haemoglobin, myoglobin or haemin, but this finding could not be repeated by SIH and TAKEGUCHI (1973).

Whilst reduced glutathione was found to stimulate the formation of all PGs (SAMUELSSON, 1969; VAN DORP, 1967), it preferentially caused a rise in PGE synthesis. Several authors (LEE and LANDS, 1972; MADDOX, 1973) have reported that PGF synthesis may be strongly stimulated by the addition of Cu^{2+} compounds. LEE and LANDS found that the addition of Cu^{2+} to vesicular gland homogenates—especially in the presence of dithiol compounds such as dihydrolipoamide—greatly stimulated the synthesis of PGF compounds at the expense of PGE compounds. The authors suggested that these copper-dithiol mixtures may favour a non-enzymic reduction to PGF compounds, a conclusion supported by the work of CHAN et al. (1975) whose results indicated that stimulation of PGF synthesis by transition metal (Cu^{2+}, Zn^{2+}, Ni^{2+}) dithiothreitol complexes was mainly due to non-enzymic reduction of the endoperoxide intermediate.

In concluding this section, it is worth noting that despite extensive work on the co-factors of prostaglandin biosynthesis, their actual role in the reaction mechanism is not clearly defined. It is unlikely that the aromatic compounds used actually act as anti-oxidants as suggested earlier (NUGTEREN et al., 1966); probably they function as electron donors for the synthetic reaction—PGF compounds requiring 2 mol and

PGE compounds requiring 1 mol of reducing equivalents per mol of product formed. The function of GSH appears to be twofold: a non-specific action—to cycle the electron donor back into a reduced state (in the absence of GSH the electron donor is rapidly oxidised, see FLOWER et al., 1973; TAKEGUCHI and SIH, 1972; SIH and TAKEGUCHI, 1973), and perhaps also as a specific co-factor in the reduction of PGG or PGH to PGE. Already mentioned is that GSH-peroxidase may be involved in this step, and that the requirement for GSH for this reaction seems to be rather specific.

III. Conditions for Optimal Activity

Several PG synthetase enzymes have been subjected to careful scrutiny and attempts have been made to delineate their optimal conditions for catalytic activity. These include enzyme preparations from spleen (FLOWER, 1974b), rabbit kidney (BLACKWELL et al., 1975c; ROSE and COLLINS, 1974), bovine thyroid gland (FRIEDMAN et al., 1975) canine myocardium (LIMAS and COHN, 1973), guinea pig lung (PARKES and ELING, 1974), sheep (WALLACH and DANIELS, 1971) and bovine seminal vesicles (FLOWER et al., 1973; TAKEGUCHI et al., 1971), and rat stomach (PACE-ASCIAK, 1972). Table 6 is a summary (necessarily simplified) of some biochemical properties from a selection of synthetase enzymes. Unfortunately, it is not always possible to draw valid comparisons between the data in this table because of the differences in enzyme preparation and assay techniques employed by each individual investigator. However, in two studies by FLOWER et al. (1973) and BLACKWELL et al. (1975c) the PG synthetase enzymes from two sources—bovine seminal vesicles and rabbit kidney—were carefully investigated using identical techniques for preparation of the crude enzyme and radiochemical assay of the products (see Figs. 13 and 14). Investigation of the bovine, seminal vesicle enzyme alone produced several interesting differences in pH, substrate, GSH and co-factor requirements, as well as optimal reaction time for each of the different products measured ($F_{2\alpha}$, F_2, D_2, and MDA) (see Table 6). Particularly interesting was the effect of increasing substrate levels on the formation of different products; for example PGE_2 synthesis was maximal at 0.5 mM and there was substrate or product inhibition at higher concentrations, whereas $PGF_{2\alpha}$ and PGD_2 synthesis was optimal at 1.5 mM substrate and MDA synthesis at 3.0 mM. Thus, at low concentrations of substrate, E_2 was exclusively formed, the other products only appearing at higher substrate concentrations. It is clear that incubation conditions have important effects, not only on the rate of PG formation but also (in some cases at least) on the type of PG produced. For example, many authors (TOMLINSON et al., 1972; CHASALOW and PHARISS, 1972; CHRIST and VAN DORP, 1972; AHERN and DOWNING, 1970; YOSHIMOTO et al., 1970; TAKEGUCHI et al., 1971) have described cyclo-oxygenase preparations that produced only E-type PGs; in many cases this result might be explained by the incubation conditions that they employed, especially the low concentrations of substrate.

As already pointed out, because of the differences in enzyme preparation and assay techniques it is generally difficult to compare the results obtained with one preparation with the results from another. However, for rabbit kidney synthetase (BLACKWELL et al., 1975c), the schedules for enzyme preparation and assay were virtually identical to those described for the bovine seminal vesicle enzyme (FLOWER et al., 1973) and a comparison is legitimate. The most striking difference between the

Table 6. Comparison of biochemical properties of some PG synthetase enzymes[a]

Enzyme source and product monitored	Optimal conditions							Initial velocity pmol/mg/min	Investigator
	Temp. °C	pH	Substrate mM	GSH mM	Co-factor mM	Max. time for which reaction is linear min	Opt. protein mg/ml		
Spleen E_2	37 (NT)	7.4 (NT)	0.05	0.1	0.09 (HQ)	10	10–20	17.5	FLOWER (1974b)
Sheep Seminal Vesicles E_2	38	8.0	2.0 (NT)	2.0	0.25–1.0 (HQ)	6	≅200	NT at least 2216 pmol/mg enz/min	WALLACH and DANIELS (1971)
Canine myocardium E_2	37 (NT)	≅8.5	≅0.05	0.8 (NT)	1.0 (AD) 1.0 (NT)	at least 10	1.21	≅10,000	LIMAS and COHN (1973)
Rat stomach E_2	37	NT	>0.01	Not used	≅1.0 (NR)	≅2	NT	NT	PACE-ASCIAK (1972)
Bovine thyroid E_2	37	7–7.3	0.163 (NT)	Had no effect	0.1–0.5 (HQ)	at least 3	20 (NT)	≅1.99 (NT)	FRIEDMAN et al. (1975)
Bovine seminal vesicles E_2	37 (NT)	8.0	≅0.5 mM	1 mM	0.2 (HQ) (NT)	≅2	12	≅7,500	YOSHIMOTO et al. (1970)
$F_{2\alpha}$	37 (NT)	7.8	1.5	1.0	5.0 (AD)	3	1.2	1,850	FLOWER et al. (1973)
E_2	37 (NT)	7.8	0.5	7.0	5.0	3	1.2	2,000	
D_2	37 (NT)	8.2	1.5	2.0	1.0	3	1.2	630	
MDA	37 (NT)	7.8	3.0	0.0	3.0	7	1.2	2,160	
Rabbit kidney $F_{2\alpha}$	37 (NT)	7.5	2.0	2.75	1.5 (AD)	8	4.5	220	BLACKWELL et al. (1975c)
E_2	37 (NT)	7.5	2.0	2.75	1.5	8	4.5	290	
D_2	37 (NT)	7.5	2.0	2.30	1.5	8	4.5	130	

[a] NT = Indicates that the particular reaction conditions used were not necessarily the optimal; no further tests had been made. HQ = Hydroquinone. AD = Adrenaline. NR = Noradrenaline.

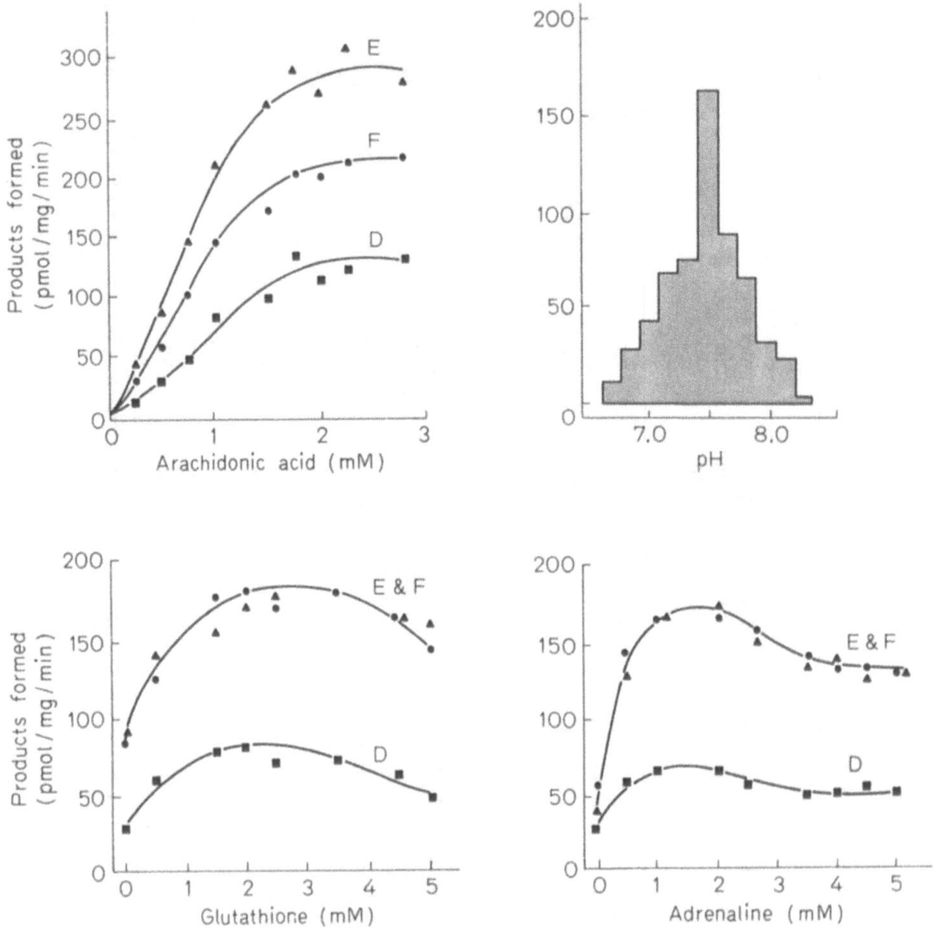

Fig. 13. Biochemical data on the rabbit kidney cyclo-oxygenase

two enzymes was in pH sensitivity. The optimal range for the bovine seminal vesicle enzyme system was between 7.8 and 8.2, and the reaction velocity was within 15% of maximal at any pH between 7.3 and 8.2. The optimal pH range for the rabbit kidney synthetase, however, was very narrow (7.5–7.6) and incubation of the reaction mixture at a pH less than 7.3 or more than 7.7 resulted in a reduction in reaction velocity of almost 45–55%. ROSE and COLLINS (1974) have compared the pH optima of the microsomal synthetase from bovine seminal vesicles and rabbit kidney and found them to be 8.5 and 7.5 respectively. These figures are in substantial agreement with those already quoted although they did not find the same sensitivity of the renal enzyme to pH variations.

Another difference between the two enzyme systems was in the shape and optima of the substrate vs. velocity curves. The optimal substrate concentration for the bovine seminal vesicle synthetase to produce PGE_2 was 0.5 mM, but it was 1.5–2.0 mM for the other products ($PGF_{2\alpha}$, PGD_2, and MDA). At this higher concentration of arachidonic acid, there was pronounced substrate (or product) inhibition of

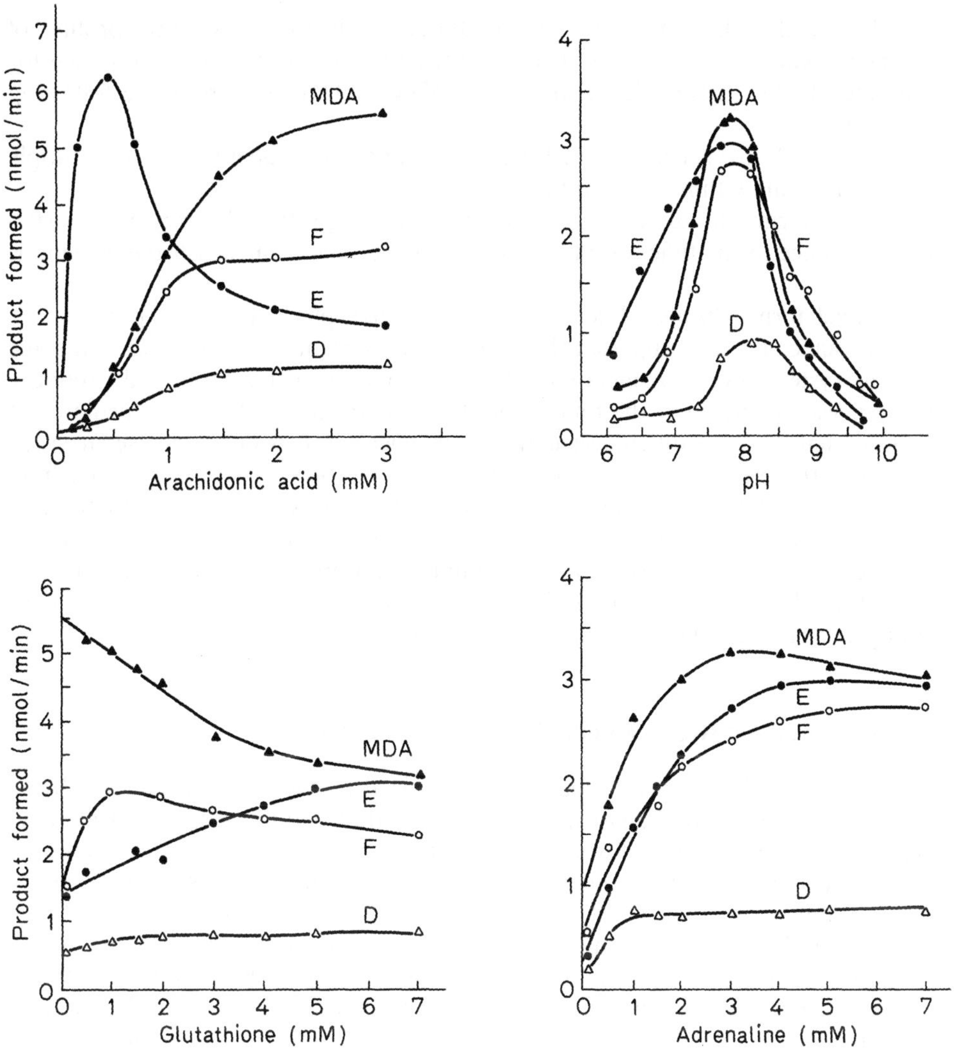

Fig. 14. Biochemical data on the bovine seminal vesicle cyclo-oxygenase

PGE_2 formation. This inhibition was not seen with the rabbit kidney synthetase, which had an optimal arachidonic concentration for all products of about 2 mM.

There were other minor differences between the optimal concentrations of glutathione, adrenaline and microsomal protein required for synthesis in these enzyme preparations, and also in the time for which the reaction was linear. Finally, the substantial differences in cyclizing capacity of the different synthetase systems should be noted; the kidney enzyme had a synthetic capability only one-tenth of that of bovine seminal vesicle enzyme.

Apart from the two enzymes described above, it may be seen that the other synthetase preparations also have different biosynthetic rates; the dog spleen enzyme (FLOWER, 1974b) is some 100-fold less active than the bovine seminal vesicle enzyme, and the bovine thyroid (FRIEDMAN et al., 1975) is some 1000 times less active.

The fact that there do appear to be differences in the biochemical profiles of synthetase enzymes (as well as their suscpetibility to inhibtion by drugs—see for example FLOWER, 1974a) led FLOWER and VANE (1974) to propose the following hypothesis:

1. the cyclo-oxygenase (or at least one component protein) exists in multiple molecular forms within the organism.
2. each form catalyzes a characteristic biochemical profile. This may be of particular relevance to the function of PGs in the tissue type from which the enzyme is derived.
3. Each form exhibits a different and characteristic pharmacological profile.

Of course, it is now apparent that one very important difference is that in some enzyme systems PGG_2 is metabolised mainly to non-prostaglandin end products, but this was unknown at the time. From the experimental data that is available, it appears that there are differences in the biochemical profiles of synthetase enzymes. However, the preparations chiefly investigated have been crude microsomal fractions, and the difficulties attending the careful characterisation of such membrane-bound multienzyme complexes are very great indeed. We shall not really know whether cyclo-oxygenase isoenzymes exist until the properties of solubilised enzymes are fully studied (see RAZ et al., 1975) and shown to be different, or until the component proteins are shown to be electrophoretically distinct.

IV. Turnover and Replacement of the Cyclo-Oxygenase

There is not much evidence germane to this topic at present. LANDS et al. (1973) has shown that the cyclo-oxygenase catalyses its own 'destruction' during substrate oxygenation in vitro. If such 'self-destruction' occurs in vivo then tissues which exhibit a high biosynthetic capacity should demonstrate continuous enzyme synthesis. To test this possibility, BLACKWELL et al. (1975a) treated rats with the protein synthesis inhibitor cycloheximide and measured biosynthetic capacity hourly for up to 7 h afterwards. Even when protein synthesis by the rat kidney tissue had fallen by an order of magnitude, PG biosynthesis had not fallen below control levels. Interestingly, although the activity of the major metabolising enzyme prostaglandin 15-hydroxy-dehydrogenase (PGDH) fell very quickly to about 25% of control levels, implying that although the cyclo-oxygenase enzyme protein was not being continuously synthesised, PGDH was. This observation poses further questions—is the synthetase enzyme really 'used up' under conditions of oxygen tension prevailing in vivo, or is it used up much more slowly than one would predict from the in vitro studies of LANDS and his co-workers.

Blockade of PG synthetase by indomethacin and some other drugs is irreversible (see FLOWER, 1974a for details), and so presumably new enzyme must be synthesised to replace the drug-inactivated molecules; perhaps this might represent a rough guide to the turnover rate of the enzyme in vivo. The data of HAMBERG (1972) suggest that the 'whole body' synthesis of PGs in man is depressed for at least 24 h (and sometimes as much as 48 h) after treatment of therapeutic doses of aspirin, indomethacin or sodium salicylate. This conclusion receives support from the work of HORTON et al. (1973) who measured the 24 h seminal PG content of two subjects before, during and after a 3 day course of aspirin treatment. The semen concentrations of PGE and PGF had returned to control levels within two days of discontinuing treatment, but the concentrations of 19-hydroxy PGA and 19-hydroxy PGB remained below control levels somewhat longer. KOCSIS et al. (1973) measured the time course of platelet PG biosynthesis inhibition following a single dose of aspirin, salicylate or indomethacin. Inhibition achieved by these compounds was variable but occurred within 1 h of oral administration of the drugs. Maximal inhibition by salicylate was maintained for less than 6 h and that of indomethacin for less than 24 h, but the effect of aspirin persisted for 2–3 days. It seems likely that this is the basis for its long-lasting action in platelets. It should be remembered, however, that the circulating platelet is only capable of restricted *de novo* enzyme biosynthesis (STEINER, 1970) and hence may be rather atypical model.

There is at the time of writing no firm evidence that the enzyme is 'inducible' in any way.

V. Miscellaneous Remarks

MARNETT et al. (1974) have observed that sheep vesicular gland microsomes emit chemiluminescence during incubation with polyunsaturated fatty acids. That the enzyme responsible was the cyclo-oxygenase was suggested by the substrate specificity of the reaction (oleic acid was without effect) and the fact that inhibitors such as indomethacin and aspirin (as well as dimercapto-propanol) blocked the effect. However, methyl arachidonate and eicosatetrynoic acid (TYA) (an acetylenic analogue of arachidonic acid) which are not oxidised by the same enzyme also produced chemiluminescence. The luminescence which was quenched by superoxide dismutase and by β-carotene, was found to be proportional to the microsome concentration and showed an initial burst of activity which decayed with a half-life of approximately 30 s. Boiled microsomes were inactive. The authors suggest that perhaps singlet oxygen is the cause of the chemiluminescence.

Another property of sheep vesicular gland cyclo-oxygenase also noted by MARNETT et al. (1975) is that, during the reaction with fatty acids, the enzyme can co-oxygenate other organic substrates. Luminol, 1,3-diphenyl-isobenzofuran and benzopyrene were oxygenated by the microsomal fraction in the presence of arachidonic acid or PGG_2 but not PGH_2. The former reaction, but not the latter, was inhibited by indomethacin and 2,3-dimercaptopropanol. This co-oxygenation was also blocked by GSH. The authors speculate that the effect arises by interaction of the organic substrates with the hydroperoxy intermediates of PG biosynthesis. At least one anti-inflammatory drug, oxyphenbutazone, is also co-oxygenated by PG synthetase (PORTOGHESE et al., 1975), a finding which may possibly have some relevance to the mode of action of some of these compounds.

LANDS and his colleagues, who have contributed significantly to the enzymology of the cyclo-oxygenase including the formulation of the kinetics (SMITH and LANDS, 1972), have reported that there are two types of fatty acid dioxygenase present in acetone powders of sheep vesicular glands. One type of activity named E_a could be distinguished by a requirement for phenol activation and the fact that it was suppressed by the enzyme glutathione peroxidase, evidence suggesting that a hydroperoxide was an obligatory intermediate. Another (slower) type of activity named E_b

was found in non-phenol-stimulated acetone powders and was not blocked by GSH peroxidase. Both types of activity were inactivated by the presence of fatty acid substrate and oxygen, and E_a was also inactivated by the presence of hydroperoxide. The phenol activation was irreversibly blocked by O-phenanthroline, as was the inhibitory action of certain aspirin-like drugs (SMITH and LANDS, 1971). Unfortunately, it is not known whether both E_a and E_b are PG-generating enzymes or not.

Before concluding this section, it is worth reflecting on the work of TAN and his colleagues (1973). Certain similarities between steroidogenesis and PG biosynthesis led these authors to speculate that cytochrome P 450 played a part in PG generation in addition to its well-established role in steroid biosynthesis. Indeed, precursor acids as well as PGs themselves were shown to bind microsomal P 450 particles from beef adrenals, as evidenced by characteristic spectral changes. Aspirin, however, had no effect on the binding of arachidonic acid to the preparation. The relevance of this finding is difficult to assess since the participation of P 450 in PG biosynthesis is by no means established; indeed it seems to be absent in preparations of seminal vesicles (POLLARD and FLOWER, 1973, unpublished observations) which are the most active enzyme sources known.

VI. Summary

The cyclo-oxygenase, although a membrane-bound enzyme, may be solubilised by a variety of detergents and purified to a certain extent thereafter. However, no entirely satisfactory methods for purification have yet been published. The enzyme seems to require GSH and a phenolic co-factor, although high concentrations of the latter are definitely inhibitory. Notwithstanding the difficulties inherent in the examination of such a membrane-bound multienzyme complex, or with the interpretation of the results, various attempts have been made to suggest differences in enzymes isolated from different anatomical sources. No reliable data are available concerning the turnover or replacement of the enzyme. Whilst catalysing the production of PGs, the enzyme also appears to co-oxygenate certain organic substrates and to chemiluminesce. Evidence suggests that there is more than one type of fatty acid oxygenase in seminal vesicle preparations.

I. Turnover of Prostaglandins

PGs are rapidly metabolised in vivo and it is impossible to obtain accurate figures for the daily PG turnover in man or animals simply by measuring PG levels in the peripheral blood. Reliable estimates of peripheral PG levels in man (obtained by radioimmunoassay) indicate concentrations of <50 pg/ml for E type PGs and <10 pg/ml for $PGF_{2\alpha}$ (DRAY and CHARBONNEL, 1974). An alternative approach is to measure the peripheral blood concentrations of the 13,14-dihydro-15-keto metabolites (see succeeding sections) (SAMUELSSON and GRÉEN, 1974; GRÉEN et al., 1974); even this metabolite, however, has a short life within the circulation (HAMBERG and SAMUELSSON, 1971). The problem has been resolved by monitoring the daily output of the major urinary metabolites of PGs. This has been carried out in two ways: by measuring the output of specific E_1 and E_2 or $F_{1\alpha}$ and $F_{2\alpha}$ metabolites and by

Table 7. Daily turnover of prostaglandins estimated from urinary metabolites

Species	Metabolite monitored	Excretion (μg/24 h)	Estimated[a] daily turnover (μg/24 h)	Reference
Human ♀	E_1+E_2	7.0	23– 48	HAMBERG and SAMUELSSON (1971)
♂		16–27	109–226	
Human ♀	E_1+E_2	2.5– 5.3	20– 40	HAMBERG (1972)
♂		6.5–46.7	50–330	
Human ♀	$F_{1\alpha}+F_{2\alpha}$	7.6–13.6	40– 60	HAMBERG (1973b)
♂		10.8–59.0	40–230	
Guinea pig ♂	E_1+E_2	1.34–2.74/kg	5– 10/kg	HAMBERG and SAMUELSSON (1972)
Rat ♀	E_1+E_2	2.16–3.93	10– 20/kg	GRÉEN and SAMUELSSON (1972)
♂		2.04–2.3		
Human ♂ or ♀	Tetranor-prostane skeleton	300.0	1000–2000	NUGTEREN (1975b)

[a] Corrected factor based on conversion of injected radioactive PGs, and efficiency of extraction etc.

determining the total output of substances yielding a tetranorprostane derivative after metabolism, i.e. the sum total of E_1, E_2, $F_{1\alpha}$ and $F_{2\alpha}$ (and D_1, D_2, A_1, A_2, B_1, B_2?).

Using the former approach, HAMBERG and SAMUELSSON (see references in Table 7) have estimated the daily turnover of E_1 and E_2 and $F_{1\alpha}$ and $F_{2\alpha}$ in the human male and female (see Table 7). A very interesting finding was the sex difference—males excreted as much as 16 times more metabolite than females. The origin of this sex difference is still unknown but could perhaps be related to the very large amounts of PGs found in male accessory sex glands. NUGTEREN (1975b) measured the total output of substances giving rise to tetranorprostane derivatives after reduction with borohydride and treatment with hydrogen iodide and zinc in methanolic HC1. He found a much greater excretion rate (1–2 mg/day) than could be accounted for by the sum total of E and F type prostaglandin output in males (max. 0.56 mg) as measured by the Swedish group, and furthermore no sex difference was observed. These findings imply that there are at least 2–4 times as many other PG metabolites as those represented by E- or F-type PGs. Perhaps they are derived from the endoperoxides themselves or from some as yet uncharacterised synthetic pathway. Assuming that an 'average' male weights 70 kg, one can calculate the 'average' human daily production rates (per kg) as follows: E-type PGs, 2.7 μg/kg, F-type PGs 1.9 μg/kg (total tetranorprostane derivatives, 214 μg/kg). These figures are low when compared with the corresponding rates in the guinea pig (5–10 μg/kg) and rat (10–20 μg/kg) (see Table 7). Compared with the average human daily production rates of other potential inflammatory mediators, such as 5-HT (114.3 μg/kg; RUTHVEN and SANDLER, 1966) and histamine (85.7 μg/kg; VARLEY, 1967), the output of PGs seems extremely low. However, the E-type PG metabolite excretion rate may be increased in the rat by cold stress (GRÉEN and SAMUELSSON, 1971) and in the guinea pig following scalding injury (HAMBERG and JONSSON, 1973) and an increase in the excretion rate of the

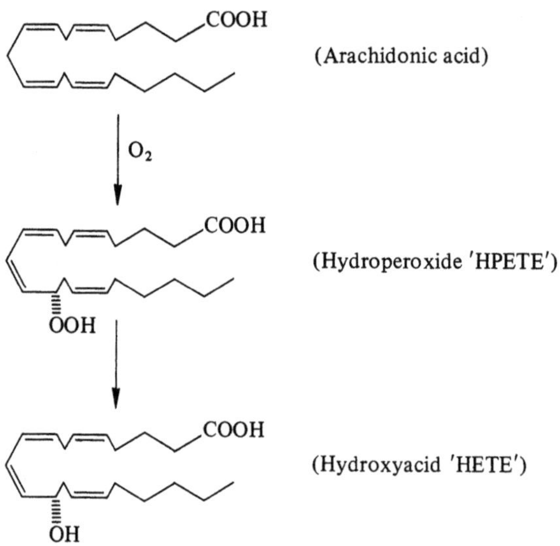

Fig. 15. Transformation by the lipoxygenase of arachidonic acid to HPETE and its subsequent reduction to HETE

F-type metabolite was observed following anaphylaxis in the guinea pig (STRANDBERG and HAMBERG, 1974), as well as pregnancy in the human (HAMBERG, 1974). As one might predict, several non-steroidal anti-inflammatory drugs block the output of urinary metabolites in man (HAMBERG, 1972) as well as guinea pig (HAMBERG and SAMUELSSON, 1972; STRANDBERG and HAMBERG, 1974).

J. Lipoxygenase

Despite extensive literature on lipid peroxidation and the identification of several plant lipoxygenases (see review by TAPPEL, 1963), the existence in mammalian tissues of enzymes catalysing the oxidation (by molecular oxygen) of polyunsaturated fatty acids to the corresponding hydroperoxides per se was only demonstrated recently (HAMBERG and SAMUELSSON, 1974a, 1974b; HAMBERG et al., 1974c; NUGTEREN, 1975a); indeed some early workers claimed that this type of enzyme was not present in mammalian cells (TAPPEL, 1953; BOYD and ADAMS, 1955).

Because of its recent discovery, no really detailed studies of this enzyme have yet been published and the brief account of the chemistry, enzymology and pharmacology of mammalian lipoxygenase which follows should be read with this fact in mind.

I. Distribution of the Enzyme

Initially, the presence of the lipoxygenase enzyme was reported in human platelets (HAMBERG and SAMUELSSON, 1974a; HAMBERG et al., 1974c) and in guinea pig lung (HAMBERG and SAMUELSSON, 1974b). In a later paper, NUGTEREN (1975a) reported the existence of lipoxygenase in platelets from horse, cow, pig, sheep and man. The enzyme was also found in lung and spleen but the presence of lipoxygenase activity in these tissues may have been due to their platelet content. At the time of writing, this point has not been adequately clarified. The product of the lipoxygenase (HETE) has, however, been identified in another tissue, psoriatic epidermis (HAMMARSTRÖM et al., 1975).

II. Nature and Location of the Enzyme

It was not clear from the initial reports of HAMBERG and SAMUELSSON (1974a, 1974b) whether the enzyme was cytoplasmic or particulate in nature like the cyclo-oxygenase. NUGTEREN (1975a), however, demonstrated that the enzyme resisted sedimentation at 100000 × *g* and was thus associated with the supernatant cytoplasmic fraction of cells, implying that it was either soluble or bound to very light particles; cyclo-oxygenase activity in these experiments sedimented at 100000 × *g*.

III. Chemical Transformations Catalysed

The enzyme catalyses the oxidation of certain polyunsaturated fatty acids by molecular oxygen. The reaction of arachidonate is used as an example (see Fig. 15).

IV. Formation of HPETE (Hydroperoxy Acid)

Using an ammonium sulphate (35% saturation) fraction of platelet 100000 × *g* supernatant, NUGTEREN (1975a) found that the 12-L-hydroperoxy derivative of arachidonic acid was formed. The corresponding hydroxy acid was also formed but more slowly. SAMUELSSON's group have named this hydroperoxy acid 'HPETE' (12-L-hydroperoxy-5,8,10,14-eicosatetraenoic acid). It can be isolated from broken platelet homogenates but was not found when intact platelets or lungs were used, presumably because of reduction to the corresponding hydroxy acid 'HETE' (12-L-hydroxy-5,8,10,14-eicosatetraenoic acid).

V. Formation of HETE (Hydroxy Acid)

Not much information is available on the transformation of HPETE into HETE. The fact that HPETE predominates in 100000 *g* supernatants or semipurified preparations, whereas only HETE is seen in intact cells, suggests the existence of a reductase enzyme located in some other cellular compartment — perhaps the membrane fraction.

VI. Enzymology of the Lipoxygenase

Using a semipurified preparation of bovine platelets, NUGTEREN (1975a) learnt that the pH optimum of the enzyme lay between 8 and 9 and that the enzyme had rather poor stability. Although the methyl ester of arachidonate was also slowly peroxidised (rate 14% of the free acid), this apparently occurred only after hydrolysis. As far as substrate specificity was concerned, arachidonic acid appeared to be the best substrate for the bovine enzyme but several other polyunsaturated fatty acids having two *cis* double bonds at the 8- or 11 position (ω-9, ω-12) were also converted to their

12-L-hydroperoxy derivatives. Fatty acids containing 18 or 22 carbons were also converted. Oxygen insertion by the mammalian lipoxygenase occurrs at C-12 (ω-9). This is in contrast to the plant lipoxygenases which have a ω-6 or ω-9 specificity (HAMBERG et al., 1974a).

An interesting case was reported recently by MALMSTEN et al. (1975). He discovered a subject who had a mild haemostatic defect and was deficient in platelet cyclo-oxygenase; platelet lipoxygenase activity was, however, normal.

K. Prostaglandin Inactivation

In addition to biosynthetic enzymes, the organism possesses extremely efficient mechanisms for the catabolism of PGs and hence their biological inactivation. The efficiency of certain vascular beds — for example, the lung—in inactivating PGs is well illustrated by the observations of FERREIRA and VANE (1967), who found that more than 95% of infused PGE_2 was inactivated during one circulation through the lungs, and by those of HAMBERG and SAMUELSSON (1971), who showed that only 3% of an intravenous bolus injection of tritiated PGE_2 remained in the plasma after 90 s. After 4.5 min there was no detectable PGE_2 at all.

Tissue or blood concentrations of PGs must therefore be regarded as a net result of the activity of two sorts of enzymes—those which biosynthesise and those which inactivate PGs. If PGs are important in inflammation or other pathological conditions, then it is clear that the activity of the catabolic enzymes could have a crucial effect on the duration and intensity of the inflammatory or other response.

I. Chemistry of Prostaglandin Catabolism

Enzymic mechanisms exist (at least for PGs of the E or F series) whereby the biological activity of the PG molecule is rapidly destroyed, the metabolite being excreted in the urine after successive modifications of the native structure. Broadly speaking, these reactions are of two types: an initial (relatively rapid) step, catalyzed by PG specific enzymes, whereby PGs lose most of their biological activity, and a second (relatively slow) step in which those metabolites are oxidised by enzyme (probably) identical to those responsible for the β- and ω-oxidation of fatty acids in general. This sequence of reactions has been investigated in man (HAMBERG and SAMUELSSON, 1971) and the degradation of PGE_2 is summarised in Figure 16.

The initial step in this degradation is the oxidation of the 15-hydroxyl group to the corresponding ketone under the influence of the enzyme PGDH (ÄNGGÅRD and SAMUELSSON, 1964, 1966; HAMBERG and SAMUELSSON, 1971). The 15-keto compound is then transformed into the 13,14-dihydro compound, a reaction catalyzed by the enzyme prostaglandin Δ^{13} reductase (ÄNGGÅRD and SAMUELSSON, 1964, 1966; ÄNGGÅRD et al., 1971). The first two reactions occur very rapidly, but subsequent steps are probably slow. These consist of oxidation of the β- and ω-side chains of the PGs giving rise to a more polar product (a dicarboxylic acid) which is excreted in the urine as the major metabolite both PGE_1 and PGE_2. The kinetics of these reactions are of interest; in the experiments of HAMBERG and SAMUELSSON (1971) only 31% of an original tritiated PGE_2 injection was present in the blood after 90 s, the bulk of

Name	Structure	Enzyme system	Chief organs in which degradation occurs
PGE_2	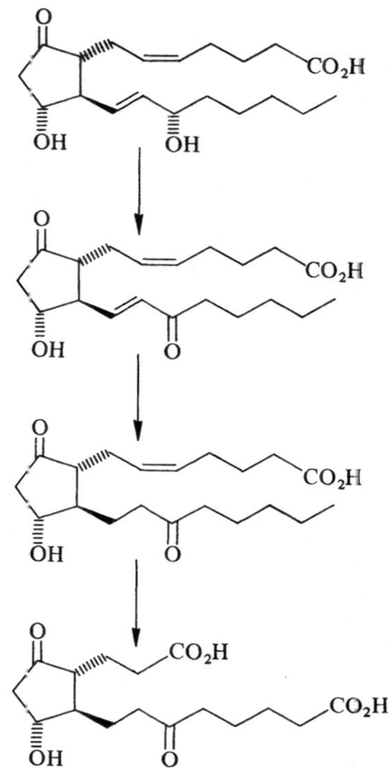		
		15–hydroxy prostaglandin dehydrogenase (PGDH)	Lung, kidney, liver, peripheral vascular beds
15–keto PGE_2			
		Prostaglandin Δ^{13} reductase	Lung, kidney, liver
13,14–dihydro– 15–keto PGE_2			
		β–and ω–Oxidizing systems	Liver
7α–hydroxy–5,11–diketo tetranor prosta 1,16 dioic acid (major urinary metabolite)			

Fig. 16. Metabolism of prostaglandin E_2 in man

the radioactivity in the plasma being present as the 13,14-dihydro-15-keto metabolite; this metabolite itself only had a half-life of some 8 min in the circulation. SAMUELSSON et al. (1971) administered tritiated $PGF_{2\alpha}$ to human subjects and measured the excretion rate of tritium (present mainly as the dioic acid metabolite) into the urine. Approximately 40% was excreted during the first 30 min, almost 80% after 2 h had maximal excretion, about 90% had occurred after 4 h. Similar studies have also been performed in the rat (GRÉEN and SAMUELSSON, 1971; SUN, 1974) and guinea pig (HAMBERG and SAMUELSSON, 1972). In each case, the initial transformations (i.e. oxidation of the C-15 hydroxy group and saturation of the 13,14 double bond) were observed but the final product of the ω- and β-oxidising systems, whilst similar to that in man, was not identical.

II. Tissue Distribution of Catabolising Enzymes

Enzymes which catalyse PG degradation are widely distributed throughout the animal body, being present in the kidney of several species (ÄNGGÅRD and SAMUELSSON, 1966; NISSEN and ANDERSEN, 1968, 1969; NAKANO, 1970a, 1970b; NAKANO and PRANGAN, 1971) and intestine (ÄNGGÅRD and SAMUELSSON, 1966), isolated rat liver and testicle (DAWSON et al., 1968; NAKANO and PRANCAN, 1971; NAKANO et al., 1971), as well as guinea pig lung (ÄNGGÅRD and SAMUELSSON, 1964). ÄNGGÅRD et al. (1971) studied the distribution of PGDH and PG-Δ^{13} reductase in swine tissue and found that both of the enzymes were located in the 100000 g supernatant of cell-free homogenates. The tissues with the highest PGDH activity were the lung, spleen and kidney. The highest reductase activity was found in the spleen, liver, kidney, adrenals and small intestine. The highest activity of PGDH per g of tissue, however, was found in adipose tissue.

The enzymes responsible for β- or ω-oxidation are found in the liver (SAMUELSSON, 1970; SAMUELSSON et al., 1971), in lung and kidney (NAKANO and MORSY, 1971) and intestine (PARKINSON and SCHNEIDER, 1969). The liver is probably the major site of side chain oxidation.

The lungs are a rich source of both the PGDH and the Δ^{13} reductase enzyme. Because of the reduction of biological activity, which is a consequence of metabolism, as well as the unique position of the lungs between venous and arterial circulation, the pulmonary circulation constitutes an important barrier through which PGs which have potent smooth muscle stimulating, cardiovascular or other actions cannot pass and are thus prevented from reaching target organs via the arterial circulation.

The significance of the pulmonary vascular bed as sites of PG inactivation in vivo was first demonstrated by FERREIRA and VANE (1967). Although stable in blood, greater than 95% of infused PGE_1 or PGE_2 (0.5–1 μg/min) were removed during one passage through cat lungs, as determined by bioassay. Similar effects were observed when the experiment was repeated in dogs and rabbits. Other vascular beds such as those of liver and hind quarters also inactivated PGs although not so effectively. The same year, MCGIFF et al. (1967), using changes in dog renal blood flow as an index of PG concentration in the arterial blood, confirmed that PGE_1 and PGE_2 were rapidly inactivated by the lung, whereas PGA_1 and PGA_2 were not. This finding was in qualitative if not quantitative agreement with the kinetic data obtained in vitro

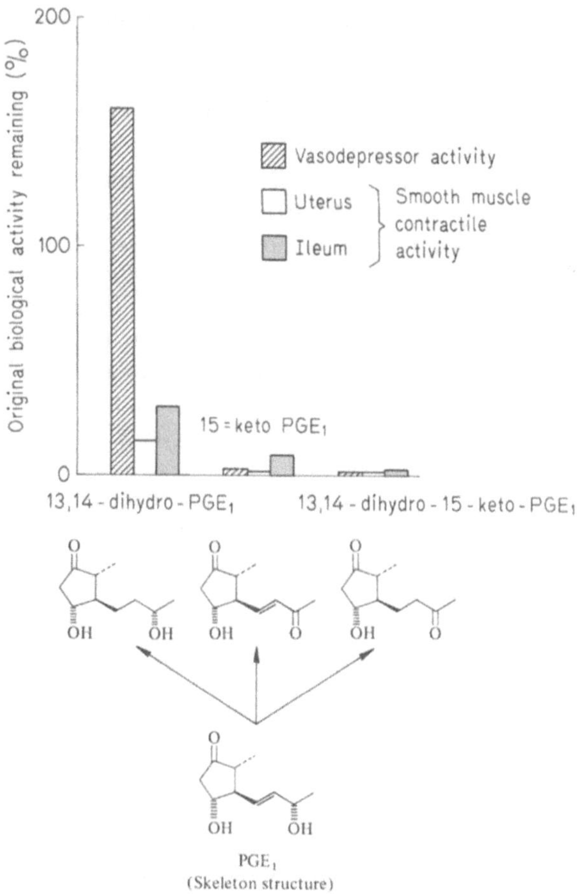

Fig. 17. Loss of vasodepressor and smooth muscle contracting activity (guinea pig), after metabolic transformation. This information is based on data published by Änggård (1966). Biological activity was assayed in the guinea pig

(Änggård and Samuelsson, 1966). The authors thus speculated that the A-series are the only PGs likely to act as circulating hormones. Horton and Jones (1969) have confirmed that a single passage through the pulmonary circulation of the cat or dog causes substantial losses of the vasodilator activity of PGE_1 but not of PGA_1. Perfused lungs in vitro can also inactivate PGs, an effect which seems to be due to the action of PGDH (Piper et al., 1970).

PGDH is apparently quite a short lived enzyme within the cell, the replacement of which depends on continual protein synthesis (Blackwell et al., 1975b). The levels of enzyme in the lung and kidney of rats or rabbits are dependent on the age of the animal (Pace-Asciak and Miller, 1973) and may alter during pregnancy or treatment with steroids (Sun and Armour, 1974; Bedwani and Marley, 1974; Blackwell and Flower, 1976a).

Because PGs possess extremely potent pharmacological activity, an important consideration is the stage of the metabolic sequence at which this loss occurs;

ÄNGGÅRD and SAMUELSSON (1967) and ÄNGGÅRD (1966) synthesised the 13,14-dihydro-PGE_1, 15-keto-PGE_1 and 15-keto-13,14-dihydro-PGE_1 and compared the biological activity (smooth muscle contractile and vasodepressor effects in the guinea pig and rabbit) with that of the parent molecule. Figure 17 shows the loss of biological activity in the guinea pig which occurs on successive modifications of the PGE_1 molecule. After saturation of the 13,14 double bond the molecule still retains a significant proportion of its biological activity, indeed, the vasodepressor effect is somewhat greater. Biological activity is, however, greatly attenuated when the 15-hydroxyl group is oxidized, and virtually disappears when both modifications are introduced. Qualitatively similar results were seen when the metabolites were tested for smooth muscle contractile and vasodepressor activity in the rabbit. NAKANO (1971) reported that the vasodilator actions of 13,14-dihydro-E_1, 15-keto-E_1 and 15-keto-13,14-dihydro-PGE_1 were approximately $^1/_4$, $^1/_{80}$ and $^1/_{100}$ of PGE_1 in dog hind limb preparations. As inhibitors of platelet aggregation, KLOEZE (1969) found that the 13,14-dihydro derivative of PGE_1 had an activity of 0.64 relative to the parent molecule and that the 15-keto compound was inactive. The 15-keto derivative of PGE_2 was likewise inactive as an inducer of platelet aggregation. 15-keto-13,14-dihydro-$PGE_{2\alpha}$ has been shown by PIKE et al. (1967) to have little spasmogenic activity on many smooth muscle preparations. 15-keto-$PGF_{2\alpha}$, however, has up to ten times the contractile activity of the parent molecule on smooth muscle preparations including human bronchial muscle and guinea pig trachea (DAWSON et al., 1974) and is also a more potent pressor agent (JONES, 1975).

III. Other Metabolic Transformations

Various other metabolic transformations of PGE have been reported. In some tissues PGE may be transformed by a '9-keto reductase' to $PGF_{2\alpha}$. LESLIE and LEVINE (1973) investigated the distribution of this enzyme in the tissues of the rat; the heart was found to contain the highest specific activity followed by the kidney, brain, liver and adrenal tissue. None was found in striated muscle, spleen or ileum. Although present in rat lung, no 9-keto reductase activity was detectable in guinea pig lung homogenates.

L. Metabolism of Other Compounds

At the time of writing, nothing is known concerning the catabolism or ultimate metabolic fate of HETE or TXB_2. Presumably, however, if the metabolic degradation could be elucidated and a urinary excretion product identified, then this could form the basis for techniques to assay whole body excretion of these potentially interesting substances.

M. Inhibition of Substrate Release From Phospholipids

From the discussion in Section D, inhibition of phospholipase enzymes would be a useful alternative means of preventing the formation of PGs and other cyclo-oxygenase products. This is a line of thought which has been somewhat neglected. The

Table 8. Inhibition of phospholipid breakdown by mepacrine

Treatment	p mol %			
	Phospholipids	Arachidonic acid	PGs	Neutral lipids
Control	77.72 (±5.27)	9.73 (±1.65)	2.10 (±0.36)	10.51 (±3.58)
Vibrated	62.35[a] (±1.09)	20.78[c] (±0.66)	5.73[b] (±0.11)	11.164 (±1.29)
Vibrated + 1 mM mepacrine	73.63 (±1.78)	14.74[b] (±0.66)	2.43 (±0.17)	9.79 (±1.19)

[a] $p<0.05$.
[b] $p<0.01$.
[c] $p<0.001$.
Data taken from FLOWER and BLACKWELL (1976).

antimalarial drug mepacrine, which possesses weak antiphospholipase activity (but unfortunately some anticyclo-oxygenase activity also), was used by VARGAFTIG and DAO HAI (1972) to provide presumptive evidence that the bradykinin-induced release of 'RCS' from guinea pig perfused lung was mediated by phospholipase A_2 stimulation. This compound was also used in the experiments of FLOWER and BLACKWELL (1976) and BLACKWELL et al. (1976). In the former experiments, mepacrine was found to block the release of labelled arachidonate from the phosphatide fraction of guinea pig spleen slices induced by mechanical vibration (see Table 8) and consequently to reduce PG biosynthesis. In the latter experiments, mepacrine was found to block the aggregation of platelets to collagen but not by arachidonic acid, whereas the cyclo-oxygenase inhibitor indomethacin blocked aggregation by both agents. Analysis of the phospholipid composition of the platelets during this experiment indicated that mepacrine blocked the collagen-induced release of arachidonate from platelet lecithin and phosphatidyl inositol. Indomethacin did not affect this step but did block the cyclo-oxygenase step. Some other drugs inhibit phospholipase A_2; SCHERPHOF et al. (1972) tested a range of procaine type local anaesthetics and found a number of compounds possessed antiphospholipase activity which parallelled their local anaesthetic potency. The drug-induced inhibition was reversed by high calcium concentrations. The descending order of potency (against pancreatic phospholipase A_2) was nupercaine > tetracaine > butacaine > lidocaine > procaine. KUNZE et al. (1974) also tested a series of local anaesthetics against the phospholipase A_2 and the cyclo-oxygenase in bovine seminal vesicles. They found that chlorpromazine, dibucaine and butacaine inhibited PG formation by blocking the cyclo-oxygenase, whereas tetracaine and procaine blocked PG generation by interference with phospholipase A_2 activity. Benzocaine acted only on PG biosynthesis. The phospholipase activity of bovine seminal vesicles was also investigated by LUCKNER and RENZ (1975). The enzyme activity was mainly associated with the microsomal fraction. Although there was a small amount in the mitochondrial fraction, none could be detected in the cytosol. Agents which inhibited the enzyme by >50% included dibutryl-cAMP (2×10^{-9}M), adrenaline (10^{-4}M), noradrenaline (10^{-4}M) and ethanol (10% v/v). PGE_2 and $PGF_{2\alpha}$ exerted 19% and 41% inhibition respectively.

The concept that the generation and release of lipid inflammatory mediators may be suppressed by antiphospholipase drugs has not been investigated in sufficient depth to decide whether or not such a technique offers any hope of success. One can, for example, foresee the potential toxicity of a compound which drastically interferes with such a dynamic process as cell membrane metabolism. However, in this connection, it may be of interest to note that the drug mepacrine—as well as its close relative chloroquine—have been used as an *ad hoc* treatment for rheumatoid arthritis; it is tempting to speculate that their action at least in part may be due to their antiphospholipase activity. Two recent papers (HONG and LEVINE, 1976; NIJKAMP et al., 1976) have proposed that anti-inflammatory corticosteroids may suppress phospholipase activity and thus inhibit the generation of PGs and other products without inhibiting the cyclo-oxygenase itself. If correct, this important idea could partially explain the anti-inflammatory actions of steroids, and could lead to the use of these drugs as pharmacological 'tools' in much the same way as VANE'S (1971) discovery led to the widespread use of aspirin-like drugs to uncover the role of PGs in physiological and pathological events.

N. Inhibition of the Cyclo-Oxygenase

This is fully dealt with in Chapters 19, 30 and 31 by GRYGLEWSKI, SHEN and FERREIRA and VANE, and will not be discussed here.

O. Inhibition of Prostaglandin Inactivation

From the foregoing discussion it is evident that agents which inhibit the metabolising enzymes could well lead to an accumulation of PGs and perhaps an exacerbation of the inflammatory response.

The concept that a specific disease state may be a reflection of diminished PG-metabolising enzyme activity is relatively new. The possibility that PGs are involved in endotoxin shock and that this is secondary to an impaired degradation mechanism has been investigated by NAKANO and PRANCAN (1973); plasma levels of PGs are elevated in endotoxin shock (SCARNES and HARPER, 1972; ANDERSON et al., 1973; KESSLER et al., 1973) and there is evidence that these increased levels of PGs could account for some of the circulatory and other changes which are a feature of this condition (PARRATT and STURGESS, 1974). NAKANO and PRANCAN (1973) investigated the hypothesis that this could be due to impaired metabolism of PGs by the lung and kidney. Eight hours after induction of endotoxin shock in rats, the lungs and kidneys were removed and the metabolism of PGE_2 measured. The capacity of the lungs (and to a lesser extent the kidneys) of these animals to metabolise PGs was greatly impaired. Inhibition of PGDH activity seemed to be caused directly or indirectly by a naturally occurring compound or bacterial endotoxin. Many attempts have, however, been made to inhibit PGDH with synthetic compounds.

NAKANO et al. (1969) found that PGDH isolated from swine lung was noncompetitively inhibited by the synthetic epimer of PGE_1, 15-R-PGE_1 and that the B type PGs (though not substrates) were also noncompetitive inhibitors; dihydro-PGE_1 and 8-iso-PGE_1 were inactive. FRIED et al. (1973) found that several PG analogues were active against a PGDH preparation isolated from human placenta. MARRAZZI and MATSCHINSKY (1972), again using the swine lung enzyme, found that a derivative of $PGF_{1\alpha}$, 7-oxy-$PGF_{1\alpha}$ (oxygen substituted at C-7), had the same V_{max} as the original substrate (but much lower affinity) and various stereoisomers of this derivative (15-epimer, the optical antipode and an analogue with both of these modifications) all showed mixed inhibition of PGDH, as did several fatty acids (arachidonic, linolenic and oleic, and their respective co-enzyme A derivatives). Polyphloretin phosphate (PPP), a high mol wt polymer of phloretin (which antagonises some of the actions of PGs on smooth muscle; see BENNETT, 1975), was also a competitive inhibitor of the enzyme whilst SC19222, (another antagonist, see BENNETT, 1975) was not.

These compounds were inhibitors at the substrate site of the enzyme. With regard to the co-factor site, MARRAZZI and MATSCHINSKY found that certain NAD^+ analogues or derivatives were inhibitory and a range of substituted pyridines were non-competitive inhibitors. Several nucleosides and nucleotides in concentrations of 3–10 mM were also active, as were the methylxanthines, caffeine and theophylline as well as aminophylline.

The aspirin-like drugs are inhibitors of PG biosynthesis, but it has been subsequently found that indomethacin inhibits the NAD^+ dependent destruction of E_1 or E_2 by the high speed supernatant of dog spleen (FLOWER, 1974a; PACE-ASCIAK and COLE, 1975), as well as the 13,14 reductase enzyme and 9-keto reductase and PGDH of rat kidney homogenates. CHEUNG and CUSHMAN (1972, unpublished observations) found that some other aspirin-like drugs also inhibited the rabbit lung dehydrogenase. Indomethacin in concentrations of 1 mM gave a 93% inhibition of PGE_2 metabolism, niflumic acid in a concentration of 0.5 mM inhibited 38% and meclofenamic acid in the same concentration inhibited 14%. Aspirin, naproxen, ibuprofen, phenylbutazone and benzydamine were inactive. According to HANSEN (1974) purified bovine lung PGDH is inhibited by both indomethacin and aspirin. Indomethacin inhibition was non-competitive.

It is not known how aspirin-like drugs inhibit PGDH. However, the salicylates are known to inhibit several dehydrogenases (SMITH and DAWKINS, 1971), probably by competing for the co-factor site, so a similar action could account for the inhibition of PGDH. The limited data available suggest that the concentrations required to inhibit the synthetase are considerably less than those which produce a corresponding inhibition of the dehydrogenase.

CRUTCHLEY and PIPER (1974) performed parallel investigations on inhibition of pulmonary inactivation of PGs by guinea pig isolated lungs, and inhibition of PG metabolism by crude guinea pig lung homogenates. Polyphloretin phosphate, as well as diphloretin phosphate, in doses of 0.1–5 μg/ml of the perfusing fluid inhibited the inactivation of PGE_2, and $PGF_{2\alpha}$ and therefore increased the amount of PGs surviving passage through the lungs. A number of metabolic inhibitors and sulphhydryl binding reagents were also tested; 2,4 dinitrophenol was inactive at doses of 0.5 mM; iodoacetate was inactive at 0.25 mM but showed weak activity (about 10%) at 0.5 mM. 2:3; dimercaptopropanol was inactive at doses of 3 mM and disulfiram showed no significant inhibition at 6 μM. Two sulphhydryl binding agents (sodium p-chloromercuri-phenylsulphonate and N-ethylmaleimide) were, however, active, having ID_{50}'s of 0.6 mM and 70 μM respectively. Both these agents were also active against the crude enzyme preparation. The same authors also tried some anti-inflammatory agents: phenylbutazone (50 μg/ml) and indomethacin (20 μg/ml) showed slight activity (a reduction of 40% and 10% respectively) but aspirin, paracetamol, ibuprofen and meclofenamic acid were inactive.

In a later paper, the same authors (CRUTCHLEY and PIPER, 1975) investigated the actions of one of these agents diphloretin phosphate, in the rabbit in vivo. By infusing PGE_2 and $PGF_{2\alpha}$ into the superior vena cava and comparing the response with that of an infusion into the aorta, a measure of pulmonary inactivation was obtained. DPP potentiated 25–100 times the depressor effects of the PGs and also the effects on gastrointestinal motility as measured by a balloon in the jejunum.

ANDERSON and ELING (1976) have suggested an interesting alternative explanation for the inhibition of lung metabolism in vivo. Presenting evidence for a PG transport system in rat lungs, they postulate that some drugs could inhibit metabolism by blocking uptake of PGs into those pulmonary cells which are responsible for their degradation.

Two diuretic agents (frusemide and ethacrynic acid) have also been shown to inhibit PGDH (PAULSRUD et al., 1974). Table 9 shows the effect of five drugs including the two diuretic agents on a PGDH preparation from rat kidney (BLACKWELL and FLOWER, 1976b).

P. Inhibition of Lipoxygenase

At the time of writing there is virtually no data available on the inhibition of the lipoxygenase beyond that which was originally published by HAMBERG and SAMUELSSON (1974a). They demonstrated that aspirin and indomethacin, which produced a good block of platelet cyclo-oxygenase, failed to inhibit platelet lipoxygenase even at doses of 100 μg/ml; thus one would not anticipate a block of this enzyme at therapeutic doses of these drugs. The acetylenic arachidonic acid analogue TYA, however, produced 70% inhibition in concentrations of 3 μg/ml. A potentially fruitful line of investigation might be to test other substrate analogues (such as those found to inhibit soyabean lipoxygenase, DOWNING et al., 1972) for inhibitory activity against the lipoxygenase. A selective inhibitor of the platelet lipoxygenase could be useful in delineating the role (if any) of HETE in platelet aggregation.

Q. Summary

The biochemistry and pharmacology of the products formed from polyunsaturated fatty acids is far from complete, but in summary we can say that the following sequence occurs is tissue or migrating cells during the inflammatory response. Fatty acids are released from the membranous fractions of cells (under the influence of phospholipase A_2) either directly or indirectly by the inflammatory agent. This substrate is rapidly transformed by a membrane bound cyclo-oxygenase into PGs, which may have a proinflammatory, hyperalgesic, febrile or bronchoconstrictor action—or to TXA_2 which is a potent platelet aggregating agent. Other compounds such as MDA or HHT generated by the cyclo-oxygenase may also have toxic effects on cells. A second transformation of unsaturated fatty acids can occur which is catalysed by an enzyme in the cell cytoplasm. This enzyme generates lipid peroxides, at least one of which has a potent stimulating effect on cell migration. The duration

Table 9. Inhibition of rat kidney PGDH

Group	p mol F_2 oxidised	% Inhibition
Control	35.13 (±1.83)	—
Frusemide	5.47 (±0.64)	84.44 (±1.82)
Ethacrynic acid	16.88 (±0.49)	51.95 (±1.39)
N-ethyl maleimide	34.58 (±1.89)	1.57 (±5.40)
Indomethacin	8.74 (±0.45)	75.13 (±1.37)
DPP	3.44 (±0.96)	90.24 (±2.74)

Data taken from BLACKWELL and FLOWER (1976b).

of action of the PGs is limited by the local levels of metabolising enzymes and the duration of action of TXA_2 is limited by its inherent lability. The metabolism of other compounds is unknown at present. Pharmacological intervention can occur at the level of the phospholipase, at the level of the cyclo-oxygenase, lipoxygenase, or (in theory at least) at the appropriate endoperoxide isomerases. Pharmacological block of tissue metabolising enzymes may exacerbate the inflammatory response by prolonging the action of PGs.

References

Aas, K. A., Gardner, F. H.: Survival of blood platelets with chromium[51]. J. clin. Invest. **37**, 1232—1257 (1958)

Ahern, D. G., Downing, D. T.: Inhibition of prostaglandin biosynthesis by eicosa-5,8,11,14-tetraynoic acid. Biochim. biophys. Acta **210**, 456—461 (1970)

Anderson, F. L., Jubiz, W., Kralios, A. C., Tsagaris, T. G.: Plasma prostaglandin E levels during endotoxin shock in dogs. Clin. Res. **21**, 194 (1973)

Anderson, M. W., Eling, T. E.: Prostaglandin removal and metabolism by isolated perfused rat lung. Prostaglandins **11**, 645—677 (1976)

Änggård, E.: The biological activities of three metabolites of prostaglandin E_1. Acta physiol. scand. **66**, 509—510 (1966)

Änggård, E., Larsson, C., Samuelsson, B.: The distribution of 15-hydroxyprostaglandin dehydrogenase and prostaglandin Δ^{13} reductase in tissues of the swine. Acta Physiol. Scand. **81**, 396—404 (1971)

Änggård, E., Samuelsson, B.: Prostaglandins and related factors. 28. Metabolism of prostaglandin E_1 in guinea pig lung: the structures of two metabolites. J. biol. Chem. **239**, 4087—4102 (1964)

Änggård, E., Samuelsson, B.: Biosynthesis of prostaglandins from arachidonic acid in guinea pig lung. Prostaglandins and related factors 38. J. biol. Chem. **240**, 3518—3521 (1965)

Änggård, E., Samuelsson, B.: Purification and properties of a 15-hydroxy prostaglandin dehydrogenase from swine lung. Prostaglandins and related factors 55. Ark. kemi **25**, 293—300 (1966)

Änggård, E., Samuelsson, B.: The metabolism of prostaglandins in lung tissue. In: Nobel Symposium 2, Prostaglandins, pp. 97—105. New York: Interscience 1967

Audet, A., Nantel, G., Proulx, P.: Phospholipase A activity in growing *Escherichia coli* cells. Biochim. biophys. Acta **348**, 334—343 (1974)

Bartels, J., Kunze, H., Vogt, W., Wille, G.: Prostaglandin: liberation from and formation in perfused frog intestine. Naunyn-Schmiedebergs Arch. Pharmacol. **266**, 199—207 (1970)

Bedwani, J. R., Marley, P. B.: Increased inactivation of prostaglandin E_2 by the rabbit lung during pregnancy. Brit. J. Pharmacol. **50**, 459P (1974)

Bennet, A.: Prostaglandin antagonists. Advanc. Drug Res. London: Academic Press (1975)
Bennett, A., Friedman, C. A., Vane, J. R.: Release of Prostaglandin E_1 from the rat stomach. Nature (Lond.) **216**, 873—876 (1967)
Bennett, J., Glavenovich, J., Liskay, R., Wulff, D. L., Cronan Jr., J. E.: Phospholipid hydrolysis in *Escherichia coli* infected with rapid lysis mutants of phage T_4. Virology **43**, 516—518 (1971)
Bergström, S., Danielsson, H., Klenberg, D., Samuelsson, B.: The enzymatic conversion of essential fatty acids into prostaglandins. J. biol. Chem. **239**, PC 4006 (1964a)
Bergström, S., Danielsson, H., Samuelsson, B.: The enzymatic formation of prostaglandin E_2 from arachidonic acid. Prostaglandins and related factors. 32. Biochim. biophys. Acta **90**, 207—210 (1964b)
Blackwell, G. J., Duncombe, W. G., Flower, R. J., Parsons, M. F., Vane, J. R.: The distribution and metabolism of arachidonic acid in rabbit platelets during aggregation and its modification by drugs (1976). Brit. J. Pharmacol. **59**, 353—366 (1977)
Blackwell, G. J., Flower, R. J.: Effects of steroid hormones on tissue levels of prostaglandin 15-hydroxydehydrogenase in the rat. Brit. J. Pharmacol. **56**, 343P (1976a)
Blackwell, G. J., Flower, R. J.: A rapid method for the estimation of prostaglandin 15-hydroxydehydrogenase activity and its application to pharmacology. Brit. J. Pharmacol. **57**, 589—598 (1976b)
Blackwell, G. J., Flower, R. J., Parsons, M. F., Vane, J. R.: Factors influencing the metabolic turnover of prostaglandin synthetase. Brit. J. Pharmacol. **53**, 467P (1975a)
Blackwell, G. J., Flower, R. J., Vane, J. R.: Rapid reduction of prostaglandin 15-hydroxy dehydrogenase activity in rat tissues after treatment with protein synthesis inhibitors. Brit. J. Pharmacol. **55**, 233—238 (1975b)
Blackwell, G. J., Flower, R. J., Vane, J. R.: Some characteristics of the prostaglandin synthesizing system in rabbit kidney microsomes. Biochim. biophys. Acta **398**, 178—190 (1975c)
Bohman, S. O., Larsson, C. A.: Prostaglandin synthesis in membrane fractions from the rabbit renal medulla. Acta physiol. scand. **94**, 244—258 (1975)
Boyd, D. H. J., Adams, G. A.: An assay method for lipoxidase in animal tissue. Canad. J. Biochem. **33**, 191—198 (1955)
Chan, J. A., Nagasawa, N., Takeguchi, C., Sih, C. J.: On agents favouring prostaglandin F formation during biosynthesis. Biochemistry **14**, 2987—2991 (1975)
Chasalow, F. I., Phariss, B. B.: Luteinizing hormone stimulation of ovarian prostaglandin biosynthesis. Prostaglandins **1**, 107—117 (1972)
Christ, E. J., Dorp, D. A. van: Comparative aspects of prostaglandin biosynthesis in animal tissues. Biochim. biophys. Acta **270**, 537—545 (1972)
Christ, E. J., Dorp, D. A. van: Comparative aspects of prostaglandin biosynthesis in animal tissue. In: Supplementum to Advances in the Biosciences. International Conference on Prostaglandins, Vienna, pp. 35—38. Braunschweig: Vieweg-Pergamon Press 1973
Coceani, F., Pace-Asciak, C., Volta, F., Wolfe, L. S.: Effect of nerve stimulation on prostaglandin formation and release from the rat stomach. Amer. J. Physiol. **213**, 1056—1064 (1967)
Cook, H. W., Lands, W. E. M.: Evidence for an activating factor formed during prostaglandin biosynthesis. Biochem. biophys. Res. Commun. **65**, 464—471 (1975)
Crutchley, D. J., Piper, P. J.: Prostaglandin inactivation in guinea pig lung and its inhibition. Brit. J. Pharmacol. **52**, 197—203 (1974)
Crutchley, D. J., Piper, P. J.: Inhibition of the pulmonary inactivation of prostaglandins in rabbit in vivo. Brit. J. Pharmacol. **53**, 467 P (1975)
Dahle, I. K., Hill, E. G., Holman, R. T.: The thiobarbituric acid reaction and the auto-oxidation of polyunsaturated fatty acid methyl esters. Arch. Biochem. **98**, 253—261 (1962)
Daniels, E. G., Krueger, W. C., Kupiecki, F. P., Pike, J. E., Schneider, W. P.: Isolation and characterization of a new prostaglandin isomer. J. Amer. chem. Soc. **90**, 5894—5895 (1968)
Danon, A., Heimberg, M., Oates, J. A.: Enrichment of rat tissue lipids with fatty acids that are prostaglandin precursors. Biochim. biophys. Acta **388**, 318—330 (1975)
Dawson, W., Lewis, R. L., Macmahon, R. E., Sweatman, W. J. F.: Potent bronchconstrictor activity of 15-keto prostaglandin $F_{2\alpha}$. Nature (Lond.) **250**, 331—332 (1974)
Dawson, W., Ramwell, P. W., Shaw, J.: Metabolism of prostaglandins by rat isolated liver. Brit. J. Pharmacol. **34**, 668—669 (1968)
Dorp, D. A. van: Aspects of the biosynthesis of prostaglandins. Progr. biochem. Pharmacol. **3**, 71—82 (1967)

Dorp, D. A. van, Beerthuis, R. K., Nugteren, D. H., Vonkeman, H.: Enzymatic conversion of all-*cis*-polyunsaturated fatty acids into prostaglandins. Nature (Lond.) **203**, 839—843 (1964a)
Dorp, D. A. van, Beerthuis, R. K., Nugteren, D. H., Vonkeman, H.: The biosynthesis of prostaglandins. Biochim. biophys. Acta **90**, 204—207 1964b
Downing, D. T., Barve, J. A., Gunstone, F. D., Jacobsberg, M., Lie, K. J.: Structural requirements of acetylenic fatty acids for inhibition of soyabean lipoxygenase and prostaglandin synthetase. Biochim. biophys. Acta **280**, 343—347 (1972)
Dray, F., Charbonnel, B.: Letter to the editor. Radioimmunoassay of PGF_α in human plasma: very low levels. Prostaglandins **5**, 173—174 (1974)
Ferreira, S. H., Vane, J. R.: Prostaglandins: their disappearance from and release into the circulation. Nature (Lond.) **216**, 868—873 (1967)
Ferreira, S. H., Vane, J. R.: Aspirin and prostaglandins. In: The Prostaglandins, Vol. II, pp. 1—34. New York: Plenum Press 1974
Flower, R. J.: Drugs which inhibit prostaglandin biosynthesis. Pharmacol. Rev. **26**, 33—67 (1974a)
Flower, R. J.: Prostaglandin synthetase and its inhibition by aspirin-like drugs. Ph.D. Thesis, London University (1974b)
Flower, R. J., Blackwell, G. J.: The importance of phospholipase A_2 in prostaglandin biosynthesis. Biochem. Pharmacol. **25**, 285—291 (1976)
Flower, R. J., Cheung, H. S., Cushman, D. W.: Quantitative determination of prostaglandins and malondialdehyde formed by the arachidonate oxygenase system of bovine seminal vesicles. Prostaglandins **4**, 325—341 (1973)
Flower, R. J., Harvey, E. A., Kingston, W. P.: Inflammatory effects of prostaglandin D_2 in rat and human skin. Brit. J. Pharmacol. **56**, 229—233 (1976)
Flower, R. J., Vane, J. R.: Some pharmacologic and biochemical aspects of prostaglandin biosynthesis and its inhibition. In: Prostaglandin Synthetase Inhibitors, pp. 9—18. New York: Raven Press 1974
Fried, J., Mehrer, M. M., Gaede, B. J.: Novel selective inhibitors of human placental PG-15-dehydrogenase. In: Supplementum to Advances in the Biosciences, International Conference on Prostaglandins, Vienna. Braunschweig: Vieweg-Pergamon Press 1973
Friedman, Y., Lang, M., Burke, G.: Further characterization of bovine thyroid prostaglandin synthetase. Biochim. biophys. Acta **397**, 331—341 (1975)
Granström, E. (1968): Quoted in: Biosynthesis of Prostaglandins by B. Samuelsson. Prog. biochem. Pharmacol. **5**, 109—128 (1969)
Gréen, K., Bygdeman, M., Toppozada, M., Wiqvist, N.: The role of prostaglandin $F_{2\alpha}$ in human parturition. Endogenous plasma levels of 15-keto-13,14-dihydro-prostaglandin $F_{2\alpha}$ during labour. Amer. J. Obstet. Gynec. **120**, 25—31 (1974)
Gréen, K., Samuelsson, B.: Quantitative studies on the synthesis in vivo of prostaglandins in the rat. Cold stress induced stimulation of synthesis. Europ. J. Biochem. **22**, 391—395 (1971)
Gryglewski, R., Vane, J. R.: The release of prostaglandins and rabbit aorta contracting substance (RCS) from rabbit spleen and its antagonism by anti-inflammatory drugs. Brit. J. Pharmacol. **45**, 37—47 (1972a)
Gryglewski, R., Vane, J. R.: The generation from arachidonic acid of rabbit aorta contracting substance (RCS) by a microsomal enzyme preparation which also generates prostaglandins. Brit. J. Pharmacol. **46**, 449—457 (1972b)
Hamberg, M.: Inhibition of prostaglandin synthesis in man. Biochem. biophys. Res. Commun. **49**, 720—726 (1972)
Hamberg, M.: A note on nomenclature. In: Advances in the Biosciences, pp. 847—850. Braunschweig: Vieweg-Pergamon Press 1973a
Hamberg, M.: Quantitative studies of prostaglandin synthesis in man. II. Determination of the major urinary metabolite of prostaglandins $F_{1\alpha}$ and $F_{2\alpha}$. Analyt. Biochem. **55**, 368—378 (1973b)
Hamberg, M.: Quantitative studies on prostaglandin synthesis in man. III. Excretion of the major urinary metabolite of prostaglandins $F_{1\alpha}$ and $F_{2\alpha}$ during pregnancy. Life Sci. **14**, 247—252 (1974)
Hamberg, M., Jonsson, C. E.: Increased synthesis of prostaglandins in the guinea pig following scalding injury. Acta physiol. scand. **87**, 240—245 (1973)
Hamberg, M., Samuelsson, B.: Novel biological transformations of 8,11,14-eicosatrienoic acid. J. Amer. chem. Soc. **88**, 2349—2350 (1966)

Hamberg,M., Samuelsson,B.: On the mechanism of the biosynthesis of prostaglandins E_1 and $F_{1\alpha}$. J. biol. Chem. **242**, 5336—5343 (1967a)
Hamberg,M., Samuelsson,B.: Oxygenation of unsaturated fatty acids by vesicular gland of sheep. J. biol. Chem. **242**, 5344—5354 (1976b)
Hamberg,M., Samuelsson,B.: On the specificity of the oxygenation of unsaturated fatty acids catalysed by the soybean lipoxidase. J. biol. Chem. **242**, 5329—5335 (1967c)
Hamberg,M., Samuelsson,B.: On the metabolism of prostaglandins E_1 and E_2 in man. J. biol. Chem. **246**, 6713—6721 (1971)
Hamberg,M., Samuelsson,B.: On the metabolism of prostaglandins E_1 and E_2 in the guinea pig. J. biol. Chem. **247**, 3495—3502 (1972)
Hamberg,M., Samuelsson,B.: Detection and isolation of an endoperoxide intermediate in prostaglandin biosynthesis. Proc. nat. Acad. Sci. (Wash.) **70**, 899—903 (1973)
Hamberg,M., Samuelsson,B.: Prostaglandin endoperoxides. Novel transformations of arachidonic acid in human platelets. Proc. nat. Acad. Sci. (Wash.) **71**, 3400—3404 (1974a)
Hamberg,M., Samuelsson,B.: Prostaglandin endoperoxides VII. Novel transformations of arachidonic acid in guinea pig lung. Biochem. biophys. Res. Commun. **61**, 942—949 (1974b)
Hamberg,M., Samuelsson,B., Björkhem,I., Danielsson,H.: Molecular mechanisms of oxygen activation. New York: Academic Press 1974a
Hamberg,M., Svensson,J., Wakabayashi,T., Samuelsson,B.: Isolation and structure of two prostaglandin endoperoxides that cause platelet aggregation. Proc. nat. Acad. Sci. (Wash.) **71**, 345—349 (1974b)
Hamberg,M., Svensson,J., Samuelsson,B.: Prostaglandin endoperoxides. A new concept concerning the mode of action and release of prostaglandins. Proc. nat. Acad. Sci. (Wash.) **71**, 3824—3828 (1974c)
Hamberg,M., Svensson,J., Samuelsson,B.: Thromboxanes: a new group of biologically active compounds derived from prostaglandin endoperoxides. Proc. nat. Acad. Sci. (Wash.) **72**, 2994—2998 (1975)
Hammarstrom,S., Hamberg,M., Samuelsson,B., Duell,E.A., Stawiski,M., Voorhees,J.J.: Increased concentrations of non-esterified arachidonic acid, 12L-hydroxy 5,8,10,14,-eicosatetraenoic acid, prostaglandin E_2 and prostaglandin $F_{2\alpha}$ in epidermis of psoriasis. Proc. nat. Acad. Sci. (Wash.) **72**, 5130—5134 (1975)
Hansen,H.S.: Inhibition by indomethacin and aspirin of 15-hydroxy prostaglandin dehydrogenase in vitro. Prostaglandins **8**, 95—105 (1974)
Haye,B., Champion,S., Jacquemin,C.: Control of TSH of a phospholipase A_2 activity, a limiting factor in the biosynthesis of prostaglandins in the thyroid. FEBS Lett. **30**, 253—260 (1973)
Hong,S.-C.L., Levine,L.: Inhibition of arachidonic acid release from cells as the biochemical action of anti-inflammatory corticosteroids. Proc. nat. Acad. Sci. (Wash.) **73**, 1730—1734 (1976)
Horton,E.W.: Hypothesis on physiological roles of prostaglandins. Physiol. Rev. **49**, 122—161 (1969)
Horton,E.W., Jones,R.L.: Prostaglandins A_1, A_2 and 19-hydroxy A_1; their actions on smooth muscle and their inactivation on passage through the pulmonary and hepatic portal vascular beds. Brit. J. Pharmacol. **37**, 705—722 (1969)
Horton,E.W., Jones,R.L., Marr,G.G.: Effects of aspirin on prostaglandin and fructose levels in human semen. J. Reprod. Fertil. **33**, 385—392 (1973)
Jones,R.L.: Actions of prostaglandins on the arterial system of the sheep: some structure-activity relationships. Brit. J. Pharmacol. **53**, 464P (1975)
Kessler,E., Hughes,R.C., Bennett,E.N., Nadella,S.M.: Evidence for the presence of prostaglandin-like material in the plasma of dogs with endotoxin shock. J. Lab. clin. Med. **81**, 85—94 (1973)
Kloeze,J.: Relationship between chemical structures and platelet-aggregation activity of prostaglandins. Biochem. biophys. Acta **187**, 285—292 (1969)
Kocsis,J.J., Hernandovich,J., Silver,M.J., Smith,J.B., Ingerman,C.: Duration of inhibition of platelet prostaglandin formation and aggregation by ingested aspirin or indomethacin. Prostaglandins **3**, 141—145 (1973)
Kunze,H., Bohn,E., Vogt,W.: The effects of local anaesthetics on prostaglandin biosynthesis in vitro. Biochim. biophys. Acta **360**, 260—269 (1974)
Kunze,H., Vogt,W.: Significance of phospholipase A for prostaglandin formation. Ann. N. Y. Acad. Sci. **180**, 123—125 (1971)

Lands, W. E. M., LeTellier, P. R., Rome, L. H., Vanderhoek, J. Y.: Modes of inhibiting the prostaglandin synthetic capacity of sheep vesicular gland preparations. Fed. Proc. **31**, 476 A (1972)

Lands, W. E. M., LeTellier, P. R., Rome, L. H., Vanderhoek, J. Y.: Inhibition of prostaglandin biosynthesis. In: Advances in the Biosciences. Bergstrom, S., Bernhard, S. (Eds.). Oxford: Pergamon Press 1973, Vol. IX, pp. 15—28

Lands, W. E. M., Samuelsson, B.: Phospholipid precursors of prostaglandins. Biochim. biophys. Acta **164**, 426—429 (1968)

Lee, R. E., Lands, W. E. M.: Cofactors in the biosynthesis of prostaglandins $F_{1\alpha}$ and $F_{2\alpha}$. Biochim. biophys. Acta **260**, 203—211 (1972)

Leslie, C. A., Levine, L.: Evidence for the presence of a prostaglandin E_2-9-keto reductase in rat organs. Biochem. biophys. Res. Commun. **52**, 717—724 (1973)

Light, R. J., Samuelsson, B.: Identification of prostaglandins in the Gorgonian *plexaura homomalla*. Europ. J. Biochem. **28**, 232—240 (1972)

Limas, C. J., Cohn, J. N.: Isolation and properties of myocardial prostaglandin synthetase. Cardiovasc. Res. **7**, 623—628 (1973)

Luckner, G., Rene, P.: On the phospholipase activity in bovine seminal vesicles and its possible role in the regulation of the prostaglandin biosynthesis. Z. Naturforsch. **30**, 429—433 (1975)

McGiff, J. C., Terragno, N. A., Strand, J. C., Lee, J. B., Lonigro, A. J., Ng, K. K. F.: Selective passage of prostaglandins across the lung. Nature (Lond.) **223**, 742—745 (1967)

Maddox, I. S.: Copper in PG synthesis. Biochim. biophys. Acta (Amst.) **306**, 74—81 (1973)

Malmsten, C., Hamberg, M., Svensson, J., Samuelsson, B.: Physiological role of an endoperoxide in human platelets: haemostatic defect due to a platelet cyclo-oxygenase deficiency. Proc. nat. Acad. Sci. (Wash.) **72**, 1446—1450 (1975)

Marcel, Y. L., Christiansen, K., Holman, R. T.: The preferred metabolic pathway from linolenic acid to arachidonic acid in vitro. Biochim. biophys. Acta **164**, 25—34 (1968)

Marnett, L. J., Wlodawer, P., Samuelsson, B.: Light emission during the action of prostaglandin synthetase. Biochem. biophys. Res. Commun. **60**, 1286—1294 (1974)

Marnett, L. J., Wlodawer, P., Samuelsson, B.: Co-oxygenation of organic substrates by the prostaglandin synthetase of sheep vesicular gland. J. biol. Chem. **250**, 8510—8517 (1975)

Marrazzi, M. A., Matschinsky, M.: Properties of 15-hydroxy prostaglandin dehydrogenase. Structural requirements for binding. Prostaglandins **1**, 373—388 (1972)

Milton, A. S., Wendlandt, S.: Effects on body temperature of prostaglandins of the A, E, and F series on injection into the third ventricle of unanaesthetised cats and rabbits. J. Physiol. (Lond.) **218**, 325—336 (1971)

Miyamoto, T., Yamamoto, S., Hayaishi, O.: Prostaglandin synthetase system-resolution into oxygenase and isomerase components. Proc. nat. Acad. Sci. (Wash.) **71**, 3645—3648 (1974)

Miyares-Cao, C. M., Menendez-Cepero, E.: Identification of prostaglandin-like substances in plants. In: Advances in Prostaglandin and Thromboxane Research. New York: Raven Press 1976, p. 877

Nakano, J.: Metabolism of prostaglandin E_1 in dog kidneys. Brit. J. Pharmacol. **40**, 317—325 (1970a)

Nakano, J.: Metabolism of Prostaglandin E_1 (PGE_1) in kidney and lung. Fed. Proc. **29**, 746 (1970b)

Nakano, J.: Effects of the metabolites of prostaglandin E_1 of the systemic and peripheral circulation in dogs. Proc. Soc. exp. Biol. (N.Y.) **136**, 1265—1268 (1971)

Nakano, J., Änggård, E., Samuelsson, B.: 15-hydroxy prostanoate dehydrogenase. Prostaglandins as substrates and inhibitors. Europ. J. Biochem. **11**, 386—389 (1969)

Nakano, J., Montague, B., Darrow, B.: Metabolism of prostaglandin E_1 in human plasma, uterus and placenta in swine ovary and in rat testicle. Biochem. Pharmacol. **20**, 2512—2514 (1971).

Nakano, J., Morsy, N. H.: Beta-oxidation of prostaglandins E_1 and E_2 in rat lung and kidney homogenates. Clin. Res. **19**, 142 (1971)

Nakano, J., Prancan, A. V.: Metabolic degradation of prostaglandin E_1 in the rat plasma and in the rat brain, heart, lung, kidney, and testicle homogenates. J. Pharm. (Lond.) **23**, 231—232 (1971)

Nakano, J., Prancan, A. V.: Metabolic degradation of prostaglandin E_1 in the lung and kidney of rats in endotoxin shock. Proc. Soc. exp. Biol. (N.Y.) **144**, 506—508 (1973)

Nelson, N. A.: Prostaglandin nomenclature. J. med. Chem. **17**, 911—918 (1974)

Niehaus, W. G., Samuelsson, B.: Formation of malondialdehyde from phospholipid arachidonate during microsomal lipid peroxidation. Europ. J. Biochem. **6**, 126—130 (1968)

Nijkamp, F. P., Flower, R. J., Moncada, S., Vane, J. R.: Partial purification of RCS-RF (rabbit aorta conctracting substance releasing factor) and inhibition of its action by anti-inflammatory steroids. Nature. (1976) (in press)
Nissen, H. M., Andersen, H.: On the localization of a prostaglandin-dehydrogenase activity in the kidney. Histochemie **14**, 189—200 (1968)
Nissen, H. M., Andersen, H.: On the activity of prostaglandin dehydrogenase system in the kidney. A histo-chemical study during hydration-dehydration and salt-repletion-depletion. Histochemie **17**, 241—247 (1969)
Nugteren, D. H.: Inhibition of prostaglandin biosynthesis by 8 *cis*, 12 *trans*, 14 *cis*-eicosatetraenoic acid. Biochim. biophys. Acta **210**, 171—176 (1970)
Nugteren, D. H.: Arachidonate lipoxygenase in blood platelets. Biochim. biophys. Acta **380**, 299—307 (1975 a)
Nugteren, D. H.: The determination of prostaglandin metabolites in human urine. J. biol. Chem. **250**, 2808—2812 (1975 b)
Nugteren, D. H., Beerthuis, R. K., van Dorp, D. A.: The enzymic conversion of all-*cis* 8, 14 eicosatrienoic acid into prostaglandin E_1. Rec. Trav. chim. Pays-Bas **85**, 405—419 (1966)
Nugteren, D. H., Hazelhof, E.: Isolation and properties of intermediates in prostaglandin biosynthesis. Biochim. biophys. Acta **326**, 448—461 (1973)
Pace-Asciak, C.: Polyhydroxy cyclic ethers formed from tritiated arachidonic acid by acetone powders of sheep seminal vesicles. Biochemistry **10**, 3664—3669 (1971)
Pace-Asciak, C.: Prostaglandin synthetase activity in the rat stomach fundus. Activation by L-norephinephrine and related compounds. Biochim. biophys. Acta **280**, 161—171 (1972)
Pace-Asciak, C., Cole, S.: Inhibitors of prostaglandin catabolism. I. Differential sensitivity of 9-PGDH, 13-PGR and 15-PGDH to low concentrations of indomethacin. Experientia (Basel) **31**, 143—145 (1975)
Pace-Asciak, C., Miller, D.: Prostaglandins during development I. Age dependent activity profiles of prostaglandin 15-hydroxy dehydrogenase and 13, 14—reductase in lung tissue of late prenatal, early postnatal and adult rats. Prostaglandins **4**, 351—362 (1973)
Pace-Asciak, C., Wolfe, L. S.: A novel prostaglandin derivative formed from arachidonic acid by rat stomach homogenates. Biochemistry **10**, 3657—3664 (1971)
Palmer, M. A., Piper, P. J., Vane, J. R.: Release of rabbit aorta contracting substance (RCS) and prostaglandins induced by chemical or mechanical stimulation of guinea-pig lungs. Brit. J. Pharmacol. **49**, 226—242 (1973)
Parkes, D. G., Eling, T. E.: Characterization of prostaglandin synthetase in guinea pig lung. Isolation of a new prostaglandin derivative from arachidonic acid. Biochemistry **13**, 2598—2604 (1974)
Parkinson, T. M., Schneider, J. C.: Absorption and metabolism of Prostaglandin E_1 by perfused rat jejunum in vitro. Biochim. biophys. Acta **176**, 78 (1969)
Parratt, J. R., Sturgess, R. M.: Evidence that prostaglandin release mediates pulmonary vascular constriction induced by endotoxin. J. Physiol. (Lond.) **84**, 41 (1974)
Patriarca, P., Beckerdite, S., Elsbach, P.: Phospholipases and phospholipid turnover in *Escherichia coli* spheroplasts. Biochim. biophys. Acta **260**, 593—600 (1972)
Paulsrud, J. R., Miller, O. N., Schlegel, W.: Inhibition of 15-OH-prostaglandin dehydrogenase by several diuretic drugs. Fed. Proc. **33**, 590 (1974)
Pike, J. E., Kupiecki, F. P., Weeks, J. R.: Biological activity of the prostaglandins and related analogies, In: Prostaglandins, Nobel Symposium, Vol. II, pp. 161—171. New York: Interscience 1967
Piper, P. J., Vane, J. R.: Release of additional factors in anaphylaxis and its antagonism by anti-inflammatory drugs. Nature (Lond.) **233**, 29—35 (1969)
Piper, P. J., Vane, J. R.: The release of prostaglandins from lung and other tissues. Ann. N.Y. Acad. Sci. **180**, 363—385 (1971)
Piper, P. J., Vane, J. R., Wyllie, J. H.: Inactivation of prostaglandins by the lungs. Nature (Lond.) **225**, 600—604 (1970)
Pollard, J., Flower, R. J.: (1973) Unpublished observations
Portoghese, P. S., Svanborg, K., Samuelsson, B.: Oxidation of oxyphenbutazone by sheep vesicular gland microsomes and lipoxygenase. Biochem. biophys. Res. Commun. **63**, 748—755 (1975)
Ramwell, P. W., Shaw, J. E.: Biological significance of the prostaglandins. Recent Progr. Hormone Res. **26**, 139—187 (1970)

Raz, A., Schwartzman, M., Gafni, Y., Kenig-Wakshal, R.: Properties of solubilized prostaglandin synthetase from sheep vesicular glands and from rabbit and rat kidney. In: Advances in Prostaglandin and Thrombosane Research, pp. 859—860. New York: Raven Press 1976

Rose, A. J., Collins, A. J.: The effect of pH on the production of prostaglandins E_2 and $F_{2\alpha}$, and a possible pH dependent inhibitor. Prostaglandins **8**, 271—283 (1974)

Roth, G. J., Stanford, N., Majerus, P. W.: Acetylation of prostaglandin synthetase by aspirin. Proc. nat. Acad. Sci. (Wash.) **72**, 3073—3076 (1975)

Ruthven, C. R. J., Sandler, M.: An improved method for the estimation of homovanillic acid in human urine. Clin. chim. Acta **14**, 511—518 (1966)

Samuelsson, B.: On the incorporation of oxygen in the conversion of 8, 11, 14-eicosatrienoic acid to prostaglandin E_1. J. Amer. chem. Soc. **87**, 3011—3013 (1965)

Samuelsson, B.: Biosynthesis of prostaglandins. Progr. biochem. Pharmacol. **5**, 109—128 (1969)

Samuelsson, B.: Structures, biosynthesis and metabolism of prostaglandins. In: Lipid Metabolism, pp. 107—153. New York-London: Academic Press 1970

Samuelsson, B.: Biosynthesis of prostaglandins. Fed. Proc. **31**, 1442—1450 (1972)

Samuelsson, B., Granström, E., Gréen, K., Hamberg, M.: Metabolism of prostaglandins. Ann. N.Y. Acad. Sci. **180**, 138—163 (1971)

Samuelsson, B., Granström, E., Hamberg, M.: On the mechanisms of the biosynthesis of prostaglandins. In: Prostaglandins, Nobel Symposium, Vol. II, pp. 31—44. Stockholm: Almqvist and Wicksell 1967

Samuelsson, B., Gréen, K.: Endogenous levels of 15-keto-dihydro prostaglandins in human plasma. Parameters for monitoring prostaglandin synthesis. Biochem. Med. **11**, 298—303 (1974)

Samuelsson, B., Hamberg, M.: Role of endoperoxides in the biosynthesis and action of Prostaglandins. In: Prostaglandin Synthetase Inhibitors, pp. 107—119. New York: Raven Press 1974

Scandella, J., Kornberg, A.: A membrane bound phospholipase A_1 purified from *Escherichia coli*. Biochemistry **10**, 4447—4456 (1971)

Scarnes, R. C., Harper, M. J. K.: Relationship between endotoxin induced abortion and synthesis of prostaglandin F. Prostaglandins **1**, 191—203 (1972)

Scherphof, G. L., Scarpa, A., Van Toorenenbergen, A.: The effect of local anesthetics on the hydrolysis of free and bound membrane phospholipids catalysed by various phospholipases. Biochim. biophys. Acta **270**, 226—240 (1972)

Schultz, H. W.: Symposium on foods: lipids and their oxidation. Westport: AVI Publ. Co. 1962

Sih, C. J., Takeguchi, C. A.: Biosynthesis. In: The Prostaglandins, pp. 83—100. New York-London: Plenum Press 1973

Smith, M. J. H., Dawkins, P. D.: Salicylate and enzymes. J. Pharm. (Lond.) **23**, 729—744 (1971)

Smith, W. L., Lands, W. E. M.: Stimulation and blockade of prostaglandin biosynthesis. J. biol. Chem. **246**, 6700—6704 (1971)

Smith, W. L., Lands, W. E. M.: Oxygenation of polyunsaturated fatty acids during prostaglandin biosynthesis by sheep seminal vesicular glands. Biochemistry **11**, 3276—3285 (1972)

Smith, J. B., MacFarlane, D. E.: Platelets. In: The Prostaglandins, pp. 293—335. New York-London: Plenum Press 1974

Sprecher, H., Lee, C. J.: The absence of an 8-desaturase in rat liver: a re-evaluation of optional pathways for the metabolism of linoleic and linolenic acids. Biochem. biophys. Acta **388**, 113—125 (1975)

Steiner, M.: Platelet protein synthesis studied in a cell-free system. Experientia (Basel) **26**, 786—789 (1970)

Strandberg, K., Hamberg, M.: Increased excretion of 5α 7α dihydroxy-11-keto tetranor prostanoic acid on anaphylaxis in the guinea-pig. Prostaglandins **6**, 159—170 (1974)

Sun, F. F., Armour, S. R.: Prostaglandin 15-hydroxy dehydrogenase and 13 reductase levels in the lungs of maternal fetal and neonatal rabbits. Prostaglandins **7**, 327—338 (1974)

Takeguchi, C., Kohno, E., Sih, C. J.: Mechanism of prostaglandin biosynthesis. I. Characterization and assay of bovine prostaglandin synthetase. Biochemistry **10**, 2372—2376 (1971)

Takeguchi, C., Sih, C. J.: A rapid spectrophotometric assay for prostaglandin synthetase: application of the study of non-steroidal, anti-inflammatory agents. Prostaglandins **2**, 169—184 (1972)

Tan, L., Wang, H. M., Lehoux, J.-G.: Binding of prostaglandins and cytochrome P-450. Prostaglandins **4**, 9—17 (1973)

Tappel, A. L.: Oxidative fat rancidity in food product: linoleate oxidation catalyzed by hemin, hemoglobin, cytochrome. Food Res. **18**, 560—573 (1953)

Tappel, A. L.: Lipoxidase. In: The Enzymes. New York: Academic Press 1963, pp. 275—283

Tomlinson, R. V., Ringold, H. J., Qureshi, M. C., Forchielli, E.: Relationship between inhibition of prostaglandin synthesis and drug efficacy: support for the current theory on mode of action of aspirin-like drugs. Biochem. biophys. Res. Commun. **46**, 552—559 (1972)

Turner, S. R., Trainer, J. A., Lynn, W. S.: Biogenesis of chemotactic molecules by the arachidonate lipoxygenase system of platelets. Nature (Lond.) **257**, 680—681 (1975)

Vane, J. R.: Inhibition of prostaglandin synthetase as a mechanism of action for aspirin-like drugs. Nature (New Biol.) **231**, 232—235 (1971)

Vane, J. R.: Prostaglandins as mediators of inflammation. In: Advances in Prostaglandin and Thromboxane Research, pp. 791—801. New York: Raven Press 1976

Vargaftig, B. B.; Dao Hai, N.: Selective inhibition by mepacrine of the release of "rabbit aorta contracting substance" evoked by the administration of bradykinin. J. Pharm. (Lond.) **24**, 159—161 (1972)

Varley, H.: Practical clinical biochemistry, 4th. ed. London: Medical Books Ltd. 1967

Vogt, W., Meyer, U., Kunze, H., Lufft, E., Babilli, S.: Entstehung von SRS-C in der durchströmten Meerschweinchenlunge durch Phospholipase A. Identifizierung mit Prostaglandin. Naunyn-Schmiedeberg's Arch. exp. Path. Pharmak. **262**, 124—134 (1969)

Vonkeman, H., van Dorp, D. A.: The action of prostaglandin synthetase on 2-arachidonyl-lecithin. Biochim. biophys. Acta **164**, 430—432 (1968)

Wallach, D. P.: Enzymatic conversion of arachidonic acid to prostaglandin E_2 with acetone powder preparations of bovine seminal vesicles. Life Sci. **4**, 361—364 (1965)

Wallach, D. P., Daniels, E. G.: Properties of a novel preparation of prostaglandin synthetase from sheep seminal vesicles. Biochim. biophys. Acta **231**, 445—457 (1971)

Willis, A. L., Comai, K., Kuhn, D. C., Paulsrud, J.: Dihomo-γ-linolenate suppresses platelet aggregation when administered in vitro or in vivo. Prostaglandins **8**, 509—519 (1974a)

Willis, A. L., Vane, F. M., Kuhn, D. C., Scott, S. G., Petrin, M.: An endoperoxide aggregator (LASS), formed in platelets in response to thrombotic stimuli. Prostaglandins **8**, 453—507 (1974b)

Wlodawer, P., Samuelsson, B.: On the organization and mechanism of prostaglandin synthetase. J. biol. Chem. **248**, 5673—5678 (1973)

Yoshimoto, A., Ito, H., Tomita, K.: Cofactor requirements of the enzyme synthesising prostaglandin in bovine seminal vesicles. J. Biochem. (Tokyo) **68**, 487—499 (1970)

Note added in proof. Since this chapter was written, a new and important pathway of arachidonic acid metabolism has been discovered (Moncada *et al.*, 1976a and b; Gryglewski *et al.*, 1976; Bunting *et al.*, 1976; Johnson *et al.*, 1976). The figure shows the transformation catalysed. The new prostaglandin, PGI_2, is a potent vasodilator and inhibitor of platelet aggregation but its significance in the inflammatory process is, as yet, undetermined.

References. Moncada, S., Gryglewski, R., Bunting, S., Vane, J. R.: An enzyme isolated from arteries transforms prostaglandin endoperoxides to an unstable substance that inhibits platelet aggregation. Nature **263**, 663—665 (1976a). — Moncada, S., Gryglewski, R. J., Bunting, S., Vane, J. R.: A lipid peroxide inhibits the enzyme in blood vessel microsomes that generates from prostaglandin endoperoxides the substance (Prostaglandin X) which prevents platelet aggregation. Prostaglandins **12**, 715—733 (1976b). — Gryglewski, R. J., Bunting, S., Moncada, S., Flower, R. J., Vane, J. R.: Arterial walls are protected against deposition of platelet thrombi by a substance (Prostaglandin X) which they make from prostaglandin endoperoxides. Prostaglandins **12**, 685—714 (1976). — Bunting, S., Gryglewski, R. J., Moncada, S., Vane, J. R.: Arterial walls generate from prostaglandin endoperoxides a substance (Prostaglandin X) which relaxes strips of mesenteric and coeliac arteries and inhibits platelet aggregation. Prostaglandins **12**, 897—913 (1976). — Johnson, R. A., Morton, D. R., Kinner, J. H., Gorman, R. R., McGuire, J. R., Sun, F. F., Whittaker, N., Bunting, S., Salmon, J. A., Moncada, S., Vane, J. R.: The chemical structure of prostaglandin X (prostacyclin). Prostaglandins **12**, 915—928.

Inflammatory Mediators Generated by Activation of Plasma Systems

CHAPTER 13

Complement*

A. NICHOLSON**, D. T. FEARON***, and K. F. AUSTEN

A. Introduction

The complement system consists of multiple serum proteins which interact sequentially to mediate a wide variety of inflammatory and immune reactions. The complement reaction consists of four segments, that is, two pathways for *recognition-activation*, the classical and alternative, a common *amplification* reaction and a single *effector* phase. Detailed studies of the human complement sequence have facilitated the demonstration of acquired abnormalities in association with disease, while an understanding of the system in certain animals has provided models for experimental studies of the role of complement in inflammation.

B. Classical Activating Pathway

Using determinants on the red-cell membrane as antigen, it has been found that one molecule of IgM, or two adjacent molecules of IgG, are sufficient to activate guinea pig C1 (BORSOS and RAPP, 1965). The relative potencies of the human Ig classes for activation of C1 are: IgM > IgG3 > IgG1 > IgG2; immune complexes containing IgG4, IgA, IgD, and IgE do not activate C1 (reviewed by MÜLLER-EBERHARD, 1969). Mixtures of polycations and polyanions, such as heparin and protamine, can also lead to C1 activation (RENT et al., 1975).

C1 is a calcium-dependent complex of a least three separate subcomponents:[1] C1q, C1r and C1s (NAFF et al., 1964). C1q, which is the subcomponent responsible

* Supported by grants AI-07722, AI-10356, AM-05577, and RR-05669 from the National Institutes of Health, Bethesda, Maryland, U.S.A.

** Intermediate Fellow, Society of Fellows, Harvard University.

*** Postdoctoral Fellow of the Helen Hay Whitney Foundation.

[1] Unless specifically indicated, the complement proteins and reactions described refer to the human system.
The nomenclature for the classical complement components conforms to that agreed upon under the auspices of the World Health Organization (1968, BULL. W. H. O. **39**, 395). The nomenclature for alternative pathway factors is that provisionally agreed upon at the Second International Congress of Immunology, 1974, Brighton, United Kingdom. *B* is the symbol for a protein that has been termed C3 proactivator (C3PA) and glycine-rich beta glycoprotein (GBG); $\bar{D}$ is the symbol for the protein that has been termed C3 proactivator convertase (C3PAse) and GBGase; P represents properdin; *C3NeF* is the abbreviation for C3 nephritic factor; *IF* is the abbreviation for initiating factor; and *C3bINA* represents the C3b inactivator. With respect to fragmentation, the larger fragment is designated *b* and the lesser fragment *a*, except for C2 where by convention *a* refers to the larger fragment. When the same letter designation is used for the precursor and active enzymatic forms of a component, a bar over the letter indicates the enzymatic form, as in D and $\bar{D}$.

for binding to Ig, has a molecular weight of 400000. Ultrastructural studies of C1q by electron microscopy have shown six peripheral globular portions joined by connecting strands to a central fibril-like region (Shelton et al., 1972); and physicochemical studies show that C1q consists of six non-covalently linked subunits (Reid et al., 1972; Yonemasu and Stroud, 1972). Each subunit consists of three different polypeptide chains covalently linked in a major triple helix, each chain having a repeating x-y-glycine sequence and a high content of hydroxylated amino acids (Reid, 1976; Reid et al., 1976). A model for C1q proposes that the six subunits are joined at their collagen-like N-terminal end to form a fibril stem from which branch the individual C-terminal globular regions carrying the immunoglobulin binding sites (Reid and Porter, 1976). Since the valency of C1q for binding to immunoglobulin is 6 (Müller-Eberhard and Kunkel, 1961; Müller-Eberhard and Calcott, 1966), it is presumed that the globular portions correspond to these binding sites. In support of this model, collagenase treatment destroys the haemolytic function of C1q but not its immunoglobulin binding capacity (Knobel et al., 1974). C1q binds to the C_H2 domain of the Fc region of IgG (Ellerson et al., 1972), and the C_H4 domain of IgM (Hurst et al., 1974). Although C1q can bind to native IgG, Fc, binding of antigen apparently increases the affinity of the Fc region for C1q and results in the structural alterations necessary for conversion of C1r to $C\bar{1}r$.

C1r is a 198000 glycoprotein with β mobility composed of two identical non-covalently linked polypeptide chains (Ziccardi and Cooper, 1976a) that convert C1s to $C\bar{1}s$. C1r can bind to sensitized erythrocytes only in the presence of C1q and Ca^{++}. $C\bar{1}s$ binds after C1r is bound, suggesting that C1r acts as the ligand between C1q and C1s. The activation of C1r to $C\bar{1}r$ involves proteolytic cleavage, which occurs spontaneously at 37° C in Ca^{++} free medium, into two disulphide-linked subunits (Ziccardi and Cooper, 1976b). The active site of $C\bar{1}r$ has been characterized as a serine esterase based on its susceptibility to inhibition by phenylmethyl sulphonyl fluoride and diisoprophylphosphofluoridate (DFP) and a capacity to hydrolyze certain synthetic amino acid esters (Naff and Ratnoff, 1968; Ziccardi and Cooper, 1976a). C1r deficiency has been described (Pickering et al., 1970; Moncada et al., 1972) and from studies of a family with multiply affected individuals it seems to be inherited as an autosomal recessive trait.

The C1s subcomponent when activated to $C\bar{1}s$ has the capacity to assemble the classical pathway C3 convertase by cleavage of C4 and C2. C1s, an α-globulin with a molecular weight of 80–100000, consists of a single polypeptide chain with intrachain disulphide bonds. Conversion to $C\bar{1}s$ occurs by cleavage of a peptide bond yielding two chains held together by disulphide bonds (Sakai and Stroud, 1973). The active site is on the smaller 37000 M.W. chain (Barkas et al., 1973) and has been characterized as a serine esterase based on its irreversible inhibition by DFP (Levine, 1955; Becker, 1956) and its capacity to cleave certain synthetic amino acid ester substrates. Normal serum contains an α-glycoprotein, the $C\bar{1}$ inhibitor ($C\bar{1}$INH), which inhibits $C\bar{1}$ or $C\bar{1}s$ stoichiometrically by irreversibly combining with the active enzymatic site (Haines and Lepow, 1964; Gigli et al., 1968); and also inhibits $C\bar{1}r$ (Ziccardi and Cooper, 1976a). C1, purified by affinity chromatography with insolubilized IgG, has an additional protein designated C1t (Assimeh et al., 1974); but this protein is not essential for $C\bar{1}$ activity. C1q, C1s and C1r concentrations vary independently of each other in some patients with severe combined immunodeficiency suggesting that the subunits are under separate synthetic control (GEWURZ et al., 1968b; STROUD et al., 1970). In vitro synthesis of haemolytically active C1 occurs in short-term cultures of tissue from the large and small intestines of humans (COLTEN et al., 1968) and guinea pigs (COLTEN et al., 1966). There is recent evidence that long-term cultures of epithelial cells derived from gut and urogenital tract tissues can produce functional C1 and C1s (BING et al., 1975).

The natural substrates of fluid phase or cell-bound $C\bar{1}$ are C4 and C2. C4, a β_1 globulin with an apparent molecular weight of 202000, consists of three polypeptide chains having molecular weights of 93000, 78000 and 33000 and α, β and γ electrophoretic mobility, respectively, which are linked by disulphide bonds. $C\bar{1}$ cleaves a 6000 M.W. fragment from the α chain to uncover a binding site on the residual C4b fragment for attachment to cell membranes (SCHREIBER and MÜLLER-EBERHARD, 1974). The site on C4b is only transiently available and if binding is not immediate, the molecule remains in the fluid phase as C4i due to irreversible decay of this site (MÜLLER-EBERHARD and LEPOW, 1965). Not all C4b bound to the membrane functions with equal efficiency for subsequent haemolytic reactions as assessed with guinea pig components (BORSOS et al., 1970; LINSCOTT, 1973a, b) and several explanations are possible: the capacity of cell-bound C4b to adsorb native C2; the ability of cell-bound C4b to retain activated C2; and the proximity of C3b binding sites in membrane for conversion of C4b2a to a C5 convertase.

Functional C4 can be synthesized in vitro by the adherent cells from guinea pig spleen and peritoneal exudates (ILGEN et al., 1974) and by the mononuclear cell fraction of human foetus (COLTEN, 1972) and guinea pig liver (ILGEN and BURKHOLDER, 1974). In humans, a complex form of genetically determined polymorphism has been found (ROSENFELD et al., 1969) and analysis of paired maternal and foetal plasma samples has provided evidence for foetal synthesis of C4 and absence of transplacental passage (BACH et al., 1971). Half-normal plasma levels of C4 in 4 of 20 individuals in a family were reported in 1969 (ROSENFELD et al., 1969). An undetectable C4 level in an individual with an illness resembling systemic lupus erythematosus has been reported (HAUPTMANN et al., 1974) and may represent a homozygous deficiency. A strain of guinea pigs has also been described which is deficient in functional and antigenic C4 (FRANK et al., 1971). When peritoneal cells from the C4-deficient guinea pigs were fused with HeLa cells, both cell types being incapable of C4 synthesis, the resulting hybrid cell could synthesize human C4 (COLTEN and PARKMAN, 1972). The C4 deficient cells produced a 45000 M.W. factor which acted like a derepressor and allowed the HeLa cells to utilize their own structural gene to synthesize human C4. Normal guinea pig peritoneal cells also produced this putative derepressor, but only in $^1/_5$–$^1/_{10}$ the quantity of C4-deficient cells (COLTEN, 1976). Cell-free synthetic studies done with polysomes isolated from liver cells of C4-deficient guinea pigs show that there is premature termination of the C4 peptide chains, as compared with C4 synthesis on polyribosomes isolated from normal guinea pigs (HALL and COLTEN, 1977).

The presence of cell-bound C4b or fluid phase C4i enhances the capacity of $C\bar{1}$ to activate its other natural substrate, C2 (GIGLI and AUSTEN, 1969a, b). C2, a single chain β-globulin with a molecular weight of 117000, is cleaved by $C\bar{1}s$ into two fragments, C2a and C2b, of 80000 and 36000 M.W., respectively (POLLEY and MÜLLER-EBERHARD, 1968). The increased rate of C2 cleavage by $C\bar{1}$ in the presence of C4b/C4i has several possible mechanisms: an allosteric modification of the enzymatic site on C$\bar{1}$ to fully uncover its C2 specificity (GIGLI and AUSTEN, 1969b; KONDO et al., 1972); localization of the substrate near C$\bar{1}$ during reversible binding of native C2 to C4b/C4i (SITOMER et al., 1966); and provision of a site for the deposition of C2a following its generation thereby freeing the active site on C$\bar{1}$s for catalysis of additional C2 (STRUNK and COLTEN, 1974).

In addition to accelerating C2 cleavage, C4b/C4i serves as an essential receptor for C2a to form the bimolecular complex, C4b2a, which is the classical C3 convertase. The active proteolytic site for both C3 and C5 cleavage resides on C2a and it is not well expressed unless C2a is bound to C4i/C4b. C4b2a exhibits temperature-dependent decay by dissociation of the bound C2a fragment and its conversion in the fluid phase to C2i; the residual C4b reforms the convertase upon interaction with additional native C2 in the presence of C$\bar{1}$. Studies on the generation and decay of the classical convertase were first conducted with guinea pig components following haemolytic activities (BORSOS et al., 1961; SITOMER et al., 1966; STROUD et al., 1965) and subsequently analyzed with specific proteins and their fragments utilizing human components (MÜLLER-EBERHARD and LEPOW, 1965; MÜLLER-EBERHARD et al., 1967).

Biosynthesis of functional C2 has been observed in the long-term cultures of normal human peripheral mononuclear cells (EINSTEIN et al., 1976), but not with monocytes from individuals with homozygous deficiency of C2 (EINSTEIN et al., 1975). Mononuclear cells from some sources are capable of synthesizing both functional C2 and C4 (WYATT et al., 1972). C2 biosynthesis has also been noted in several hepatoma cell lines (LEVISOHN and THOMPSON, 1973; STRUNK et al., 1975).

The first description of an inherited component deficiency was that of C2 in 1966 (KLEMPERER et al., 1966) and at least 11 other kindreds (RUDDY and AUSTEN, 1978) with C2 deficiency have been recognized subsequently. C2 deficiency is inherited as an autosomal recessive trait and linkage to histocompatibility antigens has been described, especially with HLA-10, W18 (FU et al., 1974). The occurrence of homozygous C2 deficiency in a normal blood donor population is reported as 1 in 10000 or less, implying heterozygosity in 1 in 100 individuals (LACHMANN, 1974).

C. Alternative Pathway

An alternative or properdin pathway of complement activation was described some twenty years ago by PILLEMER and his associates as consisting of a group of serum factors, including properdin, that interacted with complex microbial polysaccharides to form a C3-cleaving enzyme without involvement of C1, C4, and C2 (PILLEMER et al., 1954).

Factor A of the original properdin system was later shown by MÜLLER-EBERHARD and GÖTZE (1972) to be C3. Both guinea pig and human C3 have been isolated and shown to be β-globulins with a molecular weight of about 200000 (SHIN and MAYER, 1968a; BOKISCH et al., 1975; GITLIN et al., 1975; NILSSON et al., 1975). Human C3 has two polypeptide chains: α (140000 M.W.) and β (80000 M.W.) linked by disulphide bridges. Cleavage of C3 by either classical or alternative C3 convertases releases a 6000–8000 M.W. fragment, C3a, from the N-terminus of the α chain

(HUGLI et al., 1975) leaving a residual major fragment C3b. More than 24 genetically controlled electrophoretic variants of C3 have been described and all variants are allelic with no observed linkage to histocompatibility antigens (ALPER et al., 1969). Monocytes cultured in vitro synthesize antigenic C3 which has the same electrophoretic mobility as that of the cell donor's serum (EINSTEIN et al., in press). In contrast to the monocytes from homozygous C2-deficient patients, the monocytes from C3-deficient patients produce normal amounts of antigenic C3 (EINSTEIN et al., 1977). Antigenic C3 has recently been synthesized in a cell-free system and consists of a single chain of 250000 M.W. This is apparently the precursor of the 2-chain extracellular form of C3 (BRADE et al., 1977).

Factor B, which is the functional analogue of C2, consists of a single chain of 100000 M.W. with β mobility. The native molecule has some limited enzymatic activity against synthetic amino acid esters (VOGT et al., 1977). In the presence of Mg^{++}, B interacts with native C3, and more avidly with C3b, with the result that the C3 and C5 cleaving activity of B is partially unmasked (FEARON and AUSTEN, 1975b). In the presence of the specific B activating enzyme, $\bar{D}$, B is fully activated by cleavage into two fragments, Bb (80000 M.W.) which has the catalytic site and Ba (20000 M.W.) (GÖTZE and MÜLLER-EBERHARD, 1971; VOGT et al., 1974). B exhibits extensive electrophoretic polymorphism (ALPER et al., 1972a) and the responsible alleles segregate with the major histocompatibility locus in humans (ALLEN, 1974). Mouse pertioneal macrophages can synthesize B in vitro (BENTLEY et al., 1976).

$\bar{D}$, the enzymic activator of B, has been isolated from both human and guinea pig sera and has an apparent molecular weight of 25000. The isoelectric point is 7.5 for human $\bar{D}$ (FEARON and AUSTEN, 1975a) as compared with 9.4 in the guinea pig (BRADE et al., 1974a). Trypsin, pronase and plasmin can substitute for $\bar{D}$ in terms of activating guinea pig B (BRADE et al., 1974b). The active site of human $\bar{D}$ has been characterized as a serine esterase based on its irreversible inhibition by diisopropylphosphofluoridate (DFP) and competitive inhibition by P-tosyl-l-arginine methyl ester (FEARON et al., 1974; FEARON and AUSTEN, 1975d). A precursor principle termed D has been isolated from human serum and shown to be almost the same size as $\bar{D}$. D is resistant to inhibition by DFP until activated to $\bar{D}$ by trypsin (FEARON et al., 1974). The normal mechanism of converting D to $\bar{D}$ is not known, however, functional amounts of the active form $\bar{D}$ are normally present in serum and plasma.

Activated human properdin, P, is a 184000 M.W. γ-globulin with an isoelectric point of greater than 9.5 that consists of four apparently identical non-covalently linked subunits of 46000 M.W. (MINTA and LEPOW, 1973). Guinea pig P has been isolated and shown to be similar to human P in molecular weight and charge (NICHOLSON and AUSTEN, 1977). Ultracentrifugation of normal human serum shows that there are several forms of properdin, recognizable by antigenic assays, and that some of these forms are complexed with C3 or C3 fragments (CHAPITIS and LEPOW, 1976). The function of properdin is to retard the decay-dissociation of the precursor C3B and C3bB convertases and the fully activated C3bBb convertase. P does this by binding to the C3 or C3b of the convertase. A more native form of properdin has recently been purified, which fails to induce C3 and B cleavage upon addition to normal serum, and it is unable to remain bound to EAC4b3b during washing with isotonic buffers (MEDICUS et al., 1976a). This form of properdin can stabilize the convertase when bound to an intermediate (FEARON and AUSTEN, 1977a). The interconversion of the two forms of properdin is not associated with a change in size or subunit structure.

There are two naturally occurring inhibitors of the alternative pathway. The first of these is β1H, a 150000 M.W. single chain β-glycoprotein that has the capacity to bind to fluid phase or surface bound C3b and displace any factor B that may be attached. The effect of this inhibitor is to accelerate the normal dissociation-decay of the C3bBb convertase and the C3BbP stabilized convertase (WEILER et al., 1976; WHALEY and RUDDY, 1976).

The second inhibitor is the C3b inactivator (C3bINA) that consists of two β-globulin disulphide-linked polypeptide chains of 55000 and 42000 M.W., respectively (FEARON and AUSTEN, 1977a). C3bINA enzymatically cleaves the α chain of either fluid phase (RUDDY and AUSTEN, 1971) or surface bound C3b (TAMURA and NELSON, 1967) although the latter is the preferred substrate. The result of this inactivation is two haemolytically inactive fragments, C3d which remains cell bound, and C3c which is released to the fluid phase. Since the availability of C3b controls the rate of assembly of the alternative pathway convertases (NICHOLSON et al., 1974) and since neither C3c nor C3d can function to form the amplification portion of C3bBb convertase, C3bINA is a major control protein for the alternative complement pathway (ALPER et al., 1972b). Indeed, genetic deficiency of this protein is associated with in vivo hypercatabolism of C3 and B that can be blocked in vivo by administration of partially purified C3bINA (ZIEGLER et al., 1975). In vitro depletion of C3bINA from serum by immunoabsorption results in cleavage of C3 and B without a requirement for the usual activators of the alternative pathway (NICOL and LACHMANN, 1973). C3bINA also abolishes C3b-dependent immune adherence reactions (TAMURA and NELSON, 1967) and reverts the alternative C5 convertase to a C3 convertase (DAHA et al., 1976c). The α chain of C4b has also been shown to be cleaved by C3bINA into large and small fragments, C4c and C4d, respectively, that are incapable of participating in formation of the classical convertase (COOPER, 1975; NAGASAWA et al., 1976).

β1H augments the C3b inactivator by two mechanisms: first, it can dissociate the Bb from the C3bBb convertase and expose the otherwise protected C3b (WEILER et al., 1976) to inactivation by the C3bINA. Second, β1H directly accelerates the C3bINA inactivation of C3b. The mechanism of this molecular cooperation is not known, but it may involve dissociation of the enzyme from its product (WHALEY and RUDDY, 1976).

Finally, there is an active principle known as C3 nephritic factor (C3NeF), which to date has been found only in certain pathological conditions, namely hypocomplementemic membranoproliferative glomerulonephritis (SPITZER et al., 1969) and partial lipodystrophy. C3NeF was shown to be a γ-globulin with a molecular weight of 150000 and there was controversy as to whether it was (THOMPSON, 1972) or was not an immunoglobulin (VALLOTA et al., 1974). C3NeF stabilizes the convertase containing native B or Bb (DAHA et al., 1976a, b) such that it is possible to isolate the fluid phase complexes. Indeed these studies have established the molar ratio of the three components in the 10S complex composed of C3bBb(C3NeF) to be 1:1:1 (DAHA et al., 1977). Further, a surface-bound convertase stabilized by C3NeF, as opposed to properdin, is much more resistant to β1H mediated decay dissociation (WEILER et al., 1976). C3NeF is now known to be an autoantibody directed primarily against determinants on the C3bBb convertase (DAHA et al., 1978).

I. Amplification Convertase

C3b derived by either classical or alternative pathway activation interacts with B and $\bar{D}$ to generate an amplification convertase, C3bBb. This is truly an amplification convertase, because the product, C3b, can participate in the formation of more enzyme. The functional characteristics of this convertase were difficult to appreciate in the fluid phase because of its lability. Thus, erythrocyte (FEARON et al., 1973) and zymosan (BRADE et al., 1973) intermediates bearing C3b were developed which permitted measurement of the enzyme complex directly or indirectly by hemolytic assays. It was found that in the presence of Mg^{++}, native B bound to C3b prior to being cleaved by $\bar{D}$ (NICHOLSON et al., 1975). After the labile convertase, C3bBb, was formed decay was first-order with a half-life of 4 min at 30° C, secondary to loss of Bb activity (FEARON and AUSTEN, 1975c). New convertase could be formed with native B, indicating that C3b and $\bar{D}$ retained their activities. Thus, the role of B in decay and regeneration of C3bBb is analogous to that of C2 in forming the enzyme complex, C4b2a; and C3b, like C4b, serves as a binding cofactor for the protein bearing the C3-cleaving site, Bb. Direct demonstration of the contribution of both C3b and Bb to convertase function was achieved employing C3NeF for stabilization as noted above (DAHA et al., 1976a, b).

P binds to fluid phase C3, C3b, and C3c (CHAPITIS and LEPOW, 1976) and to cellular intermediates bearing C3b (EAC4b3b) in a temperature- and cation-independent reaction, while P does not fix to intermediates lacking C3b (FEARON and AUSTEN, 1975c). Further, binding of P to intermediates bearing the convertase C3bBb results, without a latent period, in a dose-related prolongation of the first-order decay of the convertase site, its half-life being extended at 30° C by as much as tenfold. Although erythrocyte-bound P is resistant to washing, P can be transferred from one intermediate (EAC4b3bP) to another (EAC4b3bBb) with consequent stabilization of the recipient convertase site (FEARON and AUSTEN, 1975c). The more native form of P described by MEDICUS et al. (1976a) which has a lower affinity for C3b, can also stabilize the amplification convertase.

Parallel experiments with C3NeF show that it also retards decay of erythrocyte-bound C3bBb (DAHA et al., 1976a), but there are two ways in which its stabilizing activity differs from that of P. First, C3NeF stabilized convertase is relatively resistant to β1H dissociation. Second, C3NeF has a dose-related latent period before expressing stabilizing activity on the sites still remaining. Interaction of C3 and B with $\bar{D}$ in the presence of C3NeF followed by sucrose density ultracentrifugation yielded a complex with a sedimentation rate of 10S that possessed C3-cleaving activity (DAHA et al., 1976b) and contained C3b,Bb,C3NeF a in 1:1:1 molar ratio (DAHA et al., 1977). The capacity of C3NeF to stabilize C3bBb in the fluid phase permitted confirmation of the bimolecular state of the convertase initially postulated on the basis of functional studies of formation, decay, and regeneration (FEARON et al., 1973). It is noteworthy that the classical convertase, C4b2a, also was not isolated as a fluid phase complex until a mechanism for stabilization of C2a was found, namely, oxidation of C2 (POLLEY and MÜLLER-EBERHARD, 1967).

II. Activation

A disparate group of substances are capable of activating the alternative pathway: complex microbial polysaccharides such as zymosan (PILLEMER et al., 1954); endotoxin (MARCUS et al., 1971); sulphated dextrans (BURGER et al., 1975); stroma of human erythrocytes (POSKITT et al., 1973) and intact rabbit erythrocytes (PLATTS-MILL and ISHIZAKA, 1974). There are two lines of evidence to suggest that activation by these substances, which leads ultimately to the formation of the amplification convertase, occurs by escape from the action of the two inhibitors, β1H and C3bINA. First, the potential for cleaving some C3 exists all the time. This concept is supported by the intense C3 and B cleavage observed in serum genetically (ALPER et al., 1972c) or immunochemically depleted (NICOL and LACHMANN, 1973) of C3bINA. The interaction of C3, B and $\bar{D}$ leads to C3 and B cleavage and the reaction is markedly facilitated by the presence of properdin (FEARON and AUSTEN, 1975a, b). Once C3b is generated, B complexes with it in preference to native C3, forming C3bBP, which in turn, the circulating $\bar{D}$ can convert to C3bBbP, the efficient C3 cleaving amplification convertase. Thus, there is the potential for continuously generating a little C3b and then forming the amplification convertase. Under normal circumstances the reaction does not advance to amplification because of the regulatory action of the two control proteins: β1H disassembles the C3 cleaving convertases and the C3bINA irreversibly inactivates the binding site for B on C3b.

The second line of evidence supporting the concept that activation of the alternative pathway occurs as a result of escape from the inhibitors comes from studies of the fate of C3b bound to the surface of "activating" and "non-activating" substances (FEARON and AUSTEN, 1977a, b). Utilizing purified C3, B, $\bar{D}$, P, β1H and C3bINA in their approximate serum ratios, it was found that the C3b deposited on the surface of rabbit erythrocytes and zymosan, both activating substances, was relatively resistant to inactivation by C3bINA. Furthermore, C3bBb convertase generated on the surface of these activating substances was also relatively resistant to the dissociation-decay action of β1H as compared to convertase on a non-activating surface such as a sheep erythrocyte. Specific activation by rabbit erythrocytes and zymosan is not detectable in the absence of the inhibitors because there is a rapid and uncontrolled turnover of components. When the reaction is limited to low-grade fluid phase turnover by the presence of regulatory proteins, introduction of an activating surface such as that of a rabbit erythrocyte results in deposition and marked accumulation of C3b, indicating that surface-dependent activation can occur by circumvention of regulation[2].

The facilitation of alternative pathway activation by antibody and an intact classical pathway (NELSON, 1958; JOHNSTON et al., 1969; ROOT et al., 1972; NICHOLSON et al., 1974) probably result from an efficient initial deposition of C3b. Once C3b is bound to the protecting surface of the activator, the reaction readily shifts to the amplification phase because of the increased rate of C3b generation and efficiency of C3b binding induced by the particle-bound C3b-dependent convertase.

The capacity of a microbial surface, by analogy to zymosan and rabbit E, to protect and thereby accumulate increasing amounts of C3b by local circumvention of the regulatory proteins is compatible with a unique role for the alternative path-

2 For references, see FEARON and AUSTEN, 1977b.

way in host defence. The specificity of the pathway resides in the capacity of certain surfaces to induce transition from constant low-grade fluid phase C3 cleavage to localized amplification because of the selective inability of C3bINA and β1H to deal with their substrates when deposited on these surface. The implication of these surface effects would hold even if initial C3 cleavage and binding was facilitated by specific antibody and classical complement or by involvement of additional principles, such as initiating factor (SCHREIBER et al., 1976).

D. Effector Sequence

The classical and alternative C3 convertases cleave the C3a peptide from the N-terminus of the α chain of C3 to generate C3b which has a labile binding site for irreversible binding to membranes. Bound C3b functions at five different steps in the haemolytic sequence. These include: 1) the binding of B to allow the formation of the C3bBb enzyme by $\bar{D}$ (FEARON et al., 1973; NICHOLSON et al., 1975); 2) the binding of P to stabilize the C3bBb convertase (FEARON and AUSTEN, 1975c); 3) the conversion of C4b2a and C3bBb to C5 convertases (SHIN et al., 1971a, b; NILSSON and MÜLLER-EBERHARD, 1965; DAHA et al., 1976c) which in the case of guinea pig classical convertase has been attributed to C3b providing a binding site for native C5 (GOLDLUST et al., 1974); 4) the provision of a binding site for the fluid phase C5b6 complex (GOLDLUST et al., 1974) thereby potentiating lysis by generating C5b67 at the membrane (HAMMER et al., 1976); 5) finally, bound C3b functions as a ligand for the immune adherence interaction with cells bearing C3b receptors as will be discussed in later sections.

The terminal complement components were first isolated in functional purity from guinea pig serum (NELSON et al., 1966). Subsequently C5 was purified from guinea pig (COOK et al., 1971) and human serum (NILSSON and MÜLLER-EBERHARD, 1965). Human C5 consists of two polypeptide chains, α (140000 M.W.) and β (83000 M.W.), held together by disulphide bridges (NILSSON et al., 1975). The in vivo synthesis of functional human C5 has been reported for lung, liver, spleen, and foetal intestine (COLTEN, 1973); and for several rat hepatoma cell clones (STRUNK et al., 1975). The human cell type(s) responsible for C5 biosynthesis have not been determined. In mice the splenic macrophage is the only cell type capable of transferring C5 biosynthetic activity to C5-deficient mice (LEVY et al., 1973).

One case of human C5 deficiency has been described and the family pedigree is consistent with an autosomal recessive mode of inheritance; heterozygotes have 34–65% of the normal haemolytic titre of C5 (ROSENFELD et al., 1974). Hybridization of cells from C5-deficient mice and chicken erythrocytes results in a cell type that produces antigenic and functional mouse C5, although neither parent cell has this capability (LEVY et al., 1973). The mechanism by which this occurs is not settled, but two possible explanations are: 1) the C5-deficient mice are missing the gene for an essential structural subunit of C5 and the sheep erythrocyte has this gene and supplies the subunit which is antigenically silent; or, 2) the C5 deficient mice have the C5 structural gene but the influence of a regulator, either the presence of a repressor of the absence of a derepressor, blocks the gene's expression. In this case, hybridization with the chicken erythrocyte would be diluting the repressor or supplying the derepressor.

Human C6 (ARROYAVE and MÜLLER-EBERHARD, 1971) has a molecular weight of 128000 and consists of a single chain (PODACK et al., 1976). Synthesis of C6 has been reported to occur in liver tissue; the cell responsible has not been identified (ROTHER et al., 1968). Microheterogeneity of human C6 that is genetically determined has been demonstrated by isoelectric focusing of plasma (HOBART et al., 1974). A proband with functional and immunochemical C6 deficiency has been described, and five of six siblings and both parents have half-normal levels of functional C6 (LEDDY et al., 1974). A strain of rabbits has been known for some time in which there is complete deficiency of C6 (ROTHER and ROTHER, 1961).

Human C7 has been purified (ARROYAVE and MÜLLER-EBERHARD, 1973) and shown to be a single polypeptide chain of 121000 M.W. (PODACK et al., 1976). There are no studies localizing the site of C7 synthesis. Two kindreds with C7 deficiency have been described, with presumed heterozygotes in both families having approximately half-normal levels of haemolytically active C7 consistent with an autosomal recessive mode of inheritance (WELLEK and OPFERKUCH, 1975; BOYER et al., 1975). The probands differed in that one persistently had no detectable C7 and the other had levels fluctuating between 0.4% and 3%.

Human C8 has a molecular weight of 174000 (MANNI and MÜLLER-EBERHARD, 1969) and is composed of three polypeptide chains: the α and γ chains are held together by disulphide bonds while the β chain is associated with the other two chains by non-covalent forces (KOLB et al., 1976). Synthesis of functional C8 has been detected from in vitro cultures of spleen, liver, lung, intestine and kidney of the foetal pig (GEIGER et al., 1972). One human has been described who is deficient in C8 (PETERSON et al., 1975).

Both human and guinea pig C9 have been isolated to functional purity (HADDING and MÜLLER-EBERHARD, 1969; TAMURA and SHIMADA, 1971). The C9 recovered from the human C5b6789 complex gives one band on SDS gels and has a molecular weight of 79000 (KOLB and MÜLLER-EBERHARD, 1975a). ROMMEL et al. (1970) have demonstrated that functional C9 can be synthesized in vitro by a rat hepatoma cell strain and the normal rat liver parenchymal cell probably synthesizes C9 (BRESLOW et al., unpublished 1975). There are no known instances of C9 deficiency in humans or animals.

Cleavage of C5 by either the classical or alternative pathway C5 convertases releases the C5a fragment (11000 M.W.) from the N-terminus of the α chain yielding the major fragment, C5b. C5b is stabilized with respect to its haemolytic potential while bound to the C3b of the C5 convertase, but once C5b dissociates it decays rapidly in the fluid phase to C5i. Under special conditions guinea pig C5b can transfer from one cell to another bearing C4b2a3b (SHIN et al., 1971b). Further, a C5b6 complex is stable in the fluid phase and has the capacity to reassociate with membrane bound C3b (GOLDLUST et al., 1974). A C5b67 complex has the capacity to interact with unsensitized membranes in a mechanism known as "reactive lysis" which extends the cytolytic effects of complement to "innocent bystander" cells that have not themselves activated either the classical or alternative pathways (THOMPSON and LACHMANN, 1970; LACHMANN and THOMPSON, 1970; GÖTZE and MÜLLER-EBERHARD, 1970; GOLDMAN et al., 1972). If C7 combines with C5b6 attached to the membrane via C3b, lysis is potentiated because the labile C5b67 complex has a greater chance of inserting into a membrane before it decays (HAMMER et al., 1976). If

C5b67 does not immediately interact with a membrane the binding site decays in about 0.1 s at 30° C (GÖTZE and MÜLLER-EBERHARD, 1970) and the complex remains in the fluid phase where it does retain chemotactic activity (WARD, 1972).

Formation of membrane-bound C5b67 is followed by binding of C8 to the complex which creates a partial membrane lesion resulting in slow cytolysis (STOLFI, 1968). Binding of C9 to C5b678 completes the lesion, accelerating the rate of lysis. Using guinea pig components one molecule of C9 for each C5b678 site is sufficient to augment lysis (ROMMEL and MAYER, 1973). In studies of human C5b6789 isolated from the fluid phase, all the components were in the molar ratio of one, except C9 which exists in a molar ratio of three (KOLB and MÜLLER-EBERHARD, 1975a). These final steps in the complement sequence do not involve cleavage reactions, but represent non-covalent assembly of a C5b-C9 multi-molecular complex. An additional serum factor distinct from the known complement components and without apparent cytolytic function has been found in the C5b-C9 complexes isolated from the fluid phase (KOLB and MÜLLER-EBERHARD, 1975a).

The mechanism of cytolysis by complement has been studied by morphological and biochemical techniques. Electron microscopy of erythrocytes that have been lysed by human complement has revealed characteristic "doughnut-shaped" lesions on the outer membrane leaflet that have a dark center of 100–110Å diameter surrounded by a lighter ring (HUMPHREY and DOURMASHKIN, 1969). The dark central area may be a depression in the membrane or a hydrophilic region, while the outer ring may be a relatively raised or hydrophobic region. Ferritin-labelled C9 has been found to be spatially associated with these lesions (RAUTERBERG and GEBEST, 1976). Incubation of sensitized erythrocytes with human serum deficient in C5, C6, C7, or C8, respectively, does not result in lysis or appearance of the ultrastructural membrane alterations, indicating that the complement reaction must proceed at least to the C8 step for these changes to occur. Extraction of membranes bearing complement lesions with chloroform-methanol results in their disappearance while trypsin-treatment has no effect, suggesting involvement of the hydrophobic lipid bilayer of the membrane (HUMPHREY and DOURMASHKIN, 1969).

Biochemical studies have focused on the interactions of the terminal five components, C5-C9, among themselves and with the membranes. Binding of C7 to C5b6 induces a conformational change which may expose hydrophobic regions on the complex which permits its partial insertion from the fluid phase into the lipophilic membrane with concomitant stabilization of the complex. These presumed hydrophobic regions would be thermodynamically unstable in an aqueous medium, and if insertion of the complex does not immediately occur these regions would be buried by an additional conformational change associated with loss of the cytolytic potential of C5b67. In support of a conformational change being induced by binding of C5b6 with C7 is the observation that this complex bears neoantigens not expressed on the individual components (KOLB and MÜLLER-EBERHARD, 1975b). The finding that C5b and C7 on the intermediate, EAC1423567, resist stripping by exposure to trypsin or high salt, while C5b on EAC142356 is removed by these procedures supports the insertion hypothesis (HAMMER et al., 1975). It is further envisioned that C8 and C9 bind to the C5b67 complex and create a hydrophilic core. When C5b6 plus C7 and C8 are reacted with planar lipid bilayers the electrical conductance increases 5–10-fold and the subsequent addition of C9 increases the conductance another 100–1000-fold (ABRAMOVITCH et al., 1976). The insertion model of a complex with a hydrophilic core creates the "holes" (MAYER, 1972) that permit the net uptake of salt and water by the cell leading to osmotic lysis.

E. Control of the Complement Reaction

Two general mechanisms limit the extent of the complement reaction. The first which has already been considered is intrinsic and is represented by the rapid decay rates of the enzymes C4b2a (BORSOS et al., 1961) and C3bBb (FEARON et al., 1973) and by the labile membrane binding sites of C4b, C3b, and C5b which localize cytolytic potential (MÜLLER-EBERHARD and LEPOW, 1965; SHIN and MAYER, 1968b; SHIN et al., 1971b). The second is extrinsic and is exemplified by four inhibitors, two of which, β1H and C3bINA, were previously discussed under Alternative Pathway (Section III).

I. C$\bar{1}$INH

C$\bar{1}$INH, an α-globulin with a molecular weight of 105000 (HARPEL and COOPER, 1975), controls the assembly of C4b2a by binding to the light chain of C$\bar{1}$s (HARPEL, 1973), and irreversibly inhibits its capacity to cleave C4 and C2. Further, C$\bar{1}$INH blocks C$\bar{1}$r activation of C1s (NAFF and RATNOFF, 1968; ZICCARDI and COOPER, 1976b), thereby controlling an even earlier step in the classical reaction sequence.

C$\bar{1}$INH also serves as a control protein in the Hageman factor initiated pathways by inhibiting active Hageman factor and its active site bearing fragments from activating prekallikrein, plasminogen proactivator, and factor XI (precursor plasma thromboplastin antecedent) (SCHREIBER et al., 1973). The kinin-generating (RATNOFF et al., 1969) and chemotactic activities of kallikrein (GOETZL and AUSTEN, 1974) are inhibited by C$\bar{1}$INH as well as by α2-macroglobulin.

II. Anaphylatoxin Inactivator (AI)

AI is an α2-globulin with a molecular weight of 310000 that consists of eight apparently identical non-covalently bound subunits of 36000 M.W. AI enzymatically cleaves the C-terminal arginine from C3a, C5a, and bradykinin to ablate their histamine-releasing and spasmogenic properties (BOKISCH and MÜLLER-EBERHARD, 1970). The enzyme is metal-dependent being inhibited by EDTA and Mg^{++}-EDTA; it is also blocked by high concentrations of EACA (VALLOTA and MÜLLER-EBERHARD, 1973).

F. Phylogeny

Studies of the phylogeny and species specificity of the complement components are difficult to interpret because the optimal reaction conditions often are lacking for examining a single step using mixed reagents. Despite the limitations imposed by using mixed reagents, these studies are of interest. Their importance resides both in analyzing the time frame in which the complement system evolved and in providing some information as to the functional compatibility of the complement components of different species.

GIGLI and AUSTEN reviewed in 1971 the phylogeny of the complement system and there have been only a few modifications since then. Adoptive immunity in terms of antibody appears first in the sea lamprey, a member of the class of Agnatha (GEWURZ et al., 1967; GREY, 1969). Although this species has a haemolysin for rabbit erythrocytes, its action seems different from the complement system because the additional factors required for haemolysis are heat stable and partially cation independent. The first definite evidence for an antibody-activatable complement system occurs in the nurse shark, an elasmobranch. A haemolytic intermediate has been prepared from antibody and complement-like components of this species (JENSEN, 1969; ROSS and JENSEN, 1973). The nurse shark has a C4 inactivator which can also cleave human C4 and may be distinct from a C1 subunit (FULLER et al., 1974).

There is evidence that the alternative pathway may occur earlier in evolution than adoptive humoural immunity. DAY et al. (1970) tested the ability of various sera to form a complex with cobra venom factor (CVF) or to react with a preformed cobra venom-serum complex to allow reactive lysis. It is now known that CVF is a form of cobra C3 (ALPER and BALAVITCH, 1976) that is resistant to the C3b inactivator of most other species and can form a stable CVF-Bb enzyme in the presence of B and $\bar{D}$. The capacity of sera to generate a CVF-Bb complex depends on the ability of native B to complex with the CVF so that $\bar{D}$ can activate it to CVF-Bb. While the ability of a sera to interact with preformed CVF-Bb and mediate reactive or indirect lysis depends on the cleavage of C5 by this enzyme and effective generation of the terminal pentamolecular complex. Of the three invertebrate species examined, the horseshoe crab and the sipunculid worm could each form a CVF complex which activated its own respective terminal components as measured by reactive lysis. Starfish sera did not support CVF-induced reactive lysis but it did form a CVF complex which activated the late complement components in frog sera. These data suggest that the alternative initiating pathway and the effector pathway are phylogenetically old and precede the appearance of a specific humoural response which is required to activate the classical pathway.

Studies of the species compatibility of complement components have been extensively reviewed by GIGLI and AUSTEN (1971). Only the studies involving mammalian complement homology will be considered here. Activated cell-bound C1, EAC$\bar{1}$, of either guinea pig or human origin can cleave the heterologous C4 and C2 efficiently enough to be of practical usefulness. However, a C$\bar{1}$4b site prepared with guinea pig components will not utilize human C2 so as to activate the terminal human complement components and permit lysis (KOETHE et al., 1972). In addition, the fluid phase inactivation of homologous C2 by human C1 is impaired by guinea pig C4 while human C4 greatly augments the inactivation rate (GIGLI and AUSTEN, 1969a). Thus, a major species incompatibility occurs when forming the bimolecular complex of the classical C3 convertase. This incompatibility is not limited to the combination described but is observed between numerous species (Table 1), and appears to reflect failure of the bound heterologous C2 to be cleaved by C$\bar{1}$ so as to form a convertase capable of activating C3. The product, designated "counterfeit convertase" (KOETHE et al., 1972) subsequently was shown to bind C3 without developing the C5 convertase activity essential for progression of the haemolytic sequence. Another step where

Table 1. Known partial or complete species incompatibilities[a] among mammalian early complement components

Index source of components	Incompatible substitions for interaction with			Source of $C_{3,5-9}$ (same as index source unless noted)	References
	Index C_1	Index C_4	Index C_2		
Human	$C4^g$ (*FP*)	$C2^R$	$C4^g$		GIGLI and AUSTEN, 1969a
	$C2^g$ (*FP*)	$C2^d$	$C4^R$		GIGLI and AUSTEN, 1971
		$C2^r$	$C4^d$		KEMPF et al., 1969
			$C4^r$		NELSON et al., 1966; SARGENT and AUSTEN, 1970
Guinea pig	$C4^h$ (*FP*)	$C2^h$	$C4^R$		GIGLI and AUSTEN, 1969a
	$C2^h$ (*FP*)	$C2^R$	$C4^d$		GIGLI and AUSTEN, 1971
		$C2^d$	$C4^r$		KEMPF et al., 1969
		$C2^r$			SARGENT and AUSTEN, 1970; CALDWELL et al., 1973
Rabbit		$C2^h$	$C4^g$		KEMPF et al., 1969
		$C2^g$	$C4^h$		NELSON and BIRO, 1968
Dog	$C4^g$	$C1^g$	$C4^h$		SARGENT and
		$C2^h$	$C4^g$		AUSTEN, 1970
		$C2^g$			
Rat			$C4^h$		
			$C4^g$		
		$C2^g$		Guinea pig	CALDWELL et al., 1972
		$C2^h$		Guinea pig	

[a]Table revised from GIGLI and AUSTEN, 1971.
Legend: Superscripts refer to species of origin: d=dog, g=guinea pig, h=human, R=rabbit, r=rat, FP=fluid phase reaction.

mixed components are often incompatible is at the C5 cleavage step of the classical pathway (Table 2). This is not surprising considering the multi-component nature of this enzyme.

Human and guinea pig P are interchangeable for stabilizing the heterologous C3bBb convertases (NICHOLSON and AUSTEN, 1977). $\bar{D}$ from either species is also able to activate the C3b-bound factor B from either species. B, however, requires homologous C3b for its binding site before it can be activated by $\bar{D}$ (BRADE et al., 1976). Thus, formation of effective convertases, classical and alternative/amplification, appears to be a step particularly susceptible to inhibition by species incompati-

Table 2.[a] Known species incompatibilities between late-acting complement components

Index Component (s)	Source of incompatible C5	Source of incompatible C6
EAC $\overline{4b2a3b}^{h}$	$C5^{d}$, $C5^{g}$	
EAC $\overline{4b2a3b}^{d}$	$C5^{h}$, $C5^{g}$	
EAC $\overline{4b2a^{g}3b}^{d}$	$C5^{d}$, $C5^{g}$	
—	$C5^{g}$	$C6^{h}$
—	$C5^{h}$	$C6^{d}$

[a] Based on a personal communication from Dr. AUSTIN SARGENT, Saskatchewan, Canada.

Legend superscripts refer to species of origin: d=dog, g=guinea pig, h=human.

bilities. Mechanistically, the incompatibilities may reflect the failure of the complement ligand interacting with the active complement enzyme to expose its catalytic site and/or the substrate binding site.

The activation of C6 by combining with C5b is, as has been discussed, a non-enzymatic step and a few incompatibilities have been noted (Table 2). There are no studies to date of species incompatibilities between C6, C7, C8, and C9. It should be noted, however, that minor incompatibilities appreciated in terms of reaction rates have not been excluded.

G. Biological Activity of Complement

Cleavage fragments generated from complement components during their interaction have the capacity to evoke an inflammatory response. This effect is achieved through alteration of local vascular permeability, chemotactic attraction of leucocytes and modulation of inflammatory cell function at the site of the complement reaction.

I. Permeability Factors

Patients with hereditary (DONALDSON and EVANS, 1963) or acquired (CALDWELL et al., 1972) deficiency of $C\bar{1}$INH have repeated attacks of localized, non-inflammatory oedema of the subcutaneous tissues and mucous membranes (SHEFFER et al., 1971). The inherited form of this disease is known as hereditary angio-oedema (HAE). Attacks involving the larynx are life-theatening due to asphyxiation while those in the gut may mimic an acute abdominal crisis. Serum taken from patients between attacks shows depressions of C4 (RUDDY et al., 1968), and during an attack, C4 and C2 levels fall even further (AUSTEN and SHEFFER, 1965) in association with detectable $C\bar{1}$ esterase activity (DONALDSON and ROSEN, 1964). Serum taken between attacks generates an activity on incubation at 37° C capable of contracting the oestrous rat uterus; and treatment of the serum with antiserum to C4 or C2, but not C3, inhibits elaboration of this activity (DONALDSON et al., 1969). Characterization of this "C-kinin" after partial purification from hereditary angio-oedema serum showed it to be heat-stable, susceptible to inactivation by trypsin, and to have an apparent molecular weight of 5000 (DONALDSON et al., 1970). Although it has been suggested that this permeability-enhancing principle is cleaved from C2 by the interaction of $C\bar{1}$ and C4 this is not an established fact (LEPOW, 1971).

Anaphylatoxin was the term applied to a toxic principle, generated during incubation of antigen-antibody complexes with guinea pig serum (FRIEDBERGER, 1909). The anaphylatoxic activity is now known to reside in two cleavage peptides, C3a and C5a, which have smooth muscle contractile activity and release histamine from mast cells (DIAS DA SILVA et al., 1967; JENSEN, 1967; COCHRANE and MÜLLER-EBERHARD, 1968). Human C3a and C5a contract the isolated guinea pig ileum at 10^{-8} and 10^{-9} M, respectively, and do not exhibit cross-tachyphylaxis indicating different spasmogenic receptors for these factors. C3a and C5a in concentrations of 10^{-12} and 10^{-15} M, respectively, cause human skin mast cell degranulation, resulting in wheal and flare reactions that are associated with pruritus and are blocked by antihistamines (DIAS DA SILVA and LEPOW, 1967; COCHRANE and MÜLLER-EBERHARD, 1968). The binding of C3a to the membrane of mast cells has been demonstrated by an immunofluorescent technique (TER LAAN et al., 1974) and the extent of uptake of C3a by mast cells is related to the amount of histamine released (JOHNSON et al., 1975). The contractile effects of C3a and C5a on guinea pig ileum (VOGT et al., 1969) and the effect of C3a on oestrous rat uterus (BOKISCH and MÜLLER-EBERHARD, 1970) are independent of histamine release. The effect of C3a on the microvasculature is also histamine independent and has recently been shown to be inhibited by the α blocker, phentolamine, suggesting that this C3a effect is mediated via α receptors (MAHLER et al., 1975). Attempts to generate and detect anaphylatoxin activity in human serum were initially unsuccessful and only C5a was recognized after activation of guinea pig serum (JENSEN, 1967). It is now known that in the human, C3a and C5a are rapidly destroyed by the anaphylatoxin inactivator (AI), while in the guinea pig AI inactivates C3a but not all of the C5a activity.

II. Chemotactic Factors

Three fluid phase products generated during the complement reaction induce directed migration of leucocytes in vitro: C3a, C5a and the haemolytically inactive fluid phase complex, C5b67i (WARD, 1972). C3a and C5a exhibit little specificity, being chemotactic for neutrophils, eosinophils and monocytes (GOETZL and AUSTEN, 1974), while C5b67i is chemotactic only for neutrophils and eosinophils (WARD, 1972). Guinea pig C3a is not chemotactic (SNYDERMAN et al., 1968) and the activity of trypsin-formed human "C3a" may reflect another peptide product. Plasmin, trypsin and a protease found in most normal tissues produce fragments from C3 that possess chemotactic activity, while trypsin and a neutral protease (elastase, kallikrein) present in lysosomal granules generate active fragments from C5 that resemble C5a (WARD, 1972). Exposure of neutrophils to one chemotactic principle renders them unresponsive to the original, as well as others, in a reaction termed "deactivation." Deactivation prevents further directed migration and may serve to hold the cells at an inflammatory focus.

In addition to these chemotactic factors which represent haemolytically inactive, non-enzymatic products of complement reactions, CVF-Bb is capable of chemotactically attracting and deactivating neutrophils (RUDDY et al., 1975a). C3bBb, which is too labile for chemotactic experiments, can deactivate neutrophils as assessed by their failure to respond to subsequent chemotactic stimulation by C5a. THEOFILOPOULOS and PERRIN (1976) have shown that Raji cells which have surface receptors for both C3 and C3b, are able to bind properdin and factor B. One wonders if, by analogy to the effect of the C3bBb convertase on chemotaxis, the functional consequences of lymphocyte-membrane assembled alternative pathway convertase relates to directed pseudopod formation.

III. Leucocyte Mobilizing Factor

An uncharacterized fragment cleaved from C3 by the classical C3 convertase releases mature polymorphonuclear leucoctyes from perfused, isolated bone marrow. Although this fragment is not chemotactic, it may set the stage for extensive accumulation of cells at sites of inflammation by inducing peripheral leucocytosis (ROTHER, 1972; McCALL et al., 1974). The in vivo activity of this fragment is suggested by the finding of leucocytosis in experimental animals after administration of CVF that induces rapid cleavage of C3 (McCALL et al., 1974), and by the absence of leucocytosis during bacterial infections in an individual with genetic deficiency of C3 (ALPER et al., 1972b).

IV. Adherence Reactions

Adherence reactions occur between C3b-coated complexes and certain cells bearing specialized membrane receptors for C3b (NELSON, 1953). Human cells that have been found to have these receptors are erythrocytes, polymorphonuclear leucocytes (neutrophilic and eosinophilic), monocytes, macrophages and B-lymphocytes. Non-primate species have the receptor on leucocytes and platelets but not erythrocytes. Although adherence may also be mediated by C4b, the C3b-dependent reaction is many times more efficient (COOPER, 1969). Treatment of erythrocyte-bound C3b with C3bINA abolishes adherence of human erythrocytes, indicating the presence on this cell of receptors only for intact C3b (GIGLI and NELSON, 1968). However, human B-lymphocytes (ROSS et al., 1973; NUSSENZWEIG, 1974), monocytes (HUBER et al., 1968) and lung macrophages have an additional receptor for C3d, the fragment remaining bound to complexes after cleavage by C3bINA. The C3b receptor has not been extensively characterized but is trypsin-sensitive and is rendered non-functional by treatment with sulphhydryl reducing agents (DIERICH et al., 1974). The biological consequences of C3b-mediated adherence depend upon the cell type involved and include enhanced phagocytosis, secretion, synthesis and blastogenesis.

Although immune complexes formed with IgG are subject to phagocytosis by polymorphonuclear leucocytes, monocytes and macrophages via their membrane receptors for the Fc region of IgG, prior interaction of the complex with complement so as to bind C3b greatly increases the rate and extent of phagocytosis (GIGLI and

NELSON, 1968). Phagocytosis in vitro can be divided into adherence and ingestion phases. The prime function of C3b is to mediate adherence, while the prime function of the Fc fragment of IgG is to stimulate ingestion (MANTOVANI, 1975). Adherence via C3b may be more important in vivo than in vitro since free Ig can block the Fc receptor on the phagocytic cell. With regard to mediating phagocytosis in the absence of IgG, this capacity of C3b may be dependent on the state of the phagocyte. "Non-activated" mouse peritoneal macrophages become adherent to C3b-coated complexes lacking IgG but do not ingest them, while "activated" peritoneal macrophages bind and phagocytose such complexes (GRIFFEN et al., 1975; BIANCO et al., 1975). The importance of enhanced phagocytosis by C3b in host defense is exemplified by patients with a genetic or acquired deficiency of C3 who experience repeated bacterial infections (ALPER et al., 1970a, b; ALPER et al., 1972b; BALLOW et al., 1975). In the case of a genetic deficiency, restoration of the C3 content in vitro with purified C3 resulted in correction of the opsonic defects (ALPER et al., 1972b).

There is experimental evidence that adherence can cause the secretion of lysosomal enzymes. Neutrophils presented with immunoglobulin and C3b-coated Millipore filters release lysosomal enzymes extracellularly, indicating that adherence in the absence of phagocytosis may trigger secretion (HENSON, 1972).

Lymphocytes derived from the bone marrow (B-lymphocytes) have membrane-associated receptors for C3, C3b and C3d, while lymphocytes derived from the thymus (T-lymphocytes) in general do not. Native C3 and C3b share a common receptor while binding via C3d occurs through a separate receptor. The functional implications for B-lymphocytes resulting from interaction with C3 and its fragments have been reviewed (NUSSENZWEIG, 1974). Incubation of B-lymphocytes with C3b results in their proliferation (HARTMAN and BOKISCH, 1975) and in secretion of a factor chemotactic for monocytes (KOOPMAN et al., 1976). Depletion of C3 in mice by treatment with CVF inhibits subsequent induction of specific IgG, IgA and IgE antibody production to T cell-dependent but not T cell-independent antigens, suggesting a role for C3 in antibody responses requiring cooperation between macrophages, B- and T-lymphocytes (PEPYS, 1974; PEPYS et al., 1976).

While the immune adherence functions of C3b described in relation to phagocytosis, secretion and B cell stimulation are terminated by the C3bINA, there are other complement dependent functions of immune complexes that appear to have another form of control that is not yet elucidated. C3b-coated immune complexes bound to B-lymphocytes are not dissociated by purified C3bINA, but are dissociated by incubation with serum in a reaction requiring Mg^{++}, B and C3. This would indicate involvement of the alternative complement pathway. Incubation of insoluble antigen-antibody aggregates with serum yields soluble immune complexes of a smaller size and this reaction also is dependent on alternative pathway factors (NUSSENZWEIG, 1974).

Studies of the interactions between the complement and coagulation pathways have focused on the aggregation of platelets with release of intracellular contents. Both lytic and non-lytic mechanisms exist by which the complement system may alter platelet homeostasis (HENSON, 1970). Lysis of platelets may occur either directly by utilization of anti-platelet antibodies (ZIMMERMAN and MÜLLER-EBERHARD, 1973), or indirectly by the reactive lysis phenomenon in the presence of an activating stimulus (GOCKE and OSLER, 1965).

Adherence of non-primate platelets to particles bearing C3b activates a non-lytic secretory response requiring energy metabolism, Ca^{++} and microtubule integrity (HENSON and COCHRANE, 1969). In another non-cytolytic reaction aggregation and release of S-HT by human platelets occurs during incubation with zymosan which had been pretreated with plasma or serum reconstituted with fibrinogen (ZUCKER and GRANT, 1974). Preparation of this active zymosan-protein complex required an intact alternative complement pathway but proceeded normally in C6-deficient human serum. Finally, assembly and binding of the C5b6789 complex to human and rabbit platelets occurred during incubation in fresh plasma in the absence of activators of either the classical or alternative complement pathways and even in the presence of EDTA (ZIMMERMAN and KOLB, 1976); this phenomenon may be related to the impaired clotting of C6-deficient rabbit blood (ZIMMERMAN et al., 1971) and to the decreased ristocetin-induced platelet aggregation and release in C5-deficient human platelet-rich plasma (GRAFF et al., 1976).

H. Complement in Experimental Tissue Injury

The role of complement in immunologically induced tissue injury has been studied using animals genetically lacking or rendered deficient in a specific component. The former is best exemplified by a strain of guinea pigs genetically deficient in C4 (ELLMAN et al., 1970) and the latter by pretreatment of animals with CVF to decrease levels of circulating C3 to less than 10% of normal (COCHRANE et al., 1970).

The Arthus reaction is that pathological process in tissue, usually cutaneous, evoked by local deposition of antigen-antibody complexes and characterized by an accumulation of neutrophils, fibrinoid necrosis of capillaries and venules, and perivascular oedema and haemorrhage. In the reverse passive Arthus reaction in which antibody is injected into the skin and antigen intravenously, immunofluorescent studies reveal the presence of immune complexes and complement components in vessel walls and in the phagosomes of neutrophils. In rabbits, rats and guinea pigs, the reaction has been diminished by depletion of neutrophils with nitrogen mustard (STETSON, 1951) or depletion of C3 with CVF pretreatment (COCHRANE et al., 1970). In the absence of neutrophils, immune complexes and C3 are deposited in vessel walls but necrosis does not occur. With C3 depletion antigen-antibody complexes are again localized in vessel walls but neutrophil accumulation and necrosis are absent (COCHRANE and JANOFF, 1974). Thus the deposition of immune complexes in the vessel wall is complement independent, but the accumulation of neutrophils, which is essential for tissue injury, is complement dependent. The reaction proceeds in C4-deficient guinea pigs (ELLMAN et al., 1971) which have been infused with γ-1-antibodies but not γ-2-antibodies, presumably due to the utilization of the alternative pathway which guinea pig γ-1-antibodies readily activate. Mice and rabbits deficient in C5 (BEN-EFRAIM and CINADER, 1964; LINSCOTT and COCHRANE, 1964) and C6 (ROTHER et al., 1964), respectively, also develop a cutaneous Arthus reaction indicating that effector complement components, other than C3, are not required for this lesion. The finding that rabbits lacking C6 showed delayed neutrophil accumulation in passive Arthus reactions in synovial tissues may indicate a role at such a site for the chemotactic activity of C5b67i which being macromolecular might not rap idly diffuse from the joint space (DE SHAZO et al., 1972a, b). The overall sequence of events in a Arthus reaction appears to be deposition of immune complexes, activation of the complement system by either the classical or alternative pathways, directed accumulation of neutrophils, immune adherence of C3b-coated complexes, enhancement of phagocytosis, and release of polymorphonuclear leucocyte lysosomal enzymes. Since the reaction occurs in animals lacking C5 and C6, but not C3, the lytic potential of complement is of less pathobiological significance than its capacity to recruit leucocytes to the site of the immunological reaction.

Acute systemic immune complex disease ("serum sickness") follows formation of circulating immune complexes. Deposition of immune complexes in arterial walls results in a severe, necrotizing arteritis which may be prevented by depletion of either neutrophils or C3, indicating a pathogenesis similar to the Arthus reaction. Mild reversible glomerular damage also occurs secondary to deposition of immune complexes but in contrast to the arterial lesions, neutrophil infiltration is not a prominent feature and proteinuria is not prevented by prior depletion of neutrophils or C3 (HENSON and COCHRANE, 1971). Thus, experimental immune complex lesions that lack leucocytic infiltration are not altered by depleting C3 to low levels.

I. Complement in Human Disease

I. Genetic Abnormalities

Genetic disorders of the complement system involve a deficiency of a specific component or a deficiency in a control factor such as C$\bar{1}$INH or C3bINA. Almost all of the complement component deficiencies are associated with pathological states and the question arises—is the pathology due to a block in the complement sequence or is the deficiency genetically linked with some other factor(s) of the immune system which might account for the abnormality? Early complement component deficiencies in C1r, C4, and C2 are associated with autoimmune diseases and this association is probably the result of genetically linked factors as opposed to causally related factors for two reasons: activation by immune complexes is partially responsible for the pathology of autoimmune diseases; and there is no evidence that a block in the complement sequence leads to abnormal activation due to loss of negative feedback. The frequency of autoimmune diseases, however, could relate to impaired clearance of an unrecognized foreign material or an antigen-antibody complex.

The complement deficiencies have provided the best in vivo information as to the significance of various components in host defence. Deficiencies of C1r, C1s, C2, and C4 are not associated with increased infections, suggesting that the classical pathway per se is not essential for host defence; but it should be emphasized that the alternative pathway is intact. C1q deficiency in patients is associated with infections, but this is probably secondary to the associated agammaglobulinaemia. There have been no descriptions of deficiencies in the alternative pathway proteins as yet. Three humans have been described with homozygous deficiency of C3 and in each case there has been an abnormal incidence of infections, especially with gram-positive pyogenic organisms. These findings corroborate the in vitro and in vivo evidence (WINKELSTEIN et al., 1975) that C3 is important as an opsonin for pyogenic microorganisms. The C5 deficient patient has had frequent pyogenic infections (ROSENFELD et al., 1974) but C5 deficient mice seem healthy and have shown only a subtle in vitro defect in opsonization (SHIN et al., 1969).

There have been multiple clinical reports of recurrent or unusually severe infections with Neisseria species occurring in humans deficient in either C6, C7, or C8. This suggests that the terminal complement sequence may have an unique role in the defence against these pathogens.

The first defect of a complement pathway control factor to be described was $C\bar{1}$INH deficiency which results in HAE (DONALDSON and EVANS, 1963). The deficiency may be due to either the absence of the protein or its presence in a non-functional state (ROSEN et al., 1965). As discussed previously, a deficiency of this protein permits the uninhibited action of episodically activated $C\bar{1}$ on its natural substracts C2 and C4, resulting in clinical attacks.

Studies of one patient with C3bINA deficiency suggest that P interacts with B and C3 to produce acquired deficiencies in B and C3 (ALPER et al., 1970b; ABRAMSON et al., 1971). The recurrent attacks of severe pyogenic infection are entirely consistent with C3 deficiency, while the urticaria appearing with plasma infusion probably reflects C3a cleavage from the sudden additional C3 source.

II. Acquired Abnormalities

Although specific activation of the complement system serves to benefit the host in terms of resistance to infectious organisms, studies of human diseases of diverse aetiologies involving multiple organs have also suggested a pathobiological role for the complement system. These diseases may be of viral, protozoal, bacterial, drug-induced or of unknown aetiology wherein the vascular system, skin, kidneys and joints seem to be particularly susceptible. Three general situations can be discerned in which the complement system may have pathobiological effects. First, specific antibody may direct the complement reaction to normal host tissues, as occurs in autoimmune haemolytic anaemia and in Goodpasture's syndrome (LERNER et al., 1967), which are diseases associated with antibodies specific for determinates on erythrocytes or glomerular and pulmonary basement membranes, respectively. Second, and most commonly, the complement system, activated by heterologous or homologous antigen-antibody complexes, may contribute to "immune-complex" diseases (LEBER and MCCLUSKEY, 1974) such as rheumatoid arthritis (RA) and systemic lupus erythematosus (SLE). Third, the alternative pathway may be involved, as in idiopathic hypocomplementemic membranoproliferative glomerulonephritis (MPGN), with or without associated partial lipodystrophy.

RA is a chronic inflammatory arthritis characterized serologically by the presence of antibodies directed against an altered form of host IgG. Although these antibodies may be of any immunoglobulin class, IgM anti-IgG ("rheumatoid factor") is generally present in such seropositive patients with a more severe form of disease. PEKIN and ZVAIFLER (1964) and HEDBERG (1967) observed that synovial fluids from patients with RA contained relatively less total haemolytic complement activity than did fluids from patients with other forms of arthritis, despite the presence of normal or elevated serum complement levels. The extent of intra-articular complement depletion was proportional to the titre of rheumatoid factor in synovial fluids (HED-

BERG, 1967), and the decreased levels of haemolytically active C1, C4, C2, and C3 compared to fluids from patients with either degenerative joint disease or seronegative RA, indicated that activation was occurring by the classical pathway (FOSTIROPOULOS et al., 1965; RUDDY and AUSTEN, 1970). Levels of C4 and C2 in seronegative patients were also depressed but to a lesser extent, presumably because their fluids lacked IgM-containing immune complexes which would be more efficient than IgG-anti-IgG complexes in the binding-activation of C1. Involvement of the amplification pathway was subsequently appreciated by the depressed levels of P and factor B in synovial fluids of patients with seropositive RA (RUDDY et al., 1975b) and the correlation of these levels with C3. That the depressions of C3 were secondary to hypercatabolism and not impaired diffusion from plasma into the joint space was shown by direct measurements of the catabolic rates of intra-articular radiolabelled C3 (RUDDY et al., 1975c), and the finding of cleavage products characteristic of the action of C3bINA on C3b in the synovial fluids (ZVAIFLER, 1969). Evidence that the complement reaction proceeded to completion included the finding of relatively depressed levels of C9 (RUDDY et al., 1971) and the detection of chemotactic factors representing C5a and the C5b67 complex (WARD and ZVAIFLER, 1971). The identification of immunoglobulins and C1q, C4 and C3 in intracytoplasmic inclusions in neutrophils (BRITTON and SCHUR, 1971) suggests that C3b-dependent immune adherence and enhanced phagocytosis of immune complexes has occurred. The presence in synovial fluids of neutrophil-derived lysosomal enzymes (HARRIS et al., 1969) may reflect this release during phagocytosis of the C3b-coated immune complexes. This description of RA in terms of the immune complexes and complement abnormalities found in synovial fluid does not account for the presence of B- and T-lymphocytes, local production of rheumatoid factor, and a proliferation of the infiltrated pannus.

Activation of the complement system by the classical pathway occurs in multiple sites in patients with SLE, a disease associated with a variety of circulating immune complexes, most characteristically DNA-anti-DNA. Depressed levels of C1q, C4, C2, and C3 have been found during episodes of arthritis (PEKIN and ZVAIFLER, 1970), pleuritis (HUNDER et al., 1972), pericarditis (HUNDER et al., 1974), cerebritis (PETZ et al., 1971) and glomerulonephritis (KOHLER and TEN BENSEL, 1969) in synovial, pleural, pericardial, and cerebrospinal fluids and serum, respectively. Deposits of complement components have been demonstrated by immunofluorescence in glomeruli of patients with SLE nephritis, and IgG specific for DNA has been eluted from renal tissue (KOHLER and TEN BENSEL, 1969). Turnover studies have shown that reductions in serum levels of C3 and C4 are secondary to hypercatabolism (HUNSICKER et al., 1972; RUDDY et al., 1975c). Furthermore, the depressions in serum levels of P and factor B correlated with reductions in C3, and the glomerular and dermal deposits of P and C3 suggest that alternative pathway amplification occurs with active SLE (GEWURZ et al., 1968a; MCLEAN et al., 1973; HUNSICKER et al., 1972).

About 10–20% of patients with chronic glomerulonephritis have markedly reduced serum levels of C3 and a characteristic morphological glomerular lesion, termed membranoproliferative (or mesangiocapillary) glomerulonephritis (MPGN). GEWURZ et al. (1968a) found that the serum levels of C1, C4, and C2 were within normal limits in these patients, despite depressions of C3, and called attention to the resemblance of this pattern of complement utilization to that induced by addition of zymosan or endotoxin to serum. Low serum levels of P (McLEAN et al., 1973) and deposits of P together with C3 occur in a high proportion of renal biopsies from patients with MPGN (WESTBERG et al., 1971) and depressed serum levels of factor B also have been found (McLEAN et al., 1973; HUNSICKER et al., 1972; WESTBERG et al., 1971). Although lowering of serum C3 levels may, in some cases, reflect hyposynthesis (ALPER and ROSEN, 1967), hypercatabolism has also been observed especially in adult patients (RUDDY et al., 1975b). Immune complexes have not been found in patients with MPGN, and immunosuppressive drugs that are effective in reversing the acute nephritis and depressions of serum complement found in SLE, do not appreciably alter the course or hypocomplementaemia of MPGN. Sera of some patients with MPGN contain a protein, C3NeF, that is capable of activating the alternative pathway when added to normal serum (SPITZER et al., 1969). C3NeF is present also in patients with partial lipodystrophy who may manifest MPGN and low serum levels of C3 with normal levels of C1, C4, and C2 (PETERS et al., 1973). The persistence of C3NeF after bilateral nephrectomy (VALLOTA et al., 1971) is compatible with it being an autoantibody to C3bBb (DAHA et al., 1978). C3b-receptors in the epithelial surface of human glomerular capillary walls (GELFAND et al., 1976) could bind C3b to localize C3bBb convertase formation, which C3NeF could stabilize, thereby permitting efficient activation of the terminal sequence. Although activation of C3-C9 in MPGN occurs predominantly by the alternative pathway, the classical pathway can be involved (WESTBERG et al., 1971; RUDDY et al., 1975d). Electron microscopy distinguishes patients with dense intramembranous deposits, who may have low serum levels of C3 and normal C4, from those with subendothelial deposits, who frequently have depressions of both components (HABIB et al., 1974).

K. Pharmacological Agents

I. Activators

Complement depletion by systemic activation might be hazardous if acute and is not currently feasible in the human. The use of reagents such as zymosan, immune aggregates and endotoxin is precluded by their systemic effects. CVF, which has been used experimentally in animals, is limited by its immunogenicity. There are several in vitro examples of pharmacological facilitators of complement function: poly-1-lysine antagonism of the C5b67 inhibitor (McLEOD et al., 1975); epsilon aminocaproic acid (EACA) inhibition of C3bINA with resultant activation of the amplification pathway (VOGT et al., 1975); and initiation of the alternative pathway by certain sulphated dextrans (BURGER et al., 1975).

II. Inhibitors

Many inhibitors of the complement pathways have been described (Table 3), but only those which have been useful in delineating the molecular mechanisms of

Table 3. Synthetic inhibitors of complement

Complement component or step in the reaction sequence inhibited	Specific inhibitor	Reference
Properdin	—	—
$\bar{\text{D}}$	$\bar{\text{D}}$FP	FEARON et al, 1974
	Cyclohexylbutylphosphonofluoridate	FEARON and AUSTEN, 1975d
	TAMe	FEARON and AUSTEN, 1975d
Activation of C1	TAMe and related esters of aromatic amino acid derivatives	STROUD et al., 1965 KONDO et al., 1972
	Antrypol	FONG and GOOD, 1972
	Maleopimaric acid and other levopimaric acid derivatives	GLOVSKY et al., 1968
C1g	Diamines	SLEDGE and BING, 1973
	Polyanions such as heparin liquoid, dextran sulfate	RAEPPLE et al., 1976
C$\bar{1}$r	DFP	BECKER, 1956
C$\bar{1}$s	DFP	BECKER, 1956
	Benzamidine and pyridinium fluorosulfonyl compounds	BAKER and CORY, 1971
C4	cinnarizine	DIPERRI and AUTERI, 1973
C2 binding	Polyanions such as heparin liquoid, dextran sulfate	—
C$\overline{462}$a	*n*-Acetyl-1-tyrosine methylester	KONDO et al., 1972
C3b binding	Phloridzin	POLLEY and MÜLLER-EBERHARD, 1968 SHIN and MAYER, 1968c
	n-Acetyl-1-tyrosyl ethylester	SHIN and MAYER, 1968c
	Salicylaldoxine	SHIN and MAYER, 1968c
B binding	Gold sodium thiomalate	BURGE et al., 1978
	Heparin	WEILER et al., 1978
C5 activation	*n*-Acetyl-1-tyrosyl ethylester	SHIN and MAYER, 1968c
C5b binding	Phloridzin	SHIN and MAYER, 1968c
C5b67	Maleopimaric acid	GLOVSKY et al., 1968
C8	C8 analogue	STOLFI, 1970
	Antrypol	STOLFI, 1970
C9	—	—

complement activation will be noted. By studying the affinity of various inhibitors for C$\bar{1}$, BECKER (1965) postulated that the C$\bar{1}$ serine esterase site must be negatively charged. BING (1969) extended these studies and found that the active site of C$\bar{1}$ is hydrophobic. FEARON and AUSTEN (1975d) found that $\bar{\text{D}}$ enzymatic activity on B is irreversibly inhibited by 10^{-3} *M* DFP and competitively inhibited with 10^{-2} *M*

TAMe (p-tosyl-1-arginine methyl ester), a synthetic substrate. Thus $\bar{D}$, like $C\bar{1}$, is a serine esterase. RAEPPLE et al. (1976) have shown that some of the polyanions such as heparin, polyvinylsulphate, dextran sulphate and liquoid which inhibit C1 do so by interfering with the ability of C1q to bind to immune complexes. In fact these substances can complex with isolated C1q and form a precipitate. Polyanions can also block the binding of native C2 to C4b prior to its cleavage-activation. This inhibition appears to depend on the ability of the polyanion to complex Mg^{++} since the addition of extra Mg^{++} can overcome the inhibition (LOOS et al., 1976). The fact that polyanions have no effect on the EAC4b2a is consistent with the fact that free Mg^{++} is not required once the C4bC2a complex is formed. Phloridzin, salicylaldoxine and several amino acid ester derivatives inhibit C3 and C5 fixation steps with little or no effect on the ability of the classical C3 and C5 convertase to cleave these components (SHIN and MAYER, 1968c). Heparin (WEILER et al., 1978) and gold sodium thiomalate (BURGE et al., 1978) interact reversibly with C3b to inhibit its interaction with B and $\bar{D}$ to form C3bBb. These inhibitors have made it possible to separate the simple enzymatic cleavage of a complement component from the more complicated haemolytic activation of the component.

Some complement inhibitors have been utilized to investigate the dependence of various biological phenomena on the complement system. The local Forssman reaction, which is essentially a tissue antigen-antibody-induced vasculitis, can be inhibited by fumaropimaric acid (FEINMAN et al., 1970) which dissociates the C5b67i chemotactic fragment but also suppresses clotting and histamine release. Cu-chlorophyllin which inhibits the in vitro sequence at the C5 activation step (NISHIOKA, 1964), has been claimed to inhibit anaphylaxis (BÜSING, 1957), allograft rejection and tumor cell killing in mice (FUJII et al., 1966). It must be noted, however, that anaphylaxis is not a complement-dependent reaction and that none of the effects were closely related to the degree of inhibition of the complement titre (FUJII et al., 1966; FRIEDBERG et al., 1969).

The use of complement inhibitors in clinical situations has been limited to the treatment of hereditary angio-oedema. EACA and a related agent, trans-4-aminomethyl-cyclohexane-1-carboxylic acid (tranexamic acid), are of prophylactic value in preventing spontaneous or post-operative attacks (FRANK et al., 1972; SHEFFER et al., 1972, 1977b). EACA inhibits the activation of $C\bar{1}s$, possibly by blocking $C\bar{1}r$ (SOTER et al., 1975) and also prevents plasminogen activation (ALKJAERSIG et al., 1958; ABLONDI et al., 1959; KAPLAN and AUSTEN, 1972) and plasmin activity (ABLONDI et al., 1959; BROCKWAY and CASTELLINO, 1971). EACA action could be at either of the latter sites since plasmin can activate C1 (RATNOFF and NAFF, 1967) and since active Hageman factor, which is inhibited by C1INH (SCHREIBER et al., 1973), activates the plasminogen pathway (KAPLAN and AUSTEN, 1972). Testosterone also has a beneficial effect in preventing spontaneous attacks (SPAULDING, 1960) by correcting the $C\bar{1}$INH deficiency (SHEFFER et al., 1977a); attenuated androgens are particularly useful in correcting the biochemical deficiency with only modest side effects (ROSSE et al., 1976). Both spontaneous attacks (JAFFE et al., 1975) and post-operative attacks have been favourably affected by infusions of $C\bar{1}$INH in whole plasma but this therapy represents a possible hazard because of the simultaneous introduction of more substrate.

References

Ablondi, F. B., Hagen, J. J., Philips, M., Derenzo, E. C.: Inhibition of plasmin, trypsin and the streptokinase-activated fibrinolytic system by ε-aminocaproic acid. Arch. Biochem. Biophys. **82**, 153—160 (1959)

Abramovitch, A. S., Michaels, D. W., Mayer, M. M.: Planar lipid bilayers as model targets for the C56-9 complement attack mechanism. Fed. Proc. **35**, 493a (1976)

Abramson, N., Alper, C. A., Lachmann, P. J., Rosen, F. S., Jandl, J. H.: Deficiency of C3 inactivator in man. J. Immunol. **107**, 19—27 (1971)

Alkjaersig, N., Fletcher, A. P., Sherry, S. J.: ε-aminocaproic acid: an inhibitor of plasminogen activation. J. Biol. Chem. **234**, 832—837 (1958)

Allen, F. H., jr.: Linkage of HL-A and GBG. Vox Sang **27**, 382—384 (1974)

Alper, C. A., Balavitch, D.: Evidence that cobra venom factor (CoF) is cobra C3. J. Immunol. **116**, 1727 (1976)

Alper, C. A., Rosen, F. S.: Studies in the in vivo behavior of human C'3 in normal subjects and patients. J. Clin. Invest. **46**, 2021—2030 (1967)

Alper, C. A., Propp, R. P., Klemperer, M. R., Rosen, F. S.: Inherited deficiency of the third component of human complement (C'3). J. Clin. Invest. **48**, 553—557 (1969)

Alper, C. A., Abramson, N., Johnston, R. B., Jandl, J. H., Rosen, F. S.: Increased susceptibility to infection associated with abnormalities of complement mediated functions and of the third component of complement (C3) N. Engl. J. Med. **282**, 349—354 (1970a)

Alper, C. A., Abramson, N., Johnston, R. B., Jandl, J. H., Rosen, F. S.: Studies in vivo and in vitro on an abnormality in the metabolism of C3 in a patient with increased susceptibility to infection. J. Clin. Invest. **49**, 1975—1985 (1970b)

Alper, C. A., Boenisch, T., Watson, L.: Genetic polymorphism in human glycine-rich beta-glycoprotein. J. Exp. Med. **135**, 68—80 (1972a)

Alper, C. A., Colten, H. R., Rosen, F. S., Rabson, A. R., MacNab, G. N., Gear, J. S. S.: Homozygous deficiency of C3 in a patient with repeated infections. Lancet II, 1179—1181 (1972b)

Alper, C. A., Rosen, F. S., Lachmann, P. J.: Inactivator of the third component of complement as an inhibitor in the properdin pathway. Proc. Natl. Acad. Sci. (Wash.) **69**, 2910—2913 (1972c)

Arroyave, C. M., Müller-Eberhard, H. J.: Isolation of the sixth component of complement from human serum. Immunochemistry **8**, 995—1006 (1971)

Arroyave, C. M., Müller-Eberhard, H. J.: Isolation of the seventh component of the complement system from human serum. J. Immunol. **111**, 302 (abstract) (1973)

Assimeh, S. N., Bing, D. H., Painter, R. H.: A simple method for the isolation of the subcomponents of the first component of complement by affinity chromatography. J. Immunol. **113**, 225—234 (1974)

Austen, K. F., Sheffer, A. L.: Detection of hereditary angioneurotic edema by demonstration of a reduction in the second component of human complement. New. Engl. J. Med. **272**, 649—655 (1965)

Bach, S., Ruddy, S., Maclaren, A. J., Austen, K. F.: Electrophoretic polymorphism of the fourth component of human complement (C4) in paired maternal and foetal plasmas. Immunology **21**, 869—878 (1971)

Baker, B. R., Cory, M.: Irreversible enzyme inhibitors 186. Irreversible enzyme inhibitors of the C'1a component of complement derived from m-(phenoxy propoxy) benzamidine by bridging to a terminal sulfonyl fluoride. J. Med. Chem. **14**, 805—811 (1971)

Ballow, M., Yang, S. Y., Day, N. K.: Complete absence of the third component of complement. Fed. Proc. **34**, 853 (abstract) (1975)

Barkas, T., Scott, G. K., Fothergill, J. E.: Purification, characterization and active site studies on human serum complement subcomponent C1s. Biochem. Soc. Trans. **1**, 1219—1220 (1973)

Becker, E. L.: Concerning the mechanism of complement action. II. The nature of the first component of guinea pig complement. J. Immunol. **77**, 469—478 (1956)

Becker, E. L.: Small molecular weight inhibitors of complement action. In: Ciba Foundation Symposium "Complement", Boston: Little Brown 1965

Ben-Efraim, S., Cinader, B.: The role of complement in the passive cutaneous reaction of mice. J. Exp. Med. **120**, 925—942 (1964)

Bentley, C., Bitter-Suermann, D., Hadding, U., Brade, V.: In vitro synthesis of factor B of the alternative pathway of complement activation by mouse peritoneal macrophages. Immunology **30**, 171—179 (1976)
Bianco, C., Griffen, F., Silverstein, S. C.: Studies of the macrophage complement receptor. Alteration of receptor function upon macrophage activation. J. Exp. Med. **141**, 1278—1290 (1975)
Bing, D. H.: Nature of the active site of a subunit of the first component of human complement. Biochemistry **8**, 4503—4510 (1969)
Bing, D. H., Spurlock, S. E., Bern, M. M.: Synthesis of the first component of complement by primary cultures of human tumors and comparable normal tissue. Clin. Immunol. Immunopathol. **4**, 341—351 (1975)
Boackle, R. J., Pruitt, K. M., Mestecky, J.: The interaction of human complement with interfacially aggregated preparations of human secretory IgA. Immunochemistry **11**, 543—548 (1974)
Bokisch, V. A., Müller-Eberhard, H. J.: Anaphylatoxin inactivator of human plasma: its isolation and characterization as a carboxypeptidase. J. Clin. Invest. **49**, 2427—2436 (1970)
Bokisch, V. A., Dierich, M. P., Müller-Eberhard, H. J.: Third component of complement (C3): structural properties in relation of functions. Proc. Natl. Acad. Sci. U.S.A. **72**, 1989—1993 (1975)
Borsos, T., Rapp, H. J.: Complement fixation on cell surfaces by 19s and 7s antibodies. Science **150**, 505—506 (1965)
Borsos, T., Rapp, H. J., Mayer, M. M.: Studies on the second component of complement. The reaction between EAC'1, 4, and C'2: evidence on the single site mechanism of immune hemolysis and determination of C2 on a molecular basis. J. Immunol. **87**, 310—325 (1961)
Borsos, T., Rapp, H. J., Colten, H. R.: Immune hemolysis and the functional properties of the second (C2) and fourth (C4) components of complement I. Functional differences among C4 sites on cell surfaces. J. Immunol. **105**, 1439—1446 (1970)
Boyer, J. T., Gall, E. P., Norman, M. E., Nilsson, U. R.: Hereditary deficiency of the seventh component of complement. J. Clin. Invest. **56**, 905—913 (1975)
Brade, V., Lee, G. D., Nicholson, A., Shin, H. S., Mayer, M. M.: The reactions of zymosan with the properdin system in normal and C4-deficient guinea pig serum. J. Immunol. **111**, 1389—1400 (1973)
Brade, V., Nicholson, A., Lee, G. D., Mayer, M. M.: The reaction of zymosan with the properdin system: isolation of purified factor D from guinea pig serum and study of its reaction characteristics. J. Immunol. **112**, 1845—1854 (1974a)
Brade, V., Nicholson, A., Bitter-Suermann, D., Hadding, U.: Formation of the C3-cleaving properdin enzyme on zymosan. Demonstration that factor D is replaceable by proteolytic enzymes: J. Immunol. **113**, 1735—1743 (1974b)
Brade, V., Dieminger, L., Schmidt, G., Vogt, W.: Incompatibility between C3b and B of guinea pig and man and its influence on the titration of the alternative pathway factors D and B in these two species. Immunology **30**, 171—179 (1976)
Brade, V., Hall, R. E., Colten, H. R.: Biosynthesis of pro-C3, a precursor of the third component of complement. J. Exp. Med. **146**, 759—765 (1977)
Breslow, J., Rothman, P., Colten, H. R.: unpublished, 1975
Britton, M. C., Schur, P. H.: The complement system in rheumatoid synovitis. II. Intracytoplasmic inclusions of immunoglobulins and complement. Arthritis Rheum. **14**, 87—95 (1971)
Brockway, W. J., Castellino, F. M.: The mechanism of the inhibition of plasmin activity by ε-aminocaproic acid. J. Biol. Chem. **246**, 4641—4647 (1971)
Büsing, K. H.: Die Hemmbarkeit des Komplements bei Antigen-Antikörper-Reaktionen in vitro und anaphylaktischen Reaktionen in vivo. Allergie Asthma **3**, 15—22 (1957)
Burge, J. J., Fearon, D. T., Austen, K. F.: Inhibition of the alternative pathway of complement by gold sodium thiomalate in vitro. J. Immunol. (in press) (1978)
Burger, R., Hadding, U., Bitter-Suermann, D.: Dextran sulfate; Influence of molecular size and degree of sulfation on the activation of complement via the alternative pathway. Fed. Proc. **34**, 981a (1975)
Caldwell, J. R., Ruddy, S., Schur, P. H., Austen, K. F.: Acquired $C\bar{1}$ inhibitor deficiency in lymphosarcoma. Clin. Immunol. Immunopathol. **1**, 39—52 (1972)
Caldwell, J., Ruddy, S., Austen, K. F.: Assay of complement components C1, C4, C2, C3, and C9 in whole rat serum. Int. Arch. Allergy Appl. Immunol. **43**, 887—897 (1973)

Chapitis, J., Lepow, I.: Multiple sedimenting species of properdin in human serum and interaction of purified properdin with the third component of complement. J. Exp. Med. **143**, 241—257 (1976)
Cochrane, C. G., Janoff, A.: The Arthus reaction: a model of neutrophil and complement-mediated injury. In: Zweifach, B. W., Grant, L., McClusky, R. T. (Eds.): The Inflammatory Process, 2nd Ed. New York: Academic Press, 1974
Cochrane, C. G., Müller-Eberhard, H. J.: The derivation of two distinct anaphylatoxin activities from the third and fifth component of human complement. J. Exp. Med. **127**, 371—386 (1968)
Cochrane, C. G., Müller-Eberhard, H. J., Aikin, B. S.: Depletion of plasma complement in vivo by a protein of cobra venom: its effect on various immunologic reactions. J. Immunol. **105**, 55—69 (1970)
Colten, H. R.: Ontogeny of the human complement system: in vitro biosynthesis of individual complement components by fetal tissues. J. Clin. Invest. **51**, 725—730 (1972)
Colten, H. R.: Biosynthesis of the fifth component of complement (C5) by human fetal tissues. Clin. Immunol. Immunopathol. **1**, 346—352 (1973)
Colten, H. R.: Biosynthesis of complement. In: Dixon, F. J., Kunkel, H. G. (Eds.): *Advances* in Immunology, Vol. 22, New York: Academic Press. 1976
Colten, H. R., Parkman, R.: Biosynthesis of C4 (fourth component of complement) by hybrids of C4-deficient guinea pig cells and HeLa cells. Science **176**, 1029—1031 (1972)
Colten, H. R., Borsos, T., Rapp, H. J.: In vitro synthesis of the first component of complement by guinea pig small intestine. Proc. Natl. Acad. Sci. U.S.A. **56**, 1158—1163 (1966)
Colten, H. R., Gordon, J. M., Borsos, T., Rapp, H. J.: Synthesis of the first component of human complement in vitro. J. Exp. Med. **128**, 595—604 (1968)
Cook, C. T., Shin, H. S., Mayer, M. M., Laudenslayer, K. A.: The fifth component of the guinea pig complement system. I. Purification and characterization. J. Immunol. **106**, 467—472 (1971)
Cooper, N. R.: Immune adherence by the fourth component of complement. Science **165**, 396—398 (1969)
Cooper, N. R.: Isolation and analysis of the mechanism of action of an inactivator of C4b in normal human serum. J. Exp. Med. **141**, 890—903 (1975)
Daha, M. R., Fearon, D. T., Austen, K. F.: C3 nephritic factor (C3NeF): stabilization of fluid phase and cell-bound alternative pathway convertase. J. Immunol. **116**, 1—7 (1976a)
Daha, M. R., Fearon, D. T., Austen, K. F.: Isolation of alternative pathway C3 convertase containing uncleaved B and formed in the presence of C3 nephritic factor (C3NeF). J. Immunol. **116**, 568—570 (1976b)
Daha, M. R., Fearon, D. T., Austen, K. F.: Additional C3 requirement for alternative pathway C5 convertase. Fed. Proc. **35**, 654 (abstract) (1976c)
Daha, M. R., Fearon, D. T., Austen, K. F.: The incorporation of C3 nephritic factor (C3NeF) into a stabilized C3 convertase, C3bBb(C3NeF), and its release after decay of convertase function. J. Immunol. **119**, 812—817 (1977)
Daha, M. R., Austen, K. F., Fearon, D. T.: Heterogeneity, polypeptide chain composition and antigenic reactivity of C3 nephritic factor. J. Immunol. (in press) (1978)
Davis, J. S., IV, Colten, H. R., Alper, C. A.: A second case of homozygous C3 deficiency (unpublished data)
Day, N. K. B., Gewurz, H., Johannsen, R., Finstad, J., Good, R. A.: Complement and complement-like activity in lower vertebrates and invertebrates. J. Exp. Med. **132**, 941—950 (1970)
DeShazo, C. V., Henson, P. M., Cochrane, C. G.: Acute immunologic arthritis in rabbits. J. Clin. Invest. **51**, 50—57 (1972a)
DeShazo, C. V., McGrade, M., Henson, P. M., Cochrane, C. G.: The effect of complement depletion on neutrophil migration in acute immunologic arthritis. J. Immunol. **108**, 1414—1419 (1972b)
Dias da Silva, W., Lepow, I. H.: Complement as a mediator of inflammation. II. Biological properties of anaphylatoxin prepared with purified components of human complement. J. Exp. Med. **125**, 921—946 (1967)
Dias da Silva, W., Eisele, I. W., Lepow, I. H.: Complement as a mediator of inflammation. III. Purification of the activity with anaphylatoxin properties generated by interaction of the first four components of complement and its identification as a cleavage product of C'3. J. Exp. Med. **126**, 1027—1048 (1967)

Dierich, M. P., Ferrone, S., Pelligrino, M. A., Reisfeld, R. A.: Chemical modulation of cell surfaces by sulphydryl components: effect on C3b receptors. J. Immunol. **113**, 940—947 (1974)

Donaldson, V. H., Evans, R. R.: A biochemical abnormality in hereditary angioneurotic edema. Absence of serum inhibitor of C'1-esterase. Am. J. Med. **35**, 37—44 (1963)

Donaldson, V. H., Rosen, F. S.: Action of complement in hereditary angioneurotic edema. The role of C'1 esterase. J. Clin. Invest. **43**, 2004—2011 (1964)

Donaldson, V. H. G., Ratnoff, O. D., Dias da Silva, W., Rosen, F. S.: Permeability-increasing activity in hereditary angioneurotic edema plasma. II. Mechanism of formation and partial characterization. J. Clin. Invest. **48**, 642—653 (1969)

Donaldson, V. H., Merler, E., Rosen, F. S., Kretschmer, K. W., Lepow, I. H.: A polypeptide kinin in hereditary angioneurotic edema plasma: role of complement in its formation. J. Lab. Clin. Med. **76**, 986—997 (1970)

Einstein, L. P., Alper, C. A., Block, K. J., Herrin, J. T., Rosen, F. S., David, J. R., Colten, H. R.: Biosynthetic defect in monocytes from human beings with genetic deficiency of the second component of complement. N. Engl. J. Med. **292**, 1169—1171 (1975).

Einstein, L. P., Schneeberger, E. E., Colten, H. R.: Synthesis of the second component of complement by long-term primary cultures of human monocytes. J. Exp. Med. **143**, 114—126 (1976)

Einstein, L. P., Hansen, P. J., Ballow, M., Davis, A. E., Davis, J. S., Alper, C. A., Rosen, F. S., Colten, H. R.: Biosynthesis of the third component of complement (C3) in vitro by monocytes from both normal and homozygous C3 deficient humans. J. Clin. Invest. **60**, 963—969 (1977)

Ellerson, J. R., Yasmean, D., Painter, R. H., Domington, K. J.: A fragment corresponding to the C_H2 region of IgG with complement fixing activity. FEBS Lett. **24**, 319—323 (1972)

Ellman, L., Green, I., Frank, M.: Genetically controlled total deficiency of the fourth component of complement in the guinea pig. Science **170**, 74—75 (1970)

Ellman, L., Green, I., Judge, F., Frank, M. M.: In vivo studies in C4-deficient guinea pigs. J. Exp. Med. **134**, 162—175 (1971)

Fearon, D. T., Austen, K. F.: Initation of C3 cleavage in the alternative complement pathway. J. Immunol. **115**, 1357—1361 (1975a)

Fearon, D. T., Austen, K. F.: Properdin: initiation of alternative complement pathway. Proc. Nat. Acad. Sci. U.S.A. **72**, 3220—3224 (1975b)

Fearon, D. T., Austen, K. F.: Properdin: binding to C3b and stabilization of the C3-dependent C3 convertase. J. Exp. Med. **142**, 856—863 (1975c)

Fearon, D. T., Austen, K. F.: Inhibition of complement-derived enzymes. Ann. N.Y. Acad. Sci. U.S.A. **256**, 441—450 (1975d)

Fearon, D. T., Austen, K. F.: Activation of the alternative complement pathway due to resistance of zymosan-bound amplification convertase to endogenous regulatory mechanisms. Proc. Natl. Acad. Sci. U.S.A. **74**, 1683—1687 (1977a)

Fearon, D. T., Austen, K. F.: Activation of the alternative complement pathway with rabbit erythrocytes by circumvention of the regulatory action of endogenous control proteins. J. Exp. Med. **146**, 22—33 (1977b)

Fearon, D. T., Austen, K. F., Ruddy, S.: Formation of a hemolytically active cellular intermediate by the interaction between properdin factors B and D and the activated third component of complement. J. Exp. Med. **138**, 1305—1313 (1973)

Fearon, D. T., Austen, K. F., Ruddy, S.: Properdin factor D: characterization of its active site and isolation of the precursor form. J. Exp. Med. **139**, 355—366 (1974)

Feinman, L., Cohen, S., Becker, E. L.: The effect of fumaropimaric acid on delayed hypersensitivity and cutaneous Forssman reaction in the guinea pig. J. Immunol. **104**, 1401—1405 (1970)

Fong, J. S. C., Good, R. A.: Suramin—a potent reversible and competitive inhibitor of complement systems. Clin. Exp. Immunol. **10**, 127—138 (1972)

Fostiropoulos, G., Austen, K. F., Bloch, K. J.: Total hemolytic complement and second component of complement ($C'2^{hu}$) activity in serum and synovial fluid. Arthritis Rheum. **8**, 219—232 (1965)

Frank, M. M., May, J., Garther, T., Ellman, L.: In vitro studies of complement function in sera of C4-deficient guinea pigs. J. Exp. Med. **134**, 176—187 (1971)

Frank, M. M., Sergent, J. S., Kane, M. A., Alling, D. W.: Epsilon aminocaproic acid therapy of hereditary angioneurotic edema: a double-blind study. N. Engl. J. Med. **286**, 808—812 (1972)

Friedberg, K. D., Garbe, G., Grützmacher, J.: Untersuchungen über die antianaphylaktische Wirkung des Chlorophyllins. Naunyn-Schmiedbergs Arch. Pharmacol. **265**, 287—300 (1969)
Friedberger, E.: Kritik der Theorien über die Anaphylaxie. Z. Immunitäetsforsch. **2**, 208—224 (1909)
Fu, S. M., Kunkel, H. G., Brusman, H. P., Allen Jr., F. H., Fotino, M.: Histocompatibility genes and those involved in the synthesis of the second component of complement. J. Exp. Med. **140**, 1108—1111 (1974)
Fujii, G., Suzuki, M., Hirose, Y., Goto, S., Ishibashi, Y., Haga, K., Sindo, T.: Effect of sodium-copper-chlorophyllin as a complement inhibitor on the allograft reaction. Jpn. J. Exp. Med. **36**, 499—507 (1966)
Fuller, L., Iglesias, E., Jensen, J. A.: Purification and properties of the C4 inactivator from nurse shark serum. Immunochemistry **11**, 93—98 (1974)
Geiger, H., Day, N., Good, R. A.: Ontogenetic development and synthesis of hemolytic C8 by piglet tissues. J. Immunol. **108**, 1092—1097 (1972)
Gelfand, M. C., Shin, M. L., Frank, M. M., Nagle, R., Green, I.: A receptor for activated C3 in the normal and abnormal human renal glomerular capillary wall. J. Immunol. **116**, 1733 (abstract) (1976)
Gewurz, H., Finstad, J., Muschel, I., Good, R. A.: In: Smith, R. T. (Ed.): Phylogeny of Immunity. Gainesville (Florida): Univ. of Florida Press 1967
Gewurz, H., Pickering, R. J., Mergenhagen, S. E., Good, R. A.: The complement profile in acute glomerulonephritis, systemic lupus erythematosus, and hypocomplementemic glomerulonephritis. Int. Arch. Allergy Appl. Immunol. **34**, 556—570 (1968a)
Gewurz, H., Pickering, R. J., Christian, C. L., Snyderman, R., Mergenhagen, S. E., Good, R. A.: Decreased C′1q protein concentration and agglutinating activity in agammaglobulinaemia syndromes: an inborn error reflected in the complement system. Clin. Exp. Immunol. **3**, 437—445 (1968b)
Gigli, I., Austen, K. F.: Fluid phase destruction of $C2^{hu}$ by $C1^{hu}$. I. Its enhancement and inhibition by homologous and heterologous C4. J. Exp. Med. **129**, 679—696 (1969a)
Gigli, I., Austen, K. F.: Fluid phase destruction of $C2^{hu}$ by $C1^{hu}$ II. Unmasking by $C4i^{hu}$ of $\overline{C1}^{hu}$ specificity for $C2^{hu}$. J. Exp. Med. **130**, 833—846 (1969b)
Gigli, I., Austen, K. F.: Phylogeny and function of the complement system. Annu. Rev. Microbiol. **25**, 309—332 (1971)
Gigli, I., Nelson, R. A.: Complement dependent immune phagocytosis. I. Requirements for C′1, C′4, C′2, and C′3. Exp. Cell Res. **51**, 45—67 (1968)
Gigli, I., Ruddy, S., Austen, K. F.: The stoichiometric measurement of the serum inhibitor of the first component of complement by the inhibition of immune hemolysis. J. Immunol. **100**, 1154—1164 (1968)
Gitlin, J. D., Rosen, F. S., Lachmann, P. J.: The mechanism of action of the C3b inactivator (conglutinogen-activating factor) on its naturally occurring substrate, the major fragment of the third component of complement (C3b). J. Exp. Med. **141**, 1221—1226 (1975)
Glovsky, M. M., Becker, E., Halbrook, N. J.: Inhibition of guinea pig complement by maleopimaric acid and other derivatives of levopimaric acid. J. Immunol. **100**, 979—990 (1968)
Gocke, D. J., Osler, A. G.: In vitro damage of rabbit platelets by an unrelated antigen-antibody reaction. I. General characteristics of the reaction. J. Immunol. **94**, 236—246 (1965)
Götze, O., Müller-Eberhard, H. J.: Lysis of erythrocytes by complement in the absence of antibody. J. Exp. Med. **132**, 898—915 (1970)
Götze, O., Müller-Eberhard, H. J.: The C3 activator system: an alternate pathway of complement activation. J. Exp. Med. **134**, 90s—108s (1971)
Götze, O., Medicus, R., Müller-Eberhard, H. J.: Comparative analysis of the properties of active and precursor properdin. J. Immunol. (abstract) **116**, 1735 (1976)
Goetzl, E. J., Austen, K. F.: Active site chemotactic factors and the regulation of the human neutrophil chemotactic response. In: Sorkin, E. (Ed.): Antibiotics and Chemotherapy, Vol. 19, pp. 218—232, Chemotaxis: Its Biology and Biochemistry. Basel: S. Karger, 1974
Goldlust, M. B., Shin, H. S., Hammer, C. H., Mayer, M. M.: Studies of complement complex C5b,6 eluted from EAC-6: reaction of C5b,6 with EAC4b, 3b and evidence on the role of C2a and C3b in the activation of C5. J. Immunol. **113**, 998—1007 (1974)

Goldman, J. N., Ruddy, S., Austen, K. F.: Reaction mechanism of nascent C$\overline{567}$ (reactive lysis). I. Reaction characteristics for production of EC$\overline{567}$ and lysis by C8 and C9. J. Immunol. **109**, 353—359 (1972)
Graff, K. S., Leddy, J. P., Breckenridge, R. T.: Platelet function in man: a requirement for C5. J. Immunol. **116**, 1735 (abstract) (1976)
Grey, H. M.: Phylogeny of immunoglobulins. In: Dixon, F. J., Kunkel, H. G. (Eds.): Advances in Immunology, Vol. X. New York-London: Academic Pr. 1969
Griffen, F. M., Bianco, C., Silverstein, S. C.: Characterization of the macrophage receptor for complement and demonstration of its functional independence from the receptor for the Fc portion of the immunoglobulin G. J. Exp. Med. **141**, 1269—1277 (1975)
Habib, R., Loirat, C., McBugler, M., Levy, M.: Morphology and serum complement levels in membranoproliferative glomerulnephritis. Adv. Nephrol. **4**, 109—136 (1974)
Hadding, U., Müller-Eberhard, H. J.: The ninth component of human complement: isolation, description and mode of action. Immunology **16**, 719—735 (1969)
Haines, A. L., Lepow, I. H.: Studies on human C'1 esterase II. function of purified C'1 esterase in the human complement system. J. Immunol. **92**, 468—478 (1964)
Hall, R. E., Colten, H. R.: Genetic deficiency of the fourth component of complement (C4). Defective translation of C4 messenger RNA (abstract). Clin. Res. **25**, 483 (1977)
Hammer, C. H., Nicholson, A., Mayer, M. M.: On the mechanism of cytolysis by complement. Evidence on insertion of the C5b and C7 subunits of the C5b,6,7 complex into the phospholipid bilayer of the erythrocyte membrane, Proc. Natl. Acad. Sci. U.S.A. **72**, 5076—5080 (1975)
Hammer, C. H., Abramovitz, A. S., Mayer, M. M.: A new activity of complement component C3: cell-bound C3b potentiates lysis of erythrocytes by C5b,6 and terminal components. J. Immunol. **117**, 830—834 (1977)
Harpel, P. C.: Studies on human plasma α2-macroglobulin interactions. Evidence of proteolytic modification of the subunit chain structure. J. Exp. Med. **138**, 508—520 (1973)
Harpel, P. C., Cooper, N. R.: Studies on human plasma C1-inactivator-enzyme interactions. I. Mechanisms of interaction with C$\overline{1}$s, plasmin and trypsin. J. Clin. Invest. **55**, 593—604 (1975)
Harris Jr., E. D., Dibona, D. R., Krane, S. M.: Collagenases in human synovial fluid. J. Clin. Invest. **48**, 2104—2116 (1969)
Hartmann, K. U., Bokisch, V. A.: Stimulation of murine B lymphocytes by purified human C3b. Fed. Proc. **34**, 854 (1975)
Hauptmann, G., Grosshans, E., Heid, E.: Lupus erythemateux aigus et deficits hereditaires en complement. A propos d'un cas par deficit complet en C4. Ann. Dermatol. Syphiligr. (Paris) **101**, 479—476 (1974)
Hedberg, H.: Studies on synovial fluid in arthritis. I. The total complement activity. Acta Med. Scand. (Suppl.) **9**, 78 (1967)
Henson, P. M.: Mechanisms of release of constituents from rabbit platelets by antigen-antibody complexes and complement I. Lytic and non lytic reactions. J. Immunol. **105**, 476—489 (1970)
Henson, P. M.: Complement-dependent adherence of cells to antigen and antibody. Mechanisms and consequences. In: Ingram, D. G. (Ed.): Biological Activities of Complement. New York: S. Karger 1972
Henson, P. M., Cochrane, C. G.: Immunological induction of increased vascular permeability. II. Two mechanisms of histamine release from rabbit platelets involving complement. J. Exp. Med. **129**, 167—184 (1969)
Henson, P. M., Cochrane, C. G.: Acute immune complex disease in rabbits. The role of complement and of a leukocyte-dependent release of vasoactive amines from platelets. J. Exp. Med. **135**, 554—569 (1971)
Hobart, K. J., Alper, C. A., Lachmann, P. J.: Polymorphism of human C6. In: Peeters, H. (Ed.): Protides of the Biologic Fluids. Amsterdam: Elsevier 1974
Huber, H., Polly, M. J., Linscott, M. D., Fudenberg, H. H., Müller-Eberhard, H. J.: Human monocytes. Distinct receptor sites for the third component of complement and for immunoglobulin G. Science **162**, 1281—1283 (1968)
Hugli, T. E., Morgan, W. T., Müller-Eberhard, H. J.: Circular dichromism of C3a anaphylatoxin. J. Biol. Chem. **250**, 1479—1483 (1975)

Humphrey, J. H., Dourmashkin, R. R.: The lesions in cell membranes caused by complement. In: Dixon, F. J., Kunkel, H. G. (Eds.): Advances in Immunology, Vol. II, pp. 75—115. New York: Academic Press 1969
Hunder, G. G., McDuffie, F. C., Hepper, N. G. G.: Pleural fluid complement in systemic lupus erythematosus and rheumatoid arthritis. Ann. Intern. Med. **76**, 357—363 (1972)
Hunder, G. G., Muller, B. J., McDuffie, F. C.: Complement in pericardial fluid of lupus erythematosus. Ann. Intern. Med. **80**, 453—458 (1974)
Hunsicker, L. G., Ruddy, S., Carpenter, C. B., Schur, P. H., Merrill, J. P., Müller-Eberhard, H. J., Austen, K. F.: Metabolism of third complement component (C3) in nephritis. N. Engl. J. Med. **287**, 835—840 (1972)
Hunsicker, L. G., Ruddy, S., Austen, K. F.: Alternate complement pathway. Factors involved in cobra venom factor activation of the third component of complement. J. Immunol. **110**, 128—138 (1973)
Hurst, M. M., Volanakis, J. E., Hester, R. B., Stroud, R. M., Bennett, J. C.: The structural basis for binding of complement by immunoglobulin M. J. Exp. Med. **140**, 1117—1121 (1974)
Ilgen, C. L., Burkholder, P. M.: Isolation of C4-synthesizing cells from guinea pig liver by ficol density gradient centrifugation. Immunology **26**, 197—203 (1974)
Ilgen, C. L., Bossen, E. H., Rowlands, Jr., D. T., Burkholder, P. M.: Isolation and characterization of C4-synthesizing cells from guinea pig spleen. Immunology **26**, 659—665 (1974)
Jaffe, C. J., Atkinson, J. P., Gelfand, A., Frank, M. M.: Hereditary angioedema: The use of fresh frozen plasma for prophylaxis in patients undergoing surgery. J. Allerg. Clin. Immunol. **55**, 386—393 (1975)
Jensen, J. A.: Anaphylatoxin and its relation to the complement system. Science **155**, 1122—1123 (1967)
Jensen, J. A.: A specific inactivator of mammalian C'4 isolated from nurse shark *(Ginglymostoma cirratum)* serum. J. Exp. Med. **130**, 217—241 (1969)
Johnson, A. R., Hugli, T. E., Müller-Eberhard, H. J.: Release of histamine from rat mast cells by the complement peptides C3a and C5a. Immunology **28**, 1069—1080 (1975)
Johnston, Jr., R. B., Klemperer, M. R., Alper, C. A., Rosen, F. S.: The enhancement of bacterial phagocytosis by serum. The role of complement components and two co-factors. J. Exp. Med. **129**, 1275—1290 (1969)
Kaplan, A., Austen, K. F.: The fibrinolytic pathway of human plasma: isolation and characterization of the plasminogen proactivator. J. Exp. Med. **136**, 1378—1393 (1972)
Kempf, R. A., Gigli, I., Austen, K. F.: Inhibition of the lytic effect of guinea pig complement by rabbit complement. J. Immunol. **102**, 795—803 (1969)
Klemperer, M. R., Woodworth, H. C., Rosen, F. S., Austen, K. F.: Hereditary deficiency of the second component of complement (C'2) in man. J. Clin. Invest. **45**, 880—890 (1966)
Knobel, H. R., Heusser, C., Rodrick, M. L., Isliker, H.: Enzymatic digestion of the first component of human complement (C1q). J. Immunol. **112**, 2094—2101 (1974)
Koethe, S. M., Austen, K. F., Gigli, I.: Differentiation of binding from complete activation by use of heterologous components of complement. J. Immunol. **108**, 1063—1072 (1972)
Kohler, P. F., Ten Bensel, R.: Serial complement component alterations in acute glomerulonephritis and systemic lupus erythematosus. Clin. Exp. Immunol. **4**, 191—202 (1969)
Kolb, W. P., Müller-Eberhard, H. J.: The membrane attack mechanism of complement. Isolation and subunit composition of the C5b-9 complex. J. Exp. Med. **141**, 724—735 (1975a)
Kolb, W. P., Müller-Eberhard, H. J.: Neoantigens of the membrane attack complex of human complement. Proc. Natl. Acad. Sci. U.S.A. **72**, 1687—1689 (1975b)
Kolb, W. P., Morgan, W. T., Müller-Eberhard, H. J.: Subunit structure and properties of human C8. J. Immunol. (abstract) **116**, 1738 (1976)
Kondo, M., Gigli, I., Austen, K. F.: Fluid phase destruction of $C2^{hu}$ by $C1^{hu}$. III. Changes in activity for synthetic substrates upon cell binding, heat inactivation and interaction with $\overline{C1}$INH. J. Immunol. **22**, 305—318 (1972)
Koopman, W. J., Sandberg, A. L., Wahl, S. M., Mergenhagen, S. E.: Activation of guinea pig lymphocytes by fragments of the third component of complement. J. Immunol. (abstract) **116**, 1739 (1976)
Lachmann, P. J.: Genetic deficiencies of the complement system. Boll. Ist. Sieroter. Milan. **53** (Suppl. No. 1), 195—207 (1974)

Lachmann, P. J., Thompson, R. A.: Reactive lysis: the complement-mediated lysis of unsensitized cells. II. The characterization of activated reactor as $C\overline{56}$ and the participation of C8 and C9. J. Exp. Med. **131**, 643—657 (1970)

Leber, P. D., McCluskey, R. T.: Immune complex diseases. In: Zweifach, B. W., Grant, L., McCluskey, R. T. (Eds.): The Inflammatory Process, Vol. III. New York: Academic Press 1974

Leddy, J. P., Frank, M. M., Gaither, T., Baum, J., Klemperer, M. R.: Hereditary deficiency of the sixth component of complement in man. I. Immunochemical, biologic and family studies. J. Clin. Invest. **53**, 544—553 (1974)

Lepow, I. H.: Permeability-producing peptide by-product of the interaction of the first, fourth and second components of complement. In: Biochemistry of the Acute Allergic Reactions, 2nd Int. Symp. London: Blackwell 1971

Lerner, R. A., Glossock, R. J., Dixon, F. J.: The role of anti-glomerular basement membrane antibody in the pathogenesis of human glomerulonephritis. J. Exp. Med. **126**, 989—991 (1967)

Levine, L.: Inhibition of immune hemolysis by diisopropylfluorophosphate. Biochim. Biophys. Acta **18**, 283—285 (1955)

Levisohn, S. R., Thompson, E. B.: Contact inhibition and gene expression in HTC/L cell hybrid lines. J. Cell. Physiol. **81**, 225—232 (1973)

Levy, N. L., Snyderman, R., Ladda, R. L.: Cytogenetic engineering in vivo: restoration of biologic complement activity to C5-deficient mice by intravenous inoculation of hybrid cells. Proc. Natl. Acad. Sci. U.S.A. **70**, 3125—3129 (1973)

Linscott, W. D.: Complement: optimal reaction conditions for guinea pig C4. J. Immunol. **111**, 189—199 (1973a)

Linscott, W. D.: Complement: A reversible temperature-dependent alteration in the reactivity of EAC1 with C4. J. Immunol. **111**, 200—211 (1973b)

Linscott, W. D., Cochrane, C. G.: Guinea pig β1C-globulin: its relationship to the third component of complement and its alteration following interaction with immune complexes. J. Immunol. **93**, 972—984 (1964)

Loos, M., Volanakis, J. E., Stroud, R. M.: Mode of interaction of different polyanions with the first (C1, $C\overline{1}$), the second (C2) and the fourth (C4) component of complement. II. Effect of polyanions on the binding of C2 to EAC4b. Immunochemistry **13**, 257—261 (1976)

McCall, C. E., Chatelet, L. R. de, Brown, D., Lachmann, P.: New biological activity following intravascular activation of the complement cascade. Nature **249**, 841—843 (1974)

McLean, R. H., Michael, A. F.: Properdin and C3 proactivator. Alternate pathway components in human glomerulonephritis. J. Clin. Invest. **52**, 634—644 (1973)

McLeod, B., Baker, P., Behrends, C., Gewurz, H.: Studies of the inhibition of $C\overline{56}$-initiated lysis (reactive lysis). IV. Antagonism of the inhibitory activity $C\overline{567}$-INH by poly-1-lysine. Immunology **28**, 379—390 (1975)

Mahler, F., Intaglietta, M., Hugli, T. E., Johnson, A. R.: Influences of C3a anaphylatoxin compared to other vasoactive agents on the microcirculation of the rabbit omentum. Microvasc. Res. **9**, 345—356 (1975)

Manni, J. A., Müller-Eberhard, H. J.: The eighth component of human complement (C8): isolation, characterization and hemolytic efficiency. J. Exp. Med. **130**, 1145—1160 (1969)

Mantovani, B.: Different roles of IgG and complement receptors in phagocytosis by polymorphonuclear leukocytes. J. Immunol. **115**, 15—17 (1975)

Marcus, R. L., Shin, H. S., Mayer, M. M.: An alternate complement pathway: C-3 cleaving activity, not due to C4,2a, on endotoxic lipopolysaccharide after treatment with guinea pig serum; relation to properdin. Proc. Natl. Acad. Sci. U.S.A. **68**, 1351—1354 (1971)

May, J. E., Frank, M. M.: Hemolysis of sheep erythrocytes in guinea pig serum deficient in the fourth component of complement. I. Antibody and serum requirements. J. Immunol. **111**, 1661—1667 (1973a)

May, J. E., Frank, M. M.: Hemolysis of sheep erythrocytes in guinea pig serum deficient in the fourth component of complement. II. Evidence for the involvement of C1 and components of the alternate complement pathway. J. Immunol. **111**, 1668—1676 (1973b)

Mayer, M. M.: Mechanism of cytolysis by complement. Proc. Natl. Acad. Sci. U.S.A. **69**, 2954—2958 (1972)

Medicus, R. G., Götze, O., Müller-Eberhard, H. J.: Alternative pathway of complement: recruitment of precursor properdin by the labile C3/C5 convertase and the potentiation of the pathway. J. Exp. Med. **144**, 1076—1093 (1976a)

Medicus, R. G., Schreiber, R. D., Götze, O., Müller-Eberhard, H. J.: A molecular concept of the properdin pathway. Proc. Natl. Acad. Sci. U.S.A. **73**, 612—616 (1976b)

Minta, J. O.: Production of antiserum to human properdin and demonstration of antigenic differences between the native and activated protein. Proc. Soc. Exp. Biol. Med. **151**, 411—414 (1976)

Minta, J. O., Lepow, I. H.: Physical and chemical studies on human properdin purified by elution from zymosan and by affinity chromatography. J. Immunol. **111**, 286 (abstract) (1973)

Moncada, B., Day, N. K. B., Good, R. A., Windhorst, D. B.: Lupus erythematosus-like syndrome associated with a familial defect of the first component of complement. N. Engl. J. Med. **286**, 689—693 (1972)

Müller-Eberhard, H. J.: Complement. Ann. Rev. Biochem. **38**, 389—414 (1969)

Müller-Eberhard, H. J., Calcott, M. A.: Interaction between Clq and γ-globulin. Immunochemistry **3**, 500—508 (1966)

Müller-Eberhard, H. J., Götze, O.: C3 proactivator convertase and its mode of action. J. Exp. Med. **135**, 1003—1008 (1972)

Müller-Eberhard, H. J., Kunkel, H. G.: Isolation of a thermolabile protein which precipitates γ-globulin aggregates and participates in immune hemolysis. Proc. Soc. Exp. Biol. Med. **106**, 291—295 (1961)

Müller-Eberhard, H. J., Lepow, I. H.: C'1 esterase effect on activity and physiochemical properties of the fourth component of complement. J. Exp. Med. **121**, 819—833 (1965)

Müller-Eberhard, H. J., Polley, M. J., Calcott, M. A.: Formation and functional significance of a molecular complex derived from the second and the fourth component of human complement. J. Exp. Med. **125**, 359—380 (1967)

Naff, G. B., Ratnoff, O. D.: The enzymatic nature of C'1r. Conversion of C'1s to C'1 esterase and digestion of amino acid esters by C'1r. J. Exp. Med. **128**, 571—593 (1968)

Naff, G. B., Pensky, J., Lepow, I. H.: The macromolecular nature of the first component of human complement. J. Exp. Med. **119**, 593—613 (1964)

Nagasawa, S., Shiraishi, S., Stroud, R. M.: The molecular structure of C4 and its cleavage products. J. Immunol. **116**, 1743 (abstract) (1976)

Nelson, R. A.: The immune adherence phenomenon. An immunologically specific reaction between microorganisms and erythrocytes leading to enhanced phagocytosis. Science **118**, 733—735 (1953)

Nelson, R. A.: An alternative mechanism for the properdin system. J. Exp. Med. **108**, 515—535 (1958)

Nelson, R. A., Biro, C. E.: Complement components of a haemolytically deficient strain of rabbits. Immunology **14**, 527—540 (1968)

Nelson, R. A., Jensen, J., Gigli, I., Tamura, N.: Methods for the separation, purification and measurement of nine components of hemolytic complement in guinea-pig serum. Immunochemistry **3**, 111—135 (1966)

Nicholson, A., Austen, K. F.: Isolation and characterization of guinea pig properdin. J. Immunol. **118**, 103—108 (1977)

Nicholson, A., Brade, V., Lee, G. D., Shin, H. S., Mayer, M. M.: Kinetic studies of the formation of the properdin system enzymes on zymosan: evidence that nascent C3b controls the rate of assembly. J. Immunol. **112**, 1115—1123 (1974)

Nicholson, A., Brade, V., Schorlemmer, H. V., Burger, R., Bitter-Suermann, D., Hadding, U.: Interaction of C3b, B, and $\bar{D}$ in the alternate pathway of complement activation. J. Immunol. **115**, 1108—1113 (1975)

Nicol, P. A. E., Lachmann, P. J.: The alternative pathway of complement activation. The role of C3b and its inactivator (KAF). Immunology **24**, 259—275 (1973)

Nilsson, U., Müller-Eberhard, H. J.: Isolation of β_{1F}-globulin from human serum and its characterization as the fifth component of complement. J. Exp. Med. **122**, 277—298 (1965)

Nilsson, U. R., Mandle, R. J., McConnell-Mapes, J. A.: Human C3 and C5: subunit structure and modification by trypsin and $C\overline{42}$–$C\overline{423}$. J. Immunol. **114**, 815—822 (1975)

Nishioka, K.: Complement in allergy. Jpn. J. Allergy **13**, 285—295 (1964) [In Japanese]

Nussenzweig, V.: Receptors for immune complexes on lymphocytes. In: Advances in Immunology, Vol. 20. New York: Academic Press 1974
Pekin, Jr., T. J., Zvaifler, N. J.: Hemolytic complement in synovial fluid. J. Clin. Invest. **43**, 1372—1382 (1964)
Pekin, Jr., T. J., Zvaifler, N. J.: Synovial fluid findings in systemic lupus erythematosus and rheumatoid arthritis. Ann. Int. Med. **76**, 357—363 (1970)
Pensky, J., Hinz, Jr., C. F., Todd, E. W., Wedgwood, R. J., Boyer, J. T., Lepow, I. H.: Properties of highly purified human properdin. J. Immunol. **100**, 142—158 (1968)
Pepys, M. B.: Role of complement in induction of antibody production in vivo. J. Exp. Med. **140**, 126—145 (1974)
Pepys, M. B., Wansbrough-Jones, M. H., Mirjah, D. D., Dash, A. C.: Complement in the induction of IgA and IgE antibody production. J. Immunol. (abstract) **116**, 1746 (1976)
Perri, T. di, Auteri, A.: Anticomplementary properties of cinnarizine. Arch. Int. Pharmacodyn. Ther. **203**, 23—29 (1973)
Peters, D. K., Williams, D. G., Charlesworth, J. A., Boulton-Jones, J. M., Sissons, J. G. P., Evans, D. J., Kourilsky, O., Marel-Morage, L.: Mesangiocapillary nephritis, partial lipodystrophy and hypocomplementemia. Lancet **1973I**, 446—449
Peterson, B. H., Graham, J. A., Brooks, G. F.: Human deficiency of the eighth component of complement: lack of bactericidal activity. Clin. Res. **23**, 295A (abstract) (1975)
Petz, L. D., Sharp, G. C., Cooper, N. R., Irwin, W. S.: Serum and cerebrospinal fluid complement and serum autoantibodies in systemic lupus erythematosus. Medicine (Baltimore) **50**, 259—275 (1971)
Pickering, R. J., Naff, G. B., Stroud, R. M., Good, R. A., Gewurz, H.: Deficiency of C1r in human serum: effects on the structure and function of macromolecular C1. J. Exp. Med. **131**, 803—815 (1970)
Pillemer, L., Blum, L., Lepow, I. H., Ross, O. A., Todd, E. W., Wardlaw, A. C.: The properdin system and immunity. I. Demonstration and isolation of a new serum protein, properdin, and its role in immune phenomena. Science **120**, 279—285 (1954)
Platts-Mills, T. A. E., Ishizaka, K.: Activation of the alternate pathway of human complement by rabbit cells. J. Immunol. **113**, 348—358 (1974)
Podack, E. R., Kolb, W. P., Müller-Eberhard, H. J.: Purification of the sixth and seventh component of human complement without loss of hemolytic activity. J. Immunol. **116**, 263—269 (1976)
Polley, M. J., Müller-Eberhard, H. J.: Enhancement of the hemolytic activity of the second component of human complement by oxidation. J. Exp. Med. **126**, 1013—1025 (1967)
Polley, M. J., Müller-Eberhard, H. J.: The second component of human complement: its isolation, fragmentation by C′1 esterase, and incorporation into C′3 convertase. J. Exp. Med. **128**, 533—551 (1968)
Poskitt, T. R., Fortwengler, Jr., H. P., Lunskis, B.: Activation of the alternate complement pathway by autologous red cell stoma. J. Exp. Med. **138**, 715—722 (1973)
Raepple, E., Hill, H. U., Loos, M.: Mode of interaction of different polyanions with the first (C1, $C\bar{1}$), the second (C2) and the fourth (C4) component of complement. I. Effect on fluid phase $C\bar{1}$ and on $C\bar{1}$ bound to EA or to EAC4. Immunochemistry **13**, 251—255 (1976)
Ratnoff, O. D., Naff, G. B.: The conversion of C′1s to C′1 esterase by plasmin and trypsin. J. Exp. Med. **125**, 337—358 (1967)
Ratnoff, O. D., Pensky, J., Ogston, D., Naff, G. B.: The inhibition of plasmin, plasma kallikrein, plasma permeability factor and the C1r subcomponent of the first component of complement by serum C′1 esterase inhibitor. J. Exp. Med. **129**, 315—330 (1969)
Rauterberg, E. W., Gebest, H. J.: Demonstration of C9 at complement induced membrane "holes" by immunoferritin electron microscopy. J. Immunol. (abstract) **116**, 1747 (1976)
Reid, K. B. M.: Isolation, by partial pepsin digestion, of the three collagen-like regions present in subcomponent C1q of the first component of human complement. Biochem. J. **155**, 5—17 (1976)
Reid, K. B. M., Porter, R. R.: Subunit composition and structure of subcomponent C1q of the first component of human complement. Biochem. J. **155**, 19—23 (1976)
Reid, K. B. M., Lowe, D. M., Porter, R. R.: Isolation and characterization of C1q, a subcomponent of the first component of complement, from human and rabbit sera. Biochem. J. **130**, 749—763 (1972)

Reid, K. B. M., Doyle, B. B., Leonard, K.: Chemical, physical and electron microscopy studies of fragments produced by limited proteolysis of human C1q by pepsin. J. Immunol. (abstract) **116**, 1747 (1976)
Rent, R., Ertel, N., Eisenstein, R., Gewurz, H.: Complement activation by interaction of polyanions and polycations. I. Heparin-protamine induced consumption of complement. J. Immunol. **114**, 120—124 (1975)
Rommel, F. A., Mayer, M. M.: Studies of guinea pig complement component C9: reaction kinetics and evidence that lysis of EAC1-8 results from a single membrane lesion caused by one molecule of C9. J. Immunol. **110**, 637—647 (1973)
Rommel, F. A., Goldlust, M. B., Bancroft, F. C., Mayer, M. M., Tashjian, A. H.: Synthesis of the ninth component of complement by a clonal strain of rat hepatoma cells. J. Immunol. **105**, 396—403 (1970)
Root, R. K., Ellman, L., Frank, M. M.: Bactericidal and opsonic properties of C4-deficient guinea pig serum. J. Immunol. **109**, 477—486 (1972)
Rosen, F. S., Charache, P., Pensky, J., Donaldson, V.: Hereditary angioneurotic edema: two genetic variants. Science **148**, 957—958 (1965)
Rosenfeld, S. I., Ruddy, S., Austen, K. F.: A familial abnormality of the concentration of the fourth component of complement (C4) in man. Clin. Res. **17**, 358 (abstract) (1969)
Rosenfeld, S. I., Kelly, M. E., Baum, J., Leddy, J. P.: Hereditary deficiency of the fifth component of complement in man. J. Clin. Invest. **53**, 67a (1974)
Ross, G. D., Jensen, J. A.: The first component (C1n) of the complement system of the nurse shark (Ginglymostoma cirratum). I. Hemolytic characteristics of partially purified C1n. J. Immunol. **110**, 175—182 (1973)
Ross, G. D., Polley, K. J., Rabelline, E. M., Grey, H. M.: Two different complement receptors on human lymphocytes. J. Exp. Med. **138**, 798—810 (1973)
Rosse, W. F., Logue, G. L., Silberman, H. R., Frank, M. M.: The effect of synthetic androgens in hereditary angioneurotic edema: alterations of $C\bar{1}$ inhibitor and C4 levels. Trans. Assoc. Amer. Phys. **89**, 122—132 (1976)
Rother, K.: Leukocyte mobilizing factor: a new biological activity derived from the third component of complement. Eur. J. Immunol. **2**, 550—558 (1972)
Rother, U., Thorbecke, G. J., Stecher-Levin, V. J., Hurlimann, J., Rother, K.: Formation of C′6 by rabbit liver tissue in vitro. Immunology **14**, 649—655 (1968)
Rother, U., Rother, K.: Über einen angeborenen Komplementdefekt bei Kaninchen. Z. Immunitaetsforsch. **121**, 224—230 (1961)
Rother, K., Rother, U., Schinders, F.: Passive Arthus-Reaktion bei Komplement-defekten Kaninchen. Z. Immunitaetsforsch. **126**, 473—488 (1964)
Ruddy, S., Austen, K. F.: Activation of the complement system in rheumatoid synovitis. I. An analysis of complement component activities in rheumatoid synovial fluids. Arthritis Rheum. **13**, 713—723 (1970)
Ruddy, S., Austen, K. F.: C3b inactivator of man. III. Fragments produced by C3b inactivator cleavage of cell-bound or fluid phase C3b. J. Immunol. **107**, 742—750 (1971)
Ruddy, S., Austen, K. F.: Inherited abnormalities of the complement system in man. In: Stanbury, J. B., Wyngarden, J. B., Frederickson, D. S. (Eds.): The Metabolic Basis of Inherited Disease, 4th Ed. New York: McGraw-Hill 1978, 1737—1754
Ruddy, S., Gigli, I., Sheffer, A. L., Austen, K. F.: The laboratory diagnosis of hereditary angioedema. In: Allergology, Proc. of the Sixth Int. Congr. of Allergology, Amsterdam: Experta Medica 1968
Ruddy, S., Everson, L. K., Schur, P. H., Austen, K. F.: Hemolytic assay of the ninth complement component: elevation and depletion in rheumatic diseases. J. Exp. Med. **134**, 259s—275s (1971)
Ruddy, S., Austen, K. F., Goetzl, E. J.: Chemotactic activity derived from interaction of factors $\bar{D}$ and B of the properdin pathway with cobra venom factor or C3b. J. Clin. Invest. **55**, 587—592 (1975a)
Ruddy, S., Fearon, D. T., Austen, K. F.: Depressed synovial fluid levels of properdin and properdin factor B in patients with rheumatoid arthritis. Arthritis Rheum. **18**, 289—295 (1975b)
Ruddy, S., Carpenter, C. B., Chin, K. W., Knostman, J. N., Soter, N. A., Götze, O., Müller-Eberhard, H. J., Austen, K. F.: Human complement metabolism: an analysis of 144 studies. Medicine **54**, 165—178 (1975c)

Ruddy,S., Fearon,D.T., Austen,K.F.: Multiple pathways of complement activation in human disease. In: Proc. of the 5th Lepetit Colloquium on the Immunol. Basis of Connective Tissue Disorders, Amsterdam: ASP Biological and Medical Press B.V. 1975d

Sakai,K., Stroud,R.M.: Purification, molecular properties and activation of C1 proesterase, C1s. J. Immunol. **110**, 1010—1020 (1973)

Sandberg,A.L., Oliveira,B., Osler,A.G.: Two complement interaction sites in guinea pig immunoglobulins. J. Immunol. **106**, 282—285 (1971)

Sargent,A.U., Austen,K.F.: The effective molecular titration of the early components of dog complement. Proc. Soc. Exp. Biol. Med. **133**, 1117—1122 (1970)

Schreiber,A.D., Kaplan,A.P., Austen,K.F.: C$\overline{1}$INH of Hageman factor fragment activation of coagulation, fibrinolysis and kinin generation. J. Clin. Invest. **52**, 1402—1409 (1973)

Schreiber,R.D., Müller-Eberhard,H.J.: Fourth component of human complement. Description of a three polypeptide chain structure. J. Exp. Med. **140**, 1324—1335 (1974)

Schreiber,R.D., Götze,O., Müller-Eberhard,H.J.: Nephritic factor and initiating factor C3/C5 convertases. Fed. Proc. **35**, 253a (1976)

Sheffer,A.L., Crait,J.M., Wilms-Kretchmer,K., Austen,K.F., Rosen,F.S.: Histopathological and ultrastructural observations on tissues from patients with hereditary angioneurotic edema. J. Allergy **47**, 292—297 (1971)

Sheffer,A.L., Austen,K.F., Rosen,F.S.: Tranexamic acid therapy in hereditary angioneurotic edema. N. Engl. J. Med. **287**, 452—454 (1972)

Sheffer,A.L., Fearon,D.T., Austen,K.F.: Methyltestosterone therapy in hereditary angioedema. Ann. Int. Med. **86**, 306—308 (1977a)

Sheffer,A.L., Fearon,D.T., Austen,K.F., Rosen,F.S.: Tranexamic acid: preoperative prophylactic therapy for patients with hereditary angioneurotic edema. J. Allergy Clin. Immunol. **60**, 38—40 (1977b)

Shelton,E., Yonemasu,K., Stroud,R.M.: Ultrastructure of the human complement component, C1q. Proc. Natl. Acad. Sci. U.S.A. **69**, 65—68 (1972)

Shin,H.S., Mayer,M.M.: The third component of the guinea pig complement system I. Purification and characterization. Biochemistry **7**, 2991—2996 (1968a)

Shin,H.S., Mayer,M.M.: The third component of the guinea pig complement system. II. Kinetic study of the reaction of EAC'4,2a with guinea pig C'3. Enzymatic nature of C'3 consumption, multiphasic character of fixation and hemolytic titration of C'3. Biochemistry **7**, 2997—3002 (1968b)

Shin,H.S., Mayer,M.M.: The third component of the guinea pig complement system. III. Effect of inhibitors. Biochemistry **7**, 3003—3006 (1968c)

Shin,H.S., Smith,M.R., Wood,W.B.: Heat labile opsonins to pneumococcus. II. Involvement of C3 and C5. J. Exp. Med. **130**, 1229—1242 (1969)

Shin,H.S., Pickering,R.J., Mayer,M.M.: The fifth component of the guinea pig complement system. II. Mechanism of SAC$\overline{1}$ 423, 5b formation and C5 consumption by EAC$\overline{1}\,\overline{423}$. J. Immunol. **106**, 473—479 (1971a)

Shin,H.S., Pickering,R.J., Mayer,M.M.: The fifth component of the guinea pig complement system. III. Dissociation and transfer of C5b, and the probable site of C5b fixation. J. Immunol. **106**, 480—493 (1971b)

Sitomer,G., Stroud,R.M., Mayer,M.M.: Reversible absorption of C'2 by EAC'4: Role of Mg^{2+}, Enumeration of competent SAC'4, two-step nature of C'2a fixation and estimation of its efficiency. Immunochemistry **3**, 57—69 (1966)

Sledge,C., Bing,D.H.: Binding properties of the human complement protein C1q. J. Biol. Chem. **248**, 2818—2823 (1973)

Snyderman,R., Gewurz,H., Mergenhagen,S.E.: Interactions of the complement system with endotoxic lipopolysaccharide. Generation of a factor chemotactic for polymorphonuclear leukocytes. J. Exp. Med. **128**, 259—275 (1968)

Soter,N.A., Austen,K.F., Gigli,I.: The complement system in necrotizing anglitis of the skin. Analysis of complement component activities in serum of patients with concomitant collagen-vascular disease. J. Invest. Dermatol. **63**, 219—226 (1974)

Soter,N.A., Austen,K.F., Gigli,I.: Inhibition of ε-amino-caproic acid of the activation of the first component of the complement system. J. Immunol. **114**, 928—932 (1975)

Spaulding,W.B.: Methyl testosterone therapy for hereditary episodic edema (hereditary angioneurotic edema). Ann. Intern. Med. **53**, 739—745 (1960)

Spitzer, R. E., Vallota, E. H., Forristal, J., Sudora, E., Stitzel, A., Davis, N C., West, C. D.: Serum C'3 lytic system in patients with glomerulonephritis. Science **164**, 436—437 (1969)

Stetson, C. A.: Similarities in the mechanisms determining the Arthus and the Shwartzman phenomena. J. Exp. Med. **94**, 349—357 (1951)

Stolfi, R.: Immune lytic transformation: a state of irreversible damage generated as a result of the reaction of the eighth component of the guinea pig complement system. J. Immunol. **100**, 46—54 (1968)

Stolfi, R. L.: An analogue of guinea pig C8: in vitro generation and inhibitory activity. J. Immunol. **104**, 1212—1219 (1970)

Stroud, R. M., Austen, K. F., Mayer, M. M.: Catalysis of C'2 fixation by C'1a. Reaction kinetics, competitive inhibition by TAMe, and transferase hypothesis of the enzymatic action of C'1a on C'2, one of its natural substrates. Immunochemistry **2**, 219—234 (1965)

Stroud, R. M., Nagaki, K., Pickering, R. J., Gewurz, H., Good, R. A., Cooper, M. D.: Subunits of the first complement component in immunologic deficiency syndromes: Independence of C1s and C1q. Clin. Exp. Immunol. **7**, 133—137 (1970)

Strunk, R., Colten, H. R.: The first component of human complement (C1): kinetics of reaction with its natural substrates. J. Immunol. **112**, 905—910 (1974)

Strunk, R. S., Tashjian, A. H., Colten, H. R.: Complement biosynthesis in vitro by rat hepatoma cell strains. J. Immunol. **114**, 331—335 (1975)

Tamura, N., Nelson, R. A.: Three naturally occurring inhibitors of components of complement in guinea pig and rabbit serum. J. Immunol. **99**, 582—592 (1967)

Tamura, N., Shimada, A.: The ninth component of guinea pig complement. Isolation and identification as an α_2-globulin. Immunology **20**, 415—425 (1971)

Ter Laan, B., Molenaar, J. L., Feltkamp-Vroom, T. M., Pondman, K. W.: Interaction of human anaphylatoxin C3a with rat mast cells demonstrated by immunofluorescence. Eur. J. Immunol. **4**, 393—395 (1974)

Theofilopoulos, A. N., Perrin, L. H.: Binding of components of the properdin system to cultured human lymphoblastoid cells and B lymphocytes. J. Exp. Med. **143**, 271—289 (1976)

Thompson, R. A.: C3 inactivating factor in the serum of a patient with chronic hypocomplementaemic proliferative glomerulo-nephritis. Immunology **22**, 147—158 (1972)

Thompson, R. A., Lachmann, P. J.: Reactive lysis: the complement-mediated lysis of unsensitized cells. I. The characterization of the indicator factor and its identification as C7. J. Exp. Med. **131**, 629—641 (1970)

Vallota, E. H., Müller-Eberhard, H. J.: Formation of C3a and C5a anaphylatoxins in whole human serum after inhibition of the anaphylatoxin inactivator. J. Exp. Med. **137**, 1109—1123 (1973)

Vallota, E. H., Forristal, J., Spitzer, R. E., Davis, N. C., West, C. D.: Continuing C3 breakdown after bilateral nephrectomy in patients with membranoproliferative glomerulonephritis. J. Clin. Invest. **50**, 552—558 (1971)

Vallota, E. H., Götze, O., Spiegelberg, H. L., Forrestal, J., West, C. D., Müller-Eberhard, H. J.: A serum factor in chronic hypocomplementemic glomerulonephritis distinct from immunoglobulins and activating the alternate pathway of complement. J. Exp. Med. **139**, 1249—1260 (1974)

Vogt, W., Zeman, N., Garbe, G.: Histaminunabhängige Wirkungen von Anaphylatoxin auf glatte Muskulatur isolierter Organe. Naunyn Schmiedebergs Arch. Pharmacol. **262**, 399—404 (1969)

Vogt, W., Dieminger, L., Lynen, R., Schmidt, G.: Formation and composition of the complex with cobra venom factor that cleaves the third component of complement. Hoppe Seylers Z. Physiol. Chem. **355**, 171—183 (1974)

Vogt, W., Schmidt, G., Lynen, R., Dieminger, L.: Cleavage of the third complement component (C3) and generation of the spasmogenic peptide, C3a, in human serum via the properdin pathway: demonstration of inhibitory as well as enhancing effects of epsilon-amino-caproic acid. J. Immunol. **114**, 671—677 (1975)

Vogt, W., Dames, W., Schmidt, G., Dieminger, L.: Complement activation by the properdin system: formation of a stoichiometric, C3 cleaving complex of properdin factor B with C3b. Immunochemistry **14**, 201—205 (1977)

Ward, P. A.: Complement-derived chemotactic factors and their interactions with neutrophilic granulocytes. In: Ingram, D. G. (Ed.): Biologic Activities of Complement. Basel: S. Karger 1972

Ward, P. A., Zvaifler, N. J.: Complement-derived leukotactic factors in inflammatory synovial fluids of humans. J. Clin. Invest. **50**, 606—616 (1971)

Weiler, J. M., Daha, M. R., Austen, K. F., Fearon, D. T.: Control of the amplification convertase of complement by the plasma protein β1H. Proc. Nat. Acad. Sci. **73**, 3268—3272 (1976)

Weiler, J. M., Yurt, R. W., Fearon, D. T., Austen, K. F.: Modulation of the formation of the amplification convertase of complement, C3b, Bb, by native and commercial heparin. J. Exp. Med. **147**, 409—421 (1978)

Wellek, B., Opferkuch, W.: A naturally occurring C7-inactivator in a case of C7 deficiency in man and in normal human serum. Clin. Exp. Immunol. **19**, 223—235 (1975)

Westberg, N. G., Naff, G. B., Boyer, J. T., Michael, A. F.: Glomerular deposition of properdin in acute and chronic glomerulonephritis with hypocomplementemia. J. Clin. Invest. **50**, 642—650 (1971)

Whaley, K., Ruddy, S.: C3b inactivator accelerator (A. C3b INA): a serum protein of the complement system required for full expression of C3b inactivator (C3b INA) activity. Fed. Proc. **35**, 654 (abstract) (1976)

Winkelstein, J. A., Smith, M. R., Shin, H. S.: The role of C3 as an opsonin in the early stages of infection. Proc. Soc. Exp. Biol. Med. **149**, 397—401 (1975)

World Health Organization: Nomenclature of Complement. Bull. Wld. Hlth Org. **39**, 935—938 (1968)

Wyatt, H. V., Colten, H. R., Borsos, T.: Production of the second (C2) and fourth (C4) components of guinea pig complement by single peritoneal cells: evidence that one cell may produce both components. J. Immunol. **108**, 1609—1614 (1972)

Yonemasu, K., Stroud, R. M.: Structural studies on human C1q: non-covalent and covalent subunits. Immunochemistry **9**, 545—554 (1972)

Ziccardi, R. J., Cooper, N. R.: Physicochemical and functional characterization of the C1r subunit of the first complement component. J. Immunol. **116**, 496—503 (1976a)

Ziccardi, R. J., Cooper, N. R.: Activation of C1r by proteolytic cleavage. J. Immunol. **116**, 504—509 (1976b)

Ziegler, J. B., Alper, C. A., Rosen, F. S., Lachmann, P. J., Sherington, L.: Restoration by purified C3b inactivator of complement-mediated function in vivo in a patient with C3b inactivator deficiency. J. Clin. Invest. **55**, 668—674 (1975)

Zimmerman, T. S., Kolb, W. P.: Human platelet-initiated formation and uptake of the C5-9 complex of human complement. J. Clin. Invest. **57**, 203—211 (1976)

Zimmerman, T. S., Müller-Eberhard, H. J.: Complement-induced platelet protein alterations. Science **180**, 1183—1185 (1973)

Zimmerman, T. S., Arroyave, C. M., Müller-Eberhard, H. J.: A blood coagulation abnormality in rabbits deficient in the sixth component of complement (C6) and its correction by purified C6. J. Exp. Med. **134**, 1591—1607 (1971)

Zucker, M. B., Grant, R. A.: Aggregation and release reaction induced in human blood platelets by zymosan. J. Immunol. **112**, 1219—1230 (1974)

Zvaifler, N. J.: Breakdown products of C'3 in human synovial fluids. J. Clin. Invest. **48**, 1532—1542 (1969)

CHAPTER 14

Bradykinin-System

J. GARCIA LEME

A. Introduction

There is general agreement that inflammation is a multimediated process. In previous chapters the participation of several endogenous substances as putative mediators of inflammatory reactions has been considered. In this chapter, evidence of the involvement of hypotensive kinins, and particularly bradykinin (Bk), in such reactions will be discussed. The main scope is to evaluate to what extent kinins are contributing to the inflammatory response, as well as to assess the significance of their participation in such a complex, multimediated process.

The term *kinin* will here denote hypotensive polypeptides which contract most smooth muscle preparations but relax the rat duodenum. We will be mainly dealing with Bk (H-Arg-Pro-Pro-Gly-Phe-Ser-Pro-Phe-Arg-OH) and the natural structurally related peptides, kallidin (Lys-Bk) and methionyl-lysyl-bradykinin (Met-Lys-Bk). They can be regarded as *plasma-kinins* in the sense that they are generated from inactive precursors present in normal plasma of higher organisms. This means that under special circumstances enzymes can be activated which release from plasma precursors, active substances capable of exerting pharmacological effects. The active substances, together with the precursors *(kininogens)*, the releasing agents *(kininogenases)* and the inactivating enzymes *(kininases)*, will be referred to as the *Bk-system.* The nomenclature for the components of the system follows the recommendations of an international meeting held in Florence in 1965 (see WEBSTER, 1970a).

Bk was first described as a hypotensive and smooth muscle-stimulating factor released from plasma globulin by snake venoms and by trypsin (ROCHA E SILVA et al., 1949). In the early sixties it was isolated, the primary structure determined and its synthesis accomplished (ELLIOTT et al., 1960a, 1961; BOISSONNAS et al., 1960a, 1963). Kallidin was obtained by PIERCE and WEBSTER (1961) from human plasma treated with human urinary kallikrein. Its structure was confirmed by synthesis (NICOLAIDES et al., 1961; PLES et al., 1962). Met-Lys-Bk was described by ELLIOTT et al. (1963) in ox blood, and its synthesis performed by SCHRÖDER (1964) and MERRIFIELD (1964). The three compounds can be differentiated by biossay (STURMER and BERDE, 1963; SCHRÖDER, 1964) and were shown to exhibit similar actions, but different potencies, depending on the assay preparation.

Synthetic Bk has been frequently used as a standard to estimate Bk-like activity appearing in biological materials. The structurally related natural peptides, kallidin and Met-Lys-Bk, may also be contributing to this activity. In most cases, however, the relative contribution of each kinin has not been assessed. A micro-analytical system using SP-Sephadex-C-25 under equilibrium chromatography conditions has recently been described for the separation of Bk, kallidin and Met-Lys-Bk. Biossay with the isolated guinea pig ileum was used to detect the peptides in the column effluent. The sensitivity for the three peptides was 0.2–4 nM (SAMPAIO et al., 1975).

Many synthetic analogues have been prepared (for a review, see SCHRÖDER, 1970), but they will be considered only when the utilization of such substances in biological models has improved the knowledge of inflammatory reactions.

Bk and the natural kininogen-derivatives are easily formed endogenously from mammalian plasma. They exhibit pharmacological properties that will induce most of the features of inflammation: vasodilation, increased vascular permeability, pain, bronchoconstriction or bronchospasm in asthmatic patients. Bk-like activity has been detected in exudates or perfusates from inflamed areas. The peptides are rapidly inactivated in the organisms. Partial depletion of the stores of the precursors, prior to the application of noxious stimuli, partially decreases the inflammatory response. These facts, which will be considered in detail, favour the participation of the Bk-system in inflammatory reactions.

B. The Bradykinin System

The general aspects of the Bk system will be briefly considered. For a comprehensive discussion of the subject the reader is referred to ERDÖS (1970), and also to ROCHA E SILVA (1970), SANDER and HUGGINS (1972), PISANO (1975) and PISANO and AUSTEN (1976).

I. Kininogens

The term kininogen covers all proteins which release a kinin by the action of proteolytic enzymes. There are phylogenetic differences and more than one kininogen may occur in the blood of the same animal.

Kininogens are acidic glycoproteins found in the globulin fraction of normal plasma. Kininogenases present in plasma (plasma kallikreins) (WEBSTER and PIERCE, 1963; HENRIQUES et al., 1966), proteases present in snake venoms (ROCHA E SILVA et al., 1949; HENRIQUES et al., 1960; HAMBERG and ROCHA E SILVA, 1957a, 1957b; HABERMANN and BLENNEMANN, 1964; SUZUKI et al., 1967), trypsin (ROCHA E SILVA et al., 1949) and plasmin (BERALDO, 1950; LEWIS and WORK, 1956; VOGT, 1964; HAMBERG, 1968) release Bk from the inactive precursor. Kininogenases of glandular origin, found in saliva, submaxillary glands, pancreas and urine (glandular kallikreins), form kallidin from the same substrates (WEBSTER and PIERCE, 1963; WERLE et al., 1961; PIERCE and WEBSTER, 1961). Plasma enzymes able to release Met-Lys-Bk in acid medium are still unknown. The active fragments corresponding to the natural hypotensive plasma kinins are retained in the precursor molecules by bonds resistant to drastic treatments (VAN ARMAN, 1955; HAMBERG and ROCHA E SILVA, 1957b; DINIZ et al., 1961). Therefore, activation of enzymic systems is an essential step for the release of the active substances in physiological or pathological processes.

Released kallidin was first shown to be converted to Bk in plasma by WEBSTER and PIERCE (1963). Kallidin and Met-Lys-Bk may be converted at a high rate into Bk by aminopeptidases found in tissues (CAMARGO et al., 1972; BORGES et al., 1974; PRADO et al., 1975) and in plasma (GUIMARÃES et al., 1973).

Trypsin and glandular kallikreins can still produce kinins from human plasma in which responses to other kinin-forming agents had been exhausted. These findings led MARGOLIS and BISHOP (1963), VOGT (1966) and EISEN (1966a) to postulate the existence of two kininogen fractions with different reactivities. At this time, it was observed that pre-incubation of rat plasma with glass only partially reduced the total kininogen level in such plasma, which nevertheless still yielded kinin activity by the action of trypsin (GARCIA LEME et al., 1967).

The heterogeneity in the amino acid sequence of the kininogen molecules has been supported by extensive experimental data. From highly purified bovine kininogen treated with pepsin, HABERMANN (1966a, 1966b), HABERMANN and coworkers (1966) and HABERMAN and HELBIG (1966) isolated two kinin-containing fragments identified as H-Met-Lys-Bk-Ser-Val-Gln-OH and H-Met-Lys-Bk-Ser-Val-Gln-Val-Met-OH. HOCHSTRASSER and WERLE (1967) obtained two kinin-containing fragments, Gly-Arg-Met-Lys-Bk and Ser-Arg-Met-Lys-Bk, from a mixture of bovine plasma Cohn fractions IV-1 and IV-4. Results obtained by SUZUKI et al. (1967), utilizing a pure kininogen preparation from bovine plasma, led to the proposition that the Bk moiety lies in the middle of a linear polypeptide chain and that the two fragments on either side of Bk are joined by a disulphide bridge.

PIERCE and WEBSTER (1966) isolated two kininogens, I and II, from human plasma (MW 50000). Carboxypeptidase B destroyed the activity of I but not that of II, indicating that the carboxy-terminal arginine of Bk is protected in II. Cyanogen bromide cleavage gave about three times as much free kinin activity from I as from II, suggesting that Bk occupies the carboxyl end of I but lies inside II. JACOBSEN (1966a) and JACOBSEN and KRIZ (1967) gave evidence for the presence in fresh human, dog, rabbit, guinea pig, and rat plasma of two main classes of kininogens: a low molecular weight (LMW) kininogen (mol. wt. around 50000), and a high molecular weight (HMW) kininogen (mol. wt. around 197000). HMW kininogen represents approximately 20% of the total kininogen content of human plasma. HMW and LMW kininogens were obtained by YANO et al. (1967) and KOMIYA et al. (1974), utilizing bovine plasma, and by HENRIQUES et al. (1967) utilizing horse plasma. In agreement with these publications are recent findings by HABAL et al. (1974). These authors isolated two functionally different kininogens from human plasma: an HMW and an LMW kininogen. In aqueous media the apparent molecular sizes were about 200000 (HMW) and 50000 (LMW). Plasma kallikrein released kinin at a much faster rate from the HMW-kininogen than from LMW-kininogen. When equipotent preparations of kininogens were incubated for 10 min with kallikrein, 60 times more enzyme was required to release the same amount of kinin from the LMW-kininogen as from the HMW-kininogen. Multiple forms of kininogens have been recently isolated from human plasma in 60% yields by a procedure involving affinity chromatography with immobilized mono-specific antibody (GUIMARÃES et al., 1974). The HMW-kininogens isolated by this procedure at concentrations higher than those found in plasma, or when mixed with prekallikrein at normal levels, formed active Hageman factor from the crude inactive form (WEBSTER et al., 1975).

Due to the relative ease with which kininogen can be manipulated in terms of its isoelectric point and electrophoretic mobility, or non-specifically modified during storage, so as to appear aggregated or to lose more of its functional responsiveness to one kininogenase relative to another, SPRAGG and AUSTEN (1971) suggested that the multiple human kininogens may represent alterations of a single plasma kininogen. These authors found only one human kininogen of mol. wt. 70000.

Though kininogens may appear aggregated in different forms, and may exhibit different structures, most of the evidence suggests the existence of at least two classes of kininogens, which include in their molecules a common amino-acid sequence released by the action of kininogenases. Further studies are required for the elucidation of still obscure aspects of the problem; for details see PIERCE (1968, 1970), HABERMANN (1970), HAMBERG et al. (1975) and PISANO (1975).

1. Kininogen Levels and Kininogen Depletion

Kininogen levels have been estimated in blood and other body fluids as the amount of kinins released after proteolysis. If trypsin is used for the digestion of the substrate, only Bk is formed. When previous contact of the fluid with glass is avoided and incubation is made after acid denaturation of the substrate, more reproducible results are obtained. The use of kininogenases other than trypsin will lead to the formation of any of the three known kinins, whose varying potencies upon test organs may interfere with the estimation of the kininogen level. Furthermore, haemodilution or haemoconcentration may introduce other causes of error due to a concomitant change in kininogen and in total plasma protein values (HABERMANN, 1970). Table 1 presents the normal values for blood kininogen in various species.

Change of kininogen levels can be observed in several physiological or pathological conditions. Kininogen depletion can be experimentally induced by purified enzymes and by substances activating the kinin system. Marked, but not total loss was observed in many species following the injection of kallikreins (WEBSTER and CLARK, 1959; DINIZ and CARVALHO, 1963; FASCIOLO and HALVORSEN, 1964; CORRADO et al., 1966), of snake venoms (DINIZ and CARVALHO, 1963; MARGOLIS et al., 1965), of trypsin (FASCIOLO and HALVORSEN, 1964; CORRADO et al., 1966; DINIZ et al., 1967), of polysaccharides such as cellulose-sulphate, carrageenin and agar (ROTHSCHILD, 1967, 1968a; ROTHSCHILD and GASCON, 1965; ROTHSCHILD and CASTANIA, 1968; GARCIA LEME et al., 1967), of ellagic acid (GAUTVIK and RUGSTADT, 1967) and of egg albumin, dextran and polyvinylpyrrolidine (LECOMTE, 1961; DINIZ and CARVALHO, 1963; CÎRSTEA et al., 1966; GREEFF et al., 1966; URBANITZ et al., 1970; ANKIER and STARR, 1967). Decrease of kininogen levels was reported in experimental haemorrhagic shock in dogs (WEBSTER and CLARK, 1959; DINIZ and CARVALHO, 1963), acute pancreatitis in dog and man (RYAN et al., 1964, 1965; DINIZ et al., 1967) and myocardial infarction in man (SICUTERI et al., 1966). However, several authors find a simultaneous decrease of kininogen with total plasma protein, as described by URBANITZ et al. (1970) for haemorrhagic and traumatic shock in the rabbit. Also, in acute pancreatitis in the dog, NUGENT et al. (1969) observed that the loss of total kininogen was equal to the loss of plasma volume.

In fact, it needs to be established that lowering of kininogen levels in pathological conditions occurs independently of loss of plasma proteins, in order to estimate the specific contribution of these substances to the pathogenesis of such conditions. An

Table 1. Kininogen content of blood of various species. Values are expressed as μg bradykinin equivalents/ml plasma or serum

Species	Range (μg/ml)
Human	
Adults	6.5–12.5 (1)
	3.0– 5.0 (2)
Men, 49–61 years	5.1– 7.3 (3)
Women, 61–85 years	6.0– 8.2 (1)
Newborn	0.7– 1.6 (1)
Cattle	10.4–14.9 (1)
	5.0–10.0 (2)
Rabbit	7.7–10.0 (1)
	6.0– 8.0 (2)
Guinea pig	6.9– 8.8 (1)
	2.0– 4.0 (2)
Rat	1.1– 2.0 (1)
	1.0– 2.0 (2)
Mouse	13.2–22.2 (1)
Dog	5.3– 5.7 (1)
Frog	2.2– 2.3 (1)
Pigeon	0.9– 1.1 (1)

References: (1) DINIZ et al., 1967; (2) HABERMAN, 1970; (3) BROCKLEHURST and ZEITLIN, 1967.

alternative possibility of increased turnover of kininogen molecules to compensate for the increased release of active kinins has not been investigated. Trauma and local inflammation lead to increased synthesis by the liver of certain plasma proteins, the acute phase reactants. Kininogen and kininogenase were shown to belong to this category. Isolated livers of injured rats perfused with a non-blood medium without recirculation produced approximately twice as much kininogen and kininogenase as livers from normal rats (BORGES and GORDON, 1976).

Though changes in total kininogen levels may point to the involvement of kinins in a pathological process, it is probably more important to look for release of kinins in the extravascular tissues from extravazated plasma proteins in order to demonstrate the participation of these substances in inflammation. Circulating kinins will mainly produce diffuse effects, which are rapidly terminated by inactivating enzymes. The persistance of the effects in a limited area of the organism requires that they be rather locally and continuously formed. This could well occur in the development of inflammatory reactions. Extravasated proteins will tend to accumulate in the injured area. Local conditions may induce a continuous formation of kinins and the active agents will thus be available for relatively long periods. Therefore, the detection of kinins in the injured area is a better parameter to judge the participation of kinins in the observed response.

2. Effect of Catecholamines on Kininogen Levels

Sympathetic stimulation, or the infusion of catecholamines into the circulation of the cat submandibular gland, led to the release of kinin-forming enzymes (HILTON and LEWIS, 1956). The process was blocked by α-adrenoceptor antagonists. Decreased kininogen content in the guinea pig plasma followed intravenous injection of adrenaline (VUGMAN, 1963). Thus, catecholamines might activate proteases which in turn would release kinin from kininogen (ROCHA E SILVA, 1968). This suggestion was questioned by BHALLA et al. (1970). However, infusion of adrenaline into rabbits led to activation of the Hageman factor (MCKAY et al., 1970) and exposure of rats to abnormally hot environment, a stress condition, resulted in kininogen breakdown (GREEFF et al., 1966). On the other hand, adrenalectomised rats had increased kininogen levels in plasma (ROSA et al., 1972) and the administration of adrenaline or noradrenaline rapidly lowered those levels (CASTANIA and ROTHSCHILD, 1974). The effect was reproduced in vitro by incubation of whole blood, but not cell-free plasma, with adrenaline for 5 min at 37° C. Propranolol or phenoxybenzamine, as well as heparin or acetylsalicylic acid, blocked the reduction of rat kininogen by adrenaline in vivo and in vitro (CASTANIA and ROTHSCHILD, 1974). Overall, these facts indicate that stress conditions lead to activation of the kinin-system, resulting in the release of active kinins.

II. Kininogenases and the Release of Kinins

Kininogenases can derive from plasma (plasma kallikreins) or from glandular sources (glandular kallikreins). Differences between both classes are summarized in Table 2. Proteolytic enzymes such as trypsin, as well as those present in snake venoms, can act as kininogenases. Also plasmin is able to release kinins from blood. Kininogenases have been the subject of a symposium (HABERLAND and ROHEN, 1973).

Table 2. Main differences between plasma and glandular kininogenases (kallikreins)

Plasma kininogenases:

- Release bradykinin from kininogens (WEBSTER and PIERCE, 1963; HABERMAN and BLENNEMANN, 1964; HABERMANN and KLETT, 1966)
- In most species utilize high molecular weight kininogens as substrates (JACOBSEN, 1966a; HENRIQUES et al., 1966, 1967; SUZUKI et al., 1967; YANO et al., 1967)
- Inhibited by SBTI (WERLE and MAIER, 1952; WEBSTER and PIERCE, 1960, 1961; HABERMANN and KLETT, 1966), and inactivated by inhibitors in plasma; (WERLE and MAIER, 1952; VOGEL and WERLE, 1970; HARPEL, 1970; MCCONNEL, 1972; RATNOFF et al., 1969; LAHIRI et al., 1974).
- Molecular weight of 97000 as calculated for kallikrein from casein-activated hog serum HABERMANN and KLETT, 1966)

Glandular kininogenases:

- Release lysyl-Bk from kininogens (PIERCE and WEBSTER, 1961; WERLE et al., 1961; WEBSTER and PIERCE, 1963; HABERMANN and BLENNEMANN, 1964)
- Not inhibited by SBTI (WERLE and MAIER, 1952; WERLE and KAUFMAN-BOETSCH, 1960; WEBSTER and PIERCE, 1961)
- Molecular weight of 33400–33800 for purified kallikrein from porcine pancreas (FRITZ et al., 1967)

1. Plasma and Glandular Kallikreins

As early as 1926 it was found that injection of urine into anaesthetised dogs produced a transient decrease of the blood pressure. This action was thought to be due to a hitherto unknown principle, which was lost by boiling but not by dialysis, and was named F-substance. Similar activity could be elicited by acidification of blood. Since great amounts of F-substance were detected in extracts of pancreas of various species, it was renamed kallikrein. Kallikrein preparations when mixed with serum stimulated the guinea pig ileum, which neither kallikrein itself or serum did not. This observation led to the conclusion that kallikrein might be acting as an enzyme releasing pharmacologically active substances (FREY, 1926; FREY et al., 1930; KRAUT et al., 1933, 1934; WERLE and VON RODEN, 1936, 1939; WERLE, 1973). In 1936, a distinction was made between plasma and glandular kallikreins (WERLE, 1936). They are now known to be limit proteases releasing kinin from kininogen and having little activity on other proteins (ZUBER and SACHE, 1974). Plasma kallikrein exists as an inactive prekallikrein which is activated by an enzymic process induced by plasma proteases or trypsin (WERLE et al., 1955). The process can also be initiated by acidification of the plasma (KRAUT et al., 1933; WERLE, 1936; EISEN, 1963). Purified plasma prekallikrein has been obtained (PIERCE, 1970; KAPLAN et al., 1972; SAMPAIO et al., 1974; HABAL et al., 1974). Pancreatic kallikrein exists in an inactive form (FIEDLER and WERLE, 1967) and its activation can be accomplished by contact with gastric juice, whereas other glandular kallikreins seem not to require a real process of activation (WEBSTER, 1970b).

Kallikrein inhibitors have been found in the blood serum of all species studied so far, in several organs of ruminants, in egg white, colostrum and in plants (for a review, see VOGEL and WERLE, 1970).

Human plasma contains inhibitory factors which are likely to be involved in the physiological regulation of kinin release. The regulatory mechanisms might be overwhelmed in pathological conditions (WERLE and VOGEL, 1960). Plasma kallikrein is inhibited by rapid interaction with human α_2-macroglobulin (HARPEL, 1970; MCCONNEL, 1972) and with serum C_1 esterase inhibitor (RATNOFF et al., 1969). Antithrombin III (LAHIRI et al., 1974) and α_1-antitrypsin produced a progressive inhibition of human plasma kallikrein.

The polyvalent inhibitor in bovine organs (aprotinin, Trasylol) takes its name from the fact that it also inhibits trypsin, chymotrypsin and plasmin. Highest concentrations are found in the lung and pancreas of cattle (WERLE and APPEL, 1959). It affects the hypotensive, esterase and kininogenase activities of most kallikreins. However, it is not detectable in the circulation.

Among the plant inhibitors, soybean trypsin inhibitor (SBTI) has been widely used. It inhibits the release of Bk by plasma kallikreins, whereas the liberation of kallidin by kallikreins from organs and urine is unaffected (WERLE and MAIER, 1952). BERALDO observed inhibition by SBTI of kinin release in peptone shock with improvement of the shock condition (BERALDO, 1950).

2. Plasmin

Plasmin was shown by BERALDO (1950) to release kinins from dog plasma globulin in vitro. His results were confirmed and extended by LEWIS and WORK (1956), SCHACH-

TER (1956) and LEWIS (1958). It was suggested that, during tissue injury, plasminogen activators can be liberated, with a subsequent release of kinins by the action of plasmin upon kininogens (LEWIS, 1960). Additional evidence for the role played by plasmin in the release of kinin was given by HAMBERG (1968), ROTHSCHILD et al. (1968) and HABAL et al. (1975). However, some dispute exists over whether plasmin can act directly as a kininogenase.

3. Other Proteolytic Enzymes

Proteolytic enzymes such as trypsin, clostripain, papain, pronase, nargase and snake venoms are able to form kinins from plasma or from partly purified globulins. When incubated with fresh plasma, appropriate doses of trypsin produced a maximal release of Bk after 1–3 min (ROCHA E SILVA et al., 1949). Crystalline trypsin releases a second hypotensive factor which remains active for a longer time than Bk and was identified with serum kallikrein (WERLE et al., 1955). Also kallidin is liberated by incubation of human plasma with crystalline trypsin (WEBSTER and PIERCE, 1963) as is Met-Lys-Bk from a kinin-yielding peptide obtained by incubation of bovine kininogen with pepsin (HABERMANN and MULLER, 1966). Clostripain, the cysteine-activated protease secreted by *Clostridium histolyticum*, was shown by PRADO et al. (1956) to exhibit kinin-forming activity when incubated with bovine plasma globulins. The peptide released was similar, if not identical, to Bk. The site of action of clostripain is suggested to be on kininogen. The proteolytic enzyme of *Streptomyces griseus* (pronase) and the crystalline proteinase from *Bacillus subtilis* (nargase), release peptide materials from blood plasma, among which one is similar to Bk. Both preparations can inactivate the released kinin, which indicates a broad proteolytic activity for the enzymes (REIS et al., 1966; PRADO, 1970). Hypotensive kinin-like principles are liberated from heat-treated horse plasma by papain and ficin (PRADO et al., 1965) and from guinea pig plasma by chymotrypsin (ROCHA E SILVA et al., 1967).

Bk-releasing activity has been found in venoms of various snakes of the genera *Bothrops*, *Agkistrodon*, *Crotalus*, *Lachesis* and *Vipera* (DEUTSCH and DINIZ, 1955; OSHIMA et al., 1969).

4. Generation of Kinins

The generation of kinins is thought to be initiated by the activation of the Hageman factor (factor XII), which also initiates the series of reactions resulting in the conversion of prothrombin to thrombin, and the activation of plasmin in vivo. Hageman factor is activated by contact with negatively charged particles, such as silica surfaces, or insoluble substances such as ellagic acid, sodium urate crystals, and also by mucopolysaccharides such as elastin and chondroitin sulphate, as well as by collagen and skin, and by fatty acid salts (MARGOLIS, 1957, 1958, 1960, 1962; ARMSTRONG et al., 1955; KEELE and ARMSTRONG, 1964; RATNOFF and MILES, 1964; MARGOLIS and BISHOP, 1962; WEBSTER and RATNOFF, 1961; see also WEBSTER, 1968). The process is known as the solid phase activation and may be particularly important when plasma come into contact with surfaces other than vessel walls and blood cells. Activation of the Hageman factor can also be achieved by enzymic pathways in a fluid phase (for reviews, see PISANO and AUSTEN, 1976). Solid phase activation may involve conformational changes in the molecule. The normal rate of activation seems to require that prekallikrein, high molecular weight kininogen and inactive Hageman factor be adsorbed to a negative surface (WEBSTER et al., 1975, 1976). Feedback loops are thus involved, as the active Hageman factor, or fragments derived therefrom, will directly activate prekallikrein (WUEPPER et al., 1970a, 1970b; KAPLAN and AUSTEN, 1971; COCHRANE and WUEPPER, 1971; OZGE-ANWAR et al., 1972; BAGDASARIAN et al., 1973; COCHRANE et al., 1973). The involvement of high molecular weight kininogen in such processes was also suggested by the findings of WUEPPER et al. (1975), who reported that blood plasma from an asymptomatic woman, surnamed Flaujeac, had prolonged activated partial thromboplastin time and inability to form plasmin, Bk and the permeability globulin factor (PF/dil). Each of these functional assays was corrected upon mixing Flaujeac trait plasma with human plasma deficient in Hageman factor or Fletcher factor. The Flaujeac factor was isolated and the activity corresponded to fractions containing high molecular weight kininogen. Flaujeac trait plasma did not release kinin upon incubation with kallikrein.

Prekallikrein is identical to the Fletcher factor, which converts the thromboplastin antecedent to thromboplastin (HATHWAY et al., 1965). The identity was suggested by the works of WUEPPER (1973) and WEISS et al. (1974). Fletcher factor-deficient plasma was found to be abnormal in tests for thromboplastin formation, plasmin formation, evolution of PF/dil or kinin generation. This plasma, but not Hageman factor-deficient plasma, was corrected by the addition of highly purified prekallikrein from human or rabbit sources or by small quantities of normal, Hageman factor- or thromboplastin antecedent-deficient plasmas. Prekallikrein antigen was not detectable in this plasma (WUEPPER, 1973). It also possessed a diminished rate of activation of the fibrinolytic pathway and was deficient in chemotactic activity. Both functions were restored by reconstitution with purified prekallikrein (WEISS et al., 1974). The ability of kallikrein to convert unactivated Hageman factor to activated Hageman factor in the fluid phase is required for the Hageman factor dependent pathways to proceed at a normal rate (WEISS et al., 1974). Therefore, blood coagulation, fibrinolysis, chemotactic functions and generation of kinins are intermingled processes.

III. Kininases

Free kinins are not easily detected in the circulation. This is mainly due to the presence of kininases, which rapidly destroy newly formed kinins. Kininases are found in tissues and biological fluids, in circulating blood cells, as well as in some micro-organisms and in snake venoms. For a detailed discussion, see ERDÖS and YANG (1970).

FERREIRA and VANE (1967a) have estimated the half-life of Bk in cat's blood to be less than 20 s. This value agrees well with that of MCCARTHY et al. (1965) for dog's blood. Despite this rapid disappearance, the removal of Bk from the circulation cannot be explained by its inactivation in blood alone. Participation by the tissues in the disappearance of Bk is an important factor. Its inactivation might be accomplished by the enzymes in the interstitial spaces, on the surface of cells, or within the cells. Up to 80% of Bk infused intravenously disappeared during passage through the pulmonary circulation. Therefore, when Bk is released into the bloodstream, the concentration will be reduced to about 1% within three circulation cycles (FERREIRA and VANE, 1967b). In perfused rat's lung, RYAN et al. (1968) studied the degradation of labelled Bk and concluded that the peptide was hydrolyzed by enzymes in or near the endothelium of the pulmonary vessels.

1. Kininases in Biological Materials

A carboxypeptidase in fraction IV-1 of human plasma, which was named carboxypeptidase N, showed kininase activity (ERDÖS, 1961; OSHIMA et al., 1974). The enzyme is a metallopeptidase which cleaves the carboxy-terminal arginine of the kinin peptides. During the process of purification of carboxypeptidase N, a second kininase was found in human plasma, which was named kininase II (YANG and ERDÖS, 1967b). It breaks a different bond from carboxypeptidase N (kininase I), cleaving the link between Pro^7 and Phe^8. This enzyme has been described in the literature as the plasma angiotensin converting enzyme (see ERDÖS, 1975). The rabbit and pigeon plasmas lack kininase II. Plasma kininases are irreversibly destroyed by heat or acid treatment (HORTON, 1959), and are inhibited by chelating agents, such as EDTA, phenanthroline, 8-hydroxyquinoline, dimercaptopropanol (BAL) (ERDÖS and SLOANE, 1962; FERREIRA and ROCHA E SILVA, 1962).

Granulocytes and erythrocytes contain kininases which differ from plasma kininases because they are blocked by different inhibitors (ERDÖS et al., 1963a; GREENBAUM and KIM, 1967; MELMON and CLINE, 1967). Kininase activity was found in urine (WERLE and ERDÖS, 1954; GADDUM and GUTH, 1960), lymph (EDERY and LEWIS, 1963; JACOBSEN, 1966b), synovial fluids (EISEN, 1966b) and saliva (AMUNDSEN and NUSTAD, 1964).

Homogenized kidney inactivated Bk and kallidin (HAMBERG and ROCHA E SILVA, 1954; CARVALHO and DINIZ, 1964). ERDÖS and YANG (1966) demonstrated that most of the activity of homogenates of rat kidney was concentrated in a fraction that sedimented with the microsomal fraction. Homogenized pancreas, lung and brain exhibited kininase activity (WERLE et al., 1950; HORI, 1968; CAMARGO and GRAEFF, 1969). The activity in pancreas was due to carboxypeptidase B, chymotrypsin and an aminopeptidase. In kidney it was attributed to an imidopeptidase, a carboxypeptidase and a kininase, named peptidase *P* (ERDÖS and YANG, 1967a). In the rabbit brain, a neutral endopeptidase and a carboxydipeptidase were partially characterized (CAMARGO et al., 1972, 1973). Cysteine-activated cathepsins from bovine spleen can inactivate kinins (GREENBAUM and YAMAFUJI, 1966).

Kininases were found in preparations from *Clostridium histolyticum* and *Pseudomonas aeruginosa* (ERDÖS and YANG, 1966; RUGSTAD, 1966). Venoms from snakes of the genera *Bothrops*, *Vipera*, *Crotalus*, *Agkistrodon* also have kininase activity (HAMBERG and ROCHA E SILVA, 1957a, 1957b; DEUTSCH and DINIZ, 1955).

2. Carboxypeptidase B and Chymotrypsin

Carboxypeptidase B is often used to identify Bk-like peptides and to investigate their participation in biological phenomena. This follows from the observation by ERDÖS and colleagues (ERDÖS et al., 1963a, b) that the enzyme rapidly and specifically hydrolyses the C-terminal arginine of Bk or kallidin molecules. Met-Lys-Bk is more resistant (ERDÖS and YANG, 1966).

Chymotrypsin splits the Phe^8-Arg^9 and the Phe^5-Ser^6 bonds of Bk (ELLIOTT et al., 1960a; BOISSONAS et al., 1960b). It had already been recognized in the early years of the Bk-system that contamination with chymotrypsin of trypsin preparations, which were used to release the peptide, resulted in a rapid destruction of the active substances (ROCHA E SILVA, 1951).

IV. Summary

Natural active polypeptides, Bk, kallidin, and methionyl-lysyl-Bk, can be enzymically released in plasma from inactive precursors, kininogens, by the action of kininogenases (kallikreins). Kininogens are found in different forms in blood and appear to belong to two main classes: high molecular and low molecular weight kininogens. The generation of kinins is thought to be initiated by the activation of Hageman factor. The process is intermingled with other Hageman factor-dependent processes, such as blood coagulation, fibrinolysis and chemotactic functions. Plasma kininogenases release Bk from kininogens; glandular kininogenases release kallidin from the same substrates. Plasma enzymes able to release methionyl-lysyl-Bk following acidification of plasma are still unknown. Released kallidin and methionyl-lysyl-Bk can be converted to the limit active polypeptide, Bk, by enzymes found in plasma and tissues. Plasma kininogenases exist in an inactive form and, therefore, require a process of activation. Human plasma contains at least four kallikrein inhibitors which are likely to be involved in the biological regulation of kinin release. Circulating free kinins are destroyed by kininases found in blood and tissues.

C. Involvement of Kinins in Inflammatory Reactions

Bk and related peptides exibit pharmacological actions which qualify them as plausible mediators of inflammatory reactions. By employing direct microscopy of mesentery and skin vessels in anaesthetized rats, guinea pigs and rabbits, ZWEIFACH (1966) observed that topical application of Bk led to a pronounced increase in flow through the capillary vessels. Venules were dilated to a proportionately greater extent than were arterioles. Amounts of Bk below 1 ng produced only vasomotor changes. When higher concentrations were added, the vasomotor changes were much more protracted and an increased permeability developed in the post-capillaries and collecting venules. The permeability-increasing action of Bk was independent of histamine release. There was a tendency for red blood cells to clump together which eventually resulted in complete stasis in such vessels. Increased sticking of leucocytes was observed with concentrations of Bk of the order of 1–10 μg. The polypeptide appeared to act on the endothelial cells, since swelling was manifest during the period of permeability changes and probably was accompanied by a separation of cells from one another.

Using the rabbit ear chamber technique, GRAHAM et al. (1965) reported that the injection of Bk elicited a vascular response characterized by arteriolar dilation which appeared within a few seconds of injection. Soon after the onset of arteriolar dilation, many leucocytes were seen rolling slowly along the vascular endothelium and, in the larger reactions, began to adhere firmly to the vessel wall. In intense reactions, migration of leucocytes was observed.

As shown by MAJNO (1964), following previous experiments by MAJNO and PALADE (1961) in which histamine and 5-hydroxytryptamine (5-HT) were used, injection of Bk in the subcutaneous tissue of the scrotum of the rat, led to a diffusion of the substance in the cremaster muscle with signs of leakage in some vessels. Electron micrographs of the leaking blood vessels showed that 5 min after the application of Bk (50 μg) and an intravenous injection of colloidal mercuric sulphide, the wall of a multiple-layered venule contained abnormal material indicating leakage: chylomicra and deposits of electron dense particles of HgS. The leakage occurred through gaps formed in the vessel walls with evidence that plasma filtered out at this site. These experiments illustrate the striking similarities in vascular changes observed in an inflammatory response to those induced by topical application of Bk. It should be recalled that histamine was first thought to act as a chemical mediator of inflammatory reactions when LEWIS (1927), observed that the triple reaction in the human skin induced by mild stimuli could be reproduced by local injection of histamine.

A relevant criterion, however, suggesting the plausibility of an endogenous substance as a mediator of inflammatory reactions concerns the duration of its effects. The endogenous permeability factors as a group increase permeability maximally in 3 min, but the effects last only 10–15 min or 20 min at the most (WILHELM, 1973). As shown by ZWEIFACH (1964), when Bk or histamine or 5-HT are administered locally on the mesentery, their effects wear off rapidly, even when the dose is several thousand times the minimal effective dose. However, although the action of Bk on vascular permeability lasted only a few minutes after its injection, salivary kallikrein was still active 45 min after its intradermal injection (LEWIS, 1970). Therefore, activation of the Bk-system when extravasated plasma comes into contact with damaged extravascular tissue seems to be a more important factor for the inflammatory events than the circulating free kinins. We (GARCIA LEME et al., 1970) observed that SBTI, infused into an inflamed rat's paw, inhibited the appearance of a Bk-like material detected in the perfusate in doses as low as 0.025 mg/ml of the perfusion fluid, whereas, when given intravenously, repeated doses of 4–5 mg/kg were required to produce some inhibition (Fig. 1). Similar results were obtained when hexadimethrine bromide was used instead of SBTI. The facts favour the possibility that irritative stimuli originate a process leading to local plasma extravazation and that the subcutaneous tissue is the chief site of formation of kinins, from the inactive precursor exuded with plasma. In fact, tying one of the iliac arteries immediately before the application of the noxious stimulus completely prevented the appearance of active material in the corresponding paw. Due to a continous activation of the system in the interstitial spaces of the affected area, the active kinins would stay relatively longer in contact with the microcirculatory bed.

Another point that has been raised in considering the significance of any active endogenous substance for the development of inflammatory reactions, and in particular for the delayed phase of the reaction, is that the blood vessels at this stage may become selectively refractory to their action (MILES, 1964). MILES and MILES (1952) found that histamine induces refractoriness of the test site to subsequent injections of

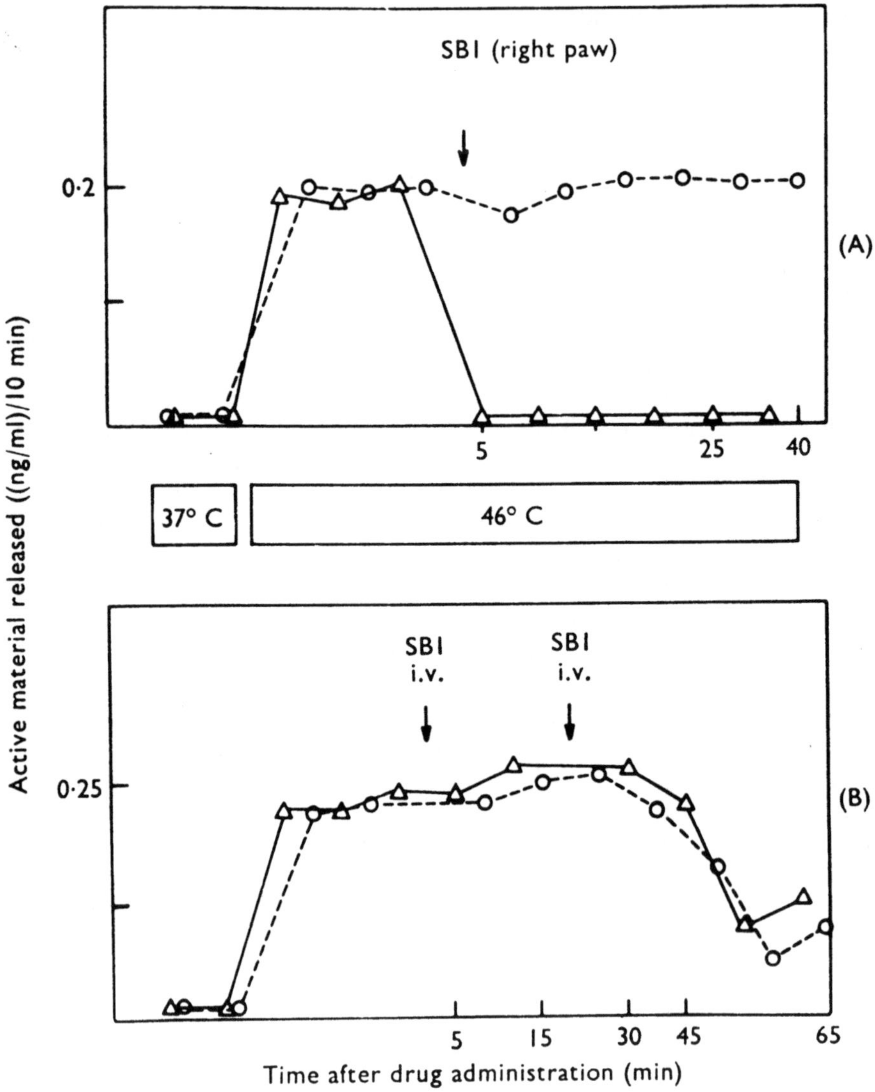

Fig. 1. Effect of soybean trypsin inhibitor (SBI) on release of active material from heated (46° C) rat hind paw. (A), 0.1 mg/ml of the substance was added to perfusion fluid reaching the right paw (—△—). Release of active material from left paw (---○---) remained unchanged. (B), Administration of 2 and 4 mg/kg SBI intravenously (*arrows from left to right, respectively*). Amount of active material released was estimated as Bk on the isolated rat uterus. According to GARCIA LEME et al. (1970) and reproduced by permission of British Journal of Pharmacology

histamine or histamine liberators. GREAVES and SHUSTER (1967) confirmed and extended this observation. In the dermal vessels of the human forearm, they observed that repeated doses of histamine or 5-HT induced tachyphylaxis to wealing, whereas Bk did not. Intracutaneous injections of Bk did not induce refractoriness of the test area to histamine, nor histamine to Bk. The results of GREAVES and SCHUSTER are also applicable to the guinea pig (BAUMGARTEN et al., 1970). Therefore, as far as the Bk system is concerned, there is no present evidence that desensitisation of blood vessels might represent an important element for the discontinuation of its effects.

In practically all species so far studied, the stores of kininogen are large enough to permit the release of significant amounts of free kinin. As shown in Table 1, values estimated for Bk equivalents in plasma or serum range between 5 and 12 µg/ml in adult humans; 6 and 10 µg/ml in the rabbit; 5 and 6 µg/ml in the dog; 1 and 2 µg/ml in the rat. Even if a small fraction were activated following plasma extravasation in an inflamed area, the newly formed kinins would be present in amounts sufficient enough to produce vascular changes. The contact of plasma proteins with extravascular tissues would favour the activation of the whole system and due to the long-lasting action of kininogenases in tissues (LEWIS, 1970) a continuous supply of active kinins would be provided.

I. Effects of Kinins Related to the Signs and Symptoms of Inflammation

1. Vasodilation

Kinins are potent vasodilating agents. The arterial injection of 2–3 ng Bk markedly increase blood flow in cat skeletal muscle (HILTON, 1960) or through the cat hind limbs (ELLIOTT et al., 1960b). In humans, regional changes in blood flow by the action of Bk were reported by FOX et al. (1961), EHRINGER et al. (1961), KONZETT (1962), COFFMAN and JAVETT (1963), MASON and MELMON (1965). The experiments by ZWEIFACH (1966), GRAHAM et al. (1965) and MAJNO (1964), referred to at the begining of this section, provided direct evidence that Bk is capable of dilating microcirculatory vessels.

2. Permeability-Increasing Action

Bk and kallidin are rated among the most effective permeability-increasing factors in most species. Concentrations of the order of 10^{-9} M of Bk are active when injected intradermally. With still impure preparations of Bk, BHOOLA and SCHACHTER (1959) reported a marked permeability-increasing effect for a circulating dye in the guinea pig following intradermal injections of the material. The results were confirmed with synthetic Bk by KONSETT and STÜRMER (1960), STÜRMER and CERLETTI (1961a) and FRIMMER (1961).

Extensive studies were made by WILHELM and colleagues to compare potencies of various factors in the skin of laboratory animals. By measuring the diameter of the lesions, the colour intensity and the amount of exuded dye, previously given by the intravenous route, accurate comparisons were made. Table 3 summarizes data from SPARROW and WILHELM (1957), MILES and WILHELM (1960), CARR and WILHELM (1965), FREUND et al. (1958) and WILHELM (1973). As shown by CARR and WILHELM (1964), the potency results are consistent with the distribution of the dye at different levels of the skin lesion. The superficial dye was most intense at the epidermo-dermal junction, the deep dye in the paniculus adiposus. The superficial dye was much more intense in Bk lesions, the deep dye in kallikrein lesions. This, in turn, raises questions concerning differences in the vasculature at various levels in the skin, as well as the

Table 3. Potency of various substances as permeability factors

Substance	Absolute potency (EBD/mg)[a]		
	Guinea pig	Rat	Rabbit
Bradykinin	2700000	9720	2330000
Kallidin	2133000	5820	769000
Kallikrein (hog)	240	70	1130
Trypsin (bovine)	2560	900	600
Histamine	32200	1400	37000
5-hydroxytryptamine	60	16200	< 20

[a] EBD, effective blueing dose, i.e., the dose in 0.1 ml that induces a mature lesion 6 mm in diameter (WILHELM et al., 1958). Data from SPARROW and WILHELM (1957), MILES and WILHELM (1960), CARR and WILHELM (1965), FREUND et al. (1958) and WILHELM (1973).

effects of permeability factors at these same levels. Also differences should be expected between organs.

Interspecies differences in permeability-increasing potencies are exhibited by the different factors (Table 3). Bk has outstanding activity in the guinea pig and rabbit, but not in the rat. Kallidin is particularly effective in the guinea pig. Bk, as well as histamine and 5—HT, induces increased vascular permeability in the synovialis of the rat. The mechanism of action is the same in the synovialis as in the skin and muscle, and the relative potency is similar in the synovialis and skin (BIGNOLD and LYKKE, 1975). Also quantitative differences were found by comparing permeability potencies with other effects of kinins. REIS et al. (1971) assayed three polypeptides with the terminal sequence of Bk: Gly-Arg-Met-Lys-Bk (GAML-Bk), Met-Lys-Bk, Lys-Bk (kallidin) and Bk itself for biological activity on the guinea pig ileum, rat uterus, rat duodenum, arterial blood pressure of the rat by venous and arterial routes and rat vascular permeability (blue test). The pharmacological actions were qualitatively similar but differed quantitatively according to the molecular weights of the peptides tested. Those with the highest molecular weights were much less active upon the smooth muscle preparations, while 10–12 times more effective in the vascular permeability test (Table 4). A situation, therefore, might arise in which a natural product, derived from kininogens, might be predominantly classified as a permeability factor. The mechanism of kinin release depends upon the prevailing test conditions and upon the nature of the enzymes involved (ELLIOTT and LEWIS, 1965; RYAN and ROCHA E SILVA, 1971). Larger polypeptides than Bk might therefore be released in the peculiar conditions of an inflammatory reaction. The polypeptide GAML-Bk in the experiments by REIS and collaborators is particularly potent as a permeability factor and much less susceptible to the action of kininases (Table 4). If similar substances occur in vivo, they would pose interesting new possibilities concerning the participation of the kinin system in phenomena of increased vascular permeability.

3. Oedema

As a direct consequence of their permeability increasing properties, kinins induce accumulation of fluid in the interstitial spaces, resulting in oedema formation. Bk is

Table 4. Ratios of potency[a] of various peptides taking bradykinin (=1.0) as standard

Peptides	Guinea pig ileum	Rat uterus	Rat duodenum	Rat's blood pressure via		Ratio B.P. Artery/vein	Vascular permeability
				Artery	Vein		
Bk	1.00	1.00	1.00	1.00	0.12	8.4 1.0[c]	1.00
Lys-Bk	0.30 (0.29–0.33)	0.88 (0.76–1.00)	1.98 (1.47–2.60)	0.91 ± 0.14 (9)	0.30 ± 0.1 (4)	3.0 1.0[c]	1.00 ± 0.5
Met-Lys-Bk	0.09 (0.08–0.10)	0.30 (0.25–0.36)	0.49 (0.46–0.52)	0.87 ± 0.13 (9)	0.43 ± 0.08 (7)	2.0 1.1[c]	10.00 ± 0.73 (6)
GAML-Bk[b]	0.063 (0.06–0.067)	0.60 (0.50–0.70)	0.72 (0.67–0.76)	1.00 ± 0.18 (7)	1.00 ± 0.05 (7)	1.0 1.0[c]	11.00 ± 0.6 (4)

[a] Ratios were calculated on molar concentrations. Pairs of figures between brackets are confidence limits obtained in 4-point assays for the 5% level of significance. For the assays on blood pressure and vascular permeability the means ± S.E. are given, and the number of experiments indicated in brackets.

[b] Corrected for 30% impurities (GAML-Bk = Gly-Arg-Met-Lys-Bk).

[c] These values were obtained by a previous treatment of the animal with BAL 20 mg/kg, i.v. According to Reis et al. (1971) and reproduced by permission of Biochemical Pharmacology.

some ten times more potent than histamine in producing swelling (STÜRMER and CERLETTI, 1961 b; VAN ARMAN et al., 1965; MALING et al., 1974). The peak is reached around 10–30 min after local injection in the rat's paw and decreases fairly rapidly (VAN ARMAN et al., 1965; VAN ARMAN and NUSS, 1969; GIORDANO and SCAPAGNINI, 1967; GARCIA LEME and WALASZEK, 1973). The intensity of localized oedema provoked by Bk in the rat's paw progressively decreases with age, being almost negligible in animals 6–8 months old, but it is indifferent with respect to sex (GIORDANO and SCAPAGNINI, 1967).

4. Production of Pain

Pain in an inflammatory focus may result from the release of algogenic substances or of substances which sensitize pain receptors to the algogenic factors. Mechanical compression of sensitive stem axons due to the accumulation of fluid in the interstitial spaces may be an additional element for pain production. However, it is questionable whether receptors for pain can be mechano-sensitive. Furthermore, pain and swelling are not related in a constant manner. When carrageenin is injected into the rat's paw, swelling is accompanied by a marked decrease in pain threshold. Dextran, on the contrary, produces oedema with an increase in pain threshold (WINTER and FLATAKER, 1965; VAN ARMAN et al., 1968). Pain receptors seem to be essentially chemoreceptors and are present in visceral as well as in cutaneous areas, being paravascularly situated. Injury or regional ischaemia may lead to the disintegration of circulating and fixed cells, release of lysosomal proteases, local acidosis, production of prostaglandins, release of vasoactive amines (histamine, 5-HT) and activation of the kinin system. All these conditions favour the stimulation and sensitization of pain receptors (LIM, 1968). Some of the produced materials or substances may directly stimulate pain receptors (algogenic factors), others behave as sensitizing factors.

ROSENTHAL and MINARD (1939) showed that threshold pain stimuli to the skin cause the release of protein split products in humans, dogs, cats, rabbits, and guinea pigs. With the blister technique, KEELE and colleagues first described the pain-producing actions of plasma kinins in human subjects (ARMSTRONG et al., 1952, 1953, 1954, 1957). The technique consists of raising a blister on the volar surface of the forearm, preferably by the use of cantharidin (KEELE and ARMSTRONG, 1964), cutting off the raised epidermis and pouring the test solutions on the denuded base. The pain thus experienced is measured subjectively with the aid of a numerical scale. Pain responses vary depending on the test substance used. Kinins produce pain which is delayed in onset by about 20–25 s, reaches a peak after about 1 min and, if left on the test area, a slow decline from peak can be traced (ARMSTRONG, 1970). High pain responses were recorded for concentrations of the order of 10^{-6} M or lower with solutions of either synthetic Bk (ELLIOTT et al., 1960b; KEELE and ARMSTRONG, 1964), kallidin (ARMSTRONG and MILLS, 1963), methionyl-lysyl-Bk (ELLIOTT and LEWIS, 1965) and glycyl-Bk (ARMSTRONG, 1970).

When Bk is injected into the human circulation, the responses vary. In the experiments by BURCH and DE PASQUALE (1962), all subjects experienced pain after intra-arterial injection of a few micrograms of Bk. Pain appeared within a period of

30 s and subsided after 60–120 s. However, only transient pain was reported in the experiments by Fox et al. (1961) with intra-arterial administration of the polypeptide. In the experiments by SICUTERI et al. (1965), no pain was produced when Bk was given into the human hand vein, unless 5-HT had been given previously.

The existence of sensitizing factors is an interesting possibility as far as inflammation is concerned. In SICUTERI's experiments, 5-HT and synthetic Bk given separately in different veins of the hand did not provoke pain. If both substances were given into the same vein, pain arose after a latent period. In 1972, FERREIRA reported that lipoperoxides and prostaglandins (PGs) cause overt pain in high concentrations. In low concentrations, likely to be present in inflammatory reactions, they sensitize the pain receptors. This sensitization can occur with minute amounts of PGs since their effects are cumulative. In the work by FERREIRA, subdermal infusions of PGs with either histamine or Bk, or both, produced pain which was more intense than with PGs alone and became continuous towards the end of the infusion. With the combination of the three substances, the removal of the needle was followed by an intense pain which lasted for about 5 min. Therefore, the combined effects of plausible mediators of inflammatory reactions can more easily produce pain by a mechanism of previous sensitization of nervous structures to the algogenic factors. This sensitization may also counteract the possibility of tachyphylaxis shown by KEELE and ARMSTRONG (1964) with Bk in the blister area.

Recently, JUAN and LEMBECK (1974) estimated the algesic effect of several substances following intra-arterial injection into the rabbit ear. The method consisted of recording action potentials of the auricular nerve in the isolated ear and also the reflex fall in systemic blood pressure elicited by the injection of the substances into the isolated perfused ear, which was still connected to the body by the nerve. The order of potency of the agents tested was: Bk, substance P > acetylcholine > ATP, histamine, 5-HT or KCl. The threshold dose for action potentials was 0.05 μg Bk, 51 μg histamine, 203 μg 5-HT, and 612 μg KCl. Eledoisin, adenosine, adrenaline, and angiotensin, among others, were inactive. PGE_1 infused into the ear, enhanced the effect of the algogenic substances. On the other hand, indomethacin inhibited the effect of the algesic substances in proportion to the dose and duration of infusion (LEMBECK and JUAN, 1974).

Bk produces effects (vocalization, hypertension, and hyperpnea) associated with pain in the dog when injected into the femoral, brachial, splenic, gastric, superior mesenteric artery, or into the portal vein, in threshold doses of 1–2 μg as compared with 50–100 μg of 5-HT and histamine, 250–500 μg of acetylcholine and 9–10 mg of KCl (GUZMAN et al., 1962). It also evoked action potentials in the splanchnic nerve when given into the splenic artery (LIM et al., 1964) (for a review, see LIM, 1968).

Intraperitoneal injection of Bk in mice produces the writhing reaction (WHITTLE, 1964), which is frequently used as a test for analgesic drugs.

Behavioural responses, including biting, scratching, backing, kicking, and squeaking, followed with reasonable frequency intradermal injection into guinea pigs of strongly anisotonic solutions, which are known to cause pain in human skin. They were also observed after intradermal injection of Bk or kallidin. This effect of Bk was depressed by pretreatment with morphine or codeine, but not with amidopyrine, calcium acetylsalicylate or phenylbutazone (COLLIER and LEE, 1963).

5. Leucocyte Accumulation

In intense reactions induced by Bk in vessels of the rabbit ear, sticking and migration of leucocytes were observed (GRAHAM et al., 1965). Although this finding is not an indication that the peptide is the causal agent, Bk promoted leucocyte accumulation in the mesentery vessels of the rat (LEWIS, 1962). SPECTOR and WILLOUGHBY (1964) and WARD (1971), however, reported that kinins were rather ineffective in causing migration of white cells.

II. Release of Kinins by Trauma

It is generally recognized that an acidic environment prevails in tissue damage and that increased proteolytic activity occurs (MÖRSDORF, 1969; MÖRSDORF et al., 1968). Various anti-inflammatory drugs, e.g. indomethacin, sodium salicylate, and phenylbutazone, can inhibit protein breakdown. The anti-proteasic action of ε-aminocaproic acid, ε-acetamidocaproic acid, aminomethylcyclohexane carboxylic acid, aprotinin, and iniprol, was studied by BERTELLI (1968) in relation to enzyme-induced rat paw oedema. The response to local injections of collagenase, pronase, plasmin, acid phosphatase, elastase, and peptidase was inhibited, indicating that proteasic activation may be present in conditions in which tissue reactivity is altered. Hydrolases believed to be involved in autolysis are not distributed freely in the cytoplasm, but are confined within the lysosomal fraction of cells, as shown by DE DUVE et al. (1955). Lysosomal rupture seems to be an early event and can be induced by acidification of the medium or anoxia. Excretion of hydrolases into extracellular spaces would lead to hydrolytic injuries to tissue components (DE DUVE, 1964). Hydrocortisone preserves lysosomes from rupture (WEISSMAN and THOMAS, 1962; WEISSMAN and DINGLE, 1961; WEISSMAN and FELL, 1962). Evidence that both collagen and protein polysaccharide complex breakdown may be mediated by lysosomal proteases was presented by WOESSNER (1969).

All these conditions may favour the activation of kallikreins and the formation of kinins, not only kallidin and Bk, but also methionyl-lysyl-Bk, the formation of which depends on an acid pH. Plasma kallikrein is activated at acid pH (WERLE, 1934). Furthermore, EDERY and LEWIS (1962) have shown that kininases are inhibited at slightly acid pH. We confirmed this finding by infusing Bk into the subcutaneous tissue of the rat's paw. When the peptide was dissolved in Tyrode's solution (pH 8) the recovery was approximately 40%. When Tyrode-Tris buffer solution adjusted to pH 3 was used as the perfusion fluid, instead of Tyrode's solution, the amount of Bk recovered was about 98–100%, as can be seen in Table 5 (GARCIA LEME et al., 1970). However, for the protection of kinins against the action of kininases it is not necessary that such an acid environment should prevail. As shown by EDERY and LEWIS, at pH 7.3 Bk is destroyed 5–10 times more rapidly than it is at pH 6. Besides that, GLADNER and colleagues (GLADNER et al., 1963; GLADNER, 1966) demonstrated the existence of naturally occurring polypeptides, released during thrombin-catalyzed conversion of fibrinogen to fibrin, which potentiated markedly some effects of Bk. These peptides occur in various species, including man, and might enhance kinin actions in inflammatory responses.

Table 5. Recovery of bradykinin in Tyrode's solution, pH 8 and pH 3, after perfusion through the subcutaneous spaces of rat paws

pH 8 Exp. No.	Response of rat uterus to bradykinin added:				Estimated recovery (%)
	(a) direct		(b) in perfusion fluid		
	ng	response (mm)	ng	response (mm)	
1	0.8	57	1.0	52	60
	1.0	63	2.0	57	40
	1.2	67	4.0	77	47
	2.0	79			
	4.0	83			
2	0.6	39	2.0	36	25
	1.0	57	4.0	56	25
	2.0	65	8.0	62	25
3	0.8	46	2.0	48	44
	1.0	51	4.0	59	38
	2.0	53	8.0	64	26
4	1.0	9	2.0	9	50
	1.6	18	4.0	22	43
	3.2	33	8.0	35	41
	4.0	47			
5	1.0	45	2.0	44	49
	2.0	52	4.0	55	51
	3.2	60	8.0	58	38
pH 3 Exp. No.					
1	2.0	47	2.0	50	106
	4.0	58	4.0	58	100
2	2.0	55	2.0	54	98
	4.0	59	4.0	58	99
3	1.0	59	1.0	61	103
	2.0	66	2.0	65	98
	4.0	70	4.0	70	100
	8.0	74	8.0	74	100
4	1.0	54	1.0	57	105
	2.0	60	2.0	61	101
	4.0	66	4.0	65	98
	8.0	70	8.0	70	100

According to GARCIA LEME et al. (1970) and reproduced, slightly modified, by permission of British Journal of Pharmacology.

Overall, a relative degree of anoxia, acidification of the medium, increased proteolytic activity, and inhibition of kininases are events which follow tissue injury. These events predispose to the activation of the kinin-system and accumulation of kinins. However, one should bear in mind that most of these conditions may also favour the release or activation of other vasoactive agents, such as histamine or PGs. Therefore sufficient identification criteria are necessary to assume the participation of a particular substance in a particular reaction.

1. Thermal Injury

In 1960, ROCHA E SILVA and ANTONIO, in the course of experiments to investigate the effect of heating to 45° C on the release of histamine by perfusion of the rat's hind legs with compound 48/80, observed that the immersion of the paws in a water bath at 45° C for 30 min caused a marked oedema, developing below the tibio-tarsal articulation. Since the heating procedure prevented the release of histamine when the paw was subsequently perfused with histamine liberators at 37° C, they excluded the participation of histamine as essential for the development of the "thermic oedema." Furthermore, antihistamine agents were ineffective in preventing the formation of such oedema, as were anti-5-HT drugs. Sympatholytic agents partially protected the animals, but no complete abolition of the reaction to heating was observed even if the rats were repeatedly given reserpine.

By perfusing the subcutaneous tissue of the rat's paw during the development of the thermic oedema and collecting the perfusion fluid (Tyrode's solution) upon ice, these authors were able to detect the presence of a principle which stimulated the isolated rat uterus. The perfusion samples collected remained inactive until the temperature inside the paw reached 43.8–44.8° C, as measured with the aid of a thermocouple. At temperatures of 48–49° C, the activity in the samples tended to disappear. The active principle was rapidly destroyed by incubation with chymotrypsin and could not be distinguished in its action upon the uterus, from Bk. In addition, 5-HT antagonists did not reduce the activity of the perfusates upon the isolated preparation. The authors concluded that Bk was released under the conditions of oedema formation. However, the identification of the principle released was only partial since the amounts obtained were too small for further types of assay.

Ten years later, in the same laboratory, an extensive study was made on the conditions and characterization of the Bk-like substance appearing during the development of thermic oedema (GARCIA LEME et al., 1970). The material stimulated the isolated rat uterus, relaxed the isolated rat duodenum, was destroyed by incubation with chymotrypsin and was potentiated by Bk-potentiating factor (BPF) (FERREIRA, 1965). Substances which interfere with the release of Bk from its inactive precursor in plasma, such as SBTI or hexadimethrine bromide (ARMSTRONG and STEWART, 1962), when added to the perfusion fluid, produced a potent and reversible inhibition of the release of the active material (Figs. 1 and 2); aprotinin caused a temporary block. Pretreatment of the animals with atropine plus diphenhydramine did not affect the release of the active kinin. The concentration released was 0.5–8 ng/ml per 10 min as estimated by comparison with responses of the isolated rat uterus to synthetic Bk. The minimal latency time for appearance of the material was 4 min in 12 rats. The estimated mean recovery of the Bk-like material was 40%. As previously discussed, much higher doses of SBTI, hexadimethrine bromide or aprotinin had to be used by the intravenous route to produce a much smaller inhibition than that obtained by local perfusion of the inhibitors through the heated paw. This fact seemed to indicate that the subcutaneous space was the chief site of activation of the material thus produced.

The release of Bk-like substances into the perfusion fluid of rat paws subjected to heat at temperatures up to 46.5° C was also detected by STARR and WEST (1967). The increases in the protein levels in the perfusates closely followed those of kinins. The

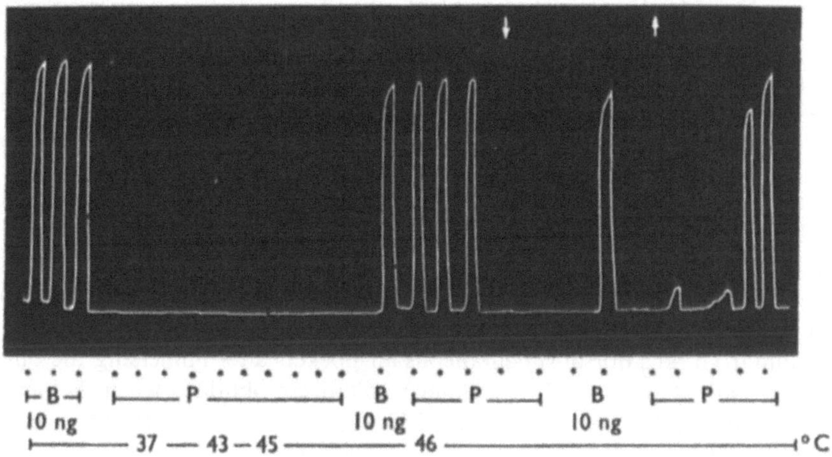

Fig. 2. Temperature dependency and effect of hexadimethrine bromide on the release of a Bk-like material from the rat's paw. The material is released when the external (water bath) temperature reached 45°–46° C (*lower scale*). Hexadimethrine bromide (0.5 mg/ml) added to the perfusion fluid (*left arrow*) completely blocked the release of such material, which reappeared after omitting the drug from the perfusion liquid (*right arrow*). *B*: standard Bk (10 ng); *P*: perfusate (0.6 ml) from the paw. Test organ: rat uterus. According to GARCIA LEME et al. (1970) and reproduced by permission of British Journal of Pharmacology

release of kininogen and of kinin-forming activity also followed a similar pattern to that of Bk, whereas the output of kininases in the perfusates was not affected by the heating procedure. The development of oedema was accompanied by marked deposition of dye, previously given intravenously, and by petechial formation. Rats which were resistant to the anaphylactoid reaction produced by dextran showed greater resistance to thermic oedema than did those giving the anaphylactoid reaction. Also lower levels of kinins, kininogen or kinin-forming enzymes were found in the perfusates from non-reacting animals.

An investigation of the effects in rats of heating up to 45° C, was undertaken by SOUZA and ROCHA E SILVA (1967, 1968). The animals were kept in an appropriate box with a double wall, where water was circulated at increasing temperatures. The whole body of the animal, with the exception of the head, was submitted to such heated environment. With the temperature in the box at 45° C, it took about 30 min for the internal (peritoneal) temperature (measured with a thermocouple) to reach 43° C. At this point, most animals died of circulatory collapse. Perfusions of the peritoneal cavity showed that exuded dye, previously given intravenously, attained higher concentrations in the period immediately preceding the lethal fall in blood pressure. The fact that kinins are released at the internal temperatures indicated, and that they produce a fall in blood pressure and increase vascular permeability, lend support to the authors' view that the kinin system is involved in this kind of heat-stroke.

Burns may increase the urinary excretion of peptides. GOODWIN et al. (1963) found that the urine of 25 severely burned patients contained kinin-like peptides in higher concentrations than those found in normal urine. SEVITT (1964) found that temperatures of 41–45° C produced a delayed and sustained increase in permeability of microcirculatory vessels of the guinea pig skin. Temperatures of 45–50° C led to an early permeability increase, associated with endothelial damage and vascular stasis. A biphasic pattern of response to heat was observed by WILHELM and MASON (1960) in guinea pigs, rats, and rabbits, and by SPECTOR and WILLOUGHBY (1959) in rats. Both groups concluded that increased vascular permeability following burns of moderate intensity is initiated by release of histamine. The latter workers suggested that the phenomenon was maintained by other endogenous mechanisms. Even when severe burns are inflicted, in which direct physical injury contributes to increasing vascular permeability, endogenous mechanisms would continue to play a role. In fact, evidence was given that histamine, Bk and adenyl compounds appeared in the wash fluid from rat's dorsal subcutaneous air pockets after immersing the outerskin in a water bath at 96° C for 15 s. Similar results were obtained when the air pocket was perfused and the skin burned by a 250-watt infrared lamp (ROCHA E SILVA and ROSENTHAL, 1961).

As shown by COTRAN and MAJNO (1964), any bacterial, physical or chemical injury, if sufficiently severe, can damage the vascular wall *directly*. This rather drastic, non-specific type of injury spares no vessels -arterioles, capillaries or venules. When thermal injury was used as a model, they observed that by applying 60° C for 20 s to depilated rat skin, the superficial capillary network, as well as the underlying vessels of all calibres were instantly affected. There was cellular injury, and gaps were formed through, as well as between, endothelial cells. Leakage occurred from vessels of all types, contrary to what is seen when mild injury is inflicted, in which venules are the predominant leaking vessels. This may be the mechanism underlying the development of a thermic oedema produced at temperatures above 45° C. In fact, however, what the thermic oedema model stresses is that active kinins can be found in the affected area. Therefore, kinins are expected to be present in adjacent areas, any time vessels start to leak in response to noxious stimuli and may contribute to the overall phenomenon. However, as noted above, reliable criteria of identification of a substance are needed for the evaluation of its participation in a phenomenon. Biological properties of extracts, changes in general conditions of the experimental animal following the application of a noxious stimulus, and increased excretion of metabolites following injury were described in this section, which might be attributed to an increased formation of kinins. Nevertheless, although these experiments suggest the participation of kinins in the phenomena considered, they should not be regarded as a demonstration that only kinins are involved.

2. Changes in Lymph Resulting From Burns

Bk and kallidin intra-arterially infused in doses of 0.005 to 1.28 μg/min over 15 min raise the flow of lymph in dogs in a reproducible and dose-dependent manner. At the same time, the total lymphocyte count and the protein content of lymph are elevated. These findings showed that plasma kinins may influence the flow and the composition of lymph (STÜRMER, 1966).

Normally, no kinin or kinin-forming activities are detected in lymph collected from the hind limbs of anaesthetised dogs and rabbits, although the samples contain the substrates for kinin-forming enzymes (JACOBSEN, 1966b). However, after scalding the limbs an increase in lymph flow and in lymph content of total proteins and of kininogens was found. This increase was supposed to reflect the increased escape of plasma proteins from leaking blood vessels into tissue spaces (JACOBSEN and WAALER, 1966). LEWIS and WAURETSCHEK (1971), found no free kinins, but an increase in the activity of acid kallikrein (EDERY and LEWIS, 1963; LEWIS and WAWRETSCHEK, 1971). The increased kinin-forming activity occurring in lymph was much higher than that present in plasma.

3. Chemical Injury

Different chemical irritants, depending on their properties, may induce inflammatory reactions by activating different mechanisms. Carrageenin releases Bk from the fresh plasma of the rat (ROTHSCHILD and GASCON, 1966; GARCIA LEME et al., 1967). As a Bk-releasing agent, carrageenin is less potent than cellulose-sulphate and more potent than dextran (GARCIA LEME et al., 1973a). However, contrary to observations with dextran, carrageenin and cellulose-sulphate are devoid of histamine-releasing properties when incubated with isolated mast cells of the rat (GARCIA LEME et al., 1973a). VAN ARMAN et al. (1965) presented evidence that yeast, but not carrageenin, incubated with peritoneal fluid from normal rats, which is rich in mast cells, released histamine and 5-HT. The irritant effect of substances with sensory nerve stimulating actions, such as xylene and mustard, which are supposed to act through the release of pro-inflammatory nerve factors, is abolished following chronic denervation, whereas that of dextran or egg-white is unaffected (JANCSO et al., 1967). However, even when the inflammatory reaction is initiated by a particular pharmacological property of the irritant, leading to the release or formation of a particular active agent, once started, other mechanisms can be activated and the reaction is frequently multimediated.

a) Macromolecular Polymers

Carrageenin, a sulphated polysaccharide extracted from seaweed, was employed by GARDNER (1960) to produce experimental arthritis in rabbits and guinea pigs. The response to this material was highly reproducible and seemed to depend entirely upon the local stimulus to an inflammatory reaction, being devoid of antigenic properties. WINTER et al. (1962) introduced carrageenin-induced oedema of the rat hind paw as an assay for anti-inflammatory drugs. A 1% suspension of the material in sterile saline injected into the subplantar tissue of the paw produced a swelling reaction reaching a peak in 3–5 h, then retaining the same degree of oedema for several hours. VAN ARMAN et al. (1965) compared the swelling induced in the rat's paw by carrageenin and by yeast and concluded that for yeast, but not for carrageenin inflammation the mast cell must be involved. Carrageenin inflammation was blocked by SBTI and the suggestion was put forward that it acted through a proteolytic process, Bk being the mediator. However, in another paper, VAN ARMAN and NUSS (1969) admitted that it was improbable that Bk could be an important mediator of the inflammatory reaction caused by carrageenin, for indomethacin, which prevents almost entirely the effects of carrageenin, did not inhibit the action of Bk or its formation from kininogen. The main argument was that intravenous injection of carrageenin lowered kininogen levels (ROTHSCHILD and GASCON, 1966; GARCIA

LEME et al., 1967) but this effect was not prevented by the anti-inflammatory drug. It is now known that Bk is an effective releaser of PG (PIPER and VANE, 1969; MCGIFF et al., 1972; MONCADA et al., 1973) and that indomethacin blocks the synthesis and release of PGs (VANE, 1971; FERREIRA et al., 1971). This might explain the apparent discrepancy shown by VAN ARMAN and NUSS and once more stresses the point that various mediators may interact in inflammatory reactions.

WILLIS (1969) studied the release of pharmacologically active substances during carrageenin inflammation by testing crude inflammatory exudates upon isolated smooth muscle preparations superfused in cascade. The exudates were obtained by the carrageenin air bleb technique in the rat. Histamine, E-type PGs, kinins, and probably 5-HT were present in the exudates. In the carrageenin-induced paw oedema reaction in the rat, BOLAM et al. (1974) observed that treatment of the animals with substances which either deplete the levels or antagonize the action of either histamine, 5-HT or kinins significantly reduced the swelling. DI ROSA and WILLOUGHBY (1971), however, found good responses to carrageenin in rats depleted of their tissue stores of histamine, 5-HT, and kininogen, whereas the oedema provoked by dextran or formalin was markedly reduced. Nevertheless, their own comments showed that there remained some points to be clarified concerning the precise role of kinins in carrageenin and other models of inflammation (DI ROSA et al., 1971), since DI ROSA and SORRENTINO (1968, 1970) had previously shown that in kininogen-depleted rats oedema induced by carrageenin was suppressed and thus was closely related to the time course of kininogen depletion. This, however, may have been due to the drop in total haemolytic complement titre induced by cellulose sulphate, the kininogen-depleting agent utilized (DI ROSA et al., 1971). Cellulose sulphate produced a transient drop in the complement titre, levels returning to normal 3 h after the injection. Carrageenin now produced a biphasic response with a small suppression of swelling at 30 min and 1 h, but a much greater suppression at $1\frac{1}{2}$–$2\frac{1}{2}$ h. The conclusion was that kinins are probably involved for this time-period of the developing oedema. In turpentine pleurisy, on the other hand, cellulose sulphate given 3 h before the intrapleural injection failed to influence the development of the inflammatory exudate.

CRUNKHORN and MEACOCK (1971) reported that intact or adrenalectomized rats which had previously been injected with ellagic acid or saliva to reduce considerably the concentration of plasma kininogens, or with antagonists of 5-HT, showed a reduced inflammatory response to carrageenin. Although rat saliva lowered complement levels by approximately 20%, ellagic acid was devoid of such an action. Mepyramine alone had no effect on oedema formation, but in combination with ellagic acid it caused a reduction. The authors concluded that kinins and 5-HT contribute significantly to oedema formation induced by carrageenin and that histamine played a minor role.

FERREIRA et al. (1974) have recently shown that carrageenin oedema in the rat's paw was potentiated by a specific Bk potentiator, BPP_{9a} (GREENE et al., 1972). This potentiation was blocked by SBTI. All animals were pretreated with indomethacin, and therefore, the contribution of PGs, in this case, was avoided. These facts suggested that Bk-like substances might be relevant in the process. Early enhancement of the oedema indicated that generation of kinins commences just after carrageenin injection. It is true that the addition of PGE_1 to the carrageenin in the indomethacin-treated rats strikingly increased the oedema formation, but as shown by THOMAS and WEST (1974), PGE_1 and Bk exhibit synergistic effects on vascular permeability in rat skin and in rat paws.

Other water-soluble sulphated polysaccharides (cellulose, starch, glycogen, dextran) promote the release of kinins when added to the plasma of the rat, guinea pig or man (ROTHSCHILD and GASCON, 1966; LECOMTE and DAMAS, 1968). Cellulose sulphate, injected into the rat's paw, produced a slow-developing oedema similar to that observed with carrageenin (GARCIA LEME et al., 1967). Previous treatment of the animals with hexadimethrine bromide, which prevents the release of kinins, markedly affected the reaction to cellulose sulphate or carrageenin (GARCIA LEME et al., 1973b) and partially reduced the response to non-sulphated dextran. On the other hand, antagonists of histamine and 5-HT, only slightly affected cellulose sulphate or carrageenin inflammation but depressed the initial response to non-sulphated dextran. Repeated administration to rats of cellulose sulphate by the intraperitoneal route, which consistently reduces kininogen levels, greatly depressed the oedema formation by subsequent injection of either cellulose sulphate or carrageenin in the paws of these animals. These findings suggest that kinins participate in the swelling reaction produced by cellulose sulphate and carrageenin, as well as in the late stages of the dextran response.

Several sulphated polymers: polyvinyl sulphate, polyethylene sulphonate, pentosan polysulphate, in the same way as carrageenin, cellulose sulphate or dextran sulphate, produced oedema in the rat's paw by local injection. They reduced the kininogen content of rat's blood when injected intravenously and when given repeatedly, by the intraperitoneal route, diminished or abolished the swelling produced in the paw by a subsequent local injection of the same or other oedema-producing polymers (ROCHA E SILVA et al., 1969).

EISEN and LOVEDAY (1971), however, observed that with a single effective intravenous dose of cellulose sulphate to rats, plasma kininogen concentrations were promptly reduced by 90% or more, complement titres fell significantly, but the oedema caused by heat or xylene was not reduced. Given over 3 days by the intraperitoneal route, cellulose-sulphate produced similar reduction of kininogen levels but reduced complement titres only slightly. Heat and xylene produced significantly less oedema than in control rats. The diminished response, however, was attributed to toxic side effects of cellulose sulphate, rather than depleted plasma kininogen, as the animals gained less weight, presented haemorrhages and impaired blood clotting.

In a series of experiments, BRISEID et al. (1971) administered intraperitoneally Bk, ellagic acid, histamine, 5-HT, aprotinin, and trypsin to unanaesthetised rats and 30 min later injected carrageenin into the plantar tissue of one hind paw. All substances tested inhibited the development of oedema, and except for aprotinin, caused a drop in total kininogen. Apart from Bk, the substances also reduced the amount of prekallikrein. There is always the possibility that these substances acted as counter-irritants, inducing the formation of endogenous anti-inflammatory factors (see Chapter 15). However, BRISEID and his colleagues showed that the substances tested exhibited an acute anti-inflammatory effect upon carrageenin, which was well correlated with actions on the kinin system.

Elevated kinin activity was found in fluids collected from paw oedema in the rat when yeast (GILFOIL and KLAVINS, 1965), 5-HT or kaolin were used as subplantar irritants, but not with polyvinylpyrrolidine (BONTA and DE VOS, 1965, 1967).

In summary, it can be said that conflicting findings exist concerning the mechanism of action of the pro-inflammatory substances discussed. Carrageenin and cellulose sulphate are not capable of releasing histamine from mast cells in vitro and are potent kinin-releasing agents. However, it is improbable that kinin release initiates their action, since kinins are mainly activated in extravascular spaces following extravazation of plasma proteins. Dextran and yeast may well initiate an inflammatory reaction through the mediation of histamine (and 5-HT). Anti-histamine drugs (and anti-5-HT drugs) are effective in reducing dextran or yeast-induced inflammatory reactions, but only slightly affect those produced by carrageenin or cellulose sulphate. Enzymes derived from cell lysis and neurogenic factors may be involved; nevertheless, as soon as plasma proteins accumulate in perivascular spaces, local conditions will favour the formation of kinins which can then participate in the phenomena described.

b) Urate Crystals

Sodium urate microcrystals added to plasma or synovial fluid activate Hageman factor (KELLERMEYER and BRECKENRIDGE, 1965) which then generates a prekallikrein activator (KAPLAN and AUSTEN, 1971), kallikrein and kinins (EISEN, 1966b; KELLERMEYER, 1967). Deposition of urates in synovial fluid is supposed to induce acute gouty attacks (MCCARTY, 1970). The participation of neutrophils seems essential (PHELPS and MCCARTY, 1966) and there are suggestions that non-steroid anti-inflammatory agents prevent the neutrophil from releasing certain enzymes after it has arrived at the site of inflammation (VAN ARMAN et al., 1970).

WEBSTER et al. (1972) used a suspension in saline of 10 mg of sodium urate microcrystals to induce oedema in one rear foot of the rat. An equal volume of saline was injected in the other pad. Six hours later, both paws were amputated at the ankle and weighed and the difference in weight between urate-injected and saline-injected paws taken as a measure of the swelling produced. Drugs were given in three separate equal doses at 0, 2, and 4 h after the subplantar injection of the urate crystals. Carboxypeptidase B, at a level of 1000 units/kg or SBTI at 80 mg/kg, for each of the three injections, partially (35%) blocked the oedema. Several antihistamine agents also partially (40%) suppressed the reaction. Two in particular, promethazine and tripelenamine, inhibited the urate-induced swelling by 75%. Complement depletion inhibited the oedema by 30%. The combination of SBTI, triprolidine and complement depletion almost completely (80%) suppressed the oedema. Antagonists of 5-HT, such as cyproheptadine and methysergide were ineffective. The conclusion was that in the rat, urate oedema appears to be mediated by the combined action of kinins, histamine, and components of complement. Microcrystalline sodium urate failed to induce detectable inflammation in leucopenic animals. Therefore, as stressed by the authors, it may well be that the first stage in the production of urate inflammation is the arrival of leucocytes. SPILBERG and OSTERLAND (1970) injected sodium urate crystals into the skin and joints of rabbits. The subcutaneous injection produced a papular area or erythema with a central focus of necrosis. Microscopic examination of the synovial inflammatory reaction induced by urate revealed oedema and mild polymorphonuclear (PMN) leucocyte infiltration in the synovium, already 5 h after the injection. Trypsin-kallikrein (T-K) inhibitor (aprotinin), a basic polypeptide extracted from bovine pancreas and lung substantially lessened the inflammatory responses. Complement depletion did not alter the joint response. In vitro testing showed that the T-K inhibitor greatly reduced the proteolytic activity of polymorphonuclear lysosomal lysates. The findings suggested that the effect of the T-K inhibitor was related to its ability to inhibit lysosomal proteases from polymorphonuclear leucocytes and to inhibit kinin-forming enzymes. Kinins have been found in synovial effusion resulting from gouty arthritis (MELMON et al., 1967). Injection of Bk into a knee joint of dogs produced warmth, swelling, and tenderness for a period of approximately 30 min (MELMON et al., 1967). Furthermore, PMN leucocytes can generate kinins (see below). Monosodium urate crystals, similar to those found in the affected joints of patients with acute gouty arthritis, enhanced clotting by activation of Hageman factor. Hageman factor and thromboplastin antecedent, primarily in inactive form, are present in normal synovial fluid in concentrations comparable to those found in plasma (KELLERMEYER and BRECKENRIDGE, 1965, 1966). However, PHELPS et al. (1966) suggested that kinins (Bk) are not mediators of the acute inflammatory response induced by urate crystals, based on experiments with carboxypeptidase B. They found that single injections of Bk into canine joints caused an abrupt, transient rise in pressure that could be greatly attenuated by prior injection of carboxypeptidase B. The enzyme, however, did not suppress the inflammation induced by urate crystals, although joints treated with carboxypeptidase were unresponsive to injected Bk even at the peak of the inflammatory response to crystals. Although this is an interesting finding, it is not evidence against the participation of kinins in urate inflammation. Furthermore, the work by WEBSTER et al. (1972), commented upon above, showed that carboxypeptidase B partially blocked the swelling induced by urate crystals in rats.

4. Electrical Stimulation and Interference of Nervous Structures

INOKI et al. (1973) reported that electrical and also thermal and mechanical stimulation of the dog's exposed dental pulp lead to the formation of a Bk-like substance in the superfusate of the pulp. Saline was placed in a well formed by a wall of dental wax surrounding the exposed pulp. Direct electrical stimulation of the pulp or electrical stimulation of the peripheral end of the cervical sympathetic nerves were used. The active principle detected in the superfusates contracted rat uterine muscle; it was heat-resistant and destroyed by incubation with chymotrypsin, but not with trypsin. When the internal carotid and occipital arteries were ligated and the pulp irrigated with Ringer-Locke's solution through a cannula interposed between the severed ends of the common carotid artery, an abolition of the activity in the superfusates was observed. The activity reappeared when irrigation with blood was restored. Therefore, the elaboration of the Bk-like factor seemed to have occurred subsequent to vasomotor responses and to originate from blood. Pretreatment of the animals with narcotic and non-narcotic analgesics abolished the release of the active principle into the superfusates, a finding difficult to interpret. Experiments of a similar nature were made by WEATHERRED et al. in 1963 (cited in INOCKI et al., 1973).

Following antidromic stimulation of alveolar nerves, these authors observed that saline samples bathing the exposed predentinal layers of the dog's pulp contained a substance which resembled kinins.

In the course of experiments on the release of a permeability factor during electric antidromic stimulation of sensory nerves of rats, GARCIA LEME and HAMAMURA (1974) found that pulses of high intensity caused the appearance of a Bk-like activity in the perfusates from the subcutaneous area supplied by the nerve. This activity was absent in animals previously treated with cellulose-sulphate. The presence of the Bk-like material was thought to be consequent to plasma extravazation following vascular alterations induced by a neurogenic factor. CHAPMAN et al. (1961), however, admitted that during the period of active vasodilation of the axon reflex flare reaction in the human skin a Bk-like substance is elaborated and that it is not a secondary consequence of vasodilation or of escape into tissue from leakage through permeable vessel walls (for a detailed dicussion of the subject, see CHAPMAN and GOODELL, 1964).

5. Micro-Organisms

Infections constitute a widespread trauma for the host. In general terms, two situations should be recognized: the infectious focus is localized in a tissue or organ causing a reaction that is restricted to the affected area; or micro-organisms may rapidly enter the circulation. Multiple reactions may then occur in different organs and the parasite or products formed as a result of its metabolism or degradation may recirculate in blood for long periods, reach other body fluids and affect the invaded organism as a whole. Endotoxins, enzymes or active substances derived therefrom, may act upon the host cells, vessels and molecular systems impairing normal homeostasis. Production of fever is a frequent symptom. To what extent do infections affect the Bk system and what is the significance of this process?

Plasma and intercellular fluid kininases increased in a non-progressive, and decreased in a progressive, bacterial infection. This is compatible with changes in a kinin-kininase system during infection (SCHWAB, 1962). The blood and urine of mice and rats infected with *Babesia rodhaini*, and the urine of mice infected with *Plasmodium berghei*, *Trypanosoma rhodesiense* and *Streptococcus pyogenes*, contain substances which stimulate the isolated guinea pig ileum and rat duodenum. The amount of active material excreted increased as the infection increased (GOODWIN and RICHARDS, 1960). The active substances were destroyed rapidly by papain and less rapidly by chymotrypsin, but were unaffected by trypsin or pepsin. Their action on smooth muscle was not influenced by atropine, eserine, antihistamines, iproniazid, bretylium or lysergic acid diethylamide. They are probably a mixture of peptides, some of which relaxed and some of which contracted the rat duodenum. In mice infected with *Trypanosoma brucei*, RICHARDS (1965) observed increasing amounts of pharmacologically active peptides and histamine in the urine as the infection progressed. Rabbits and rats were similarly affected (BOREHAM, 1968). Kinins in plasma and leucocytes increased during the infection and kininogen levels decreased. This indicates that several micro-organisms can release kinins from their precursors, directly or indirectly. However, intact or ultrasonically treated *Escherichia coli*, *Pseudomonas aeruginosa* or β-haemolytic streptococci, as well as the media from their cultures, revealed no kinin-forming activity, whereas marked kininase activity was seen after ultrasonic treatment of all three types of microbial sediments (AMUNDSEN and RUGSTAD, 1965). The purified enzyme isolated from *Pseudomonas aeruginosa* inactivates Bk, kallidin and Bk-isoleucyl-tyrosine. Increased levels of kallikrein, measured in terms of Bk equivalents, and increased kininase activity were shown to be present in the systemic circulation of monkeys infected with *Plasmodium knowlesi*. This was concomitant with a remarkable fall in the kininogen content of the infected animal, thus suggesting a large turnover of kinins in these animals (ONABANJO and MAEGRAITH, 1970; ONABANJO et al., 1970).

With so few observations, conclusions are necessarilly limited. The presence of parasites in blood or tissue may generate kinins. Degradation products exibit kininase activity. However, circulating free kinins will be rapidly destroyed, as previously noted and their presence in increased amounts in urine as the infection progresses may be consequent to increased metabolic rates of the host organism, a condition that frequently accompanies infections.

In our laboratory a circumstance was investigated where a pure strain of *Staphylococcus aureus* was injected into the subplantar tissues of the rat's paw; 0.1 ml of suspensions containing from 1.25×10^8 to 10×10^8 cells/ml induced a biphasic oedema, the first peak appearing 30 min after injection, the second peak at 4 h. The reaction subsided in 24–48 h, except that elicited by suspensions containing 10×10^8 cells/ml, which partially persisted after 72 h. The effects were investigated of previous treatments of the animals with hexadimethrine bromide, or with antagonists of histamine (diphenhydramine) or 5-HT (methysergide) using suspensions of 2.5×10^8 cells/ml. Hexadimethrine given intraperitoneally in two separate doses of 20 and 10 mg/kg, the first 30 min before, the second 90 min after the plantar injection, markedly reduced the swelling. Diphenydramine, injected by the same route in two separate doses of 25 and 5 mg/kg, the first 30 min before, the second 150 min after the micro-organism, was practically ineffective (Fig. 3). Methysergide, injected in the same way as diphenhydramine, in two doses of 3 mg/kg, was also ineffective. On the basis of these results, it was suggested that kinins participate in the reaction. Hexadimethrine, a potent inhibitor of plasma kinin formation (ARMSTRONG and STEWART, 1962), was shown by KELLETT (1965) to block oedema formation induced in the rat by kaolin, dextran, formaldehyde, silver nitrate, 5-HT and histamine. It suppressed the tuberculin reaction in BCG-sensitized guinea pigs and given locally, it partially prevented the increase in vascular permeability produced by intradermal injection of histamine and Bk. Although part of the oedema-suppressing effect of hexadimethrine may be due to a direct release of catecholamines from the adrenal medulla (KELLETT, 1966), its strong capacity to inhibit kinin generation should be taken into account to explain the reduction of the response to *Staphylococcus* in the rat's paw.

6. Anaphylaxis

The immune response involves the recognition of a non-self, antigenic substance and its elimination. This is performed through the production of antibodies (immunoglobulins) by adapted cells, with which the challenging antigen can combine (anaphylaxis); or through the direct intervention of specific sensitized cells capable of interacting with the antigen (cellular immunity). The antigen-antibody complex or

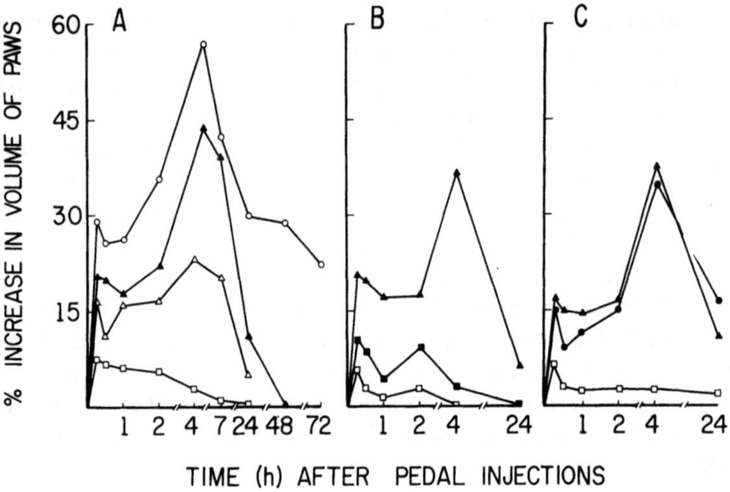

Fig. 3. (A) Oedema formation in rat hind paws after local injection of 0.1 ml of suspensions of *Staphylococcus aureus* containing 1.25 (–△–), 2.5 (–▲–) and 10 (–○–) microorganisms × 10^8/ml, or of 0.1 ml of saline (–□–). (B) Effect of hexadimethrine bromide on the development of the oedema induced by the local injection of 0.1 ml of a suspension of *S. aureus* containing 2.5×10^8 micro-organisms/ml (–■–), or of 0.1 ml of saline (–□–). Drug was given intraperitoneally in two separate doses of 20 and 10 mg/kg, 30 min before and 90 min after the injections in the paws. (C) Oedema induced by the same number of microorganisms (—●—), or the same volume of saline (—□—), as in (B), in animals treated with diphenylhydramine. Two separate doses of 25 and 5 mg/kg were given intraperitoneally, 30 min before and 150 min after the pedal injections. In (B) and (C), —▲— represents responses of untreated controls to 0.1 ml of a suspension containing 2.5×10^8 micro-organisms/ml. Each point is mean value of six rats

antigen-sensitized cell complex can react with the complement system of plasma proteins. If the reaction takes place on the surface of cells, lysis of the cells may occur. Endogenous substances, such as histamine, 5-HT or slow reacting substance-A (SRS-A) are released by immunologic pathways. The Bk-system is also activated. The whole subject has been extensively dealt with in Chapters 7 and 13, and sections of Chapters 10, 11, 23, 33, and 36. We will, therefore, restrict ourselves to brief comments on experimental findings relating the kinin system to anaphylaxis.

BERALDO (1950) presented evidence that in addition to histamine a Bk-like substance was formed during the course of anaphylactic shock in dogs. He assumed, however, that the material thus released was not a very important factor in the overall mechanisms of such shock, but only an aggravating one. This was due to the finding that blood samples withdrawn 90 min after the injection of the antigen showed maximum activity, in terms of equivalents of Bk, which did not coincide with the maximal drop in blood pressure.

Increased levels of kinins during anaphylaxis were detected in the rat, guinea pig, rabbit, and dog (BROCKLEHURST and LAHIRI, 1962; DAWSON et al., 1966; COLLIER and JAMES, 1966; STARR and WEST, 1969; BACK et al., 1963). If rats were given antagonists of histamine and 5-HT, the antigen still caused a marked fall in blood pressure, which could be mimicked by the injection of Bk (BROCKLEHURST and LAHIRI, 1962).

Decreased kininogen levels associated with anaphylactic responses were shown in rabbits (LECOMTE, 1960a, 1961; CÎRSTEA et al., 1965, 1966), in two out of seven guinea pigs tested (CÎRSTEA et al., 1966), in mice (LIMA, 1967) and in rats submitted to passive cutaneous anaphylaxis (ROTHSCHILD, 1968b). In dogs, CÎRSTEA et al. (1965, 1966) failed to demonstrate a fall. Elevation was reported by DAWSON et al. (1966) and STARR and WEST (1969) in rat plasma after challenge with the specific antigen.

Evidence was presented that the addition of antigen-antibody complexes to guinea pig or rabbit serum is followed by complement fixation, activation of Hageman factor and of kinin-forming enzymes, resulting in the generation of kinins. The serum thus treated acquired the property of increasing vascular permeability when injected into animals previously given anti-histamine drugs; of contracting guinea pig ileum in the presence of anti-histamine; and of causing a fall in blood pressure of anaesthetised rabbits (MOVAT, 1967). However, fresh blood drawn from sensitized guinea pigs and then challenged with the antigen showed no increase in Bk content (BROCKLEHURST and LAHIRI, 1962).

D. Intervention of Cells in the Release and Destruction of Kinins

An integral part of inflammatory reactions is the migration of cells to the affected area. Suspensions of whole or disintegrated leucocytes had no effect on vascular permeability or on the isolated guinea pig ileum. This might indicate that there is no readily available kinin in the cells (SCHWAB, 1962).

A series of experiments were carried out to investigate whether or not migrating cells were capable of producing kinins from specific substrates, or to destroy them. PMN leucocytes, harvested from peritoneal exudates of rabbits were lysed and the lysate subjected to differential centrifugation (GREENBAUM et al., 1967, 1969; GREENBAUM and KIM, 1967). The lysosomal and extra-lysosomal fractions so obtained were tested for kinin-forming and kinin-inactivating enzymes. The presence of a kinin-forming activity in the lysosomal fraction was considered conclusive. The incubation of this fraction with human kininogen slowly yielded, over a period of time, increasing quantities of a kinin-like material detected by bioassay. The maximal activity was produced in the acid range at about pH 5, a sharp drop occurring if the pH of the reaction was raised to near 6. Aprotinin or SBTI had no effect on the kinin-forming activity of this fraction. The activity was resistant to heating to 50° C for 30 min, but was destroyed by boiling for 10 min. Similar results were obtained with the extra-lysosomal fraction. With this fraction however, the possibility exists that leakage from the lysosomes occurred during fractionation. The peptide released was named PMN-kinin and differed from Bk in that it was six times more active on the rat uterus than on the guinea pig ileum, when indices of discrimination were calculated with the Bk index set at 1. In comparison with Bk and kallidin, PMN-kinin had a greater index in causing the relaxation of the rat duodenum and in its hypotensive activity in the rabbit. It increased vascular permeability and caused joint pain in dogs. It was destroyed by chymotrypsin, carboxypeptidase B and by kininases from plasma and from the PMN cells themselves. Its molecular weight is in the range of 1700, more of the order of that of methionyl-lysyl-Bk, which it resembles in some biological aspects. Unlike methionyl-lysyl-Bk, however, PMN-kinin was not affected by the action of trypsin.

The relative amounts of PMN-kinin and Bk-like peptides produced by kinin-forming enzymes of PMN cells depended on the species of substrate and species of the cell used. Human cell enzymes catalysed the formation of more Bk-like material than PMN-kinin, when human kininogen was the substrate. The rabbit enzymes acting on rabbit kininogen appeared to produce about equal quantities of the two peptides. Rabbit enzymes acting on human substrate produced larger concentrations of PMN-kinin.

Kininase activity was demonstrated by incubating Bk with the extra-lysosomal fraction of the lysate of PMN leucocytes. The optimum pH for the kininase activity was pH 8.5, although a considerable amount of enzyme activity was present at neutrality. Its characteristics differed from those observed for kininases in blood and other body fluids (ERDÖS et al., 1964). Leucocyte kininases were also described by SCHWAB (1962).

MELMON and CLINE (1967, 1968) studied human cells. Granulocytes generated and destroyed kinins, whereas lymphocytes were devoid of such properties. The cells, obtained from heparinized venous blood, were suspended in a minimal essential medium and added to homologous or heterologous plasma, free of leucocyte antibodies, or to human globulin. Increased concentrations of kinins were observed within 10 min and this was associated with a 30–50% depletion of kininogen levels. Myeloblasts, obtained from patients with leucemia, had an activity similar to that of the adult cells. Kinin production by whole cells was greatest at physiological pH. The total sonicate of cells exhibited two peaks of activity, at pH 4, which is probably the same enzyme as that defined by GREENBAUM and colleagues, and at pH 7.4. Kininase activity was also demonstrated in intact or disrupted granulocytes and in lysates of red blood cells, but not in lymphocytes. By increasing the time of incubation to 3 h at pH 4.0 with purified human kininogen, kinin-forming activity was detected in the whole lysate and in subcellular fractions of human lymphocytes (ENGLEMAN and GREENBAUM, 1971). More recently, MILLER et al. (1975) suggested that a plasminogen activator is present on the human leucocyte surface. This activates plasminogen to form plasmin which in turn acts on kininogen to release kinins.

Lysosomal and extra-lysosomal fractions of rabbit macrophages contain enzymes that formed kinins from purified kininogen substrates at acid pH (GREENBAUM et al., 1969). The activity was of the same level or greater than that demonstrated in PMN leucocytes. Aprotinin did not inhibit the kinin-forming activity of these cells, but did inhibit the kininases present in the extra-lysosomal fraction.

Cells harvested from the peritoneal cavity of the rat released kinin and lowered kininogen after brief incubation with rat plasma in the presence of adrenaline. These effects were not reproduced when either cells or the catecholamine were incubated alone with plasma. Previous incubation of peritoneal cells with adrenaline enabled these cells to reduce kininogen in adrenaline-free plasma. Peritoneal cavity washings which contained no mast cells, but were normal in their lymphocyte and eosinophil content had no effect on plasma kininogen in the presence of adrenaline. Approximately 3×10^6 cells containing 100000 ± 10000 mast cells/ml plasma were required to produce a significant effect on kininogen over a 5-min incubation period in the presence of adrenaline (ROTHSCHILD et al., 1974a). In parallel experiments, catecholamines decreased the kininogen content of rat blood in vivo and in vitro. Blood cells were also required for this effect; these were neither erythrocytes, lymphocytes, eosinophils nor platelets (ROTHSCHILD et al., 1974b). The remaining major cell group is formed by the neutrophils. In view of the ability demonstrated by these cells to release kinins from specific substrates, as noted above, they could be the target of the action of catecholamines. However, monocytes and basophils cannot be excluded, though they are rather rare in rat's blood (less than 10% and 1%, respectively). From the results with peritoneal cavity washings, ROTHSCHILD and collaborators could not exclude that mast cells, which are in many respects similar to blood basophils, may be the mediators of the effects of catecholamines on plasma kininogen. Accordingly, more than one cell type may be involved in the phenomenon.

Kinins, therefore, may be released and destroyed by enzymes present in cells. These cells are present at different stages of an inflammatory reaction. Some of the cell enzymes require an acid pH to act (GREENBAUM'S experiments) some do not (MELMON and CLINE'S experiments). It has been recognized that there is an increased lactic acid formation resulting from alterations in leucocyte metabolism wich accompanies ingestion of particles. The pH within the cytoplasma of PMN leucocytes may be as low as 5 after phagocytosis (ROGERS, 1964). The cells which migrated may even disintegrate, liberating their lysosomal enzymes and cytoplasmic materials into the inflamed area.

These are local conditions favouring the activation of cell enzymes capable of forming kinins. Migrating cells may, therefore, contribute to the production of active polypeptides in an inflammatory focus. Acid environment on the other hand, may inhibit kininases (EDERY and LEWIS, 1962; GARCIA LEME et al., 1970). Even if kininases are concomitantly activated with cell kininogenases, it is reasonable to suppose that kinins will tend to accumulate in an inflamed area. Furthermore, adrenaline-activated cells (mast cells?) are able to release Bk-like substance from kininogens. These findings open new possibilities for the local activation of kinin in inflamed areas. However, in vitro conditions may be consistently different from those which occur in vivo. Though potentially interesting and suggestive, the findings described in this section will necessarily allow limited extrapolations.

E. Cell Proliferation and Tissue Repair

Bk stimulated mitotic activity in rat thymocyte populations suspended in vitro. The effect was calcium dependent and probably mediated by cAMP, as it was potentiated by caffeine and inhibited by imidazole (PERRIS and WHITFIELD, 1969; WHITFIELD et al., 1970). Also kallikrein stimulated mitotic activity in the thymus and bone marrow of rats (RIXON et al., 1971). The mitogenic activity resembles that of growth hormone, parathyroid hormone and vasopressin, and might have significance for post-injury stimulation of cell proliferation and repair. As shown by RIXON and WHITFIELD (1973), exposure of thymus lymphocytes to low concentrations of Bk (1–4 μM) in a serum free medium initiates a virtually immediate mitogenic response of these cells. Within 1 h the number of cells synthesizing deoxyribonucleic acid (DNA) is maximal and nearly double the number normally synthesizing DNA in control, non-stimulated populations. Kallikrein given to rats in a single intraperitoneal dose of 3 units/

100 g body weight initiated events which about 3 h later caused increased mitosis of thymic lymphoblasts and marrow cells. The effect was probably indirect through the liberation of kinins, and the suggestion was advanced that kinins might act as "wound hormones", initiating tissue regeneration. Similar results were obtained by ROHEN and PETERHOFF (1973) in the intestinal epithelium of rats and by LÖBBECKE (1973) in various tissues.

F. Kinins and Disease

"The occurrence of kinins in tissues affected by a wide range of diseases has naturally evoked considerable interest in their pathogenic role. However, the presence of kinins does not warrant the conclusion that they are prime causal factors of these diseases, although, in some cases at least, the evidence suggests that the association has a meaningful relation" (WILHELM, 1971).

It is beyond the purpose of this chapter to discuss clinical evidence suggesting the involvement of kinins in human diseases (for reviews, see EISEN, 1969; KEELE, 1969; WILHELM, 1971). We will merely enumerate some inflammatory conditions, important for human pathology, in which kinins might play a role. Most of the information, however, derives from experimental findings in laboratory animals.

I. Rheumatoid Arthritis

The immune diseases of connective tissue, among them rheumatoid arthritis (RA), have features suggesting the formation of antibodies or of antibody-forming cells reacting with the patient's native antigens (GARDNER, 1965). This condition, as previously mentioned, may well favour the release of kinins. RA begins as an acute inflammation of the smaller joints. Acute synovitis presents itself with the cardinal signs of inflammation. Material with the staining characteristics of fibrin accumulates within the inflamed synovial tissues and there is aggregation of proteins derived from the plasma. The volume of synovial fluid increases. Many cells are present, predominantly neutrophil granulocytes (GARDNER, 1965). Synovial fluid from patients with RA contained kinins in concentrations ranging from 1.6 to 58 ng/ml (MELMON et al., 1967). Similar findings were reported by EISEN (1969) who examined 82 effusions from 73 patients with a diagnosis of RA. A kinin-like substance was found in 33 effusions, in concentrations high enough to produce inflammatory signs and symptoms. EISEN suggested that complexes of rheumatoid factor and aggregated γ-globulin may be directly involved in the kinin formation in the rheumatoid joint. The complex was prepared from sera, plasmas or synovial effusions from patients and incubated with suitable substrates, revealing kinin-forming activity. A Bk-like, pain-producing substance activated by contact with glass or certain other foreign surfaces, was detected in RA fluids applied to a blister area (ARMSTRONG et al., 1957).

II. Acute Gouty Arthritis

In a previous section of this chapter, evidence was given which suggested the involvement of kinin in inflammations produced by urate crystals (see also Chapter 22). Primary gout is characterized by a genetic predisposition leading to excessive formation and decreased destruction and excretion of uric acid. This eventually results in deposit of urates in connective tissue. Where these deposits occur in articular cartilage or in para-articular connective tissue, gouty arthritis develops (GARDNER, 1965). Deposition of urates in synovial fluid is supposed to induce gouty attacks (MCCARTY, 1970). The participation of neutrophils seems essential (PHELPS and MCCARTY, 1966). Urate crystals activate Hageman factor and this is probably the mechanism behind kinin formation in synovial exudates (KELLERMEYER and BRECKENRIDGE, 1965). The presence of kinins has been demonstrated in effusions of joints of patients with gout (MELMON et al., 1967).

III. Bronchial Asthma

Inhalation of Bk induced bronchoconstriction in asthmatic patients (HERXHEIMER and STRESEMAN, 1963). The effect appeared more rapidly than with the inhalation of ten fold histamine concentrations (LECOMTE et al., 1962). Kinin activity in peripheral venous blood of asthmatic patients was ten times greater than in blood of healthy persons (ABE et al., 1967).

Bk has a potent contracting effect upon the bronchiolar muscles of the guinea pig (COLLIER et al., 1960). This effect can be observed in vivo by registering the variations of the pumping pressure needed to force air into the bronchiolar tree. Doses of 0.5–1.0 μg/kg injected intravenously were effective. This effect is blocked by several non-steroid anti-inflammatory drugs. Bk produces only a slight bronchoconstriction in rabbits and cats (KONZETT and STÜRMER, 1960). Dogs are insensitive (WAALER, 1961). Kinins and other mediators of anaphylaxis are produced in the lungs. Prostaglandins are released from lungs by Bk. Interaction between them and other endogenous substances is a probable occurrence in asthma. These findings, which greatly helped the development of research on the pathophysiology of bronchial asthma, are treated in detail in Chapter 24.

IV. Pancreatitis

Acute pancreatitis is characterized by local inflammatory reactions with systemic repercussions of varying intensity, that, at least partially, might depend on the action of proteolytic enzymes, resulting in the formation of kinins (POWERS et al., 1955; BERNARD, 1959; FORELL, 1963; HUREAU et al., 1968; POPIERAITIS and THOMPSON, 1969; ANDERSON et al., 1969); for a review of the experimental aspects of pancreatitis, see SCHILLER et al. (1974). Kinin-like substances were found in plasma of patients with pancreatitis. The levels of the active materials correlated well with the clinical state of the disease (THAL et al., 1963). In experimental pancreatitis, kinin levels in plasma and lymph increased significantly 3 h after induction (SATAKE et al., 1973). Decreased kininogen levels were found in experimental conditions (RYAN et al., 1964, 1965; DINIZ et al., 1967; CASTELFRANCHI and CORRADO, 1971) and in man (GREEFF, 1966). However, it is disputable whether or not kallikrein inhibitors are therapeutically effective. Beneficial effects were suggested by the works of NUGENT et al. (1969), FORELL (1963), MORGAN et al. (1968) and CASTELFRANCHI and CORRADO (1971). In a recent double blind controlled clinical trial, to investigate the effectiveness of aprotinin in acute pancreatitis, 105 patients were studied. They provided uniform clinical material and all were managed on an identical strict procedure except that patients received either the drug or a placebo. The trial showed that mortality was significantly lower in the group treated with the drug (TRAPNELL et al., 1974).

V. Miscellaneous

For the involvement of the kinin system in injuries provoked by burns or in infectious states, see previous sections in this chapter. Suggestions were made that kinins might participate in migraine and fever production (SICUTERI, 1970; PELÁ et al., 1975). A new orthostatic syndrome due to hyperbradykininism was described by Streeten et al. (1972).

G. Effect of Drugs on Kinin System and Consequences in Inflammatory Reactions

The release of kinins has been demonstrated during the development of inflammatory reactions induced by varying noxious stimuli, as discussed above. This means that among the series of events characterising inflammation, activation of the kinin-system is a frequent finding. However, the real significance of active kinins present in an inflamed area cannot be fully established until specific antagonists for their effects are found. Not before potent anti-histamine agents were synthesized was it possible to show that inhibition of the actions of histamine was not closely associated with anti-inflammatory activity. Similar conclusions derived from the use of antagonists of 5-HT. These results, nevertheless, by no means imply that histamine or 5-HT are not involved in an inflammatory response. They only emphasize the usefulness of specific inhibitors in assessing the relative degree of participation of endogenous substances in physiological or pathological phenomena. For further information on the subject of drugs affecting the kinin system, the reader is referred to ERDÖS (1968), LEWIS (1970) and ROCHA E SILVA and GARCIA LEME (1972).

I. Interference With the Actions of Kinins

Synthetic analogues of Bk, obtained by altering the position of the amino acid residues in the polypeptide chain, were tested as antagonists of the active peptide. Only a few compounds displayed low anti-Bk effects (NICOLAIDES et al., 1963; SCHRÖDER and LÜBKE, 1966; STEWART and WOOLEY, 1967). An attempt to find anti-Bk agents led us to investigate a large series of compounds chemically related to phenothiazines, as well as flavonoids, which were reported to result in beneficial effects in some inflammatory conditions. The guinea pig ileum and rabbit duodenum were used as test preparations in vitro. Antagonistic action was observed with some compounds, most of them acting as non-competitive inhibitors. The inhibition, however, was not specific, for the actions of angiotensin, eledoisin, and histamine were also reduced. In vivo, partial protection was noted against the increase of vascular permeability induced by Bk, and against the development of oedema induced by heating the rat's paw, or by injecting carrageenin or Bk itself (ROCHA E SILVA and GARCIA LEME, 1965, 1972; GARCIA LEME and ROCHA E SILVA, 1965; GARCIA LEME and WALASZEK, 1973). These results are compatible with anti-inflammatory activity partially associated with anti-Bk effects of the substances tested.

COLLIER and collaborators have studied the effects of non-steroid anti-inflammatory drugs upon bronchoconstriction induced by Bk in the guinea pig. Calcium-acetylsalicylate, amidopyrine, phenazone, mefenamic and flufenamic acids, and sodium meclofenamate produced an antagonistic action. Atropine, mepyramine or LSD-25 were ineffective. On the other hand, responses to histamine, 5-HT or acetylcholine remained intact after these agents (COLLIER et al., 1960; COLLIER and SHORLEY, 1960, 1963; COLLIER, 1961; see also Chapter 24). AARSEN (1966), however, could only partially confirm these findings, using the perfused isolated lung of guinea pigs.

Aspirin, methdilazine, and phenylbutazone caused a partial inhibition of the Bk permeability effect (LISH and MCKINNEY, 1963). Phenylbutazone also reduced the hypotensive actions of the peptide (LECOMTE, 1960b; LECOMTE and TROQUET, 1960). On the other hand, NORTHOVER and SUBRAMANIAN(1961), observed that the fall in blood pressure of anesthetised dogs produced by Bk, kallidin, and also histamine, acetylcholine or 5-HT was either unaffected or very slightly reduced by several anti-inflammatory drugs, whereas that produced by human salivary kallikrein was abolished. Similarly, rabbits infused with these drugs had the accumulation of protein-bound dye at the site of injection of salivary kallikrein nearly abolished, while that induced by local injection of Bk was only slightly affected.

Inhibitory effects towards the algogenic action of Bk in dogs were displayed by anti-inflammatory drugs such as acetylsalicylate, sodium salicylate, acetaminophen, aminopyrine or phenylbutazone in experiments in which potentials evoked in splenic nerves were recorded, or in experiments of cross perfusion of dog spleens (GUZMAN et al., 1964; LIM et al., 1964; LIM, 1968). Salicylates, however, did not reduce the algogenic activity of Bk in man, when the blister base test was used (KEELE and ARMSTRONG, 1964); the same applied to indomethacin, when the venous constriction test was employed (SICUTERI et al., 1965). In experiments by FERREIRA et al. (1973), the reflex rise in blood pressure induced by intra-arterial Bk injections into the spleen of lightly anaesthetised dogs was used as an indication of sensory stimulation. Doses of Bk that released prostaglandins from the spleen gave positive responses in proportion to the dose used and the response was reduced by indomethacin. Also LEMBECK and JUAN (1974), with the technique of the isolated perfused rabbit ear connected to the body by its nerve only, observed that the algesic effect of Bk was enhanced by PGE_1 and inhibited by indomethacin. The factor by which the algesic effect was reduced by the anti-inflammatory agent, and the factor by which it was enhanced by the sensitizing PG were found to be correlated, thus showing the dependence on the presence of PGE_1 of the response induced by Bk. However, when additional amounts of PGE_1 were infused, indomethacin was still able to reduce the algesic effect of Bk to some extent. This cannot be explained by blockade of PG synthesis, only. The idea that PGs may modulate the pain-producing activity of Bk was suggested as well by the results of COLLIER and SCHNEIDER (1972). These authors reported that there was a delay in the mouse writhing responses to Bk, but not to PGE_1, and that aspirin-like drugs did not affect the response induced by the last, but inhibited Bk effects.

II. Interference With the Generation of Kinins

Substances which interfere with the release of kinin from its inactive precursor in plasma may affect inflammatory reactions. Several anti-inflammatory drugs have been claimed to block the formation of kinins by some research workers, and have been denied by others.

The antiheparin agents, protamine sulphate and hexadimethrine bromide, are potent in vitro inhibitors of the activation of kinins induced by procedures such as dilution of plasma or serum, or contact with glass (ARMSTRONG and STEWART, 1962). Hexadimethrine strongly blocked the development of oedema in the rat's paw by yeast (KELLETT, 1965), carrageenin and by heating (GARCIA LEME et al., 1967, 1973b). Part of its anti-inflammatory effect, however, may be due to the release of catecholamines from the adrenal medulla (KELLETT, 1966). SBTI, which blocks kinin formation, suppressed kaolin oedema in the rat's paw (HLADOVEC et al., 1958), reduced the haemorrhagic necrosis following the intradermal injection of a mixture of bacterial endotoxin and adrenaline (ZWEIFACH et al., 1961), and inhibited carrageenin, trypsin, urate crystals or yeast-induced oedemas in the rat's paw (VAN ARMAN et al., 1965; WEBSTER et al., 1972). Also aprotinin was found to be effective in counteracting inflammatory responses (KALLER et al., 1966). Hexadimethrine, SBTI and aprotinin blocked the release of a Bk-like substance during heating of rat paws (GARCIA LEME et al., 1970).

Locally injected sodium salicylate completely suppressed the permeability response to intradermal kallikrein in guinea pigs (SPECTOR and WILLOUGHBY, 1962). Inhibition of kinin-forming enzymes by sodium salicylate, acetylsalicylic acid, phenylbutazone and related anti-inflammatory drugs was reported by NORTHOVER and SUBRAMANIAN (1961), but not confirmed by HEBBORN and SHAW (1963). As shown by DAVIES et al. (1966), indomethacin, flufenamic acid, phenylbutazone, ibufenac, chloroquine, acetylsalicylic acid and paramethasone at a concentration of 100 μg/ml did not inhibit the release of kinin, whereas aprotinin and SBTI were effective. Plasmin was partially inhibited by salicylates, amidopyrine and cinchophen (UNGAR et al., 1952), and is able to release kinin under certain circumstances. Hydrocortisone suppressed the release of kinins by interfering with the kinin-forming system (CLINE and MELMON, 1966). This finding was not supported by EISEN et al. (1968) who examined the action of three glucocorticoids, hydrocortisone, dexamethasone, and prednisolone, demonstrating that even at high concentrations they had little or no effect on kinin activity or kinin formation. Furthermore, they also showed that plasma from patients receiving corticosteroids released quantities of kinins similar to those from the plasma of normal subjects.

Another point that should be considered is that depletion of the labile pool of kininogen, potentially decreases the supply of active kinins for an inflammatory reaction. Various aspects have already been discussed in previous sections of this chapter. In summary, it can be said that decreased inflammatory reactions were observed following kininogen depletion (GARCIA LEME et al., 1967; DI ROSA and SORRENTINO, 1970; CRUNKHORN and MEACOCK, 1971; DI ROSA et al., 1971; EISEN and LOVEDAY, 1971). This finding, however, is open to criticism. In many instances, the treatments employed to deplete the animals of their kininogen stores produced side effects that might interfere with the developing reaction (EISEN and LOVEDAY,

1971; Di Rosa et al., 1971). Some anti-inflammatory drugs, which prevent almost entirely several symptoms of inflammation, did not prevent the lowering of kininogen levels induced by effective agents (Van Arman and Nuss, 1969). Increased kininogen was found in some experimental inflammatory conditions, such as adjuvant arthritis (Van Arman and Nuss, 1969) or anaphylaxis (Dawson et al., 1966; Starr and West, 1969). Good responses to irritative stimuli were observed in animals partially depleted of their kininogen (Di Rosa and Willoughby, 1971).

Nevertheless, changes in kininogen levels is only one parameter in assessing the activation of the kinin-system. Furthermore, a complete depletion is almost impracticable and any negative result based on decreased levels is always disputable. In spite of this, small amounts of plasma proteins leaving the circulation in an inflamed area may lead to a reasonable production of kinins in the interstitial spaces and this is expected to occur any time a vessel starts to leak.

III. Potentiating and Destroying Agents

Carboxypeptidase B, when injected immediately before a standard dose of Bk, abolished or diminished its action on the blood pressure of the cat (Erdös and Yang, 1967b). Some kininases have the specificity of carboxypeptidases which are metalloenzymes and, therefore, chelating agents such as thioglycolic acid, 8-hydroxyquinoline, EDTA, and dimercaptopropanol (BAL), can prevent the rapid destruction of newly formed kinins. The bradykinin-potentiating factor (BPF), a mixture of polypeptides extracted from *Bothrops jararaca* venom (Ferreira, 1965), potentiates Bk mainly by interfering with the activity of destroying enzymes. All these agents offer interesting possibilities for the investigation of the involvement of kinins in physiological or pathological phenomena.

BPF was utilized to identify a hypotensive agent released under conditions of shock by trypsin, nargase and by animal venoms (Ferreira and Rocha e Silva, 1969). As previously noted, the swelling response to carrageenin in the rat's paw was potentiated by one of the peptides, BPP_{9a}, extracted from the venom of *B. jararaca* (Ferreira et al., 1974), thus suggesting that this might have resulted from the persistance of the kinin action, as BPP_{9a} is a fairly specific potentiator of Bk.

On the other hand, carboxypeptidase B strongly diminished carrageenin oedema in the rat's paw, and partially blocked the swelling caused by sodium urate crystals (Van Arman et al., 1968; Webster et al., 1972). Mailing et al. (1974), however, did not observe inhibition when the oedema was induced by Bk itself.

It should be expected that substances capable of restricting the duration of the effects of kinins will lead to a restricted manifestation of the processes involving kinins. Intraperitoneal administration of α-chymotrypsin blocked oedema induced by Bk and formalin in the rat and partially affected the responses to dextran and carrageenin (Giordano and Scapagnini, 1967). Studies involving rabbit ear cellulitis and venous thrombosis demonstrated marked regression of inflammatory infiltration following proteolytic enzyme therapy (Innerfield, 1957). As it was later shown (Innerfield et al., 1963), an antagonism is observed after oral protease therapy for the enhancement of vascular permeability, hypotension, and smooth muscle contraction induced by Bk. Therefore, it is possible that the inflammatory condition observed in the rabbit involved the participation of kinins.

IV. Anti-Inflammatory Drugs and Experimental Inflammation

Cyproheptadine was fairly potent in reducing the development of thermic oedema of the rat's paw (45° C for 30 min), in which the release of kinins was clearly observed (ROCHA E SILVA and GARCIA LEME, 1965). On the other hand, VAN ARMAN et al. (1965) reported its ineffectiveness in preventing carrageenin-induced or Bk-induced swelling, while reducing greatly the oedema caused by 5-HT. These authors also confirmed the findings of WINTER et al. (1962) that acetylsalicylic acid and phenylbutazone are fairly good antagonists of carrageenin. Sodium salicylate (ROCHA E SILVA and ANTONIO, 1960) and indomethacin (GARCIA LEME et al., 1973b) had no inhibitory effect upon the development of thermal oedema in rat's paw. Sodium salicylate, however, reduced dye-leakage into the skin of rats submitted to burns of moderate intensity (55° C for 27 s), as shown by SPECTOR and WILLOUGHBY (1959). Acetylsalicylic acid and indomethacin were effective in reducing swelling and dye-leakage when given before the injection of carrageenin into the rat's paw, but much less effective when given 30 or 60 min after carrageenin. Combined administration of diphenhydramine and methysergide before carrageenin caused only a slight reduction in oedema and dye-leakage (GARCIA LEME et al., 1973b). Indomethacin is known to diminish inflammation produced by either carrageenin (WINTER et al., 1962), adjuvant (WINTER and NUSS, 1966), sodium urate or ellagic acid (VAN ARMAN et al., 1970). However, it did not prevent foot-swelling caused by Bk nor by trypsin (VAN ARMAN and NUSS, 1969), neither did it prevent Bk formation from plasma by trypsin, nor kallidin formation in vitro by kallikrein (VAN ARMAN et al., 1968; DAVIES et al., 1966). GIORDANO and SCAPAGNINI (1967), however, observed inhibition by indomethacin of the Bk-induced swelling in the rat's paw. Also effective were aminopyrine and polymethylene-salicylic acid. These drugs also reduced the responses to formalin, dextran, carrageenin, and egg-white.

These facts indicate that many anti-inflammatory drugs, as tested clinically, apparently do not interfere with the Bk system, in a direct way. On the other hand, however, several substances may partially antagonize the pharmacological actions of plausible mediators of inflammation without greatly restricting the development of an inflammatory reaction. That is the case when one considers the effects of specific antagonists of histamine or 5-HT.

GUNNAR and WEEKS (1949) observed in rabbits the failure of tripelennamine to alter the intensity of the concentration of trypan blue following burns and injections of turpentine, while completely blocking reactions following the injections of histamine. In man, antihistamine agents were unable to influence the course of experimental burns (60° C for 15 s) (SEVITT et al., 1952). Significant delay in the development of cutaneous blue-staining at 30 min was shown by previous administration of mepyramine to rats submitted to thermal injury (55° C for 27 s). The drug, however, was ineffective in reducing dye-leakage after that time (SPECTOR and WILLOUGHBY, 1959). The delaying effect of anti-histamine drugs was also observed by WILHELM and MASON (1960) in rabbits and guinea pigs submitted to thermal stimulus (54° C for 20 s). Repeated injections of promethazine, alone or associated with a 5-HT antagonist, had no effect upon oedema induced by carrageenin or cellulose-sulphate into the rat's paw and had only a delaying effect when dextran was used as an irritant (GARCIA LEME et al., 1967).

5-HT is an important permeability factor only in rodents (SPARROW and WILHELM, 1957). Specific antagonists of its actions, however, are usually ineffective in inflammatory reactions in these animals, with the possible exception of anaphylactoid reactions, such as those induced by dextran or egg-white (PARRAT and WEST, 1957; SPECTOR and WILLOUGHBY, 1957, 1959; ROCHA E SILVA and ANTONIO, 1960; GARCIA LEME et al., 1967).

Overall, the results discussed in this section suggest that alternative mechanisms may be involved in the development of an inflammatory reaction. Different irritants might activate different mechanisms to start the reaction, whose final manifestation is, nevertheless, a pattern response. Many of these mechanisms can intermingle in the phenomenon. Therefore, it is not surprising that anti-inflammatory drugs may exhibit so many and apparently unrelated properties. Assuming that they can act at different steps of this complex, multimediated reaction, it is reasonable to admit that this is done through different pathways.

H. Conclusions

Kinins are involved in inflammatory reactions. They have been detected in inflammatory perfusates and exudates in sufficient concentrations to produce signs and symptoms associated with inflammation: vasodilation, increased vascular permeability, pain, and oedema. Diminished inflammatory reactions can be observed when the generation of kinins is impaired, for example, by the use of kallikrein inhibitors. Depletion of the labile pool of kininogens in many instances led to partially reduced inflammatory reactions. Kinin-destroying agents, such as carboxypeptidase B, may interfere with inflammation. Furthermore, some pharmacological effects of kinins, for instance bronchoconstriction, are inhibited by several anti-inflammatory drugs.

Relevant kinins in an inflammatory reaction seem to be locally formed and must derive from proteins extravazated from circulation. Extravascular conditions prevail, during the development of inflammatory responses, which favour their generation. A persistant activation of the kinin-system will result in the maintainance of the effects of the peptides. The acidic environment helps its accumulation in the affected area through the inhibition of kininases. Besides that, migrating cells, such as PMN leucocytes and macrophages can contribute to the formation of kinins. These conclusions, however, should not imply that the development of inflammatory reactions might strictly depend on the activation of the kinin system.

Inflammation is a complex process. Several endogenous systems can be activated following injury and this leads to the release or formation of pharmacologically active agents, capable of promoting the development of the reaction. The relative degree of participation of each of the known agents is not easy to assess. They act synergistically to ensure the development of inflammatory reactions. Kinins are amongst these endogenous, pro-inflammatory agents.

Finally, it should be said that several aspects of the problem are still disputable. It has been my intention, when writing this chapter, to expose them clearly, instead of presenting a personal view of the facts. This was done with the hope that they will stimulate further research on the subject.

Acknowledgments. I would like to thank Drs. S. H. Ferreira, L. S. Greene, and A. C. M. Camargo for profitable discussions during the preparation of the text and for critical reading of the manuscript. Mrs. Solange Jorge and Miss Célia Santos accurately typed this work.

References

Aarsen, P. N.: The influence of analgesic antipyretic drugs on the responses of guinea-pig lungs to bradykinin. Brit. J. Pharmacol. **27**, 196—204 (1966)

Abe, K., Watanabe, N., Kumagai, N., Mouri, T., Seki, T., Yoshinaga, K.: Circulating plasma kinin in patients with bronchial asthma. Experientia (Basel) **23**, 626—627 (1967)

Amundsen, E., Nustad, K.: Kinin-forming and destroying activities of saliva. Brit. J. Pharmacol. **23**, 440—444 (1964)

Amundsen, E., Rugstad, H. E.: Influence of some pathogenic bacteria on kinin formation and destruction. Brit. J. Pharmacol. **25**, 67—73 (1965)

Anderson, M. C., Schiller, W. R., Gramatica, L.: Alterations of portal venous and systemic arterial pressure during experimental acute pancreatitis. Amer. J. Surg. **117**, 715—720 (1969)

Ankier, S. I., Starr, M. S.: The importance of plasma kinins in the anaphylactoid reaction in rats. Brit. J. Pharmacol. **31**, 331—339 (1967)

Armstrong, D.: Pain. In: Erdös, E. G. (Ed.): Bradykinin, Kallidin, and Kallikrein. Handbook of Experimental Pharmacology, Vol. XXV, pp. 434—481. Berlin-Heidelberg-New York: Springer 1970

Armstrong, D., Dry, R. M. L., Keele, C. A., Markham, J. W.: Pain-producing substances in blister fluid and in serum. J. Physiol. (Lond.) **117**, 4 P—5 P (1952)

Armstrong, D., Dry, R. M. L., Keele, C. A., Markham, J. W.: Observation on chemical excitants of cutaneous pain in man. J. Physiol. (Lond.) **120**, 326—351 (1953)

Armstrong, D., Jepson, J. B., Keele, C. A.: Activation by glass of pharmacologically active agents in blood various species. J. Physiol. (Lond.) **129**, 80 P—81 P (1955)

Armstrong, D., Jepson, J. B., Keele, C. A., Stewart, J. W.: Developing of pain-producing substance in human plasma. Nature (Lond.) **174**, 791—792 (1954)

Armstrong, D., Jepson, J. B., Keele, C. S., Stewart, J. W.: Pain producing substance in human inflammatory exudates and plasma. J. Physiol. (Lond.) **135**, 350—370 (1957)

Armstrong, D., Mills, G. L.: Chemical characterization of kinins of human plasma. Nature (Lond.) **197**, 490 (1963)

Armstrong, D. A., Stewart, J. W.: Anti-heparin agents as inhibitors of plasma kinin formation. Nature (Lond.) **194**, 689 (1962)

Back, N., Munson, A. E., Guth, P. S.: Anaphylactic shock in dogs. J. Amer. med. Ass. **183**, 260—263 (1963)

Bagdasarian, R. A., Talamo, R. C., Colman, R. W.: Isolation of high molecular weight activators of human plasma kallikrein. J. biol. Chem. **248**, 3456—3463 (1973)

Baumgarten, A., Melrose, G. J. H., Vagg, W. J.: Interactions between histamine and bradykinin assessed by continuous recording of increased vascular permeability. J. Physiol. (Lond.) **208**, 669—675 (1970)

Beraldo, W. T.: Formation of bradykinin in anaphylactic and peptone shock. Amer. J. Physiol. **163**, 283—289 (1950)

Bernard, A.: La pancréatite aigüe. Toxémie enzymatique. Presse méd. **67**, 2351—2353 (1959)

Bertelli, A.: Proteases and anti-proteasic substances in the inflammatory response. Biochem. Pharmacol. Spec. Suppl., 229—240 (1968)

Bhalla, T. N., Sinha, J. N., Tangri, K. K., Bhargava, K. P.: Role of catecholamines in inflammation. Europ. J. Pharmacol. **13**, 90—96 (1970)

Bhoola, K. D., Schachter, M.: A comparison of serum kallikrein, bradykinin, and histamine on capillary permeability. J. Physiol. (Lond.) **149**, 80 P—81 P (1959)

Bignold, L. P., Lykke, A. W. J.: Increased vascular permeability induced in synovialis of the rat by histamine, serotonin, and bradykinin. Experientia (Basel) **31**, 671—672 (1975)

Boissonas, R. A., Guttmann, S., Jaquenoud, P. A.: Synthèse de la L-arginyl-L-prolyl-prolyl-glycyl-L-phénylalanyl-L-séryl-L-prolyl-L-phénylalanyl-L-arginine, un nonapeptide présentant les proprietés de la bradykinine. Helv. chim. Acta **43**, 1349—1358 (1960a)

Boissonnas, R. A., Guttmann, St., Jaquenoud, P. A., Konzett, H., Sturner, E.: Synthesis and biological activity of peptides related to bradykinin. Experientia (Basel) **16**, 326 (1960b)

Boissonas, R. A., Guttmann, S., Jaquenoud, P. A., Pless, J., Sandrin, E.: The synthesis of bradykinin and of related peptides. Ann. N.Y. Acad. Sci. **104**, 5—14 (1963)

Bolam, J. P., Elliott, P. N. C., Ford-Hutchinson, A. W., Smith, M. J. H.: Histamine, 5-hydroxytryptamine, kinins, and the anti-inflammatory activity of human plasma fraction in carrageenan-induced paw oedema in the rat. J. Pharm. (Lond.) **26**, 434—440 (1974)

Bonta, I. L., De Vos, C. J.: Presence of a slow-contraction inducing material in fluid collected from the rat paw oedema induced by serotonin. Experientia (Basel) **21**, 34—38 (1965)

Bonta, I. L., De Vos, C. J.: Significance of the kinin system in rat paw oedemas and drug effects on it. Europ. J. Pharmacol. **1**, 222—225 (1967)

Boreham, P. F. L.: In vitro studies on the mechanism of kinin formation by trypanosomes. Brit. J. Pharmacol. **34**, 598—603 (1968)

Borges, D. R., Gordon, A. H.: Kininogen and kininogenase synthesis by the liver of normal and injured rats. J. Pharm. (Lond.) **28**, 44—48 (1976)

Borges, D. R., Prado, J. L., Guimarães, J. A.: Characterization of a kinin-converting arylamino peptidase from human liver. Naunyn-Schmiedebergs Arch. Pharmacol. **281**, 403—414 (1974)

Briseid, K., Arntzen, F. C., Dyrud, O. K.: Inhibition of carrageenin-induced rat paw-oedema by substances causing a reduction of kininogen and prekallikrein in plasma. Acta pharmacol. (Kbh.) **29**, 265—274 (1971)

Brocklehurst, W. E., Lahiri, S. C.: The production of bradykinin in anaphylaxis. J. Physiol. (Lond.) **160**, 15P—16P (1962)

Brocklehurst, W. E., Zeitlin, I. J.: Determination of plasma kinin and kininogen levels in man. J. Physiol. (Lond.) **191**, 417—426 (1967)

Burch, G. E., De Pasquale, N. P.: Bradykinin, digital blood flow, and the arteriovenous anastomoses. Circulat. Res. **10**, 105—115 (1962)

Camargo, A. C. M., Graeff, F. G.: Subcellular distribution and properties of the bradykinin inactivation system in rabbit brain homogenates. Biochem. Pharmacol. **18**, 548—549 (1969)

Camargo, A. C. M., Ramalho-Pinto, F. J., Greene, L. J.: Brain peptidases: conversion and inactivation of kinin hormones. J. Neurochem. **19**, 37—49 (1972)

Camargo, A. C. M., Shapanka, R., Greene, L. J.: Preparation, assay, and partial characterization of a neutral endopeptidase from rabbit brain. Biochemistry **12**, 1838—1844 (1973)

Carr, J., Wilhelm, D. L.: The evaluation of increased vascular permeability in the skin of guinea-pigs. Aust. J. exp. Biol. med. Sci. **42**, 511—522 (1964)

Carr, J., Wilhelm, D. L.: Interspecies differences in response to polypeptides as permeability factors. Nature (Lond.) **208**, 653—655 (1965)

Carvalho, I. F., Diniz, C. R.: Kinin forming enzyme (kininogenin) in rat kidney. Ann. N.Y. Acad. Sci. **116**, 912—917 (1964)

Castania, A., Rothschild, A. M.: Lowering of kininogen in rat blood by adrenaline and its inhibition by sympatholytic agents, heparin, and aspirin. Brit. J. Pharmacol. **50**, 375—389 (1974)

Castelfranchi, P. L., Corrado, A. P.: Variações do bradicininógeno plasmático e efeitos de um inhibidor enzimático em pancreopatias agudas experimentais. Ciênc. Cult. **23**, 505—514 (1971)

Chapman, L. F., Goodell, H.: The participation of the nervous system in the inflammatory reaction. Ann. N.Y. Acad. Sci. **116**, 990—1017 (1964)

Chapman, L. F., Ramos, A. O., Goodell, H., Wolff, H. G.: Neurohumoral features of afferent fibers in man. Arch. Neurol. **4**, 617—650 (1961)

Cîrstea, M., Suhaciu, G., Butculescu, I.: Bradykinin and anaphylactic shock in dogs. Int. Arch. Allergy **26**, 356—361 (1965)

Cîrstea, M., Suhaciu, G., Butculescu, I.: Evaluation du rôle de la bradykinine dans le choc anaphylactique. Arch. int. Pharmacodyn. **159**, 18—33 (1966)

Cline, M. J., Melmon, K. L.: Plasma kinins and cortisol: a possible explanation of the anti-inflammatory action of cortisol. Science **153**, 90—92 (1966)

Cochrane, C. G., Revak, S. D., Wuepper, K. D.: Activation of Hageman factor in solid and fluid phases. A critical role of kallikrein. J. exp. Med. **138**, 1564—1583 (1973)

Cochrane, C. G., Wuepper, K. D.: The first component of the kinin-forming system in human and rabbit plasma. Its relationship to clotting factor XII (Hageman factor). J. exp. Med. **134**, 986—1004 (1971)

Coffman, J. D., Javett, S. L.: Calf blood flow and oxygen usage during bradykinin infusions. J. appl. Physiol. **18**, 1003—1007 (1963)
Collier, H. O. J.: La bradykinin et ses antagonists. Actualités pharmacol. **14**, 51—74 (1961)
Collier, H. O. J., Holgate, J. A., Schachter, M., Shorley, P. G.: The bronchoconstrictor action of bradykinin in the guinea-pig. Brit. J. Pharmacol. **15**, 290—297 (1960)
Collier, H. O. J., James, G. W. L.: Bradykinin and slow reacting substance in anaphylactic bronchoconstriction of the guinea pig in vivo. J. Physiol. (Lond.) **185**, 71 P—72 P (1966)
Collier, H. O. J., Lee, I. R.: Nociceptive responses of guinea-pigs to intradermal injections of bradykinin and kallidin-10. Brit. J. Pharmacol. **21**, 155—164 (1963)
Collier, H. O. J., Schneider, C.: Nociceptive response to prostaglandins and analgesic actions of aspirin and morphine. Nature (New Biol.) **236**, 141—143 (1972)
Collier, H. O. J., Shorley, P. G.: Analgesic antipyretic drugs as antagonists of bradykinin. Brit. J. Pharmacol. **15**, 601—610 (1960)
Collier, H. O. J., Shorley, P. G.: Antagonism by mefenamic and flufenamic acids of the bronchoconstrictor action of kinins in the guinea-pig. Brit. J. Pharmacol. **20**, 345—351 (1963)
Corrado, A. P., Reis, M. L., Carvalho, I. F., Diniz, C. R.: Bradykininogen and bradykinin in the cardiovascular shock produced by proteolytic enzymes. Biochem. Pharmacol. **15**, 959—970 (1966)
Cotran, R. S., Majno, G.: A light and electron microscopic analysis of vascular injury. Ann. N.Y. Acad. Sci. **116**, 750—764 (1964)
Crunkhorn, P., Meacock, S. C. R.: Mediators of the inflammation induced in the rat paw by carrageenin. Brit. J. Pharmacol. **42**, 392—402 (1971)
Davies, G. E., Holman, G., Johnston, T. P., Lowe, J. S.: Studies on kallikrein: failure of some anti-inflammatory drugs of affect release of kinin. Brit. J. Pharmacol. **28**, 212—217 (1966)
Dawson, W., Starr, M. S., West, G. B.: Inhibition of anaphylactic shock in the rat by antihistamines and ascorbic acid. Brit. J. Pharmacol. **27**, 249—255 (1966)
De Duve, C.: Lysosomes and cell injury. In: Thomas, L., Uhr, J. W., Grant, L. (Eds.): Injury, Inflammation, and Immunity, pp. 283—311. Baltimore: Williams & Wilkins Comp. 1964
De Duve, C., Pressman, B. C., Gianetto, R., Wattiaux, R., Appelmans, F.: Tissue fractionation studies: intracellular distribution patterns of enzymes in rat liver tissue. Biochem. J. **60**, 604—617 (1955)
Deutsch, H. F., Diniz, C. R.: Some proteolytic activities of snake venoms. J. biol. Chem. **216**, 17—26 (1955)
Diniz, C. R., Carvalho, I. F.: A micromethod for determination of bradykininogen under several conditions. Ann. N.Y. Acad. Sci. **104**, 77—89 (1963)
Diniz, C. R., Carvalho, I. F., Reis, M. L., Corrado, A. P.: Bradykininogen in some experimental conditions. In: Rocha e Silva, M., Rothschild, H. A. (Eds.): Int. Symp. on Vaso-Active Polypeptides: Bradykinin and Related Kinins, pp. 15—20. São Paulo: Edart 1967
Diniz, C. R., Carvalho, I. F., Ryan, J., Rocha e Silva, M.: A micromethod for the determination of bradykininogen in blood plasma. Nature (Lond.) **192**, 1194—1195 (1961)
Di Rosa, M., Giroud, J. P., Willoughby, D. A.: Studies on the mediators of the acute inflammatory response induced in rats in different sites by carrageenin and turpentine. J. Path. **104**, 15—29 (1971)
Di Rosa, M., Sorrentino, L.: The mechanism of the inflammatory effect of carrageenin. Europ. J. Pharmacol. **4**, 340—342 (1968)
Di Rosa, M., Sorrentino, L.: Some pharmacodynamic properties of carrageenin in the rat. Brit. J. Pharmacol. **38**, 214—220 (1970)
Di Rosa, M., Willoughby, D. A.: Screens for anti-inflammatory drugs. J. Pharm. (Lond.) **23**, 297—298 (1971)
Edery, H., Lewis, G. P.: Inhibition of plasma kininase activity at slightly acid pH. Brit. J. Pharmacol. **19**, 299—308 (1962)
Edery, H., Lewis, G. P.: Kinin-forming activity and histamine in lymph after tissue injury. J. Physiol. (Lond.) **169**, 568—583 (1963)
Ehringer, H., Herzog, P., Konzett, H.: Über die Wirkung von synthetischem Bradykinin auf die Durchblutung der Extremitäten des Menschen. Helv. physiol. pharmacol. Acta **19**, C66—C68 (1961)

Eisen, V.: Kinin formation and fibrinolysis in human plasma. J. Physiol. (Lond.) **166**, 514—529 (1963)
Eisen, V.: Kinin forming enzymes and substrates in human plasma. J. Physiol. (Lond.) **186**, 133P (1966a)
Eisen, V.: Urates and kinin formation in synovial fluid. Proc. roy. Soc. Med. **59**, 302—307 (1966b)
Eisen, V.: Kinin formation in human diseases. In: Basis Med. Ann. Rev., pp. 146—165. London: Athlone 1969
Eisen, V., Greenbaum, L., Lewis, G.P.: Kinins and anti-inflammatory steroids. Brit. J. Pharmacol. **34**, 169—176 (1968)
Eisen, V., Loveday, C.: In vivo effects of cellulose sulphate on plasma kininogen, complement, and inflammation. Brit. J. Pharmacol. **42**, 383—391 (1971)
Elliott, D.F., Horton, E.W., Lewis, G.P.: Actions of pure bradykinin. J. Physiol. (Lond.) **153**, 473—480 (1960b)
Elliott, D.F., Horton, E.W., Lewis, G.P.: The isolation of bradykinin. A plasma kinin from ox blood. Biochem. J. **78**, 60—65 (1961)
Elliott, D.F., Lewis, G.P.: Methionyl-lysyl-bradykinin, a new kinin from ox blood. Biochem. J. **95**, 437—447 (1965)
Elliott, D.F., Lewis, G.P., Horton, E.W.: The structure of bradykinin—a plasma kinin from ox blood. Biochem. biophys. Res. Commun. **3**, 87—91 (1960a)
Elliott, D.F., Lewis, G.P., Smyth, D.C.: A new kinin from ox blood. Biochem. J. **87**, 21P (1963)
Engleman, E.G., Greenbaum, L.M.: Kinin-forming activity of human lymphocytes. Biochem. Pharmacol. **20**, 922—924 (1971).
Erdös, E.G.: Enzymes that inactivate active polypeptides. Biochem. Pharmacol. **8**, 112 (1961)
Erdös, E.G.: Effect of nonsteroidal anti-inflammatory drugs in endotoxin shock. Biochem. Pharmacol. Suppl., 283—291 (1968)
Erdös, E.G. (Ed.): Bradykinin, Kallidin, and Kallikrein. Handbook of Experimental Pharmacology, Vol. XXV. Berlin-Heidelberg-New York: Springer 1970
Erdös, E.G.: Angiotensin I converting enzyme. Circulat. Res. **36**, 247—255 (1975)
Erdös, E.G., Renfrew, A.G., Sloane, E.M., Wohler, J.R.: Enzymatic studies on bradykinin and similar peptides. Ann. N.Y. Acad. Sci. **104**, 222—235 (1963a)
Erdös, E.G., Sloane, E.M.: An enzyme in human blood plasma that inactivates bradykinin and kallidin. Biochem. Pharmacol. **11**, 585—592 (1962)
Erdös, E.G., Sloane, E.M., Wohler, I.M.: Carboxypeptidase in blood and other fluids. I. Properties, distribution, and partial purification of the enzyme. Biochem. Pharmacol. **13**, 893—905 (1964)
Erdös, E.G., Whohler, J.R., Levine, M.I.: Blocking of the in vivo effects of bradykinin and kallidin with carboxypeptidase B. J. Pharmacol. exp. Ther. **142**, 327—334 (1963b)
Erdös, E.G., Yang, H.Y.T.: Inactivation and potentiation of the effects of bradykinin. In: Erdös, E.G., Back, N., Sicuteri, F. (Eds.): Hypotentive Peptides, pp. 235—251. Berlin-Heidelberg-New York: Springer 1966
Erdös, E.G., Yang, H.Y.T.: An enzyme in microsomal fraction of kidney that inactivates bradykinin. Life Sci. **6**, 569—574 (1967a)
Erdös, E.G., Yang, H.Y.T.: Metabolism of bradykinin and related peptides. In: Rocha e Silva, M., Rothschild, H.A. (Eds.): International Symposium on Vaso-Active Substances: Bradykinin and Related Kinins, pp. 239—246. São Paulo: Edart 1967b
Erdös, E.G., Yang, H.Y.T.: Kininases. In: Erdös, E.G. (Ed.): Bradykinin, Kallidin, and Kallikrein. Handbook of Experimental Pharmacology, Vol. XXV, pp. 289—323. Berlin-Heidelberg-New York: Springer 1970
Fasciolo, J.C., Halvorsen, K.: Specificity of mammalian kallidinogen. Amer. J. Physiol. **207**, 901—905 (1964)
Ferreira, S.H.: A bradykinin-potentiating factor (BPF) present in the venom of *Bothrops Jararaca*. Brit. J. Pharmacol. **24**, 163—169 (1965)
Ferreira, S.H.: Prostaglandins, aspirin-like drugs, and analgesia. Nature (New Biol.) **240**, 200—203 (1972)
Ferreira, S.H., Moncada, S., Vane, J.R.: Indomethacin and aspirin abolish prostaglandin release from the spleen. Nature (New Biol.) **231**, 237—239 (1971)

Ferreira, S. H., Moncada, S., Vane, J. R.: Prostaglandins and the mechanism of analgesia produced by aspirin-like drugs. Brit. J. Pharmacol. **49**, 86—97 (1973)
Ferreira, S. H., Moncada, S., Vane, J. R.: Prostaglandins and signs and symptoms of inflammation. In: Robinson, H. J., Vane, J. R. (Eds.): Prostaglandin Synthetase Inhibitors, pp. 175—187. New York: Raven 1974
Ferreira, S. H., Rocha e Silva, M.: Potentiation of bradykinin by dimercaptopropanol (BAL) and other inhibitors of its destroying enzyme in plasma. Biochem. Pharmacol. **11**, 1123—1128 (1962)
Ferreira, S. H., Rocha e Silva, M.: Liberation of bradykinin in the circulating blood of dogs by trypsin, chymotrypsin, and nagarse. Brit. J. Pharmacol. **36**, 611—622 (1969)
Ferreira, S. H., Vane, J. R.: The disappearance of bradykinin and eledoisin in the circulation and vascular beds of the cat. Brit. J. Pharmacol. **30**, 417—424 (1967a)
Ferreira, S. H., Vane, J. R.: Half-lives of peptides and amines in the circulation. Nature (Lond.) **215**, 1237—1240 (1967b)
Fiedler, F., Werle, E.: Vorkommen zweier Kallikreinogene im Schweinepankreas und Automation der Kallikrein- und Kallikreinogenbestimmung. Hoppe-Seyler's Z. physiol. Chem. **348**, 1087—1089 (1967)
Forell, M. M.: Therapy with kallikrein and protease inhibitors. Ann. N.Y. Acad. Sci. **104**, 368—375 (1963)
Fox, R. H., Goldsmith, R., Kidd, D. J., Lewis, G. P.: Bradykinin as a vasodilator in man. J. Physiol. (Lond.) **157**, 589—602 (1961)
Freund, J., Miles, A. A., Mill, P. J., Wilhelm, D. L.: Vascular permeability factors in the secretion of the guinea pig coagulating gland. Nature (Lond.) **182**, 174—175 (1958)
Frey, E. K.: Zusammenhänge zwischen Herzarbeit und Nierentätigkeit. Langenbecks Arch. klin. Chir. **142**, 663—669 (1926)
Frey, E. K., Kraut, H., Schultz, F.: Über eine nerveninnersekretorische Funktion des Pankreas. Naunyn-Schmiedeberg's Arch. exp. Path. Pharmak. **158**, 334—347 (1930)
Frimmer, M.: Beeinflussung der Durchlässigkeit von Blut-Cappilaren der Kaninchenhaut für Makromoleküle durch einige biogene, gefäßaktive Substanzen. Naunyn-Schmiedeberg's Arch. exp. Path. Pharmak. **242**, 390—395 (1961)
Fritz, H., Eckert, I., Werle, E.: Isolierung und Charakterisierung von sialinsäurehaltigem und sialinsäurefreiem Kallikrein aus Schweinepankreas. Hoppe-Seyler's Z. physiol. Chem. **348**, 1120—1132 (1967)
Gaddum, J. H., Guth, P. S.: A comparison of the kallikrein-kinin system in sheep and dogs. Brit. J. Pharmacol. **15**, 181—184 (1960)
Garcia Leme, J., Hamamura, L.: Formation of a factor increasing vascular permeability during electrical stimulation of the saphenous nerve in rats. Brit. J. Pharmacol. **51**, 383—389 (1974)
Garcia Leme, J., Hamamura, L., Leite, M. P., Rocha e Silva, M.: Pharmacological analysis of the acute inflammatory process induced in the rat's paw by local injection of carrageenin and by heating. Brit. J. Pharmacol. **48**, 88—96 (1973b)
Garcia Leme, J., Hamamura, L., Migliorini, R. H., Leite, M. P.: Influence of diabetes upon the inflammatory response of the rat. A pharmacological analysis. Europ. J. Pharmacol. **23**, 74—81 (1973a)
Garcia Leme, J., Hamamura, L., Rocha e Silva, M.: Effect of anti-proteases and hexadimethrine bromide on the release of a bradykinin-like substance during heating (46° C) of rat paws. Brit. J. Pharmacol. **40**, 294—309 (1970)
Garcia Leme, J., Rocha e Silva, M.: Competitive and non-competitive inhibition of bradykinin on the guinea-pig ileum. Brit. J. Pharmacol. **25**, 50—58 (1965)
Garcia Leme, J., Schapoval, E. E. S., Rocha e Silva, M.: Factors influencing the developement of local swelling induced in the rat's paw by macromolecular compounds and heating. In: Rocha e Silva, M., Rothschild, H. A. (Eds.): International Symposium on Vaso-Active Polypeptides: Bradykinin and Related Kinins, pp. 213—221. São Paulo: Edart 1967
Garcia Leme, J., Walaszek, E. J.: Antagonists of pharmacologically active peptides. Effect on guinea pig ileum and inflammation. In: Proceedings 5th International Congress Pharmacology, Vol. V, pp. 328—335. Basel-München-Paris-London-New York-Sidney: Karger 1973
Gardner, D. L.: Production of arthritis in the rabbit by the local injection of the mucopolysaccharide caragheenin. Ann. rheum. Dis. **19**, 369—376 (1960)

Gardner, D. L.: Pathology of the connective tissue diseases. London: Edward Arnold 1965

Gautvik, K. M., Rugstad, H. D.: Kinin formation and kininogen depletion in rats after intravenous injection of ellagic acid. Brit. J. Pharmacol. **31**, 390—400 (1967)

Gilfoil, T. M., Klavins, I.: 5-hydroxytryptamine, bradykinin, and histamine as mediators of inflammatory hyperesthesia. Amer. J. Physiol. **208**, 867—876 (1965)

Giordano, F., Scapagnini, U.: L'oedème localisé par bradykinine synthétique chez le rat comme test pour l'évaluation de médicaments anti-inflammatoires. Med. Pharmacol. exp. **17**, 445—465 (1967)

Gladner, J. A.: Potentiation of the effect of bradykinin. In: Erdös, E. G., Back, N., Sicuteri, F. (Eds.): Hypotensive Peptides, pp. 344—355. Berlin-Heidelberg-New York: Springer 1966

Gladner, J. A., Murtaugh, P. M., Folk, J. E., Laki, K.: Nature of peptides released by thrombin. Ann. N.Y. Acad. Sci. **104**, 47—52 (1963)

Goodwin, L. G., Jones, C. R., Richards, W. H. G., Kohn, J.: Pharmacologically active substances in the urine of burned patients. Brit. J. exp. Path. **44**, 551—560 (1963)

Goodwin, L. G., Richards, W. H. G.: Pharmacologically active peptides in the blood and urine of animals infected with *Babesia Rodhaini* and other pathogenic organisms. Brit. J. Pharmacol. **15**, 152—159 (1960)

Graham, R. C., Erbert, R. H., Ratnoff, O. D., Moses, J. M.: Pathogenesis of inflammation. II. In vivo observations of the inflammatory effects of activated Hageman factor and bradykinin. J. exp. Med. **121**, 807—818 (1965)

Greaves, M., Schuster, S.: Responses of skin blood vessels to bradykinin, histamine, and 5-hydroxytryptamine. J. Physiol. (Lond.) **193**, 255—267 (1967)

Greeff, K., Lühr, R., Strobach, H.: Die Abnahme des Kininogengehaltes des Plasmas beim toxischen, anaphylaktischen und anaphylaktoiden Schock. Naunyn-Schmiedeberg's Arch. exp. Path. Pharmak. **253**, 235—239 (1966)

Greenbaum, L. M., Freer, R., Chang, J., Semente, G., Yamafuji, K.: PMN-kinin metabolizing enzymes in normal and malignant leucocytes. Brit. J. Pharmacol. **36**, 623—634 (1969)

Greenbaum, L. M., Kim, K. S.: The kinin-forming and kininase activities of rabbit polymorphonuclear leukocytes. Brit. J. Pharmacol. **29**, 238—247 (1967)

Greenbaum, L. M., Yamafuji, K.: The in vitro inactivation and formation of plasma kinins by spleen cathepsins. Brit. J. Pharmacol. **27**, 230—238 (1966)

Greenbaum, L. M., Yamafuji, K., Kim, K. S.: Studies on the kinin-forming and inactivating enzymes in tissues and leucocytes. In: Rocha e Silva, M., Rothschild, H. A. (Eds.): International Symposium on Vaso-active Polypeptides: Bradykinin and Related Kinins, pp. 21—25. São Paulo: Edart 1967

Greene, L. J., Camargo, A. C. M., Krieger, E. M., Stewart, J. M., Ferreira, S. H.: Inhibition of the conversion of angiotensin I to II and potentiation of bradykinin by small peptides present in *Bothrops jararaca* venom. Circulat. Res. XXX, Suppl. **II**, 62—71 (1972)

Guimarães, J. A., Borges, D. R., Prado, E. S., Prado, J. L.: Kinin-converting aminopeptidase from human serum. Biochem. Pharmacol. **22**, 3157—3172 (1973)

Guimarães, J. A., Chen-Lu, R., Webster, M. E., Pierce, J. V.: Multiple forms of human plasma kininogen. Fed. Proc. **33**, 641 (1974)

Gunnar, R. M., Weeks, R. E.: Effect of tripelennamine hydrochloride on burn shock. Arch. Path. (Chicago) **47**, 594—597 (1949)

Guzman, F., Braun, C., Lim, R. K. S.: Visceral pain and the pseudoaffective response to intraarterial injection of bradykinin and other algesic agents. Arch. int. Pharmacodyn. **136**, 353—384 (1962)

Guzman, F., Braun, C., Lim, R. K. S., Potter, G. D., Rodgers, D. W.: Narcotic and non-narcotic analgesics which block visceral pain evoked by intraarterial injection of bradykinin and other algesic agents. Arch. int. Pharmacodyn. **149**, 571—588 (1964)

Habal, F. M., Burrowes, C. E., Movat, H. Z.: Generation of kinin by plasmin. Fed. Proc. **34**, 859 (1975)

Habal, F. M., Movat, H. Z., Burrowes, C. E.: Isolation of two functionally different kininogens from human plasma—separation from proteinase inhibitors and interaction with plasma kallikrein. Biochem. Pharmacol. **23**, 2291—2303 (1974)

Haberland, G. L., Rohen, J. W., Eds.: Kininogenases. First Symposium on Physiological Properties and Pharmacological Rational. Stuttgart-New York: F. K. Schattauer 1973

Habermann, E.: Enzymatic kinin release from kininogen and from low-molecular compounds. In: Erdös, E. G., Back, N., Sicuteri, F. (Eds.): Hypertensive Peptides, pp. 116—129. Berlin-Heidelberg-New York: Springer 1966a

Habermann, E.: Struktur auf Klärung kininliefernder Peptide aus Rinderserum-Kininogen. Naunyn-Schmiedeberg's Arch. exp. Path. Pharmak. **253**, 474—483 (1966b)

Habermann, E.: Kininogens. In: Erdös, E. G. (Ed.): Bradykinin, Kallidin, and Kallikrein. Handb. Exp. Pharmakol., Vol. XXV, pp. 250—288. Berlin-Heidelberg-New York: Springer 1970

Habermann, E., Blennemann, G.: Über Substrate und Reaktionsprodukte der kininbildenden Enzyme Trypsin, Serum- und Pankreaskallikrein sowie von Crotalusgift. Naunyn-Schmiedeberg's Arch. exp. Pathol. Pharmakol. **249**, 357—373 (1964)

Habermann, E., Blennemann, G., Müller, B.: Charakterisierung und Reinigung peptischer kininliefernder Fragmente (PKF) sowie von „Pepsitocin" aus Rinderserumkininogen. Naunyn-Schmiedeberg's Arch. exp. Path. Pharmak. **253**, 444—463 (1966)

Habermann, E., Helbig, J.: Cleavage of kininogen by cyanogen bromide and enzymes: a procedure for determining position and structure of the kinin-yielding sequence. Naunyn-Schmiedeberg's Arch. exp. Path. Pharmak. **255**, 20 (1966)

Habermann, E., Klett, W.: Reinigung und einige Eigenschaften eines Kallikreins auf Schweineserum. Biochem. Z. **346**, 133—158 (1966)

Habermann, E., Müller, B.: Zur enzymatischen Spaltung peptischer kininliefernder Fragmente (PKF) sowie von Rinderserumkininogen. Naunyn-Schmiedeberg's Arch. exp. Path. Pharmak. **253**, 464—473 (1966)

Hamberg, U.: Plasma protease and kinin release with special reference to plasmin. Ann. N.Y. Acad. Sci. **146**, 517—526 (1968)

Hamberg, U., Elg, P., Nissingen, E., Stelwagen, P.: Purification and heterogeneity of human kininogen. Int. J. pept. prot. Res. **7**, 261—280 (1975)

Hamberg, U., Rocha e Silva, M.: Studies on the enzymatic inactivation of bradykinin. Acta physiol. scand. **30**, 215—225 (1954)

Hamberg, U., Rocha e Silva, M.: On the release of bradykinin by trypsin and snake venom. Arch. int. Pharmacodyn. **110**, 222—238 (1957a)

Hamberg, U., Rocha e Silva, M.: Release of bradykinin as related to the esterase activity of trypsin and the venom of *Bothrops jararaca*. Experientia (Basel) **13**, 489—490 (1957b)

Harpel, P. C.: Human plasma alpha-2-macroglobulin. An inhibitor of plasma kallikrein. J. exp. Med. **132**, 329—352 (1970)

Hathway, W. E., Belhasen, L. P., Hathway, H. S.: Evidence for a new plasma thromboplastin factor. I. Case report, coagulation studies and physicochemical properties. Blood **26**, 521—532 (1965)

Hebborn, P., Shaw, B.: The action of sodium salicylate and aspirin on some kallikrein systems. Brit. J. Pharmacol. **20**, 254—263 (1963)

Henriques, O. B., Fichman, M., Beraldo, W. T.: Bradykinin-releasing factor from *Bothrops jararaca* venom. Nature (Lond.) **187**, 414—415 (1960)

Henriques, O. B., Kauritcheva, N., Kuznetsova, V., Astrakan, M.: Substrates of kinin-releasing enzymes isolated from horse plasma. Nature (Lond.) **215**, 1200—1201 (1967)

Henriques, O. B., Lavras, A. A. C., Fichman, M., Picarelli, Z. P.: Plasma enzymes that release kinins. Biochem. Pharmacol. **15**, 31—40 (1966)

Herxheimer, H., Streseman, E.: Bradykinin and ethanol in bronchial asthma. Arch. int. Pharmacodyn. **144**, 315—318 (1963)

Hilton, S. M.: Plasma kinin and blood flow. In: Schachter, M. (Ed.): Polypeptides Which Affect Smooth Muscles and Blood Vessels, pp. 258—265. Oxford: Pergamon 1960

Hilton, S. M., Lewis, G. P.: The relationships between glandular activity, bradykinin formation and functional vasodilatation in the submandibular salivary gland. J. Physiol. (Lond.) **134**, 471—478 (1956)

Hladovéc, J., Mansfeld, V., Horáková, Z.: Inhibitory action of trypsin and trypsin-inhibitors on experimental inflammation in rats. Experientia (Basel) **14**, 146—147 (1958)

Hochstrasser, K., Werle, E.: Über kininliefernde Peptide aus pepsinverdautem Rinderplasmaprotein. Hoppe-Syler's Z. physiol. Chem. **348**, 177—182 (1967)

Hori, S.: The presence of bradykinin-like polypeptides, kinin-releasing and—destroying activity in brain. Jap. J. Physiol. **18**, 772—787 (1968)

Horton, E. W.: The estimation of urinary kallikrein. J. Physiol. (Lond.) **148**, 267—282 (1959).
Hureau, J., Forlot, P., Raby, C., Vairel, E.: Évidence de la présence de trypsine dans le sang périphérique au cours des pancréatites aigües hemorrhagiques. Son rôle dans le dévelopment du choc. Rev. franç. Êt. clin. biol. **13**, 80—82 (1968)
Innerfield, I.: The anti-inflammatory effect of parenterally administered proteases. Ann. N.Y. Acad. Sci. **68**, 167—177 (1957)
Innerfield, I., Bundy, R. E., Hochberg, R.: Bradykinin antagonism following oral protease therapy. Proc. Soc. exp. Biol. (N.Y.) **112**, 295—297 (1963)
Inoki, R., Toyoda, T., Yamamoto, I.: Elaboration of a bradykinin-like substance in dog's canine pulp during electrical stimulation and its inhibition by narcotic and nonnarcotic analgesics. Naunyn-Schmiedeberg's Arch. Pharmacol. **279**, 387—398 (1973)
Jacobsen, S.: Substrates for plasma kinin-forming enzymes in human, dog, and rabbit plasmas. Brit. J. Pharmacol. **289**, 64—72 (1966a)
Jacobsen, S.: Observations on the content of kininogen, kallikrein, and kininase in lymph from hind limbs of dogs and rabbits. Brit. J. Pharmacol. **27**, 213—221 (1966b)
Jacobsen, S., Kriz, M.: Some data on two purified kininogens from human plasma. Brit. J. Pharmacol. **29**, 25—36 (1967)
Jacobsen, S., Waaler, B. A.: The effect of scalding on the content of kininogen and kininase in limb lymph. Brit. J. Pharmacol. **27**, 222—229 (1966)
Jancsó, N., Jancsó-Gábor, A., Szolcsányi, J.: Direct evidence for neurogenic inflammation and its prevention by denervation and by pretreatment with capsaicin. Brit. J. Pharmacol. **31**, 138—151 (1967)
Juan, H., Lembeck, F.: Action of peptides and other algesic agents on paravascular pain receptors of the isolated perfused rabbit ear. Naunyn-Schmiedeberg's Arch. Pharmacol. **283**, 151—164 (1974)
Kaller, H., Hoffmeister, F., Kroneberg, G.: Die Wirkung von Trasylol auf verschiedene Ödemformen der Rattenpfote. Arch. int. Pharmacodyn. **161**, 398—409 (1966)
Kaplan, A. P., Austen, K. F.: A prealbumin activator of prekallikrein. II. Derivation of activators of prekallikrein from active Hageman factor by digestion with plasmin. J. exp. Med. **133**, 696—712 (1971)
Kaplan, A. P., Kay, A. B., Austen, K. F.: A prealbumin activator of prekallikrein. III. Appearance of chemotactic activity for human neutrophils by the conversion of human prekallikrein to kallikrein. J. exp. Med. **135**, 81—97 (1972)
Keele, C. A.: Clinical and pathological aspects of kinins in man. Proc. roy. Soc. B, **173**, 361—369 (1969)
Keele, C. A., Armstrong, D.: Substances producing pain and itch. London: Edward Arnold Ltd. 1964
Kellermeyer, R. W.: Inflammatory process in acute gouty arthritis. III. Vascular permeability-enhancing activity in normal human synovial fluid; induction by Hageman factor activators; and inhibition by Hageman factor antiserum. J. Lab. clin. Med. **70**, 372—383 (1967)
Kellermeyer, R. W., Breckenridge, R. T.: The inflammatory process in acute gouty arthritis. I. Activation of Hageman factor by sodium urate crystals. J. Lab. clin. Med. **65**, 307—315 (1965)
Kellermeyer, R. W., Breckenridge, R. T.: The inflammatory process in acute gouty arthritis. II. The presence of Hageman factor and plasma thromboplastin antecedent in synovial fluid. J. Lab. clin. Med. **67**, 455—460 (1966)
Kellett, D. N.: On the anti-inflammatory activity of protamine sulphate and of hexadimethrine bromide, inhibitors of plasma kinin formation. Brit. J. Pharmacol. **24**, 705—713 (1965)
Kellett, D. N.: On the mechanism of the anti-inflammatory activity of hexadimethrine bromide. Brit. J. Pharmacol. **26**, 351—357 (1966)
Komiya, M., Kato, H., Suzuki, T.: Bovine plasma kininogens. I. Further purification of high molecular weight kininogen and its physic-chemical properties. J. Biochem. (Tokyo) **76**, 811—822 (1974)
Konzett, H.: Some properties of synthetic bradykinin-like polypeptides. Biochem. Pharmacol. **10**, 39—45 (1962)
Konzett, H., Stürmer, E.: Synthetic bradykinin: its biological identity with natural pure trypsin bradykinin. Nature (Lond.) **188**, 998 (1960)

Kraut, H., Frey, E. K., Werle, E.: Über den Nachweis und das Vorkommen des Kallikreins in Blut. VIII. Mitteilung über Kallikrein. Hoppe-Seyler's Z. physiol. Chem. **222**, 73—99 (1933)
Kraut, H., Frey, E. K., Werle, E., Schultz, F.: Nachweis und Vorkommen des Kallikreins in Harn. IX. Mitteilung über Kallikrein. Hoppe-Seyler's Z. physiol. Chem. **230**, 259—277 (1934)
Lahiri, B., Rosenberg, R., Talamo, R. C., Mitchell, B., Bagdasarian, A., Colman, R. W.: Antithrombin III, an inhibitor of human plasma kallikrein. Fed. Proc. **33**, 642 (1974)
Lecomte, J.: Bradykinine et réactions anaphylactiques du lapin. C.R. Soc. Biol. (Paris) **154**, 1118—1120 (1960a)
Lecomte, J.: Antagonisme entre bradykinin synthétique et phénylbutazone chez le lapin. C.R. Soc. Biol. (Paris) **154**, 2389—2391 (1960b)
Lecomte, J.: Consommation des kininogènes plasmatiques an cours du choc anaphylactique du lapin. C.R. Soc. Biol. (Paris) **155**, 1411—1413 (1961)
Lecomte, J., Damas, J.: Formation de kinines in vivo lors de l'administration de sulfate de dextran chez le rat. C.R. Soc. Biol. (Paris) **162**, 2055—2057 (1968)
Lecomte, J., Petit, J. M., Mélon, J., Troquet, J., Marcelle, R.: Proprietés broncho-constrictrices de la bradykinine chez l'homme asthmatique. Arch. int. Pharmacodyn. **137**, 232—235 (1962)
Lecomte, J., Troquet, J.: Antagonisms entre bradykinine et phénylbutazone chez le lapin. C.R. Soc. Biol. (Paris) **154**, 1115—1117 (1960)
Lembeck, F., Juan, H.: Interaction of prostaglandins and indomethacin with algesic substances. Naunyn-Schmiedeberg's Arch. Pharmacol. **285**, 301—313 (1974)
Lewis, G. P.: Formation of plasma kinins by plasmin. J. Physiol. (Lond.) **140**, 285—300 (1958)
Lewis, G. P.: Active polypeptides derived from plasma proteins. Physiol. Rev. **40**, 647—676 (1960)
Lewis, G. P.: Bradykinin-biochemistry, pharmacology, and its physiological role in controlling local blood flow. Sci. Basis Med. **14**, 242—258 (1962)
Lewis, G. P.: Kinins in inflammation and tissue injury. In: Erdös, E. G. (Ed.): Bradykinin, Kallidin, and Kallikrein, Handb. exp. Pharmakol., Vol. XXV, pp. 516—530. Berlin-Heidelberg-New York: Springer 1970
Lewis, G. P., Wawretscheck, W. A.: Effect of thermal injury on the kinin system in rabbit hind limb lymph. Brit. J. Pharmacol. **43**, 127—139 (1971)
Lewis, G. P., Work, T.: Formation of bradykinin or bradykinin-like substances by the action of plasmin on plasma proteins. J. Physiol. (Lond.) **135**, 7 P (1956)
Lewis, T.: The blood vessels of the human skin and their responses. London: Shaw & Sons Ltd. 1927
Lim, R. K. S.: Neuropharmacology of pain and analgesia. In: Lim, R. K. S., Armstrong, D., Pardo, E. G. (Eds.): Pharmacology of Pain, pp. 169—217. Oxford: Pergamon Press 1968
Lim, R. K. S., Guzman, F., Rodgers, D. W., Gotto, K., Braun, C., Dickerson, G. D., Engle, R. J.: Site of action of narcotic and non-narcotic analgesics determined by blocking bradykinin evoked visceral pain. Arch. int. Pharmacodyn. **152**, 25—58 (1964)
Lima, A. O.: Pharmacologically active substances released during anaphylactic shock in the mouse. Int. Arch. Allergy **32**, 46—54 (1967)
Lish, P. M., McKinney, G. R.: Pharmacology of methdilazine. II. Some determinants and limits of action on vascular permeability and inflammation in model systems. J. Lab. clin. Med. **61**, 1015—1027 (1963)
Löbbecke, E. A.: Effect of kallikrein on the proliferation of various cell systems. In: Haberland, G. L., Rohen, J. W. (Eds.): Kininogenases. First Symp. on Physiological Properties and Pharmacological Rational, pp. 161—169. Stuttgart-New York: F. K. Schattauer 1973
McCarthy, D. A., Potter, D. E., Nicolaides, E. D.: An in vivo estimation of the potencies and half-lives of synthetic bradykinin and kallidin. J. Pharmacol. exp. Ther. **148**, 117—122 (1965)
McCarty, D. J., Jr.: Cristal-induced inflammation of the joints. Ann. Rev. Med. **21**, 357—366 (1970)
McConnell, D. J.: Inhibitors of kallikrein in human plasma. J. clin. Invest. **51**, 1611—1623 (1972)
McGiff, J. C., Terragno, A. M., Malik, K. U., Lonigro, A. J.: Release of a prostaglandin E-like substance from canine kidney by bradykinin. Circulat. Res. **31**, 36—43 (1972)
McKay, D. G., Lactour, J. G., Parrish, M. H.: Activation of Hageman factor by alpha-adrenergic stimulation. Thrombos. Diathes. haemorrh. (Stuttg.) **23**, 417—422 (1970)
Majno, G.: Mechanisms of abnormal vascular permeability in acute inflammation. In: Thomas, L., Uhr, J. W., Grant, L. (Eds.): Injury, Inflammation, and Immunity, pp. 58—93. Baltimore: The Williams & Wilkins Company 1964

Majno, G., Palade, G. E.: Studies on inflammation. I. The effect of histamine and serotonin on vascular permeability: An electron microscopic study. J. biophys. biochem. Cytol. **11**, 571—605 (1961)

Maling, H. M., Webster, M. E., Williams, M. A., Saul, W., Anderson, Jr., W.: Inflammation induced by histamine, serotonin, bradykinin, and compound 48/80 in the rat: antagonists and mechanisms of action. J. Pharmacol. exp. Ther. **191**, 300—310 (1974)

Margolis, J.: Initiation of blood coagulation by glass and related surfaces. J. Physiol. (Lond.) **137**, 95—109 (1957)

Margolis, J.: Activation of plasma by contact with glass. Evidence for a common reaction which releases plasma-kinin and initiates coagulation. J. Physiol. (Lond.) **144**, 1—22 (1958)

Margolis, J.: The mode of action of Hageman factor in the release of plasma kinin. J. Physiol. (Lond.) **151**, 238—252 (1960)

Margolis, J.: Activation of Hageman factor by saturated fatty acids. Aust. J. exp. Biol. med. Sci. **40**, 505—513 (1962)

Margolis, J., Bishop, E. A.: Interrelations between different mechanisms of release of biologically active peptides from blood plasma. Nature (Lond.) **194**, 749—751 (1962)

Margolis, J., Bishop, E.: Studies on plasma kinins. I. The composition of kininogen complex. Aust. J. exp. Biol. med. Sci. **41**, 293—306 (1963)

Margolis, J., Bruce, S., Starzecki, B., Horner, G. J., Halmagyi, D. F. J.: Release of bradykinin-like substance (BKLS) in sheep by venom of *Crotalus atrox*. Aust. J. exp. Biol. med. Sci. **43**, 237—244 (1965)

Mason, D. T., Melmon, K. L.: Effects of bradykinin in forearm venous tone and vascular resistance in man. Circulat. Res. **17**, 106—113 (1965)

Melmon, K. L., Cline, M. J.: Kallikrein activator and kininase in human granulocytes: a model of inflammation. In: Rocha e Silva, M., Rothschild, H. A. (Eds.): Int. Symp. on Vaso-active kinins: Bradykinin and Related Kinins, pp. 223—228. São Paulo: Edart 1967

Melmon, K. L., Cline, M. J.: The interaction of leucocytes on the kinin system. Biochem. Pharmacol. Suppl., 271—281 (1968)

Melmon, K. L., Webster, M. E., Goldfinger, S. E., Seegmiller, J. E.: The presence of a kinin in inflammatory synovial effusion from arthritides of varying etiologies. Arthr. Rheum. **10**, 13—20 (1967)

Merrifield, R. H.: Solid-phase peptide synthesis. IV. The synthesis of methionyl-lysyl-bradykinin. J. org. Chem. **29**, 3100—3102 (1964)

Miles, A. A.: Large molecular substances as mediators of the inflammatory reaction. Ann. N.Y. Acad. Sci. **116**, 855—865 (1964)

Miles, A. A., Miles, E. M.: Vascular reactions to histamine-liberator and leukotaxine in the skin of guinea-pigs. J. Physiol. (Lond.) **118**, 228—257 (1952)

Miles, A. A., Wilhelm, D. L.: The activation of endogenous substances inducing pathological increases of capillary permeability. In: Stoner, H. B. (Ed.): The Biochemical Response to Injury, pp. 51—79. Oxford: Blackwell 1960

Miller, R. L., Webster, M. E., Melmon, K. L.: Interaction of leukocytes and endotoxin with the plasmin and kinin systems. Europ. J. Pharmacol. **33**, 53—60 (1975)

Moncada, S., Ferreira, S. H., Vane, J. R.: Prostaglandins, aspirin-like drugs and the oedema of inflammation. Nature (Lond.) **246**, 217—219 (1973)

Morgan, A., Robinson, L. A., White, T. T.: Postoperative changes in the trypsin inhibitor activities of human pancreatic juice and the influence of infusion of trasylol on the inhibitor activity. Amer. J. Surg. **115**, 131—135 (1968)

Mörsdorf, K.: The inhibition of protein catabolism by anti-inflammatory drugs. In: Bertelli, A., Houck, J. C. (Eds.): Inflammation Biochemistry and Drug Interaction, pp. 255—260. Amsterdam: Excerpta Medica 1969

Mörsdorf, K., Marten, S., Purchert, I.: Ein Beitrag zur antiproteolytischen Wirkungsqualität von Phenylbutazon, Oxyphenbutazon und Natriumsalicylat. Arzneimittel-Forsch. **18**, 1516—1520 (1968)

Movat, H. Z.: Activation of the kinin system by antigen-antibody complexes. In: Rocha e Silva, M., Rothschild, H. A. (Eds.): Int. Symp. on Vaso-Active Polypeptides: Bradykinin and Related kinins, pp. 177—188. São Paulo: Edart 1967

Nicolaides, E. D., De Wald, H. A., McCarthy, D. S.: The synthesis of a biologically active decapeptide having the structure proposed for kallidin II. Biochem. biophys. Res. Commun. **6**, 210—212 (1961)
Nicolaides, E. D., De Wald, H. A., McCarthy, D. A.: The synthesis of kinin analogs. Ann. N.Y. Acad. Sci. **104**, 15—23 (1963)
Northover, B. J., Subramanian, G.: Analgesic-antipyretic drugs as inhibitors of kallikrein. Brit. J. Pharmacol. **17**, 107—115 (1961)
Nugent, F. W., Zuberi, S., Bulan, M. B.: Kinin precurssor in experimental pancreatitis. Proc. Soc. exp. Biol. (N.Y.) **130**, 566—567 (1969)
Onabanjo, A. O., Bhabani, A. R., Maegraith, B. G.: The significance of kinin-destroying enzymes activity in *Plasmodium knowlesi* malarial infection. Brit. J. exp. Path. **51**, 534—540 (1970)
Onabanjo, A. O., Maegraith, B. G.: Kallikrein as a pathogenic agent in *Plasmodium knowlesi* infection in *Macaca mulatta*. Brit. J. exp. Path. **51**, 523—533 (1970)
Oshima, G., Kato, J., Erdös, E. G.: Subunits of human plasma carboxypeptidase N (Kininase I; anaphylatoxin inactivator). Biochem. biophys. Acta. **365**, 344—348 (1974)
Oshima, G., Sato-Omori, T., Suzuki, T.: Distribution of proteinase, arginine-ester hydrolase and kinin releasing enzyme in various kinds of snake venoms. Toxicon **7**, 229—234 (1969)
Özge-Anwar, A. H., Movat, H. Z., Scott, J. G.: The kinin system of human plasma. IV. The interrelationship between the contact phase of blood coagulation and the plasma kinin system in man. Thrombos. Diathes. haemorrh. (Stuttg.) **27**, 141—158 (1972)
Parrat, J. R., West, G. B.: 5-hydroxytryptamine and the anaphylactoid reaction in the rat. J. Physiol. (Lond.) **139**, 27—41 (1957)
Pelá, I. R., Gardey-Levassort, C., Lechat, P., Rocha e Silva, M.: Brain kinins and fever induced by bacterial pyrogens in rabbits. J. Pharm. (Lond.) **27**, 793—794 (1975)
Perris, A. D., Whitfield, J. F.: The mitogenic action of bradykinin on thymic lymphocytes and its dependence on calcium. Proc. Soc. exp. Biol. (N.Y.) **130**, 1198—1201 (1969)
Phelps, P., McCarty, D. J., Jr.: Crystal-induced inflammation in canine joints. II. Importance of polymorphonuclear leukocytes. J. exp. Med. **124**, 115—126 (1966)
Phelps, P., Prockop, D. J., McCarty, D. J.: Crystal induced inflammation in caninine joints. III. Evidence against bradykinin as a mediator of inflammation. J. Lab. clin. Med. **68**, 433—444 (1966)
Pierce, J. V.: Structural features of plasma kinins and kininogens. Fed. Proc. **27**, 52—57 (1968)
Pierce, J. V.: Purification of mammalian kallikrein, kininogens, and kinins. In: Erdös, E. G. (Ed.): Bradykinin, Kallidin, and Kallikrein, Hand. exp. Pharmak., Vol. XXV, pp. 21—51. Berlin-Heidelberg-New York: Springer 1970
Pierce, J. V., Webster, M. E.: Human plasma kallidins; isolation and chemical studies. Biochem. biophys. Res. Commun. **5**, 353—357 (1961)
Pierce, J. V., Webster, M. E.: The purification and some properties of two different kallidinogens from human plasma. In: Erdös, E. G., Back, N., Sicuteri, F. (Eds.): Hypotensive Peptides, pp. 130—138. Berlin-Heidelberg-New York: Springer 1966
Piper, P. J., Vane, J. R.: Release of aditional factors in anaphylaxis and its antagonism by anti-inflammatory drugs. Nature (Lond.) **223**, 20—35 (1969)
Pisano, J. J.: Chemistry and biology of the kallikreins-kinin system. In: Reich, E., Rifkin, D. B., Shaw, E. (Eds.): Proteases and Biological Control, pp. 199—222. Cold Spring Harbor Laboratory 1975
Pisano, J. J., Austen, K. F. (Eds.): Chemistry and biology of the kallikrein-kinin system in health and disease. Fogarty Int. Center Proc. 27. Washington, D.C.: U.S. Gov. Printing Office 1977
Pless, J., Stürmer, E., Gutmann, S., Boissonnas, R. A.: Kallidin, Synthese und Eigenschaften. Helv. chim. Acta **45**, 394—396 (1962)
Popieraitis, A. A., Thompson, A. G.: The site of bradykinin release in acute experimental pancreatitis. Arch. Surg. (Chicago) **98**, 73—77 (1969)
Powers, S. R., Brown, H. H., Stein, A.: The pathogenesis of acute and chronic pancreatitis. Ann. Surg. **142**, 690—697 (1955)
Prado, J. L.: Proteolytic enzymes as kininogenases. In: Erdös, E. G. (Ed.): Bradykinin, Kallidin, and Kallikreins. Handb. exp. Pharmakol., pp. 156—192. Berlin-Heidelberg-New York: Springer 1970

Prado, J. L., Limãos, E. A., Roblero, J., Freitas, J. O., Prado, E. S., Paiva, A. C. M.: Recovery and conversion of kinins in exsanguinated rat preparations. Naunyn-Schmiedeberg's Arch. Pharmacol. **290**, 191—205 (1975)

Prado, J. L., Mendes, J., Rosa, R. C.: On the kininogenic activity of ficin, with a note on papain. An. Acad. bras. Cienc. **37**, 295—301 (1965)

Prado, J. L., Monier, R., Prado, E. S., Fromageot, C.: Pharmacologically active polypeptide formed from blood globulin by a cysteine-activated protease from *Clostridium histolyticum*. Biochim. biophys. Acta **22**, 87—95 (1956)

Ratnoff, O. D., Miles, A. A.: The induction of permeability-increasing activity in human plasma by activated Hageman factor. Brit. J. exp. Path. **45**, 328—345 (1964)

Ratnoff, O. D., Pensky, J., Ogston, D., Naff, G. B.: The inhibition of plasmin, plasma kallikrein, plasma permeability factor, and the C_{1r} subcomponent of the first component of complement by serum C'1 esterase inhibitor. J. exp. Med. **129**, 315—332 (1969)

Reis, M. L., Medeiros, M. C., Rocha e Silva, M.: Release and destruction of kinins by a proteolytic enzyme (Pronase) derived from a fungus *Streptomyces griseus*. In: Abstracts III International Pharmacology Congress. São Paulo: Abs. 485, 1966

Reis, M. L., Okino, L., Rocha e Silva, M.: Comparative pharmacological actions of bradykinin and related kinins of larger molecular weights. Biochem. Pharmacol. **20**, 2935—2946 (1971)

Richards, W. H. G.: Pharmacologically active substances in the blood and urine of mice infected with *Trypanosoma brucei*. Brit. J. Pharmacol. **24**, 124—131 (1965)

Rixon, R. H., Whitfield, J. F.: Kallikrein, kinin, and cell proliferation. In: Haberland, G. L., Roten, J. W. (Eds.): Kininogenases, First Symposium on Physiological Properties and Pharmacological Rational, pp. 131—145. Stuttgart-New York: F. K. Schattauer 1973

Rixon, R. H., Whitfield, J. F., Bayliss, J.: The stimulation of mitotic activity in the thymus and bone marrow of rats by kallikrein. Horm. Metab. Res. **3**, 279—284 (1971)

Rocha e Silva, M.: Bradykinin-mechanism of its release by trypsin and kallikrein. Arch. int. Pharmacodyn. **88**, 271—282 (1951)

Rocha e Silva, M.: On the participation of polypeptides and biogenic amines in the acute inflammatory reactions. In: Jasmin, G. (Ed.): Endocrine Aspects of Disease Processes, pp. 74—95. St. Louis: Warren H. Green, Inc. 1968

Rocha e Silva, M.: Kinin Hormones. Springfield: Charles C. Thomas 1970

Rocha e Silva, M., Antonio, A.: Release of bradykinin and the mechanism of production of a "thermic edema (45° C)" in the rat. Med exp. **3**, 371—382 (1960)

Rocha e Silva, M., Beraldo, W. T., Rosenfeld, G.: Bradykinin, a hypotensive and smooth muscle stimulating factor released from plasma globulin by snake venoms and by trypsin. Amer. J. Physiol. **156**, 261—273 (1949)

Rocha e Silva, M., Cavalcanti, R. Q., Reis, M. L.: Anti-inflammatory actions of sulfated polysaccharides. Biochem. Pharmacol. **18**, 1285—1295 (1969)

Rocha e Silva, M., Garcia Leme, J.: Studies on the antagonists of bradykinin. In: Garattini, S., Dukes, M. N. G. (Eds.): Non steroidal anti-inflammatory drugs, pp. 120—133. Amsterdam: Excerpta Medica 1965

Rocha e Silva, M., Garcia Leme, J.: Chemical mediators of the acute inflammatory reaction. Oxford: Pergamon 1972

Rocha e Silva, M., Reis, M. L., Ferreira, S. H.: Release of kinins from fresh plasma under varying experimental conditions. Biochem. Pharmacol. **16**, 1665—1676 (1967)

Rocha e Silva, M., Rosenthal, S. R.: Release of pharmacologically active substances from the rat skin in vivo following thermal injury. J. Pharmacol. exp. Ther. **132**, 110—116 (1961)

Rogers, D. E.: Intracellular inflammation: dynamics and metabolic changes in polymorphonuclear leukocytes participating in phagocytosis. In: Thomas, L., Uhr, J. W., Grant, L. (Eds.): Injury, Inflammation, and Immunity, pp. 110—126. Baltimore: Williams & Wilkins Comp. 1964

Rohen, J. W., Peterhoff, I.: Stimulation of mitotic activity by kallikrein in the gastrointestinal tract of rats. In: Haberland, G. L., Rohen, J. W. (Eds.): Kininogenases. First Symp. on Physiological Properties and Pharmacological Rational, pp. 147—157. Stuttgart-New York: F. K. Schattauer 1973

Rosa, A. T., Rothschild, Z., Rothschild, A. M.: Fibrinolytic activity evoked in the plasma of the normal and adrenalectomized rat by cellulose sulfate. Brit. J. Pharmacol. **45**, 470—475 (1972)

Rosenthal, S. R., Minard, D.: Experiments on histamine as the chemical mediator for cutaneous pain. J. exp. Med. **70**, 415—425 (1939)
Rothschild, A. M.: Pharmacodynamic properties of cellulose sulfate and related polysaccharides—a group of bradykinin-releasing compounds. In: Rocha e Silva, M., Rothschild, H. A. (Eds.): Int. Symp. on Vaso-Active Polypeptides: Bradykinin and Related Kinins, pp. 197—203. São Paulo: Edart 1967
Rothschild, A. M.: Some pharmacodynamic properties of cellulose sulfate, a kininogen-depleting agent in the rat. Brit. J. Pharmacol. **33**, 501—512 (1968a)
Rothschild, A. M.: Role of anaphylatoxin and of bradykinin in passive cutaneous anaphylaxis against heterologous precipitating antibody in the rat. In: Schild, H. O. (Ed.): Immunopharmacology, pp. 83—89. Oxford: Pergamon 1968b
Rothschild, A. M., Castania, A.: Endotoxin shock in dogs pretreated with cellulose sulfate, an agent causing partial plasma kininogen depletion. J. Pharm. (Lond.) **20**, 77—78 (1968)
Rothschild, A. M., Castania, A., Cordeiro, R. S. B.: Consumption of kininogen, formation of kinin and activation of arginine ester hydrolase in rat plasma by rat peritoneal fluid cells in the presence of l-adrenaline. Naunyn-Schmiedeberg's Arch. Pharmacol. **285**, 243—256 (1974a)
Rothschild, A. M., Cordeiro, R. S. B., Castania, A.: Lowering of kininogen in rat blood by catecholamines. Involvement of non-eosinophil granulocytes and selective inhibition by trasylol. Naunyn-Schmiedebergs Arch. Pharmacol. **282**, 323—326 (1974b)
Rothschild, A. M., Gascon, L. A.: Effect of agar on bradykininogen levels and esterolytic activity in rat plasma. Experientia (Basel) **21**, 208—209 (1965)
Rothschild, A. M., Gascon, L. A.: Sulphuric esters of polysaccharides as activators of a bradykinin-forming system in plasma. Nature (Lond.) **212**, 1364 (1966)
Rothschild, Z., Rosa, A. T., Rothschild, A. M.: On a plasminogen activator induced in rat plasma by cellulose sulfate, an activator of the kinin-generating system. Acta physiol. lat.-amer. **18**, 199 (1968)
Rugstad, H. E.: Kininase production by some microbes. Brit. J. Pharmacol. **28**, 315—323 (1966)
Ryan, J. W., Moffat, J. G., Thompson, A. G.: Role of bradykinin in the development of acute pancreatitis. Nature (Lond.) **204**, 1212—1213 (1964)
Ryan, J. W., Moffat, J. G., Thompson, A. G.: Role of bradykinin system in acute hemorrhagic pancreatitis. Arch. Surg. (Chicago) **91**, 14—24 (1965)
Ryan, J. W., Roblero, J., Stewart, J. M.: Inactivation of bradykinin in the pulmonary circulation. Biochem. J. **110**, 795—797 (1968)
Ryan, J. W., Rocha e Silva, M.: Release of kinins by acidified bovine pseudoglobulin. Biochem. Pharmacol. **20**, 459—462 (1971)
Sampaio, M. U., Reis, M. L., Fink, E., Camargo, A. C. M., Greene, L. J.: Chromatographic systems for desalting and separating kinins: application to trypsin-treated human plasma. Life Sci. **16**, 796 (1975)
Sampaio, C., Wong, S. C., Show, E.: Human plasma kallikrein. Arch. Biochem. **165**, 133—139 (1974)
Sander, G. E., Huggins, C. G.: Vasoactive peptides. Ann. Rev. Pharmacol. **12**, 227—264 (1972)
Satake, K., Rozmanith, J. S., Appert, H., Howard, J. M.: Hemodynamic change and bradykinin levels in plasma and lymph during experimental acute pancreatites in dogs. Ann. Surg. **178**, 659—662 (1973)
Schachter, M.: A delayed slow contracting effect of serum and plasma due to the release of a substance resembling kallidin and bradykinin. Brit. J. Pharmacol. **11**, 111—118 (1956)
Schiller, W. R., Suriyapa, C., Anderson, M. C.: A review of experimental pancreatitis. J. surg. Res. **16**, 69—90 (1974)
Schröder, E.: Über Peptidsynthesen. Synthese von Methionyl-Lysyl-Bradykinin, einem Kinin aus Rinderblut. Experientia (Basel) **20**, 39 (1964)
Schröder, E.: Structure-activity relationships of kinins. In: Erdös, E. G. (Ed.): Bradykinin, Kallidin, and Kallikrein. Handb. exp. Pharmakol., Vol. XXV, pp. 324—350. Berlin-Heidelberg-New York: Springer 1970
Schröder, E., Lübke, K.: The peptides, Vol. II. New York-London: Academic Press 1966
Schwab, J.: Kininases in leucocytes and other tissues. Nature (Lond.) **195**, 345—347 (1962)

Sevitt, S.: Inflammatory changes in burned skin: Reversible and irreversible effects and their pathogenesis. In: Thomas, L., Uhr, J. W., Grant, L. (Eds.): Injury, Inflammation, and Immunity, pp. 183—210. Baltimore: The Williams & Wilkins Comp. 1964

Sevitt, S., Bull, J. P., Cruikshank, C. N. D., Jackson, D. M., Lowbury, E. J. L.: Failure of an antihistamine drug to influence the course of experimental human burns. Brit. med. J. **1952 II**, 57—59

Sicuteri, F.: Bradykinin and intracranial circulation in man. In: Erdös, E. G. (Ed.): Bradykinin, Kallidin, and Kallikrein. Handb. exp. Pharmakol., Vol. XXV, pp. 482—515. Berlin-Heidelberg-New York: Springer 1970

Sicuteri, F., Franchi, G., Bianco, P. L. D., Fanciollacci, M.: Some physiological and pathological roles of kininogen and kinins. In: Erdös, E. G., Back, N., Sicuteri, F. (Eds.): Hypotensive Peptides, pp. 522—535. Berlin-Heidelberg-New York: Springer 1966

Sicuteri, F., Franchi, G., Fanciullacci, M., Del Bianco, P. L.: Serotonin-bradykinin potentiation of the pain-receptors in man. Life Sci. **4**, 309—316 (1965)

Souza, J. M., Rocha e Silva, M.: Possivel participação de cinina (bradicinina) no mecanismo do choque térmico em ratos. Ciênc. Cult. **19**, 396 (1967)

Souza, J. M., Rocha e Silva, M.: Novas evidências de participação da bradicinina no choque térmico de ratos. Ciênc. Cult. **20**, 405 (1968)

Sparrow, E. M., Wilhelm, D. L.: Species differences in susceptibility to capillary permeability factors histamine, 5-hydroxytryptamine and compound 48/80. J. Physiol. (Lond.) **137**, 51—65 (1957)

Spector, W. G., Willoughby, D. A.: Histamine and 5-hydroxytryptamine in acute experimental pleurisy. J. Path. Bac. **74**, 57—65 (1957)

Spector, W. G., Willoughby, D. A.: Experimental supression of the acute inflammatory changes of thermal injury. J. Path. Bact. **78**, 121—132 (1959)

Spector, W. G., Willoughby, D. A.: Salicylate and increased vascular permeability. Nature (Lond.) **196**, 1104 (1962)

Spector, W. G., Willoughby, D. A.: The effect of vascular permeability factors on emigration of leukocytes. J. Path. Bact. **87**, 341—346 (1964)

Spilberg, I., Osterland, C. K.: Anti-inflammatory effect of the trypsin-kallikrein inhibitor in acute arthritis induced by urate crystals in rabbits. J. Lab. clin. Med. **76**, 472—479 (1970)

Spragg, J., Austen, K. F.: The preparation of human kininogen. II. Further characterization of purified human kininogen. J. Immunol. **107**, 1512—1519 (1971)

Starr, M. S., West, G. B.: Bradykinin and oedema formation in heated paws of rats. Brit. J. Pharmacol. **31**, 178—187 (1967)

Starr, M. S., West, G. B.: Further evidence for the involvement of kinin in anaphylactic shock in the rat. Brit. J. Pharmacol. **37**, 178—184 (1969)

Stewart, J. M., Woolley, D. W.: Bradykinin analogs. In: Rocha e Silva, M., Rothschild, H. A. (Eds.): International Symposium on Vaso-Active Polypeptides: Bradykinin and Related Kinins, pp. 7—13. São Paulo: Edart 1967

Streeten, D. H. P., Kerr, C. B., Kerr, L. P., Prior, J. C., Dalakos, T. G.: Hyperbradykininism: a new orthostatic syndrome. Lancet **18**, 1048—1053 (1972)

Stürmer, E.: The influence of intra-arterial infusions of synthetic bradykinin on flow and composition of lymph in dogs. In: Erdös, E. G., Back, N., Sicuteri, F. (Eds.): Hypotensive Peptides, pp. 368—374. Berlin-Heidelberg-New York: Springer-Verlag 1966

Stürmer, E., Berde, B.: A pharmacological comparison between synthetic bradykinin and kallidin. J. Pharmacol. exp. Ther. **139**, 38—41 (1963)

Stürmer, E., Cerletti, A.: Bradykinin. Amer. Heart J. **62**, 149—154 (1961 a)

Stürmer, E., Cerletti, A.: Das Bradykinin-Oedem der Rattenpfote. Helv. physiol. pharmacol. Acta **19**, C 32—C 35 (1961 b)

Suzuki, T., Iwanaga, S., Sato, T., Nagasawa, S., Kato, H., Yano, M., Horiuchi, K.: Biochemical properties of kininogens and kinin-releasing enzymes. In: Rocha e Silva, M., Rothschild, H. A. (Eds.): International Symposium on Vaso-Active Polypeptides: Bradykinin and Related Kinins, pp. 27—33. São Paulo: Edart 1967

Thal, A. P., Kobold, E. E., Holenberg, M. J.: The release of vasoactive substances in acute pancreatitis. Amer. J. Surg. **105**, 708—713 (1963)

Thomas, G., West, G. B.: Prostaglandins, kinin and inflammation in the rat. Brit. J. Pharmacol. **50**, 231—235 (1974)
Trapnell, J. E., Righby, C. C., Talbot, C. H., Duncan, H. L.: A controlled trial of trasylol in the treatment of acute pancreatitis. Brit. J. Surg. **61**, 177—182 (1974)
Ungar, G., Damgaard, E., Hummel, F. P.: Action of salicylates and related drugs on inflammation. Amer. J. Physiol. **171**, 545—553 (1952)
Urbanitz, D., Sailer, R., Habermann, E.: In vivo investigations on the role of the kinin system in tissue injury and shock syndromes. In: Sicuteri, E., Rocha e Silva, M., Back, N. (Eds.): Bradykinin and Related Kinins: Cardiovascular, Biochemical, and Neural Actions, pp. 343—354. New York-London: Plenum Press 1970
Van Arman, C. G.: Interrelationship among some peptide precursors. In: Gaddum, J. H. (Ed.): Polypeptides Which Stimulate Plain Muscle, pp. 103—114. Edinburgh-London: Livingstone 1955
Van Arman, C. G., Begany, A. J., Miller, L. M., Pless, H. H.: Some details of the inflammations caused by yeast and carrageenin. J. Pharmacol. exp. Ther. **150**, 328—334 (1965)
Van Arman, C. G., Carlson, R. P., Risley, E. A., Thomas, R. H., Nuss, G. W.: Inhibition effects of indomethacin, aspirin, and certain other drugs on inflammations induced in rat and dog by carrageenan, sodium urate and ellagic acid. J. Pharmacol. exp. Ther. **175**, 459—468 (1970)
Van Arman, C. G., Nuss, G. W.: Plasma bradykininogens levels in adjuvant arthritis and carrageenan inflammation. J. Path. **99**, 245—250 (1969)
Van Arman, C. G., Nuss, G. W., Winter, C. A., Flataker, L.: Proteolytic enzymes as mediators of pain: In: Lim, R. K. S., Armstrong, D., Pardo, E. G. (Eds.): Pharmacology of Pain, pp. 25—32. Oxford: Pergamon 1968
Vane, J. R.: Inhibition of prostaglandin synthesis as a mechanism of action for aspirin-like drugs. Nature (New Biol.) **231**, 232—235 (1971)
Vogel, R., Werle, E.: Kallikrein inhibitors. In: Erdös, E. G. (Ed.): Bradykinin, Kallidin, and Kallikrein. Handbook experimental Pharmacology, Vol. XXV, pp. 213—249. Berlin-Heidelberg-New York: Springer 1970
Vogt, W.: Kinin formation by plasmin, an indirect process mediated by activation of kallikrein. J. Physiol. (Lond.) **170**, 153—166 (1964)
Vogt, W.: Demonstration of the presence of two separate kinin-forming systems in human and other plasma. In: Erdös, E. G., Back, N., Sicuteri, F. (Eds.): Hypotensive Peptides, pp. 185—197. Berlin-Heidelberg-New York: Springer 1966
Vugman, I.: Alterações no teor de bradicininogênio do plasma do cobaio induzidas por choque adrenalínico. Ciênc. Cult. **15**, 259—260 (1963)
Waaler, B. A.: The effect of bradykinin in an isolated perfuzed dog lung preparation. J. Physiol. (Lond.) **157**, 475—483 (1961)
Ward, P. A.: Chemotactic factors for neutrophils, eosinophils, mononuclear cells and lymphocytes. In: Austen, K. F., Becker, E. L. (Eds.): Biochemistry of Acute Allergic Reaction, pp. 229—241. Oxford: Blackwell Scientific 1971
Webster, M. E.: Human plasma kallikrein, its activation and pathological role. Fed. Proc. **27**, 84—89 (1968)
Webster, M. E.: Recommendations for nomenclature and units. In: Erdös, E. G. (Ed.): Bradykinin, Kallidin, and Kallikrein. Handb. exp. Pharmacology, Vol. XXV, pp. 659—665. Berlin-Heidelberg-New York: Springer 1970a
Webster, M. E.: Kallikreins in glandular tissues. In: Erdös, E. G. (Ed.): Bradykinin, Kallidin, and Kallikrein. Handb. exp. Pharmakol. Vol. XXV, pp. 131—155. Berlin-Heidelberg-New York: Springer 1970b
Webster, M. E., Clark, W. R.: Significance of the kallikrein-kallidinogen-kallidin system in shock. Amer. J. Physiol. **197**, 406—412 (1959)
Webster, M. E., Guimãraes, J. A., Kaplan, A. P., Colman, R. W., Pierce, J. V.: Activation of surface-bound Hageman factor: pre-eminent role of high molecular weight kininogen and evidence for a new factor. Advanc. exp. Med. Biol. (1976) (in press)
Webster, M. E., Guimãraes, J. A., Pierce, J. V.: High molecular weight kininogen: its role in activation of Hageman factor. In: Abstracts International Symposium on Vaso-peptides, Kinin 75, Fiesole: 1975

Webster, M. E., Maling, H. M., Zweig, M. H., Williams, M. A., Anderson, W., Jr.: Urate crystal induced inflammation in the rat: evidence for the combined actions of kinins, histamine, and components of complement. Immunol. Commun. **1**, 185—198 (1972)
Webster, M. E., Pierce, J. V.: Studies on plasma kallikrein and its relationship to plasmin. J. Pharmacol. exp. Ther. **130**, 484—491 (1960)
Webster, M. E., Pierce, J. V.: Action of the kallikreins on synthetic ester substrates. Proc. Soc. exp. Biol. (N.Y.) **107**, 186—191 (1961)
Webster, M. E., Pierce, J. V.: The nature of the kallidins released from human plasma by kallikreins and other enzymes. Ann. N.Y. Acad. Sci. **104**, 91—107 (1963)
Webster, M. E., Ratnoff, O. D.: Role of Hageman factor in the activation of vasodilator activity in human plasma. Nature (Lond.) **192**, 180—181 (1961)
Weiss, A. S., Gallin, J. I., Kaplan, A. P.: Fletscher factor deficiency. A diminished rate of Hageman factor activation caused by absence of prekallikrein with abnormalities of coagulation, fibrinolysis, chemotactic activity, and kinin generation. J. clin. Invest. **53**, 622—633 (1974)
Weissmann, G., Dingle, J.: Release of lysosomal protease by ultraviolet irradiation and inhibition by hydrocortisone. Exp. Cell Res. **25**, 207—210 (1961)
Weissmann, G., Fell, H. B.: The effect of hydrocortisone on the response of fetal rat skin in culture to ultraviolet irradiation. J. exp. Med. **116**, 365—380 (1962)
Weissmann, G., Thomas, L.: Studies on lysosomes. I. The effects of endotoxin, endotoxin tolerance, and cortisone on the release of acid hydrolases from a granular fraction of rabbit liver. J. exp. Med. **116**, 433—450 (1962)
Werle, E.: Über die Inaktivierung des Kallikreins. Biochem. Z. **273**, 291—305 (1934)
Werle, E.: Über Kallikrein aus Blut. Biochem. Z. **287**, 235—261 (1936)
Werle, E.: History of kallikrein and some aspects of its chemistry and physiology. In: Haberland, G. L., Rohen, J. W. (Eds.): Kininogenases. First Symposium on Physiological Properties and Pharmacological Rational, pp. 7—22. Stuttgart-New York: F. K. Schattauer 1973
Werle, E., Appel, W.: Über einen Hemmkörper für Kallikrein und verschiedene Proteinasen aus Rinderleben. II. Z. Naturforsch. **14B**, 385—392 (1959)
Werle, E., Erdös, E. G.: Über eine neue blutdrucksenkende, darm- und uteruserregende Substanz im menschlichen Urin. Naunyn-Schmiedeberg's Arch. exp. Path. Pharmak. **223**, 234—243 (1954)
Werle, E., Forell, M. M., Maier, L.: Zur Kenntnis der blutdrucksenkenden Wirkung des Trypsins. Naunyn-Schmiedeberg's Arch. exp. Path. Pharmak. **225**, 369—380 (1955)
Werle, E., Kaufmann-Boetsch, B.: Über esteratische Wirkungen von Kallikrein und Trypsin und ihre Hemmung durch Kallikrein- und Trypsininhibitoren. Hoppe-Seyler's Z. physiol. Chem. **319**, 52—63 (1960)
Werle, E., Kehl, R., Koebke, K.: Über Trypsin, Chymotrypsin, Kallidin, und Bradykinin. Biochem. Z. **321**, 213—220 (1950)
Werle, E., Maier, L.: Über die chemische und pharmakologische Unterscheidung von Kallikreinen verschiedener Herkunft. Biochem. Z. **323**, 279—283 (1952)
Werle, E., Roden, P. von: Über das Vorkommen von Kallikrein in den Speicheldrüsen und im Mundspeichel. Biochem Z. **286**, 213—219 (1936)
Werle, E., Roden, P. von: Über das Vorkommen von Kallikrein in den Speicheldrüsen und im Mundspeichel und über eine blutdrucksteigernde Substanz in der Submaxillarisdrüse des Hundes. Biochem. Z. **301**, 328—337 (1939)
Werle, E., Trautschold, I., Leysath, G.: Isolierung und Struktur des Kallidins. Hoppe-Seyler's Z. physiol. Chem. **326**, 174—176 (1961)
Werle, E., Vogel, R.: Über die Kallikreinausscheidung im Harn nach experimenteller Nierenschädigung. Arch. int. Pharmacodyn. **126**, 171—186 (1960)
Whitfield, J. F., MacManus, J. P., Gillan, D. J.: Ciclic AMP mediation of bradykinin-induced stimulation of mitotic activity and DNA synthesis in thymocytes. Proc. Soc. exp. Biol. (N.Y.) **133**, 1270—1274 (1970)
Whittle, B. A.: Release of a kinin by intraperitoneal injection of chemical agents in mice. Int. J. Neuropharmacol. **3**, 369—371 (1964)
Wilhelm, D. L.: Kinins in human disease. Ann. Rev. Med. **22**, 63—84 (1971)

Wilhelm, D. L.: Chemical mediators. In: Zweifach, B. W., Grant, L., McCluskey, R. T. (Eds.): The Inflammatory Process, 2nd Ed., Vol. II, pp. 251—301. New York-London: Academic Press 1973
Wilhelm, D. L., Mason, B.: Vascular permeability changes in inflammation: The role of endogenous permeability factors in mild thermal injury. Brit. J. exp. Path. **41**, 487—506 (1960)
Wilhelm, D. L., Mill, P. J., Sparrow, E. M., MacKay, M. E., Miles, A. A.: Enzyme-like globulins from serum reproducing the vascular phenomena of inflammation. IV. Activable permeability factor and its inhibitor in the serum of the rat and the rabbit. Brit. J. exp. Path. **39**, 228—250 (1958)
Willis, A. L.: Release of histamine, kinin, and prostaglandins during carrageenin-induced inflammation in the rat. In: Mantegazza, P., Horton, E. W. (Eds.): Prostaglandins, peptides and amines, pp. 31—38. New York: Academic 1969
Winter, C. A., Flataker, L.: Reaction thresholds to pressure in edematous hindpaws of rats and responses to analgesic drugs. J. Pharmacol. exp. Ther. **150**, 165—171 (1965)
Winter, C. A., Nuss, G. W.: Treatment of adjuvant arthritis in rats with anti-inflammatory drugs. Arthr. Rheum. **9**, 394—404 (1966)
Winter, C. A., Risley, E. A., Nuss, G. W.: Carrageenin-induced edema in hindpaw of the rat as an assay for anti-inflammatory drugs. Proc. Soc. exp. Biol. (N.Y.) **111**, 544—547 (1962)
Woessner, J. F. Jr.: Lysosomal enzymes and connective tissue breakdown. In: Bertelli, A., Houck, J. C. (Eds.): Inflammation Biochemistry and Drug Interaction, pp. 122—130. Amsterdam: Excerpta Medica Foundation 1969
Wuepper, K. D.: Prekallikrein deficiency in man. J. exp. Med. **138**, 1345—1355 (1973)
Wuepper, K. D., Lawrence, T. G., Cochrane, C. G.: Proenzyme components of the plasma kinin system. J. clin. Invest. **49**, 105a (1970a)
Wuepper, K. D., Miller, D. R., Lacombe, M. J.: Flaujeac trait: deficiency of kininogen in man. Fed. Proc. **34**, 859 (1975)
Wuepper, K. D., Tucker III., E. S., Cochrane, C. G.: Plasma kinin system: Proenzyme components. J. Immunol. **105**, 1307—1311 (1970b)
Yang, H. Y. T., Erdös, E. G.: Second kininase in human blood plasma. Nature (Lond.) **215**, 1402—1403 (1967)
Yano, M., Nagasawa, S., Horiuchi, K., Suzuki, T.: Separation of a new substrate, kininogen I, for plasma kallikrein in bovine plasma. J. Biochem. (Tokyo) **62**, 504—506 (1967)
Zuber, M., Sache, E.: Isolation and characterization of porcine pancreatic kallikrein. Biochemistry **13**, 3098—3110 (1974)
Zweifach, B. W.: Microcirculatory aspects of tissue injury. Ann. N.Y. Acad. Sci. **116**, 831—838 (1964)
Zweifach, B. W.: Microcirculatory effects of polypeptides. In: Erdös, E. G., Back, N., Sicuteri, F. (Eds.): Hypotensive Polypeptides, pp. 451—462. Berlin-Heidelberg-New York: Springer 1966
Zweifach, B. W., Nagler, A. L., Troll, W.: Some effects of proteolytic inhibitors on tissue injury and systemic anaphylaxis. J. exp. Med. **113**, 437—450 (1961)

CHAPTER 15

Endogenous Modulators of the Inflammatory Response

I. L. BONTA

"Pus bonum atque laudabile"

A. New Look at an Old Phenomenon

At the outset of an article like this, one thing useful to be said is what it is not. Certainly it is not another historical survey of inflammation, not even of some aspects of it, despite the fact that the reader might get this impression from the citation. The reason for choosing as a motto the wise banality "pus has beneficial properties" is that the quoted phrase has some, albeit purely phenomenological, bearing on one of the two guidelines of this chapter: (1) inflammation has a built-in homeostatic function, (2) fulfilment, at least partially, of this function might, amongst others, be exerted through materials which occur at the site of acute or subacute tissue injury. Without going into any details of the controversial preoccupation of ancient physicians about the beneficial properties of pus—recently denoted as "the most pernicious concept that ever sullied medicine" (LONG, 1965)—the reader is reminded that in venerable texts pus has a manifold meaning and is certainly not always used in the same sense as presently. To those educated in the medical profession in this century, pus has the unambiguous meaning of that particular kind of exudate which is "thick and yellowish due to the presence of large number of white cells" (WARD, 1967). This however, has little resemblance to the laudable pus, which is characterised for example by FRANCESCO PECCETTI (a 17th century physician of the Tuscan town of Volterra) as "excrementum, quod ex ulceribus emanat, quod est album, mediocriter crassum, leve, aequale et quamminime foetidum" (PECCETTI, 1619). The beneficial pus is thus a colourless, transparant, aqueous product, in this respect resembling the clear exudate originating from sites of acute inflammation. The evidence, to be shown later, indicates that such exudates (amongst others) are sources of substances which have anti-inflammatory properties and accordingly are beneficial. Debatable as it is, to what extent the similarities between the favourable properties of medieval pus and contemporary exudate are valid, the ancient classification of inflammatory excretes in good and bad ones can be considered as an instinctive recognition that endogenous substances might give a good or bad turn to tissue injury.

I. Terminology: By Way of Questioning What is a Modulator?

The purpose of this chapter is to survey the present knowledge about endogenous modulators of the inflammatory response. While the term modulator is rapidly becoming used in the literature, it does not appear superfluous to define exactly what it covers. No investigator in the medical-biological field will nowadays encounter

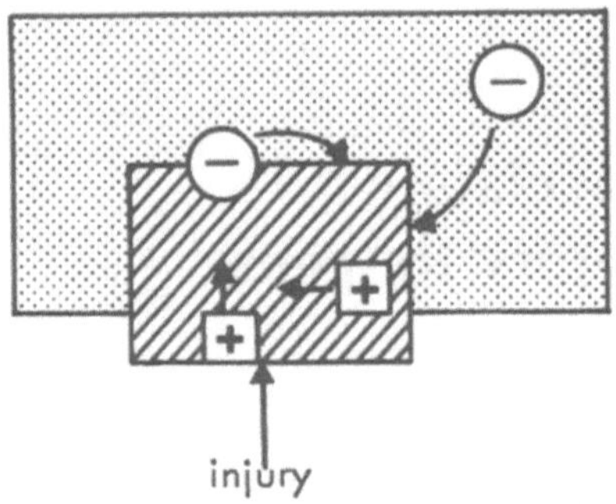

Fig. 1. The concept of mediators ⊞ and modulators ⊖. Mediators invariably occur at site of inflammation and promote it. Modulators may occur at site of inflammation or remote from it and mostly inhibit it. In this and other figures shaded areas symbolise local inflammatory reaction

difficulties with the term *mediator*. Although in certain texts the class of these endogenous substances is variously called "humoral mediators", "local hormones" or "autacoids" (COLLIER, 1971), the interchangeability of these terms is common knowledge. The subclassification to differentiate between "mediator" or "immediator" (ROCHA E SILVA, 1972) refers to the role in time sequence rather than to the qualitative characteristics of the substance. The four minimal criteria which a substance must fulfil to be identified as an inflammatory mediator are clearly set (MILLER and MELMON, 1970). By contrast, we may search in vain for the definition, let alone the criteria, of what should be understood as a *modulator*. In fact, this term is not even listed in the subject index of books on inflammation. Lacking an orthodox definition, one has the freedom to define a concept and to this end a semantic approach might be helpful. Dictionaries will tell us that modulation is the process of altering, adjusting, regulating or shifting an already existing object or ongoing event. Particularly well known is the concept of modulation in the musical world, where it means regulation of the pitch in sound or changing the key of a theme. Modulation is also a familiar term for radio engineers, who will interpret it as altering the amplitude or frequency of a wave by a frequency of a different order. When applying these definitions to the field of biology in general and to inflammation in particular, a modulator might mean anything which changes in magnitude or quality an event which has already been started. Using the concept of *modulator* in such a sense is convenient, because it sharply differentiates it from *mediators*, which are involved in generating or triggering inflammation rather than changing it. Another important difference between modulators and mediators is by definition inherent to the very first criterion of a mediator: occurrence in abnormally large quantities at the site of inflammation (MILLER and MELMON, 1970). Having still in mind our approach of semantics—indeed for the present we have no better substitute for it—there is no reason to restrict the occurrence of a modulator to the site of event which it does change. In fact, evidence will be presented in this review that modulators may occur both locally and at sites remote to the injured tissue (Fig. 1).

Notwithstanding the differences, the families of mediators and modulators have one characteristic in common: involvement in the biological event of inflammation.

Thus, in the context of the present review, any kind of endogenous factor, irrespective of chemical property or location of occurrence, which might cause a shift either in vehemence or in quality of inflammation will be considered a putative modulator.

II. Homeostatic Function and Self-Limiting Nature of Inflammation

Present-day research differs essentially from that of half a century ago; whereas new observations are seldom being made, efforts to find interrelationships between earlier described phenomena are promoted. The Nobel laureate ALBERT SZENTGYÖRGYI formulated this by saying that "research is to see what everybody has seen and think what nobody has thought." We put this forward by way of apology for presenting some time-honoured statements about inflammation and trying to look at them from an angle which is, as yet, a little bit less crowded than others. The reason why this particular angle attracted researchers less than others may be because the viewpoint it offers is seemingly too evident. What then are those scattered truisms on inflammation which the modulator concept may help us to assemble?

Any kind of local injury is followed by a defensive reaction on the part of the tissues. This is what we call inflammation and should be *eo ipso* seen as a purposeful phenomenon, designed to rid the body either from the noxious agent itself (e.g. in case of infection) or from the primary damage caused by the deleterious influence (e.g. thermal or chemical burn). Next to inflammation the process of tissue repair ensues, but this latter cannot effectively proceed unless the field is cleared from the hostile act and the devastation produced by it. Inflammation and repair are thus closely interwoven themes in the story of the response of cells and tissues to injury. When inflammation fails in its task to control and neutralise the hostile influence, failure to repair will be unavoidable. Putting things in this way, we ascribe to inflammation a purposeful function, which is rather unscientific, because it is a wholly teleological view. Nevertheless, it is compatible with what we would call homeostatic function, and then the untasteful bolus becomes more palatable. What is homeostasis aiming at: to ensure that the response is limited both in duration and in physical extent. The purposeful element of homeostasis is even more apparent if one considers that the inflammatory reaction is a peculiar blend of beneficial elements and of unwanted ones which cause discomfort. Further, provided that inflammation is essentially a protective response—an axiom since time immemorial—it should not last longer than necessary to achieve its objective, which is the green light for the initiation of the repair process.

In fact, acute inflammation is the trivial example of the presence of a self-curtailing element. In other cases, however, a chronic course prevails and intermediate situations, showing a fluctuating character with spontaneous remissions and exacerbations, are sometimes seen (certain skin conditions, like psoriasis, have this character). Thus, inflammations pass from a transient reaction to sustained events. Although efforts were made to explain this alternating course of inflammation, many earlier investigators satisfied themselves by describing the features of acute and chronic inflammation. Others still offered the trivial (and in a certain sense obviously valid) explanation that when tissue injury is caused by a single finite event—a non-replicating agent—the process progresses smoothly to an end. By contrast, when the injurious agent is persistent, the response will be long lasting and continue for as long as the agent is there. For some situations, however, this is an oversimplified view. Although a single stimulus, e.g. application of a chemical irritant, triggers a chain of endogenous events, in some cases the response will be longer lasting than in others. This variability may depend, apart from the nature of the noxa, on endogenous factors such as the site of injury (carrageenin causes a shorter inflammation in the hind foot of the rat than in the back part of the animal). Other factors, like endocrine hormones or stress, may regulate this process as well. When substances were recovered at the injured site which mimicked at least some components of the reaction (MENKIN, 1939), speculations were made about the existence at the injured location of other materials which would have opposite effects. The postulate that inflammation when left to itself displays a short course because of the local presence of anti-inflammatory factors led to the first convincing demonstration that the self-limiting character has a biochemical background (RINDANI, 1956). This evidence, followed by many other demonstrations of the presence of similar factors at the site of the injury and remote from it, shows even more: it pinpoints the inflammatory reaction as a potentially perfectly functioning homeostatic event. The noxious influence initiates a reaction which, while containing protective (beneficial) elements and harmful ones, has a built-in capacity only to last as long and be as vehement as needed. Malfunctioning of the system may then be expected to cause an "unnecessary" chronic course of inflammation. Recently, it was proposed that defective homeostasis is the underlying factor in chronicity of rheumatoid arthritis (MORLEY, 1974).

Generation of anti-inflammatory substances at the spot is only one example of how inflammation may trigger its self-limiting character, and in fact the ideally functioning homeostasis of inflammation probably results from a delicate interaction of a multiplicity of endogenous modulators. Besides reviewing these modulators, another main concern in this chapter is an effort to define whether, and to what extent, the inflammatory reaction itself has a regulatory role in triggering the participation of such modulators. Hopefully, this might help to obtain better insight into the delicately functioning balance between the good and bad sides of inflammation.

B. Counter-Irritation

When defining the term modulation in the sense used in radio technology, namely altering a wave frequency by interfering with a wave frequency of a different order, then the counter irritation phenomenon, i.e. the ability of irritation to interfere with another simultaneously ongoing irritation, fits well into what we should understand as a modulation of the inflammatory reaction. The first work of true scientific value on *counter-irritation* was written 80 years ago (GILLIES, 1895), but the procedure itself, to combat inflammation and/or pain at one site of the organism by irritating a remote site of the same organism, is perhaps the oldest of all methods used for relieving pain. It is not unintentional when we write relief of pain rather than of inflammation. It appears that there is some contradiction between the observations referring to the medical use (i.e. the therapeutical use on patients) of counter-irritation and the data emerging from experimental studies on animals. In fact, there is some confusion about the purpose of applying counter-irritation. In his monograph,

GILLIES claimed that irritants applied at some distance from the inflamed joints in rheumatism can cause absorption of the exudation (GILLIES, 1895). However, in recent therapeutically oriented literature, including textbooks of medical pharmacology, counter-irritation is advocated for antinociceptive purposes. On the other hand, the majority of experimental studies on animals are designed to assess the extent to which counter-irritation can suppress inflammation. The source of this schism may be in the inadequacy of earlier methods to measure inflammation in humans and the difficulties in measuring the pain component separately from other constituents of inflammation in animals. Another explanation is masked by the variety of counter-irritants, the site and the manner of their application. For human use, chemical irritants are believed to be less purposeful than physical means (GOODMAN and GILMAN, 1970; MACARTHUR and ALSTEAD, 1953). On the other hand, there is a paucity of animal experimental data on the effect of physical counter-irritation. Also, it appears that besides the kind of irritant and the way or site of application, the type of inflammation or the species on which it is measured are determinant factors for the effect. Doubtlessly, however, the phenomenon as such is not limited to a certain species and is operant in mice, rats, guinea pigs, dogs, and humans. Differences between rat strains, however, have been reported (HITCHENS et al., 1967). The animal data on counter-irritation have been recently reviewed (ATKINSON and HICKS, 1975a), but the analgesic effects, although belonging to the entirety of anti-inflammation, were disregarded. In the present chapter, counter-irritation will be highlighted from other angles than in the paper mentioned and the discussion of antinociceptive aspects will also be included.

I. Inflammations Responsive and Non-Responsive to Counter-Irritation

One of the obstacles to obtaining a coherent picture on counter-irritation is implicit in the complex nature of inflammation itself. The difficulties in explaining the suppressing effect of counter-irritation on inflammation are thus essentially similar to those involved in the pharmacology of conventional anti-inflammatory drugs. This is obvious because of the similarities in experimental situations used for the purpose. At present most of the data on counter-irritation are derived from experiments on rat hind paw oedema, a frequently used prototype model representing acute inflammation. Depending, however, on the subplantarly administered provoking agent, rat paw oedema displays a shorter (1–3 h) or longer (up to 8–10 h) time course, reflecting the participation of various endogenous mediators. Even within the long-lasting type of rat hind limb oedemas, different phases can be distinguished (BONTA, 1969; DI ROSA et al., 1971; VINEGAR et al., 1969). While not entering into details of this extensively investigated phenomenon, we just remind the reader that in short-lasting oedemas and in the early phase of long-lasting ones, 5-hytroxytryptamine (5-HT) and/or histamine are probably involved, whereas in the later phase prostaglandins play an important role (DI ROSA et al., 1971). Kinins appear to participate throughout the whole course of the rat paw oedema, at least when carrageenin is used as the inducer (FERREIRA et al., 1974). As for the suppressing effect of counter-irritation, there is agreement that irrespective of the irritant, inhibition of the carrageenin oedema can be achieved (ATKINSON, 1971; ATKINSON and HICKS, 1971; GARATTINI et al., 1965; JORI and BERNARDI, 1966; NOORDHOEK and BONTA, 1974). This is also true when kaolin is used as the oedema provoker (BÜCH and WAGNER-JAUREGG, 1960; BONTA and DE VOS, 1969; VINEGAR et al., 1974). Since these two types of oedemas have many aspects in common, their similar sensitivity towards counter irritation is not surprising. It was even shown with both types of oedemas that counter-irritation inhibits the delayed phase without any effect on the initial phase (NOORDHOEK and BONTA, 1974; VINEGAR et al., 1974). Other oedemas with uniformity of data regarding suppression by counter-irritation include those induced by yeast, dextran and filipin (ATKINSON, 1971; BÜCH and WAGNER-JAUREGG, 1960; DOMENJOZ et al., 1955; GOLDSTEIN et al., 1967). It should be remarked that the antagonistic profiles of these oedemas with respect to conventional anti-inflammatory drugs are dissimilar (GARATTINI et al., 1965), and the observations that they are sensitive to suppression by counter-irritation indicate that in the latter process the mechanism involved is different from that of existing drugs. Still considering the oedemas with a longer time course, the data reported on counter-irritation and formol oedema are less uniform than with the oedemas mentioned above. Some investigators showed that formol oedema was sensitive to suppression by counter-irritation (BÜCH and WAGNER-JAUREGG, 1960; DOMENJOZ et al., 1955). In another study, however, the remote irritant, in a strength which inhibited the carrageenin oedema, did not inhibit the effect of formol (ATKINSON, 1971).

When counter-irritation was induced by wound healing instead of a chemical, the formol oedema was inhibited by a wound produced on the same day, but not if the wound was made two days earlier (RUDAS and STOKLASKA, 1967). This was also found with dextran oedema. While this may indicate that the counter-irritation-sensitive components are similar in formol and dextran oedema, nevertheless the remote stimulus which proved unable to inhibit formol inflammation markedly suppressed dextran oedema as well as carrageenin oedema (ATKINSON, 1971). With short-term oedemas provoked by chemicals other than dextran, inhibition by counter-irritation was observed when the mast cell degranulator compound 48/80 was the oedema inducer (GARATTINI et al., 1965; GOLDSTEIN et al., 1967) or when ovalbumin served this purpose (BÜCH and WAGNER-JAUREGG, 1960). In both of the latter rat paw oedemas, local discharge of 5-HT has been implicated, so it is even more peculiar that the hind limb oedema provoked by 5-HT itself is resistant to inhibition by counter-irritation (BONTA and DE VOS, 1969), although in another study this was not found to be the case (HORAKOVA and MURATOVA, 1965). In the latter two studies, counter-irritation was produced by different means and this in turn may have influenced the results, as will be shown later. Thus, the data show that in most studies acute rat paw oedema was susceptible to modulation by counter-irritation; there are exceptions. Further, there is little to explain the anti-inflammatory mechanism of counter-irritation. Although the results with dextran, ovalbumin, and compound 48/80 may indicate that counter-irritation interferes with the release or effect of 5-HT as a mediator, it is not understandable that the early phase of carrageenin oedema—in which participation of 5-HT has been proposed (DI ROSA et al., 1971)—is non-responsive.

In the delayed phase of kaolin or carrageenin oedema (which is susceptible to counter-irritation) complement activation and subsequent leucotaxis has been proposed to play a role. Anticipating the discussion that release of a humoral factor is a possible explanation for the anti-inflammatory effect of counter-irritation, it is relevant to mention that a material extracted from inflamed tissue inhibited complement and suppressed the delayed phase of kaolin and carrageenin oedema (BONTA and NOORDHOEK, 1973). Again with rat paw oedema, counter-irritation induced by kaolin suppressed the oedema provoked by polyvinylpyrrolidone (PVP) (BÜCH and WAGNER-JAUREGG, 1961), although this swelling is non-inflammatory, its mechanism being colloid osmotic imbalance (WINNE, 1964). The PVP oedema, however, is resistant to the anti-inflammatory effect evoked by counter-irritation due to intraperitoneal administration of phenylquinone (BONTA and DE VOS, 1969).

Other acute types of inflammation, in which inhibition through counter-irritation was shown, include pleural exudation (LADEN et al., 1958), bradykinin-induced skin permeability change in rats (BONTA and DE VOS, 1969) and conjunctival sac inflammation of rabbits (AMBERG et al., 1917; WINTERNITZ, 1901). However, skin erythema produced by ultraviolet (UV) irradiation in guinea pigs is not suppressed by counter-irritation induced either by intraperitoneal administration of phenylquinone (BONTA and DE VOS, 1969) or by subcutaneous injection of an irritant copper salt (BONTA, 1969). Only one other counter-irritation study has been reported in the guinea pig (GAUGAS et al., 1970), and the influence of counter-irritation on irradiation-induced erythema has not been studied on other animals. Thus, it is not possible to conclude whether there is a species difference or whether skin erythema represents an exception to other acute inflammations. A clarification of this question would be of considerable interest, since the endogenous mediator involved in the skin erythema is most probably prostaglandin (in this respect resembling other acute inflammations) and the clinical efficacy of non-steroid anti-inflammatory drugs is fairly well correlated with their potency in either guinea pig erythema or carrageenin rat paw oedema, the latter being sensitive and the former non-sensitive to counter-irritation.

Suppression of inflammation by remote site irritation is not limited to acute phenomena. Proliferation of granulation tissue was shown to be sensitive to counter-irritation as measured by the cotton-pellet test (CYGIELMAN and ROBSON, 1963; GOLDSTEIN et al., 1967; HICKS, 1969; ROBINSON and ROBSON, 1964), by a carrageenin-induced abcess (GOLDSTEIN et al., 1967) or by wound healing (RUDAS and STOKLASKA, 1967; SELYE et al., 1969). Particular importance should be attached to studies in which counter-irritation prevented the development (VINEGAR and TRUAX, 1970) or mitigated the severity of the already developed (ATKINSON, 1971) arthritis component of the Freund's adjuvant-induced autoimmune disease of the rat. The value of these observations is evident: this type of rat arthritis resembles in several aspects (immune mechanism, bone changes, cellular events, sensitivity to drugs) clinical rheumatoid arthritis, and thus its susceptibility to counter-irritation suggests that the modulating mechanisms—whatever they may be—inherent to counter-irritation might also be operant in human pathology.

II. Components of Inflammation Susceptible and Non-Susceptible to Counter-Irritation

In the previous section, the discussion was centered around the type of inflammatory models that have been studied for inhibitory modulating effects by counter-irritation. Inflammation, however, is the end result of the interaction of a number of either sequentially or simultaneously ongoing events, and present research trends are characterised by efforts to analyse these events separately before building up the integral image. Accordingly, in this section the data will be arranged from such a viewpoint. To this end, whilst aware that this is an oversimplified approach, the following elements of inflammation will be considered: cellular reaction, mediator release, microvascular alterations, local pain component and connective tissue proliferation. Having in mind that in counter-irritation humoral factors most probably play a significant role, some of the following comments will be related to data born out of experiments with exudates from the counter-irritant site.

The direct or indirect participation of neutrophilic leucocytes as a prerequisite for the development of the acute phase of certain hind paw oedemas has been demonstrated recently (VINEGAR et al., 1974), although others challenged this view (DI ROSA et al., 1971). It was shown, however, that counter-irritation achieved through intraperitoneal injection of carrageenin results in marked inhibition of the same phase of the kaolin-induced rat hind limb oedema which is also suppressed in severely granulocytopenic rats (VINEGAR et al., 1974). This might indicate that counter-irritation can inhibit the migration of leucocytes to the remote site damaged tissue area. The experiments in which inhibition of complement activation was shown with a factor recovered from irritated tissue (BONTA and NOORDHOEK, 1973; NOORDHOEK and BONTA, 1974) are also in favour of this assumption, since leucotactic substances are known to be generated from the C_3 part of the complement system. Local production of a leucopenic factor as a consequence of tissue irritation had been shown earlier (MENKIN and DURHAM, 1946). Thrombocytes form another cell population to which a putative role as a source of prostaglandins in acute inflammation has been recently attributed (GLATT et al., 1974), but whether counter-irritation has any influence on them has not been studied. Regarding the macrophages—the cell system having a function in chronic inflammation—it was suggested that the chronic type of counter-irritation may through competition limit their availability at another site of inflammation (CYGIELMAN and ROBSON, 1963), although in a subsequent study (ROBINSON and ROBSON, 1966) this possibility was made less probable.

The various systems of mediators obviously attracted the attention of investigators of the counter-irritation phenomenon, particularly because materials, e.g. kaolin or carrageenin, frequently used to provoke counter-irritation are themselves known to trigger processes finally leading to release of mediators. Apart from the proposals that mediator discharge at one site of inflammation may exhaust the available quantity of the endogenous substance participating at another site of inflammation (competition mechanism of counter-irritation, to be discussed in Sect. B.IV.), there is little information at hand to show that counter-irritation would inhibit the direct effects of putative mediators. In one study, it was argued that inhibition rather than exhaustion of complement might be the underlying effect of counter-irritation (NOORDHOEK and BONTA, 1974). Counter-irritation was shown to inhibit the effect of bradykinin (BONTA and DE VOS, 1969; HORAKOVA and MURATOVA, 1965), histamine and 5-HT (HORAKOVA and MURATOVA, 1965). In these studies, however, the vascular permeability effect of these mediators was measured and this may interfere with the possibility that counter-irritation affected permeability as such, rather than specifically the activity of any one of the mediators. Unfortunately, no study has been devoted to a resolution of the problem of whether counter-irritation antagonises some effect of these mediators other than the permeability change.

Concerning the vascular component of tissue damage, in the majority of counter-irritant studies no attempts have been made to observe the hyperaemia (i.e. vasodilation) separately from the permeability process. In most of the commonly used inflammatory models, the permeability change follows so closely the initial vasodilation that it is hardly possible sharply to separate them. An exception is the dermal response to UV irradiation. In this situation, at least when guinea pigs are used, there is a time lag of several hours between erythema and plasma leakage as measured by protein-bound dye escape (WINTER et al., 1958). The erythema of UV irradiation remained unaffected when counter-irritation was evoked either by an irritant copper salt or by phenylquinone (BONTA and DE VOS, 1969; BONTA, 1969). There is no information available whether the permeability change as a delayed response to UV irradiation is influenced by remote site irritation.

As remote-site irritation does not seem to inhibit all kinds of rat paw oedemas to the same extent and local oedema is by definition a process that, irrespective of the causative mechanism, is characterised by fluid extravasation one is apt to conclude that the microvessel alteration as such is not a susceptible target of counter-irritation. Although in a few studies efforts were made to establish the effect separately on local oedema and plasma-bound dye leakage (BONTA and DE VOS, 1969; JORI and BERNARDI, 1966; ROBINSON and ROBSON, 1966), the results are rather inconclusive. At present the most appropriate method for determining microvascular permeability is the carbon particle labelling technique on the vessels of the cremaster in rats, and this should be used in counter irritation studies.

There is little doubt that the tissue proliferation component of inflammation, either measured by granuloma formation (CYGIELMAN and ROBSON, 1963; DI PASQUALE et al., 1963; GOLDSTEIN et al., 1967; ROBINSON and ROBSON, 1966) or by tensile strength of healing wounds (HIGHTON, 1963; ROBINSON and ROBSON, 1966; RUDAS and STOKLASKA, 1967), is markedly reduced by simultaneous or foregoing inflammation at another site of the organism.

Suppression of *local inflammatory pain* by application of an irritant at a remote site is well documented in humans (GAMMON et al., 1936; HARDY et al., 1940; MACARTHUR and ALSTEAD, 1953; PARSONS and GOETZI, 1945), but these studies do not define whether the same irritant which provoked elevation of pain threshold concomitantly inhibited inflammation. In rats, however, intraperitoneal injection of phenylquinone, which inhibits some types of inflammation (BONTA and DE VOS, 1969), induced antinociception as measured by the tail pinch method (WINTER and FLATAKER, 1965). In another study on rats chemical irritants reduced pain of inflammation caused by phenylquinone (abdominal writhing) and by pressure and the hot plate test (HITCHENS et al., 1967). From the antinociceptive profile of the irritants, the conclusion was drawn that their mode of action is dissimilar to that of peripherally acting anti-inflammatory analgesic (aspirin-like) drugs and resembled the centrally acting (morphine-like) pain suppressing agents. In the same study, data derived from parabiotic rats indicated that the analgesic effects produced by the irritants were not due to a humoral factor released at the site of irritation. In a series of unpublished experiments from our own department, we observed that a factor extracted from granuloma pouch exudate—and proven strongly to inhibit certain types of rat paw oedemas (BONTA et al., 1970)—was unable to produce analgesia in the phenylquinone writhing test. The quoted study on parabiotic rats (HITCHENS et al., 1967) together with our observations indicate that counter-irritation produces analgesic and anti-inflammatory actions by two separate mechanisms: the humoral pathway appears to be involved in suppressing certain events while leaving the pain component unaffected, whereas the latter seems to be susceptible to a nervous pathway. A non-humoral mechanism of counter-irritation might be less selective, as the possibility is open that it may additionally contribute to the anti-inflammatory effect.

III. Stimulants and Tissue Sites to Trigger Counter-Irritation

The means to inhibit inflammation at one site of the organism by irritating a remote site can roughly be divided into chemical and non-chemical stimuli. There is a long and varied list of chemicals which act as counter-irritants. These substances include: hypertonic saline, 0.1 N sodium hydroxide, capsaicin, all of which produce very transient tissue irritation; materials such as carrageenin, kaolin, formol, animal charcoal, mustard oil, turpentine, dextran, acetic acid, phenylquinone, compound 48/80, which after single administration provoke local inflammation lasting from 1 h up to 6–8 h; substances such as croton oil, santal oil, metal compounds, silver nitrate, soluble and insoluble copper chelates, which are very strong irritants leading to necrotizing inflammation; inflammatory mediators like histamine, 5-HT and bradykinin. A number of these substances inhibit inflammation provoked by themselves at another site (AMBERG et al., 1917; ATKINSON, 1971; BONTA and NOORDHOEK, 1974; HORAKOVA and MURATOVA, 1965; NOORDHOEK and BONTA, 1974; ROCHA E SILVA et al., 1969). In fact, counter-irritation triggered by carrageenin was found more active against inflammation induced by itself than by other agents (ATKINSON, 1971) but this did not hold for histamine or 5-HT (HORAKOVA and MURATOVA, 1965). In a careful study (ATKINSON, 1971) measuring the inhibition of carrageenin-induced rat paw oedema, the intraperitoneal potency was carrageenin > acetic acid > kaolin. When, however, the anticarrageenin ED_{50} of each irritant was tested against rat paw oedemas by mustard, yeast or dextran, the order of activities was acetic acid > kaolin > carrageenin, whereas with the same dose but measuring inhibition of established rat adjuvant arthritis, kaolin was more active than either carrageenin or acetic acid, the latter two not differing from each other. The fact that equi-effective anticarrageenin doses of the three irritants showed different degrees of activity on other inflammatory models was considered by the authors to be an argument that the anti-inflammatory actions of each of these counter-irritants is exerted through different mechanisms. Provided, however, that the counter-irritation exerted by these materials was associated with the presence of an endogenous humoral anti-inflammatory factor—one of the major putative mechanisms (Sections B.IV. and C.I.) to explain by a common denominator the counter-irritation phenomenon—it is conceivable that the anti-inflammatory potency of such a natural factor depends on the inflammation it should inhibit.

Local application of tetrahydrofurfuryl nicotinate (THFN) on the forearm, despite causing intense flushing of the skin, was an ineffective counter-irritant, at least when pain production due to irritation by hypertonic NaCl injection was measured (MACARTHUR and ALSTEAD, 1953). Under the same conditions, however, counter-irritation by mustard oil caused analgesia. The skin irritant property of THFN is rather similar to that of UV irradiation (HAINING, 1963), i.e. the effect is limited to hyperaemia. However, the inflammation due to UV irradiation was resistant to suppression by counter-irritation. It appears that stimuli provoking only the vasodilation component of inflammation cannot suppress remote site tissue irritation; furthermore the vasodilation element of tissue injury is not susceptible to inhibition by counter-irritation. Whether these two aspects, vasodilation being their common denominator, are interrelated cannot be judged from the available data. If, however, one accepts the competitive exhaustion of inflammatory mediator(s) as a possible mechanism (Section B.IV.) of modulation by counter-irritation, the quantities of endogenous mediators which cause hyperaemia are so minimal that mutual exhaustion at two simultaneously involved tissue sites does not seem to play a role.

Amongst non-chemical counter-irritants, implantation of a foreign body, e.g. cotton-pellet or polyester foam, has been succesfully used (BILLINGHAM et al., 1969a; CYGIELMAN and ROBSON, 1963; ROBINSON and ROBSON, 1964), suggesting that tissue granulation triggers anti-inflammation at a remote site. The observation, however, that inhibition of rat paw oedema was only achieved by wound infliction on the animal's back on the same day, but not two days before oedema induction (RUDAS and STOKLASKA, 1967), indicates that an earlier phase than granulation is involved in counter-irritation. Further procedures to inhibit remote site inflammation and/or pain include rubber band tourniquet application (LADEN et al., 1958; HARDY et al., 1940) and major abdominal surgery (BILLINGHAM et al., 1969b). Galvanic stimulation of less than a minute, but sufficient in strength to produce severe skin irritation, suppressed remote site nociception following irritation by hypertonic saline injection (MACARTHUR and ALSTEAD, 1953). Regretfully, there is nothing known about whether remote site anti-inflammation can also be achieved by galvanic stimulation as a trigger of counter-irritation.

Possibly this is the appropriate place to mention the rather controversial matter of *acupuncture*. The value of this ancient "Far Eastern" medical art is highly disputable. Except for yellow press articles and make-believe scientific papers—largely contributing to the malreputation of this treatment—there is hardly any access to reliable literature in Western European languages on acupuncture. Obviously, this makes it exceptionally difficult to separate chaff from wheat. It is believed that antinociception is one of the domains where acupuncture is of benefit. As the practise of acupuncture—when stripped of the hocus-pocus around it—consists of placing needles subcutaneously at certain body sites remote from those at which pain suppression is aimed, the resemblence to counter-irritation is striking. According to a recent paper (KAADA, 1974) reviewing the literature critically, a humoral analgesic agent is possibly liberated in the brain during prolonged acupuncture, but no such substance is produced at the site of stimulation. The nature of the postulated humoral factor is unknown, although reserpine augments acupuncture analgesia. The author of the paper postulated that the brain-midraphe 5-HT system may be involved in acupuncture analgesia. A workshop on the use of acupuncture in rheumatic diseases discussed some tentative claims for the anti-inflammatory effects of acupuncture (PLOTZ et al., 1974). Most participants believed that there is no realistic basis for anti-inflammatory effects of the acupuncture art, so that the possible pain-relieving effect would be best studied in non-inflammatory arthritis, such as osteoarthritis. The

Chinese claim that needling certain points on the body of normal persons or animals increases phagocytosis led to reappraisal of this question (BROWN et al., 1974). The latter study showed that in normal healthy male volunteers acupuncture resulted in an increase in blood leucocyte count. The writer of the present chapter agrees with the conclusion drawn elsewhere (LEWIN, 1974) that until acupuncture has been more extensively investigated under stringent scientific conditions, any other word about its mechanism would increase rather than diminish the existing confusion about it.

As already discussed, counter-irritation works in a variety of inflammation models, has different effects on different components of inflammation and can be provoked by different irritating stimuli. Besides these factors, the efficacy also depends on the site of applying the stimulus. In the majority of studies, chemical irritants were injected either intraperitoneally or subcutaneously. Other routes by which counter-irritation was successful include administration into the knee joint (LADEN et al., 1958), intravenous injections (GOLDSTEIN et al., 1967; HORAKOVA and MURATOVA, 1965) and oral treatment (BONTA, 1969; GOLDSTEIN et al., 1967; HITCHENS et al., 1967; JORI and BERNARDI, 1966; WINTERNITZ, 1901). In fact, the oral administration of santal oil (WINTERNITZ, 1901) was the first experimental demonstration of an anti-inflammatory effect following irritation of a remote tissue, although the gastric mucosa irritating property of santal oil was only shown a couple of years after WINTERNITZ's studies. Although practically any kind of irritant seems suitable to achieve remote anti-inflammation, there are some scattered data to indicate that the kind of tissue which is irritated might be one of the factors determining the extent of remote suppression of inflammation and/or pain. GOLDSTEIN et al. (1967) found no difference between intraperitoneal, subcutaneous, and oral administration of formol and croton oil, but carrageenin was only effective when given by the first two routes and kaolin only when injected intraperitoneally. The latter observation was confirmed in another work (HITCHENS et al., 1967), in which, however, formol was ineffective orally. Oral formol exerted effective counter-irritation in a study by JORI and BERNARDI (1966). However, the oral effectiveness of formol, was assessed by anti-inflammation, whereas oral ineffectiveness was measured by analgesia. The different pathways possibly involved in counter-irritation for anti-inflammation and analgesia have been mentioned earlier. It is conceivable that only peritoneal, but not gastric mucosa irritation, is suitable to trigger the postulated nervous mechanism involved in remote site analgesia. This interpretation might, however, only be part of the truth, because it does not explain the oral analgesic efficacy of croton oil (HITCHENS et al., 1967). The latter is an exceptionally strong irritant and it is possible that the discrepent results reflect irritation threshold or even simplier, irritated tissue surface differences between the intragastric and intraperitoneal cavities. Counter-irritation by carrageenin through intraperitoneal administration was also found more effective than deep subcutaneous injection into the forepaws (BONTA and NOORDHOEK, 1973; NOORDHOEK and BONTA, 1974). Still returning to the question of the gastric mucosa as a site to trigger counter-irritation, two remarks seem of relevance. Macroscopically observable irritation does not appear a *conditio sine qua non* for effective counter-irritation, since orally administered croton oil exerted remote anti-inflammation even at concentrations below those which caused visible changes in stomach mucosa (GOLDSTEIN et al., 1967). On the other hand, while investigating a series of copper chelates we observed (BONTA, 1969) that there was a good correlation between the irritating and anti-inflammatory properties of these compounds when administered subcutaneously, but not when given orally, even though on the stomach mucosa harsh irritation was manifest. Unpublished data with the same compounds however, suggested that in guinea pigs the situation was reversed: remote anti-inflammation was seen after oral administration but not after subcutaneous treatment. If at least one mechanism of counter-irritation depends on the presence of some endogenous anti-inflammatory factors at the irritated tissue site, one cannot rule out the possibility that a species-dependent variation plays a role in this respect. For example, in the guinea pig, gastric but not subcutaneous tissue may produce such a factor, while in other species this may be the reverse. Unfortunately, scarcity of data prevents any conclusion, except that more attention than hitherto should be given to this aspect.

IV. Modulating Mechanisms Triggered by Counter-Irritation

The previous sections described the conditions under which counter-irritation operates and now we consider, the mechanisms involved. In this context we wish to discuss counter-irritation as a model situation which illustrates that *inflammation* possesses the potentiality of *anti-inflammation* and *eo ipso* should have built in a triggering step for modulation. This consideration will thus be the background against which the mechanisms of counter-irritation will be projected. Furthermore, a variety of mechanisms probably operate simultaneously and the involvement of one of them does not exclude a role for others. Also it should be clear from the foregoing sections that the processes involved seem to be highly dependent on the kind of inflammations in which both the inducing counter-irritant and the process that is influenced by this phenomenon have to be considered.

Competitive exhaustion of components of tissue damage is a factor to be taken into account when two inflammatory processes are turned on simultaneously. In this context, the term *component* is meant in a grossly generalised sense: tissue constituents either non-cellular (plasma) or cellular, enzymes to activate mediators, the substrates of such enzymes and the mediators themselves. Extensive fluid and protein extravasation (i.e. oedema) at one site may cause major disturbance of osmotic pressure balance, thus preventing plasma leakage at a remote site. Indeed, the non-inflammatory rat paw oedema caused by polyvinylpyrrolidone (PVP) was prevented by intraperitoneal administration of other oedema-causing, but not necessarily irritant, substances (BÜCH and WAGNER-JAUREGG, 1961). However, an intraperitoneal injection of the true irritant phenylquinone, known to cause massive peritoneal fluid accumulation, failed to prevent the PVP induced paw oedema (BONTA and DE VOS, 1969), confirming the validity of observations under reversed circumstances: prevention of plasma loss at the counter-irritated (silver nitrate) knee articulation did not turn off the remote site (pleural cavity) anti-inflammation (LADEN et al., 1958). In the same study, non-inflammatory paw oedema failed to exert inhibition of pleural inflammation. Two-sited plasma loss can thus be discarded as a mechanism of counter-irritation.

Exhaustion of the macrophage population by invasion at the chronically counter-irritated site, thus leaving an insufficient number of these cells for a remote chronic inflammation site, was proposed as a mechanism (CYGIELMAN and ROBSON,

1963), but the same group rejected this possibility in a following paper (ROBINSON and ROBSON, 1964), in which they also showed that competitive limitation of granulation tissue does not explain counter-irritation.

Concerning the mediator systems, it was proposed that the anti-inflammatory action of carrageenin could be explained by depletion of bradykininogen, leaving insufficient substrate for the cleaving enzyme activated at a remote site by tissue damage (ROCHA E SILVA et al., 1969). The tenability of this explanation, however, has been rebuffed, as the counter-irritant effect of carrageenin was still present after doses that do not cause kinin release, and because the delayed (4-h) phase of the carrageenin oedema, in which kinin mediation is of subordinate importance, can still be suppressed by remote site carrageenin pretreatment (NOORDHOEK and BONTA, 1972).

The enzyme cascade of *complement* is another mediator system which might be exhausted by simultaneous inflammations. Tissue irritation by carrageenin or turpentine resulted in local fixation of C′1 (DI ROSA et al., 1971; WILLOUGHBY et al., 1969), thus rendering it no longer available for turning on subsequent constituents of the complement cascade at another damaged tissue site. Systemic depletion of complement occurred after injection of carrageenin intraperitoneally or into the hind limbs of rats (NOORDHOEK and BONTA, 1974), although with some other counter-irritants this was not the case. Besides local fixation, viz. depletion of complement, carrageenin also inhibits C′1 (DAVIES, 1963). Anticomplement activity was also suggested to mediate the counterirritant effect of compound 48/80 (GIROUD and TIMSIT, 1970). Thus, competition for the complement system may play a role in counter-irritation. Since turning on the complement cascade may lead to release of other mediators (kallikrein activation resulting in kinin release and leucotaxis to provide a source wherefrom prostaglandins may be discharged), non-availability of complement at a tissue site remote from the counter-irritated location may have the ultimate consequence that the entirety of the vicious circle of mediators will not operate. Without evidence, however, this remains speculative. Until proof is available, it is questionable if not improbable that the competitive exhaustion of two simultaneous tissue damage sites can adequately explain a homeostatic modulation of a single inflammation. Depletion is at its best a limiting rather than an actively modulating factor.

Another process, not only more likely than competitive exhaustion to operate during counter-irritation, but also satisfying our image of active modulation of a single inflammation, is the participation of anti-inflammatory *humoral factors*. The train of thought behind this concept is briefly that, during counter-irritation, not only are inflammatory mediators produced but also anti-inflammatory materials discharged, which through the bloodstream arrive at the remote site inflammation and suppress it. Ever since this idea was first suggested (LADEN et al., 1958), it intrigued those researchers who observed counter-irritation either casually or during deliberate experiments. Subsequently, efforts were made first to prove or disprove the presence of a natural anti-inflammatory factor in response to tissue irritation. To indicate the condition associated with the occurrence of such factor(s), we introduce the term *irritated tissue anti-inflammatory factor* (ITAIF). Secondary to this, and obviously if ITAIF is a reality, come a series of other questions: what is the source of ITAIF; is it a homogenous material or a complex mixture of substances; can these be separately identified or is it a recognised hormone not presently known to have the function of ITAIF; and last but not least what is its mode of action.

Regarding the first question, it was plausible that the evidence should come either from the presence of ITAIF in tissues or extracts thereof collected from inflamed sites, or from the existence of ITAIF in blood of an organism afflicted with inflammatory sites. Fortunately, both approaches turned out to be fertile and there is now a large body of evidence accumulating for the existence of ITAIF. Nevertheless, a number of controversial observations still await clarification. The methodological principle in the first kind of approach to furnish corroboration of ITAIF is essentially similar: irritated tissue or some part of it (mostly exudate) is submitted to some kind of chemical procedure (basically extraction, dialysis, chromatography, lyophilization) and the product is injected into animals to observe its anti-inflammatory effects. In the ensuing part, methodological aspects will be largely omitted. Instead of mentioning them, the reader is once more reminded of what has been discussed in the foregoing sections: the counter-irritation phenomenon depends much on the kind of inflammations at *both sites*, the counter-irritated and the remote one. *Mutatis mutandis* the same is valid for ITAIF. All these circumstances should be considered as potential sources of some of the still existing controversies. A further element leading to contradictions, not playing part in the counter-irritation phenomenon itself but not to be underestimated with regard to ITAIF, is the chemical purification.

Keeping the foregoing warnings in mind, an account of data on ITAIF will be given briefly. A favoured source of ITAIF is the granuloma pouch exudate or what is somewhat akin to it, the exudate around or in polyester foam implanted subcutaneously. The first demonstration (RINDANI, 1956) of ITAIF from such a source—in fact, the first report on ITAIF whatever the source—was not prompted by investigating counter irritation but by the concept to which counter-irritation is merely a model tool, namely modulation of inflammation. In honour of two decades of RINDANI'S work, a few sentences from his original paper will be quoted:

> Since inflammatory reaction, left to itself, sometimes undergoes complete resolution, ... the validity of a biochemical theory of inflammation would be further re-inforced if the presence of anti-inflammatory substances also could be demonstrated in the exudate. ... The recovery of biochemical fraction, from the exudate having anti-inflammatory action is significant as it may contribute to the understanding of the mechanism of inflammation... (RINDANI, 1956).

Although RINDANI ascribed the anti-inflammatory effect of his ITAIF to the presence of corticosteroid, in the light of present views, discarding adrenocortical materials as part of ITAIF (see evidence later in this section), his fraction might have contained other materials as well. The presence of ITAIF from granuloma exudate source has subsequently been demonstrated by a number of investigators (ATKINSON et al., 1969; ATKINSON and HICKS, 1971; BILLINGHAM et al., 1969a; BONTA et al., 1970; BONTA and NOORDHOEK, 1973; DI PASQUALE and GIRERD, 1961; DI PASQUALE et al., 1963; ROBINSON and ROBSON, 1964), several of them using adrenalectomized donor rats. ITAIF from rats is not species specific, since it displays anti-inflammatory effect when administered to mice (BONTA and NOORDHOEK, 1974). Other sources from which ITAIF was recovered include oedema fluid extruded from inflamed rat hind paws or irritated peritoneal cavity exudates from rats (BONTA and DE VOS, 1969) or rabbits (BONTA and DE VOS, 1968), mesenchymal cells of Arthus reactions in rabbits (HAYASHI et al., 1964) and gastric surgery exudates from humans (BILLINGHAM et al., 1969b).

It would be an oversimplification to conclude that if ITAIF was recovered from inflamed sites, the latter are necessarily the sites of production. Indeed, there is circumstantial evidence to suggest that subcutaneous foreign body implantation may set the liver to synthesize a protein, which after having been carried in the blood stream is trapped at the injured site from where it can be recovered as ITAIF (BILLINGHAM et al., 1969a, 1971; BILLINGHAM and GORDON, 1976a, 1976b). The proposal of BILLINGHAM remains speculative, albeit intriguing, at present. An intimate connection between tissue injury and the liver will be discussed in Section C.III.

Counter-irritation studies also generated a series of observations in which the presence of ITAIF was shown in the blood of organisms bearing inflammation. The first studies of this kind consisted of demonstrating the anti-inflammatory effect of whole blood taken from locally injured rats (LADEN et al., 1958). Although these were intact animals, the role of the pituitary-adrenal axis in counter-irritation was convincingly excluded in another part of the same study, thus indirectly suggesting that the anti-inflammatory activity of blood was not due to corticosteroids. Subsequent studies succeeded in demonstrating anti-inflammatory effect of plasma and serum gained from animals—including adrenalectomized ones—subjected to chronic (BILLINGHAM et al., 1969a; ROBINSON and ROBSON, 1964) or acute (BONTA and DE VOS, 1969) irritation. Elegant experiments on parabiotic rats have shown that the counter-irritant effect was associated with ITAIF carried in the blood stream from one rat to the attached partner (GOLDSTEIN et al., 1967). In these experiments the plasma and/or serum from non-irritated animals was either devoid of (BILLINGHAM et al., 1969a) or contained little (BONTA and DE VOS, 1969) anti-inflammatory action. Particularly interesting are the results in which the lysosome stabilising—in extrapolation anti-inflammatory—activity of sera from adjuvant arthritis rats was demonstrated (PERSELLIN, 1972), since these experiments are closely related to studies showing the animal anti-inflammatory effect of sera from patients with rheumatoid arthritis (HIGHTON, 1963). In contrast to the above data two groups of researchers failed to detect anti-inflammatory activity in sera or in blood of rats bearing chronic inflammations (ATKINSON and HICKS, 1975a; DI PASQUALE et al., 1963).

All the facts mentioned above seem to indicate that the formation of ITAIF is a prerequisite for anti-inflammation during counter-irritation. There is, however, one methodological flaw in this concept: in testing the ITAIF materials, of whatever origin, for anti-inflammatory activity, the possibility that they themselves act as counter-irritants has not always been excluded. To discard such a possibility, oral administration of ITAIF may lead to erroneous results, since many irritants provoke anti-inflammation when given orally. Therefore, it was advocated that tissue extracts suspected of having ITAIF activity should be administered locally into the site where suppression of inflammation is expected. Indeed, it was shown that irritants promoted the inflammation after administration into the same site, while substances having genuine anti-inflammatory effect but devoid of irritancy did not display the proinflammatory profile (GOLDSTEIN et al., 1966; SHANAHAN, 1968) (Fig. 2). Not even such an approach is watertight, however, when dealing with materials having a mechanism of competitive mediator exhaustion (activation, i.e. proinflammation preceeding the depletory phase). For such types of materials intravenous administration might be preferred, as such a route causes the least possible tissue irritation. At least for one kind of ITAIF, its anti-inflammatory activity was not different when administered either intraperitoneally or intravenously (BONTA and NOORDHOEK, 1974; NOORDHOEK and BONTA, 1974). The intravenous route to discriminate between genuine anti-inflammation and counter-irritancy has been criticised, however (AT-

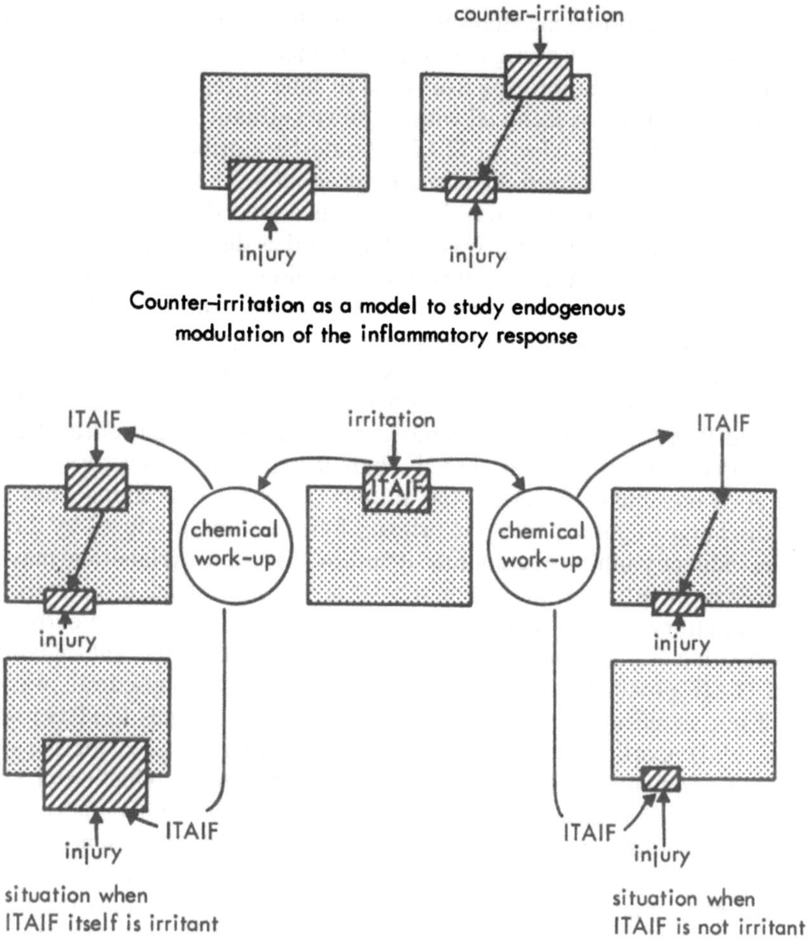

Fig. 2. ITAIFs may have irritant properties, in which case they themselves may act as counter-irritants when injected. Other ITAIFs may be devoid of irritancy. The latter type of ITAIFs when injected locally are anti-inflammatory, but the former type are proinflammatory

KINSON and HICKS, 1975b). In some reports it was shown that with improved dialysis methods it is possible to separate, at least partially, the irritant and anti-inflammatory properites of ITAIF (BILLINGHAM and ROBINSON, 1972; NOORDHOEK and BONTA, 1974). ATKINSON showed that both activities of ITAIF from a polyester sponge exudate were retained after dialysis (ATKINSON et al., 1969; ATKINSON and HICKS, 1971) and he concluded that, at least with respect to ITAIF from chronic exudate origin, the anti-inflammatory action after exogenous administration is due to counter-irritation rather than inherent suppression of inflammation.

It is not unintentional that we emphasised exogenous administration, because separation of irritancy and genuine anti-inflammation might be of great importance when attempts are made to arrive at an ITAIF for eventual therapeutic use, although it might be a less critical point when using ITAIF as a mechanism to explain endogenous modulation of the inflammatory response. In the latter context the parabiotic approach is more relevant (GOLDSTEIN et al., 1967) to demonstrate the presence of a blood-borne mechanism, which might operate irrespective of whether the organism is afflicted by a single or two simultaneous inflammations.

Another question, reappearing from time to time in reports, concerns the possibility of whether ITAIF is identical with a known substance or whether at least part of the anti-inflammatory effect of ITAIF should be ascribed to the presence of a *hormone recognised for its anti-inflammatory properties*. The latter possibility, showing the presence of corticosteroids, has been suggested (RINDANI, 1956). It might have been a coincidental finding, because later studies discarded the possibility that stress stimulus and subsequent stimulation of the pituitary-adrenal system should be considered as playing a major role in counter-irritation. Anti-inflammatory effect of remote site irritant injection was demonstrated in hypophysectomized and/or adrenalectomized animals (ATKINSON and HICKS, 1975b; CYGIELMAN and ROBSON, 1963; GOLDSTEIN et al., 1967; HORAKOVA and MURATOVA, 1965; LADEN et al., 1958; ROBINSON and ROBSON, 1964). In one study it was even shown that adrenalectomy in rats reinforced rather than abolished counter-irritation (ATKINSON and HICKS, 1975a). As a possible explanation, the authors proposed that endogenous corticosteroid discharge might suppress the primary inflammation produced by the irritant and thus indirectly inhibit the counter-irritation. Such an explanation may not be valid, since corticosterone, the major steroid of the rat adrenal, has a rather feeble anti-inflammatory effect. Whatever the interpretation might be, the correctness of the observation is relevant to another work showing that the anti-inflammatory effect of ITAIF obtained from pouch exudates of adrenalectomised rats was consistently, if not significantly, larger than that from intact animals (DI PASQUALE and GIRERD, 1961). Corticosteroid discharge is thus neither required for the counter-irritation phenomenon itself, nor is it a prerequisite for the production of ITAIF at the irritated site. Nevertheless, it was shown that the anti-inflammatory effect of ITAIF obtained from irritated rat paw perfusates required the presence of adrenals in the test animals (GARCIA-LEME and SCHAPOVAL, 1975). In other works, however, there was either circumstantial or direct evidence that anti-inflammation by ITAIF from rat paw oedema, rat peritoneal fluid, implanted sponge exudate or granuloma pouch exudate did not require mediation through an adrenocortical mechanism (BILLINGHAM et al., 1969a; BONTA and DE VOS, 1969; BONTA and NOORDHOEK, 1973). However, irritation may result in the occurrence of multiple ITAIF at the inflamed site and it cannot be excluded that one of them acts through intervention of adrenals, though others may not. In fact GARCIA-LEME and SCHAPOVAL (1975) proposed that the ITAIF recovered by them is not identical to that found by others.

Apart from endogenous corticosteroid in humoral pathway of counter-irritation, adrenaline may participate as a locally released substance (GOLDSTEIN et al., 1967; HORAKOVA and MURATOVA, 1965; SPECTOR and WILLOUGHBY, 1960). Although adrenaline undoubtedly has anti-inflammatory properties (BROWN and WEST, 1965; GREEN, 1972), it is unlikely that it contributes to counter-irritation. Firstly adrenergic mechanisms do not play a significant role in counter-irritation, at least not in the one induced by intraperitoneally administered acetic acid and measured on suppression of the carrageenin rat paw oedema (ATKINSON and HICKS, 1974). Secondly the anti-inflammatory activity of ITAIF from various sources was associated with a macromolecule of a size between gamma globulins and albumins (BILLINGHAM et al., 1969a, 1969b; BONTA et al., 1970; BONTA and NOORDHOEK, 1974). While this finding does not necessarily exclude that the active anti-inflammatory agent is a protein-bound non-protein substance, we discarded the presence of adrenaline on the basis of bioassay (BONTA and DE VOS, 1968).

No indication is found in the literature that a *neurogenic* pathway is involved in the anti-inflammatory component of counter-irritation. Participation of neurogenic factors was excluded by the demonstration that the anti-inflammatory effect of intraperitoneal administration of an irritant was not reduced after sectioning the main innervation of the rat hind paw (ATKINSON and HICKS, 1974). Non-humoral (thus neurogenic?) mechanisms may, however, significantly contribute to the antinociceptive component of counter-irritation (HITCHENS et al., 1967).

In finishing the section on counter-irritation, a few concluding remarks seem appropriate. Counter-irritation is observed under extremely artificial conditions. Animal models are poor imitations of human disease conditions anyway and care is required in interpreting them. This applies particularly to the counter-irritation phenomenon, as *eo ipso* it implicates the involvement of two model inflammations on the same animal. Models are seldom good enough to deliver us the philosopher's stone and we have little reason to expect that counter-irritation would do so. Provided that we are ready to accept the participation of endogenous humoral anti-inflammatory factors, then it is plausible to imagine that in the natural situation when the organism is afflicted by only a single inflammation, a humoral mechanism essentially identical to the one in counter-irritation may also operate, for the materials carried in the blood would reach any place, irrespective of whether one or two inflammations are present. In this respect, the counter-irritation appears to provide the optimal conditions to identify such factors and isolate them in such quantities as would allow more accurate studies on their chemical nature and pharmacological properties. Besides the methodological problems which should be surmounted (improvement of biochemical techniques for separation and pharmacological methods for testing), more attention than hitherto should be payed to studying the separate influences of counter-irritation, viz. the humoral factors involved in it, on individual components of inflammation. Implicit in this is that the mechanisms of counter-irritation in suppressing acute or chronic inflammation may not necessarily be identical. It is conceivable that one source of controversy is hidden by the frequently used practice that the exudate to obtain ITAIF was collected from a chronically irritated site but was pharmacologically tested in acute inflammation models or vice versa. Work on counter-irritation as a genuinely useful model in search of natural humoral modulators of inflammation has two obvious limitations which should be kept in mind: (1) humoral mechanisms may still turn out only partially to account for counter-irritation; (2) counter-irritation does not cover all endogenous modulating factors of inflammation.

C. Humoral Factors as Modulators

I. Local Tissue Factors

The previous section has shown the circumstances which led to the finding that irritated tissue is a source of factors having anti-inflammatory properties, collectively called ITAIF. Most reports went no farther than demonstrating the existence of

ITAIF, but some groups made attempts to characterise these factors chemically or pharmacologically. The most thorough chemical work was achieved by BILLINGHAM and his colleagues who, using either sponge exudates of rats or abdominal surgery exudates of humans as sources, adapted a combination of Sephadex G-150 gel filtration and cellulose ion exchange chromatography for purification (BILLINGHAM et al., 1969a, 1969b). Inhibition of the carrageenin rat paw oedema served to monitor the activity. For the purest material obtained, the purification factor was approximately 24, yielding a protein in molecular size between the α-globulins and the albumins, and which on a weight basis was approximately as active as hydrocortisone. However, even the most concentrated material was by no means pure, producing after electrophoresis several bands. In further work using preparative polyacrylamide electrophoresis, a material was obtained which was devoid of irritancy and still retained the anti-inflammatory effect following subcutaneous administration (BILLINGHAM and ROBINSON, 1972). The mode of action of BILLINGHAM'S ITAIF was not studied, apart from the observation that it did not require the presence of the adrenals.

Another group used the carrageenin granuloma pouch exudate of rats as starting material and gel filtration on Sephadex and Sepharose columns partially to purify the non-dialysable portion of the exudate, the activity being monitored on the kaolin rat paw oedema after subcutaneous administration (BONTA et al., 1970; BONTA and NOORDHOEK, 1973). This ITAIF contained at least two anti-inflammatory materials, one of them having a mol wt somewhat below 200000 and the other closer to 1000000 (NOORDHOEK and BHARGAVA, unpublished data); no further chemical work on it was made. Instead however, the pharmacological mode of action of this ITAIF was studied to some extent (BONTA and NOORDHOEK, 1973, 1974; NOORDHOEK and BONTA, 1974; DE VOS, unpublished data). This ITAIF was hardly irritant in the rat paw assay and was anti-inflammatory after intravenous administration. It inhibited the kaolin rat and mouse paw oedema and the carrageenin rat paw oedema, did not require the presence of adrenals, but was unable to suppress histamine, 5-HT or PVP rat paw oedemas. Neither trypsin nor kallikrein activity were inhibited by this ITAIF. The material did not prevent the UV irradiation-induced dermal erythema, which involves prostaglandin release and thus this ITAIF may not have interfered with the prostaglandin system. It was not antipyretic in rats and was not antinociceptive in the phenylquinone writhing test (BONTA, unpublished data). However, in vitro and in vivo it inhibited complement, the effect being reversible, lasting approximately 4 h (NOORDHOEK and BONTA, 1974). Two fold evidence was also furnished for a correlation between complement inhibitory and anti-inflammatory activity of this ITAIF (Fig. 3). Firstly, amongst the various tissue extract batches prepared, only those which inhibited complement were anti-inflammatory. Secondly, this ITAIF preferentially inhibited those kinds of rat paw inflammations, viz. induced by kaolin and carrageenin, in which complement activation is involved as a trigger. During activation of complement, chemotaxis leads to leucocytosis in the damaged tissue area, and so it is conceivable that an ITAIF which inhibits complement indirectly prevents the migration of leucocytes. Complement activation might also cause release of prostaglandins (GIROUD and WILLOUGHBY, 1970), and in this context it is relevant that the complement inhibitory ITAIF prevented those kind of rat paw inflammations which were shown to be suppressed in animals depleted by dietary

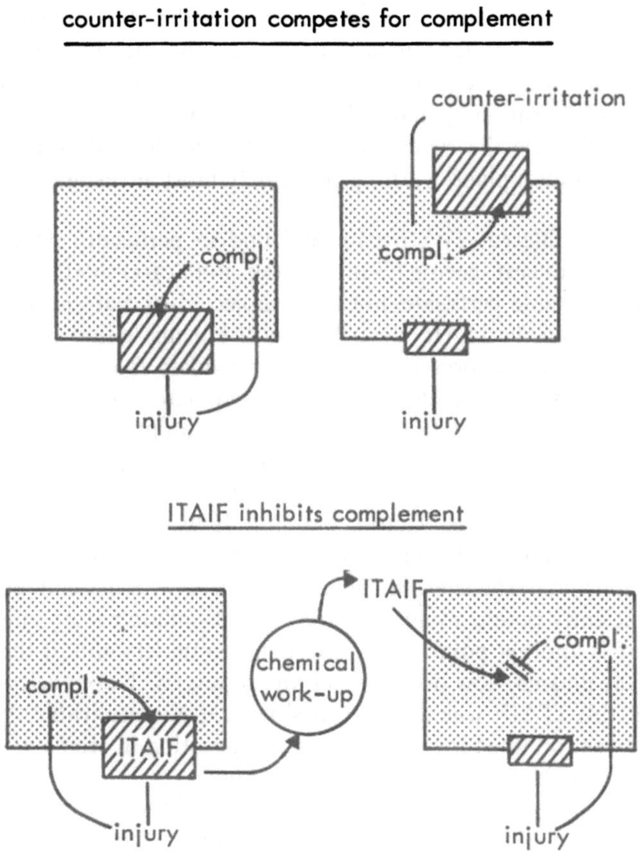

Fig. 3. Differences in complement-mediated anti-inflammatory mechanisms involved in action of counter-irritation and of an ITAIF obtained from granuloma pouch exudate (NOORDHOEK and BONTA, 1974)

means of precursors of prostaglandins (BONTA et al., 1974). Release of prostaglandins, however, can be achieved by a variety of mechanisms and as complement has not been shown to play a role in the dermal erythema response, this might explain that this particular type of inflammation was resistant to ITAIF, the latter probably not inhibiting the prostaglandin synthetase enzymes, but interfering with another mediator system.

Whereas the presence of leucocytosis-promoting factors in inflammatory exudates was one of the first indications of the humoral mediator concepts (MENKIN, 1939), several years later the peritoneal exudates of dogs were shown by MENKIN to contain a *leucopenic factor* (MENKIN and DURHAM, 1946). Although not defining it more closely chemically, he found indications of the probable polypeptide nature of this factor. He proposed further that the balance of release of the leucocytotic and leucopenic factor determines the final picture of inflammation. In this view, the local automodulating mechanism of inflammation is obviously implicit.

At present, it is not possible to conclude whether the above-mentioned preparations are camouflaged manifestations of the same substance having similar actions (like the situation with some mediators). This problem, however, is not unusual in the early phases of examining natural materials, and to emphasise the stringent necessity to standardise the biochemical or pharmacological conditions is just a repetition of a commonplace warning, to which most investigators will not pay attention anyway.

An apparently different ITAIF can be found in perfusates collected 2 h after treating rat paws with carrageenin (GARCIA-LEME and SCHAPOVAL, 1975). Apart from the fact that it is a crude perfusate, not even subjected to dialysis, it differed in two essential aspects from the ITAIF described by the teams either of BILLINGHAM or BONTA. Firstly, it was not present in the plasma taken from donor rats, whereas under the conditions in which the above-discussed factors were collected, the anti-inflammatory activity was detected in the donor animal plasma (BILLINGHAM, 1969a). Secondly, the ITAIF recovered by GARCIA-LEME required for its anti-inflammatory effect the intactness of the hypothalamo-pituitary-adrenal cortex axis, whereas the earlier-mentioned factors did not. It was also shown that the paw perfusate stimulated the median eminence of the hypothalamus to effect a discharge of corticotrophin and corticosteroid. Debatable as it is, whether endogenous corticosterone is sufficiently potent to account for the anti-inflammatory effect of the paw perfusate, there is another point which is difficult to understand. If the factor is not detectable in the plasma, how does it reach the pituitary? Nevertheless, since it was proposed that this ITAIF was discharged slowly, it is conceivable that its plasma concentration was too low for exerting anti-inflammation in recipient rats, but high enough to stimulate the hypothalamus in the donors.

Another type of local tissue factor, distinct from ITAIF, is represented by the *chalones* (BULLOUGH, 1968). There are several chalones, the one prepared from pig skin epithelium is known as a glycoprotein but others are chemically poorly defined. The chalones are produced within the tissue and are tissue-specific, but not species-specific. They are antimitotic agents and an epithelial chalone from pig skin origin will inhibit the proliferation of epithelial cells from another species, but display no inhibition of mitosis on cells from another tissue of pigs. Chalones are not anti-inflammatory in conventional animal models, but since hypermitosis is characteristic for some inflammatory conditions, e.g. represented by gouty arthritis or psoriasis, an agent with antimitotic property should be considered as potentially anti-inflammatory, though restricted for certain types. Whereas chalones have been prepared from normal (i.e. unirritated) tissues and are considered homeostatic regulators of normal cell proliferation, it would be of interest to study whether tissue injury, particularly one leading to increased mitosis, is a condition to stimulate their production. Although this is speculative, we might cautiously credit a modulator function of inflammation to chalones.

Recently, it was shown that rheumatoid arthritis patients have a markedly elevated *gastrin* level in their plasma (ROONEY et al., 1974). In the study the question was raised, but remained unanswered, whether gastrin is involved as a proinflammatory factor in rheumatoid arthritis or whether it is elevated secondary to the disease. In a certain sense, this study anticipates a role, still to be established, of gastrin as a proinflammatory modulator.

II. Plasma Factors

It has been mentioned already that tissue irritation is not only a condition which leads to occurrence of anti-inflammatory factors at the injured site, but that the blood or plasma of injured organisms contain such factors as well. It is just too obvious to suppose that the two sites reflect each others content of the same factors, also because in some papers similar anti-inflammatory profiles of ITAIF on the one hand and of the plasma factor on the other were found (BILLINGHAM et al., 1969a; BONTA and DE VOS, 1969). The anti-inflammatory tests used for the purpose are not very discriminative and do not allow far-reaching conclusions. Nevertheless, it was proposed that these factors might be identical and regarding their origin two alternatives were considered (BILLINGHAM et al., 1969a). Firstly, the anti-inflammatory factor may be produced at the inflamed site by the invading cells and the inflammation suppressing activity in plasma represent the removal transport of ITAIF. Secondly, the factor may be synthesized remote (possibly in the liver) from the injured site and while travelling in the circulation might be sequestered at an inflammatory site. Neither possibility has been satisfactory excluded, although BILLINGHAM argued in favour of the second, mainly on the basis that the ITAIF being a protein, its major site of synthesis should be hepatic. This circumstance will be discussed in the ensuing section. We turn now to other plasmatic modulators of inflammation. *Antilymphocytic serum*, known to suppress cell-mediated immunity, also inhibited the non-immune inflammation provoked by carrageenin, and the anti-inflammatory fraction of antilymphocytic serum was not associated with lymphocytotoxic activity (BILLINGHAM and ROBINSON, 1970). The Sephadex chromatography elution pattern of the anti-inflammatory fraction of antilymphocytic serum was similar to that of ITAIF isolated from different exudates (BILLINGHAM et al., 1969a, 1969b; GAUGAS et al., 1970).

Rheumatoid arthritis is a major injury to the human organism and the observation that sera of arthritic patients exerted anti-inflammatory effects (HIGHTON, 1963) is analogous to the above-discussed finding with sera of injured animals. The arthritic sera inhibited production of granulation tissue and reduced the tensile strength of healing wounds in rats. Both effects were most probably associated with decreased collagen formation. The sera of injured rats, however, were effective in acute inflammatory models (BILLINGHAM et al., 1969a). Since the rat sera might have contained the same ITAIF, which was earlier shown to inhibit granulation tissue formation (ROBINSON and ROBSON, 1964), it appears possible that the anti-inflammatory factor of sera from injured rats and arthritic patients is identical. Unfortunately, the work demonstrating the anti-inflammatory effect of rheumatoid sera did not give any clue as to the chemical nature of the active factor. However, during turpentine-induced subcutaneous inflammation (ASHTON et al., 1970) or polyvinyl sponge implantation (SARCIONE and BOGDEN, 1966), the synthesis of certain serum glycoproteins is increased. Similar changes were also observed during Freund's adjuvant-induced arthritis of rats (BILLINGHAM and GORDON, 1975a). In the latter study, the peak of *α-2-glycoprotein* synthesis fell simultaneously with the maximum of disorder in afflicted hind limbs, the latter subsiding thereafter in swelling. The time correlates suggested that the production of α-2-glycoprotein was a consequence of maximal injury, whereas the reduction of inflammation was a sequel to the protein's presence.

This type of mechanism has also been shown with respect to foetal α-2-globulin, suggested to be identical with α-2-glycoprotein. Foetal α-2-globulin is anti-inflammatory in the carrageenin rat paw oedema test, in addition to protecting against a cutaneous inflammatory response induced by bradykinin (VAN GOOL and LADIGES, 1969; VAN GOOL et al., 1974). The presence of foetal α-2-globulin in irritated tissue exudates has also been shown by VAN GOOL and his colleagues. The data are thus converging to indicate that at least one type of ITAIF might be identical with one of the plasmatic anti-inflammatory factors and that this material is likely to be the glycoprotein, also recognised as foetal α-2-globulin. There is also agreement amongst the authors that the occurrence of this substance after injury forms part of a homeostatic control system which with other mechanisms assists to curtail the progress of certain inflammatory reactions. It is by no means certain, however, that other ITAIF materials, having a similar function, are chemically identical with the plasma factor. For example, the ITAIF recovered from paw perfusates (GARCIA-LEME and SCHAPOVAL, 1975) was not detected in plasma, but stimulated the pituitary-adrenal system, while foetal α-2-globulin does not seem to do so (VAN GOOL et al., 1974). The ITAIF found by our group, though showing certain similarities, may still not be identical with the foetal α-2-globulin; the latter inhibits the whole course of the carrageenin rat paw oedema (VAN GOOL et al., 1974), while the ITAIF recovered by us preferentially suppresses the delayed phase leaving the first 2 h unaffected (NOORDHOEK and BONTA, 1974).

Amongst plasma factors able to participate as modulators of inflammation, the α-2-glycoprotein is only one of the major possibilities. Two others are interesting enough to be discussed here. In a study aimed at unravelling the anti-inflammatory effect of chymotrypsin it was found that the globulin fraction of chymotrypsin-treated rats inhibited an exudative pleural inflammation (SARKAR and FOSDICK, 1964). The fraction appeared to be an *anti-enzyme*, because it did not occur in sera of animals bearing pleural inflammation but untreated with chymotrypsin. Subsequently, it was shown that such anti-enzyme was also present in human plasma of subjects treated with chymotrypsin (HAKIM et al., 1965) and that this plasma factor was anti-inflammatory on the granuloma pouch of adrenalectomized rats. Although this material was formed in response to an exogenously administered enzyme, the possibility that anti-enzymes activated towards endogenous enzymes during tissue injury may also play a homeostatic modulating function is suggested. Two other aspects of these studies are worth mentioning. Firstly, the inflammation suppressing activity was associated with a dialyzable fraction of plasma (HAKIM et al., 1965), thus discriminating it from other anti-inflammatory plasma factors. Secondly, the anti-inflammatory globulin fraction was not only found in chymotrypsin-treated rats, but in normal rats as well, albeit to a lesser extent (SARKAR and FOSDICK, 1964). The latter finding leads us to take up the subject of anti-inflammatory factors in plasma of non-injured organism.

As early as 1968 we observed that the serum of normal rats exerted inhibition of the kaolin rat paw oedema after intraperitoneal administration (BONTA and DE VOS, 1969), and we found that the effect was present in the non-dialyzable, but to some extent also in the dialyzable, portion of serum (BONTA and DE VOS, 1968). The effect was marginally significant and we payed little attention to it, being at that time more preoccupied with the counter-irritation phenomenon. The credit of finding and—

even more important—properly appreciating the anti-inflammatory effect of a *low molecular weight constituent of normal plasma* should be given to SMITH and colleagues, who after first having described this effect with normal human serum (MCARTHUR et al., 1972), reported a simple method to recover the active principle from citrated human plasma (FORD-HUTCHINSON et al., 1973). Subsequently, they studied the properties of this factor in detail. An extensive treatise of the factor is to be found in Chapter 37 (SMITH, 1977) of this book, but for the sake of comparison with plasma factors of injured organisms some aspects will be mentioned here. The anti-inflammatory activity of this factor remained stable towards acid and proteolytic digestion, ultrafiltration indicated 1000 mol wt or less and it is believed not to be a linear peptide (FORD-HUTCHINSON et al., 1973). It is anti-inflammatory in the carrageenin rat paw test when administered intravenously (FORD-HUTCHINSON et al., 1974), and even when given orally (ELLIOTT et al., 1974b). It did not affect granuloma formation, but suppressed adjuvant arthritis and passive cutaneous anaphylaxis (FORD-HUTCHINSON et al., 1975; ELLIOT et al., 1974a; BOLAM et al., 1974b). In addition, the plasma factor inhibits leucocyte migration, but the mechanism does not involve complement depletion or specific interference with the prostaglandin system or inhibition of the action of SRS-A (FORD-HUTCHINSON et al., 1975; SMITH et al., 1974b). Nevertheless, these explanations of the mode of action were not maintained in another paper, in which interference with histamine, 5-HT or bradykinin were excluded (BOLAM et al., 1974a). Neither antinociception, nor antipyresis belong to the properties of this plasma factor (SMITH et al., 1974a). In view of its mol wt and non-peptide character, it is not likely that it has relevance to either of the factors discussed in the foregoing, although the possibility that an ITAIF macromolecule may have the carrier function to transport a non-protein substance has been mentioned in one paper (BONTA and NOORDHOEK, 1973). The need to investigate the binding of the small-sized anti-inflammatory plasma factor to a carrier protein has also been pointed out (FORD-HUTCHINSON et al., 1973). The pharmacological profile of the low mol wt plasma factor is dissimilar to any of the putative modulators as discussed. Furthermore, the postulation that this factor, present in normal plasma, may be an integral part of a natural defensive system against inflammation (ELLIOTT et al., 1974b; FORD-HUTCHINSON et al., 1973) has still to be proven. It is difficult to understand how a preformed factor should have a defensive function towards inflammation, itself a genuinely defencive reaction.

III. Hepatic Factors

The findings that one of the plasma anti-inflammatory factors of inflammation-bearing animals is most probably α-2-glycoprotein and furthermore, the hepatic synthesis of this protein in perfused livers of acutely injured rats (SARCIONE and BOGDEN, 1966) led to speculations that the liver may participate in the homeostatic control of inflammation. In favour of this argument were experiments showing that livers from polyester sponge implanted rats, when perfused with blood of normal animals produced an anti-inflammatory plasma factor. Livers from normal rats failed to do so (BILLINGHAM et al., 1971). Moreover, the chromatographical elution pattern of the plasma from perfusates of inflammation-bearing rat liver was similar to exudates from which ITAIF was recovered (BILLINGHAM et al., 1969a, 1969b), thus suggesting the hepatic origin of this ITAIF. Treatment of the animals with the protein synthesis inhibitor actinomycin D suppresses the occurrence of this type of ITAIF and also that of foetal α-2-globulin in the plasma of traumatized rats (BILLINGHAM et al., 1971; VAN GOOL et al., 1974). In two recent papers (BILLINGHAM and GORDON, 1976a, 1976b), it was suggested that the so-called acute phase reactant protein—known to be of hepatic origin in response to major systemic inflammation (GLENN et al., 1968)—may have the function of endogenously curtailing inflammation. The role of acute phase reactants is treated in more detail in Chapter 23 (BILLINGHAM and DAVIES, 1977) of this book. However, it has been proposed earlier that while the local phase of inflammation is primarily destructive, the systemic phase—of which the liver is a part—may be genuinely protective (GLENN et al., 1968). There are some discrepancies for example the observation that adrenalectomy suppresses the occurence of α-2-glycoprotein (GLENN et al., 1968) but does not abolish the presence of that particular ITAIF which is supposed to be identical to α-2-glycoprotein. Nevertheless, the concept of hepatic synthesis of this anti-inflammatory protein being part of the homeostatic modulation of tissue injury remains a valuable one. The connecting pathway between the inflamed area and the liver is, however, unexplained. The proposal that a triggering substance (of unknown nature) is released from the injured area and stimulates the liver to produce the anti-inflammatory protein (VAN GOOL et al., 1974) awaits definite proof, although this will not be an easy task. It is conceivable that ITAIF represents two materials: one of them *travelling to the liver* to trigger it and thus indirectly anti-inflammatory; the *other coming from the liver* and directly anti-inflammatory (Fig. 4). It was indicated that ITAIF of granuloma pouch origin may have contained two anti-inflammatory principles, largely differing in mol wt (BONTA and NOORDHOEK, 1973), but no attempts were made to differentiate their action.

Besides the materials proven to be related to counter-irritation, the liver may have additional functions in modulating inflammation. It is an old clinical experience that during hepatitis and/or jaundice a rheumatoid arthritis may improve. A speculative explanation was given that bilirubin has the ability to displace corticosteroids from sites of transport protein binding (BRODIE, 1965). Subsequently, it was shown that in rats ligature of the bile duct caused inhibition of the carrageenin paw oedema, either in normal or in adrenalectomized animals, but the granuloma formation around a cotton-pellet remained unaffected (SILVESTRINI et al., 1968). In the same study, however, bile duct ligation resulted in thymolysis, a characteristic response to endogenous discharge of adrenal steroids or to administration of corticosteroids. It might have been that the thymus involution was caused by bilirubin competition with corticosterone at the protein binding site, although corticosteroid displacement by other drugs (e.g. phenylbutazone) does not usually lead to thymus atrophy. Finally, the study showed that bile duct ligation led to protection of serum proteins from heat denaturation (the anti-inflammatory Mizushima test) and that bilirubin, sodium cholate and sodium deoxycholate also displayed the antidenaturant effect when added to bovine serum albumin. While there is indeed a correlation between the Mizushima test and antirheuma efficacy of drugs, the rationale behind this is not really known. In this respect, the above experiments do little to explain the association between jaundice and improvement of rheumatic condition.

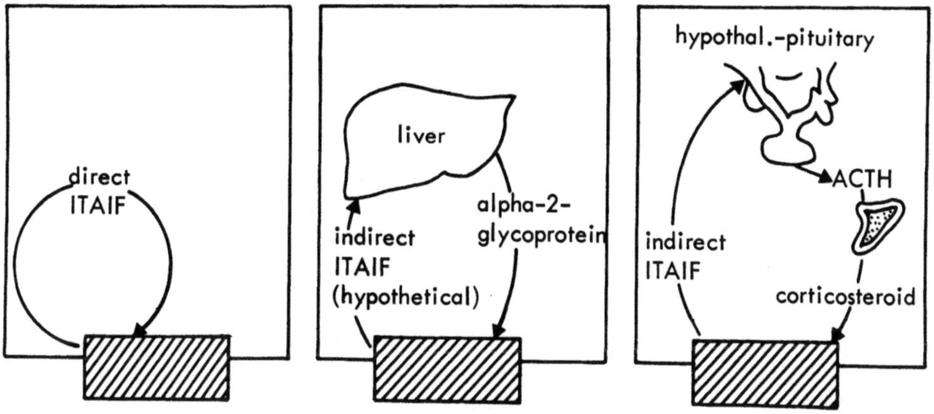

Fig. 4. Putative pathways in the action of different ITAIFs

In adjuvant-induced arthritis of rats, bile duct ligation did not change the incidence of the disease, although it inhibited the severity (GLENN and GRAY, 1965). On the other hand, during adjuvant arthritis there is a marked impairment in the drug-metabolizing capacity of the liver (WHITEHOUSE, 1973). The effect was manifest with hexobarbital and trichloroethanol, the former being metabolized through cytochrome P 450, but the latter not. Therefore, reduction in the synthesis of cytochrome P 450 does not provide a sufficient explanation. WHITEHOUSE has speculated that a messenger molecule passes from the site of inflammation and triggers in the liver an adaptive syndrome, involving depression of the level of some proteins (e.g. drug hydroxylating enzymes), while stimulating the synthesis of others (e.g. acute phase reactants). It is possible that there is question about the same (hypothetical) substance mentioned above in connection with ITAIF and liver relation, but there might be more than one factor involved in the mechanism by which the liver is programmed to respond to a distant inflammation.

Bovine liver served as a source to isolate the anti-inflammatory metalloprotein known as *orgotein* (HUBER et al., 1968). Following the initial studies indicating the inhibiting property of orgotein on a variety of inflammatory responses in rats, guinea pigs and rabbits, it recently underwent a preliminary evaluation in clinical osteoarthritis (LUND-OLFSEN and MENANDER, 1974). Orgotein contains both copper and zinc, the role of which in inflammatory disorders has been discussed in a recent paper (WHITEHOUSE, 1976). The liver is possibly not the only source of orgotein, because it might be identical to proteins known as hepatocuprein, erythrocuprein or cerebrocuprein (WHITEHOUSE, 1976). Therefore, these data do not allow conclusions on eventual relationship of orgotein to other hepatic factors discussed above. For more details about orgotein the reader is referred to Chapter 37 (SMITH, 1977).

IV. Endocrine Factors (Adrenal Steroids, Oestrogens, Insulin)

This section is not intended as a repetition of hackneyed text book knowledge. Instead, a brief attempt will be made to raise some new questions on old facts. Starting with the *adrenal steroids*, the arrival of an uninterrupted flow of synthetic glucocorticosteroids nearly overshadowed the potential role of the adrenal cortex as an endogenous modulator of inflammation, although in the original discovery of HENCH this was implicit (HENCH et al., 1949). One of the difficulties in properly evaluating the function of endogenous adrenal steroids is methodologically linked to a species difference. In the rat, frequently used for inflammation model studies and easily subjected to manipulations for selective exclusion of any part of the hypothalamic-pituitary-adrenal system, the end product of this system is corticosterone which has hardly any detectable anti-inflammatory effect. Therefore, results obtained on rats in favour of or against the modulating function of adrenocortical steroid can only be extrapolated with the greatest caution to man, whose adrenocortical product is largely cortisol, the latter having pronounced anti-inflammatory properties. Nevertheless, even in the rat acute hind limb oedema is believed to involve a series of modulating events in which the final member may be corticosterone (GARCIA-LEME and SCHAPOVAL, 1975). Injury produced by endotoxin was also associated with elevated blood level of adrenocortical steroid (MELBY et al., 1960; MOBERG, 1971). More important, however, than demonstrating the injury-triggered discharge of adrenal steroid, would be the study of a correlation with a conceivable subsequent curtailing of inflammation. In the latter context, however, not so much the blood level but other pharmacokinetic parameters (bioavailability at the injury site, displacement from transport protein) are relevant. These in turn depend on extra-adrenal factors (i.e. the liver); the hurdles to be surmounted for pinpointing the modulating function of adrenal steroids should thus not be underestimated. That this should happen to the first product of major therapeutic anti-inflammatory use of endogenous origin is rather ironical.

A natural situation, long clinically recognised to be associated with improvement of certain inflammatory conditions—particularly rheumatoid arthritis—is the state of *pregnancy*. The great many changes which the body undergoes during pregnancy render it exceptionally difficult to select the ones which can be considered as modulating a tissue injury. It is common knowledge that pregnancy is associated with an increased discharge of adrenocortical steroids and in fact HENCH in his discovery was guided by the belief that the temporary remission which arthritic patients experienced during pregnancy was due to a metabolite (HENCH, 1938). His bet was cortisol, which indeed became a winner, even though its role as an endogenous modulator of inflammation is still unclear, as pointed out above. Two other hormones which display a grossly elevated plasma level during pregnancy are progesterone and oestrogens. There are no data which point in the direction that progesterone might be anti-inflammatory. Such an effect with *oestrogens* was, however, demonstrated in several ways. Oestriol dihemisuccinate inhibits rat paw oedemas, irrespective of the inducer irritant (BONTA and DE VOS, 1965). In the same study, oestrogen equally suppressed the early and delayed phase of acute rat paw inflammation. This, together with other arguments to be read in the original paper, led to the interpretation that oestrogen did not interfere with either the release or the action of one particular mediator, but exerted a direct effect on the microvessels, the latter being the final target organs of inflammatory oedema (BONTA, 1969). Other investigators have also shown the antipermeability effect of oestrogens on skin vessels (ISHIOKA et al., 1969). The vessel protecting activity of oestrogens seems to be independent of a systemic endocrine effect for two reasons. Firstly, oestriol dihemisuccinate, as used in the above studies, has a particularly feeble effect on female sex organs. Secondly, the vessel protecting effect of oestrogens is also demonstrable when directly applied to the pulmonary tissue (BONTA et al., 1965, 1969) in an orthodox heart-lung preparation in which the target tissue is not in circulatory contact with other parts of the body. In a recent paper, it was argued that the experimental conditions, under which the vascular anti-inflammatory effect of oestrogens is readily demonstrable, represent an unconventional model of acute inflammation in which substances like indomethacin, antihistamine agents or corticosteroids are ineffective, inhibitory efficacy being confined to agents "protecting" the tissues (BONTA and VARGAFTIG, 1976). The mechanism of the vascular anti-inflammatory effect of oestrogens is far from clear. Some investigators considered that they exerted such an effect through influencing the acid mucopolysaccharides in the perivascular ground substance (for references see VINCENT et al., 1970), but more recently it was proposed that activation of the adenylcyclase system played a role in the effect of oestrogens on the microvessels (VINCENT et al., 1970). As the adenylcyclase-cAMP system is the chief regulator of lysosomal enzyme release, results demonstrating that oestrogens have a membrane stabilising effect on liposomes are somewhat in this line (WEISSMANN and RITA, 1972), because liposomes are artificial models akin to lysosomes. Leucocytic lysosomal enzyme release was also counteracted by pregnancy sera and a large mol wt protein with lysosomal stabilising activity was present in serum of oestrogen treated women (HEMPEL et al., 1970; PERSELLIN and PERRY, 1972). The oxygen consumption of phagocytotic leucocytes is inhibited by oestrogens, and a similar effect was also observed with leucocytes obtained from pregnant women (BODEL et al., 1972). Some inhibition of prostaglandin biosynthesis has been recently described with non-steroidal oestrogens (LERNER et al., 1975). Whereas the above effects of oestrogens are related to the acute phase of inflammation, anti-inflammation by oestrogens was also shown in the adjuvant arthritis of rats (GLENN, 1966; MUELLER and KAPPAS, 1964). In these studies, progesterone was without effect and although the effect of oestrogens was associated with tissue catabolism (TOIVANEN et al., 1967), it was suggested that they may have acted by suppressing the capacity of the tissues to react to the immunologic inflammatory stimulus in the disorder (MUELLER and KAPPAS, 1964). In man, oestrogens have been reported to benefit some cases of rheumatoid arthritis (SPANGLER et al., 1969). Whatever might be the mechanism, it is likely that oestrogens are contributory (if not more) to the modulating influence of pregnancy on inflammation (Fig. 5).

Last but not least, it is possible that foetal α-2-globulin, known to be present in amniotic fluid (VAN GOOL et al., 1974), also assists in pregnancy temporarily to suppress inflammation. However, it is uncertain whether foetal α-2-globulin also occurs in the maternal circulation. As in pregnancy there is in any case a peculiar immunological tolerance towards the foetus, it is likely that a coincidence of several immune mechanisms results in remission of rheumatoid arthritis.

It has been known for some time that *hormonal influences on carbohydrate metabolism* are associated with aberrant inflammatory reactions. This appeared particularly true with respect to the anaphylactoid type of reactions (for literature before 1972 see ROCHA E SILVA and GARCIA-LEME, 1972). Briefly, it was shown that hyperglycemia, due to overdosage of glucose, cortisol, adrenaline or diabetes, attenuated the anaphylactoid reactions and that hypoglycemic states sensitized the animals. In

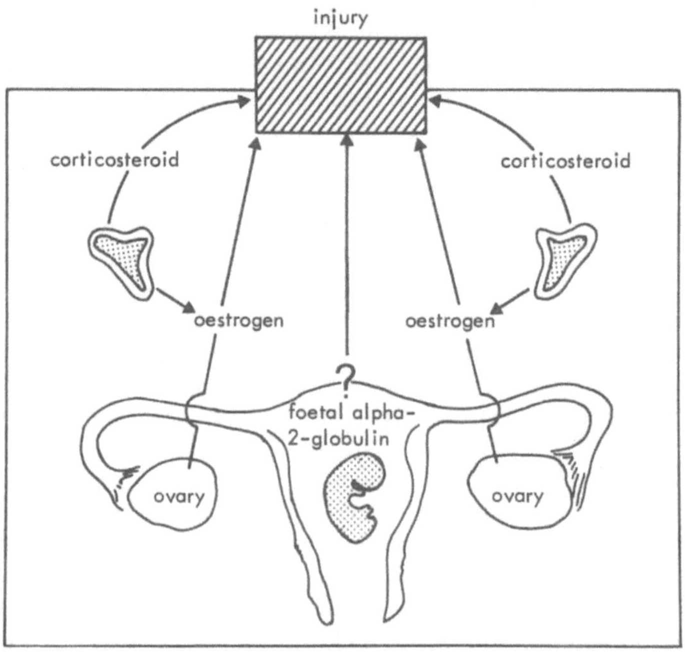

Fig. 5. During the state of pregnancy adrenal corticosteroids, oestrogens and possibly also foetal α-2-globulin may have the role of modulators of inflammation

two recent studies, however, strong evidence was furnished that not so much the blood glucose, but rather the presence or absence of *insulin* is the factor that upsets the balance, at least with some type of inflammations (GARCIA-LEME et al., 1973, 1974). In rat paw oedema induced by dextran or carrageenin, the inflammatory response was still inhibited in diabetic animals rendered normoglycemic by fasting but such inhibition was readily reversed by insulin. Diabetic animals displayed decreased responses to intradermally injected histamine, 5-HT or bradykinin, although the in vitro release of the mediators was not influenced by diabetes. It was concluded that not the release of mediators but their final effect upon vessels is reduced during diabetes and indications were found that insulin exerts a local influence in the control of vascular permeability. Electron microscopic studies revealed that endothelial gap opening might, at least partially, depend on the local availability of insulin (GARCIA-LEME et al., 1974). A proinflammatory effect of insulin was also observed with respect to granuloma formation (NAGY et al., 1961). These findings themselves, though of great interest, are very difficult to interpret, because insulin directly and indirectly (through metabolic feedback) has a profound influence on the adenylcyclase-cAMP system which itself is much involved in regulating several steps of the inflammatory response. It is likely therefore that the available data on insulin as a potential modulator of inflammation are just showing us the top of the iceberg. The value of the above studies is all the greater, because they may herald even more important future findings.

V. Mediators as Modulators: Role of the Cyclic Nucleotides

Evidence is accumulating that some mediators not only have proinflammatory but anti-inflammatory effects as well. It would be an intrusion into other chapters of this book to discuss such effects in detail, but some examples will be given to support the view that a mediator may have the inherent function of modulating the inflammatory response. The idea that a balance between the intracellular levels of the cyclic nucleotides cAMP and cGMP will determine the secretory activity of cells which are present in or migrating to the inflammatory area is gaining more and more acceptance. This metabolism of cyclic nucleotides, the levels of which amongst other factors depend on membrane-bound cyclases which can be activated by mediators such as histamine or prostaglandins, is the subject of several reviews (e.g. BOURNE, 1972; WEISSMANN et al., 1973) and will not be covered in this section. Furthermore, viewing the problem in generalised terms, no difference will be made as to whether the secretory cell activity comprises the discharge of a preformed mediator stored in granules or the release of a lysosomal enzyme which will contribute to the synthesis or cleavage of a mediator. For allergic inflammation the twofold—mediator and modulator—function of *histamine* was first indicated by the finding that this amine blocks its own release (BOURNE et al., 1971). The mechanism involved became clearer after H_2-receptor antagonists were used for such studies. The data reported show that the mediator function comprises cGMP in the release and H_1-receptors at the target organs, whereas the modulator function involves H_2-receptors on the surface of immune-challenged histamine releasing cells themselves and further cAMP for retaining histamine and lysosome enzymes (LICHTENSTEIN, 1975). The same paper also indicates that during the allergic type of antigen-antibody interaction, a transient fall in the intracellular cAMP level will cause a predominance in the release. The decrease in cAMP level can be restored and the release process short-circuited by any agent, also histamine itself, which activates adenylcyclase. Obviously this is an oversimplified view, but it may serve as a blueprint for other inflammatory processes being modulated by mediators.

The data emerging from the literature indicate that *prostaglandins* may have a modulator function as well. One difficulty in studies aimed to show such a function is the lack of powerful antagonists to prostaglandins. There are other obstacles, amongst which are the plurality of prostaglandins, their simultaneous release and their actions opposite to each other. Nevertheless, the activating function of prostaglandins on cell membrane-bound cyclases and the subsequent build-up of cAMP to retain lysosomal enzymes led to studies in which the anti-inflammatory effect of prostaglandins has been demonstrated. Such investigations comprised acute situations like the carrageenin or egg-white-induced rat paw oedema (DI PASQUALE et al., 1973) chronic inflammations represented by the granuloma pouch and adjuvant arthritis of rats (DI PASQUALE et al., 1973; GLENN and ROHLOFF, 1972; ZURIER et al., 1973). The doses to obtain anti-inflammations by prostaglandins were in all studies exceptionally high; nevertheless the results prompted other investigators to find explanations for such effects in terms of endogenous prostaglandins. Whereas the earlier workers offered inhibition of lysosomal enzyme release as the underlying mechanism of prostaglandins as pharmacological agents (i.e. administered), the more recent studies of MORLEY and his colleagues indicate that an interaction between two different cell populations in the tissue damage area is an additional factor to be taken into account for understanding a putative regulating function of prostaglandins. The data in these studies indicate that E-type prostaglandins suppress the lymphokine discharge by lymphocytes and the possibility was suggested that endogenous prostaglandins of macrophage origin may have this role (BRAY et al., 1976; MORLEY et al., 1975; MORLEY, 1976). In agreement with this was the proposal that the key defect leading to chronicity of inflammation in rheumatoid arthritis is loss of responsiveness of immune activated lymphocytes to the suppressing function of endogenous prostaglandins on lymphokine secretion (MORLEY, 1974). Many gaps in this intriguing concept need to be filled. Particularly, we do not know whether inhibition by prostaglandins of lymphokine secretion involves the intracellular cyclic nucleotide mechanism. There are, however, data indicating that through elevation of cAMP not only allergic type of inflammations, but also those involving chronic granulomatous inflammations can be inhibited (ICHIKAWA et al., 1972). Furthermore, it was recently shown that theophylline, an inhibitor of cAMP breakdown, potentiates the PGE_1-induced suppression of the adjuvant arthritis in rats and the suppressant effect of jointly administered PGE_1 and theophylline parallelled the inhibition of splenomegaly (BONTA et al., 1977a). These observations led to the proposal that the PGE_1 plus theophylline-induced suppression of adjuvant arthritis is probably related to cAMP mediated events in splenic lymphocytes (BONTA et al., 1977a). The data converge thus that the modulator function of some mediators is exerted through the feed-back which involves the cyclic nucleotides. There is no pretention of originality in this statement, because it has been advocated earlier (GLENN, 1974).

Endogenous prostaglandins may exert their anti-inflammatory modulator function by other mechanisms as well. In essential fatty acid deficient (EFAD) rats, which are deprived of endogenous prostaglandin precursors, the carrageenin-induced granuloma formation was increased (BONTA et al., 1977b) and the increased granuloma formation, in absence of endogenous prostaglandins, is associated with increased collagen synthesis (PARNHAM et al., 1977). Thus, in the proliferative phase of inflammation the endogenous prostaglandins may exert their modulator function through inhibition of collagen synthesis.

In the light of recent data (KUEHL et al., 1977) it appears justified to attribute a pivotal mediator, i.e. pro-inflammatory, function to the cyclic endoperoxide PGG_2 and to ascribe the modulator function to the end products of arachidonate conversion, i.e. the prostaglandins themselves. This modulator function appears to be partly exerted through the cyclic nucleotide system, partly through an influence on collagen synthesis of proliferating tissue.

It would be an attractive hypothesis to attribute *mediator function to the cycloendoperoxides formed* in the biosynthesis of prostaglandins from arachidonic acid and *modulator functions to the end products, i.e. the prostaglandins themselves.* No data are as yet available on this matter.

D. Neurogenic Factors as Modulators

In studies aimed at unravelling nervous interactions with the inflammatory response sometimes potent neuropharmacologic agents (including neuroleptics or antidepressants) were used as experimental tools. Such drugs have a broad spectrum of activity, exerting effects centrally and peripherally. Furthermore the mechanism of action of such neuropharmacologic agents include simultaneous actions on neurochemical processes at nerve terminals releasing noradrenaline, 5-HT and dopamine. Investigations using such drugs, though important for their own merrit, do not allow to draw conclusions as to the role of endogenous nervous function in inflammation and will be disregarded in the present review.

I. Peripheral Nervous System: Neurotransmitters and Other Factors

In the counter irritation situation the possibility that the release of *adrenergic* substances may account for the anti-inflammatory effect has been postulated (HORAKOVA and MURATOVA, 1965; GOLDSTEIN et al., 1967), but more recent studies appeared to exclude this (ATKINSON and HICKS, 1974). The counter irritation model represents an extreme artificial condition in which the release of other endogenous anti-inflammatory factors (ITAIF, hepatic proteins etc.) may overshadow the effect of the adrenergic substance. However, the latter may still have a role as modulator when the organism is only afflicted by a single inflammation. Indeed it was indicated earlier that locally produced catecholamines, either adrenaline (SPECTOR and WILLOUGHBY, 1960), but possibly also noradrenaline (BROWN and WEST, 1965) may act as endogenous anti-inflammatory substances. One argument in favour of an adrenaline-like substance having the function of endogenous inhibitor of inflammation was that monoamine oxidase inhibition led to suppression of inflammation (SPECTOR and WILLOUGHBY, 1960). It was proposed in the study that the adrenaline like substance was not produced by adrenergic nerve terminals. The anti-inflammatory effect of adrenaline has been reported in various acute situations, including rat paw oedema induced by carrageenin, formol or yeast, and also in the peritoneal cavity and paw inflammation in mice (ARNTZEN and BRISEND, 1973; BROWN et al., 1968b; GREEN, 1972; KELLET, 1965). In contrast, proinflammatory effects of adrenaline have been shown in thermal paw oedema and various other (calciphylaxis, anaphylactoid oedema, ischemic necrosis, thrombohaemorrhagic syndrome) tissue injury situations in the rat (GREEN, 1974a; SELYE et al., 1968). The contradiction may be only seeming, however, because adrenaline has affinity for, and intrinsic activity on, both types of adrenoceptors, the α and the β ones. Stimulation of each of these adrenoceptors results in different events, having in turn different consequences on the inflammation, and the end effect of adrenaline may thus depend on which receptor stimulation predominates. As for the potential mechanisms underlying the pro-, viz. anti-inflammatory effect of adrenaline, a number of possibilities are discussed in the literature.

Concerning the *proinflammatory* effect: adrenaline was supposed to activate the kallikrein-kinin system (ROCHA E SILVA, 1964), but other studies did not confirm this (ARNTZEN and BRISEND, 1973). It is now accepted that bradykinin leads to release of adrenaline (PIPER et al., 1967). More recently, it was shown that local administration of adrenaline resulted in decreased output of bradykinin from perfusates of thermal rat paw oedema (GREEN, 1974a). Nevertheless, adrenaline was proinflammatory in the latter situation and reduced blood flow in the paw resulted in a rise of paw temperature, thus potentiating the injury. This proinflammatory effect of adrenaline was antagonised by phenoxybenzamine and by phentolamine, but not by propranolol. It was concluded that the proinflammatory effect of adrenaline is associated with stimulation of α-adrenoceptors (GREEN, 1974a).

Regarding the *anti-inflammatory* effect of adrenaline, in a careful study it was concluded that β-adrenoceptor stimulation was involved (GREEN, 1972). Somewhat in line with this is the earlier finding that the anti-inflammatory effect of adrenaline entirely depended on its hyperglycemic property (KELLET, 1965). In this respect again, the system of the intracellular cyclic nucleotides emerges. Evidence is steadily growing that β-adrenoceptor stimulation leads to an increase of cAMP, whereas cholinergic activation results in elevation of cGMP (WEISSMANN et al., 1973; IGNARRO and GEORGE, 1974). Grossly extrapolating from lysosomal release to tissue injury, cGMP is proinflammatory and cAMP anti-inflammatory. Adrenaline was shown to increase cAMP and to inhibit lysosomal enzyme release which effects were counteracted by the β-adrenoceptor blocking agent propranolol (IGNARRO and GEORGE, 1974). Therefore, it is conceivable that the anti-inflammatory effect of adrenaline should be interpreted in terms of shifting the intracellular balance of the two cyclic nucleotides. Adrenaline is believed to strengthen the action of chalones (BULLOUGH, 1968). Still it is questionable whether *endogenous* catecholamines are indeed involved in shifting tissue injury. Although α-adrenoceptor blocking agents did show an anti-inflammatory effect (GREEN, 1974b), this might have been secondary due to their hypotensive effect. On the other hand, the findings that β-adrenoceptor blocking agents did not markedly potentiate various forms of inflammation (BROWN et al., 1968b; RIESTERER and JAQUES, 1968) suggest that endogenous catecholamines may not play an important role in reducing the inflammatory response. This points in the same direction as found in counter-irritation studies, also rendering unlikely that adrenoceptor mechanisms are involved in the remote anti-inflammatory effect of a tissue injury (ATKINSON and HICKS, 1974). This supports the view that counter-irritation is a useful situation to study endogenous modulating factors of inflammation.

Concerning other neurotransmitters, *acetylcholine* was shown to elevate intracellular cGMP level and this effect was associated with promotion of lysosomal enzyme release (IGNARRO and GEORGE, 1974). This property of acetylcholine is associated with activation of muscarinic receptors, because it is inhibited by atropine but not by hexamethonium. Increase of endogenous acetylcholine by subcutaneous administration of physostigmine inhibited the formol induced rat paw oedema (BROWN et al., 1968a). However, subcutaneous injection of a cholinesterase inhibitor might have caused too many systemic effects, e.g. pronounced hypotension to interfere with inflammation. It is not known to what extent a *local endogenous imbalance between cholinergic and adrenergic* predominance is involved in modulating a tissue injury.

Not only humoral neurotransmission but also *other peripheral neurogenic* effects were studied on inflammation. Acute denervation of the rat paw by sectioning the sciatic nerve did not prevent anti-inflammation provoked through counter-irritation (ATKINSON and HICKS, 1974). Blood pressure rise induced by local application of an irritant was, however, abolished after acute or chronic denervation of the injured area (FEARN et al., 1965). These experiments together indicate that long neurogenic reflexes are involved in some systemic events associated with acute tissue injury, but such reflexes are not involved in modulation of the inflammatory reaction itself. Infiltration of a local anaesthetic into the hind paw inhibited the early phase of the formol oedema (BROWN et al., 1968a). Local axon reflexes have a definite role in acute inflammation. Antidromic stimulation of sensory nerves was shown to elicit arteriolar vasodilatation, enhanced vascular permeability and deposition of injected colloidal particles on to the walls of venules (JANCSO et al., 1968). It was proposed that a humoral agent was released, but acetylcholine, histamine, 5-HT, adrenaline, and noradrenaline were excluded. Subsequent studies showed that inflammation induced by neurogenically-acting irritants (capsaicin, xylol) was not abolished by application of tetrodotoxin, but surgical denervation prevented the effect (JANCSO-GABOR and SZOLCSANYI, 1969). The most recent development shows that during antidromic stimulation of the saphenous nerve, a permeability increasing factor is released and this agent, though still unidentified, was distinguishable from acetylcholine, histamine, 5-HT, plasma kinins, substance P, prostaglandins and high mol wt proteins (GARCIA-LEME and HAMAMURA, 1974). The factor, however, led to indirect activation of the kinin system, through plasma exudation and dilution. The role of this factor as an endogenous modulator which reinforces inflammation needs to be established.

II. Central Nervous Influences

Characteristic for this question is the paucity of relevant data. Thalamic or spinothalamic lesions in patients were associated with a decreased flare response to histamine, indicating that the vasodilator component of inflammation is modulated by the CNS (APPENZELLER and MCANDREWS, 1966). The dextran oedema of rats was attenuated immediately after decerebration, pithing or spinal transection, but 3 h after surgery the inflammatory reaction was again normal (FEARN et al., 1965). In adrenalectomized rats, however, the neurosurgical procedures were without influence on the hind paw inflammation, showing that these CNS manipulations must have acted as acute stress. Midspinal transection abolished the early phase of carrageenin or formol-induced rat hind paw oedema, but in the fore paws (above the transection) the reaction remained unaffected (BROWN et al., 1968a). The same study showed that morphine when administered subcutaneously caused a similar effect as did midspinal transection; however, local administration of morphine was without effect. Concerning chronic inflammations, in Freund's adjuvant-treated rats which were daily submitted to cold stress, there was marked inhibition of the arthritis (GLENN and GRAY, 1965). Swimming stress, however, was a less effective influence. A role of the adrenals was likely, but was not evaluated because adrenalectomised rats did not survive the adjuvant disease. In all the above studies the central influences on inflammation were investigated by rather harsh methods. Except for showing that the CNS *can* modulate a local inflammation, the studies did not contain a clue to the way it does so. Future investigations with presently available refined neurophysiological or neuropharmacological approaches are thus awaited.

It would be naive to think that a modulating connection between a local inflammation and the CNS is restricted to one-way traffic. An interesting step in exploring a mutual interrelation was made recently: cortical potentials evoked by electrical stimulation of the dental pulp in the rat were decreased following stimulation of the peripheral cut end of the saphenous nerve (GARCIA-LEME and LICA, 1974). The permeability-increasing factor recovered from the subcutaneous tissues in the vicinity of the stimulated saphenous nerve (GARCIA-LEME and HAMAMURA, 1974) also inhibited the cortical potentials. Recognised inflammatory mediators were devoid of this property, and it was suggested that a chemically unidentified proinflammatory humoral factor released during antidromic sensory nerve stimulation may help to modulate the processing of afferent inputs from nociceptive stimuli.

E. Automodulation and Therapy

The following, last section of this chapter neither pretends to be another effort to explain the mode of action of existing anti-inflammatory drugs (AID) nor is it a copyright repertory of hints for drug design. Rather it is some kind of enumeration of fragmentary questions or ideas which arose in the course of writing.

I. Automodulation and Present Drugs

When judging the merits and disadvantages of presently used anti-inflammatory drugs from the angle of automodulation the puzzle is, are they doing too little or too much? In other words, do these drugs, or at least some of them, have any aspect in their mode of action which assists the organism's modulating mechanisms or are they so anti-inflammatory that they suppress not merely the adverse components of inflammation but the self-curtailing elements of it as well? Concerning the first part of the question, in the literature there are indeed theories which attribute the efficacy of some anti-inflammatory drugs to their ability to activate or displace one or the other endogenous modulating substance. It was suggested that aspirin, which unlike other anti-inflammatory drugs damages the stomach mucosa by contact, not only has a direct anti-inflammatory effect but also acts by virtue of gastric site counter-irritation (JORI and BERNARDI, 1966). As it appears that macroscopically observable damage is not necessary for counter-irritation from a gastric site (see Section B.III.), it is conceivable that some orally administered anti-inflammatory proteolytic enzyme preparations (bromelain, ficin, chymotrypsin), besides other actions, elicit counter-irritation without themselves being "irritant" in the usual sense (PAULUS and WHITEHOUSE, 1973).

For antirheumatic drugs it was proposed that part of their effect might be due to displacement of an anti-inflammatory peptide (present in normal serum) from its albumin binding (MCARTHUR et al., 1971). Although later studies showed that the referred endogenous substance is a low-molecular weight non-peptide material, the proposal was essentially maintained (FORD-HUTCHINSON et al., 1973). Somewhat in the same line is the possibility that anti-inflammatory drugs displace an endogenous anti-inflammatory factor of hepatic origin from transport protein binding. Vice versa a hepatic anti-inflammatory factor (bilirubin?) may displace corticosteroids (or also non-steroid anti-inflammatory drugs?) from sites of transport protein binding (BRODIE, 1965).

Corticosteroids and ACTH might reinforce the effect of that particular ITAIF which acts by stimulation of the hypothalamo-pituitary-adrenal axis (GARCIA-LEME and SCHAPOVAL, 1975). This proposal is not likely to be valid insofar as the corticosteroids are concerned, which themselves suppress the discharge of ACTH, although for the latter substance the validity of the postulate cannot be ruled out.

In recent years, data have been accumulating that those anti-inflammatory drugs, to which inhibition of prostaglandin biosynthesis is credited as the key mechanism are by virtue of phosphodiesterase inhibition elevators of intracellular cAMP level. Through the latter mechanism, paradoxical as it sounds, such drugs may assist the anti-inflammatory modulator function of prostaglandins. This point obviously brings us to the shadowy side of anti-inflammatory drugs: suppression of the organism's automodulation function. Inhibition of prostaglandin biosynthesis might be expected to produce dramatic relief of, e.g. arthritis, if prostaglandins were only mediators, viz. proinflammatory. However, neither are the prostaglandins only proinflammatory, nor is the benefit of the prostaglandin release inhibitors too dramatic. It is possible that these anti-inflammatory drugs are in a certain sense camouflaged traitors, suppressing the production of the modulator, thereby (partially) annihilating the benefit of counteracting the release of the mediator. Recently it was tried to reconcile this paradox (MORLEY et al., 1975), but the final solution of this complex question is still awaited. Another way in which anti-inflammatory drugs may jeopardise the natural modulation of the inflammatory reaction is suppression of the hepatic synthesis of α-2-glycoprotein. Suppression of α-2-glycoprotein may be a sensitive index of the "anti-inflammatory" action of non-steroid anti-inflammatory drugs (GLENN et al., 1968). This proposal was made shortly before recognition of α-2-glycoprotein itself being anti-inflammatory and does not appear tenable at present. The above data, selected a little arbitrarily, were meant to exemplify that in the light of our increasing knowledge on inflammation itself the task of explaining the mode of action of some type of anti-inflammatory drugs does not really become easier.

II. Automodulation: A Possible Guide to New Drugs?

At the end of review articles it is customary to anticipate future developments of the subject or to make proposals about the direction likely to be rewarding in future research. Predictions have the inherent danger (for the author) that soon after they were made they might turn out to be wrong, unmasking the writer as having misjudged the situation. This seems unattractive and no anticipations will be made here. Research proposals from a pharmacologist might mean ways potentially leading to better drugs. Fundamentally, new drugs are still mostly found through unexpected discoveries and paperproposals run the risk of being discarded. This is likely to be the fate of the few ensuing points.

Further studies of the counter-irritation model may offer a few interesting possibilities. One of them comprises non-humoral mechanism(s), the existence of which has not been substantially excluded. Understanding of such pathways may indicate mechanisms to be synergistically influenced or mimicked by putative drugs. Secondly, identification, purification and preparation of humoral anti-inflammatory factors from the inflamed site is necessary for mode of action studies. Only such studies will tell us whether such ITAIF preparations are differing enough from synthetic drugs, either by an alternate mode of action or through lack of side-effects, to warrant therapeutic evaluation. Proteins have only a small chance to be developed into clinically useful drugs, but their mode of action might serve as a blueprint for synthetic drugs. Also it has not yet been ruled out that one of the ITAIFs is a complex molecule consisting of a small active core bound to a carrier protein. A third possibility arising from counter-irritation would be to recover from the irritated area the substance which boosts the liver to increase its output of anti-inflammatory protein.

The story of one plasma anti-inflammatory factor in response to chymotrypsin treatment tells us that anti-enzymes should not necessarily be such giant molecules as to exclude their clinical use. The problem is more to pinpoint the enzyme to be counteracted, but this is outside the scope of this article.

Oestrogens are not new drugs and in this respect they would not belong in this section. It is felt, however, that in face of the more recent data they warrant re-evaluation as potential anti-inflammatory drugs. Their potent hormonal activity is an obvious major hindrance in their use in males. There are some indications that their hormonal and anti-inflammatory properties are less firmly interlinked than is commonly believed, and the concept of a "non-oestrogenic" oestrogen is a time-honoured idea. Besides having a mode of action completely different from existing anti-inflammatory drugs, in contrast to the latter they may lack gastrotoxicity entirely. In fact, they may be of benefit in certain gastric conditions (LAURENCE, 1966). As rheumatoid arthritic patients have, according to some opinions, a vulnerable gastric mucosa, a drug being anti-inflammatory and gastro-protective might be of potential interest.

Last but not least the cAMP pathway in the modulator function of mediators invites speculation as follows. If the loss of responsiveness of lymphocytes to prostaglandin-suppressed lymphokine secretion (MORLEY, 1974) might turn out to reflect a refractory adenylcyclase, then the defective homeostasis might be corrected through activating another adenylcyclase, insensitive to prostaglandins but susceptible to other substances.

Most of the above points in all probability also occurred to several inflammation researchers and therefore can be considered truisms. This chapter started with truisms and ends with them. In this way it remained faithful to itself.

Acknowledgements. I am grateful to my colleague and friend Dr. J. E. Vincent for devoting his time to comment on the text. Mr. M. J. Van Lieburg, a medical student in our faculty, furnished original literature on laudable pus. Dr. H. S. Verbrugh (Pathology Department of this University) kindly gave permission to select from his collection of articles on acupuncture. Mr. C. J. De Vos (Organon Laboratories, Oss, The Netherlands) was my main co-worker in earlier experiments on counter-irritation and on oestrogens and it is still pleasant to recall the time he assisted me. Mrs. B. H. Magda Busscher-Lauw typed the manuscript and helped compile the list of references.

References

Amberg, S., Loevenhart, A. S., McClure, W. B.: The influence of oxygen upon inflammatory reactions. J. Pharmacol. exp. Ther. **10**, 209—235 (1917)

Appenzeller, O., McAndrews, E. J.: The influence of the central nervous system on the triple response of Lewis. J. nerv. ment. Dis. **143**, 190—194 (1966)

Arntzen, F. C., Brisend, K.: Inhibition of carrageenin-induced paw oedema by catecholamines and amine-depleting drugs. Acta Pharmacol. (Kbh.) **32**, 193—204 (1973)

Ashton, F. E., Jamieson, J. C., Friesen, A. D.: Studies on the effect of inflammation on rat serum proteins. Canad. J. Biochem. **48**, 841—850 (1970)

Atkinson, D. C.: A comparison of the systemic anti-inflammatory activity of three different irritants in the rat. Arch. int. Pharmacodyn. **193**, 391—396 (1971)

Atkinson, D. C., Boura, A. L. A., Hicks, R.: Observations on the pharmacological properties of inflammatory exudate. Europ. J. Pharmacol. **8**, 348—354 (1969)

Atkinson, D. C., Hicks, R.: Relationship between the anti-inflammatory and irritant properties of inflammatory exudate. Brit. J. Pharmacol. **41**, 480—487 (1971)

Atkinson, D. C., Hicks, R.: Possible role of adrenergic mechanisms in the systemic anti-inflammatory activity of acetic acid in rats. Europ. J. Pharmacol. **26**, 158—165 (1974)

Atkinson, D. C., Hicks, R.: The possible occurrence of endogenous anti-inflammatory substances in the blood of injured rats. Brit. J. Pharmacol. **53**, 85—91 (1975a)

Atkinson, D. C., Hicks, R.: The anti-inflammatory activity of irritants. Agents Actions **5**, 239—249 (1975b)

Billingham, M. E. J., Davies, G. E.: Inhibition of inflammatory responses induced by a allergic reaction. In: Vane, J. R., Ferreira, S. H. (Eds.): Inflammation and Anti-Inflammatory Drugs. Handbook of Experimental Pharmacology, Vol. 50. Berlin-Heidelberg-New York: Springer 1977

Billingham, M. E. J., Gordon, A. H.: Changes in concentration and synthesis rates of plasma proteins during experimental arthritis. In: Peeters, H. (Ed.): Protides of Biological Fluids, pp. 451—454. Oxford: Pergamon Press 1976a

Billingham, M. E. J., Gordon, A. H.: The role of the acute reaction in inflammation. Agent Actions **6**, 195—200 (1976b)

Billingham, M. E. J., Gordon, A. H., Robinson, B. V.: Role of the liver in inflammation. Nature (New Biol.) **231**, 26—27 (1971)

Billingham, M. E. J., Robinson, B. V.: Two anti-inflammatory components in antilymphocytic serum. Nature (Lond.) **227**, 276—277 (1970)

Billingham, M. E. J., Robinson, B. V.: Separation of irritancy from the anti-inflammatory component of inflammation exudate. Brit. J. Pharmacol. **44**, 317—320 (1972)

Billingham, M. E. J., Robinson, V. B., Robson, J. B.: Partial purification of the anti-inflammatory factor(s) in inflammatory exudate. Brit. J. Pharmacol. **35**, 543—557 (1969a)

Billingham, M. E. J., Robinson, B. V., Robson, J. M.: Anti-inflammatory properties of human inflammatory exudate. Brit. med. J. **2**, 93—96 (1969b)

Bodel, P., Dillard, G. M., Kaplan, S. S., Malawista, S. E.: Anti-inflammatory effects of estradiol on human blood leucocytes. J. Lab. clin. Med. **80**, 373—384 (1972)

Bolam, J. P., Elliott, P. N. C., Ford-Hutchinson, A. W., Smith, M. J. H.: Histamine, 5-hydroxytryptamine, kinins, and the anti-inflammatory activity of human plasma fraction in carrageenan-induced paw oedema in the rat. J. Pharm. Pharmacol. **26**, 434—440 (1974a)

Bolam, J. P., Ford-Hutchinson, A. W., Elliott, P. N. C., Smith, M. J. H.: Effects of a human plasma fraction on skin reactions in the rat and rabbit. J. Pharm. Pharmacol. **26**, 660—661 (1974b)

Bonta, I. L.: Microvascular lesions as a target of anti-inflammatory and certain other drugs. Acta physiol. pharmacol. neerl. **15**, 188—222 (1969)

Bonta, I. L., Bhargava, N., De Vos, C. J.: Specific oedema-inhibiting property of a natural anti-inflammatory factor collected from inflamed tissue. Experientia (Basel) **26**, 759—760 (1970)

Bonta, I. L., Chrispijn, H., Noordhoek, J., Vincent, J. E.: Reduction of prostaglandin-phase in hind-paw inflammation and partial failure of indomethacin to exert anti-inflammatory effect in rats on essential fatty acid deficient diet. Prostaglandins **5**, 495—503 (1974)

Bonta, I. L., De Vos, C. J.: Report of work done at Organon Laboratories. Unpublished (1968)

Bonta, I. L., De Vos, C. J.: The effect of estriol-16,17-dihemisuccinate on vascular permeability as evaluated in the rat paw oedema test. Acta endocr. (Kbh.) **49**, 403—411 (1965)

Bonta, I. L., De Vos, C. J.: A natural anti-inflammatory response evoked by acute experimental inflammation. In: Bertelli, A., Houck, J. C. (Eds.): Inflammation Biochemistry and Drug Interaction, pp. 118—121. Amsterdam: Excerpta Medica 1969

Bonta, I. L., De Vos, C. J., Delver, A.: Inhibitory effects of estriol-16,17-disodium succinate on local haemorrhages induced by snake venom in canine heart-lung preparations. Acta endocr. (Kbh.) **48**, 137—146 (1965)

Bonta, I. L., Noordhoek, J.: Anti-inflammatory mechanism of inflamed-tissue factor. Agents Actions **3**, 348—356 (1973)

Bonta, I. L., Noordhoek, J.: Inflamed-tissue factor(s): an autoregulatory mechanism of some acute inflammatory responses. Experientia (Basel) **30**, 419—422 (1974)

Bonta, I. L., Parnham, M. J., Van Vliet, L., Vincent, J. E.: Mutual enhancement of the effects of prostaglandin E_1 and theophylline on the Freund adjuvant-induced arthritis syndrome of rats. Brit. J. Pharmacol. **59**, 438 P—439 P (1977 a)

Bonta, I. L., Parnham, M. J., Adolfs, M. J. P.: Reduced exudation and increased tissue proliferation during chronic inflammation in rats deprived of endogenous prostaglandin precursors. Prostaglandins **14**, 295—307 (1977 b)

Bonta, I. L., Vargaftig, B. B.: Cobra venom induced pulmonary vessel lesion: An unconventional model of acute inflammation. Bulletin Inst. Pasteur. **74**, 131—136 (1976)

Bonta, I. L., Vargaftig, B. B., De Vos, C. J., Grijsen, H.: Haemorrhagic mechanisms of some snake venoms in relation to protection by estriol succinate of blood vessel damage. Life Sci. **8**, 881—888 (1969)

Bourne, H. R.: Leucocyte cyclic AMP: Pharmacological regulation and possible physiological implications. In: Ramwell, P. W., Pharris, B. B. (Eds.): Prostaglandins in Cellular Biology, pp. 151—170. New York: Plenum Press Publ. 1972

Bourne, H. R., Melmon, K. L., Lichtenstein, L. M.: Histamine augments leucocyte cyclic AMP and blocks antigemic histamine release. Science **173**, 743—745 (1971)

Bray, M. A., Gordon, D., Morley, J.: Regulation of lymphokine secretion by prostaglandins. Agents Actions **6**, 171—175 (1976)

Brodie, B. B.: Displacement of one drug by another from carrier or receptor sites. Proc. roy. Soc. Med. **58**, 946—954 (1965)

Brown, R. A., West, G. B.: Sympathomimetic amines and vascular permeability. J. Pharm. Pharmacol. **17**, 119—120 (1965)

Brown, J. H., Kissel, J. W., Lish, P. M.: Studies on the acute inflammatory response. I. Involvement of the central nervous system in certain models of inflammation. J. Pharmacol. exp. Ther. **160**, 231—242 (1968 a)

Brown, J. H., Mackey, H. K., Riggild, D. A., Schwartz, N. L.: Studies on the acute inflammatory response. II. Influences of antihistamines and catecholamines on formaldehyde induced oedema. J. Pharmacol. exp. Ther. **160**, 243—248 (1968 b)

Brown, M. L., Ulett, G. A., Stern, J. A.: The effects of acupuncture on white cell counts. Amer. J. clin. Med. **2**, 383—398 (1974)

Büch, O., Wagner-Jauregg, Th.: Hemmung des Polyvinylpyrrolidon-Oedems der Rattenpfote durch intraperitoneale Injection Oedem-erzeugender Substanzen. Arzneimittel Forsch. **12**, 639—640 (1961)

Büch, O., Wagner-Jauregg, Th.: Zur Problematik antiphlogistischer Teste. Arzneimittel Forsch. **10**, 834—836 (1960)

Bullough, W. S.: The control of tissue growth. In: Bittar, E. E., Bittar, N. (Eds.): The Biological Basis of Medicine, Vol. I, pp. 311—333. London: Academic Press 1968

Collier, H. O. J.: Introduction to the actions of kinins and prostaglandins. Proc. roy. Soc. Med. **64**, 1—4 (1971)

Cygielman, S., Robson, J. M.: The effect of irritant substances on the deposition of granulation tissue in the cotton pellet test. J. Pharm. Pharmacol. **15**, 794—797 (1963)

Davies, G. E.: Inhibition of guinea-pig complement in vitro and in vivo by carrageenin. Immunology **6**, 561—568 (1963)

Di Pasquale, G., Girerd, R. J.: Anti-inflammatory properties of lyophilized inflammatory exudates. Amer. J. Physiol. **201**, 1155—1158 (1961)

Di Pasquale, G., Girerd, R. J., Beach, V. L., Steinetz, B. G.: Antiphlogistic action of granuloma pouch exudates in intact or adrenalectomized rats. Amer. J. Physiol. **205**, 1080—1082 (1963)

Di Pasquale, G., Rassaert, G., Richter, R., Welaj, P., Tripp, L.: Influence of prostaglandins (PG) E_2 and $F_{2\,alpha}$ on the inflammatory process. Prostaglandins **3**, 741—757 (1973)

Di Rosa, M., Giroud, J. P., Willoughby, D. A.: Studies of the mediators of the acute inflammatory response induced in rats in different sites by carrageenan and turentone. J. Path. **104**, 15—29 (1971)

Domenjoz, R., Theobald, W., Mörsdorf, K.: Die Beeinflussung der an der Ratte gleichzeitig gesetzten Formalin- und Dextranentzündung. Arzneimittel-Forschung **5**, 488 (1955)

Elliott, P. N. C., Bolam, J. P., Ford-Hutchinson, A. W., Smith, M. J. H.: The effects of a human plasma fraction on adjuvant arthritis and granuloma pellet reactions in the rat. J. Pharm. Pharmacol. **26**, 751—752 (1974 a)

Elliott, P. N. C., Ford-Hutchinson, A. W., Smith, M. J. H.: Anti-inflammatory and irritant effects of a fraction from normal human plasma. Brit. J. Pharmacol. **50**, 253—257 (1974b)
Fearn, H. J., Karady, S., West, G. B.: The role of the nervous system in local inflammatory responses. J. Pharm. Pharmacol. **17**, 761—765 (1965)
Ferreira, S. H., Moncada, S., Parsons, M., Vane, J. R.: The concomitant release of bradykinin and prostaglandin in the inflammatory response to carrageenin. Brit. J. Pharmacol. **52**, 108 P—109 P (1974)
Ford-Hutchinson, A. W., Elliott, P. N. C., Bolam, J. P., Smith, M. J. H.: The effects of a human plasma fraction on carrageenan-induced paw oedema in the rat. J. Pharm. Pharmacol. **26**, 878—881 (1974)
Ford-Hutchinson, A. W., Insley, M. Y., Elliott, P. N. C., Srurges, E. A., Smith, M. J. H.: Anti-inflammatory activity in human plasma. J. Pharm. Pharmacol. **25**, 881—886 (1973)
Ford-Hutchinson, A. W., Smith, M. J. H., Elliott, P. N. C., Bolam, J. P., Walker, J. R., Lobo, A. A., Badcock, J. K., Colledge, A. J., Billimoria, F. J.: Effects of a human plasma fraction on leucocyte migration into inflammatory exudates. J. Pharm. Pharmacol. **27**, 106—112 (1975)
Gammon, G. D., Starr, I., Jr., Bronk, D. W.: The effect of counterirritation upon pain produced by cutaneous injury. Amer. J. Physiol. **116**, 56 (1936)
Garattini, S., Jori, A., Bernardi, D., Carrara, C., Paglialunga, S., Segre, D.: Sensitivity of local oedemas to systemic pharmacological effects. In: Garattini, S., Dukes, M. N. G. (Eds.): Non-steroidal Anti-Inflammatory Drugs, pp. 151—161. Amsterdam: Excerptia Medica 1965
Garcia-Leme, J., Bohm, G. M., Migliorini, H., De Souza, Z. A.: Possible participation of insulin in the control of vascular permeability. Europ. J. Pharmacol. **29**, 298—306 (1974)
Garcia-Leme, J., Hamamura, L.: Formation of a factor increasing vascular permeability during electrical stimulation of the saphenous nerve in rats. Brit. J. Pharmacol. **51**, 383—389 (1974)
Garcia-Leme, J., Hamamura, L., Migliorini, R. H., Leite, M. P.: Influence of diabetes upon the inflammatory response of the rat. A pharmacological analysis. Europ. J. Pharmacol. **23**, 74—81 (1973)
Garcia-Leme, J., Lica, M.: Cortical potentials evoked by nociceptive stimuli: their depression by a factor released during saphenous nerve stimulation in the rat. Brit. J. Pharmacol. **51**, 491—496 (1974)
Garcia-Leme, J., Schapoval, E. E. S.: Stimulation of the hypothalamo-pituitary-adrenal axis by compounds formed in inflamed tissue. Brit. J. Pharmacol. **53**, 75—83 (1975)
Gaugas, J. M., Billingham, M. E. J., Rees, R. J. W.: Suppressive effect of homologous and heterologous inflammatory exudate on tuberculin sensitivity in the guinea-pig. Amer. Rev. resp. Dis. **101**, 432—434 (1970)
Gillies, C. H.: The theory of practice of counter-irritation. London: Macmillan & Co. 1895
Giroud, J. P., Timsit, J.: Activité anticomplémentaire et anti-inflammatoire du 48/80. C.R. Soc. Biol. (Paris) **164**, 2219—2224 (1970)
Giroud, J. P., Willoughby, D. A.: The interrelations of complement and a prostaglandin-like substance in acute inflammation. J. Path. **101**, 241—248 (1970)
Glatt, M., Peskar, B., Brune, K.: Leucocytes and prostaglandins in acute inflammation. Experientia (Basel) **30**, 1257—1259 (1974)
Glenn, M. E.: Adjuvant-induced arthritis: effects of certain drugs on incidence, clinical severity and biochemical changes. Amer. J. vet. Res. **27**, 339—352 (1966)
Glenn, M. E.: Chairman's closing remarks. In: Velo, G. P., Willoughby, D. A., Giroud, J. P. (Eds.): Future Trends in Inflammation, pp. 61—68. Padua-London: Piccin Medical Books 1974
Glenn, M. E., Bowman, B. J., Koslowske, T. C.: The systemic response to inflammation. Biochem. Pharmacol. Suppl. March, 27—49 (1968)
Glenn, M., Gray, J.: Adjuvant-induced polyarthritis in rats: biologic and histologic background. Amer. J. vet. Res. **26**, 1180—1194 (1965)
Glenn, M. E., Rohloff, N.: Antiarthritic and antiinflammatory effects of certain prostaglandins. Proc. Soc. exp. Biol. (N.Y.) **139**, 290—294 (1972)
Goldstein, S., Demeo, R., Shemano, I., Beiler, J. M.: A method for differentiating nonspecific irritants from anti-inflammatory agents using the carrageenin abcess test. Proc. Soc. exp. Biol. (N.Y.) **123**, 712—715 (1966)
Goldstein, S., Shemano, I., de Meo, R., Beiler, J. M.: Anti-inflammatory activity of several irritants in three models of experimental inflammation in rats. Arch. int. Pharmacodyn. **167**, 39—53 (1967)

Goodman, L. S., Gilman, A.: The pharmacological basis of therapeutics, 4th. Ed., p. 993. London: MacMillan & Co. 1970
Green, K. L.: The anto-inflammatory activity of catecholamines in the peritoneal cavity and hind paw of the mouse. Brit. J. Pharmacol. **45**, 322—332 (1972)
Green, K. L.: Mechanism of the pro-inflammatory activity of sympathomimetic amines in thermic oedema of the rat paw. Brit. J. Pharmacol. **50**, 243—251 (1974 a)
Green, K. L.: Role of endogenous catecholamines in the anti-inflammatory activity of alpha-adrenoceptor blocking agents. Brit. J. Pharmacol. **51**, 45—53 (1974 b)
Haining, C. J.: Effects of anti-rheumatic compounds and pyridine derivatives on the cutaneous response to thurfyl nicotinate in the guinea-pig. Brit. J. Pharmacol. **21**, 104—112 (1963)
Hakim, A. A., Dailey, J. P., Lesh, J. B.: Mechanism of action of certain enzymes: mediators of anti-inflammatory effects of chymotrypsin, trypsin, and pancreatic collagenase. In: Gavattini, S., Dukes, M. N. G. (Eds.): Non-Steroidal Anti-Inflammatory Drugs, pp. 265—269. Amsterdam: Excerpta Medica Foundation 1965
Hardy, J. D., Wolff, H. G., Goodell, H.: Studies on pain. A new method for measuring pain threshold: observations on spatial summation of pain. J. clin. Invest. **19**, 649—657 (1940)
Hayashi, H., Yoshinaga, M., Koono, M., Miyoshi, H., Matsumura, M.: Endogenous permeability factors and their inhibitors affecting vascular permeability in cutaneous arthus reactions and thermal injury. Brit. J. exp. Pathol. **45**, 419—435 (1964)
Hempel, K. H., Fernandez, L. A., Persellin, R. H.: Effect of pregnancy sera on isolated lysosomes. Nature (Lond.) **225**, 955—956 (1970)
Hench, P. S.: The ameliorating effect of pregnancy on chronic atrophic (infections rheumatoid) arthritis, fibrositis and intermittent hydrarthrosis. Proc. Mayo Clin. **13**, 161—167 (1938)
Hench, P. S., Kendall, E. C., Slocumb, C. H., Polley, H. F.: The effect of a hormone of the adrenal cortex (17-hydroxy-11-dehydrocorticosterone: compound (E) and of pituitary adrenocorticotrophic hormone on rheumatoid arthritis. Proc. Mayo Clin. **24**, 181—197 (1949)
Hicks, R.: The evaluation of inflammation induced by material implanted subcutaneously in the rat. J. Pharm. Pharmacol. **21**, 581—588 (1969)
Highton, T. C.: The effect of sera from patients with rheumatoid arthritis on carrageenin granuloma pouches, skin wounds and weight gain in rats. Brit. J. exp. Pathol. **44**, 137—144 (1963)
Hitchens, J. T., Goldstein, S., Shemano, I., Beiler, J. M.: Analgesic effects of irritants in three models of experimentally-induced pain. Arch. int. Pharmacodyn. **169**, 384—393 (1967)
Horakova, Z., Muratova, J.: Means of influencing the oedematous component of inflammation. In: Garattini, S., Dukes, M. N. G. (Eds.): Non-steroidal Anti-Inflammatory Drugs, pp. 237—244. Amsterdam: Excerpta Medica Foundation 1965
Huber, W., Schulte, T. L., Carson, S., Goldhamer, R. E., Vogin, E. E.: Some chemical and pharmacologic properties of a novel anti-inflammatory protein. Toxicol. appl. Pharmacol. **12**, 308 (1968)
Ichikawa, A., Nagasaki, M., Umezu, K., Hayashi, H., Tomita, K.: Effect of cyclic 3′,5′-monophosphate on oedema and granuloma induced by carrageenin. Biochem. Pharmacol. **21**, 2615—2626 (1972)
Ignarro, L. J., George, W. J.: Hormonal control of lysosomal enzyme release from human neutrophils. Elevation of cyclic nucleotide levels by autonomic neurohormones. Proc. nat. Acad. Sci. (Wash.) **71**, 2027—2031 (1974)
Ishioka, T., Honda, Y., Sagara, A., Shimamoto, T.: The effect of oestrogens on blueing lesions by bradykinine and histamine. Acta endocr. (Kbh.) **60**, 177—183 (1969)
Jancso, N., Jancso-Gabor, A., Szolcsanyi, J.: The role of sensory nerve endings in neurogenic inflammation induced in human skin and in the eye and paw of the rat. Brit. J. Pharmacol. **32**, 32—41 (1968)
Jancso-Gabor, A., Szolcsanyi, J.: The mechanism of neurogenic inflammation. In: Bertelli, A., Houck, J. C. (Eds.): Inflammation Biochemistry and Drug Interaction, pp. 210—217. Amsterdam: Excerpta Med. Publ. 1969
Jori, A., Bernardi, D.: Presence of a general irritation and inhibition of a local inflammation. MEd. Pharmacol. Exp. **14**, 500—506 (1966)
Kaada, B.: Mechanisms of acupuncture analgesia. T. norske Laegeforen. **94**, 422—431 (1974)
Kellet, D. N.: The relationship of adrenaline and carbohydrate metabolism to inflammation. In: Garattini, S., Dukes, M. N. G. (Eds.): Non-steroidal Anti-Inflammatory Drugs, pp. 203—206. Amsterdam: Excerpta Medica Foundation 1965

Kuehl,F.A., Humes,J.L., Egan,R.W., Ham,E.A., Beveridge,G.C., Van Arman,C.G.: Role of prostaglandin endoperoxide PGG_2 in inflammatory processes. Nature **265**, 170—173 (1977)
Laden,C., Quentin,B., Fosdick,L.S.: Anti-inflammatory effects of counterirritants. Amer. J. Physiol. **195**, 712—718 (1958)
Laurence,D.R.: Clinical Pharmacology, 3rd Ed. London: Churchill Ltd. Publ. 1966
Lerner,L.J., Carminati,P., Schiatti,P.: Correlation of anti-inflammatory activity with inhibition of prostaglandin synthesis activity of nonsteroidal anti-estrogens and estrogens. Proc. Soc. exp. Biol. (N.Y.) **148**, 329—332 (1975)
Lewin,A.J.: Acupuncture and its role in modern medicine. West. J. Med. **120**, 27—32 (1974)
Lichtenstein,L.M.: Sequential analysis of the allergic Response: cyclic AMP, Calcium and Histamine. Int. Arch. Allergy appl. Immun. **49**, 143—154 (1975)
Long,E.R.: The history of pathology. New York: Dover Publ. 1965
Lund-Olfsen,K., Menander,K.B.: Orgotein: a new anti-inflammatory metalloprotein drug: preliminary evaluation of clinical efficacy and safety in degenerative joint disease. Curr. ther. Res. **16**, 706—717 (1974)
Macarthur,J.G., Alstead,S.: Counter-irritants: a method of assessing their effect. Lancet **11**, 1060—1062 (1953)
McArthur,J.N., Dawkins,P.D., Smith,M.J.H., Hamilton,E.B.D.: Mode of action of antirheumatic drugs. Brit. med. J. **1971 II**, 677—679
McArthur,J.N., Smith,M.J.H., Freeman,P.C.: Anti-inflammatory substance in human serum. J. Pharm. Pharmacol. **24**, 669—671 (1972)
Melby,J., Egdahl,R., Spink,W.: Secretion and metabolism of cortisol after injection of endotoxin. J. Lab. clin. Med. **56**, 50—62 (1960)
Menkin,V.: Presence of a leucocytosis-promoting factor in inflammatory exudates. Science **90**, 237—238 (1939)
Menkin,V., Durham,N.C.: Leukopenia and inflammation. Arch. Path. **41**, 50—62 (1946)
Miller,R.L., Melmon,K.L.: The related roles of histamine, serotonin, and bradykinin in the pathogenesis of inflammation. Ser. Haematol. **3**, 5—38 (1970)
Moberg,G.P.: Site of action of endotoxins on hypothalamic pituitary-adrenal axis. Amer. J. Physiol. **220**, 397—400 (1971)
Morley,J.: Prostaglandins and lymphokines in arthritis. Prostaglandins **8**, 315—326 (1974)
Morley,J.: Prostaglandins as regulators of lymphoid cell function in allergic inflammation: a base for chronicity in rheumatoid arthritis. In: Dumonde,D.C. (Ed.): Infection and Immunity in Arthritis. Oxford-Edinburg: Blackwell 1976. In press
Morley,J., Bray,M.A., Gordon,D., Kennedy,W.P.: Interaction of prostaglandins and lymphokines in arthritis. In: Silvestrini,L.G. (Ed.): The Immunological Basis of Connective Tissue Disorders, pp. 129—140. Amsterdam: North Holland Publ. 1975
Mueller,M.N., Kappas,A.: Estrogen pharmacology II. Suppression of experimental immune polyarthritis. Proc. Soc. exp. Biol. (N.Y.) **117**, 845—847 (1964)
Nagy,S., Redei,A., Karady,S.: Studies on granulation tissue production in alloxan-diabetic rats. J. Endocr. **22**, 143—146 (1961)
Noordhoek,J., Bonta,I.L.: The mechanism of the anti-inflammatory and hypotensive effect of carrageenin. Arch. int. Pharmacodyn. **197**, 385—386 (1972)
Noordhoek,J., Bonta,I.L.: Mechanism of the anti-inflammatory effect of carrageenin pouch exudate. In: Velo,G.P., Willoughby,D.A., Giroud,J.P. (Eds.): Future trends in inflammation, pp. 249—259. Padua-London: Piccin Med. Books Publ. 1974
Parnham,M.J., Shoshan,S., Bonta,I.L., Neiman-Wollners,S.: Increased collagen synthesis in granulomata induced by carrageenan in rats which lack endogenous prostaglandin precursors Prostaglandins **14**, 709—714 (1977)
Parsons,C.M., Goetzi,F.R.: Effect of induced pain on pain threshold. Proc. Soc. exp. Biol. (N.Y.) **60**, 327—329 (1945)
Paulus,H.E., Whitehouse,M.W.: Non-steroid anti-inflammatory agents. Ann. Rev. Pharmacol. **13**, 118 (1973)
Peccetti,F.: Opera chirurgica. Lib. III. Francofurti (1619). In: Gurlt,E. (Ed.): Geschichte der Chirurgie und ihrer Ausübung, Vol. III, p. 598. Hildesheim: Georg Olms Verlagsbuchhandlung 1964
Persellin,R.H.: Lysosome stabilization by adjuvant arthritis serum. Arthr. and Rheum. **15**, 144—152 (1972)

Persellin, R. H., Perry, A.: Effect of pregnancy serum on experimental inflammation. Clin. Res. **20**, 49 (1972)
Piper, P. J., Collier, H. O. J., Vane, J. R.: Release of catecholamines in the guinea-pig by substances involved in anaphylaxis. Nature (Lond.) **213**, 838—840 (1967)
Plotz, C. M., Plotz, P. H., Lamont-Havers, R. W.: Workshop on the use of acupuncture in the rheumatic diseases. Arthr. and Rheum. **17**, 939—942 (1974)
Riesterer, L., Jaques, R.: Interference by beta-adrenoceptor blocking agents, with the antiinflammatory action of various drugs. Helv. physiol. pharmacol. Acta **26**, 287—293 (1968)
Rindani, T. H.: Recovery of an anti-inflammatory fraction from inflammatory exudate. Indian. J. med. Res. **44**, 673—675 (1956)
Robinson, B. V., Robson, J. M.: Production of an anti-inflammatory substance at a site of inflammation. Brit. J. Pharmacol. **23**, 420—432 (1964)
Robinson, B. V., Robson, J. M.: Further studies on the anti-inflammatory factor found at a site of inflammation. Brit. J. Pharmacol. **26**, 372—384 (1966)
Rocha e Silva, M.: Chemical mediators of the acute inflammatory reaction. Ann. N.Y. Acad. Sci. **116**, 899—911 (1964)
Rocha e Silva, M.: The possible kinin function in the acute inflammatory reaction. Pharmacology and the future of man. Proceedings 5th International Congress Pharmacology, San Francisco **5**, 320—327 (1972)
Rocha e Silva, M., Cavalcanti, R. Q., Reis, M. L.: Anti-inflammatory action of sulfated polysaccharides. Biochem. Pharmacol. **18**, 1285—1295 (1969)
Rocha e Silva, M., Garcia-Leme, J.: Chemical mediators of the acute inflammatory reaction. Oxford: Pergamon Press 1972
Rooney, P. J., Hayes, J. R., Webb, J., Lee, P., Carson, R. W.: Is gastrin involved in the inflammatory responses. In: Velo, G. P., Willoughby, D. A., Giroud, J. P. (Eds.): Future Trends in Inflammation, pp. 277—281. Padua-London: Piccin Medical Books 1974
Rudas, B., Stoklaska, E.: Wechselbeziehungen von Pfotenödemen und Wundheilung bei Ratten. Med. Pharmacol. Exp. **16**, 57—65 (1967)
Sarcione, E. J., Bogden, A. E.: Hepatic synthesis of alpha$_2$ (acute phase)-globulin of rat plasma. Science **153**, 547—548 (1966)
Sarkar, N., Fosdick, L. S.: Mode of action of chymotrypsin on pleural inflammation. J. Pharmacol. exp. Ther. **146**, 258—264 (1964)
Selye, H., Cunnington, J., Somogyi, A., Cote, G.: Acceleration and inhibition of wound healing by topical treatment with different types of inflammatory irritants. Amer. J. Surg. **117**, 610—614 (1969)
Selye, H., Somogyi, A., Vegh, P.: Inflammation topical stress and the concept of pluricausal diseases. In: Honck, J. C., Forscher, B. K. (Eds.): Chemical Biology of Inflammation, pp. 107—122. Oxford: Pergamon Press 1968
Shanahan, R. W.: Local activity of anti-inflammatory and irritant agents on rat paw oedema induced by carrageenin. Arch. int. Pharmacodyn. **175**, 186—192 (1968)
Silvestrini, B., Burberi, S., Catanese, B.: Inflammatory responses in normal and adrenalectomized rats during obstructive jaundice. Jap. J. Pharmacol. **18**, 421—429 (1968)
Smith, M. J. H.: Antiinflammatory Agents of Animal Origin. In: Vane, J. R., Ferreira, S. H. (Eds.): Inflammation and Anti-Inflammatory Drugs. Handbook of Experimental Pharmacology, Vol. 50. Berlin-Heidelberg-New York: Springer 1977
Smith, M. J. H., Colledge, A. J., Elliott, P. N. C., Bolam, J. P., Ford-Hutchinson, A. W.: A human plasma fraction with anti-inflammatory but without either analgesic or antipyretic properties. J. Pharm. Pharmacol. **26**, 836—837 (1974a)
Smith, M. J. H., Ford-Hutchinson, A. W., Elliott, P. N. C., Bolam, J. P.: Prostaglandins and the anti-inflammatory activity of a human plasma fraction in carrageenan-induced paw oedema in the rat. J. Pharm. Pharmacol. **26**, 692—698 (1974b)
Spangler, A. S., Antoniades, H. N., Sotman, S. L.: Enhancement of the anti-inflammatory action of hydrocortisone by estrogen. J. clin. Endocr. **29**, 650—655 (1969)
Spector, W. G., Willoughby, D. A.: The enzymic inactivation of an adrenaline-like substance in inflammation. J. Path. Bact. **80**, 271—280 (1960)
Toivanen, P., Maatta, K., Suolanen, R., Tykkylainen, R.: Effect of estrone and progesterone on adjuvant arthritis in rats. Med. Pharmacol. **17**, 33—42 (1967)

Van Gool, J., Ladiges, N. C. J. J.: Production of foetal globulin after injury in rat and man. J. Path. **97**, 115—126 (1969)
Van Gool, J., Schreuder, J., Ladiges, N. C. J. J.: Inhibitory effect of foetal α_2 globulin, an acute phase protein, on carrageenin oedema in the rat. J. Path. **112**, 245—262 (1974)
Vincent, J. E., Bonta, I. L., De Vries-Kragt, K., Bhargava, N.: L'influence des oestrogènes sur la perméabilité de la paroi vasculaire. Steroidologia **1**, 367—377 (1970)
Vinegar, R., Macklin, A. W., Truax, J. F., Selph, J. L.: Pedel edema formation in normal and granulocytopenic rats. In: Van Arman, G. C. (Ed.): White Cells in Inflammation, pp. 111—130. Springfield: C. C. Thomas 1974
Vinegar, R., Schreiber, W., Hugo, R.: Biphasic development of carrageenin edema in rats. J. Pharmacol. exp. Ther. **166**, 96—103 (1969)
Vinegar, R., Truax, J. F.: Some characteristics of the anti-inflammatory activity of carrageenin in rats. Pharmacologist **12**, 202 (1970)
Ward, F. A.: A primer of pathology, p. 43. London: Butterworth 1967
Weissmann, G., Rita, G. A.: Molecular basis of gouty inflammation. Interaction of monosodium urate crystals with lysosomes and liposomes. Nature (New Biol.) **240**, 167—172 (1972)
Weissmann, G., Zurier, R. B., Hoffstein, S.: Leucocytes as secretory organs of inflammation. Agents Actions **3**, 370—379 (1973)
Whitehouse, M. W.: Abnormal drug metabolism in rats after an inflammatory insult. Agents Actions **3**, 312—316 (1973)
Whitehouse, M. W.: Ambivalent role of copper in inflammatory disorders. Symposium. Agents Actions **6**, 201—206 (1976)
Willoughby, D. A., Coote, E., Turk, J. L.: Complement in acute inflammation. J. Path. **97**, 295—307 (1969)
Winder, C. V., Wax, J., Burr, V., Been, M., Rosiere, C. E.: A study of pharmacological influences on ultraviolet erythema in guinea-pigs. Arch. int. Pharmacodyn. **116**, 261—292 (1958)
Winne, D.: Die Bildung des Rattenpfotenödems durch Polyvinylpyrrolidon. Arzneimittel-Forsch. **14**, 1290—1294 (1964)
Winter, Ch. A., Flataker, L.: Nociceptive thresholds as affected by parenteral administration of irritants and of various antinoceptive drugs. J. Pharmacol. exp. Ther. **148**, 373—379 (1965)
Winternitz, R.: Über die entzündungswidrige Wirkung ätherischer Öle. Naunyn-Schmiedeberg's Arch. exp. Path. Pharmak. **46**, 163—180 (1901)
Zurier, R. B., Hoffstein, S., Weissmann, G.: Suppression of acute and chronic inflammation in adrenalectomized rats by pharmacologic amounts of prostaglandins. Arthr. and Rheum. **16**, 606—619 (1973)

Contribution of the Inflammatory Mediators to the Signs and Symptoms of Inflammation

CHAPTER 16

Inflammatory Mediators and Vascular Events

L. J. F. YOULTEN

A. Introduction

The phenomena of the early stages of inflammation include obvious changes in the microcirculation. Most of the classic "cardinal signs" of acute inflammation can be ascribed to these microvascular changes. The redness and increase in local temperature reflect vasodilatation and consequent increase in blood flow; the swelling results from increased filtration of fluid due to increase in both the hydrostatic pressure within, and the permeability to macromolecules of, the small blood vessels. Another phenomenon, the invasion of the inflamed tissues by phagocytic cells from the circulating blood, also involves a change in the endothelial cells of the same vessels, leading to sticking and subsequent extravascular migration of leucocytes. These vascular events are observed in many different experimental forms of inflammation and represent an intrinsic part of the early inflammatory response. There is considerable evidence that some at least of these vascular phenomena of inflammation are mediated through endogenous chemical agents.

Unfortunately, damaged tissues are embarrassingly rich in substances with pharmacological effects that suggest they may be mediators of the vascular events of inflammation. In this chapter, we examine how the involvement of particular mediators may be established or excluded. The pharmacological properties of individual mediators are dealt with in detail in their respective sections elsewhere in this book. The examples chosen to illustrate this chapter concern almost exclusively those chemical mediators whose chemical structure is known and which are available in pure form, namely histamine, bradykinin (Bk), 5-hydroxytryptamine (5-HT), and prostaglandins (PGs). This is not because other substances are thought to be less important, but because it is difficult to argue from incomplete data. When substances such as lymph node or spleen permeability factor (WILLOUGHBY et al., 1962; HARTLEY et al., 1973) or neurogenic factor (HAMMAMURA and GARCIA LEME, 1973) have their structures identified and are available in pure form, the same criteria as are described here may be applied to assess whether or not they play an important role in natural or experimental inflammation.

The other limitation accepted in this chapter is that most of the phenomena described are those of the acute inflammatory response. Although there is a vascular component to chronic inflammation, other aspects are probably more important. Little work appears to have been published on the responses of the blood vessels in chronically inflamed tissues to the known mediators of vascular effects. These may well be different from those of normal tissues. In general, the investigations in chronic inflammation of the mechanisms leading to tissue destruction have received more attention than has the role of the early mediators in the later phases. This is understandable, since although suppression of the pain, swelling and joint stiffness of rheumatoid disease can be achieved by a number of effective anti-inflammatory drugs, the eventual outcome in the form of tissue destruction and deformity appears to be mediated by some process not susceptible to such drugs, and presumably involving separate mechanisms.

B. Criteria for Implicating a Particular Mediator in the Production of Specific Effects

The criteria put forward by DALE, which should be satisfied to establish a role for a particular substance as a chemical transmitter, have been adapted, as suggested by VANE (1972), to the field of inflammatory mediators. Unfortunately, for most of the suggested and even some of the well-established mediators, the criteria are far from fully met. In some cases only one criterion has been met, and that not rigorously, before a substance has been suggested as a mediator. This is partly because of the nature of the inflammatory process. As it is essentially a connective tissue phenomenon with an important vascular component, it is not possible to study it in isolation. The early phenomena of inflammation still need to be studied in living, preferably unanaesthetised, whole animals, with all the attendant disadvantages of such studies.

The criteria, which are dealt with in detail below, are as follows:

1. The mediator should be detectable at the right place, at the right time, in amounts adequate to account for the effect in question.
2. The mediator, when administered in concentrations of the order of those found in the lesion, should produce the observed effects, and no others.
3. Specific blocking agents or antagonists of the effects of the postulated mediator should prevent or attenuate the effect.
4. Prevention of release of the mediator should abolish or prevent the effect.
5. Agents or procedures preventing the breakdown or removal of the mediator should prolong or potentiate the effect.

I. Mediator Released in Adequate Amounts at Right Time

This is a difficult matter to assess clearly. If mediators are present in a preformed state, ready for release by an appropriate stimulus to be followed by destruction or removal, then their release may be deduced from a declining tissue content of the mediator. Such an approach, for example, may demonstrate the release of histamine from mast cells in tissues (RILEY and WEST, 1955). Another approach involves the detection of mediators in increased amounts either in inflamed tissues or in perfusates (ROCHA E SILVA and ROSENTHAL, 1961; GREAVES and SØNDERGAARD, 1970) or exudates (WILLIS, 1969) from them. Possibly easier to detect and localise in tissue by, for example, histochemical techniques, are enzymes able to synthesise particular mediators. Detection of such enzymes in increased amounts in inflamed tissues (SCHAYER, 1963) is only of indirect significance, and the assumption that such increases are necessarily associated with increased release or production of the mediator concerned is not necessarily valid.

It is difficult to estimate accurately the amounts of mediators present in tissues, and for this reason various techniques have been developed to produce inflammation experimentally in natural cavities such as joints, the pleural space or the peritoneal cavity, or in artificially produced air pockets, blisters or implanted capsules or sponges. In this way, a fluid exudate can be obtained which is convenient for sampling and analysis. All these techniques involve some local trauma in creating the lesion, which must be allowed for by using proper controls. There may be important differences between these sites, depending on the permeability of the local blood vessels, their reactions to different mediators and the types of cell present in the area at the time of introduction of the inflammatory stimulus. It may be unwise to extrapolate too freely between one site and another, even within a single species.

Techniques involving extraction of tissues do not always differentiate between mediators present in the tissue and those released during the extraction procedure, and are therefore often open to misinterpretation. The role of histamine as a chemical mediator of vascular reactions in traumatised skin was first suggested by LEWIS (1927). Certainly histamine has been identified in many tissues in many species; a comprehensive list is to be found in VUGMANN and ROCHA E SILVA (1966). The amount varies according to the species, the tissue and even the region. A positive correlation has been found between histamine content and blueing in response to histamine liberators in different regions of skin in rats and guinea pigs (FELDBERG and MILES, 1953; BERALDO and DIAS DA SILVA, 1966). The histamine content usually parallels the number of the mast cells, the granules of which have been shown to contain histamine but some, at least, of the histamine in skin appears not to be associated with granules. Some inflammatory stimuli are followed by mast cell degranulation.

Although 5-HT is present in many tissues, and sometimes associated with histamine in mast cell granules, no definite role in inflammation has been established for 5-HT except in rats and mice (WILHELM, 1962).

Unlike the previous two mediators, the peptide Bk has as its inactive precursor a plasma protein or kininogen. In theory, therefore, there is no difficulty in its being formed in inflamed tissues, since the precursor is present throughout the plasma and interstitial space. Bk is rapidly destroyed, however, and this makes its detection or measurement difficult in inflamed tissues or exudates. Measuring the levels of the enzymes (kininogenases) (LEWIS, 1959) or converting the inactive precursor (kininogen) to kinin, or estimation of the precursor itself have all been used as alternative approaches.

The first lipid substances to be suggested as inflammatory mediators were PGE_2 and $PGF_{2\alpha}$ (WILLIS, 1969). They fulfilled the criterion of being present in inflammatory exudates.

II. Mediator Produces Effect When Administered in Reasonable Concentration

Many substances are active vasodilators or produce other signs associated with inflammation when topically applied or injected. Since there is usually little information available about the concentration of the proposed mediator in inflamed tissues, it is difficult to decide what is a reasonable dose or concentration to apply; some mediators are destroyed or removed rapidly from tissues. Another problem is how to measure the inflammatory effect of the administered mediator. Sometimes effects take minutes or hours to develop, and only one estimation of effect can be made. Methods which have been commonly used for assessing the vascular effects of mediators include the blueing of skin or other tissues after intravenous injection of protein-bound dyes, or similar techniques using proteins or other macromolecules labelled with radioisotopes. In general, pharmacologists have not been sufficiently critical of their own techniques in this field. Much published work is at best only semiquantitative, and some authors do not seem to appreciate that changes in such measurements may not be due to changes in vascular permeability. The problem is that since the haemodynamic status of the inflamed tissue is altered, increased flow and pressures may themselves lead to increases in the volume of the local extravascular space and produce apparent changes in extravascular label, which may have little or nothing to do with changes in permeability of the vessel wall. Similarly, an agent which produced only an increase in permeability might not produce a marked increase in extravascular label unless blood flow and pressure were also increased locally. To take an extreme case, if an agent produced an increase in protein permeability accompanied by profound local vasoconstriction, then the techniques mentioned above would not detect the permeability change. Such changes are most obvious when, as is usually the case, they are accompanied by increased blood flow and filtration. This problem is discussed in more detail below.

The effects of histamine on the vessels of human skin were carefully studied and described by LEWIS and GRANT (1924) and LEWIS (1927). They include both vasodilatation and oedema. The same effects have been found in many other species and other tissues, and in many situations have been associated with increased vascular permeability as judged by dye or labelled protein extravasation. Like the effects of 5-HT and Bk, vascular structural changes associated with application of histamine to tissues, namely disruption of inter-endothelial cell junctions, or labelling of vessels with colloidal carbon, are seen only in the venous segments of the microcirculation, not in the true capillaries or arterioles (MAJNO et al., 1961). 5-HT can itself produce vascular changes indistinguishable from those caused by histamine in rats and mice.

The main justification for considering Bk as an important inflammatory mediator is its extremely potent inflammatory effects on injection. It is a potent vasodilator in animals (HOLTON and HOLTON, 1952; ELLIOTT et al., 1960) and in man (FOX et al., 1961; BURCH and DE PASQUALE, 1962) at concentrations as low as 10^{-10} g/ml applied locally or 10^{-7} g intra-arterially. Intense blueing, interpreted as evidence of increased vascular permeability, is also seen (HOLDSTOCK et al., 1957) on intradermal injection. PGs reproduce features of inflammation when injected into normal skin (CRUNKHORN and WILLIS, 1971).

III. Effect Blocked by Specific Blocking Agents

In some cases, more or less specific pharmacological antagonists are available which abolish or attenuate the inflammatory effects of administered agents. These agents may then be used in experimental inflammation to discover whether or not the particular agonist is involved. While of undoubted help, the contribution made by this approach to the understanding of inflammatory mechanisms has been disappointingly limited. Abolition of an effect by an antagonist is not, of course, itself very strong evidence of the involvement of the agonist in causing the effect. A so-called antihistamine, for example, may have many actions other than antagonism of the actions of histamine, including the possibility of antagonising the actions of other, possibly unknown mediator substances, potentiating natural anti-inflammatory mechanisms or having a direct effect (ALTURA, 1970). A negative result, too, may be misleading. The subdivision of the receptors for catecholamines into α and β, and for histamine into H_1 and H_2 types, respectively, each with specific groups of antagonist drugs, demonstrates the difficulties of interpreting the failure of an antagonist to block an inflammatory response. Unless the antagonist can be demonstrated to block the particular response which is being studied, when produced by the injected agonist, doubt will always be present that one is dealing with a different class of effect. It has also been suggested that mediator released at or within effector cells is not susceptible to the action of blocking drugs. Relatively specific antagonists are known only for histamine and 5-HT.

The use of antihistamine drugs has both supported a role for histamine early in acute inflammation and also shown that its importance is limited. In several forms of acute inflammation antihistamine agents, in doses known to abolish the vascular effects of injected histamine, considerably reduce the initial phases of hyperaemia, oedema and increased vascular permeability (SPECTOR and WILLOUGHBY, 1959; WILHELM and MASON, 1960). Unless the drug has some anti-inflammatory action independent of histamine (which is by no means unlikely), this supports the idea that histamine is involved. Even more significant, however, is the fact that antihistamine drugs, when effective, only modify the initial phase of inflammation. This demonstrates both that the later phases of inflammation can proceed in the absence of a histamine-mediated, antihistamine susceptible, effect and also that the early histamine effect is not essential for the development of the subsequent phases.

An effective antagonist of the inflammatory actions of 5-HT (BOL 148), has some anti-inflammatory action in certain forms of inflammation (PARRATT and WEST, 1957) but not in others (SPECTOR and WILLOUGHBY, 1959), not even in rats—one of the few species in which 5-HT has inflammatory actions.

One of the difficulties in clearly defining the importance of Bk and of PGs as mediators of acute inflammation is the lack of effective or specific antagonists to their action.

IV. Prevention of Release Prevents Effects

This approach has been somewhat more fruitful than that mentioned in the previous section. Prevention of release of mediators may be achieved either by previous depletion of stores of precursors or of ready formed mediator, as in the case of histamine release by mast cell degranulating agents, or by interfering with the enzymic synthesis of newly formed mediators. A good example of the latter approach was the discovery that many non-steroid anti-inflammatory drugs were powerful inhibitors of PG synthesis (VANE, 1971; SMITH and WILLIS, 1971; FERREIRA et al., 1971). Since histamine and 5-HT antagonists, such as mepyramine and methysergide, had only very limited effects in most forms of inflammation, this new discovery about the mode of action of the aspirin-like drugs suggested that endogenous PGs played an important role in those types of inflammation in which such drugs were effective. This in turn greatly increased interest in the possible involvement of PGs in inflammation.

For some mediators, specific measures to prevent release are not available, but the mediators or putative mediators for which such an approach may be used include kinins, histamine and complement. Usually, release is prevented by prior depletion of the mediator or of a precursor. Reducing the levels of cells thought to act as a source of mediator, such as polymorphonuclear leucocytes, lymphocytes or platelets, also falls within this category. With all these measures for both humoral and cellular factors, the main problem is knowing how specific the procedure is. Many depleting agents and cytotoxic agents have more than one known effect. Inhibitors of proteinases prevent the formation of kinins from kininogens and should be able to eliminate the component of inflammation or of other pathological processes due to kinins. In fact, such enzyme inhibition, for example with soya bean trypsin inhibitor, does have some anti-inflammatory effect, as shown in the case of carrageenin oedema (VAN ARMAN et al., 1965). Other processes involving proteinases, such as blood coagulation, fibrinolysis and complement activation are also likely to be affected by this class of inhibitor, so making it less specific as a test of kinin involvement.

V. Prevention of Breakdown of Mediator Enhances Effect

Although in theory this approach could be applied to many mediators of inflammation, there are at present relatively few methods for interfering with the breakdown of specific mediators. One such method involves the use of Bk potentiating peptide (FERREIRA et al., 1974) which could be expected to potentiate any effects produced by endogenous Bk production. It acts by inhibiting kininase, but is not completely specific having at least one other important biological action, namely the inhibition of conversion of angiotensin I to angiotensin II. Another substance which inhibits kininase, 1, 10-phenanthroline, has also been reported to enhance foot oedema caused by carrageenin or cellulose sulphate, but not that induced by egg albumin or dextran (CAPASSO et al., 1975).

C. Difficulties With the Above

All the above five approaches have their shortcomings, more or less serious. Most concern lack of specificity: artefacts are common in the measurements of mediators in tissues; potent mediators may be short-lived; blocking agents may not block the effect under observation because it is mediated through different receptors. Some of these and other problems are mentioned below, with examples.

I. Limitations of Methods of Detection and Identification

For some mediators, established or putative, chemical or physical methods of a high degree of specificity are available. Some colorimetric tests, and even more so such techniques as gas chromatography—mass spectrometry, give a certainty of identification that is hard to challenge. When such methods are available, the investigator's problems are those of devising suitable preparative procedures for samples. The problem is at least halved; the identity is settled but the question of whether it was present in active form in the inflamed tissue remains. Careful controls are necessary to exclude artefacts of extraction.

Almost by definition, inflammatory mediators are potent compounds, and for some of them chemical methods are just not sensitive enough. Bioassay still has a part to play in the discovery and characterisation of inflammatory mediators, particularly when made selective by the use of several tissues in parallel and by the use of blocking drugs in the superfusing fluid. The most commonly used bioassay method is, of course, the measurement of contraction of isolated strips of smooth muscle. Remarkably, many of the postulated inflammatory mediators are agents contracting or relaxing various smooth muscle preparations. This may, of course, just be a reflection of the popularity of this technique as a screening test when searching for possible inflammatory mediators. It certainly makes more sense to use microvascular effects as a test for putative mediators of such effects, but these are less widely used than muscle strip bioassay. PGs not readily measurable by smooth muscle bioassay, such as PGD_2, have been comparatively neglected until recently, even though it is now apparent that some of them have significant and interesting biological activity on such systems as platelets (MILLS and MACFARLANE, 1974) and small blood vessels (FLOWER et al., 1976).

II. Ubiquity of Mediators, Extraction Artefacts

Some inflammatory mediators are stored ready for rapid release, as in the granules of mast cells, or formed from precursors present in plasma and interstitial fluid, such as kininogens. This makes it rather easy to extract such substances from tissues, but difficult to interpret the presence of such substances, once found. Since release or formation of mediators may be triggered by such non-specific measures as mechanical trauma, cooling, dilution or contact with foreign surfaces, all possible precautions must be taken to avoid artefacts in the preparation of the samples. The use of uninflamed tissues as controls can be helpful when negative, but when mediators are extracted from such tissues in similar amounts to those found in inflamed areas, the involvement of the mediator concerned cannot be definitely excluded or established.

In those few cases where potent inhibitors of synthesis or release are available, they may be used to halt production of mediator during tissue preparation or extraction. Addition of indomethacin, for example, can prevent the PG production which may occur during the homogenisation of many normal uninflamed tissues. Where specific chemical methods of preventing synthesis or release are not available, such measures as rapid chilling, homogenisation of deep-frozen samples and protein precipitation may be helpful, provided the mediator can be shown to survive such treatment in measurable form.

III. Possible Involvement of Potent Short-Lived Compounds

There are also problems in interpreting the absence of a particular mediator, since potent destructive and de-activating mechanisms exist for the removal of various active compounds in living tissue. Potent compounds whose biological half-life is short may be very important, but difficult to detect. Knowledge of the biochemical pathways of degradation may be useful in suggesting ways of preventing breakdown or of identifying biologically less active breakdown products. As well as PGs, other products of unsaturated fatty acids such as hydroxy eicosatetraenoic acid and thromboxanes may also be involved. The short biological half-life of some of these compounds makes it difficult to investigate them by direct methods.

IV. Interactions Between Mediators, Dual Mechanisms, Release One by Another

The investigation of mediators of inflammation is bedevilled by the existence of several systems by which similar vascular effects may be produced. Histamine, Bk and E-type PGs, for example, can produce very similar vascular effects upon local injection. The fact that these different compounds can also interact, in some cases potentiating, in others inhibiting each other's actions, can make interpretation of experiments very difficult. The fact, for example, that neither an antihistamine drug nor a PG synthetase inhibitor has much effect on a particular inflammatory phenomenon does not mean that neither histamine nor PGs are involved. It may be that they are both involved, particularly if one agent has some suppressive effect on the production of another. The only ways to deal with this very difficult problem are to use blockers and inhibitors in combination as well as separately, and to work on inflammatory lesions which are submaximal, so that any potentiating effects will be apparent.

The release of one mediator by another may also complicate the picture. If, for example, PGs were to cause their inflammatory effects by releasing histamine in a particular inflammatory model, then either antihistamine drugs or PG synthetase inhibitors might have an anti-inflammatory effect. This could be difficult to interpret if the possibility of sequential release were not borne in mind.

The observation that some of the vascular effects of histamine can be potentiated by PGs raises the interesting question of how important such interactions between mediators may be. The position of 5-HT as a mediator has been complicated by the discovery that it may release histamine (FELDBERG and SMITH, 1953) and potentiate some of the effects of Bk (SICUTERI et al., 1965). DI ROSA and SORRENTINO (1970) have argued from the modification of the time-course of carrageenin inflammation over the first 6 h by various antagonists or depletors, that a sequential release of mediators is involved. They suggest that histamine and 5-HT are responsible for the early phase, succeeded by kinins and later followed by PGs. Complement activation is said to occur throughout. Much more direct evidence is needed to show that this is the case, since other interpretations of their data are possible. A fading vascular response, or tachyphylaxis to histamine, known to occur from experiments in which histamine is applied continuously (see below), could account for the failure of antihistamine drugs to modify inflammation after the first 90 min, while the responding tissues may become more sensitive to other mediators later. Another possibility is that the "late-phase" mediator, PG, although being continually produced from the beginning, takes time to reach levels at which it has an effect.

V. Effect of Other Factors

Both blood pressure and body temperature are likely to be low in an animal anaesthetised for a long period, and this no doubt explains, at least in part, why acute inflammatory lesions do not develop so well in the anaesthetised animal (MILES and MILES, 1952). Also, drugs with an apparent anti-inflammatory effect may be acting non-specifically, by an effect on blood pressure or skin blood flow.

One interesting field, which has not been fully investigated, is the relationship between the early phases of acute inflammation and the later phases. If non-specific or specific measures prevent the full development of the early phases of acute inflammation, is the progression to later phases or to chronic inflammation affected? Treatment of burns by local cooling or by dropping the local blood pressure, as by elevation of a burned limb, may have some rational basis of this type. Effective suppression of the histamine phase of acute thermal injury, however, does not seem to modify the later events (SPECTOR and WILLOUGHBY, 1959; WILHELM and MASON, 1960).

VI. Specificity of Different Inflammatory Models, Difficulties in Extrapolation

The literature on inflammation is notable for the variety of experimental models which have been used by different workers. Many different agents—physical, bacterial, chemical, and immunological irritants—have been used to induce experimental lesions, and the choice of method is apparently often made on grounds of expediency. A worker interested in the mode of action of a particular anti-inflammatory drug must obviously choose an inflammatory model against which the drug is effective. The method chosen must also be convenient for the measurement of the changes which are of special interest. Swelling or oedema is most easily followed by measuring the changes in volume of the paws of small animals. Vascular permeability changes are most easily measured in skin. Cellular infiltration is easier to investigate in exudates than in tissues. Thus, methods chosen for a particular study may be quite unsuitable for use in another.

Different inflammatory models have been to some extent classified into groups, such as complement-dependent, nerve supply-dependent, neutrophil-dependent, and so on. Such categorisation of the existing methods is still incomplete, but it would be helpful if any investigator introducing a new inflammatory model were to take the trouble of identifying as far as possible which of the existing models it resembled. The existence of so many different models, between which comparison is often difficult, is a major problem in this area of research.

VII. Species Variation, Strain, Site, etc.

Not only the agent used to cause experimental inflammation but also the species and even the site, may be critical. It is thought, for example, that the mediators involved in local and systemic anaphylaxis in the rat and mouse include 5-HT (WILHELM, 1962). This substance is not of great importance in other species. Dextran induces an anaphylactic syndrome, with snout and paw swelling, in some strains of rats but not in others (HARRIS and WEST, 1963). Just as certain smooth muscle preparations may be particularly sensitive to specific mediators, so certain strains may be particularly sensitive to such mediators or to inflammatory models involving them.

VIII. Doubts on Specificity of Blockers

In the case of many of the postulated mediators of vascular events in inflammation, no method of blocking their effects pharmacologically is yet known. This is particularly true of the, as yet, chemically undefined compounds. Specific blocking agents for the inflammatory effects of such mediators would be very useful, not only in defining the role of such substances in inflammation, but also for their possible therapeutic use. Much effort by the pharmaceutical industry is still expended on finding variations on existing drugs, such as the non-steroid group of aspirin-like drugs, now widely believed to act by inhibiting prostaglandin synthetase. Since many of the toxic side-effects of such drugs may also be due to inhibition of PG synthesis, it is very likely that further investigation in this field will produce only marginal improvements in therapeutic ratio, since only those aspects of inflammation mediated or modulated through PGs will be suppressed by such drugs, and a similar spectrum of toxic effects will be likely to occur. Rather, the search should be for specific antagonists of the harmful actions of PG and other mediators. A good analogy here is the H_1 antihistamine group of drugs, which block the inflammatory effects of histamine but not its stimulation of gastric acid secretion. More characterisation of the receptors of the inflammatory mediators would be useful.

D. Vascular Events Possibly Mediated by Endogenous Agents and Methods of Measuring Them

In this section some of the methods which have been adopted for measuring vascular aspects of inflammation will be briefly described and some comments made on their usefulness, accuracy and merits. In some cases, techniques which are relatively crude have been adopted because they are fast and convenient for screening procedures. Such methods are often not suitable when the fundamental processes involved in inflammation are being investigated.

I. Vasoconstriction, Vasodilatation, Changes in Blood Flow

Alterations in blood flow in inflamed tissues are common and a prominent feature of microscopical observation of suitably thin inflamed tissues. When the skin is the site of inflammation, the colour of the skin—provided it is not darkly pigmented or covered with fur, hair, feathers or scales—is easy to observe, particularly when surrounded by normal skin. Blanching or reddening of the skin, though reasonably interpreted as evidence of vasoconstriction or vasodilatation respectively, does not in itself give any information about the blood flow changes occurring in the area. For the latter, the temperature of the skin may be a more reliable index of blood flow than its colour. Skin with normal or reduced blood flow may appear red because of venous dilatation. Since most of the skin's blood volume is contained in small veins and venules, it is changes in these which make most difference to skin colour.

Many methods used in physiological measurements of blood flow are not applicable to inflamed lesions. Venous occlusion plethysmography, or the use of electromagnetic flow meters, for example, are able to measure flow to fairly substantial masses of tissue, such as a segment of a limb or an extremity. Inflaming such a large piece of tissue might well confuse the picture by producing such systemic effects as a fall in blood pressure. A small inflammatory lesion, however, might not produce enough of a change to be measurable by such techniques. Temperature measurement and heat clearance methods can be used to measure blood flow, as can the technique of intra-arterial injection of microspheres labelled with radio-isotopes, which gives a measure of relative blood flow distribution. In transparent tissues such as mesentery, hamster cheek pouch or rabbit ear chamber, techniques measuring blood velocity in small vessels can be used to give an estimate of blood flow. The absence of convenient methods probably accounts for the small number of published quantitative measurements of blood flow in inflammation. A more satisfactory technique is probably one of those involving clearance of a locally injected radioisotope. This method, using xenon-133, has recently been used by WILLIAMS (1976) to measure blood flow simultaneously with permeability increases (using intravenously injected radio-iodinated serum albumin). Using a rabbit's back, up to 36 sites can be injected and the blood flow estimated by punching out the injection site some 20–30 min later, and counting skin from untreated and treated areas. The fall in ^{133}Xe in inflamed skin in comparison with that in the control area gives a measure of comparative blood flow.

II. Pressure Changes in the Microcirculation, Filtration, Oedema, Stasis

Measurement of the pressures in capillaries and other small vessels is a specialised technique, the use of which has been mainly confined to physiological studies. However, some workers, including the originator of this method (LANDIS, 1928), have used it to study the changes in pressure and in hydraulic conductance associated with the application to living thin sheets of tissue of injuries or possible inflammatory mediators. More recent studies by VERRINDER et al. (1974), using an indirect method in rat cremasteric vessels, have included measurement of the effect on the filtration coefficient in single vessels of inflammatory mediators. Among their findings was confirmation that the effect of histamine was confined to venules and small veins, as proposed on the basis of combined light and electron microscopical studies by MAJNO and PALADE (1961) and MAJNO et al. (1961). A surprising amount of information can be obtained from studies on single vessels, using the movement of red cells to measure filtration from or absorption into a blocked segment of blood vessel at different intraluminal pressures (CURRY et al., 1974). Hydraulic conductivity (filtration coefficient) and the osmotic reflection coefficient for various solutes (a measure of the vessel wall's retentivity) can be estimated by this technique. Due to their larger size, frog capillaries are technically easier to investigate by these techniques, whereas mammalian vessels require a more indirect approach, as used for the vessels in the rat cremaster muscle. Only a few studies have used this kind of preparation to investigate the changes in vessels affected by damage or inflammatory mediators. For those with the patience to master the techniques, there is still a lot of interesting work to be done on the basic mode of action of inflammatory mediators on single vessels. In this type of preparation it is possible to make a more direct correlation with ultrastructural changes than in any other (CURRY et al., 1973). It is a pity that some doubt must always remain about how far one can extrapolate findings on frog blood vessels to mammals, and in particular, man.

More frequently used is the assessment of swelling in an inflamed area. This can be measured by skinfold callipers or micrometer, by amputation and weighing (ROCHA E SILVA, and ANTONIO, 1960), or by displacement plethysmography (WINDER et al., 1957). A popular method is to dip the inflamed part into mercury and measure the pressure rise resulting from the rise in mercury level.

Such techniques can only give information about increase in volume, and do not differentiate between purely haemodynamic causes for increased filtration and those due to changes in the hydraulic conductance or colloid permeability of the vessel wall. In many situations, both types of change may be involved, and to differentiate between them a technique measuring protein permeability is needed. The displacement plethysmograph has the considerable advantage over other methods that repeated measurements of volume can be made, and the time course of the development of the swelling followed. It has been an extremely useful technique as applied to the inflamed rat paw.

Direct microscopical observation of transparent tissues, unless combined with micropipette cannulation of small vessels, can show little quantitative information about increased filtration, short of the stasis associated with extreme degrees of filtration. Increases in filtration coefficient or in hydrostatic pressure alone are unlikely to lead to stasis, as filtration will lead to a concentration of the plasma protein within the blood vessel and the consequent reaching of a new equilibrium position, with an increased haematocrit of the blood. Frank stasis must always imply a degree of increased permeability of the vessel wall to colloids or an abnormal rise of the extravascular fluid colloid content for some other reason, such as breakdown of hyaluronic acid matrix into soluble macromolecules.

III. Permeability Changes

One of the most widely used indices of inflammation in response to experimental procedures or to administration of mediators is the accumulation in the affected tissue of plasma protein. This is commonly taken as an indication of increased vascular permeability and can be measured either by a protein-bound dye, or by an isotopically labelled protein, injected intravenously and subsequently more or less quantitatively estimated in samples of tissue, often skin, taken at different times or observed in situ. Since the widespread introduction of methods of radioactive counting, the most popular indicator has been ^{131}I or ^{125}I-labelled serum albumin (MACFARLANE, 1957). By timing the induction of the inflammatory lesion in relation to the injection of labelled protein, a time course of "permeability change" may be obtained. Addition of an intravascular marker, such as ^{51}Cr-labelled erythrocytes, enables correction to be made for the amount of intravascular label in the tissue sample. It is even possible to use this kind of technique to measure protein accumulation continuously in certain tissues (WILLIAMS and MORLEY, 1974).

Such techniques are probably most useful in obtaining a quick assessment of the microvascular changes occurring in inflamed tissues, or in screening anti-inflammatory compounds. They give us little precise information, however, about the mechanisms involved. As pointed out by ASCHEIM (1965) in one of the few studies trying to deal with this difficulty, extravasation of plasma proteins into inflamed tissues depends not only on the permeability of the local blood vessels to macromolecules but also on blood flow, hydrostatic pressure and the volume of extravascular interstitial fluid. Lymph drainage is yet another variable which may affect the picture. By comparing blood and tissue content of two markers, one a large molecule (albumin), the other much smaller (^{86}Rb), and also water content, it was found that changes in blood flow made a big difference to the amount of extravascular albumin. Most studies before and since have made no attempt to separate these two factors, namely changes in haemodynamics and changes in the permeability of the vessel walls to macromolecules. Microscopic and ultra-structural investigations, with which attempts are made to correlate the permeability studies, are not likely to give any information relevant to blood flow or pressures. Recently, WILLIAMS (1976) has introduced a technique in which the blood flow in an inflamed area of skin is measured by the clearance rate of locally injected ^{133}Xe, during simultaneous measurement of labelled protein accumulation. It has been found possible using this method to dissociate to some extent the two phenomena, and more studies using this technique should bring a better understanding of the mechanism of altered vascular protein leakage in inflammation. So far, PGs seem to exert their permeability-increasing and histamine- or Bk-potentiating effects by increasing blood flow. Histamine and Bk themselves may have some genuine permeability-increasing effect.

To demonstrate such an effect unequivocally, more than one large molecule should be used as a marker. For normal skin blood vessels there is a considerable restriction to transcapillary passage with increasing molecular size in the Stokes-Einstein radius range 2.0–4.0 nm (RENKIN, 1964). Such information is based largely on studies of steady state lymph-plasma ratios after injection intravenously of dextrans of various molecular sizes (GROTTE, 1956). Recently, lymph studies of macromolecular passage out of blood vessels have included experiments on the effects of inflammatory mediators, particularly histamine (RENKIN et al., 1974). Unfortunately, it takes a relatively long time to achieve a steady state lymph-plasma ratio, and short-lasting changes cannot be studied by this technique. This is a particularly important point in trying to correlate structural changes with changes in vascular permeability. MAJNO and PALADE (1961) and MAJNO et al. (1961) suggested that carbon labelling of small blood vessels was a good guide to the presence of gaps between endothelial cells, and demonstrated that such gaps appeared in venules in response to locally applied histamine or 5-HT. Several authors since then have assumed that the opening of endothelial gaps is the anatomical basis of the increased permeability of blood vessels in response to inflammatory mediators. However, it has recently been reported that these endothelial gaps close within 30 min, even in the continued presence of histamine (CASLEY-SMITH and WINDOW, 1976). In the early phase there is an obvious increase in extravasation of large molecules, but no information is available about changes in relation to molecular size, i.e. diminution in selectivity. It would seem likely that such a decrease in selectivity would be present in the early, endothelial gap, phase. Lymph studies (JOYNER et al., 1974) show a prolonged diminution of selectivity to passage of dextrans and proteins in the dog paw, long outlasting the phase of closure of the gaps. It has been suggested that the mechanism for this is an increase in micropinocytotic vesicle size, but this has not been observed in a recent quantitative electron microscopic study (CASLEY-SMITH and WINDOW, 1976). This study did show, however, a persistent increase in the number of large vacuoles observed in endothelial cells up to 90 min after burning or histamine administration, and these may account for the increase in permeability which outlasts the endothelial gaps.

IV. Leucocyte/Endothelium and Platelet/Endothelium Interactions

The only way in which these important interactions have been directly studied is microscopically (MARCHESI and FLOREY, 1960). Many features of the later phases of the inflammatory response are modified in the absence of leucocytes, particularly neutrophil polymorphonuclear leucocytes. The tissue damage which features in some sorts of inflammation may be mediated through substances, such as lysosomal enzymes, originating from these cells. In teleological terms, the other vascular changes observed in inflammation may be interpreted as having the function of bringing phagocytic cells to the site of injury, and enhancing their function by increased delivery to the inflamed area of humoral agents such as antibodies and opsonins. The role of platelets in inflammation is less clearly defined. Although they have releasable stores of inflammatory mediators, and also possess the enzyme systems capable of synthesising active substances, such as PGs and other possibly even more active lipid compounds such as thromboxanes, it appears that some forms at least of inflammation can progress in the absence of platelets. An in vitro method of investigating the function of platelets exists, in the form of the aggregometer (BORN and CROSS, 1963) and this technique has been widely used for the investigation of biochemical and structural aspects of platelet function. Platelet-platelet interaction in the form of aggregation may be analogous to platelet-endothelium interactions.

Both platelet and leucocyte interactions with the vascular wall have been studied in vivo (BEGENT and BORN, 1970; ATHERTON and BORN, 1972) and it appears that the mechanisms underlying such interactions differ. Information from such studies currently in progress should improve our knowledge of this critical step in the development of the inflammatory process.

E. Summary and Conclusion

Even for the "well-established" chemical mediators of the vascular changes of acute inflammation, such as histamine, there remains some doubt about their importance in different types of inflammation and about the mechanism by which the effects are produced. Among the obvious gaps in our knowledge of this phenomenon are the nature of the receptors involved in the vascular effects of such mediators as PGs and other, less well-identified substances. New blocking agents, as effective against the other mediators as are the antihistamines against the vascular effects of histamine, might bring new therapeutic possibilities. More work is needed, too, on the endothelial changes leading to cell migration into inflamed tissues.

References

Altura, B. M.: Contractile responses of microvascular smooth muscle to antihistamines. Amer. J. Physiol. **218**, 1082—1091 (1970)

Ascheim, E.: Kinetic characterisation of the terminal vascular bed during inflammation. Amer. J. Physiol. **208**, 270—274 (1965)

Atherton, A., Born, G. V. R.: Quantitative investigations of the adhesiveness of circulating polymorphonuclear leucocytes to blood vessel walls. J. Physiol. (Lond.) **222**, 447—474 (1972)

Begent, N. A., Born, G. V. R.: Quantitative investigation of intravascular platelet aggregation. J. Physiol. (Lond.) **210**, 40—41 P (1970)

Beraldo, W. T., Dias da Silva, W.: Release of histamine by animal venoms and bacterial toxins. In: Rocha e Silva, M. (Ed.): Histamine and Antihistamines. Handbook of Exptl. Pharmacology, Vol. XVIII/I, pp. 334—366. Berlin-Heidelberg-New York: Springer 1966

Born, G. V. R., Cross, M. J.: The aggregation of blood platelets. J. Physiol. (Lond.) **168**, 178—195 (1963)

Burch, G. E., de Pasquale, N. P.: Bradykinin, digital flow and the arteriovenous anastomoses. Circulat. Res. **10**, 105—115 (1962)

Capasso, F., Balestrieri, B., di Rosa, M., Persico, P., Sorrentino, L.: Enhancement of carrageenin foot oedema by 1, 10-Phenanthroline and evidence for the bradykinin as endogenous mediator. Agents Actions **5**, 359—363 (1975)

Casley-Smith, J. R., Window, J.: Quantitative morphological correlations of alterations in capillary permeability, following histamine and moderate burning, in the mouse diaphragm, and the effects of benzpyrones. Microvasc. Res. **11**, 279—306 (1976)

Crunkhorn, P., Willis, A. L.: Cutaneous reactions to intradermal prostaglandins. Brit. J. Pharmacol. **41**, 49—56 (1971)

Curry, F. E., Mason, J. C., Michel, C. C.: The measurement in a single capillary of the filtration coefficient and the permeability and the osmotic reflection coefficient to sucrose. J. Physiol. (Lond.) **242**, 111—112 P (1974)

Curry, F. E., Mason, J. C., Michel, C. C., White, I. F.: A method for investigating the ultrastructure of a single capillary of known permeability properties. J. Physiol. (Lond.) **234**, 24—25 P (1973)

Di Rosa, M., Sorrentino, L.: Some pharmacodynamic properties of carrageenin in the rat. Brit. J. Pharmacol. **38**, 214—220 (1970)

Elliott, D. F., Horton, E. W., Lewis, G. P.: Actions of pure bradykinin. J. Physiol. (Lond.) **153**, 437—480 (1960)

Feldberg, W., Miles, A. A.: Regional variations of increased permeability of skin capillaries induced by histamine liberator and their relation to histamine content of skin. J. Physiol. (Lond.) **120**, 205—213 (1953)

Feldberg, W., Smith, A. N.: Release of histamine by tryptamine and 5-hydroxytryptamine. Brit. J. Pharmacol. **8**, 406—411 (1953)

Ferreira, S. H., Moncada, S., Parsons, M., Vane, J. R.: The concomitant release of bradykinin and prostaglandin in the inflammatory response to carrageenin. Brit. J. Pharmacol. **52**, 108—109 P (1974)

Ferreira, S. H., Moncada, S., Vane, J. R.: Indomethacin and aspirin abolish prostaglandin release from the spleen. Nature (New Biol.) **231**, 237—239 (1971)

Flower, R. J., Harvey, E. A., Kingston, W. P.: Inflammatory effects of prostaglandin D_2 in rat and human skin. Brit. J. Pharmacol. **56**, 229—233 (1976)

Fox, R. H., Goldsmith, R., Kidd, D. J., Lewis, G. P.: Bradykinin as a vasodilator in man. J. Physiol. (Lond.) **157**, 589—602 (1961)

Greaves, M. W., Søndergaard, J. S.: Pharmacologic agents released in ultraviolet inflammation studied by continuous skin perfusion. J. invest. Derm. **54**, 365—367 (1970)

Grotte, G.: Passage of dextran molecules across the blood-lymph barrier. Acta chir. scand. Suppl. 211 (1956)

Hammamura, L., Garcia Leme, J.: Neurogenic inflammation in the rat. Evidence for the release of a permeability factor from sensory nerves following electrical stimulation. Agents Actions **3**, 381—382 (1973)

Harris, J. M., West, G. B.: Rats resistant to the dextran anaphylactoid reaction. Brit. J. Pharmacol. **20**, 550—562 (1963)

Hartley, R. E., Davies, H. T. S., Schild, H. O.: The isolation from spleen tissue of high molecular weight proteins which alter vascular permeability: investigations of their chemical and pharmacological properties. Agents Actions **3**, 307—311 (1973)
Holdstock, D. J., Mathias, A. P., Schachter, M.: A comparative study of kinin, kallidin, and bradykinin. Brit. J. Pharmacol. **12**, 149—158 (1957)
Holton, F. A., Holton, P.: Vasodilator activity of spinal roots. J. Physiol. (Lond.) **118**, 310—327 (1952)
Joyner, W. L., Carter, R. D., Raizes, G. S., Renkin, E. M.: Influence of histamine and some other substances on blood-lymph transport of plasma protein and dextran in dog paw. Microvasc. Res. **7**, 19—30 (1974)
Landis, E. M.: Microinjection studies of capillary permeability. III. The effect of lack of oxygen on the permeability of the capillary wall to fluid and to the plasma proteins. Amer. J. Physiol. **83**, 528—542 (1928)
Lewis, G. P.: Plasma kinin forming enzymes in body fluids and tissues. J. Physiol. (Lond.) **147**, 458—468 (1959)
Lewis, T.: The blood vessels of the human skin and their responses. London: Shaw and Sons, Ltd. 1927
Lewis, T., Grant, R. T.: Vascular reactions of the skin to injury. Heart **11**, 119—209 (1924)
Macfarlane, A. S.: The behaviour of ^{131}I labelled plasma proteins in vivo. Ann. N.Y. Acad. Sci. **70**, 19—25 (1957)
Majno, G., Palade, G. E.: Studies on inflammation. I. The effect of histamine and serotonin on vascular permeability: an electron microscopic study. J. biophys. biochem. Cytol. **11**, 571—605 (1961)
Majno, G., Palade, G. E., Schoefl, G. I.: Studies on inflammation. II. The site of action of histamine and serotonin along the vascular tree: a topographic study. J. biophys. biochem. Cytol. **11**, 607—626 (1961)
Marchesi, V. T., Florey, H. W.: Electron micrographic observations on the emigration of leucocytes. Quart. J. exp. Physiol. **45**, 343—348 (1960)
Miles, A. A., Miles, E. M.: Vascular reactions to histamine, histamine liberator, and leukotaxine in the skin of guinea-pigs. J. Physiol. (Lond.) **118**, 228—257 (1952)
Mills, D. C. B., Macfarlane, D. E.: Stimulation of human platelet adenyl cyclase by prostaglandin D_2. Thromb. Res. **5**, 401—412 (1974)
Parratt, J. R., West, G. B.: 5-Hydroxytryptamine and the anaphylactoid reaction in the rat. J. Physiol. (Lond.) **139**, 27—41 (1957)
Renkin, E. M.: Transport of large molecules across capillary walls. Physiologist **7**, 13—28 (1964)
Renkin, E. M., Carter, R. D., Joyner, W. L.: Mechanism of the sustained action of histamine and bradykinin on transport of large molecules across capillary walls in the dog paw. Microvasc. Res. **7**, 49—60 (1974)
Riley, J. F., West, G. B.: Histamine liberation in the rat and mouse. Arch. int. Pharmaçodyn. **102**, 304—313 (1955)
Rocha e Silva, M., Antonio, A.: Release of bradykinin and the mechanism of production of a "Thermic edema (45° C)" in the rat's paw. Med. exp. **3**, 371—382 (1960)
Rocha e Silva, M., Rosenthal, S. R.: Release of pharmacologically active substances from the rat skin in vivo following thermal injury. J. Pharmacol. exp. Ther. **132**, 110—116 (1961)
Schayer, R. W.: Induced synthesis of histamine, microcirculatory regulation and the mechanism of action of the glucocorticoid hormones. Progr. Allergy **1**, 187—212 (1963)
Sicuteri, F., Fanciullacci, M., Franchi, G., Del Bianco, P. L.: Serotonin-bradykinin potentiation on the pain receptors in man. Life Sci. **4**, 309—316 (1965)
Smith, J. B., Willis, A. L.: Aspirin selectively inhibits prostaglandin production in human platelets. Nature (New Biol.) **231**, 235—237 (1971)
Spector, W. G., Willoughby, D. A.: Experimental suppression of the acute inflammatory changes of thermal injury. J. Path. Bact. **78**, 121—132 (1959)
Van Arman, C. G., Begany, A. J., Miller, L. M., Pless, H. H.: Some details of the inflammation caused by yeast and carrageenin. J. Pharmacol. exp. Ther. **150**, 328—334 (1965)
Vane, J. R.: Inhibition of prostaglandin synthesis as a mechanism of action for aspirin-like drugs. Nature (New Biol.) **231**, 232—235 (1971)

Vane, J. R.: Prostaglandins in the inflammatory response. In: Lepow, I. H., Ward, P. A. (Eds.): Inflammation: Mechanisms and Control, pp. 261—279. New York-London: Academic Press 1972

Verrinder, A., Fraser, P., Smaje, L. M.: Effect of drugs on mass transport across venular walls. Biorheology **11**, 387 (1974)

Vugman, I., Rocha e Silva, M.: Biological determination of histamine in living tissues and body fluids. In: Rocha e Silva, M. (Ed.): Histamine and Antihistamines. Handbook of Experimental Pharmacology, Vol. XVIII/I, pp. 367—385. Berlin-Heidelberg-New York: Springer 1966

Wilhelm, D. L.: The mediation of increased vascular permeability in inflammation. Pharmacol. Rev. **14**, 251—280 (1962)

Wilhelm, D. L., Mason, B.: Vascular permeability changes in inflammation: the role of endogenous permeability factors in mild thermal injury. Brit. J. exp. Path. **41**, 487—506 (1960)

Williams, T. J.: Simultaneous measurements of local plasma exudation and blood flow changes induced by intradermal injection of vasoactive substances, using ^{131}I albumin and ^{133}Xe. J. Physiol. (Lond.) **254**, 4—5 P (1976)

Williams, T. J., Morley, J.: Measurement of rate of extravasation of plasma protein in inflammatory responses in guinea pig skin using a continuous recording method. Brit. J. exp. Path. **55**, 1—12 (1974)

Willis, A. L.: Parallel assay of prostaglandin-like activity in rat inflammatory exudate by means of cascade superfusion. J. Pharm. (Lond.) **21**, 126—128 (1969)

Willoughby, D. A., Boughton, B., Spector, W. C., Schild, H. O.: A vascular permeability factor extracted from normal and sensitized guinea pig lymph node cells. Life Sci. **1**, 347—353 (1962)

Winder, C. V., Wax, J., Been, M. A.: Rapid foot volume measurements on anaesthetised rats and the question of anaphylactoid edema. Arch. int. Pharmacodyn. **112**, 174—187 (1957)

CHAPTER 17

Pain and Inflammatory Mediators

S. MONCADA, S. H. FERREIRA, and J. R. VANE

A. Introduction

Pain and hyperalgesia are common features of the inflammatory process. Some pain arises as an immediate sensation after tissue injury, due to direct stimulation of sensory nerve endings. Another component arises with the inflammation which ensues after injury; the pain which then develops is a combination of mechanical and chemical stimulation due to the vascular changes inherent to the inflammatory process and due to direct chemical stimulation by the pain producing substances released.

We do not intend to deal with the central components or psychic aspects of pain, nor will we analyse in detail the physiological aspects of the transmission of pain by different types of nerve fibres or different types of receptors involved in the perception of pain. We are mainly concerned with the neurohumoral aspects of the peripheral mechanism through which information develops which is recognised by the CNS as pain and/or hyperalgesia, as a common component of the reaction to injury called inflammation.

We shall discuss the involvement of chemical mediators in the induction of inflammatory pain in order to explain the analgesia caused by anti-inflammatory agents.

B. Measurement of Pain in Inflammation

Pain is difficult to study. The most reliable way is to use man's description of the subjective experience of pain under controlled experimental conditions (LEWIS, 1942; BEECHER, 1957; KEELE and ARMSTRONG, 1964). However, the study of reflex reactions in laboratory animals has been widely accepted. Throughout the years, many methods for studying pain and analgesia in laboratory animals have been developed; almost as many as the research workers or laboratories that have been interested in the problem. Extensive reviews on the subject are available (BEECHER, 1957; LIM, 1968; COLLIER, 1969a; SWINGLE, 1974). As in any other scientific field, the multitude of different techniques has been in part a consequence of the lack of precise definition of the parameters being measured; in this instance, pain and analgesia. This has been especially true in relation to the mechanism of action of the "mild" analgesics.

The standard way of studying these substances by measuring the type of energy used to induce pain, whether it is mechanical, thermal, electrical or chemical, has not led to an understanding of the mechanism of action of mild analgesics, for these types of stimulation can vary from mild to severe, short to long lasting or non-damaging to traumatic. Moreover, the integrity of the tissue to which any type of stimulation is applied was not considered as a factor of primary importance. The ability of specific stimuli to induce damage or not, and the nature of the tissue being stimulated, were realised more recently as basic points of reference in the analysis of pain and analgesia (RANDALL and SELITTO, 1957; LIM, 1968).

There are few methods sensitive to aspirin-like drugs. The most popular assays are those derived from RANDALL and SELITTO's technique (1957) and the stretching assays in rodents (SIEGMUND et al., 1957). Other tests, though not widely used in screening of aspirin-like drugs, include the study of the pseudoeffective response after intraarterial injection of pain producing substances described by GUZMAN et al. (1962) and recently developed by FERREIRA et al. (1973), the induction of inflammation subcutaneously (HESS et al., 1930), in the foot joint of the rat (MARGOLIN, 1965) or in physiological cavities such as the knee joint of dogs (PHELPS et al., 1966; PARDO and RODRIGUEZ, 1966) or pigeons (BRUNE et al., 1974). Aspirin-like drugs also inhibit the generation of impulses from heat stimulation of the dental receptors of the cat (SCOTT, 1968), the hypertensive reflex induced by bradykinin (Bk) injections into the knee joint of dogs (MONCADA et al., 1975) and the affective response after intra-abdominal injections in humans (LIM et al., 1967).

In tests which involve short lasting stimulation with any type of energy or in which there is no delay between the stimulus and the response, aspirin-like drugs are either inactive or only active when used in very high concentrations (see COLLIER, 1969a).

WOODWORTH and SHERRINGTON (1904) and SHERRINGTON (1906) described the pseudoaffective response in the decerebrated cat. This response consisted of flexion of the ipsilateral and extension of the contralateral limb after noxious stimulation of the foot. There were also autonomic reflexes such as tachycardia, hypertension, hypernea, and the more complex response of vocalisation.

These responses were observed after mechanical or electric stimulation of different cutaneous, muscular or visceral nerves (WOODWORTH and SHERRINGTON, 1904). MOORE and MOORE (1933), MOORE and SINGLETON (1933) and MOORE (1938) observed this response in lightly anaesthetized dogs and cats when irritants were injected intra-arterially to different areas of the body, and showed that they were mediated by afferent pathways entering the medulla via the dorsal roots. Using and developing this technique, GUZMAN et al. (1962) and LIM et al. (1964) demonstrated in dogs the pain producing ability of several vasoactive substances released during inflammation; moreover, they demonstrated that the analgesic activity of aspirin-like drugs was a peripheral effect. These observations had been made also in man by KEELE and ARMSTRONG (see review, 1964).

GOETZL et al. (1943) stated that theoretically any reflex response could serve as a measure of pain provided that only pain nerve endings are stimulated. The selected standard response should be:

1. Clearly perceptible to the observer;
2. Of such a character as to allow a clear distinction to be made between minimal and sub-minimal stimuli;
3. Constant in its appearance when a stimulus of identical intensity is applied repeatedly;
4. Definite in its onset

Using the criteria proposed by GOETZL et al. (1943) and taking into consideration the difficulties of measuring analgesia induced by aspirin-like drugs in laboratory models, two approaches have been used when studying pain and analgesia and its relationship to prostaglandin (PG) release. Firstly, experiments were carried out using human volunteers and analysing the verbal reports (FERREIRA, 1972) and secondly, experiments using the hypertensive reflex induced by pain producing substances in lightly anaesthetized dogs (FERREIRA et al., 1973; MONCADA et al., 1974, 1975). These later models were chosen because of their comprehensive previous analysis as models for studying pain and because of the clarity with which LIM and co-workers (1964) showed the peripheral effect of aspirin and analgesia.

Due to the developing concept that PGs act as modulators of algesic substances, the study of a more complicated response, like vocalisation, which many authors agree is the nearest to the human response to pain (LIM, 1968), was not used. This was because this complex response which involves higher centres in the CNS, although clearly observable, is not as sensitive to slight changes in the intensity of the stimulus and would not allow the study of a "sensitizing effect" which would need quantitation and a clear difference between minimal and subminimal stimuli (GOETZL et al., 1943). The study of the hypertensive reflex induced by pain producing substances fulfills the proposed criteria.

With the dog spleen preparation (FERREIRA et al., 1973), it has been widely recognised (GUZMAN et al., 1962; DELLA BELLA and BENELLI, 1969; TALLARIDA et al., 1970) that reflex hypertension induced by bradykinin is due to the stimulation of pain receptors rather than the mechanical contraction of the spleen (GUZMAN et al., 1962). Moreover, this response disappears after dorsal root gangliectomy and can be abolished by applying local anaesthesia to the splanchnic nerve.

We confirmed some of these observations and have noted that the reflex effect depends on the depth of the anaesthesia; in deeply anaesthetized dogs, the vasodilatory action of Bk injected intra-arterially into the spleen is similar to the response produced by an intravenous injection.

In the knee joint cavity it has been observed by others (PHELPS et al., 1966; MELMON et al., 1967) that in high concentrations, Bk induces a reflex response compatible with that due to the stimulation of pain receptors. This response is not caused by leakage of the Bk into the general circulation as this would result in a hypotensive rather than a hypertensive response. We have shown that this response depends, as does the one obtained from the spleen, on the level of the anaesthesia, and that it can be blocked by local application of an anaesthetic such as lignocaine (MONCADA et al., 1975). Besides, injections potassium chloride into the synovial cavity, which stimulate pain nerve endings, produce the same reflex hypertension (MONCADA et al., 1975). Thus, our experiments using two quantitative models for studying pain and analgesia have allowed us to re-analyse the mechanisms of analgesia induced by aspirin-like drugs.

C. Pain Receptors

Two types of skin pain have been accepted since their first description by LEWIS and POCHIN (1937). One type, evoked by a brisk needle jab into the skin, is well localized, appearing and disappearing quickly, with a low potential for eliciting visceral or somatic reflexes. The second type is described as a burning pain with a slow onset and a more generalised effect which often persists after the initial stimulus has disappeared. The latter evokes the characteristic cardiovascular and respiratory reflexes which are associated with pain. Present evidence supports the view that these two types of pain are served by two specific sets of peripheral nerve fibres. The pricking pain with its short latency period is transmitted by certain δ fibres; burning pain with its long latency period is transmitted by certain C fibres (BISHOP and LANDAU, 1958; SINCLAIR and STOKES, 1967; COLLINS et al., 1966). Pain of a severe and aching quality is evoked by injury to deep structures of the body, especially in muscle fascia, joints, and tendons. The δ and C fibres which occur in the skin are also present in these structures (IGGO, 1962; PAINTAL, 1960; GARDNER, 1950). LIM (1960) proposed that both types of fibres are present in cutaneous as well as visceral or deep areas and that the difference between cutaneous and visceral pain was due to a preponderance of fast "pricking" pain fibres serving the skin and slow "aching" pain fibres serving the deep structures. He suggested that this difference would tend to disappear according to the severity or the duration of the injury leading to inflammation.

The identification of pain receptors, as such, has eluded more than seventy years of research. The theories have varied from the original which proposed modality specificity (VON FREY, 1922), suggesting the existence of histologically distinguishable nerve endings considered to serve separate sensory modalities, to the more recent pattern theory proposed by WEDDELL (1962), in which the pain sensation depends on central decoding of the information travelling through the afferent nerves. SHERRINGTON (1906) proposed that any type of energy which threatened damage would produce pain. He recognised the lack of stimulus specificity of the nerve endings subserving pain and suggested the use of the word "nociceptive" to describe stimuli which elicited pain. The description of thermosensitive pain receptors which elicit pain in skin and visceral surfaces when exposed to temperatures of 45° C or more is in accord with this proposition (HARDY et al., 1968; DICKERSON et al., 1965). On the other hand, PERL and associates (1968) have described skin receptors which are specific in that they respond only to noxious deformation; neither damaging heat nor noxious concentrations of sulphuric acid or bradykinin elicited discharge.

In 1952, HARDY et al. discussed the role of tissue damage in the production of pain by heat. The threshold temperature for noxious stimulation of the skin required to evoke pain in man or reflex activity in animals is about 45° C. This is the temperature at which denaturation of cellular protein begins (HENRIQUEZ, 1947; MORITZ and HENRIQUEZ, 1947). HARDY et al. (1952) proposed that noxious stimulation caused partial denaturation of the cellular proteins of the nerve endings and thus led to pain. However, tissue damage leads to plasma leakage and activation of factors which result in the release of kinins and other vasoactive substances. The finding by ARMSTRONG et al. (1952, 1953) that vasoactive substances, especially kinins, are potent inducers of pain in man and animals (ARMSTRONG et al., 1952, 1953, 1957; GUZMAN et al., 1962; KEELE and ARMSTRONG, 1964) led them to propose that pain receptors in general were chemoreceptors and not nociceptors as suggested by SHERRINGTON (1906).

The only sensory endings with a sufficient widespread distribution to fulfill the role of pain chemoreceptors are the free terminals of C fibres which have profuse branchings in cutaneous and visceral surfaces extending over all the tegumental areas (FITZGERALD, 1968). These terminals accompany blood vessels (LIM et al., 1962; MILLER, 1948) almost everywhere to end in the skin (WEDDELL et al., 1954), intertegumental cavities like the joints (GARDNER, 1950) or internal viscera (LIM et al., 1962).

Whether pain chemoreceptors can be excited directly, either by thermal or mechanical stimulation, is still unresolved. The common characteristic of both types of stimulation is that they become adequate pain-producers after tissue damage is produced. It is possible that both stimuli act through the release of a chemical mediator. Certainly, tissue injury releases potent vasoactive and pain producing substances. The fact that in some instances Bk, one of the most potent pain producing substances released during inflammation, does not produce pain when applied alone (SICUTERI et al., 1965), or activate sensory non-myelinated fibres (FJALLBRANT and IGGO, 1961), does not exclude the possibility that pain receptors are chemoreceptive. However, this does strengthen the view that, like other signs of inflammation, the origin of pain is multicausal and requires the development of a sensitized state, as well as a combination of different substances.

Corroborating the idea of multiple mediation of pain, we have observed instances in which Bk fails to elicit a pain response but becomes active in the presence of small amounts of 5-HT or PGs either exogenously applied or endogenously released (FERREIRA et al., 1973; MONCADA et al., 1975). In this context, it is important to note the observations of BISHOP and LANDAU (1958) who studied production of pain in subdermal areas and analysed the responses by selective blockade of different nerve fibres. Certain nerve fibres in the subcutaneous tissue of humans responded to ordinary stimuli only under conditions of inflammation. They concluded that such endings register the sequelae of tissue damage rather than the initial injurious incident. They proposed that inflammatory subcutaneous pain is assignable almost entirely to activation of C fibres which seem to be specifically sensitized during the inflammatory process.

Thus, thermal, mechanical and chemoreceptors may be involved in the transmission of pain during inflammation and the inflammatory process specifically sensitizes them to stimuli which are normally subthreshold.

D. Chemical Stimulation of Pain Receptors

Elemental ions and endogenous vasoactive substances are released after almost any kind of damaging stimulation, provided this stimulation is maintained for long enough, leading many investigators to search for a chemical which stimulates pain receptors. One of the first studies orientated to the discovery of such a substance was by LEWIS (see LEWIS, 1942). He described the development of pain in the forearm of a subject gripping an ergograph once every second during occlusion of the circulation. The time of onset of pain was fairly constant (60–90 s). The pain remained unchanged after the exercise was stopped for as long as the circulation was occluded and disappeared only when the circulation was restored.

LEWIS thought that this pain was due to the release of a "factor P" during muscle exercise which stimulated pain endings but only accumulated during circulatory occlusion in high enough concentrations to produce this effect. This work was extended by DORPAT and HOLMES (1955) who demonstrated that "factor P" could not be just lactic acid or carbon dioxide accumulation or a depression of pH of the muscle, but thought that it might be potassium released from the muscle cells.

The role of potassium ions as activators of the pain receptors during inflammation or ischaemia has been discussed by several authors. Certainly, potassium is released when tissue is damaged or exposed to anoxic conditions (BOMMER, 1924; BENJAMIN, 1959) and might accumulate at the inflammatory site. Furthermore, potassium salts induce pain when given intra-arterially (BOMMER, 1924) or into the skin (SKOUBY, 1953) in human subjects or intra-arterially in experimental animals (MOORE and MOORE, 1933; GUZMAN et al., 1962). BENJAMIN (1959) thought that the release of intracellular potassium could be the stimulus of pain and later (BENJAMIN and HELVEY, 1963) described the production of pain in human skin when potassium was applied by iontophoresis. In all these experiments, however, the concentration of potassium needed to produce pain was so high that it is unlikely to be achieved during inflammation and thus will have little significance as a mediator of pain. This conclusion is reinforced by the work of LINDAHL (1962). He used a vaccine pistol for intradermal injections and found that potassium induced only slight pain at concentrations as high as 31.8 mM and was much weaker than acid solutions. He showed that pain occurred when the pH fell to 6.2 and was maximal at 3.2. As the pH of inflamed tissues is low he proposed that an increase in hydrogen ion concentration was the chemical factor in pain. Activation of pain receptors by hypertonic salt solutions or injections of acids and alkalis has been described in man (ODERMATT, 1922; FROLICH and MEYER, 1922; BROOKS, 1924; SINGLETON, 1928) and in animals (MOORE and MOORE, 1933; MOORE and SINGLETON, 1933; GUZMAN et al., 1962). The possibility that hydrogen concentration is in part responsible for pain during inflammation has not been completely settled and more recent workers strongly argue in favour of this possibility (see below).

Induction of pain by several endogenous vasoactive substances has been studied for many years (see FELDBERG, 1956), but their pain producing properties were mostly established by KEELE and his colleagues (ARMSTRONG et al., 1952, 1953, 1957; KEELE and ARMSTRONG, 1964). They applied substances to the denuded base of the cantharidin-induced blister and showed that pain was induced by amines like acetylcholine, 5-HT and histamine; peptides like angiotensin, substance P and Bk; plasma activated by glass, serum, and various inflammatory exudates. Later, LIM and coworkers (GUZMAN et al., 1962) showed that these substances induced physiological responses indicative of pain when injected into different arteries of lightly anaesthetized dogs. Of all the substances tested, however, only Bk and later, substance P (POTTER et al., 1962) produced pain in submicrogram concentrations. All the other substances required concentrations 10–100 times higher. However, claims for one or another substance as a potential mediator of pain are frequently observed. Histamine (ROSENTHAL, 1949, 1950, 1964) has been regarded as a mediator of cutaneous pain and referred pain in the skin of visceral origin. Similarly, it has been proposed that 5-HT (see SICUTERI, 1968) is involved in the pain of thrombo-embolic disorders and migraine.

The pain-producing actions of the plasma kinins and later Bk were first described by ARMSTRONG et al. (1952, 1953, 1957). The high potency of Bk in relation to other endogenous vasoactive substances, coupled with the discovery of its formation from kininogens in plasma by a kinin forming enzyme (ROCHA E SILVA, 1964), led to the proposal that Bk could be the mediator of pain during the inflammatory process (see LIM, 1968). This proposition was supported by the fact that Bk is released during several inflammatory conditions (see ROCHA E SILVA and GARCIA LEME, 1972) and that local acidosis characteristic of the acute inflammatory process leads to accumulation of Bk in the inflamed site (EDERY and LEWIS, 1962).

Bk produces pain when injected intradermally (CORMIA and DOUGHERTY, 1960; LIM et al., 1967; FERREIRA, 1972) intra-arterially (BURCH and DE PASQUALE, 1962; COFFMAN, 1966) or intra-abdominally (LIM et al., 1967) in humans and intra-arterially (GUZMAN et al., 1962; HASHIMOTO et al., 1964; FERREIRA et al., 1973) or intra-articularly (MELMON et al., 1967; MONCADA et al., 1975) in dogs. However, not all workers found that Bk induces pain and sometimes a main sensation of warmth is described (FOX et al., 1961). SICUTERI et al. (1965) found that Bk induced pain only when the area had been previously sensitized by 5-HT. Moreover, in the blister base, Bk-induced pain is tachyphylactic (KEELE and ARMSTRONG, 1964), a phenomenon which is not observed when Bk is injected into a vein previously sensitized by 5-HT (SICUTERI et al., 1965) or when injected intra-arterially in dogs (GUZMAN et al., 1962).

All these observations, coupled with the facts that recoverable kinins from inflammatory exudates in man and animals are very low (MELMON et al., 1967) and that their concentration does not correlate with the severity of the symptoms in rheumatoid arthritis (MELMON et al., 1967) strongly suggest that Bk is not the sole mediator of pain during inflammation but one of the contributors to the pain sensation.

The complexities of the inflammatory response and the nature of the substances involved lead to the conclusion that several mediators, either together or in sequence, contribute to the production of pain. The synergism between these substances means that they are not all necessary, nor in any special combination. This has been suggested in recent years by CHAPMAN et al. (1961), KEELE and ARMSTRONG (1964) and ROCHA E SILVA and GARCIA LEME (1972), although they emphasise the role that kinins might play.

In LIM's view, tissue damage or ischaemia leading to acidosis and production of H+ and K+, which in turn favours the formation of plasma kinins, explains not only the pain but also the hyperalgesia during inflammation. From his results in dogs and man, LIM (1968) suggested that excitation of pain chemoreceptors was unlikely to depend on specific chemical configuration because a wide variety of substances with different chemical structures were able to induce pain, but would rather be the result of electrophilic interaction between an electronegative receptor and molecules with a positive charge. Although structural fit at receptor sites might not be necessary for algesic activity, he thought that steric hindrance might prevent some agents from acting at these sites.

A recurrent proposition in the literature is, however, that there is a selective sensitization to pain-producing substances during inflammation because of a background of injury to the tissue (LEWIS, 1942; LANDAU and BISHOP, 1953; GUZMAN et al., 1962).

This concept, which is qualitatively different from the one postulating the simple interaction of chemical mediators, has been developed by SICUTERI et al. (1965) and

SICUTERI (1968) in relation to 5-HT, as a possible substance responsible for this sensitization, and by FERREIRA (1972), FERREIRA et al. (1973) and MONCADA et al. (1975) in relation to the sensitizing effects of PGs.

E. Sensitization of Pain Receptors: Hyperalgesia

Apart from the presence of overt pain during inflammation, there is also a state of hyperalgesia (LEWIS and HESS, 1933; LEWIS, 1942), defined as a reduced pain threshold to stimuli which are normally non-painful. For example, after sunburn, gentle rubbing of the skin by the clothes can be painful. In fact, HARDY et al. (1950) found that after UV light irradiation the skin pain threshold was reduced by 50%. LEWIS and HESS (1933) showed that immersing hyperalgesic areas of the body in warm water (40° C), which is usually not painful, evokes pain within 2–3 s and reaches a peak after 10 s. As the hyperalgesia state increases, lower temperatures provoke pain.

Pain can also be evoked in sensitive skin by near-zero temperatures. Even stretching sunburnt skin, as caused by the increased hydrostatic pressure associated with moving the leg from a horizontal to a hanging position, sometimes induces pain. A similar effect is seen when the leg is maintained in a horizontal position and venous pressure is increased by inflating a cuff round the thigh (LEWIS and HESS, 1933; KEELE and ARMSTRONG, 1964).

When inflammation occurs in closed cavities such as the tooth pulp, joint cavities or the external auditory meatus, increased tissue tension is one of the causes of pain. This is clearly shown by the relief that is obtained when the cavity is drained. Tension by itself, however, does not necessarily cause pain; in some conditions like burning the skin, pain develops before the swelling and there are some clinical conditions in which there is swelling without pain. Urticarial wheals have as much tension as sunburnt skin and instead of pain they produce itch (LEWIS, 1942).

LEWIS (1936, 1942) recognised two distinct areas of hyperalgesia. One, which he called "erythalgia" was localized near the site of injury; this was probably due to the spreading of pain products formed in the injured area. The other, which he named "nocifensor" was a more widespread tenderness and possibly due to axon reflexes. HARDY et al. (1950) confirmed and extended this observation. They showed that at the site of injury there was a reduced pain threshold to previously non-noxious stimuli; they called this "increased sensitivity". There was also an increased response to previously painful stimulation which they called "increased sensibility". These two conditions occurred in the area of primary hyperalgesia. Secondary hyperalgesia, in which only increased sensibility was observed, corresponded to the widespread area of hyperalgesia described by LEWIS.

The explanation of the pathophysiological process underlying these two types of hyperalgesia has varied. Most authors agree that primary hyperalgesia is due to vasoactive, pain producing substances spreading from the site of injury through the lymphatic system (LEWIS, 1942; HARPMAN and WHITEHEAD, 1955). The secondary hyperalgesia has been explained in terms of a nervous mechanism which through an axon reflex releases pain producing substances (LEWIS, 1942; CHAPMAN et al., 1961), or alternatively creates a hyperexcitable state maintained by a network of internuncial neurones in the posterior horn of the spinal cord (HARDY et al., 1950).

Several authors have concluded that the substance responsible for primary hyperalgesia is the same one that determines pain but present in lower concentrations (LEWIS, 1942). Others suggest that hyperalgesia is caused by a mixture of different substances synergizing with each other (KEELE and ARMSTRONG, 1964). There is also the possibility that the substance that sensitizes pain nerve endings is not the same substance or mixture of substances that stimulates them. A vasodilator, for instance, can lead to increased capillary permeability and thus to the formation of pain producing substances like Bk (KEELE, 1960). LIM (1966, 1968, 1970) discussed this possibility and concluded that sensitization of pain receptors was a non-specific state due to subthreshold stimulation of pain receptors by hydrogen or potassium ions. This idea extends the same author's concept (already discussed) of an electrophilic interaction of the pain agent with the pain receptor.

Sensitization of pain receptors to mechanical stimulation has been recognised since the classical description by LEWIS et al. in 1931 of the development of sensitization during muscular exercise in condition of ischaemia. This type of sensitization has been used by DENEAU et al. (1953) and SMITH et al. (1966) to assess pain and analgesia. Sensitization of pain receptors by ischaemia has been described by SICUTERI (1966) who observed in humans the development of pain to a subthreshold dose of Bk injected into the carotid artery after occlusion and by LIM and GUZMAN (1968) in dogs.

Synergism between chemical substances which activate pain receptors has been observed by several authors. Sensitization of pain receptors to chemical and mechanical stimulation has been described for histamine (LEWIS, 1942; EMMELIN and FELDBERG, 1947), for acetylcholine (SKOUBY, 1953) and for Bk (SONINA and KHAITIN, 1967). SICUTERI et al. (1965) showed that 5-HT sensitizes pain receptors in the veins of the dorsal surface of the hand to a previously subthreshold dose of Bk. He proposed that the release of a Bk-like peptide causing vasodilatation in some cranial vessels, and the liberation of 5-HT from blood platelets, may explain headaches related to migraine. More recently, sensitization by 5-HT to the pain induced by Bk was observed by FERREIRA et al. (1973) using the dog spleen preparation described by GUZMAN et al. (1962).

By far the most frequently observed sensitization to pain is the one which develops after tissue injuries which lead to inflammation. To quote LEWIS (1942): "The hyperalgesic skin, according to my theory is one which has been brought to this state by the action of certain tissue substances upon the pain nerve endings, the latter being rendered hyperexcitable. It is suggested that these substances are the outcome of processes following at varying intervals according to the nature and severity of tissue injury; the interval is short after cut or burn and long after ultraviolet light." LEWIS thought that the product of the injury that induced the hyperalgesia was a stable pain substance spreading from the injury area through the lymphatic channels. HARDY et al. (1950) agreed with LEWIS' concept that after tissue injury, agents were released which excited the terminal nerve endings.

Inflammatory sensitization in man and animals has been used for the study of pain and for assessment of analgesia by several workers. KEELE and associates (see KEELE and ARMSTRONG, 1964) used the denuded base of a cantharadin-induced blister, combining an inflammatory sensitization with the exposure of free nerve endings. Inflammatory sensitization of pain receptors was also used by HESS et al. (1930) and LA BELLE and TISLOW (1950). However, it was RANDALL and SELLITO (1957) who clearly recognised inflammatory sensitization and successfully used it in animals for the assessment of algesia. Later, several other experimental models were developed (GILFOIL et al., 1963; WINTER and FLATAKER, 1965; PARDO and RODRIGUEZ, 1966; MARGOLIN, 1965).

The concept of hyperalgesia as a state which develops at different intervals after tissue injury and involves the release of chemical mediators has been generally accepted (LEWIS, 1942; HARDY et al., 1950; LIM, 1966). GILFOIL and KLAVINS (1965) made the important observation that in the rat paw hyperalgesia induced by 5-HT, Bk or histamine, given alone or in combination, was somewhat delayed and concluded that the effect was indirect. A delay between the stimulation and the painful response has also been observed in experimental models which do not involve the induction of an inflammatory state.

In 1962, GUZMAN et al. found that there was delay between injection of a pain producing substance intra-arterially and the development of the pseudoeffective response in lightly anaesthetized dogs. The delay was much longer than that normally required for somatic reflexes or even the most complicated central pathways and they concluded that changes were necessary at the receptor level before its excitation. Similar delays were observed by FERREIRA et al. (1973) using the same experimental model and by MONCADA et al. (1975) using the cavity of the knee joint of the dog. Moreover, we observed that the latency shortened as the intensity of the stimulus increased and that aspirin-like drugs increased the latency, suggesting that they acted on this intermediate step. Another experimental model in which a lag time occurs between stimulation and effect is the "stretching reflex" of mice or rats, after intraperitoneal injection of pain producing substances (VAN DER WENDE and MARGOLIN, 1956; SIEGMUND et al., 1957). Some substances such as hypertonic saline induce an early stretch reflex (10–30 s) whereas others like phenylbenzoquinone take about 2 min. Aspirin-type drugs are more effective against the longer latency reflex and COLLIER (1969a) suggested (as did WINDER in 1959) that there might be an intermediate step between the application of the stimulus and the stimulation of pain receptors. WINDER called this the development of a pre-inflammatory state and COLLIER suggested that it was due to the release of a pain producing substance. Later, COLLIER (1969b) suggested that this could be rabbit aorta contracting substance (RCS) (PIPER and VANE, 1969), a factor released from the lungs during anaphylaxis and the release of which is inhibited by aspirin-like drugs.

From our discussion it may be concluded that during inflammation there is a sensitization of pain receptors (hyperalgesia) which ensues after the initial trauma and is probably due to the release of inflammatory mediators. There is also a delay period between stimulation and "pain" response in those tests in which (as in inflammation) weak analgesic agents such as aspirin or paracetamol display analgesic effect. This delay in response may be due to the noxious stimulus releasing pain mediators or substances which sensitize the pain receptor to normally subthreshold stimulation; weak analgesics possibly act by preventing the generation or release of such mediator(s). We shall now discuss the evidence that one specific inflammatory, an E-type PG, is the substance which causes hyperalgesia.

F. Prostaglandin Release During Inflammation

Prostaglandin release has been observed, by a variety of stimuli, from all cells so far studied. Distortion or trauma of the cell membrane is common to the different PG-releasing stimuli which can be mechanical, chemical or pathological (FERREIRA and VANE, 1967; PIPER and VANE, 1971). Generation of PGs in inflammation and its contribution to vasodilatation, oedema and fever is discussed in Chapters 16, 18 and 31.

I. Prostaglandins and Pain

HORTON (1963) found that PGE did not produce pain when instilled onto a blister base. Similarly, CRUNKHORN and WILLIS (1969, 1971) reported that intradermal injections of microgram doses of PGE_1, PGE_2 or $PGF_{2\alpha}$ did not produce pain. However, SOLOMON et al. (1968) and JUHLIN and MICHAELSSON (1969) found that the oedematous area caused by intradermal injections of microgram doses of PGE_1 was tender or hypersensitive to touch. In fact, JUHLIN and MICHAELSSON observed hyperalgesia after injections of PGE_1 in doses as low as 10 ng. Moreover, intra-arterial, intravenous or intramuscular injections of PGs of the E series were variously reported to produce pain and headache (BEVERGARD and ORO, 1969; KARIM, 1971; COLLIER et al., 1972; GILLESPIE, 1972). Bk, in contrast, produces systemic and intracranial vasodilatation without pain (SICUTERI et al., 1966). In high concentrations, PGs of the E series produce pain when injected intra-arterially into the spleen of anaesthetized dogs (MONCADA, 1974). In dogs, injections into the knee joint of PGs of the E and F series induced, after a delay, an incapacitation which was untouched by treatment with aspirin-like drugs (ROSENTHAL et al., 1972). COLLIER and SCHNEIDER (1972) found that PGs injected into the peritoneal cavity of mice elicited the stretching response and this was not antagonised by aspirin-like drugs. COLLIER and SCHNEIDER (1972) suggested that PGs could be one of the pain mediators released by noxious stimulation or even the final link between the stimulus and the activation of pain receptors. Thus, apart from the work of SOLOMON et al. (1968) and JUHLIN and MICHAELSSON (1969) there is general agreement that PGs in high concentrations produce pain.

II. Prostaglandins and Hyperalgesia

In 1972, FERREIRA observed that subdermal infusions in man of PGs in low concentrations produced hyperalgesia. Infusions were used to mimic the continuous release of mediators at the site of an injury. The hyperalgesic effect of PGs was cumulative, since it depended not only on the concentration, but also on the duration of the infusion. Neither Bk nor histamine showed this property.

During separate subdermal infusions of PGE_1, Bk and histamine (or a mixture of Bk and histamine) there was no pain, but when PGE_1 was added to Bk or histamine or a mixture of both, strong pain occurred. Furthermore, in areas made hyperalgesic by an infusion of PGE_1, a second infusion either of histamine or Bk caused pain which gradually increased in intensity. However, at the site where Bk or histamine had been previously infused (without producing hyperalgesia) an infusion of PGE_1 caused little or no pain.

FERREIRA concluded that inflammatory mediators such as Bk or histamine had a direct pain producing action only when the chemical receptors were sensitized by PGs. Another possibility was an indirect action of the sensitized receptors due to the oedema they produced.

FERREIRA also found that histamine, Bk or PGE_1 infusions by themselves did not cause itch. However, when PGE_1 was infused with histamine, itching always preceded pain. PGE_1 infused together with Bk only caused pain. These observations have been confirmed by GREAVES and MCDONALD-GIBSON (1973) who showed that PGE_1 lowers the threshold of human skin to histamine-evoked itching.

PGs also sensitize pain nerve endings in the spleen of lightly anaesthetized dogs (FERREIRA et al., 1973). In this preparation, it is widely accepted (GUZMAN et al., 1962; DELLA BELLA and BENELLI, 1969) that Bk induces reflex hypertension due to stimulation of pain receptors and not due to the mechanical contraction of the spleen (GUZMAN et al., 1962). The response disappears after dorsal root gangliectomy and is abolished by applying local anaesthesia to the splenic nerve.

We confirmed some of these results and observed sensitization when an E-type PG was infused in low concentrations into the splenic artery (Fig. 1). We also noted, that the hypertensive reflex depends on the depth of the anaesthesia; in deeply anaesthetized dogs, intra-arterial injections of Bk into the spleen induce only a fall in blood pressure similar to that caused by an intravenous injection.

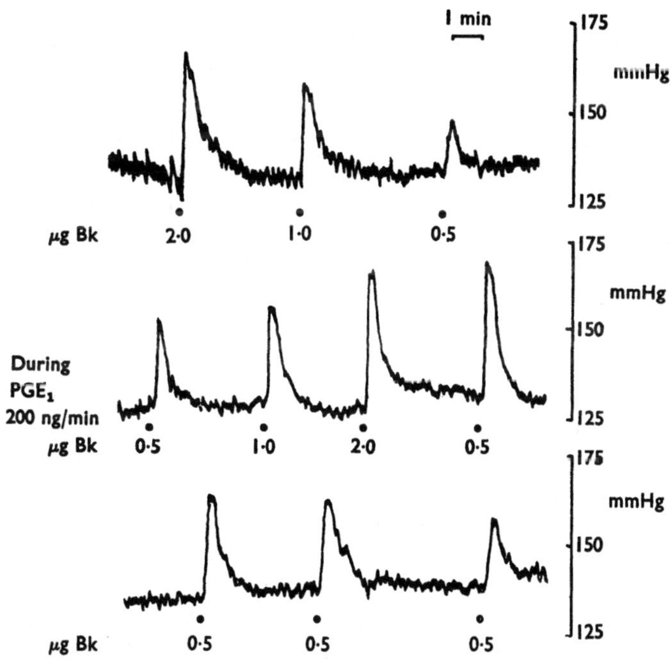

Fig. 1. Prostaglandin E_1 *(PGE_1)* potentiates the reflex effect of bradykinin. A continuous tracing of the blood pressure of a dog is shown arranged in three panels. In the upper one, the hypertensive responses to 2.0, 1.0, and 0.5 μg of bradykinin are shown; in the second tracing the same injections are repeated during infusion of prostaglandin E_1 (200 ng/min). After the infusion (third tracing) the pressor effects of 0.5 μg of bradykinin gradually declined towards pre-treatment levels. Time 1 min; vertical scales; mm Hg. (Data taken from, FERREIRA et al., 1973)

Interestingly enough, the spleen generates and releases an E-like PG continuously into the venous outflow, and this release is readily increased by intra-arterial Bk (FERREIRA et al., 1973). Thus, it is possible that there is already a background of sensitization and pain producing substances injected will always find an appropriate environment in which to act. This might be why LIM and co-workers (LIM et al., 1964) found it a suitable model for studying pain and analgesia induced by mild analgesics.

It is important to stress that in this preparation the pain producing substance must act on a background sensitization caused by spontaneous or induced release of PGs. The released PG is not itself a "classical" pain mediator, for intra-arterial adrenaline injections do not cause pain but release PGs in similar amounts to Bk injections.

Bk injected in high doses into the knee joint cavity induces a reflex response compatible with stimulation of pain receptors (PHELPS et al., 1966; MELMON et al., 1967). The response depends on the level of anaesthesia and is blocked by a local anaesthetic. Potassium chloride also elicits a similar reflex rise in blood pressure (MONCADA et al., 1975). In this preparation, E-type PGs also have the same sensitizing effect to the pain producing effects of Bk (MONCADA et al., 1974, 1975). In contrast to the spleen, which has a continuous basal release of PGs, normal synovial fluid does not contain PGs (HERMAN and MONCADA, 1975). This correlates well with our observation that the responses to Bk injected into the dog's knee joint were more reproducible after PG release had been induced by a continuous infusion of saline into the joint (MONCADA et al., 1975).

Sensitization of pain receptors by PGs has also been described by KUHN and WILLIS (1973) and WILLIS and CORNELSON (1973), who showed the development of hyperalgesia in the rat paw after single or repeated injections of an E-type PG; JUAN and LEMBECK (1974) observed a similar effect of PGE_1 in the circulation of the rabbit ear, potentiating the pain response induced by several substances. STASZEWSKA-BARCZAK et al. (1976) found that E-type PGs sensitized the surface of the dog's heart to the reflex rise in blood pressure induced by Bk topically applied to the surface, and HANDWERKER (1975) showed sensitization to thermally induced discharge of sensory nerves by E-type PGs.

The use of infusions (FERREIRA, 1972; FERREIRA et al., 1975; MONCADA et al., 1975) allowed us to study the characteristics of PG-induced hyperalgesia, two important features of which are its cumulative nature and the long duration of the action. The cumulative nature of the PG-induced hyperalgesia was defined by FERREIRA (1972) who showed that the hyperalgesic effect of E-type PGs depended not only on the concentration infused but also on the duration of the infusion. Later, we showed that even very small amounts of PGs infused into the knee joint of the dog were able to induce hyperalgesia provided they were maintained for long enough (MONCADA et al., 1975).

Similar cumulative effects have been described by WILLIS and CORNELSON (1973) in the rat paw, and by JUAN and LEMBECK (1974) in the arterial circulation of the rabbit's ear. As a pain producing substance, Bk does not share this property.

The second feature of PG hyperalgesia is its long duration (JUHLIN and MICHAELSSON, 1969; FERREIRA, 1972; MONCADA et al., 1975). This characteristic, which is such that the effect outlasts the presence of PGs in the sensitized area, is shared by 5-HT (SICUTERI, 1968) and is poorly understood. Other authors have described the same phenomenon (WILLIS and CORNELSON, 1973; JUAN and LEMBECK, 1974). WILLIS and CORNELSON (1973) hypothesized that the long lasting hyperalgesia could be due to the accumulation of PG metabolites sharing with the parent PGs their sensitizing activity. Recent experiments (MONCADA and PONTIERI, 1975) have shown that PG metabolites have sensitizing activity on the pain nerve endings; however, they are several-fold less active than the parent PGs.

It is possible that other products of the metabolism of arachidonic or dihomo-γ-linoleic acids have a role to play in pain production. These include RCS (PIPER and VANE, 1969), thought to be an unstable intermediate in the synthesis of PGs (GRYGLEWSKI and VANE, 1972). RCS is now known to be a mixture of PG endoperoxides and thromboxane A_2 (SVENSSON et al., 1975; NEEDLEMAN et al., 1976; MONCADA et al., 1976). Not much is known about the pharmacology of these substances (WILLIS et al., 1974; HAMBERG et al., 1975; BUNTING et al., 1976), but they could well contribute to the local pharmacological effects during continued PG synthesis in inflammation. Certainly, fatty acid hydroperoxides can cause pain in man (FERREIRA, 1972). Intensity of pain produced by intradermal injections of fatty acid hydroperoxides was greater than that induced by either the parent fatty acid, or acetylcholine, Bk, histamine or PGE_1. This pain producing activity of fatty acid hydroperoxides needs to be further explored.

From all these results, it is clear that PGs (and perhaps some of the unstable intermediates), released in almost any form of tissue damage, sensitize the pain receptors to different types of stimulation (chemical, thermal, mechanical). Other mediators released during the inflammation process interact to stimulate the pain receptors but at the concentrations present, their activity is probably effective only against a background of sensitization induced by the presence of PGs.

G. Aspirin-Like Drugs and Their Mechanism of Analgesia

Aspirin-like drugs are weak analgesics in contrast to the "strong" narcotic analgesics like morphine. Several differences separate the groups. Strong analgesics induce tolerance and addiction. They block inhibitory pathways controlling muscle tones, giving rise to the phenomena described as "plastic rigidity" or "straub tail" in mice and rats. They relieve pain through an effect on the CNS independent of the aetiology of pain. Aspirin-like drugs, on the other hand, do not induce tolerance and addiction. They do not affect central inhibitory pathways and are selective analgesics against pain produced in some clinical or experimental conditions.

This selectivity of aspirin-like drugs against pain in certain pathological states and in some experimental models but not in others (COLLIER, 1969a), coupled with the fact that the increase in pain threshold they produce is not greater than 50% (WOLFF et al., 1941; WINDER et al., 1946; WINDER, 1947; DENEAU et al., 1953; SHERMAN et al., 1963) made difficult the assessment of aspirin-like drugs as analgesics and gave rise to a great number of papers with conflicting results (for reviews see GOETZL, 1946; BEECHER, 1952; COLLIER, 1969a), and a discussion which lasted for over 50 years. It was not until 1953 that BEECHER et al. recognised the placebo effect and, using the double blind technique, demonstrated that aspirin relieves post-operative pain, being approximately 10 times less potent than codeine and 60 times less potent than morphine. Later studies have confirmed and extended this observation (SHERMAN et al., 1963; BEAVER, 1965).

Conditions in clinical experience in which aspirin-like drugs are effective as analgesics include pain of low and moderate intensity but not of high intensity (WOODBURY, 1970; LIM, 1966). The pain is usually associated with inflammatory tissue damage, or processes in which the involvement of chemical mediators have been suggested, like post-operative pain, osteo-arthritis, rheumatoid arthritis, ankylosing spondilitis, and some forms of headache (LIM, 1966). Aspirin-like drugs have no measurable activity against pain of high intensity due to muscular spasm, distension of a hollow viscera, acute noxious stimulation of the skin or pain in which nerve trunks are involved.

Aspirin-like drugs are effective in experimental models involving the induction of a previous inflammatory state (HESS et al., 1930; RANDALL and SELLITO, 1957; PARDO and RODRIGUEZ, 1966; MARGOLIN, 1965; GILFOIL et al., 1963; WINTER, 1965; WINTER and FLATAKER, 1965). When there is no previous inflammation, aspirin-like drugs are effective analgesics only when there is a delay between the application of the stimulus and the development of the "pain response". For instance there is a delay between the injection of phenylbenzoquinone and the production of the stretching response (KEITH, 1960). Aspirin and other aspirin-type drugs block this delayed stretching response but have low activity against the almost immediate stretching response induced by hypertonic saline (COLLIER et al., 1968). They have low activity against the early stretching induced by Bk (COLLIER et al., 1968) but are very active against the delayed response of Bk (EMELE and SHANAMAN, 1963). Aspirin-like drugs are not effective against nociception of short duration induced by pinching or stimulating the tail or toes of mouse, rat or guinea pig (COLLIER and CHESHER, 1956; WINTER and FLATAKER, 1965).

The site of action and the mechanism by which aspirin-like drugs produce analgesia has been the subject of much discussion. An action on the CNS was claimed by DRESER as early as 1899 and throughout the years it has been maintained as the most plausible explanation, despite increasing evidence for a peripheral mode of action (WOODBURY, 1970).

There are several experimental animal models in which inflammation is able to sensitize pain receptors to mechanical and chemical stimulation. Always, hyperalgesia occurs after a latent period, generally when other inflammatory signs or symptoms are developing; but there does not seem to be a strict correlation between oedema and pain (VAN ARMAN et al., 1968; FERREIRA et al., 1976). Figure 2 illustrates that in the same rat, carrageenin causes greater hyperalgesia than dextran although the oedema produced by the latter was much more, intense.

The observation that anti-inflammatory and analgesic activity run parallel in many cases (RANDALL, 1963) led several authors to believe that at least part of the analgesic activity was peripheral (RANDALL and SELLITO, 1957; SIEGMUND et al., 1957; WINDER, 1959). Some authors suggested that analgesia was an indirect action produced as a consequence of the anti-inflammatory properties (HARRIS and FOSDICK, 1952; RANDALL and SELLITO, 1957; SMITH, 1960). This proposition does not explain the results of GUZMAN et al. (1962) in which aspirin-like drugs antagonised pain induced by Bk in conditions in which there is no inflammation. Nor does it

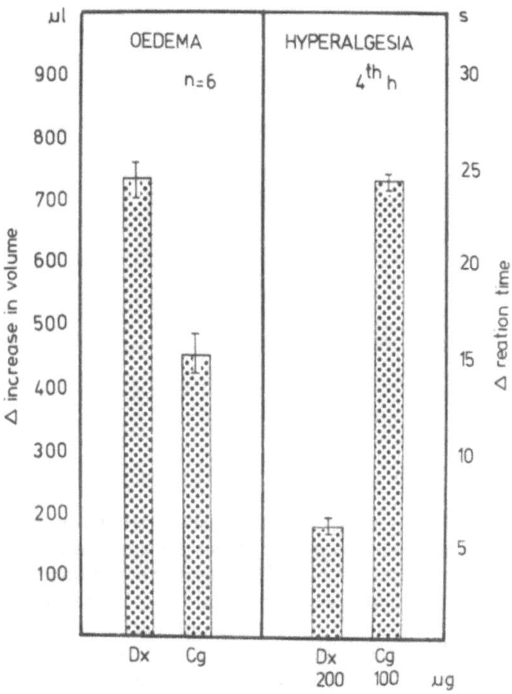

Fig. 2. Comparison of rat paw oedema and hyperalgesia induced by dextran *(Dx)* and carrageenin *(Cg)* in the same animal. Injections of Cg (100 µg) and Dx (200 µg) were made in different paws at 0 and 3 h respectively and measurements of oedema (pletysmography) and hyperalgesia (Randall-Sellito technique) were made at 4 h. Dextran produced a much greater oedema than carrageenin but there was a much smaller hyperalgesia (FERREIRA, unpublished observations)

explain the fact that in several models aspirin-like drugs are effective as analgesics in doses at which they do not exert anti-inflammatory activity (WHITTLE, 1964; GILFOIL et al., 1963; WINTER, 1965; WINTER and FLATAKER, 1965). GUZMAN et al. (1964) and LIM et al. (1964) provided definitive evidence which showed the peripheral analgesic activity of aspirin-like drugs. Other authors (WHITTLE, 1964; SCOTT, 1968) using other models have confirmed this concept.

As a mechanism for this peripheral activity LIM et al. (1964) and LIM (1968) claimed a direct antagonism at a receptor level between algesic substances (believed to be electropositive; see above) and aspirin-like drugs. However, the repeated observation that some sort of inflammation or damage of the tissue needs to be present in order to observe the analgesic effect of aspirin-like drugs (WINDER, 1959; RANDALL, 1963; COLLIER, 1969a) led several authors to suggest that analgesia was produced as a result of an action against pain producing substances released during inflammation (e.g. Bk, as is inferred from the work of GUZMAN et al., 1962; and LIM et al., 1964) or against the release of an intermediary substance responsible in the final step for the action of several mediators in inflammation (COLLIER, 1969a, 1969b) or as WINDER (1959) put it, the suppression of some "pre-inflammatory process" in the course of the reaction by tissues to injury. The same process could lead both to stimulation of pain endings and eventually to frank inflammation.

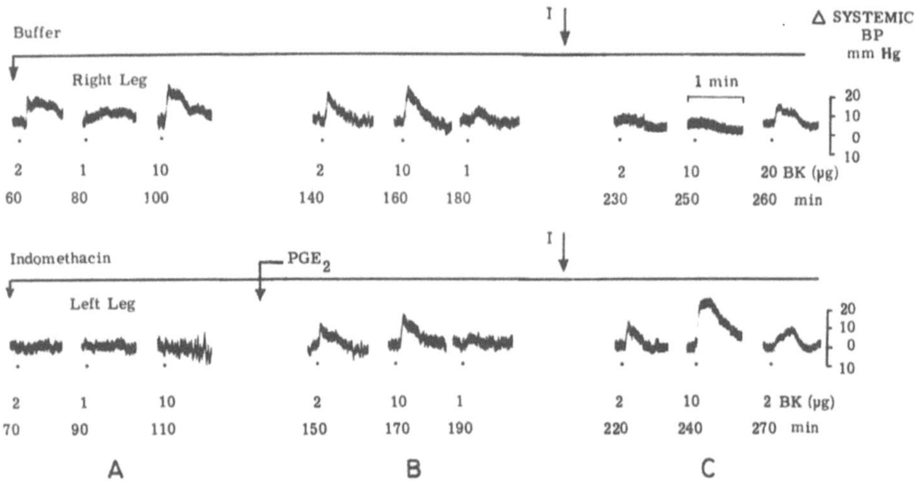

Fig. 3. Indomethacin fails to antagonise the hypertensive response induced by bradykinin injections in a dog knee joint which is receiving exogenous prostaglandin E_2. The tracings show the changes in systemic blood pressure (mm Hg) of the dog and are arranged in three panels. Panel A *(upper part)* shows the rise in blood pressure induced by 2, 1, and 10 μg of bradykinin injected into the right knee joint (receiving a Tris-buffer infusion); Panel A *(lower part)* shows the lack of effect of bradykinin in the left knee joint (receiving an infusion of indomethacin at 1 μg/min). Panel B shows the responses to the same doses of bradykinin 30 min after adding PGE_2 (50 ng/min) to the infusion into the left knee joint. This increased the sensitivity so that both joints responded similarly to bradykinin. Panel C shows the responses 30 min after each knee joint received an injection of 1 mg of indomethacin (I). In the right joint *(upper part)* receiving Tris-buffer, the responses to 2 and 10 μg bradykinin were blocked, and 20 μg only produced an effect similar to that of 2 μg in the left joint, receiving prostaglandin E_2. In this joint, the responses to bradykinin were not inhibited after local indomethacin treatment. The numbers below the doses of bradykinin indicate the time at which each injection was made after the start of the experiment. Time 1 min; vertical scales, variation of blood pressure mm Hg. (Data taken from MONCADA et al., 1975)

Three main findings allowed the development of our concept of the mechanism of analgesia induced by aspirin-like drugs. First there was the observation that PGs are released during inflammation (WILLIS, 1969). Next came the discovery that aspirin-like drugs inhibit PG biosynthesis (VANE, 1971) and third, the finding that PGs induce hyperalgesia rather than pain in concentrations likely to be present in inflammatory exudates (FERREIRA, 1972; FERREIRA et al., 1973; MONCADA et al., 1975).

We have, therefore, proposed that PGs sensitize rather than stimulate sensory nerve endings to the pain producing activity of other stimuli. The pain producing activity of Bk in the presence of exogenous PGs is unaffected by aspirin-like drugs (MONCADA et al., 1975; Fig. 3). This rules out a possible antagonism between Bk and aspirin at a receptor level as proposed by LIM (1966, 1968).

The mechanism by which PGs sensitize sensory nerve endings remains unknown; however, in other systems several authors have demonstrated lowering of threshold and increased response to electrical stimulation (CLEGG et al., 1966; KHAIRALLAH et al., 1967; STRONG and BOHR, 1967). Potentiation of the action of other agonists has been explained in terms of hypopolarization of the cell membrane probably by decreasing calcium (Ca^{++}) at sites which normally fix Ca^{++} (KHAIRALLAH et al., 1967; STRONG and BOHR, 1967).

Numerous workers have shown an inter-relationship between PGs and calcium ions. In fact, the actions of PGs vary inversely with the concentration of calcium ions in the media or the effects of PGs can be antagonised by addition of calcium (MANTEGAZZA, 1965; CLEGG et al., 1966; FASSINA and CONTESSA, 1967; FASSINA et al., 1969; HEDQVIST, 1973). In this context it is interesting to note that recently OLGART et al. (1974) have demonstrated, using the tooth pulp preparation for the study of pain, that lowering of extracellular calcium by addition of sodium citrate or EDTA leads to electrical discharge and to lowering of the threshold for heat-induced stimulation. This effect was readily antagonised by addition of calcium ions.

If the general mechanism of action of PGs is a lowering of the membrane potential due to an effect on calcium ions this could be the basis for the explanation of the sensitizing ability on sensory nerve endings. On the other hand, such a mechanism could explain the findings by LEVITAN and BARKER (1972) who demonstrated that the overall effect of salicylates on the nerve cells of the buccal ganglion of a mollusc was an increase in the membrane potential and suggested that this effect could be the basis for the analgesic effect of these drugs.

Aspirin-like drugs increase the pain threshold by no more than 50% (WOLFF et al., 1974; WINDER et al., 1946; WINDER, 1947; DENEAU et al., 1953) in experimental models, and in clinical conditions they are ineffective against pain of high intensity (see above). This fits with our proposed mechanism of action, for a removal of a sensitization would explain why this analgesic activity can be overcome by increasing the original stimulus and would explain why direct immediate damage of the nerve ending or trunks or, on the other hand, extensive damage leading to massive concentration of pain producing substances, is unlikely to be affected by aspirin-like drugs.

There are then three possibilities. Firstly, as in the spleen model (GUZMAN et al., 1962; FERREIRA et al., 1973), the increased basal release and any stimulated release of PGs is readily blocked by aspirin-like drugs thus allowing an immediate observation of their analgesic effect. Secondly, there are models in which the stimulus leads to PG release; an example would be the delayed stretching response induced by phenylbenzoquinone or Bk (KEITH, 1960; EMELE and SHANAMAN, 1963). Thirdly, in models like the skin or knee joint, an inflammatory state has to develop, leading to PG release, and only then can the analgesic effects of aspirin-like drugs be observed.

The knee joint of the dog becomes sensitive to the analgesic effects of aspirin-like drugs when inflammation is induced (PARDO and RODRIGUEZ, 1966; ROSENTHALE et al., 1966). We have observed the release of PGs during carrageenin-induced inflammation in this model and the sensitization by PGs to the pain induced by Bk. More recently, HERMAN and MONCADA (1975) have observed a close correlation between PG concentration and degree of incapacitation during endotoxin-induced inflammation in the knee joint of the dog.

Experimental models in which PGs do not seem to be involved like dextran-induced rat paw oedema or passive cutaneous anaphylaxis (PCA) develop much less hyperalgesia (VAN ARMAN et al., 1968; FERREIRA et al., 1975). Conversely, sunburn hyperalgesia (an example used by LEWIS in 1942 to suggest the presence of a factor specifically sensitizing nerve endings) is effectively inhibited by aspirin-like drugs

(HSIA et al., 1974) and is a model in which the presence of PGs has been firmly established (GREAVES and SONDERGAARD, 1970).

SICUTERI et al. (1968) suggested that 5-HT (released from platelets) is involved in the genesis of migraine headache by sensitizing the pain receptors to the action of Bk. PGs can also be released by platelets (SMITH and WILLIS, 1970) and perhaps by an intense contraction of vascular smooth muscle. This release would create a state of hyperalgesia and later could also be responsible for the vasodilatation by abolishing sympathetic tone. The overt pain felt by the patient suffering from migraine could be due to a mechanical factor acting in a hyperalgesic area, such as the pulsatile dilatation of blood vessels. Changes in the intensity of the migraine headache are related to changes in amplitude of the pulsations of the cranial arteries. Factors which decrease the amplitude of the pulsation also decrease the intensity of the headache (WOLFF, 1943). Such an interpretation may explain why aspirin-like drugs, some 5-HT antagonists and ergotamine derivatives, have a therapeutic effect in migraine.

Patients suffering from chronic headaches are very sensitive to spinal injections of Bk, and the intracranial pain receptors of rabbits display high sensitivity to Bk (SICUTERI et al., 1966). Interestingly enough, indomethacin is an effective inhibitor of this pain producing activity of Bk in both man and rabbit. The blockade indicates an involvement of the PG system, probably in the same way as in the dog spleen (FERREIRA et al., 1973). Thus, the local release of PG by injected Bk sensitizes the pain receptors to the pain producing activity of Bk. Certainly, both in vitro and in vivo, Bk is an effective stimulus for PG release (PIPER and VANE, 1971; MCGIFF et al., 1972; MONCADA et al., 1972; FERREIRA et al., 1973).

We can conclude that the anti-inflammatory acids do not reduce the effect of PGs but reduce only those effects caused by inflammatory substances or stimuli that induce generation of PGs. Such a conclusion depends upon the specific activity of the anti-inflammatory compound on the synthetase rather than on the PG receptor. However, with fenamates, which are among the most potent synthetase inhibitors, some receptor antagonism may also occur (COLLIER and SWEATMAN, 1968). Such an effect is likely to be additive to the analgesia caused by synthetase inhibition.

Our proposition explains the difference between experimental pain and pathological pain (BEECHER, 1952; LIM, 1966), explains the specific sensitization described by LANDAU and BISHOP (1953) during inflammation and explains the effectiveness of aspirin-like drugs in experimental models which lead to pathological pain (WINDER, 1959; LIM, 1966; COLLIER, 1969a). As shown in Figure 4 aspirin-like drugs which act peripherally will be active as analgesics only against those forms of pain in which PG release is involved: however, we suggest that conditions in which a massive release of other mediators is enough to produce a strong stimulation of pain receptors, the presence or absence of modulator PGs will not affect the sensation of pain. In these conditions, aspirin-like drugs will not have analgesic activity.

One of the main arguments put forward against the PG theory for explaining analgesia is the existence of aspirin-like drugs which have weak analgesic activity without conspicuous anti-inflammatory activity in man, and paracetamol (acetaminophen) is given as an example. In fact, paracetamol is as effective as aspirin in blocking hyperalgesia in the RANDALL and SELLITO (1958) test, but it should not be overlooked that paracetamol in higher doses also inhibits carrageenin oedema.

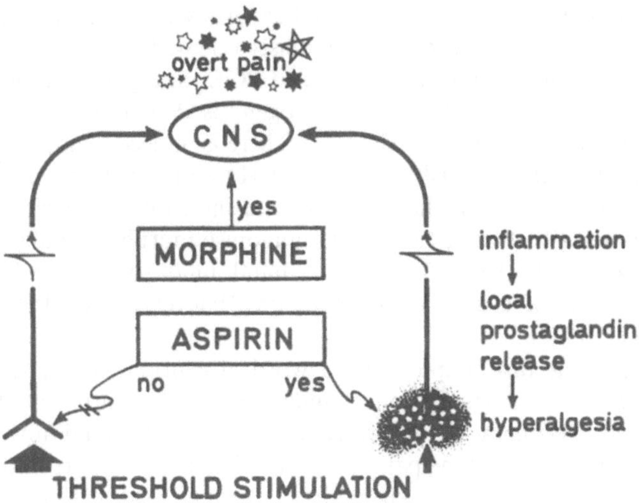

Fig. 4. An explanation of the analgesic action of aspirin. For details, see text. (From FERREIRA and VANE, 1974)

Paracetamol or dipyrone (FLOWER and VANE, 1972; DEMBINSKA-KIEC et al., 1976) were compared with aspirin-like drugs against PG synthetase of several tissues. They were relatively inactive on all but nervous tissue, where paracetamol was as active as aspirin and dipyrone was 4 times more potent. Our suggestion is that weak analgesics which display more intense analgesic and antipyretic than anti-inflammatory activity are mainly effective against nervous tissue synthetase, or have an easier access to the nervous system as in the case of paracetamol (DAVISON et al., 1961).

The evidence that the analgesic action of aspirin-like drugs is dependent on a central action is meagre and difficult to interpret. In some cases, the observed analgesic effect could easily be a consequence of a peripheral effect since the type of stimulation used could lead to trauma, i.e. radiant energy and electrical shock through chronically implanted electrodes in the brain (BONNYCASTLE et al., 1953; DUBAS and PARKER, 1971). Against this possibility is the fact that morphine blocks Bk-evoked potentials in the CNS after an intrasplenic injection while aspirin has no effect (LIM et al., 1969).

Undoubtedly aspirin-like drugs act in vivo against PG synthetase in the brain as demonstrated by their antipyretic activity (see Chapter 18). If PG synthetase in sensory nerves is as sensitive as brain synthetase to drugs like paracetamol and dipyrone and hyperalgesia is a consequence of PGs released within the nerves themselves, then a selective inhibition of that synthetase could explain analgesia by a peripheral mechanism. If, however, there is a central component to the analgesic action of aspirin-like drugs, it could also involve the PG system, for electrical stimulation of the hind paws of frogs (RAMWELL et al., 1966) or the radial nerves of cats (RAMWELL and SHAW, 1966) release PGs in the spinal cord and sensory cortex. Moreover, some PGs can facilitate polysynaptic reflexes (SIGGINS et al., 1971).

Thus, aspirin-like drugs might act by removing PG facilitation produced by centrally released PGs. An attractive hypothesis suggested recently by COLLIER and

ROY (1974) proposes that morphine-induced analgesia is the result of a blockade in the increase of cAMP induced by endogenously released PGE. This has been substantiated by the finding that centrally applied PGE_1 antagonises morphine analgesia (FERRI et al., 1974). The absence of endogenous PGs after synthesis inhibition would have the same effect on cAMP levels. There is, indeed, evidence which shows that cAMP injected intravenously induces pain (LEVINE, 1970) and that drugs which inhibit cAMP breakdown by phosphodiesterase increase the sensitivity of rats to painful stimulation (PAALZOW, 1975) and antagonise morphine analgesia (HO et al., 1973; CONTRERAS et al., 1972). On the other hand, imidazole-induced analgesia can be explained in terms of its ability to decrease cAMP levels (PUIG MUSET et al., 1972; CONTRERAS et al., 1972).

We may conclude this chapter with a word of caution. It is a step forward to understand the diverse participation of inflammatory mediators in the genesis of hyperalgesia and overt pain. However, we still do not understand how PGs produce a long lasting sensitization of the pain receptors when their half-life in the circulation and in most vascular beds is so short (FERREIRA and VANE, 1967). Furthermore, drugs such as corticosteroids and colchicine do not interfere with the release of PGs in exudates but nevertheless display an analgesic effect. We discard the simplistic idea that the analgesic effect is a consequence of reduced inflammation, because we are convinced that the action of drugs on inflammatory signs or symptoms can ultimately be explained either by an interference with genesis of mediators or with the responsiveness of the effector cells (Chapter 31). There is general agreement that inflammatory signs and symptoms derive from the multiple action of mediators and a symptom such as pain results (as do other symptoms) from a fine balance between the actions of these mediators. As a result of this, removal of one of them may cause analgesia.

Corticosteroids might stabilise the pain receptor or block the release or antagonise the action of unknown inflammatory mediators. Although corticosteroids can interfere with PG release (see Chapters 31 and 37), the clinical usefulness of corticosteroids indicates a much more diverse mechanism of action.

There are many candidates for the honorary title of inflammatory mediators whose role in inflammatory pain is not yet defined. These include lymph node permeability factor, slow reacting substance A, substance P, leucocytic inflammatory substance, etc. It is improbable that any one of them will be the "pain mediator", if active, they will almost certainly be classified either as pain-triggering substance (like Bk or histamine), or as pain-sensitizing substances (like PGs and 5-HT).

References

Armstrong, D., Dry, R. M. L., Keele, C. A., Markham, J. W.: Pain producing substances in blister fluid and in serum. J. Physiol. (Lond.) **117**, 4 P (1952)

Armstrong, D., Dry, R. M. L., Keele, C. A., Markham, J. W.: Observations on chemical excitants of cutaneous pain in man. J. Physiol. (Lond.) **120**, 326—351 (1953)

Armstrong, D., Jepson, J. B., Keele, C. A., Stewart, J. W.: Pain producing substance in human inflammatory exudate and plasma. J. Physiol. (Lond.) **135**, 350—370 (1957)

Beaver, W. T.: Mild analgesics, a review of their clinical pharmacology. Amer. J. med. Sci. **250**, 577—604 (1965)

Beecher, H. K.: Experimental pharmacology and measurements of the subjective response. Science **116**, 157—162 (1952)
Beecher, H. K.: The measurement of pain. Prototype for the quantitative study of subjective responses. Pharmacol. Rev. **9**, 59 (1957)
Beecher, H. K., Keats, A. S., Mosteller, F., Lasagna, L.: The effectiveness of oral analgesics (morphine, codeine, acetyl-salicylic acid) and the problem of placebo "reactors" and "non-reactors". J. Pharmacol. **109**, 393—400 (1953)
Benjamin, F. B.: Release of intracellular potassium as a physiological stimulus for pain. J. appl. Physiol. **14**, 643—646 (1959)
Benjamin, F. B., Helvey, W. M.: Iontophoresis of potassium for experimental determination of pain endurance in man. Proc. Soc. exp. Biol. (N.Y.) **113**, 566—568 (1963)
Bevegard, S., Oro, L.: Effect of prostaglandin E_1 on forearm blood flow. Scand. J. clin. Lab. Invest. **23**, 347—352 (1969)
Bishop, G. H., Landau, W.: Evidence for a double peripheral pathway for pain. Science **128**, 712—713 (1958)
Bommer, S.: Neutrale Salzreaktionen auf der Haut. Klin. Wschr. **3**, 1758—1760 (1924)
Bonnycastle, D. D., Cook, L., Ipsen, J.: The actions of some analgesic drugs in intact and chronic spinal rats. Acta Pharmacol. (Kbh.) **9**, 331—336 (1953)
Brooks, B.: Intra-arterial injection of sodium iodide. J. Amer. med. Ass. **82**, 1016—1019 (1924)
Brune, K., Bucher, K., Walz, D.: The avian micro-crystal rthritis. II. Central versus peripheral effects of sodium salicylate, acetaminophen, and colchicine. Agents Actions **4**, 27—33 (1974)
Bunting, S., Moncada, S., Vane, J. R.: The effects of prostaglandin endoperoxides and thromboxane A_2 on strips of rabbit coeliac artery and certain smooth muscle preparations. Brit. J. Pharmacol. **57**, 426 P (1976)
Burch, G. E., Pasquale, N. P. de: Bradykinin, digital blood flow, and the arteriovenous anastomoses. Circulat. Res. **10**, 105—115 (1962)
Chapman, L. F., Ramos, A. O., Goodell, H., Wolff, H. G.: Neurohumoral features of afferent fibres in man. Their role in vasodilation inflammation and pain. Arch. Neurol. (Chic.) **4**, 617—650 (1961)
Clegg, P. C., Hall, W. F., Pickles, V. R.: The action of ketonic prostaglandins on guinea pig myometrium. J. Physiol. (Lond.) **183**, 123—144 (1966)
Coffman, J. D.: The effect of aspirin on pain and hand blood flow responses to intra-arterial injection of bradykinin in man. Clin. Pharmacol. Ther. **7**, 26—37 (1966)
Collier, H. O. J.: A pharmacological analysis of aspirin. Advanc. Pharmacol. Chemother. **7**, 333—405 (1969 a)
Collier, H. O. J.: New light on how aspirin works. Nature (Lond.) **223**, 35—37 (1969 b)
Collier, H. O. J., Chesher, G. B.: Antipyretic and analgesic properties of 2 hydroxyisophthalic acids. Brit. J. Pharmacol. **11**, 20—26 (1956)
Collier, H. O. J., Dineen, L. C., Johnson, C. A., Schneider, C.: The abdominal constriction response and its suppression by analgesic drugs in the mouse. Brit. J. Pharmacol. **32**, 295—310 (1968)
Collier, H. O. J., Hammond, A. R., Horwood-Barrett, S., Schneider, C.: Rapid induction by acetylcholine, bradykinin, and potassium of a nociceptive response in mice and its selective antagonism by aspirin. Nature (Lond.) **204**, 1316—1318 (1964)
Collier, H. O. J., Roy, A. C.: Inhibition of E prostaglandin-sensitive adenyl cyclase as the mechanism of morphine analgesia. Prostaglandins **7**, 361—376 (1974)
Collier, H. O. J., Schneider, C.: Nociceptive response to prostaglandins and analgesic actions of aspirin and morphine. Nature (New Biol.) **236**, 141—143 (1972)
Collier, H. O. J., Sweatman, W. J. F.: Antagonism by fenamates of $PGF_{2\alpha}$ and of slow reacting substances on human bronchial muscle. Nature (Lond.) **219**, 864—865 (1968)
Collier, H. O. J., Warner, B. T., Skerry, R. J.: Multiple toe-pinch method for testing analgesic drugs. Brit. J. Pharmacol. **17**, 28—40 (1961)
Collier, J. G., Karim, S. M. M., Robinson, B., Somers, K.: Action of prostaglandins A_2, B_1, E_2 and $F_{2\alpha}$ on superficial hand veins of man. Brit. J. Pharmacol. **44**, 374—375 (1972)
Collins, W. F., Nulsen, F. E., Sheally, C. N.: Electrophysiological and central pathways conducting pain. In: Pain. Boston: Little Brown & Co. 1966
Contreras, E., Castilli, S., Quijada, L.: Effect of drugs that modify 3′, 5′-AMP concentrations on morphine analgesia. J. Pharm. Pharmacol. **24**, 65—66 (1972)

Cormia, F. E., Dougherty, J. W.: Proteolytic activity in development of pain and itching. Cutaneous reactions to bradykinin and kallikrein. J. invest. Derm. **35**, 21—26 (1960)
Crunkhorn, P., Willis, A. L.: Actions and interactions of prostaglandins administered intradermally in rat and in man. Brit. J. Pharmacol. **36**, 216P—217P (1969)
Crunkhorn, P., Willis, A. L.: Cutaneous reactions to intradermal prostaglandins. Brit. J. Pharmacol. **41**, 49—56 (1971)
Davison, C., Guy, J. L., Levitt, M., Smith, P. K.: The distribution of certain non-narcotic agents in the CNS of several species. J. Pharmacol. exp. Ther. **134**, 176—183 (1961)
Della Bella, D., Bennelli, G.: Bradykinin and the spleen: different reaction *in vitro* and *in vivo*. In: Mantegazza, P., Horton, E. W. (Eds.): Prostaglandins Peptides an Amines, pp. 99—107. London: Academic Press 1969
Dembinska-Kiec, A., Zmuda, A., Krupinska, J.: Inhibition of prostaglandin synthetase by aspirin-like drugs in different microsomal preparations. In: Samuelsson, B., Paoletti, R. (Eds.): Advances in Prostaglandins and Thromboxane Research, pp. 99—103. New York: Raven Press 1976
Deneau, G. A., Waud, R. A., Gowdey, C. W.: A method for the determination of the effects of drugs on the pain threshold of human subjects. Can. J. med. Sci. **31**, 387—393 (1953)
Dickerson, G. D., Engle, R. J., Guzman, F., Rodgers, D. W., Lim, R. K. S.: The intraperitoneal bradykinin-evoked pain test for analgesia. Life Sci. **4**, 2039—2069 (1965)
Dorpat, T. L., Holmes, T. H.: Mechanism of skeletal muscle pain and fatigue. Arch. Neurol. Psychiat. (Chic.) **77**, 628—640 (1955)
Dreser, H.: Pharmakologisches über Aspirin (Acetylsalicylsäure). Pflügers Arch. ges. Physiol. **76**, 306—318 (1899)
Dubas, T. C., Parker, J. M.: A central component in the analgesic action of sodium salicylate. Arch. int. Pharmacodyn. **194**, 117—122 (1971)
Edery, H., Lewis, G. P.: Inhibition of plasma kininase activity at slight acid pH. Brit. J. Pharmacol. **19**, 299—305 (1962)
Emele, J. F., Shanaman, J.: Bradykinin writhing: method for measuring analgesia. Proc. Soc. exp. Biol. (N.Y.) **114**, 680—682 (1963)
Emmelin, N., Feldberg, W.: The mechanism of the sting of the common nettle *(Urtica urens)*. J. Physiol. (Lond.) **106**, 440—455 (1947)
Fassina, G., Carpenedo, F., Santi, R.: Effect of prostaglandin E_1 on isolated short circuted frog skin. Life Sci. **8**, 181—187 (1969)
Fassina, G., Contessa, A. R.: Digitoxin and prostaglandin E_1 as inhibitors of catecholamine-stimulated lipolysis and their interaction with Ca^{++} in the process. Biochem. Pharmacol. **16**, 1447—1453 (1967)
Feldberg, W.: The role of mediators in the inflammatory tissue response. Int. Arch. Allergy **8**, 15—31 (1956)
Ferreira, S. H.: Prostaglandins, aspirin-like drugs and analgesia. Nature (New Biol.) **240**, 200—203 (1972)
Ferreira, S. H., Harvey, E. A., Vane, J. R.: Hyperalgesia, inflammatory oedema and prostaglandins. Proceedings of the VI International Congress of Pharmacology, 1976 (in press)
Ferreira, S. H., Moncada, S., Vane, J. R.: Prostaglandins and the mechanism of analgesia produced by aspirin-like drugs. Brit. J. Pharmacol. **49**, 86—97 (1973)
Ferreira, S. H., Vane, J. R.: Prostaglandins: their disappearance from and release into the circulation. Nature (Lond.) **216**, 868—873 (1967)
Ferreira, S. H., Vane, J. R.: New aspects of the mode of action of non-steroid anti-inflammatory drugs. Ann. Rev. Pharmacol. **14**, 57—73 (1974)
Ferri, S., Sangostino, A., Braga, P. C., Galatulas, I.: Decreased antinociceptive effect of morphine in rats treated intraventricularly with prostaglandin E_1. Psychopharmacologia (Berl.) **39**, 231 (1974)
Fitzgerald, M. J. T.: The innervation of the epidermis. In: Kenshalo, D. R. (Ed.): The Skin Senses, pp. 61—83. Illinois: Springfield 1968
Fjallebrant, N., Iggo, A.: The effect of histamine, 5-hydroxytryptamine and acetylcholine on cutaneous afferent fibres. J. Physiol. (Lond.) **156**, 578—590 (1961)
Flower, R. J., Vane, J. R.: Inhibition of prostaglandin synthetase in brain explains the anti-pyretic activity of paracetamol (4-Acetamidophenol). Nature (Lond.) **240**, 410—411 (1972)

Fox,R.H., Goldsmith,R., Kidd,D.J., Lewis,G.P.: Bradykinin as a vasodilator in man. J. Physiol. (Lond.) **157**, 589—602 (1961)
Frolich,A., Meyer,H.H.: Visceral sensibility. Klin. Wschr. **1**, 1368—1369 (1922)
Gardner,E.: Physiology of movable joints. Physiol. Rev. **30**, 127—176 (1950)
Gilfoil,T.M., Klavins,I.: 5-hydroxytryptamine, bradykinin, and histamine as mediators of inflammatory hyperesthesia. Amer. J. Physiol. **208**, 867—876 (1965)
Gilfoil,T.M., Klavins,I., Grumbach,L.: Effects of acetylsalicylic acid on the oedema and hyperesthesia of the experimentally inflamed rat's paw. J. Pharmacol. exp. Ther. **142**, 1—5 (1963)
Gillespie,A.: Prostaglandin-oxytocin enhancement and potentiation and their clinical applications. Brit. med. J. **1**, 150—152 (1972)
Goetzl,F.R.: The experimental evidence for analgesic properties of antipyretic drugs. Permanente Fdn. med. Bull. **4**, 49—83 (1946)
Goetzl,F.R., Burrill,D.Y., Ivy,A.C.: A critical analysis of algesimetric methods with suggestions for a useful procedure. Quart. Bull. Northw. Univ. med. Sch. **17**, 280—291 (1943)
Greaves,M.W., McDonald-Gibson,W.: Itch: role of prostaglandins. Brit. Med. J. **3**, 608—609 (1973)
Greaves,M.W., Sondergaard,J.: Urticaria pigmentosa and factitious urticaria. Direct evidence for release of histamine and other smooth muscle contracting agents in dermographic skin. Arch. Derm. **101**, 418—425 (1970)
Gryglewski,R., Vane,J.R.: The release of prostaglandins and rabbit aorta contracting substance (RCS) from rabbit spleen and its antagonism by anti-inflammatory drugs. Brit. J. Pharmacol. **45**, 37—47 (1972)
Guzman,F., Braun,C., Lim,R.K.S.: Visceral pain and the pseudaffective response to intraarterial injection of bradykinin and other algesic agents. Arch. int. Pharmacodyn. **136**, 353—384 (1962)
Guzman,F., Braun,C., Lim,R.K.S., Potter,G.D., Rodgers,D.W.: Narcotic and non-narcotic analgesics which block visceral pain evoked by intra-arterial injections of bradykinin and other algesic agents. Arch. int. Pharmacodyn. **149**, 571—588 (1964)
Hamberg,M., Hedqvist,P., Strandberg,K., Svensson,J., Samuelsson,B.: Prostaglandin endoperoxides. IV. Effects on smooth muscle. Life Sci. **16**, 451—462 (1975)
Handwerker,H.O.: Influence of prostaglandin E_2 on the discharge of cutaneous nociceptive C-fibres induced by radiant heat. Pflügers Arch. ges. Physiol. **355**, Suppl., R 116 (1975)
Hardy,J.D., Stolwijk,J.A.J., Hoffman,D.: Pain following step increase in the skin temperature. In: Kenshalo,D.R. (Ed.): The Skin Senses, pp. 444—457. Illinois: Springfield 1968
Hardy,J.D., Wolff,H.G., Goodell,H.: Experimental evidence on the nature of cutaneous hyperalgesia. J. clin. Invest. **29**, 115—140 (1950)
Hardy,J.D., Wolff,H.C., Goodell,H.: Pain Sensations and Reactions. Baltimore: Williams & Wilkins 1952
Harpman,J.A., Whitehead,T.P.: Observations on chemical and neural mechanisms of cutaneous hyperalgesia, flare, and inflammation. Brain **78**, 634—660 (1955)
Harris,S.C., Fosdick,L.S.: Theoretical considerations of the mechanism of antipyretic analgesia. Bull. Northw. Univ. dent. Res. grad. Study **53**, 6—9 (1952)
Hashimoto,K., Kumakura,S., Taira,N.: Vascular reflex responses induced by an intra-arterial injection of aza-azepinophenothiazine, andromedotoxin, veratridine, bradykinin, and kallikrein and blocking action of sodium salicylate. Jap. J. Physiol. **14**, 299—308 (1964)
Hedqvist,P.: Autonomic neurotransmission. In: Ramwell,P.W. (Ed.): The Prostaglandins, Vol. I, pp. 101—131. New York-London: Plenum Press 1973
Henriquez,F.C.: Studies of thermal injury. V. The predictability and the significance of thermally induced rate processes leading to irreversible epidermal injury. Arch. Path. **43**, 489—502 (1947)
Herman,A.G., Moncada,S.: Release of prostaglandins and incapacitation after injection of endotoxin in the knee joint of the dog. Brit. J. Pharmacol. **53**, 465 P (1975)
Hesse,E., Roesler,G., Bühler,F.: Zur biologischen Wertbestimmung der Analgetika und ihrer Kombinationen. Naunyn-Schmiedeberg's Arch. expt. Path. Pharmak. **158**, 247—253 (1930)
Ho,I.K., Loh,H.H., Leong Way,E.: Cyclic adenosine monophosphate antagonism of morphine analgesia. J. Pharmacol. exp. Ther. **185**, 336—346 (1973)

Horton, E. W.: Action of prostaglandin E_1 on tissues which respond to bradykinin. Nature (Lond.) **200**, 892—893 (1963)
Hsia, S. L., Ziboh, V. A., Snyder, D. S.: Naturally occurring and synthetic inhibitors of prostaglandin synthetase in the skin. In: Robinson, H. J., Vane, J. R. (Eds.): Prostaglandin Synthetase Inhibitors, pp. 353—361. New York: Raven Press 1974
Iggo, A.: Non-myelinated visceral muscular and cutaneous afferent fibres and pain. In: Keele, C. A., Smith, R. (Eds.): The Assessment of Pain in Man and Animals, pp. 74—87. Edinburgh: Livingstone 1962
Juan, H., Lembeck, F.: Action of peptides and other algesic agents on paravascular pain receptors of the isolated perfused rabbit ear. Naunyn-Schmiedeberg's Arch. exp. Path. Pharmak. **283**, 151—164 (1974)
Juhlin, L., Michaelsson, G.: Cutaneous vascular reactions to prostaglandins in healthy subjects and in patients with urticaria and atopic dermatitis. Acta. derm.-venereol. (Stockh.) **49**, 251—261 (1969)
Karim, S.: Action of prostaglandin in the pregnant woman. Ann. N.Y. Acad. Sci. **180**, 483—498 (1971)
Keele, C. A.: Polypeptides which affect smooth muscles and blood vessels. New York: Pergamon Press 1960
Keele, C. A., Armstrong, D.: Substances producing pain and itch. London: Edward Arnold 1964
Keith, E. F.: Evaluation of analgesic substances. Amer. J. Pharm. **132**, 202—230 (1960)
Khairallah, P. A., Page, I. H., Turker, R. K.: Some properties of prostaglandin E_1 action on muscle. Arch. int. Pharmacodyn. **169**, 328—341 (1967)
Kuhn, D. C., Willis, A. L.: Prostaglandin E_2, inflammation and pain threshold in rat paws. Brit. J. Pharmacol. **49**, 183 P—184 P (1973)
La Belle, A., Tislow, R.: A method of evaluating analysis of the anti-arthralgic type in the laboratory animal. J. Pharmacol. exp. Ther. **98**, 19—20 (1950)
Landau, W., Bishop, G. H.: Pain from dermal periostal and fascial endings and from inflammation. Arch. Neurol. Psychiat. (Chic.) **69**, 490—504 (1953)
Levitan, H., Barker, J. L.: Effect of non-narcotic analgesics on membrane permeability of molluscan neurones. Nature (New Biol.) **239**, 55—57 (1972)
Levine, R. A.: Effects of exogenous adenosine 3′, 5′-monophosphate in man. III. Increased response and tolerance to the dibutyryl derivative. Clin. Pharmacol. Ther. **11**, 238—243 (1970)
Lewis, T.: Experiments relating to cutaneous hyperalgesia and its spread through somatic nerves. Clin. Sci. **2**, 373—417 (1936)
Lewis, T.: Pain. New York: MacMillan 1942
Lewis, T., Hess, W.: Pain derived from the skin and the mechanism of its production. Clin. Sci. **1**, 39—61 (1933)
Lewis, T., Pickering, G. W., Rotschild, P.: Observations upon muscular pain in intermittent claudication. Heart **15**, 359—383 (1931)
Lewis, T., Pochin, E. E.: The double pain response of human skin to a single stimulus. Clin. Sci. **3**, 67—76 (1937)
Lim, R. K. S.: Visceral receptors and visceral pain. Ann. N.Y. Acad. Sci. **86**, 73—89 (1960)
Lim, R. K. S.: Salicylate analgesia. In: Smith, M. J. H., Smith, P. K. (Eds.): The Salicylates, p. 155. New York-London-Sydney: Smith Interscience Publishers 1966
Lim, R. K. S.: Neuropharmacology of pain and analgesia. In: Lim, R. K. S., Armstrong, D., Pardo, E. G. (Eds.): Pharmacology of Pain, pp. 169—217. Oxford: Pergamon Press 1968
Lim, R. K. S.: Pain. Ann. Rev. Physiol. **32**, 269—288 (1970)
Lim, R. K. S., Guzman, F.: Manifestations of pain in analgesic evaluation in animals and man. In: Soulairac, A., Cahn, J., Chartentier, J. (Eds.): Pain, pp. 119—152. London-New York: Academic Press 1968
Lim, R. K. S., Guzman, F., Rodgers, D. W., Goto, K., Braun, C., Dickerson, G. D., Engle, R. J.: Site of action of narcotic and non-narcotic analgesics determined by blocking bradykinin-evoked visceral pain. Arch. int. Pharmacodyn. **152**, 25—58 (1964)
Lim, R. K. S., Lin, G. N., Guzman, F., Braun, C.: Visceral receptors concerned in visceral pain and the pseudoaffective response to intra-arterial injections of bradykinin and other algesic agents. J. comp. Neurol. **118**, 269—293 (1962)

Lim, R. K. S., Krathamer, G., Guzman, F., Fulp, R.: Central nervous system activity associated with pain evoked by bradykinin and its alteration by morphine and aspirin. Proc. nat. Acad. Sci. **63**, 705—712 (1969)
Lim, R. K. S., Miller, D. G., Guzman, F., Rodgers, D. W., Wang, R. W., Chao, S. K., Shih, T. Y.: Pain and analgesia evaluated by intraperitoneal bradykinin-evoked pain method in man. Clin. Pharmacol. Ther. **8**, 521—542 (1967)
Lindahl, O.: Pain: a chemical explanation. Acta. rheum. scand. **8**, 161—169 (1962)
McGiff, J. C., Terragno, N. A., Malik, K. U., Lonigro, A. J.: Release of prostaglandin E like substance from canine kidney by bradykinin. Circulat. Res. **31**, 36—43 (1972)
Mantegazza, P.: La prostaglandina E_1 come sostanza sensibilizzatrice per il calcio a livello del cuore isolato di cavia. Atti. Accad. med. lombarda **20**, 66—72 (1965)
Margolin, S.: A simple method for the simultaneous determination of the anti-inflammatory and analgesic properties of drugs. In: Garattini, S., Dukes, M. N. G. (Eds.): Non-Steroidal Anti-Inflammatory Drugs, pp. 214—217. Amsterdam: Excerpta Medica 1965
Melmon, K. L., Webster, M. E., Goldfiner, S. E., Seegmiller, J. E.: The presence of a kinin in inflammatory synovial effusion from arthritides of varying etiologies. Arthr. and Rheum. **10**, 13—20 (1967)
Miller, J. W.: Observations on the innervation of blood vessels. J. Anat. (Lond.) **82**, 68—80 (1948)
Moncada, S.: Inhibition by aspirin-like drugs of prostaglandin release in the spleen and its effect on the functioning of efferent and afferent nerve fibres. University of London, Thesis, 1974
Moncada, S., Ferreira, S. H., Vane, J. R.: Does bradykinin produce pain through prostaglandin production? In: Abstracts of the V. International Congress of Pharmacology, p. 160. San Francisco: 1972
Moncada, S., Ferreira, S. H., Vane, J. R.: Sensitization of pain receptors of dog knee joint by prostaglandins. In: Robinson, H. J., Vane, J. R. (Eds.): Prostaglandin Synthetase Inhibitors, pp. 189—195. New York: Raven Press 1974
Moncada, S., Ferreira, S. H., Vane, J. R.: Inhibition of prostaglandin biosynthesis as the mechanism of analgesia of aspirin-like drugs in the dog knee joint. Europ. J. Pharmacol. **31**, 250—260 (1975)
Moncada, S., Needleman, P., Bunting, S., Vane, J. R.: Prostaglandin endoperoxides and thromboxane generating systems and their selective inhibition. Prostaglandins **12**, 323—336 (1976)
Moncada, S., Pontieri, V.: Are prostaglandin metabolites sensitizers of pain nerve-endings? In: Abstracts of the VI. International Congress of Pharmacology, p. 330, Helsinki, 1975
Moore, R. M.: Some experimental observations relating to visceral pain. Surgery **3**, 534—545 (1938)
Moore, R. M., Moore, R. E.: Studies on the pain sensibility of arteries. I. Some observations on the pain sensibility of arteries. Amer. J. Physiol. **104**, 259—266 (1933)
Moore, R. M., Singleton, A. O.: Studies on pain sensibility of arteries. II. Peripheral paths of afferent neurones from the arteries of the extremities and of the abdominal viscera. Amer. J. Physiol. **104**, 267—275 (1933)
Moritz, A. R., Henriquez, F. C.: Studies of thermal injury. II. The relative importance of time and surface temperature in the causation of cutaneous burns. Amer. J. Path. **23**, 695—720 (1947)
Needleman, P., Moncada, S., Bunting, S., Vane, J. R., Hamberg, M., Samuelsson, B.: Identification of an enzyme in platelet microsomes which generates thromboxane A_2 from prostaglandin endoperoxides. Nature (Lond.) **261**, 558—560 (1976)
Odermatt, W.: Sensitivity of blood vessels. Bruns' Beitr. klin. Chir. **127**, 1—84 (1922)
Olgart, L., Haugertam, G., Edwall, L.: The effect of extracellular calcium on thermal excitability of the sensory units in the tooth of the cat. Acta. physiol. scand. **91**, 116—122 (1974)
Paalzow, L. K.: Pharmacokinetics of theophylline in relation to increased pain sensitivity in the rat. J. Pharm. Biopharm. **3**, 25 (1975)
Paintal, A. S.: Functional analysis of group III afferent fibres in mammalian muscles. J. Physiol. (Lond.) **52**, 250—270 (1960)
Pardo, E. G., Rodriguez, R.: Reversal by acetylsalicylic acid of pain induced functional impairment. Life Sci. **5**, 775—781 (1966)
Perl, E. R.: Relation of cutaneous receptors to pain. Proc. Int. Union. Pysiol. Sci. **6**, 235—236 (1968)

Phelps, P., Prockop, D. J., McCarty, D. J.: Crystal induced inflammation in canine joints. III. Evidence against bradykinin as a mediator of inflammation. J. Lab. clin. Med. **68**, 433—444 (1966)
Piper, P. J., Vane, J. R.: Release of additional factors in anaphylaxis and its antagonism by anti-inflammatory drugs. Nature (Lond.) **223**, 29—35 (1969)
Piper, P. J., Vane, J. R.: The release of prostaglandins from lung and other tissues. Ann. N.Y. Acad. Sci. **180**, 363—385 (1971)
Potter, G. D., Guzman, F., Lim, R. K. S.: Visceral pain evoked by intra-arterial injection of substance P. Nature (Lond.) **193**, 983—984 (1962)
Puig Muset, P., Puig Parellada, P., Martin Esteve, J.: Biochemical and pharmacological aspects of imidazole. In: Puig Muset, P., Puig Parellada, P., Martin Esteve, J. (Eds.): Biochemical and Pharmacological Aspects of Imidazole. Barcelona: JIMS 1972
Ramwell, P. W., Shaw, J. E.: Spontaneous and evoked release of prostaglandins from cerebral cortex of anaesthetized cats. Amer. J. Physiol. **211**, 125—134 (1966)
Ramwell, P. W., Shaw, J. E., Jessup, R.: Spontaneous and evoked release of prostaglandins from frog spinal cord. Amer. J. Physiol. **211**, 998—1004 (1966)
Randall, L. O.: Non-narcotic analgesics. In: Root, W. S., Hofmann, F. G. (Eds.): Physiological Pharmacology, The Nervous System, Vol. 1, part A, pp. 313—416. New York: Academic Press 1963
Randall, L. O., Selitto, J. J.: A method for measurement of analgesic activity on inflamed tissue. Arch. int. Pharmacodyn. **111**, 409—419 (1957)
Randall, L. O., Selitto, J. J.: Anti-inflammatory effects of Romilar CF. J. Amer. pharmac. Ass. **47**, 313—314 (1958)
Rocha e Silva, M.: The participation of substances of low molecular weight in inflammation with special reference to histamine and bradykinin. In: Thomas, L., Uhn, J. W., Grant, L. (Eds.): Injury, Inflammation, and Immunity, p. 220. Baltimore: Williams & Wilkins 1964
Rocha e Silva, M., Garcia Leme, J.: Chemical Mediators of the Acute Inflammatory Reaction. Oxford: Pergamon Press 1972
Rosenthal, S. R.: Histamine as possible chemical mediator of cutaneous pain: painful responses to intradermal injections of perfusates from stimulated human skin. J. appl. Physiol. **2**, 348—354 (1949)
Rosenthal, S. R.: Histamine as possible chemical mediator for cutaneous pain: dual pain response to histamine. Proc. Sco. exp. Biol. (N.Y.) **74**, 167 (1950)
Rosenthal, S. R.: Histamine as chemical mediator for cutaneous pain. Fed. Proc. **23**, 1109—1111 (1964)
Rosenthale, M. E., Dervinis, A., Massarich, J., Singer, S.: Prostaglandins and anti-inflammatory drugs in the knee joint. J. Pharm. Pharmacol. **24**, 149—150 (1972)
Rosenthale, M. E., Kassarich, J., Schneider, F. Jr.: Effect of anti-inflammatory agents on acute experimental synovitis. Proc. Soc. exp. Biol. (N.Y.) **122**, 693—696 (1966)
Scott, D., Jr.: Aspirin action on receptor in the tooth. Science **161**, 180—181 (1968)
Sherman, H., Fiasconaro, J. E., Grundfest, H.: Laboratory evaluation of analgetic effectiveness in human subjects. Exp. Neurol. **7**, 435—456 (1963)
Sherrington, C. S.: The integrative actions of the central nervous system. London: Constable 1906
Sicuteri, F.: Vasoneuroactive substances in migraine. Headache **6**, 109—126 (1966)
Sicuteri, F.: Sensitization of nociceptors by 5-hydroxytryptamine in man. In: Lim, R. K. S., Armstrong, D., Pardo, E. G. (Eds.): Pharmacology of Pain, pp. 57—86. Oxford: Pergamon Press 1968
Sicuteri, F., Franchi, P. L. del B., Franciulacci, M.: Peptides and Pain. In: Rocha e Silva, M., Rothschild, H. A. (Eds.): International Symposium on Vasoactive Polypeptides, Bradykinin, and Related Kinins, pp. 255—261. Brazil: Edat Sao Paulo 1966
Sicuteri, F., Franciullacci, M., Franchi, G., Del Bianco, P. L.: Serotonin-bradykinin potentiation on the pain receptors in man. Life Sci. **4**, 309—316 (1965)
Siegmund, E. A., Cadmus, R. A., Lu, G.: A method for evaluating both non-narcotic and narcotic analgesics. Proc. Soc. exp. Biol. (N.Y.) **95**, 729—731 (1957)
Siggins, G., Hoffer, B., Bloom, F.: Prostaglandin-norepinephrine interactions in brain: microelectrophoretic and histochemical correlates. Ann. N.Y. Acad. Sci. **180**, 302—323 (1971)

Sinclair, D. C., Stokes, B. A. R.: The production and characterisation of "Second Pain". Brain **87**, 609 (1967)

Singleton, A. O.: Use of intra-arterial injections of sodium iodide in determining conditions of circulation in extremities. Report of cases. Arch. Surg. **16**, 1232—1241 (1928)

Skouby, A. P.: The influence of acetylcholine curarine and related substances on the threshold for chemical pain stimuli. Acta. physiol. scand. **29**, 340—352 (1953)

Smith, G. M., Egbert, L. D., Markowitz, R. A., Mosteller, F., Beecher, H. K.: An experimental pain method sensitive to morphine in man: the submaximum effort tourniquet technique. J. Pharmacol. exp. Ther. **154**, 324—332 (1966)

Smith, J. B., Willis, A. L.: Formation and release of prostaglandins by platelets in response to thrombin. Brit. J. Pharmacol. **40**, 545 P (1970)

Smith, P. K.: The pharmacology of salicylates and related compounds. Ann. N.Y. Acad. Sci. **86**, 38—63 (1960)

Solomon, L. M., Juhlin, L., Kirschbaum, M. B.: Prostaglandin on cutaneous vasculature. J. invest. Derm. **51**, 280—282 (1968)

Sonina, R. S., Khaitin, V. M.: Exaggeration of sensitivity of afferent fibres to irritatory action of potassium ions induced by bradykinin, chemoreaction, and pain-inducing substances. Sechenov physiol. J. U.S.S.R. **53**, 291 (1967)

Staszewska-Barczak, J., Ferreira, S. H., Vane, J. R.: An excitatory nociceptive cardiac reflex elicited by bradykinin and potentiated by prostaglandins and myocardial ischemia. Cardiovasc. Res. **10**, 314 (1976)

Strong, C. G., Bohr, D. F.: Effects of prostaglandins E_1, E_2, A_1, and F_1 on isolated vascular smooth muscle. Amer. J. Physiol. **213**, 725—733 (1967)

Svensson, J., Hamberg, M., Samuelsson, B.: Prostaglandin endoperoxides. IX. Characterization of rabbit aorta contracting substance (RCS) from guinea pig lung and human platelets. Acta. physiol. scand. **94**, 222—228 (1975)

Swingle, K. F.: Evaluation for antiinflammatory activity. In: Scherrer, R. A., Whitehouse, M. W. (Eds.): Anti-Inflammatory Agents, Vol. II, pp. 33—122. New York: Academic Press 1974

Tallarida, G., Cassone, R., Semprini, A., Condorelli, M.: Systemic arterial pressure variations induced by the stimulation of bradykinin-sensitive vascular receptors. In: Sicuteri, F., Rocha e Silva, M., Back, N. (Ed.): Bradykinin and Related Kinins, pp. 201—212. London: Plenum Press 1970

Van Arman, C. G., Nuss, G. W., Winter, C. A., Flataker, L.: Proteolytic enzymes as mediators of pain. In: Lim, R. K. S., Armstrong, D., Pardo, E. G. (Eds.): Pharmacology of Pain, pp. 25—32. Oxford: Pergamon Press 1968

Vander Wende, C., Margolin, S.: Analgesic test based upon experimentally induced acute abdominal pain in rats. Fed. Proc. **15**, 494 (1956)

Vane, J. R.: Inhibition of prostaglandin synthesis as a mechanism of action for aspirin-like drugs. Nature (New Biol.) **231**, 232—235 (1971)

Von Frey, M.: Versuche über schmerzerregende Reize. Z. Biol. **76**, 1—24 (1922)

Weddell, A. G. M.: Observations on the anatomy of pain sensibility. In: Keele, C. A., Smith, R. (Eds.): The Assessment of Pain in Man and Animals, pp. 47—59. Edinburgh: Livingstone 1962

Weddell, G., Pallie, W., Palmer, E.: The morphology of peripheral terminations in the skin. Quart. J. micr. Sci. **95**, 483—501 (1954)

Whittle, B. A.: The use of changes in capillary permeability in mice to distinguish between narcotic and non-narcotic analgesics. Brit. J. Pharmacol. **22**, 246—253 (1964)

Willis, A. L.: Release of histamine, kinin, and prostaglandins during carrageenin induced inflammation in the rat. In: Mantegazza, P., Horton, E. W. (Eds.): Prostaglandins, Peptides, and Amines, pp. 31—38. London: Academic Press 1969

Willis, A. L., Cornelsen, M.: Repeated injection of prostaglandin E_2 in rat paws induces chronic swelling and a marked decrease in pain threshold. Prostaglandins **3**, 353—357 (1973)

Willis, A. L., Vane, F. M., Kuhn, D. C., Scott, C. G., Petrin, M.: An endoperoxide aggregator (LASS), formed in platelets in response to thrombotic stimuli. Purification, identification, and unique biological significance. Prostaglandins **8**, 453—507 (1974)

Winder, C. V.: A preliminary test for analgesic action in guinea-pigs. Arch. int. Pharmacodyn. **74**, 176—192 (1947)

Winder, C. V.: Aspirin and algesimetry. Nature (Lond.) **184**, 494—497 (1959)
Winder, C. V., Pfeiffer, C. C., Maison, G. L.: The nociceptive contraction of the cutaneous muscle of the guinea pig as elicited by radiant heat, with observations on mode of action of morphine. Arch. int. Pharmacodyn. **72**, 329—359 (1946)
Winter, C. A.: The physiology and pharmacology of pain and its relief. In: Stevens, G. (Ed.): Medicinal Chemistry: Analgesics, pp. 9—74. New York-London: Academic Press 1965
Winter, C. A., Flataker, L.: Nociceptive thresholds as affected by parental administration of irritants and of various anti-nociceptive drugs. J. Pharmacol. exp. Ther. **148**, 373—379 (1965)
Wolff, H. G., Hardy, J. D., Goodell, H.: Measurement of the effect on the pain threshold of acetylsalicylic acid, acetanilid, acetophenetidin, aminopyrine, ethylalcohol, trichlorethylene, a barbiturate, quinine, ergotamine tartrate, and caffeine: an analysis of their relation to pain experience. J. clin. Invest. **20**, 63—80 (1941)
Wolff, H. G.: Headache mechanisms. In: Wolff, H. G., Gasser, H. S., Hinsey, C. J. (Eds.): Pain, Proceedings of the Association, pp. 173—184. Baltimore: Williams & Wilkins 1943
Woodbury, D. M.: Analgesic-antipyretics, anti-inflammatory agents, and inhibitors of uric acid synthesis. In: Goodman, L. S., Gilman, A. (Eds.): The Pharmacological Basis of Therapeutics, pp. 314—347. London: Collier-Macmillan Ltd. 1970
Woodworth, R. S., Sherrington, C. S.: A pseudoaffective reflex and its spinal path. J. Physiol. (Lond.) **31**, 234—243 (1904)

CHAPTER 18

Prostaglandins and Body Temperature

W. FELDBERG and A. S. MILTON

The prostaglandins were introduced into the field of thermoregulation in 1970 by MILTON and WENDLANDT when they found that prostaglandin E_1 (PGE_1) injected into the third ventricle of unanaesthetized cats produced fever. The effect has been confirmed and extended to other species. It was found to be due to an action on the pre-optic anterior hypothalamic area and to be resistant to the action of those antipyretics which were shown to inhibit prostaglandin synthesis (VANE, 1971) and to bring down fever produced by endotoxins and endogenous pyrogens. These findings provided the first evidence for the theory that prostaglandins of the E series are the mediators of the fever produced by endotoxins, endogenous pyrogens, and perhaps of the fever of all infectious diseases (FELDBERG and SAXENA, 1971a; MILTON and WENDLANDT, 1971b; VANE, 1971).

There is little doubt that the site of action of endotoxins and endogenous pyrogens lies within the brain and is centred in the region concerned with the control of thermoregulation, the pre optic and the anterior hypothalamic area. The problem at present is whether pyrogen molecules act directly on neurones in these areas or whether the action involves a mediator such as a prostaglandin of the E series.

A. An Introduction on Fever

With these introductory remarks it is intended not to compete with the many reviews on fever, but merely to give a background for the understanding of the prostaglandin theory of fever. For a recent comprehensive review, see ATKINS and BODEL (1974).

Fever may be produced by a wide variety of organisms including both Gram-negative and Gram-positive bacteria, viruses, fungi, yeasts, and protozoa and by many inflammatory and related reactions such as tissue damage and necrosis, malignancy, antigen antibody reactions and tissue graft rejection.

Fever which occurs as a result of changes in the central control of deep body temperature produced by pyrogenic substances released following infection and inflammation, differs from the hyperthermia associated, for example, with exposure to a hot environment or following heavy exercise. These hyperthermias result from the inability of the body to balance heat loss with heat gain, whereas in fever the balance is maintained, but at a higher temperature than normal.

The causative agents of fever are referred to as pyrogens. Many different pyrogens are known. Unfortunately the nomenclature which has been used during the past 100 years is confusing. Pyrogens may be divided into exogenous and endogenous: exogenous pyrogens are external to the body and endogenous pyrogens are produced by the body. According to present views, the exogenous pyrogens act through the formation and release into the circulation of an endogenous pyrogen.

I. Exogenous Pyrogens

A large group of exogenous pyrogens is represented by the endotoxins often loosely referred to as bacterial pyrogens: they are the toxic principle produced by Gram-negative bacteria. There is no evidence for the presence of endotoxins in Gram-positive bacteria (WESTPHAL, 1957). For the present purpose it is necessary to discuss merely the endotoxins, since they are practically the only exogenous pyrogens used for investigating the role of prostaglandin in fever.

Endotoxins are lipopolysaccharides comprising three separate regions of the bacterial wall (LÜDERITZ et al., 1971). The outermost region I comprises the O-specific chain which is specific for each organism and responsible for its immunological properties. It is composed of repeating groups of oligosaccharides differing from species to species. The middle region II comprises the basal core which is also polysaccharide in nature and includes 2-β-3-deoxyoctonic acid (KDO) as well as attached phosphate groups and ethanolamine. The innermost region III is known as lipid A. It is attached to the basal core by a link to KDO (LÜDERITZ, 1970; WORK, 1971). By hydrolysis and other degradation studies it has been shown that lipid A "is a highly substituted long-chain fatty acid derivative of a phosphorylated hexosamine disaccharide backbone: 4 phospho-glucosaminyl-β 1.6 glucasamine-1-phosphate" (RIETSCHEL et al., 1972; LÜDERITZ et al., 1973; WESTPHAL, 1975). Its molecular weight is about 2000. Practically the whole toxicity, including the pyrogenicity, of an endotoxin resides in the lipid A moiety (GALANOS et al., 1972; LÜDERITZ et al., 1973).

The dose of endotoxin required to produce fever is extremely low. Measurable fevers are produced in the rabbit with doses between 0.1 and 1.0×10^{-9} g $\cdot$ kg^{-1} (LANDY and JOHNSON, 1955) and in man with doses between 1.0 and 10×10^{-9} g $\cdot$ kg^{-1} (VAN MIERT, 1971). After an intravenous injection of endotoxin there is a delay of between 20 and 30 min before fever begins to develop. The fever generally lasts for several hours and, if sufficient endotoxin is given, the fever is biphasic with maxima at approximately 1 and 3 h. The delay in onset of fever is consistent with the view that the endotoxin itself is not directly responsible for fever but acts by promoting synthesis and release of endogenous pyrogen. Some species, for example guinea pigs, mice, rats, and certain primates (not including man), do not readily develop fever following intravenous injections of endotoxins.

II. Endogenous Pyrogens

The theory that exogenous pyrogens act not directly but through endogenous pyrogen, which is considered to be the essential intermediary of endotoxin fever (see ATKINS, 1960), is based on the original observations of BEESON (1948) and BENNETT and BEESON (1953) that endogenous pyrogens are produced by the action of endotoxins on granular leucocytes (neutrophils) of rabbits. Saline extracts prepared from such leucocytes were found to be pyrogenic when injected intravenously into rabbits. The pyrogenic material from the leucocytes differed from endotoxin in that it was heat labile, that the onset of fever was more rapid, that no tolerance developed with repeated administration, and that the fever was of equal magnitude in untreated and endotoxin-tolerant animals. Since the first endogenous pyrogens were obtained from leucocytes, the term leucocyte pyrogen has often been used synonymously with endogenous pyrogen. However, leucocytes are no longer regarded as the only source of endotoxin-induced pyrogen (see SNELL, 1971). Endogenous pyrogens may be derived from a variety of cells of the reticulo-endothelial system, from Kupffer cells in the liver and from mononuclear cells of spleen, lung, and lymph nodes (ATKINS et al., 1967; DINARELLO et al., 1968; GANDER and GOODALE, 1975).

It is generally accepted (see ATKINS and BODEL, 1974) that the cells capable of producing endogenous pyrogen are activated either by exogenous pyrogens or such endogenous factors as inflammation or tissue damage, and that the activation consists in the synthesis and subsequent release into the circulation of endogenous material, which is the common mediator of fever.

Characterisation studies by MURPHY et al. (1971) as well as by GANDER and GOODALE (1962), RAFTER et al. (1960) and BODEL et al. (1969), indicate that endogenous pyrogen is a protein with a molecular weight in the order of 10000–20000 and with an isoelectric point of approximately pH 7.0. It is a heat labile substance readily inactivated by alkali. Activity lost during purification can often be restored by the addition of mercapto ethanol, suggesting that free sulphhydryl groups are necessary for pyrogenicity.

Recently, GANDER and GOODALE (1975) have investigated the release of endogenous pyrogen from various cells of the body. They found that the origin of the endogenous pyrogen differed according to whether bacteria and influenza virus or endotoxins were injected intravenously. Bacteria and influenza virus stimulated the spleen and liver, whereas endotoxin was more active in stimulating neutrophils and monocytes in the blood. GANDER and GOODALE interpret their results by saying that although Kupffer cells, spleen and blood monocytes, as well as neutrophils, are all able to synthesize and release endogenous pyrogen following stimulation either as a result of phagocytosis or by bacterial endotoxin, only the cells which are most capable of removing exogenous pyrogen from the blood normally release endogenous pyrogen. Consequently, since the fixed cells of the reticular endothelial system are most efficient in removing foreign particulate matter from the circulation, these cells will be mainly responsible for the release of endogenous pyrogen. However, as was shown by ATKINS (1960), endotoxin binds most readily with the circulating neutrophils and this explains why endotoxin is most effective in activating neutrophils to produce endogenous pyrogen.

GANDER and GOODALE conclude that in many naturally occurring fevers the fixed cells of the reticular endothelial system are the source of the circulating endogenous pyrogen causing the rise in temperature, while the neutrophils may be of little importance in these fevers. The neutrophil leucocytes, on the other hand, may be activated to produce endogenous pyrogen by circulating endotoxins as well as in acute inflammatory reactions. Yet the leucocytes do not appear to be the sole source of endogenous pyrogen, even in endotoxin fever. GREISMAN and WOODWARD (1970) have convincingly shown that the second peak of the biphasic fever produced by a first injection of endotoxin into rabbits, is hepatic in origin.

III. Pyrogen Injections Into the Liquor Space or Into Discrete Regions of the Brain

Both exogenous and endogenous pyrogens produce fever not only when injected intravenously but also when injected into the cisterna magna, into the cerebral ventricles, or directly into the pre-optic anterior hypothalamic region. This region is thought to be the site in the brain where pyrogens act. ROSENDORFF and MOONEY (1971) found in rabbits an additional secondary site in the mid-brain where pyrogen (they used purified leucocyte pyrogen) acts. This finding has not been confirmed either in rabbits or in cats. However, fever obtained in rabbits with pyrogen injected into the lateral ventricles after bilateral destruction of the pre-optic anterior hypothalamic region (see page 61), suggests the existence of a secondary pyrogen sensitive site in the brain, at least in the rabbit (VEALE and COOPER, 1975).

With injection into the liquor space or directly into the pre-optic anterior hypothalamic region, the fever is monophasic, no tolerance develops with repeated injection, the doses required to produce fever are much smaller and the onset of fever occurs earlier than with intravenous injection. Further, the latency is shorter following the injections of endogenous rather than exogenous pyrogen, and the shortest latencies occur on injection of endogenous pyrogen into the pre-optic anterior hypothalamic region.

The first observations with injections of pyrogens into the liquor space were those of BENNET et al. in 1957, who used injections of typhoid vaccine into the cisterna magna in rabbits and dogs, those of KING and WOOD in 1958 with similar injections of endogenous pyrogen into rabbits, and those of SHETH and BORISON in 1960 with injections of endotoxin into the lateral cerebral ventricles of cats. BENNET et al., also pointed out that following the cisternal injections of typhoid vaccine, no leucopenia developed during the fever and no endogenous pyrogen was detected in the serum of the animals.

The first observations with injections into the anterior hypothalamus were those of VILLABLANCA and MYERS in 1965, when they found that in cats fever is readily produced on injection of endotoxin not only into the lateral cerebral ventricles but also into the anterior hypothalamus. No pyrexia occurred with the endotoxin injections into other areas of the brain, unless very large doses were injected. Subsequently, in 1967, three publications appeared—those of COOPER et al., of JACKSON and of REPIN and KRATSKIN—in which the pre-optic anterior hypothalamic region was firmly established as the site where pyrogens act when producing fever. COOPER et al., who made the most extensive investigation, used endogenous pyrogen prepared from rabbit peritoneal exudate and injected it into selected areas of the brain. Fever occurred only when the pyrogen was injected into the pre-optic or into the anterior hypothalamic region, but not when injected into the posterior hypothalamus, mid-brain, pons, cerebellum or cerebral cortex. The mean onset time for fever was 7.8 min with leucocyte pyrogen, compared with 24.8 min with endotoxin injected into the anterior hypothalamus. JACKSON mentions in his publication a fever that occurred after a long latency following the injection of sterile saline solution into the anterior hypothalamus. This appears to be the first observation of the "non-specific fever" described on page 642.

Since then, the methods for producing fever by injection of pyrogens either into the cerebral ventricles or directly into the pre-optic anterior hypothalamic region have been widely used. To a certain extent, this is due to the discovery of the pyrogenic action of prostaglandins, because to obtain hyperthermia with prostaglandins these two routes of administration are required; in many instances the effects of prostaglandins have been compared with those of endotoxins, lipid A or endogenous pyrogen. The two routes of administration have been used to produce fever with these pyrogens not only in rabbits (ROSENDORFF and MOONEY, 1971; LIN and CHAI, 1972; EISENMAN, 1974; CRANSTON et al., 1975a, 1975b; KANDASAMY et al., 1975; TANGRI et al., 1975) and cats (MILTON and WENDLANDT, 1968, 1971c; CLARK, 1970; FELDBERG et al., 1973; SCHOENER and WANG, 1974; DEY et al., 1975; MILTON and HARVEY, 1975), but also in monkeys (CHAI et al., 1971; MYERS et al., 1971a, 1971b, 1973, 1974; LIPTON and FOSSLER, 1974), newborn lambs (PITTMAN et al., 1975), rats (BOROS-FARKAS and ILLEI-DONHOFFER, 1969; MILTON and WENDLANDT, 1971a; LIPTON et al., 1973; FELDBERG and SAXENA, 1975; VEALE and COOPER, 1975) and birds (ARTUNKAL et al., 1975).

Antipyretics now known to inhibit prostaglandin synthesis have also been shown to be antagonist to the fever produced by endotoxins, lipid A or endogenous pyrogen when injected into the cerebral ventricles or into the pre-optic anterior hypothalamic region. This was first shown by MILTON and WENDLANDT (1968) with intraperitoneal paracetamol on the fever produced by an injection of endotoxin into the cerebral ventricles of cats. Since then, this finding has been extended to other antipyretics when applied not only systemically but also when injected either into the cerebral ventricles or into the anterior hypothalamus of rabbits (CRANSTON et al., 1971; CRANSTON and RAWLINS, 1972), cats (CLARK, 1970; FELDBERG et al., 1973; SCHOENER and WANG, 1974; DEY et al., 1975), rabbits (LIN and CHAI, 1972), monkeys (CHAI et al., 1971; MYERS et al., 1971a, 1971b, 1974) and rats (FELDBERG and SAXENA, 1975).

IV. The Problem of Pyrogens Entering the CNS

Although endotoxins and endogenous pyrogens injected into the cerebral ventricles or directly into the anterior hypothalamus produce fever, evidence is sadly lacking to show how they enter the CNS when injected intravenously. All the experimental evidence is against endotoxin crossing the blood-brain barrier. In 1956, ROWLEY, HOWARD, and JENKIN were unable to detect any radioactivity in the brains of either mice or guinea pigs following the peripheral administration of ^{32}P labelled bacterial lipopolysaccharide. Similarly BRAUDE et al. (1955), using very large (lethal) doses of endotoxin prepared from *E. coli* and labelled with ^{51}Cr, found no radioactivity in the brains of rabbits following parenteral administration. Further, COOPER and CRANSTON (1963), using ^{131}I labelled endotoxin, also failed to find any activity in the brain. The only claim for endotoxin passing into the CNS was made by BENNETT et al. (1957), who found that animals made tolerant to endotoxin by repeated administration would still respond to a large dose of endotoxin by developing fever. Their suggestion that this was due to leakage of small amounts of endotoxin into the CNS, where tolerance does not develop, is not convincing. It now seems probable that tolerance is never complete, and the finding of these authors may be explained as a residual effect due to the large dose of endotoxin used. There are virtually no studies on the passage of other exogenous pyrogens into the CNS.

Evidence for endogenous pyrogen passing the blood-brain barrier is also lacking. ALLEN (1965) prepared serum from afebrile and febrile rabbits and labelled the total serum proteins with ^{131}I. The labelled serum was injected into the carotid arteries of recipient rabbits; the animals were subsequently killed and autoradiographs were prepared from brain slices. In rabbits receiving labelled serum from afebrile donors, no radioactivity was found in any of the brain slices, whereas in animals receiving labelled serum from febrile donors radioactivity was detected in the posterior hypothalamus in 4 out of 5 animals, but not in any other areas of the brain including the pre-optic anterior hypothalamic region. Recently, GANDER and MILTON (personal communication) labelled endogenous pyrogen prepared from rabbit neutrophils (peritoneal exudate cells) with ^{125}I and injected this material intravenously into unanaesthetized rabbits. No significant amounts of radioactivity were detected in any areas of the brain.

If endogenous pyrogen does not enter the CNS, and if it is the mediator of pyrogen fever, it must be initiating events outside the brain tissue, perhaps at the level of the brain capillaries, or it must enter the CSF and act on the brain tissue surrounding the walls of the cerebral ventricles in the same way as when injected into the cerebral ventricles.

To find out whether leucocyte pyrogen injected intravenously reaches the hypothalamus directly from the blood stream or passes into the CSF either through the ependyma or by being excreted through the choroid plexus, COOPER and VEALE (1972a, 1972b) investigated in unanaesthetized rabbits the effect of two procedures on fever produced by intravenous injection or infusion of leucocyte pyrogen: the effect of rapid washing of the ventricular system and the effect of filling the ventricular system with inert oil. The results obtained are contradictory and provide no clear answer.

The first procedure consisted in rapid perfusion of the ventricular system, from lateral ventricle to cisterna magna, with artificial CSF. This did not alter the onset, magnitude and duration of the leucocyte pyrogen fever, suggesting that the hypothalamic tissue is reached directly via the blood stream (FELDBERG et al., 1971).

The second procedure consisted in filling the entire ventricular system with sterile paraffin oil, which did not affect the normal body temperature, nor did it alter the time of onset of the leucocyte pyrogen fever, again suggesting that the ventricular system is of little importance for the entry of leucocyte pyrogen into the hypothalamus. However, the height and duration of the fever were greatly increased when the pyrogen was injected after the ventricles had been filled with the oil. When the procedure was reversed, the pyrogen being infused first to reach a steady state of fever and the ventricles subsequently filled with the oil, the body temperature began to climb again and continued to climb considerably thereafter. The explanation given for this exaggeration of the fever response is that the leucocyte pyrogen, or a substance released by it, may pass through the ependyma into the CSF and that the contact of the oil with the ventricular walls would prevent this route of excretion (COOPER and VEALE, 1972a, 1972b; VEALE and COOPER, 1974b). It could well be that it is the prostaglandin synthesized and then released by the pyrogen which is prevented from being removed by the oil (see page 646).

B. Temperature Responses to Prostaglandins in Different Species

The effects of PGE_1 and PGE_2 differ from those of the monoamines, with regard to body temperature, in several ways. On intraventricular injection, micrograms of the monoamines are required to be effective, whereas the E prostaglandins act in nanograms. Further, the monoamines affect body temperature differently in different species, whereas the E prostaglandins raise temperature in cats, rabbits, monkeys, rats, mice, and birds, though not in echidna.

I. Temperature Responses in Cats

On injection of PGE_1 into the third ventricle of unanaesthetized cats, MILTON and WENDLANDT (1970, 1971 b) obtained a rise in rectal temperature dependent on doses between 10 ng and 10 µg. Temperature began to rise after a latency of between 30 s and 3 min. The fever was associated with skin vasoconstriction and vigorous widespread shivering, and after the larger doses with piloerection, somnolence and stupor. Piloerection was also observed in experiments by BAIRD et al. (1974). The upper record of Figure 1 is from the paper by MILTON and WENDLANDT (1971 b) and shows the graded rises in temperature produced by 10, 100, and 1000 ng of PGE_1. The lower record, from FELDBERG and SAXENA (1971 a), illustrates the temperature re-

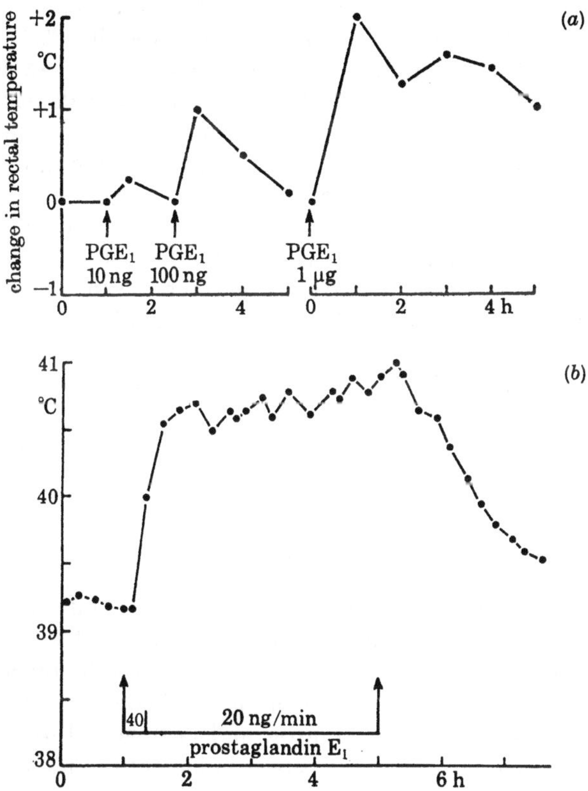

Fig. 1

sponse of a continuous PGE_1 infusion into a lateral cerebral ventricle. It shows the steep rise shortly after the onset of infusion, the persistent elevation during infusion and the relatively rapid return to nearly normal after the infusion.

Fever was also obtained on injection of 1 and 5 μg of PGE_2 into the third ventricle, but the other prostaglandins ($PGF_{1\alpha}$, $PGF_{2\alpha}$, and PGA_1), when injected in these doses, produced either no immediate rise in temperature, or small rises only (MILTON and WENDLANDT, 1971 b). For PGE_1, it was shown that its action is on the anterior hypothalamus. Injected into this part of the brain, PGE_1 produced a rise in temperature which was dose-dependent between 2 and 100 ng, but no effect was obtained with injections of 100 ng into the posterior hypothalamus (FELDBERG and SAXENA, 1971 b).

II. Temperature Responses in Rabbits

An injection of PGE_1 into a lateral ventricle or into the third cerebral ventricle of unanaesthetized rabbits produces a rise in temperature (FELDBERG and SAXENA, 1971 a; MILTON and WENDLANDT, 1971 b). The rise was found to be dose-dependent between 20 ng and 2.5 μg and was attributed mainly to skin vasoconstriction. There was also increased muscle tone but shivering was slight and not regularly seen. On injection of 1 μg of $PGF_{2\alpha}$ or PGA_1, MILTON and WENDLANDT obtained no effect on rectal temperature. STITT (1973) confirmed in rabbits the findings obtained in cats, that the anterior hypothalamus is a specific locus for the PGE_1 febrile activity. Microinjections of 20–1000 ng into this region produced a dose-dependent hyperthermia, whereas similar injections into the posterior hypothalamus or into the midbrain reticular formation did not affect rectal temperature. On injection into the anterior hypothalamus, decrease in heat loss and increase in heat production were detectable within 1 to 2 min, and temperature began to rise within 2 to 4 min. There was no difference in the degree of fever when the microinjections were made either uni- or bilaterally. HORI and HARADA (1974) showed that not only PGE_1 but also PGE_2 produced fever on injection into a lateral cerebral ventricle and that there was no significant difference in the hyperthermic responses of the two prostaglandins in terms of magnitude and time course.

VEALE and COOPER (1974 a) perfused the pre-optic anterior hypothalamic region simultaneously on both sides with labelled PGE_1-^3H. During the perfusion, which produced fever, between 2 and 8 ng of the labelled PGE_1 were retained in the hypothalamic tissues.

III. Temperature Responses in Monkeys

Some primates such as the rhesus monkey, baboon, and chimpanzee, are relatively insensitive to endotoxins injected intravenously. Often hypothermia is produced and fever only with very high doses. The squirrel monkey on the other hand, responds with fever to intravenous injections of small doses of endotoxins; a dose-dependent monophasic fever was obtained by LIPTON and FOSSLER (1974) in response to between 0.08 and 1 μg/kg. This difference between different species of monkey does not exist when the endotoxins are injected into the cerebral ventricles, or into the pre-optic anterior hypothalamic region. Fever is produced both in the squirrel monkey

(LIPTON and FOSSLER, 1974) and in the rhesus monkey (MYERS et al., 1971a, 1971b; 1974) by small doses of endotoxins injected into the pre-optic anterior hypothalamic region. There also appears to be no difference between different monkeys in the sensitivity to PGE_1 similarly injected.

In squirrel monkeys weighing 400–600 g, LIPTON and FOSSLER (1974) obtained fever on injection of PGE_1 into the pre-optic anterior hypothalamic region. The threshold was 10 ng, but 500 to 750 ng were required to produce reliable fevers. Temperature began to rise after a much shorter latency (5–10 min) than after similar injections of endotoxins. Other sites in the diencephalon that were insensitive to endotoxin were found to be insensitive to PGE_1 as well. In somewhat larger squirrel monkeys (800–1200 g), CRAWSHAW and STITT (1975) obtained dose-dependent rises in rectal temperature on injection of between 20 and 500 ng of PGE_1 into the pre-optic anterior hypothalamic region. These rises, obtained at an ambient temperature of 22° C, which is below the thermoneutral zone of the squirrel monkey (STITT and HARDY, 1971), were produced entirely by increase in metabolic rate. In Rhesus monkeys, fever produced on injection of PGE_1 into the pre-optic anterior hypothalamic region was shown by WALLER and MYERS (1973), and on injection of PGE_1 into the cerebral ventricles of the Japanese Macaque and the crab-eating Macaque by HORI and HARADA (1974).

In behavioural experiments in which the monkey can vary the ambient temperature of the chamber in which it is sitting on a restraining chair, it activates heat lamps more frequently or selects warm air following injections of PGE_1 into the pre-optic anterior hypothalamic area, thereby increasing the heat storage. This was shown for the Rhesus monkey by WALLER and MYERS (1973) and for the squirrel monkey by CRAWSHAW and STITT (1975).

IV. Temperature Responses in Humans

When examining the efficacy of intravenous infusions of prostaglandins for induction of abortion and for stimulation of uterine contractions, HENDRICKS et al. (1973) found that fever occurred in all five women in whom 200 µg/min of $PGF_{2\alpha}$, was infused, but in only one woman out of five in whom 20 µg/min of PGE_2 was infused.

V. Temperature Responses in Sheep

In Welsh mountain sheep, BLIGH and MILTON (1973) found that at thermoneutral temperature (18° C) infusions of 2 µg/min of PGE_1 into a lateral cerebral ventricle produced rises in rectal temperature associated with violent bursts of shivering, vasoconstriction in the skin (ear) and a great decrease in respiratory frequency. HALES et al. (1973) also found in male adult Merino sheep that at thermoneutral temperature (18/22° C) not only PGE_1 but also PGE_2, $PGF_{1\alpha}$, and $PGF_{2\alpha}$ produced hyperthermia on injection into a lateral ventricle. The dose routinely used was 100 µg but much smaller doses, down to 0.5 µg, were effective. Of the four prostaglandins tested, PGE_1 and PGE_2 were the most effective ones, $PGF_{2\alpha}$ was slightly, and $PGF_{1\alpha}$ considerably less effective. The rises were due to shivering and skin vasoconstriction; at thermoneutral temperature there was no change in the respiratory rate which was slow. The latent period varied between 5 and 60 min which is longer than that in cats, rabbits, and rats. This may be due to the fact that the body weight (32–40 kg) of the sheep used was about 15–350 times greater than that of these animals.

MARTIN and BAILE (1973) did not obtain any significant changes in body temperature on injection of PGE_1 into the anterior hypothalamus of sheep, but as BAILE et al. (1971) had also failed to obtain hyperthermia in rats on injection of PGE_1 into the anterior hypothalamus (see page 627), the value of their negative findings is doubtful.

In newborn lambs, varying in age between 4 and 168 h, PITTMAN et al. (1975) investigated the effect on rectal temperature of varying doses of PGE_1 injected into a lateral cerebral ventricle. A dose of 2 or 20 μg produced a rise in temperature in 40% of the experiments; in the remaining experiments 2 μg had no effect and 20 μg had either no effect or produced a fall in temperature; a dose of 100 or 200 μg produced a fall.

VI. Temperature Responses in Rats

The situation resembles that described for certain primates (page 624) in that the effects of endotoxins on body temperature is different when injected intravenously or into the cerebral ventricles. On intravenous injection, the usual response of rats to bacterial pyrogens is hypothermia although hyperthermic responses have been reported (see VAN MIERT and FRENS, 1968). Lipid A, the lipopolysaccharide in which the pyrogenic property of endotoxins resides, also produces hypothermia on intravenous injection, but both endotoxins and lipid A regularly produce hyperthermia on injection into the cerebral ventricles (FELDBERG and SAXENA, 1975). This is also the action of prostaglandins injected intraventricularly or directly into the pre-optic anterior hypothalamic region.

In the unanaesthetized rat kept at an ambient temperature of 20–25° C, injections of 5 ng to 5 μg of PGE_1 into a lateral cerebral ventricle were found to produce sharp rises in rectal temperature in restrained (FELDBERG and SAXENA, 1971 a) and unrestrained (MILTON and WENDLANDT, 1971 a) rats. Hyperthermia was also obtained with PGE_2 on injection into a lateral cerebral ventricle of restrained rats (POTTS and EAST, 1972). The hyperthermias were associated with vasoconstriction, shivering, and piloerection (BAIRD et al., 1974). It was shown later (FELDBERG and SAXENA, 1975) that hyperthermia associated with sedation was produced not only by the E but also by the F prostaglandins when injected into a lateral cerebral ventricle of restrained rats. When comparing their potencies, PGE_2 was found to be the most potent hyperthermic prostaglandin, followed in descending order by PGE_1, $PGF_{2\alpha}$, and $PGF_{1\alpha}$. A dose of 20 ng which was subthreshold for the F prostaglandins, produced hyperthermia with the E prostaglandins. The temperature effect of the E prostaglandins differed further from that of the F prostaglandins in being followed by a fall to below the pre-injection level. As in other species, the hyperthermia appears to result from an action on the pre-optic anterior hypothalamic region: LIPTON et al. (1973) obtained large rises in rectal temperature on injection of 1 μg of PGE_1 into this region, the effect being maximal when the injections were made within 0.8 mm of the mid-line. Smaller doses (0.01–0.5 μg) produced smaller and less reliable rises. RUDY and VISWANATHAN (1975) obtained a mean rise in temperature of 1.3° C (+0.12° C) on unilateral injection of 100 ng of PGE_1 into the pre-optic anterior hypothalamic region. Even smaller doses were effective in the experiments of VEALE and WHISHAW (1974). In the unrestrained rat, microinjections of 5 ng into this region produced rises of about 2° C; microinjections of this dose of PGE_1 into the lateral or posterior hypothalamus did not affect temperature. On injection into the pre-optic anterior hypothalamic region, rises in temperature of 1° C or more were obtained with as little as 100 pg. It is, therefore, not clear why BAILE et al. (1971) had observed no changes in body temperature on injection of 1 μg of PGE_1 into the anterior hypothalamic region of rats.

LIPTON et al. (1973) found that the same doses of PGE_1 that produced hyperthermia on injection into the pre-optic anterior hypothalamic region, caused a pronounced fall in rectal temperature when injected into the medulla oblongata in a region below the fourth ventricle, although cooling or heating this region had the same effect on rectal temperature as cooling and heating the pre-optic anterior hypothalamic region (LIPTON, 1973). It is possible that the hypothermia following the hyperthermia produced by larger doses of the E prostaglandins injected into a lateral cerebral ventricle (FELDBERG and SAXENA, 1975), results from an action on this region.

With intraperitoneal injection, POTTS and EAST (1972) found that PGE_2 lowered rectal temperature, but much larger doses were required than those affecting body temperature on injection into the cerebral ventricles or into the pre-optic anterior hypothalamic region. A dose-related hypothermia was produced on intraperitoneal injection of 0.035–9 mg/kg; a hypothermia of over 2.5° C occurred on injection of about 2 mg/kg. It is suggested that the hypothermia results from intense vasodilatation, since intravenous injections of PGE_1 have a strong hypotensive action in unanaesthetized rats (WEEKS and WINGERSON, 1964).

VII. Temperature Responses in Mice

WILLIS et al. (1972) found that injections of 0.6 μg of either PGE_1 or PGE_2 into the cerebral ventricles of mice produced fever.

VIII. Temperature Responses in Echidna (Tachyglossus aculeatus)

This monotreme is the only species so far examined in which, at thermoneutral temperature, injections into a lateral cerebral ventricle of PGE_1 and of PGE_2 (2 μg) produce large falls in deep body temperature (BAIRD et al., 1974). The hypothermia was mainly due to skin vasodilatation, but there was also some decrease in metabolic rate, and shivering, when present—as in a cold environment—was abolished. The effects of PGE_2 were of shorter duration than those of PGE_1. In this species not only the E prostaglandins but also noradrenaline, 5-hydroxytryptamine (5-HT) and acetylcholine produced hypothermia on injection into the cerebral ventricles.

IX. Temperature Responses in Birds

In the unanaesthetized adult fowl, NISTICO and MARLEY (1973) found that at an environmental temperature of 20–25° C, i.e. within the thermoneutral range for adult fowls (BAROTT and PRINGLE, 1946), PGE_1 injected into the third ventricle in doses of 1–10 μg, or infused into the hypothalamus in doses of 150–2300 ng, produced a dose-dependent rise in temperature associated with sedation and sleep. Following the intraventricular injections of 5 or 10 μg, the temperature remained elevated for some 5 h. In general, the rise was uninterrupted but after the intraventricular injections of the larger doses, the fever curve sometimes showed two peaks. During the rise in temperature there was abduction of the wings from the trunk, erection of body and tail feathers, and occasionally shivering. Infusions of PGE_1 into other brain areas, such as the paleostriatum augmentatum, telencephalon or mesencephalon, did not affect body temperature.

In young chicks at thermoneutral temperature (31° C), infusions of PGE_1 (14.3 nmol) into the hypothalamus raised body temperature and produced, electrocortical sleep (ARTUNKAL and MARLEY, 1974). Unexpectedly, the rise was associated with a decrease in carbon dioxide elimination and with vasodilatation; the rise was therefore attributed to behavioural changes. Arterial or intravenous injections of PGE_1 (16.0 nmol/100 g) also caused a rise in temperature, but after an initial fall.

C. Temperature Effects of Prostaglandins at Different Ambient Temperatures

The hyperthermic effect of PGE_1 was obtained not only at thermoneutral but also at low and high ambient temperature. In all these conditions, fevers of similar magnitude were generated, but, as CRAWSHAW and STITT (1975) expressed it, "the ambient temperature does determine the relative extent by which heat conservation and production mechanisms are increased and heat loss mechanisms decreased." In other words, it depends on whether, at the respective ambient temperature, shivering or panting is present and on whether the skin vessels are dilated or constricted.

In cats, MILTON and WENDLANDT (1971 b) showed that 0.5 μg of PGE_1 injected into the third ventricle also produced hyperthermia when the cat was exposed to an ambient temperature of 36° C, although the rise developed more gradually and shivering was less pronounced. In rabbits, STITT (1973) tested the effect of 0.2 μg of PGE_1 injected into the anterior hypothalamus at ambient temperatures of 24, 10, and 32° C. The sharp rises obtained were about the same in all three conditions. However, whereas at 24° C the hyperthermia was due partly to increased heat production and partly to inhibition of heat loss, that obtained at 10° was essentially due to increased heat production with scarcely any inhibition of heat loss, which was already minimal before the injection. The hyperthermia obtained at 32° C was essentially due to inhibition of heat loss with scarcely any increase in heat production. HORI and HARADA (1974) compared the hyperthermic effect of 20 μg of PGE_1 injected into a lateral cerebral ventricle in the same rabbit during exposure to an environmental temperature of 7, 20, and 32° C. Again, there was no great difference in magnitude and time course between the responses in the three conditions. At 7° C, however, the hyperthermia was mainly brought about by increased shivering and at 20° C by shivering and vasoconstriction. At 32° C, it was brought about by vasoconstriction without shivering; in addition, there was inhibition of the panting which occurred at this temperature. At 32° C the hyperthermic effect was therefore solely due to inhibition of heat loss. PGE_1 was shown to produce fever on injection into the pre-optic anterior hypothalamic region of rabbits even at an ambient temperature of −5° C (STITT et al., 1974).

Essentially the same results were obtained in sheep. In Welsh mountain sheep, BLIGH and MILTON (1973) obtained hyperthermia on infusion of PGE_1 into a lateral ventricle at thermoneutral temperature (18° C), and at a cold (10° C) and hot (40–45° C) ambient temperature. At 18° C, the rise was partly due to increased shivering, skin vasoconstriction and slowing of respiration. At 10° C, it was mainly due to increased shivering and at 40–45° C mainly to vasoconstriction and to slowing of respiration. In Merino sheep, HALES et al. (1973) obtained rises in rectal temperature of 22° C, 9° C, and 37° C with injections of PGE_1, PGE_2, $PGF_{1\alpha}$, and $PGF_{2\alpha}$, into a lateral ventricle. At 22° C, the rise was due to shivering and vasoconstriction; at 9° C mainly to shivering with only slight vasoconstriction, and at 37° C there was no shivering but there was slight vasoconstriction and cessation of panting. The respiratory rate decreased from 100–120/min to 30/min.

In rats, VEALE and COOPER (1974b) found that the magnitude of the febrile response to a microinjection of a few nanograms of PGE_1 into the pre-optic anterior hypothalamic region was the same at an ambient temperature of 3 and 40° C.

In the squirrel monkey, CRAWSHAW and STITT (1975) examined the hyperthermic effect of 0.25 µg of PGE_1 injected into the pre-optic anterior hypothalamic region at 22° C, which is below the thermoneutral zone, and at 32° C which is at the upper end of the thermoneutral zone for this monkey (STITT and HARDY, 1971). The hyperthermia was similar in both conditions, but at 22° C it resulted entirely from increased metabolic rate, whereas at 32° C it resulted from both increased metabolic rate and vasoconstriction.

The effect of infusion of PGE_1 into the hypothalamus of young chicks was examined by ARTUNKAL and MARLEY (1974) at thermoneutrality (31° C) and below, at 16° C. At 31° C the PGE_1 produced a rise in body temperature and at 16° C a fall in body temperature. Electrocortical sleep occurred in both conditions, and in both the carbon dioxide elimination decreased and the vessels dilated, although these two effects were more pronounced at 16° C than at 31° C. The rise at thermoneutrality was accounted for by behavioural changes. The effect of infusions of PGE_2 was examined at 16° C only; they caused a fall in body temperature (ARTUNKAL et al., 1975).

In Echidna, in which injections of PGE_1 and PGE_2 into a lateral cerebral ventricle cause hypothermia mainly due to skin vasodilatation, the hypothermia was accentuated in a cold environment, because in the cold Echidna shivers and the PGE injections abolished the shivering. On the other hand, the fall was attenuated (PGE_1) or abolished (PGE_2) in a warm environment as the skin vessels were already greatly dilated (BAIRD et al., 1974).

D. Effect of Prostaglandins on Thermosensitivity of the Anterior Hypothalamus and on the Firing Rate of its Neurones

Several investigations have shown that endotoxins, given systemically, can alter the characteristics of the temperature-sensitive neurones in the anterior hypothalamus. In anaesthetized cats and rabbits, warm-sensitive neurones (those whose activity is greatly increased by warming the brain) have their sensitivity depressed by pyrogen, while the cold-sensitive neurones become more sensitive (WIT and WANG, 1968;

CABANAC et al., 1968; EISENMAN, 1969; SCHOENER and WANG, 1974). A group of cold-sensitive neurones in the mid-brain reticular formation of rabbits has also been found to have their sensitivity increased by the administration of pyrogen systemically (NAKAYAMA and HORI, 1973). These actions of pyrogen seem to be specific for the temperature-sensitive neurones, since the activity of other neurones was unaffected.

In another type of experiment on unanaesthetized animals, local hypothalamic temperature has been changed and some effector response measured. Some of these results (GRANT and ADLER, 1967; EISENMAN, 1974) are in agreement with the neuronal studies just mentioned, in that the temperature sensitivity of the hypothalamus to warming is depressed in pyrogen fever. In others (ANDERSEN et al., 1961; SHARP and HAMMEL, 1972) no such depression was found.

During the fever produced in unanaesthetized animals by prostaglandins, the anterior hypothalamus retained its sensitivity to warming and cooling. This was shown in rabbits by HORI and HARADA (1974) for PGE_1 and PGE_2 injected into a lateral cerebral ventricle, and by STITT (1973) for PGE_1 injected into the pre-optic anterior hypothalamic region. STITT et al. (1974) showed that the same result was obtained when the rabbits were exposed to low ambient temperatures (17° C, 5° C, and −5° C). Warming this region counteracted or attenuated the hyperthermic effect of the prostaglandins and cooling this region had the opposite effect and accentuated the prostaglandin fever.

The effect of PGE_1 on the firing rate of single hypothalamic neurones was examined by FORD (1974b) in his diencephalic island preparation of the decerebrate cat (FORD, 1974a). The effect of PGE_1, applied iontophoretically from multi-barrelled pipettes, was studied on 46 hypothalamic neurones which were either firing spontaneously or activated by iontophoretically applied glutamate. Of the 32 neurones which were not affected by either local warming or cooling 1 was excited, 3 were suppressed and 28 did not respond to PGE_1. Of the 9 excited by warming, 2 were suppressed and 7 did not respond, but all 5 that were excited by cooling were excited by PGE_1. Thus, the main effect of PGE_1 in this condition was not inhibition of warm-sensitive but excitation of cold-sensitive neurones which are presumed to drive heat production and heat conservation.

Recently STITT and HARDY (1975) examined in anaesthetized rabbits the effect of microelectrophoretic application of PGE_1 onto single units in the pre-optic anterior hypothalamic region. The firing rate changed in less than 9% of a total population of 138 units but in contrast to the finding of FORD, no specific unit type (thermosensitive or insensitive) appeared to be selectively affected and the change was invariably one of mild facilitation.

E. Effects of Drugs on Prostaglandin Fever

I. Antipyretics

In their first publication on the fever-producing effect of PGE_1 injected into the third cerebral ventricle of cats, MILTON and WENDLANDT (1970) showed that PGE_1 fever, in contrast to the fever produced by endotoxins or 5-HT, is not prevented or abolished by 4-acetamidophenol (paracetamol) injected intraperitoneally[1]. They therefore speculated "that PGE_1 may be acting as a modulator in temperature regulation and that the action of antipyretics may be to interfere with the release of PGE_1 by 5-hydroxytryptamine or pyrogens." From the work of VANE (1971) and co-workers, we know that it is not the release but the synthesis of prostaglandins which is inhibited by antipyretics. However, "prostaglandin release," as pointed out by PIPER and VANE (1971), "can often be equated with prostaglandin synthesis; for many tissues can be provoked to release more prostaglandin than they contain." The resistance of prostaglandin fever to the action of antipyretics has been confirmed and extended to other species, to prostaglandins other than PGE_1 and to antipyretics other than paracetamol.

In *cats* MILTON and WENDLANDT (1971b) showed that the fever which, after a short latency, follows injection of PGE_1 and PGE_2 into the third cerebral ventricle is not inhibited by paracetamol given intraperitoneally, whereas the late secondary fever which is often observed after such PGE injections and which is probably an unspecific effect of intraventricular injections (see unspecific fever, page 643), is abolished by paracetamol. MILTON (1972) later found that fever produced by PGE_1 injected into the third ventricle of cats was resistant not only to paracetamol but also to indomethacin and acetylsalicylic acid injected intraperitoneally. SCHOENER and WANG (1974) found that sodium acetylsalicylate injected intravenously did not prevent the fever produced by an injection of PGE_1 into the third ventricle and CLARK and CUMBY (1975b) found the same for intravenous indomethacin on the fever produced by PGE_1 injected into a lateral ventricle.

In *rabbits*, MILTON and WENDLANDT (1971a) found that intraperitoneal paracetamol did not affect the fever produced by injection of PGE_1 into the third ventricle and KANDASAMY et al. (1975), found that subcutaneous injections of indomethacin (10 and 30 mg/kg) and of the even more potent ketoprofen (1, 3, and 10 mg/kg) had no effect, or only a dubious one, on the fever produced by injection of PGE_1 into the cerebral ventricles. Similarly WOOLF et al. (1975) showed that intravenous infusions of sodium salicylate did not affect the febrile response to a subsequent unilateral injection of PGE_1 into the anterior hypothalamus.

In *rats*, the resistance of prostaglandin fever to intraperitoneally injected paracetamol was observed by MILTON and WENDLANDT (1971a) with injections of PGE_1 into a lateral cerebral ventricle.

In *mice*, WILLIS et al. (1972) found that the fever produced by PGE_1 or PGE_2 injected into a lateral cerebral ventricle was not affected by oral administration of either paracetamol or acetylsalicylic acid.

In *young chicks*, ARTUNKAL and MARLEY (1974) and ARTUNKAL et al. (1975) found that intravenous indomethacin prolonged and intensified the temperature responses to PGE_1 and PGE_2 infused into the hypothalamus or injected intravenously or intra-arterially. The temperature responses varied according to the ambient temperature. Indomethacin enhanced and prolonged both the hyperthermia obtained at thermoneutrality (31° C) and the hypothermia obtained below thermo-

[1] The apparent antipyretic action of paracetamol on the hyperthermias produced by $PGF_{1\alpha}$ and PGA_1 is equivocal as it is not certain whether the small hyperthermias observed were due to the prostaglandins injected or were of a non-specific nature.

neutrality (16° C). Two possibilities were considered to explain the enhancement of the prostaglandin fever—supersensitivity to prostaglandins as a result of the inhibition of prostaglandin synthesis, and retardation of the breakdown of prostaglandin because indomethacin also inhibits prostaglandin dehydrogenase. This latter possibility was excluded when it was found that pre-treatment with 3, 8, 11, 14-eicosatetraynoic acid, an arachidonic acid analogue which selectively inhibits prostaglandin synthetase (FLOWER, 1974), produces the same potentiation as indomethacin (ARTUNKAL et al., 1975). We should therefore expect inhibitors of prostaglandin synthesis to potentiate the febrile responses to prostaglandins in other species as well, and MILTON and WENDLANDT (1971 b) when examining the effect of paracetamol on the PGE fever in cats stated that "in fact, the hyperthermias induced by PGE_1 appeared to be accentuated."

II. Prostaglandin Antagonist

The compound 1-acetyl-2(8-chloro-10,11-dihydrodibenz-(b,f)-(1,4)-oxazepine-10 carbonul) hydrazine (SC. 19220, Searle) is considered to be the most specific antagonist to prostaglandin in the dibenzoxazepine series. Although it acts as a competitive antagonist to prostaglandins on a variety of smooth muscle preparations (SANNER, 1969), it does not block a number of prostaglandin effects on other preparations (BENNET and POSNER, 1971; SANNER, 1974). Its intravenous injection into cats results in a fall in body temperature and during this hypothermia the temperature raising effects of PGE_1 injected into a lateral cerebral ventricle and of leucocytic pyrogen injected intravenously are attenuated (CLARK and CUMBY, 1975a), but it is not certain whether this is the result of a specific prostaglandin antagonism or whether it is due to an unspecific action. Once the hypothermic effect of SC.19220 has subsided, the effects of PGE_1 and of leucocytic pyrogen are no longer attenuated. In rats, SC.19220 is hypothermic according to SANNER (1974), and POTTS (1974) found that large doses injected intraperitoneally inhibited the hyperthermia induced by PGE_2 injected into the cerebral ventricles. In rabbits, CRANSTON et al. (1976) found that the prostaglandin fever was inhibited by SC.19200 when the antagonist and prostaglandin were injected together into the cerebral ventricles, but leucocyte pyrogen fever was not inhibited when the antagonist and the pyrogen were injected together in this way. (This discrepance is discussed on page 649).

III. Drugs Which Deplete the Stores of the Monoamines or Block Their Actions

The prostaglandins produce fever in cats, rabbits, monkeys, sheep, rats, and birds when acting on the pre-optic anterior hypothalamic region. The monoamines noradrenaline and 5-HT when acting in this way, affect body temperature differently in these species (see HELLON, 1974; FELDBERG, 1975). This makes it unlikely that prostaglandin fever is mediated by the monoamines, but it would not exclude the possibility of a contributory effect through stimulation or inhibition of monoaminergic neurones ending in the anterior hypothalamus. In order to find out whether alterations in their activities influence prostaglandin fever, the effect on this fever of drugs which either deplete the stores of the monoamines or block their actions has been examined.

COOPER and VEALE (1974) and VEALE and COOPER (1975) showed in rabbits that monoamine depletion of the hypothalamus produced by *reserpine* injected into the cerebral ventricles did not render the anterior hypothalamus insensitive to PGE_1 or to leucocyte pyrogen. An injection of 100 ng of PGE_1 into the pre-optic anterior hypothalamic region or of leucocyte pyrogen intravenously produced fever also after such monoamine depletion, although the fevers appeared to be delayed and attenuated in each case.

LABURN et al. (1974, 1975) found that in rabbits selective destruction of the noradrenergic terminals in the pre-optic anterior hypothalamic region by *6-hydroxydopamine* significantly reduced the hyperthermic effect of PGE_1 (0.5 μg) injected into this region from 1.07° C (S.E. ±0.09° C) to 0.50° C (S.E. ±0.12° C). In rabbits, noradrenaline and PGE_1 act synergistically, in cats they act antagonistically. Although no corresponding experiments have been carried out in cats with PGE_1, it was shown by MILTON and HARVEY (1975) that fever produced in this species by a bacterial pyrogen was considerably greater after pre-treatment with injections of 6-hydroxydopamine into the third ventricle.

LABURN et al. (1974, 1975) also found that the fever produced by injections of PGE_1 into the pre-optic anterior hypothalamic region became attenuated when the PGE_1 was injected together with 50 μg *phenoxybenzamine*. *Propranolol* did not have this action. No conclusions, however, can be drawn from the attenuating effect of phenoxybenzamine on the PGE_1 fever because 50 μg of phenoxybenzamine injected alone into the cerebral ventricles of rabbits caused a pronounced fall in body temperature (FELDBERG and SAXENA, 1971c). In their own experiments, LABURN et al. (1975) found that as little as 25 μg of phenoxybenzamine injected into the anterior hypothalamus had a slight hypothermic effect. Intravenous phenoxybenzamine (1 mg/kg) also abolished the fever produced by PGE_1 injected into the cerebral ventricle of rabbits, whereas *phentolamine* (10 mg/kg) delayed, but did not reduce, the fever (KANDASAMY et al., 1975). The results of the temperature effects produced by the intravenous injections of these adrenoreceptor blocking agents by themselves are not given.

HARVEY and MILTON (1974) and MILTON and HARVEY (1975) found that in cats depletion of the central stores of 5-HT by *p-chlorophenyl-alanine* (pCPA), a tryptophan hydroxylase inhibitor, reduced pyrogen fever as well as the hyperthermic responses to 50–150 ng of PGE_1, but scarcely affected those to 250–500 ng PGE_1 injected into the third ventricle. SINCLAIR and CHAPLIN (1974) found that pre-treatment with pCPA or with *o-methyl-p-tyrosine*, a tyrosine hydroxylase inhibitor given intraperitoneally, had no effect on the hyperthermia produced by either 0.5 or 5 μg PGE_1 injected into the lateral cerebral ventricles of cats. According to VEALE and COOPER (1975), the febrile response of pCPA-treated cats to injections of PGE_1 into the pre-optic anterior hypothalamic region was of slower onset, but of similar magnitude to that seen in control cats. The fever in response to leucocyte injections into the same region was scarcely affected by the treatment. Since pCPA was given orally, its effect need not have been confined to the pre-optic anterior hypothalamic region.

In rabbits, the hyperthermic effect of PGE_1 injected into a lateral cerebral ventricle was not affected by a preceding intravenous injection of the 5-HT neuronal blocker *chlorimiprazine* (5 mg/kg) or of the 5-HT antagonist *methysergide* bimaleate (1 mg/kg) (SINCLAIR and CHAPLIN, 1974). On the other hand, KANDASAMY et al. (1975) found that under similar conditions the antagonist *cyproheptadine* (3 mg/kg) abolished the PGE_1 hyperthermia whilst the antagonist *cinanserin* (3 mg/kg) slightly increased it.

IV. Atropine, Benztropine, Mecamylamine, and (+)-Tubocurarine

Results obtained on rabbits and rats provide no evidence in favour of the view that prostaglandins produce fever by an action on acetylcholine release from cholinergic nerve endings in the anterior hypothalamic region. SINCLAIR and CHAPLIN(1974) found in rabbits that an intravenous injection of benztropine mesylate (0.2 mg/kg) had no effect on the hyperthermia produced by a subsequent injection of PGE_1 into a lateral cerebral ventricle. Stronger evidence is provided by the results of RUDY and VISWANATHAN (1975) who showed in rats that injections of atropine into the pre-optic anterior hypothalamic region (blocking the muscarinic receptors), or of mecamylamine (blocking the nicotinic receptors), produced long-lasting hyperthermias, but the fevers produced and superimposed on these hyperthermias by subsequent injections of PGE_1 into this region were of the same magnitude as the fever produced by PGE_1 injections without pre-treatment with either atropine or mecamylamine. Microinjections of non-convulsive doses of d-tubocurarine into the pre-optic anterior hypothalamic region also had no pronounced effect on the fever produced by a subsequent injection of PGE_1 into the same region.

Atropine sulphate injected intraperitoneally (80 mg/kg) had the same effect on the PGE_1 fever in rats as its injection into the pre-optic anterior hypothalamic region (VISWANATHAN and RUDY, 1974).

COOPER and VEALE (1974) and VEALE and COOPER (1975) made the interesting observation in rabbits that atropine sulphate (200 μg) injected into the pre-optic anterior hypothalamic region did not affect the fever produced by PGE_1 also injected into this region, or by leucocyte pyrogen injected intravenously. However, when the atropine was injected into a lateral ventricle, it delayed and greatly reduced the PGE_1 and pyrogen fever when injected 15 min before, and abolished these fevers when injected 15 min after the injection of PGE_1 or pyrogen into the pre-optic anterior hypothalamic region. This suggests that atropine acts caudal to this region on some cholinergic synapses in the efferent pathways involved in the febrile responses and reached by intraventricular injections.

V. Morphine and Chlorpromazine

SINCLAIR and CHAPLIN (1974) found in rabbits that an intravenous injection of either morphine sulphate (10 mg/kg) or of chlorpromazine (5 mg/kg) reduced the hyperthermic effect of 5 μg of PGE_1 injected 15 min later into a lateral cerebral ventricle. Yet the intravenous injections of those substances alone lowered body temperature. The authors discuss the different possibilities of how these two drugs may act, but point out that their mechanisms of action are unknown.

VI. Anaesthetics

The effects of anaesthetics on the prostaglandin hyperthermia have not been systematically investigated. Only two observations have been made, one on cats and one on rats, both with pentobarbitone sodium.

When a cat is anaesthetized with an intraperitoneal injection of pentobarbitone sodium and not kept warm, body temperature decreases and may fall to low levels (about 32° C) during the following 1–2 h. During this time, the cat is unable to maintain body temperature. Later on, whilst the cat is still deeply anaesthetized, the vessels of the pinna constrict, the cat begins to shiver vigorously and temperature rises steeply, sometimes to beyond the pre-anaesthesia level. This rise is due to a hyperthermic action of pentobarbitone sodium on the pre-optic anterior hypothalamic region. LIPTON and FOSSLER (1974) showed that 1 μg of pentobarbitone sodium injected into this region produced fever in unanaesthetized rats.

FELDBERG and SAXENA (1971b) examined the effect of PGE_1 injected into a lateral cerebral ventricle of cats during the initial and during the later phase of pentobarbitone sodium anaesthesia. In the initial phase, when body temperature was falling, a large dose of PGE_1 (8 μg) had no effect on the body temperature which continued to fall. During the later phase, when temperature began to rise and the sensitivity of the pre-optic anterior hypothalamic region to PGE_1 began to return, a relatively large dose of PGE_1 (0.8 μg) accentuated the rise.

In rats, POTTS and EAST (1972) showed that injections of PGE_2 into the cerebral ventricles in doses which in the unanaesthetized animal resulted regularly in sharp rises in body temperature, produced only slight and doubtful rises when the rat was anaesthetized with an intraperitoneal injection of pentobarbitone sodium (50 mg/kg).

VII. Theophilline and Nicotinic Acid

The effect of these drugs on prostaglandin fever was examined to discover whether this fever, and pyrogen fever as well, is mediated by cAMP (see page 636), since theophilline inhibits and nicotinic acid activates nucleotide phosphodiesterase, the enzyme which degrades cAMP. In rabbits, LABURN et al. (1974) and WOOLF et al. (1975) found that the addition of theophilline to the PGE_1 solution injected into the pre-optic anterior hypothalamus accentuated the febrile response to PGE_1, whilst the addition of nicotinic acid attenuated the response. Both theophilline and nicotinic acid injected alone produced slight fever. This could account for the potentiating effect of theophilline but not for the attenuating effect of nicotinic acid. In the dose used, however, nicotinic acid is cytotoxic and WOOLF et al. point out that in view of the non-specific effects of both theophilline and nicotinic acid, their results must be interpreted with caution.

F. Prostaglandin Fever and Cyclic AMP

Since prostaglandins stimulate the formation of cAMP in brain tissue, the possibility had to be considered that prostaglandin fever may be mediated by activation of cAMP. The effect on body temperature of cAMP, its more soluble dibutyryl derivative (Db-cAMP) and other adenine nucleotides, has therefore been examined in various species, by injection either into the cerebral ventricles or into the pre-optic anterior hypothalamic region. The weight of evidence suggests that prostaglandin fever is not mediated through activation of cAMP, although the cAMP level in the CSF of cats was found to increase during endotoxin fever, but remained high when the fever was brought down by antipyretics (Dascombe and Milton, 1975a).

In *rats*, Breckenridge and Lisk (1969) found that implants into the anterior hypothalamus of cAMP, AMP, and Db-cAMP produced fever, but also produced hyperactivity and aggressive behaviour. The rises in temperature may therefore have been brought about indirectly by these behavioural changes.

In *cats*, Varagic and Beleslin (1973) were the first to examine the effect on body temperature of injections of cAMP, ATP (adenosinetriphosphate), Db-cAMP, and butyrate itself into a lateral cerebral ventricle. Long-lasting hyperthermias (more than 12 h) were produced by all of these substances. With Db-cAMP, the hyperthermia was sometimes preceded by transient hypothermia. The authors considered the possibility that the hyperthermias were unspecific effects and that only the hypothermia produced by Db-cAMP was a specific action. A biphasic effect on body temperature on injection of Db-cAMP into a lateral cerebral ventricle of the cat was obtained also by Clark et al. (1974). Not only the long duration of the hyperthermia (10–12 h) was stressed but also the long latency—temperature began to rise about 3 h after the injection. Clark et al. further showed that the hyperthermia was reduced by indomethacin and paracetamol. They therefore concluded that cAMP could not mediate prostaglandin fever, but that it might induce prostaglandin synthesis. It is more likely that the late rise represents the unspecific fever often seen when a physiological salt solution is injected into the cerebral ventricles or into the anterior hypothalamus, and that it is due to a disturbance or tissue damage produced by the injection and initiating prostaglandin synthesis (see page 643). This is the view expressed by Dascombe and Milton (1975b). They also found that Db-cAMP and cAMP applied by microinjection to the pre-optic anterior hypothalamic region of cats regularly produced hypothermia, which was dose-dependent; between 50 and 500 μg, as did AMP, ATP, and ADP (adenosine diphosphate) similarly applied. In those cats in which the injections produced a long-lasting rise as well, a rise was also obtained on microinjection of 0.9% NaCl solution into this region. All of these rises were reduced or abolished by paracetamol. Since the genuine or specific effect of cAMP and Db-cAMP acting on the pre-optic anterior hypothalamus of the cat appears to be a fall in temperature, the authors concluded "that it is unlikely that endogenous cAMP in this region mediates the hyperthermic response to pyrogens or to prostaglandins."

In *rabbits*, an injection of cAMP or Db-cAMP (20–500 μg) into a lateral cerebral ventricle produced a significant fall in body temperature according to Duff et al. (1972). When a rise occurred after larger doses, it did not appear within 90 min of the injection, and may therefore represent the unspecific rise which sometimes follows intraventricular injections. In contrast with these findings are those of Laburn et al. (1974) and Woolf et al. (1975) who obtained dose-dependent rises with a mean latency of approximately 3.5 min after injection of Db-cAMP (between 2.5 and 10 μg) into the pre-optic anterior hypothalamic region. In three rabbits a microinjection of 0.5 and 1 μg produced hyperexcitability and fatal hyperpyrexia.

In *squirrel monkeys*, in which injections of PGE_1 and of bacterial endotoxin into the pre-optic anterior hypothalamic region produced rises in rectal temperature, the injection of Db-cAMP in doses of 500–750 ng produced no rise in temperature. In one monkey even the bilateral application of 75 μg was ineffective (LIPTON and FOSSLER, 1974).

G. Prostaglandin in CSF and Fever

The theory that prostaglandins of the E series are the final mediator of the fever response to endotoxins, was put forward when it was found that these prostaglandins produce fever on injection into the cerebral ventricles or into the pre-optic anterior hypothalamic region and that non-steroid antipyretics inhibit prostaglandin synthesis (FELDBERG and SAXENA, 1971a, 1971b; MILTON and WENDLANDT, 1971b; VANE, 1971).

The evidence for the fever-producing effect of prostaglandins has been summarized in the previous paragraphs and the action of antipyretics on pyrogen fever is dealt with in a separate chapter by ROSENDORFF (Chapter 28). This section deals with further evidence brought forward in favour of the theory, i.e. the appearance of increased prostaglandin activity in CSF during fevers produced by exogenous and endogenous pyrogens, and its disappearance or the prevention of its appearance by antipyretics which inhibit prostaglandin synthesis and bring down or prevent these fevers.

The idea that an increased prostaglandin content in CSF indicates stimulation of prostaglandin synthesis in parts of the brain which, like the pre-optic anterior hypothalamic region, lie in close proximity to the liquor space, presupposes that the prostaglandin synthesized and released in these parts of the brain escapes into the CSF. Evidence for a transport of prostaglandin from the hypothalamic region to the liquor space was provided by VEALE and COOPER (1974a, 1974b). Using a double perfusion method, i.e. perfusing the pre-optic anterior hypothalamic regions on both sides with labelled PGE_1-^3H by means of push-pull cannulae and at the same time perfusing the ventricular system from a lateral ventricle to cisterna magna, they were able to detect some of the labelled PGE_1 in the cisternal effluent.

Before a connection between prostaglandins and pyrogen fever was suspected, prostaglandin activity had been detected in the CSF or, rather, in the perfusate from the perfused cerebral ventricles. FELDBERG and MYERS (1966) found an hydroxy acid, resembling prostaglandins, in the effluent from the perfused cerebral ventricles, particularly from the perfused inferior horn of anaesthetized cats. In the light of the present knowledge, this unidentified hydroxy acid was probably PGE_2. A few years later, HOLMES (1970) identified PGE_1, PGE_2, $PGF_{1\alpha}$, and $PGF_{2\alpha}$ in the effluent from the perfused cerebral ventricles in anaesthetized dogs. He also found a fourfold increase in the release of E prostaglandins on perfusion of a high concentration of 5-HT (1 in 50000) through the ventricles.

I. Endotoxin Fever

The first evidence of increased prostaglandin activity in CSF during fever produced by an endotoxin was obtained by FELDBERG and GUPTA (1972, 1973). In unanaesthetized cats, CSF from a Collison cannula implanted into the third ventricle was found to contain some prostaglandin activity, but the activity increased greatly in CSF collected during fever produced by an injection of the endotoxin of *Shigella dysenteriae* into the third ventricle and became low again in CSF collected when the fever was brought down by an intraperitoneal injection of paracetamol. Twenty-four hours later, when the effect of the paracetamol had subsided and the fever returned, prostaglandin activity in the CSF was again high. The activity was assayed on the rat fundic preparation rendered insensitive to 5-HT, and then expressed in ng PGE_1/ml. CSF. We know now, however, that the activity was probably due to PGE_2.

FELDBERG and GUPTA pointed out that the prostaglandin in the ventricular CSF need not have been derived solely from the anterior hypothalamic regions. Subsequent experiments, also on unanaesthetized cats, showed that there was no need to have been so cautious about the origin of the CSF since the same results were obtained with CSF collected from the cisterna magna, and not only when the endotoxin of *Shigella dysenteriae* was injected into the third ventricle but also when it was injected into the cisterna magna or intravenously (FELDBERG et al., 1972, 1973; DEY et al., 1974a). Further, the effect of bringing down the endotoxin fever and reducing the high prostaglandin activity of the CSF was shown for intraperitoneal injections not only of paracetamol but also of indomethacin and aspirin. Figure 2 illustrates experiments on two cats in which the intravenous injection of the endotoxin of *Shigella dysenteriae* produced fever with a rise in PGE activity in the CSF (expressed as PGE_1 in ng/ml.). In the lower record, the effect of indomethacin is shown, reducing both the fever and PGE activity.

The prostaglandin activity was again routinely assayed on the rat fundic preparation, but when the samples were subjected to thin layer chromatography the activity was found mainly or solely in the zone corresponding to the E prostaglandins. When, in addition, the method of radioimmunoassay was applied to pooled non-fever and to pooled fever samples, it became clear that the activity was due to PGE_2. Thus in cats bacterial endotoxins appear to stimulate the synthesis and release of this prostaglandin. In experiments in which indomethacin and paracetamol were injected before the endotoxin, the fever and high PGE activity in the cisternal CSF were prevented or greatly delayed and attenuated.

In *rabbits*, PHILIPP-DORMSTON and SIEGERT (1974a, 1974b) produced fever by the endotoxin of *E. coli* and collected samples of CSF by puncturing the cisterna magna immediately following a light pentobarbital anaesthesia. The samples, when extracted with an organic solvent, chromatographed and analyzed by radioimmunoassay, were shown to contain prostaglandins of the E and F series. A distinction between the numbers in the prostaglandin series, for example between PGE_1 and PGE_2, was not possible because the antisera exhibited no specificity for the aliphatic side chains in the prostaglandin molecule. In the samples of CSF collected during fever produced by the intravenous injection of 10 μg/kg of the endotoxin of *E. coli*, the concentration of PGE was more than twice that in the samples collected in untreated control rabbits. It increased from between 0.24 and 2.8 ng/ml (mean 1.87 ng/ml) to between 2.01 and 4.98 ng/ml (mean 4.11 ng/ml). There was no increase in the concentration of PGF. The method used by HARVEY et al. (1975) was slightly different. They collected their samples of CSF from the cisterna magna immediately after killing the rabbits by injection of air into the heart and assaved the samples

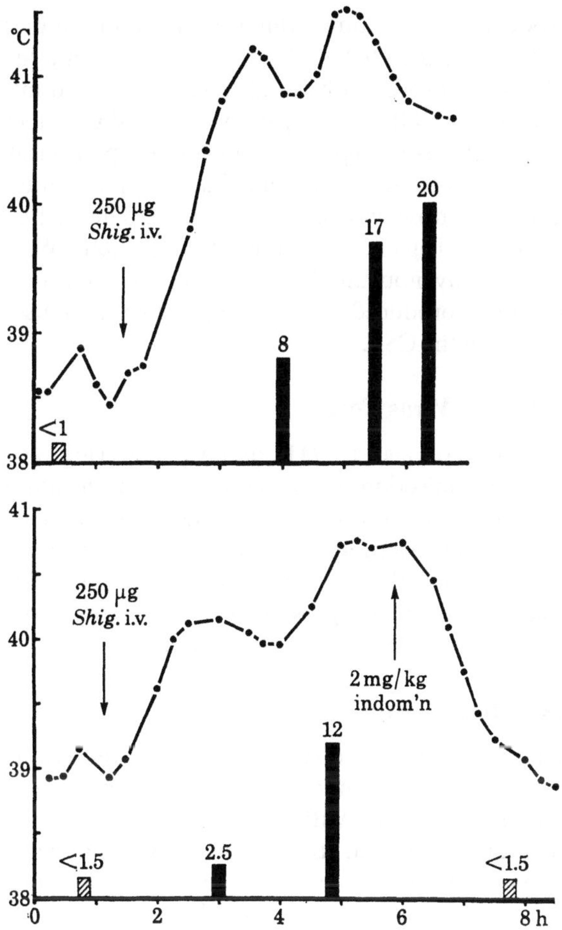

Fig. 2

against PGE_2 on the rat fundic preparation. In the samples collected from control rabbits, the activity corresponded to less than 1 ng/ml. PGE_2; in those collected from rabbits killed during fever produced by intravenous injection of the endotoxin of *Shigella dysenteriae* or of purified *proteus* endotoxin (pyrogen E), it varied between 4.5 and 60 ng/ml, and in those killed during the fever produced by an injection of the endotoxin of *Shigella dysenteriae* into the cerebral ventricles it varied between 31 and 85 ng/ml. On the other hand, the PGE_2 activity was again low in the CSF collected from those rabbits in which the fever was either prevented or abolished by an intraperitoneal injection of acetylsalicylic acid, paracetamol or indomethacin.

II. Lipid A Fever

Since the pyrogenic property of endotoxin resides almost entirely in the lipid A moiety of the lipopolysaccharide, the finding that lipid A fever, too, is associated with increased prostaglandin E_2 activity in the CSF suggests that all endotoxins act in the same way and produce fever by stimulating prostaglandin synthesis in the pre-optic anterior hypothalamic region. DEY et al. (1974b, 1975), found in non-anaesthetized cats that during the fever produced by lipid A, either injected intravenously or into the cerebral ventricles, the PGE_2 activity in the cisternal CSF increased but became low again when the fever was brought down by an intraperitoneal injection of either acetyl salicylic acid, paracetamol or indomethacin. Lipid A was more potent than endotoxin. The threshold dose was between 0.1 and 0.3 μg/kg for intravenous injections and between 5 and 20 ng for intraventricular injections. When the cat had been rendered tolerant to intravenous lipid A by its repeated intravenous injection and such injections no longer produced a rise in temperature, they also ceased to produce a rise in PGE_2 activity of the CSF.

III. Newcastle Disease Virus Fever

PHILIPP-DORMSTON and SIEGERT (1974b) found that during the fever produced in rabbits with intravenous injections of this virus, the concentration of PGE in cisternal CSF increased about twofold whereas there was no increase in the concentration of PGF. The prostaglandins were identified by chromatographic separation and by radioimmunoassay. But since the antisera used for this assay exhibited no specificity of the aliphatic side chains in the prostaglandin molecule, it was not possible to distinguish between the members of prostaglandin series.

IV. Endogenous Pyrogen Fever

From the two assumptions that endogenous pyrogens released into the circulation are the essential intermediary of endotoxin fever (see page 418) and that this fever results from stimulation of PGE synthesis in the region of the pre-optic anterior hypothalamus, it would follow that stimulation of PGE synthesis is an effect not of the endotoxins themselves, but of circulating endogenous pyrogen. Consequently, fever produced by endogenous pyrogen should also be associated with increased PGE activity in CSF and in three independent series of experiments this was shown to be so.

PHILIPP-DORMSTON and SIEGERT (1974b) found that during the fever produced in rabbits by intravenous injection of endogenous pyrogen, the PGE content of CSF increased about twofold. The identification of the prostaglandins was the same as in their experiments with *E. coli* endotoxin and with Newcastle Disease virus (see page 438). As endogenous pyrogen, they used serum obtained from other rabbits by sterile heart puncture at the height of fever produced by intravenous injection of Newcastle Disease virus. Further experiments on rabbits with endogenous pyrogen were carried out by CRANSTON et al. (1975a, 1975b) who produced a steady state of fever by continuous infusion of endogenous pyrogen prepared from rabbit blood incubated with purified *Proteus* endotoxin. Samples of CSF were collected from the cisterna magna at hourly intervals and assayed on the rat fundic preparation against PGE_2; the activity was identified as PGE by thin layer chromatography and radioimmunoassay. During the steady fever produced by the pyrogen, the PGE content of CSF was found to be increased to 3.6 ± 0.5 ng/ml PGE_2. When the pyrogen infusion was preceded by a continuous infusion of sodium salicylate, a weak antipyretic in rabbits (GRUNDMANN, 1969; CRANSTON et al., 1970; VAN MIERT et al.,

1972) especially if administered early in the course of fever (CRANSTON et al., 1971), the PGE in the CSF remained low although the pyretic action of the pyrogen persisted and was not even attenuated. This discrepancy led the authors to conclude "that the idea that prostaglandin synthesis forms an essential link in the action of pyrogen on the brain, must be called into question." This problem is dealt with on page 648.

In cats, HARVEY and MILTON (1975) collected samples of CSF from the cannulated cisterna magna and assayed them against PGE_2 on the rat fundic preparation. The endogenous pyrogen they used was either peritoneal exudate prepared from a cat or plasma obtained from cats during fever produced by intravenous injection of endotoxin of *Shigella dysenteriae*. The intravenous injection or infusion of these pyrogens produced fever associated with a rise in the PGE_2 content of the CSF, both being dependent on the amount of pyrogen administered. Further, intraperitoneal injections of acetylsalicylic acid, paracetamol or indomethacin, inhibited or abolished the rise in body temperature and PGE_2 content of the CSF. A convincing control experiment was carried out with intravenous injection of plasma obtained during fever produced by an injection of 0.1 µg of endotoxin of *Shigella dysenteriae* into the cerebral ventricles. This plasma, which should not contain circulating endogenous pyrogen, produced neither fever nor a rise in the PGE_2 content of CSF. On the other hand, plasma obtained from a cat during a post-operative fever and infused into a recipient cat, produced fever with an increased PGE_2 activity in the CSF (from <1 to 3.8 ng/ml). A subsequent intraperitoneal injection of paracetamol brought down both fever and PGE_2 activity. Thus, in these experiments with endogenous pyrogen on cats, there was no discrepancy between the action of antipyretics on the fever and the high PGE activity of CSF.

V. Variations in Increased Prostaglandin Activity During Endotoxin Fever and the Effect of Pentobarbitone Sodium Anaesthesia

Large variations were found in the increase of prostaglandin activity in the cisternal CSF during fever produced by intravenous injections of endotoxin or endogenous pyrogen, not only between results obtained by different authors using different methods of collecting CSF but also by the same authors without varying the procedure of CSF collection. For example, FELDBERG et al. (1973) found in cats that after intravenous injection of the same dose of endotoxin, the activity expressed as PGE_1 in ng/ml rose in eight experiments only to between 0.8 and 3 ng; in nine experiments to between 8 and 29 ng, in one experiment to 60 and in another to 195 ng. Two factors may account for these wide variations. (1) The very low values may indicate that in these experiments only a particularly small fraction of the prostaglandin released from the pre-optic anterior hypothalamus has reached the cisterna magna. Since the prostaglandin released into the ventricular CSF reaches the subarachnoid space near the ventral surface of the brain stem, passes into this space through the lateral recesses and the main stream of CSF and then flows in rostral direction along this ventral surface, many conditions such as movements of the head or of the whole body may influence the flow of the CSF to different parts of the subarachnoid space. (2) The very high values may result from prostaglandin synthesis in inflammatory or injured tissue near the site where the hollow needle used for collecting the CSF pierces the atlanto-occipital membrane. Apart from the initial piercing by the needle, further injury of the membrane may be brought about at the injection site by head movements of the unrestrained cat. This may result in a widening of the hole in the membrane allowing fluid from the injured or inflammatory tissue surrounding the dura to seep into the liquor space. Alternatively, the position of the needle may have to be readjusted necessitating re-puncturing and thereby setting up further injury of the membrane or even inadvertently producing a slight injury at the surface of the brain stem. Such injuries stimulating prostaglandin synthesis may be responsible for the high prostaglandin activity occasionally obtained in control samples of CSF collected without any pyrogen injections. The local inflammatory processes following these injuries may then become activated by the pyrogen injection, the activation consisting in further stimulation of prostaglandin synthesis resulting in particularly high PGE activity in the CSF. It is known that endotoxin may activate existing silent focal infections and this provocative reaction has in fact been proposed and used as a diagnostic search for focal injections (see WESTPHAL, 1975).

It became possible to avoid these complications when it was found that the effect of endotoxin in increasing the PGE_2 activity in the CSF was not suppressed in pentobarbitone sodium anaesthesia, which rendered the anterior hypothalamus relatively insensitive to the hyperthermic action of prostaglandins (see page 635). In anaesthesia, the cat lies quietly on its side without moving its head, and further injury to the dura during the course of the experiment was prevented by rigidly fixing the hollow needle used for collecting the CSF, once it had pierced the membrane, with dental cement to the guide cannula. Under these conditions, the variations in the increase of PGE_2 activity in the CSF were greatly reduced. In cats anaesthetized with pentobarbitone sodium, DASHWOOD and FELDBERG (1976) found that following intravenous injections of the endotoxin of *Salmonella abortus equi*, the increases in PGE_2 activity of the cisternal CSF varied only little. They further showed that by fixing the hollow needle with dental cement in a short-lasting Althesin anaesthesia and then allowing the cat to recover from the anaesthesia before injecting the endotoxin, the same result was obtained. The rises in PGE_2 activity were of the same order, although the fevers were naturally more pronounced. On the basis of these results they concluded that pentobarbitone anaesthesia does not, or does not appreciably depress the stimulation of prostaglandin synthesis produced by endotoxin, and further, that movements of the cat have apparently no great influence on the flow of CSF from beneath the ventral surface of the brain stem to the cisterna magna.

VI. An Unspecific Fever

It has been pointed out (FELDBERG et al., 1970; FELDBERG and SAXENA, 1970, 1971b; MILTON and WENDLANDT, 1971b) that an injection of a small amount of 0.9% NaCl solution or of artificial CSF into the cerebral ventricles, or their perfusion with artificial CSF into the cerebral ventricles, can produce prolonged fever after a latency of varying duration, sometimes as long as several hours. This happens also, though not as frequently, with injections into the cisterna magna. DEY et al. (1974a) showed in cats that such fever is associated with increased PGE_2 activity in cisternal CSF and that antipyretics which inhibit prostaglandin synthesis bring down the fever and the high PGE_2 content in the CSF. DASCOMBE and MILTON (1975b) also obtained such fever with microinjections into the region of the pre-optic anterior hypothalamus, and showed that the fever was brought down by paracetamol. They made the pertinent observation that the latency of the rise was dependent upon the exact placement of the injection cannula, being shorter at sites nearer the pre-optic anterior hypothalamus. This suggests that it is initiated from this region.

These fevers can be considered to be prostaglandin fevers. They are explained on the assumption that such injections or perfusions produce a disturbance in the ventricular walls or in surface structures of the brain stem, resulting in increased synthesis and release of PGE. This would imply that at least in some parts of the brain, for example in the pre-optic anterior hypothalamic region, increased synthesis and release of prostaglandin represents the response to the mildest "injury", in the same way as release of histamine with the ensuing "triple response" represents the first defence mechanism of the human skin to stimuli which are not sufficiently harmful to set in motion the whole range of inflammatory reactions (DEY et al., 1974a). When, on investigation of temperature effects of drugs injected into the cerebral ventricles or into the pre-optic anterior hypothalamic region, a late long-lasting hyperthermia is obtained—although not consistently—and when this effect is sensitive to non-steroid antipyretics, the probability is great that it represents the unspecific fever and not a drug effect. The long-lasting fever of the biphasic febrile response to intraventricular injections of 5-HT (FELDBERG and MYERS, 1964) may be accounted for in this way, although 5-HT may be capable of stimulating prostaglandin synthesis. This is suggested from the experiments of HOLMES (1970) in which 5-HT perfused through the cerebral ventricles was found to increase the prostaglandin content in the effluent (see page 637). On the other hand, the prolonged hyperthermic response frequently obtained by VARAGIC and BELESLIN (1973) in cats with intraventricular injections of Db-cAMP, ATP, and butyrate and which, as shown for Db-cAMP, is sensitive to indomethacin and paracetamol (CLARK et al., 1974), is obviously such an unspecific fever. This was proposed by VARAGIC and BELESLIN and strongly supported by DASCOMBE and MILTON (1975a, 1975b), who also obtained such antipyretic sensitive hyperthermias with the nucleotides when injected into the pre-optic anterior hypothalamic region.

One condition under which the unspecific fever was only rarely observed following intraventricular injections, was after pre-treatment with intramuscular chloromycetin (DEY et al., 1974a).

VII. Sodium Fever

Perfusing the cerebral ventricles of unanaesthetized cats with a 0.9% NaCl solution rather than with artificial CSF results in a high fever, known as a sodium fever. Under physiological conditions, the hyperthermic effect of the sodium ions is checked by the calcium ions. The sodium fever is therefore prevented when the cerebral ventricles are perfused with physiological salt solutions containing calcium ions (FELDBERG et al., 1970). The sodium fever is independent of prostaglandin synthesis since it is not prevented by antipyretics which inhibit prostaglandin synthesis, nor is it associated with the appearance of PGE activity or its increased activity in the effluent on perfusion of the cerebral ventricles with 0.9% NaCl solution (DEY et al., 1974a).

H. Febrile Episodes in Schizophrenia

The prostaglandin in CSF withdrawn from the cisterna magna during a fever produced by a bacterial or endogenous pyrogen or by lipid A is probably derived to only a small extent from the pre-optic anterior hypothalamic region. Most of it may be released from other parts of the brain which also border the liquor space. Structures near the ventral surface of the brain stem are apparently a main source, as suggested from results obtained by DASHWOOD and FELDBERG (1976) in experiments on cats. They collected the CSF from that part of the liquor space which lies beneath this ventral surface and found that its PGE_2 content rose much higher during endotoxin fever than in experiments in which the CSF was collected from the cisterna magna. If the high PGE_2 content during fever results from increased prostaglandin synthesis—and there is scarcely any reason to assume otherwise—this would imply that the property of pyrogens to stimulate synthesis and release of prostaglandin occurs in many parts of the brain and that it is not a specific property of the pre-optic anterior hypothalamic region, although to produce fever the prostaglandin has to act on this region. The property of pyrogens to stimulate prostaglandin synthesis may be more widespread, not even confined to the synthetase of the brain.

The idea that stimulation of prostaglandin synthesis by pyrogen in the brain may not only occur in the pre-optic anterior hypothalamic region, poses the intriguing question of whether some of the symptoms of high fever, such as malaise, are really the result of high temperature. Instead they may be effects produced by prostaglandins acting on other parts of the brain. Stupor and delirium, when they develop during high fever, may be accounted for in this way (FELDBERG et al., 1973; DEY and FELDBERG, 1975; FELDBERG, 1975). High fever produced by severe muscular exercise, that is, when it occurs independently of prostaglandin synthesis in the brain, is not associated with these symptoms. Marathon runners develop extremely high temperatures during running as a result of the tremendous heat production; the temperature regulating mechanisms may actually break down and yet these athletes show no signs of malaise, stupor or delirium (personal communication by Dr. R.H. FOX).

On the other hand, injections of endotoxin or lipid A produced a stuporous state in which the animal (cat) did not react to events in its environment; frequently a condition of real catalepsy developed. For instance, when the cat was placed in an upright posture by putting its paws across the rung of an inverted stool, it retained this position without struggling, but when it sagged down after a while and moved away, its movements were not impaired. The development of cataleptic features during fever often foretold high PGE_2 activity in the CSF (FELDBERG et al., 1973; DEY et al., 1975b). The same conditions—a stuporous state (MILTON and WENDLANDT, 1971b) and, with doses larger than those required to produce fever, catalepsy (HORTON, 1964; HOLMES and HORTON, 1968)—are produced by PGE_1 injected into the cerebral ventricles of cats.

Catatonia, the equivalent of catalepsy in humans, and stupor, are characteristic features of certain forms of schizophrenia and it has been suggested (FELDBERG, 1975) that this disease may be due to a disturbance of the prostaglandin metabolism in the brain or, to be more precise, in the diencephalon. There is also an association between schizophrenia and fever. "We would not expect fever to be a constant feature of the disease since it should only occur when the released prostaglandin reaches the anterior hypothalamus. But fever is a genuine syndrome of schizophrenia, even if not a frequent occurrence ..." (FELDBERG, 1975). The main publications appeared in the thirties by GJESSING (1939) in Oslo, and by SCHEID in Munich. SCHEID wrote a monograph in 1937, and gave a lecture in 1938, with the title "Febrile episodes in schizophrenia". According to both authors, a periodic exacerbation of the disease is often associated with fever or subfebrile episodes; according to SCHEID, every fourth or fifth admission to his hospital occurred during a subfebrile or febrile episode.

There is another, more severe and critical form of fever associated with schizophrenia which was well known to the psychiatrists at the beginning of the century. A sudden onset of very high, often lethal fever, with an exacerbation of the psychosis. Hyperthermia can be so extreme that temperature can no longer be measured with the normal fever thermometer. Psychiatrists not aware that such a fever is a syndrome of the psychosis, go on looking for a bacterial origin, then for a virus infection, and finally for tuberculosis. In the meantime, they treat the patient with antibiotics. But if the fever were due to increased prostaglandin synthesis near the anterior hypothalamus, treatment of choice would be large doses of antipyretics (FELDBERG, 1975).

The antipyretic of choice would be paracetamol because it inhibits more or less specifically the synthetase in brain (WILLIS et al., 1972; FLOWER and VANE, 1972, 1974).

If schizophrenia were due to a disturbance in the prostaglandin metabolism of the brain, one would expect psychotropic drugs which have a therapeutic effect in schizophrenia to be inhibitors of the prostaglandin synthetase. So far, the effects of such drugs have been examined in vitro on the synthetase system of either the guinea pig lung (LEE, 1974) or the bovine seminal vesicle (KRUPP and WESP, 1975). From results obtained with paracetamol, however, we know that an inhibitor which has little effect on the enzyme system in such peripheral tissues may be a potent inhibitor of brain synthetase. LEE found that chlorpromazine and tricyclic anti-depressants strongly inhibited the synthetase in his system. KRUPP and WESP confirmed these findings in their synthetase system, but found little inhibitory effect with haloperidol, which is reported to have great therapeutic value in schizophrenia.

I. The Evidence for and Against the Prostaglandin Theory of Fever

The theory that fever produced by pyrogens is mediated by a prostaglandin of the E series presupposes that they induce prostaglandin synthesis in the pre-optic anterior hypothalamic region and that the final mediator of the febrile response is an E prostaglandin. Direct experimental evidence that pyrogens stimulate the prostaglandin synthetase in the brain is still lacking. At present, the main evidence for the theory centres on the following three findings: (1) that prostaglandins of the E series which are natural constituents of hypothalamic tissue produce fever when injected in minute amounts into the cerebral ventricles or directly into the pre-optic anterior hypothalamic region; (2) that antipyretics which inhibit prostaglandin synthesis prevent and abolish the pyrogen fever, and (3) that during such fever the PGE activity of CSF collected either from the third cerebral ventricle or from the cisterna magna increases but that antipyretics which inhibit prostaglandin synthesis prevent and bring down both the fever and the high PGE activity in CSF.

The theory is further strengthened by the fact that the pre-optic anterior hypothalamic region which is the only site on which the prostaglandins act in the brain when producing fever, is apparently also the only site where bacterial and endogenous pyrogens act when producing fever, although a secondary leucocyte pyrogen sensitive site in the mid-brain has been described by ROSENDORFF and MOONEY (1971) in the rabbit. The existence of this secondary site, however, has so far not been confirmed. Another prerequisite of the theory is met by the finding that antipyretics which inhibit the synthetase do so not only in peripheral tissues but also in brain, as shown in homogenates of mouse and gerbil brain for paracetamol (WILLIS et al., 1972) and in homogenate of rabbit and dog brain for paracetamol, indomethacin and sodium acetyl salicylate (FLOWER and VANE, 1972).

VEALE and COOPER (1974 b) have listed a number of additional facts in support of the theory. *Firstly*, the latency of the febrile response to PGE_1 is shorter than that to pyrogens injected directly into the pre-optic anterior hypothalamic region. *Secondly* and *thirdly*, the febrile response to intravenous leucocyte pyrogen is interfered with when conjugated antibody to PGE_1 is placed in the pre-optic anterior hypothalamic region, but potentiated when the ependymal wall becomes coated with oil following the injection of paraffin oil into the cerebral ventricles (COOPER and VEALE, 1972a, 1972 b). The oil is thought to prevent the egrees of the synthesized PGE into the CSF of the ventricles from whence it would otherwise be carried away into the subarachnoid space and then absorbed into the blood stream. This idea is based on their own finding that ^3H PGE_1 placed in the tissue of the pre-optic anterior hypothalamic region passes into the fluid perfusing the cerebral ventricles. *Fourthly*, reserpine which interferes with thermoregulation does not prevent the febrile response to either PGE_1 or intravenous leucocyte pyrogen. *Fifthly*, atropine, when acting caudal to the pre-optic anterior hypothalamic region, i.e. when injected not into this region itself but into the cerebral ventricles, blocks the febrile response to both PGE_1 and intravenous leucocyte pyrogen (see page 634).

There are differences between the temperature effects of prostaglandins and of pyrogens, which are readily explained without creating difficulties for the prostaglandin theory. A difference in the effects on these fevers of antipyretics which inhibit prostaglandin synthesis would be expected since they do not inhibit the action of the prostaglandins, but only their synthesis. Another difference which is readily accounted for is observed in rats and in certain primates. Their temperature response to intravenous injections of bacterial pyrogens is not usually fever, and yet the prostaglandins, when injected into the cerebral ventricles or directly into the pre-optic anterior hypothalamus, do produce fever. The explanation may be that the endotoxin or the endogenous pyrogen produced by them cannot pass the blood-brain barrier (FELDBERG and SAXENA, 1975) since in these species, too, pyrogens produce fever on injection into the cerebral ventricles or into the pre-optic anterior hypothalamic region.

It is not certain how pyrogens produce fever through increased prostaglandin synthesis in the pre-optic anterior hypothalamic region when they are injected into this region or into the cerebral ventricles. Various possibilities have been suggested by DEY et al. (1975) when discussing the action of lipid A administered in this way. Endotoxins may initiate the local formation and release of endogenous pyrogen from leucocytes which, as shown by COOPER et al. (1967), invade the injection site, or from leucocytes that accumulate in the ventricular walls. This explanation is favoured by SNELL (1971). Another source of the endogenous pyrogen could be the microglia which is thought by various authors to be related to the reticulo-endothelial system (HORTEGA, 1932; FLEISCHHAUER, 1964; CAMMERMEYER, 1965; FEIGIN, 1969). Alternatively, when the endotoxins are not applied via the blood stream, they may directly stimulate prostaglandin synthesis in the CNS without involvement of endogenous pyrogen.

Recently, five publications have appeared in which the validity of the prostaglandin theory is questioned. ARTUNKAL et al. (1975) found that in young chicks the temperature response to prostaglandins, but not that to bacterial pyrogen, changed with the ambient temperature. PGE_1 and PGE_2 infused into the hypothalamus produced hyperthermia at 31° C but at 16° C hypothermia was produced. The endotoxin of *Shigella dysenteriae* (1 µg) similarly infused produced fever at both ambient temperatures. At present it is not possible to explain this difference by the prostaglandin theory. Their other finding, however, that indomethacin potentiated the prostaglandin responses but not the endotoxin fever, creates no difficulty for the theory, as the authors seem to assume, since indomethacin, even if potentiating the prostaglandin responses, should prevent or bring down endotoxin fever.

PITTMAN et al. (1975) found in newborn lambs a certain, though not an absolute, dissociation between the action of endotoxin and PGE_1. In ten lambs sensitized to endotoxin, a subsequent challenge with an intravenous injection of 0.3 µg of the endotoxin of *Salmonella abortus equi* resulted in fever, but in only two of them did the injection of PGE_1 into the cerebral ventricles produce hyperthermia. On the other hand, in three other sensitized lambs in which the intravenous injection of the endotoxin gave no febrile response, the injection of PGE_1 into the cerebral ventricles resulted in fever. Injected into the cerebral ventricles, the endotoxin seemed to be rather insensitive—a dose of 3 ng did not produce hyperthermia, but fever was produced with 0.3 µg. Since this dose was usually also effective on intravenous injection, the response obtained on intraventricular administration may have been due to absorption of the endotoxin into the bloodstream. The authors themselves leave open the question whether their results indicate that the febrile response to bacterial pyrogens in the newborn lambs is independent of prostaglandin, or whether in these animals the method of intraventricular injection is not suitable to obtain evidence of prostaglandin involvement in the febrile response to endotoxins.

VEALE and COOPER (1975) found that in rabbits in which the entire pre-optic anterior hypothalamic region had been destroyed bilaterally, PGE_1 and leucocyte pyrogen no longer produced fever when injected into this region. In this respect, there was no discrepancy. However, when the injections were made into the cerebral ventricles, PGE_1 remained inactive but leucocyte pyrogen still produced fever. This was also the case when injections were made intravenously, and although temperature then rose more gradually, it reached the same end point as in control rabbits. This result can only be explained on the assumption that, at least in the rabbit, there is in addition to the pre-optic anterior hypothalamic region another secondary site (or secondary sites) on which pyrogen can act and produce fever. The difference in effectiveness between prostaglandin and leucocyte pyrogens on intraventricular injection would mean that, with this method of application, the secondary site is not reached by the prostaglandin but by the pyrogen. The reason may be that it lies some distance away from the ventricular lumen and that the prostaglandin when penetrating the wall is destroyed before reaching the site, whereas the pyrogen is not. If pyrogens act on the pre-optic anterior hypothalamic region through prostaglandin, the same mechanism of action would be expected at the secondary site. From the results so far obtained therefore, it does not follow that the pyrogen fever is independent of prostaglandin, as suggested by the authors. This suggestion would only be valid if it were shown that this fever is resistant to antipyretics which inhibit prostaglandin synthesis. This was not shown and is unlikely. In fact, if the site is identical with the secondary leucocyte pyrogen-sensitive site in the mid-brain described by Rosendorff and Mooney (1971), its sensitivity to antipyretics is as good as established. Cranston and Rawlins (1972) made bilateral microinfusions of salicylate into different regions of the rabbit's brain during fever produced by intravenous infusion of leucocyte pyrogen. A defervescence was obtained from two sites and from two sites only—when the infusions were made into the pre-optic anterior hypothalamic areas and when they were made into the mid-brain in or near the periaqueductal grey matter.

Cranston et al. (1975, 1976a) examined in rabbits the effect of salicylate on pyrogen fever and PGE content of cisternal CSF. When a steady-state fever was produced with intravenous infusion of leucocyte pyrogen, the PGE level in the cisternal CSF increased and remained high during the fever. The ability of leucocyte pyrogen to stimulate prostaglandin synthesis is thus not denied. On the contrary, the authors state "that throughout the fever there was a release of prostaglandin into the CSF." However, these authors have denied or "called into question" the idea that prostaglandin synthesis forms an essential link in the action of pyrogens on the brain, because on infusion of salicylate the fever produced by the leucocyte pyrogen infusion was not affected, neither its latency nor its rate of rise and the final level attained. Yet the appearance of PGE activity in the CSF was prevented. Salicylate has only weak antipyretic action in rabbits and the dose used was submaximal but the "partial inhibition of prostaglandin might have been expected to cause partial abatement of the fever; none was observed." Therefore it was thought that the pyrogens act directly on the brain.

These observations with salicylate on rabbits are at variance with the numerous results obtained in rabbits and cats with endotoxins, lipid A and endogenous pyrogen and described in section G, in which the high PGE content of CSF and the fever were brought down together by antipyretics, including salicylate. There are two ways of explaining the dissociation found by Cranston et al. without having to question the role of prostaglandins as mediators of pyrogen fever.

1. The prostaglandin which appears in the cisternal CSF represents only the "tip of the iceberg." Pyrogens stimulate prostaglandin synthesis, probably not only in the pre-optic anterior hypothalamic region. Of the prostaglandin synthesized in this region, however, only a small fraction will appear in the cisternal CSF owing to the absence of a foramen of Magendie, as has been pointed out elsewhere (page 641). In the experiments of Cranston et al., the level of prostaglandin in the cisternal CSF during fever was very near to the threshold of sensitivity of their assay method, the rat fundic strip (it was lower than in corresponding experiments on cats); a slight reduction in prostaglandin synthesis might have been sufficient to give negative results when assaying the CSF, but insufficient to bring about a perceptible effect on the fever.

2. The PGE detected in the cisternal CSF may have been derived to a great extent from synthesis, activated by the pyrogen, in injured or inflammatory tissue near the site where the hollow needle used for the CSF collection pierced the atlanto-occipital membrane. Such extraneous sources of PGE were suggested as responsible for the great variations in PGE activity of cisternal CSF observed in cats after intravenous endotoxin injections (see page 641). It was pointed out that as long as such extraneous sources are not rigidly excluded, a high PGE level in cisternal CSF is not always a sign of increased prostaglandin synthesis in the pre-optic anterior hypothalamic region. The results obtained by CRANSTON et al. underline this view, particularly since in rabbits the synthetase of peripheral tissue may well be more sensitive to salicylate than that of the brain.

Perhaps the strongest evidence so far brought forward against the prostaglandin theory is the latest finding by CRANSTON et al. (1976b) that when the prostaglandin antagonist SC.19220 was injected into the cerebral ventricles of the rabbit together with either prostaglandin or leucocyte pyrogen, it prevented the prostaglandin but not the pyrogen fever. This is yet another instance in which the actions of prostaglandins and pyrogen differ on injection into the cerebral ventricles. The root of this difference may again lie in differences of penetration into the brain tissue and of destruction during this process.

Thus, in spite of the many findings in favour of the prostaglandin theory, there are a few observations which at the moment are not consistent with it. Each of them is a challenge and will have to be satisfactorily explained before the theory is firmly established and accepted without reservation.

Acknowledgement. We would like to thank Dr. R. F. Hellon for the many valuable suggestions he made when reading through the manuscript.

References

Allen, L. V.: The cerebral effects of endogenous serum and granulocytic pyrogen. Brit. J. exp. Path. **46**, 25—34 (1965)

Andersen, H. T., Hammel, H. T., Hardy, J. D.: Modifications of the febrile response to pyrogen by hypothalamic heating and cooling in the unanaesthetized dog. Acta physiol scand. **53**, 247—254 (1961)

Artunkal, A. A., Marley, E.: Hyper- and hypothermic effects of prostaglandin E_1 (PGE_1) and their potentiation by indomethacin, in chicks. J. Physiol. (Lond.) **242**, 141—142P (1974)

Artunkal, A. A., Marley, E., Stephenson, J. D.: Dissociation of bacterial pyrexia from prostaglandin E activity. Brit. J. Pharmacol. **54**, 250—251 P (1975)

Atkins, E.: Pathogenesis of fever. Physiol. Rev. **40**, 580—646 (1960)

Atkins, E., Bodel, P. T.: Fever. In: Grant, L., McClusky, R. T. (Eds.): The Inflammatory Process, 2nd Ed., Vol. III, pp. 467—514. New York: Academic Press 1974

Atkins, E., Bodel, P. T., Francis, L.: Release of an endogenous pyrogen in vitro from rabbit mononuclear cells. J. exp. Med. **126**, 357—383 (1967)

Baile, C. A., Simpson, C. W., Bean, S. M., Jacobs, H. J.: Feeding effects of hypothalamic injections of prostaglandin. Fed. Proc. **30**, 375 (1971)

Baird, J. A., Hales, J. R. S., Lang, W. J.: Thermoregulatory responses to the injection of monoamines, acetylcholine, and prostaglandins into a lateral cerebral ventricle of the echidna. J. Physiol. (Lond.) **236**, 539—548 (1974)

Barott, H. G., Pringle, E. M.: Energy and gaseous metabolism of the hen as affected by temperature. J. Nutr. **31**, 35—50 (1946)

Beeson, P. B.: Temperature elevating effect of a substance obtained from polymorphonuclear leucocytes. J. clin. Invest. **27**, 524 (1948)

Bennet, A., Posner, J.: Studies on prostaglandin antagonists. Brit. J. Pharmacol. **42**, 584—594 (1971)

Bennett, I. L., Beeson, P. B.: Studies in the pathogenesis of fever. II. Characterisation of fever producing substances from polymorphonuclear leucocytes, and from the fluid of sterile exudates. J. exp. Med. **98**, 493—508 (1953)

Bennet, J. L. Jr., Petersdorf, R. C. Jr., Keene, W. R.: Pathogenesis of fever, evidence for direct cerebral action of bacterial endotoxins. Trans. Ass. Amer. Physcns **70**, 64—71 (1957)

Bligh, J., Milton, A. S.: The thermoregulatory effects of prostaglandin E_1 when infused into a lateral cerebral ventricle of the Welsh Mountain sheep at different ambient temperatures. J. Physiol. (Lond.) **229**, 30—31 P (1973)

Bodel, P. T., Wechsler, A., Atkins, E.: Comparison of endogenous pyrogens from human and rabbit leucocytes utilizing Sephadex filtration. Yale J. Biol. Med. **41**, 376—387 (1969)

Boros-Farkas, M., Illei-Donhoffer, A.: The effect of hypothalamic injections of noradrenaline, serotonin, pyrogen, γ-amino-N-butyric acid, triiodothyronine, triiodothyroacetic acid, DL-phenylalamine, DL-alanine, and DL-γ-amino-β-hydroxybutyric acid on body temperature and oxygen consumption in the rat. Acta physiol. Acad. Sci. hung. **36**, 105—116 (1969)

Braude, A. I., Carey, F. J., Zalesky, M.: Studies with radioactive endotoxin. II. Correlation of physiological effects with distribution of radioactivity in rabbits injected with lethal doses of *E. coli* endotoxin labelled with radioactive sodium chromate. J. clin. Invest. **34**, 858—866 (1955)

Breckenridge, B. McL., Lisk, R. D.: Cyclic adenylate and hypothalamic regulatory functions. Proc. Soc. exp. Biol. (N.Y.) **131**, 934—935 (1969)

Cabanac, M., Stolwijk, J. A. J., Hardy, J. D.: Effect of temperature and pyrogens on single-unit activity in the rabbit's brain stem. J. appl. Physiol. **26**, 645—652 (1968)

Cammermeyer, J.: The hypependymal microglia cell. Z. Anat. Entwickl.-Gesch. **124**, 543—561 (1965)

Chai, L. Y., Lin, M. T., Chen, N. I., Wang, S. C.: The site of action of leukocytic pyrogen and antipyresis of sodium acetylsalicylate in monkeys. Neuropharmacology **10**, 715—723 (1971)

Clark, W. G.: The antipyretic effects of acetaminophen and sodium salicylate on endotoxin induced fevers in cats. J. Pharmacol. exp. Ther. **175**, 469—475 (1970)

Clark, W. G., Cumby, H. R.: Effects of prostaglandin antagonist SC.19220 on body temperature and on hyperthermic responses to prostaglandin E_1 and leucocytic pyrogen in the cat. Prostaglandins **9**, 361—368 (1975a)

Clark, W. G., Cumby, H. R.: The antipyretic effect of indomethacin. J. Physiol. (Lond.) **248**, 625—638 (1975b)

Clark, W. G., Cumby, H. R., Davis, I. V., Henry, E.: The hyperthermic effect of intracerebroventricular cholera toxin in the unanaesthetized cat. J. Physiol. (Lond.) **240**, 493—504 (1974)

Cooper, K. E., Cranston, W. I.: Clearance of radioactive bacterial pyrogen from the circulation. J. Physiol. (Lond.) **166**, 41 P (1963)

Cooper, K. E., Cranston, W. I., Honour, A. J.: Observations on the site and mode of action of pyrogens in the rabbit brain. J. Physiol. (Lond.) **191**, 325—337 (1967)

Cooper, K. E., Veale, W. L.: Potentiation of fever produced by intravenous leucocyte pyrogen following the injection of paraffin oil into the cerebral ventricles of the unanaesthetized rabbit. Experientia (Basel) **28**, 917—918 (1972a)

Cooper, K. E., Veale, W. L.: The effect of an inert oil in the cerebral ventricular system upon fever produced by intravenous pyrogen. Canad. J. Physiol. **50**, 1066—1071 (1972b)

Cooper, K. E., Veale, W. L.: The effects of reserpine and atropine, injected into the lateral cerebral ventricle, on fever due to intravenous leucocyte pyrogen and hypothalamic injection of prostaglandin E_1 in the unanaesthetised rabbit. J. Physiol. (Lond.) **241**, 25P—26P (1974)

Cranston, W. I., Duff, G. W., Hellon, R. F., Mitchell, D.: Effect of a prostaglandin antagonist on the pyrexias caused by PGE_2 and leucocyte pyrogen in rabbits. J. Physiol (Lond.) **256**, 120P—121P (1976)

Cranston, W. I., Hellon, R. F., Mitchell, D.: Fever and brain prostaglandin release. J. Physiol. (Lond.) **248**, 27P—28P (1975a)

Cranston, W. I., Hellon, R. F., Mitchell, D.: A dissociation between fever and prostaglandin concentration in cerebrospinal fluid. J. Physiol. (Lond.) **253**, 583—592 (1975b)

Cranston, W. I., Luff, R. H., Rawlins, M. D., Rosendorff, C.: The effects of salicylate on temperature regulation in the rabbit. J. Physiol. (Lond.) **208**, 251—259 (1970)
Cranston, W. I., Luff, R. H., Rawlins, M. D., Wright, V. A.: Influence of the duration of experimental fever on salicylate antipyresis in the rabbit. Brit. J. Pharmacol. **41**, 344—351 (1971)
Cranston, W. I., Rawlins, M. D.: Effects of intracerebral microinjection of sodium salicylate on temperature regulation in the rabbit. J. Physiol. (Lond.) **222**, 257—266 (1972)
Crawshaw, L. I., Stitt, J. T.: Behavioural and autonomic induction of prostaglandin E_1 fever in squirrel monkeys. J. Physiol. (Lond.) **244**, 197—206 (1975)
Dascombe, M. J., Milton, A. S.: Cyclic adenosine-3′,5′-monophosphate in cerebrospinal fluid during fever and antipyresis. J. Physiol. (Lond.) **247**, 29—31 P (1975a)
Dascombe, M. J., Milton, A. S.: The effects of cyclic adenosine 3′,5′-monophosphate and other nucleotides on body temperature. J. Physiol. (Lond.) **250**, 143—160 (1975b)
Dashwood, M., Feldberg, W.: Unpublished experiments (1976)
Dey, P. K., Feldberg, W., Gupta, K. P., Milton, A. S., Wendlandt, S.: Further studies on the role of prostaglandin in fever. J. Physiol. (Lond.) **241**, 629—646 (1974a)
Dey, P. K., Feldberg, W., Wendlandt, S.: Lipid A and prostaglandin. J. Physiol. (Lond.) **239**, 102—103 P (1974b)
Dey, P. K., Feldberg, W., Gupta, P. K., Wendlandt, S.: Lipid A fever in cats. J. Physiol. (Lond.) **253**, 103—119 (1975)
Dinarello, C. A., Bodel, P. T., Atkins, E.: The role of the liver in the production of fever and in pyrogenic tolerance. Trans. Ass. Amer. Physcns **81**, 334—344 (1968)
Duff, G. W., Cranston, W. I., Luff, R. H.: Cyclic 3′,5′adenosine monophosphate in central control of body temperature. Fifth Int. Congr. Pharmacol. (1972)
Eisenman, J. S.: Pyrogen-induced changes in the thermosensitivity of septal and pre-optic neurons. Amer. J. Physiol. **216**, 330—334 (1969)
Eisenman, J. S.: Depression of pre-optic thermosensitivity by bacterial pyrogen in rabbits. Amer. J. Physiol. **227**, 1067—1073 (1974)
Feigin, I.: Mesenchymal tissues of the nervous system. The indigenous origin of brain macrophages in hypoxic states and in multiple sclerosis. J. Neuropath. exp. Neurol. **26**, 6—23 (1969)
Feldberg, W.: Body temperature and fever: changes in our views during the last decade. Proc. roy. Soc. B **191**, 199—229 (1975)
Feldberg, W., Gupta, K. P.: Sampling for biological assay of cerebrospinal fluid from the third ventricle in the unanaesthetized cat. J. Physiol. (Lond.) **222**, 126—129 P (1972)
Feldberg, W., Gupta, K. P.: Pyrogen fever and prostaglandin activity in cerebrospinal fluid. J. Physiol. (Lond.) **228**, 41—53 (1973)
Feldberg, W., Gupta, K. P., Milton, A. S., Wendlandt, S.: Effect of bacterial pyrogen and antipyretics on prostaglandin activity in cerebrospinal fluid of unanaesthetized cats. Brit. J. Pharmacol. **46**, 550—551 P (1972)
Feldberg, W., Gupta, K. P., Milton, A. S., Wendlandt, S.: Effect of pyrogen and antipyretics on prostaglandin activity in cisternal CSF of unanaesthetized cats. J. Physiol. (Lond.) **234**, 279—293 (1973)
Feldberg, W., Myers, R. D.: Effect on temperature of amines injected into the cerebral ventricles. A new concept of temperature regulation. J. Physiol. (Lond.) **173**, 226—237 (1964)
Feldberg, W., Myers, R. D.: Appearance of 5-hydroxytryptamine and an unidentified pharmacologically active lipid acid in effluent from perfused cerebral ventricles. J. Physiol. (Lond.) **184**, 837—855 (1966)
Feldberg, W., Myers, R. D., Veale, W. L.: Perfusions from cerebral ventricle to cisterna magna in the unanaesthetized cat. Effect of calcium on body temperature. J. Physiol. (Lond.) **207**, 403—417 (1970)
Feldberg, W., Saxena, P. N.: Mechanism of action of pyrogen. J. Physiol. (Lond.) **211**, 245—261 (1970)
Feldberg, W., Saxena, P. N.: Fever produced by prostaglandin E_1. J. Physiol. (Lond.) **217**, 547—556 (1971a)
Feldberg, W., Saxena, P. N.: Further studies on prostaglandin E_1 fever in cats. J. Physiol. (Lond.) **219**, 739—745 (1971b)
Feldberg, W., Saxena, P. N.: Effects of adrenoceptor blocking agents on body temperature. Brit. J. Pharmacol. **43**, 543—554 (1971c)

Feldberg, W., Saxena, P. N.: Prostaglandins, endotoxin and lipid A on body temperature in rats. J. Physiol. (Lond.) **249**, 601—615 (1975)
Feldberg, W., Veale, W. L., Cooper, K. E.: Does leucocyte pyrogen enter the hypothalamus via the cerebrospinal fluid. 25th International Congress of Physiological Sciences, Vol. **IX**, p. 175 (1971)
Fleischhauer, K.: Über die Fluoreszens perivasculärer Zellen im Gehirn der Katze. Z. Zellforsch. **64**, 140—152 (1964)
Flower, R. J.: Drugs which inhibit prostaglandin biosynthesis. Pharmacol. Rev. **26**, 33—67 (1974)
Flower, R. J., Vane, J. R.: Inhibition of prostaglandin synthetase in brain explains the anti-pyretic activity of paracetamol (4-acetamidophenol). Nature (Lond.) **240**, 410—411 (1972)
Flower, R. J., Vane, J. R.: Some pharmacological and biochemical aspects of prostaglandins biosynthesis and its inhibition. In: Robinson, H. J., Vane, J. R. (Eds.): Prostaglandin Synthetase Inhibitors, pp. 9—18. New York: Raven Press 1974
Ford, D. M.: A diencephalic island for the study of thermally responsive neurones in the cat's hypothalamus. J. Physiol. (Lond.) **239**, 67—68 P (1974a)
Ford, D. M.: A selective action of prostaglandin E_1 on hypothalamic neurones in the cat which respond to brain cooling. J. Physiol. (Lond.) **242**, 142—143 (1974b)
Galanos, C., Rietschel, E. T., Lüderitz, O., Westphal, O., Kim, Y. B., Watson, D.: Biological activities of lipid A complexes to bovine-serum albumin. Europ. J. Biochem. **31**, 230—233 (1972)
Gander, G. W., Goodale, F.: Chemical properties of leucocytic pyrogen. I. Partial purification of rabbit leucocytic pyrogen. Exp. molec. Path. **1**, 417—426 (1962)
Gander, G. W., Goodale, F.: The role of granulocytes and mononuclear leucocytes in fever. In: Temperature Regulation and Drug Action Symposium, Paris, pp. 51—58. Basel: Karger 1975
Gjessing, R.: Beiträge zur Kenntnis der Pathophysiologie des katatonen Stupors. Mitteilungen I—IV. Arch. Psychiat. Nervenkr. **96**, 318—392; 393—474 (1932); **104**, 354—416 (1935); **109**, 525—595 (1939)
Grant, R., Adler, R. D.: Responses to leucocytic pyrogen (LP) in hyperthermic and hypothalamus-heated rabbits: a challenge to "reset" hypothesis of fever. Physiologist **10**, 186 (1967)
Greisman, S. E., Woodward, C. L.: Mechanism of endotoxin tolerance. VII. The role of the liver. J. Immunol. **105**, 1468—1476 (1970)
Grundmann, M. J.: Studies on the action of antipyretic substances. D. Phil. Thesis, University of Oxford (1969)
Hales, J. R. S., Bennett, J. W., Baird, J. A., Fawcett, A. A.: Thermo-regulatory effects of prostaglandins E_1, E_2, $F_{1\alpha}$, and $F_{2\alpha}$ in the sheep. Pflügers Arch. ges. Physiol. **339**, 125—133 (1973)
Harvey, C. A., Milton, A. S.: The effect of parachlorophenylalanine on the response of the conscious cat to intravenous and intraventricular bacterial pyrogen and to intraventricular prostaglandin E_1. J. Physiol. (Lond.) **236**, 14—15 P (1974)
Harvey, C. A., Milton, A. S.: Endogenous pyrogen fever, prostaglandin release and prostaglandin synthetase inhibitors. J. Physiol. (Lond.) **250**, 18—20 P (1975)
Harvey, C. A., Milton, A. S., Straughan, D. W.: Prostaglandin E levels in cerebrospinal fluid of rabbits and the effects of bacterial pyrogen and antipyretic drugs. J. Physiol. (Lond.) **248**, 26—27 P (1975)
Hellon, R. F.: Monoamines, pyrogens, and cations; their actions on central control of body temperature. Pharmacol. Rev. **26**, 290—321 (1974)
Hendricks, C. H., Brenner, W. E., Ekbladh, L., Brotanek, V., Fisburne, J. I.: Efficacy and tolerance of intravenous prostaglandins $F_{2\alpha}$ and E_2. Amer. J. Obstet. Gynec. **111**, 564—579 (1973)
Holmes, S. W.: The spontaneous release of prostaglandins into the cerebral ventricles of the dog and the effect of external factors on this release. Brit. J. Pharmacol. **38**, 653—658 (1970)
Holmes, S. W., Horton, E. W.: The distribution of tritium labelled prostaglandin E_1 in amounts sufficient to produce central nervous effects in cats and chicks. Brit. J. Pharmacol. **34**, 32—37 (1968)
Hori, T., Harada, Y.: The effects of ambient and hypothalamic temperatures on the hyperthermic responses to prostaglandins E_1 and E_2. Pflügers Arch. ges. Physiol. **350**, 123—134 (1974)
Hortega, P. De Rio X.: Microglia. In: Penfield, W. (Ed.): Cytology and Cellular Pathology of the Nervous System, pp. 481—534. New York: P. P. Hoeber 1932

Horton, E. W.: Actions of prostaglandin E_1, E_2, and E_3 on the central nervous system. Brit. J. Pharmacol. **22**, 189—192 (1964)

Jackson, D. L.: A hypothalamic region responsive to localized injection of pyrogens. J. Neurophysiol. **30**, 586—602 (1967)

Kandasamy, B., Girault, J. M., Jacob, J.: Central effects of a purified bacterial pyrogen, prostaglandin E_1 and biogenic amines on the temperature in the awake rabbit. In: Lomax, P., Schönbaum, E., Jacob, J. (Eds.): Temperature Regulation and Drug Action, pp. 124—132. Basel: S. Karger 1975

King, M. K., Wood, W. B. Jr.: Studies on the pathogenesis of fever. IV. The site of action of leucocytic and circulating endogenous pyrogen. J. exp. Med. **107**, 291—303 (1958)

Krupp, P., Wesp, M.: Inhibition of prostaglandin synthetase by psychotropic drugs. Experientia (Basel) **31**, 330—331 (1975)

Laburn, H. P., Rosendorff, C., Willies, G., Woolf, C.: A role for noradrenaline and cyclic AMP in prostaglandin E_1 fever. J. Physiol. (Lond.) **240**, 49—50 P (1974)

Laburn, H., Woolf, C. J., Willies, G. H., Rosendorff, C.: Pyrogen and prostaglandin fever in the rabbit. II. Effects of noradrenaline depletion and adrenergic receptor blockade. Neuropharmacology **14**, 405—411 (1975)

Landy, M., Johnson, A. G.: Studies on O antigen of *Salmonella typhosa*. IV. Endotoxic properties of the purified antigen. Proc. Soc. exp. Biol. (N.Y.) **90**, 57—62 (1955)

Lee, R. E.: The influence of psychotropic drugs on prostaglandin synthesis. Prostaglandins **5**, 63—68 (1974)

Lin, M. T., Chai, C. Y.: The antipyretic effect of sodium acetyl-salicylate on pyrogen-induced fever in rabbits. J. Pharmacol. exp. Ther. **180**, 603—609 (1972)

Lipton, J. M.: Thermosensitivity of medulla oblongata in control of body temperature. Amer. J. Physiol. **224**, 890—897 (1973)

Lipton, J. M., Fossler, D. E.: Fever produced in the squirrel monkey by intravenous and intracerebral endotoxin. Amer. J. Physiol. **226**, 1020—1027 (1974)

Lipton, J. M., Welch, J. P., Clark, W. G.: Changes in body temperature produced by injecting prostaglandin E_1, EGTA and bacterial endotoxins into the POPO/AH region and the medulla oblongata of the rat. Experientia (Basel) **29**, 806—808 (1973)

Lüderitz, O.: Recent results on the biochemistry of the cell wall lipopolysaccharides of *Salmonella* bacteria. Angew. Chemie **9**, 649—663 (1970)

Lüderitz, O., Galanos, C., Lehmann, V., Nurminen, M., Rietschel, E. T., Rosenfelder, G., Simon, M., Westphal, O.: Lipid A. J. infect. Dis. **128** (suppl.), 17—29 (1973)

Lüderitz, O., Westphal, O., Staub, A. M., Nicaido, H.: Isolation and chemical and immunological characterisation of bacterial lipopolysaccharides. In: Weinbaum, G., Kadis, S., Ajl, S. T. (Eds.): Bacterial Endotoxins, Vol. IV, pp. 145—233. New York-London: Academic Press 1971

Martin, F. H., Baile, C. A.: Feeding elicited in sheep by intrahypothalamic injections of PGE_1. Experientia (Basel) **29**, 306—307 (1973)

Milton, A. S.: Prostaglandin E_1 and endotoxin fever, and the effects of aspirin, indomethacin, and 4-acetamidophenol. In: Advanc. Biosci. **9**, 495—500 (1972)

Milton, A. S., Harvey, C. A.: Prostaglandins and monoamines in fever. In: Lomax, P., Schönbaum, E., Jacob, J. (Eds.): Temperature Regulation and Drug Action, pp. 133—142. Basel: S. Karger 1975

Milton, A. S., Wendlandt, S.: The effect of 4-acetamidophenol in reducing fever produced by the intracerebral injection of 5-hydroxytryptamine and pyrogen in the conscious cat. Brit. J. Pharmacol. **34**, 215—216 P (1968)

Milton, A. S., Wendlandt, S.: A possible role for prostaglandin E_1 as a modulator for temperature regulation in the central nervous system of the cat. J. Physiol. (Lond.) **207**, 76—77 P (1970)

Milton, A. S., Wendlandt, S.: The effects of 4-acetamidophenol (paracetamol) on the temperature response of the conscious rat to the intracerebral injection of prostaglandin E_1 adrenaline and pyrogen. J. Physiol. (Lond.) **217**, 33 P (1971 a)

Milton, A. S., Wendlandt, S.: Effects on body temperature of prostaglandins of the A, E, and F series on injection into the third ventricle of unanaesthetized rats and rabbits. J. Physiol. (Lond.) **218**, 325—336 (1971 b)

Milton, A. S., Wendlandt, S.: The effect of different environmental temperatures on the hyperpyrexia produced by the intraventricular injection of pyrogen, 5-hydroxytryptamine and prostaglandin E_1 in the conscious cat. J. Physiol. (Paris) **63**, 340—342 (1971 c)
Murphy, P. A., Chesney, P. T., Wood, W. B. Jr.: Purification of an endogenous pyrogen with an appendix on assay methods. In: Wolstenholme, G. E. W., Birdh, T. (Eds.): Pyrogen and Fever. Ciba Foundation Symposium, pp. 59—72. London: Churchill Livingston 1971
Myers, R. D., Rudy, T. A., Yaksh, T. L.: Fever in the monkey produced by the direct action of pyrogen on the hypothalamus. Experientia (Basel) **27**, 160—161 (1971 a)
Myers, R. D., Rudy, T. A., Yaksh, T. L.: Effect in the rhesus monkey of salicylate on centrally induced endotoxin fever. Neuropharmacology **10**, 775—778 (1971 b)
Myers, R. D., Rudi, T. A., Yaksh, T. L.: Evocation of a biphasic febrile response in the rhesus monkey by intracerebral injection of bacterial endotoxins. Neuropharmacology **12**, 1195—1198 (1973)
Myers, R. D., Rudy, T. A., Yaksh, T. L.: Fever produced by endotoxin injected into the hypothalamus of the monkey and its antagonism by salicylate. J. Physiol. (Lond.) **243**, 167—193 (1974)
Nakayama, T., Hori, T.: Effects of anaesthetic and pyrogen on thermally sensitive neurons in the brain stem. J. appl. Physiol. **34**, 351—355 (1973)
Nistico, G., Marley, E.: Central effects of prostaglandin E_1 in adult fowls. Neuropharmacology **12**, 1009—1016 (1973)
Philipp-Dormston, W. K., Siegert, R.: Identification of prostaglandin E by radio-immunoassay in cerebrospinal fluid during endotoxin fever. Naturwissenschaften **61**, 134—135 (1974 a)
Philipp-Dormston, W. K., Siegert, R.: Prostaglandins of the E and F series in rabbits cerebrospinal fluid during fever induced by Newcastle disease virus, *E. coli*-Endotoxin or endogenous pyrogen. Med. Microbiol. Immunol. **159**, 279—284 (1974 b)
Piper, P., Vane, J.: The release of prostaglandin from lung and other tissues. Ann. N.Y. Acad. Sci. **180**, 363—385 (1971)
Pittman, Q. J., Veale, W. L., Cooper, K. E.: Temperature responses of lambs after centrally injected prostaglandins and pyrogens. Amer. J. Physiol. **228**, 1034—1038 (1975)
Potts, W. J.: Quoted from Sanner, J. H. Substances that inhibit the actions of prostaglandins. Arch. intern. Med. **133**, 133—146 (1974)
Potts, W. J., East, P. F.: Effects of prostaglandin E_2 on body temperature of conscious rats and cats. Arch. int. Pharmacodyn. **197**, 31—36 (1972)
Rafter, G. W., Collins, R. D., Wood, W. B. Jr.: Studies on the pathogenesis of fever. VIII. Preliminary chemical characterization of leucocytic pyrogen. J. exp. Med. **111**, 831—840 (1960)
Repin, I. S., Kratskin, I. L.: An analysis of hypothalamic mechanisms of fever. Fiziol. Zh. (Mosk.) **53**, 1206—1211 (1967)
Rietschel, E. T., Gottert, H., Lüderitz, O., Westphal, O.: Nature and linkages of the fatty acids present in the lipid A component of *Salmonella* lipopolysaccharides. Europ. J. Biochem. **28**, 166—173 (1972)
Rosendorff, C., Mooney, J. J.: Central nervous system sites of action of a purified leucocyte pyrogen. Amer. J. Physiol. **220**, 597—603 (1971)
Rowley, D., Howard, J. G., Jenkin, C. R.: The fate of ^{32}P-labelled bacterial lipopolysaccharide in laboratory animals. Lancet **1956 I**, 336—367
Rudy, Th. A., Viswanathan, C. T.: Effect of central cholinergic blockade on the hyperthermia evoked by prostaglandin E_1 injected into the rostral hypothalamus of the rat. Canad. J. Physiol. Pharmacol. **53**, 321—324 (1975)
Sanner, J. H.: Anatagonism of prostaglandin E_2 by 1-acetyl-2(8-chloro-10,11-dihydrodibenz[b,f][1,4]oxazepine-10 carbonyl) hydrazine (SC.19220). Arch. int. Pharmacodyn. **180**, 46—56 (1969)
Sanner, J. H.: Substances that inhibit the actions of prostaglandins. Arch. intern. Med. **133**, 133—146 (1974)
Scheid, K. F.: Febrile Episoden bei schizophrenen Psychosen. Leipzig: Georg Thieme 1937
Scheid, K. F.: Die Symptomatologie der Schizophrenie. Z. Neurol. **163**, 585—603 (1938)
Schoener, E. P., Wang, S. C.: Sodium acetylsalicylate effectiveness against fever induced by leukocytic pyrogen and prostaglandin E_1 in the cat. Experientia (Basel) **30**, 383—384 (1974)
Sharp, F. R., Hammel, H. T.: Effect of fever on salivation response in the resting and exercising dog. Amer. J. Physiol. **223**, 77—82 (1972)

Sheth, U.K., Borison, H.L.: Central pyrogenic action of *Salmonella Typhosa* lipopolysaccharide injected into the lateral cerebral ventricle in cats. J. Pharmacol. exp. Ther. **130**, 411—417 (1960)

Sinclair, J.G., Chaplin, M.F.: Effect of p-chlorophenylalanine, α-methyl-p-tyrosine, morphine, and chloropromazine on prostaglandin E_1 hyperthermia in the rabbit. Prostaglandins **25**, 117—124 (1974)

Snell, E.S.: Endotoxin and the pathogenesis of fever. In: Kadis, W., Weinbaum, G., Ajl, S.J. (Eds.): Microbial Toxins, Vol. V, pp. 277—340. New York-London: Academic Press 1971

Stitt, J.T.: Prostaglandin E_1 fever induced in rabbits. J. Physiol. (Lond.) **232**, 163—179 (1973)

Stitt, J.T., Hardy, J.D.: Thermoregulation in the squirrel monkey in relation to body weight. J. appl. Physiol. **31**, 48—54 (1971)

Stitt, J.T., Hardy, J.D.: Microelectrophoresis of PGE_1 onto single units in the rabbits hypothalamus. Amer. J. Physiol. **229**, 240—245 (1975)

Stitt, J.T., Hardy, J.D., Stolwijk, A.J.: PGE_1 fever: its effect on thermoregulation at different low ambient temperatures. Amer. J. Physiol. **227**, 622—629 (1974)

Tangri, K.K., Bhargava, A.K., Bhargava, K.P.: Significance of central cholinergic mechanism in pyrexia induced by bacterial pyrogen in rabbits. In: Lomax, P., Schönbaum, E., Jacob, E. (Eds.): Temperature Regulation and Drug Action, pp. 65—74. Basel: S. Karger 1975

Vane, J.R.: Inhibition of prostaglandin synthesis as a mechanism of action for aspirin-like drugs. Nature (New Biol.) **231**, 232—235 (1971)

Van Miert, A.S.: Inhibition of gastric motility by endotoxin (bacterial lipopolysaccharide) in conscious goats and modification of their response by a splanchnectomy, adrenalectomy or adrenergic blocking agents. Arch. int. Pharmacodyn. **193**, 405—414 (1971).

Van Miert, A.S., Frens, J.: The reaction of different animal species to bacterial pyrogens. Zbl. vet. Med. **15**, 532—543 (1968)

Van Miert, A.S., Van Essen, J.A., Thorp, G.A.: The antipyretic effect of pyrazolone derivatives and salicylates on fever induced with leukocytic or bacterial pyrogen. Arch. int. Pharmacodyn. **197**, 388—391 (1972)

Varagic, V.M., Beleslin, D.B.: The effect of cyclic N-2-O-dibutyryl-adenosine-3',5-monophosphate, adenosine triphosphate and butyrate on the body temperature of conscious cats. Brain Res. **57**, 252—254 (1973)

Veale, W.L., Cooper, K.E.: Prostaglandin in cerebrospinal fluid following perfusion of hypothalamic tissue. J. appl. Physiol. **37**, 942—945 (1974a)

Veale, W.L., Cooper, K.E.: Evidence for the involvement of prostaglandins in fever. In: Recent Studies of Hypothalamic Function. Int. Symp., Calgary 1973, pp. 359—370. Basel: Karger 1974b

Veale, W.L., Cooper, K.E.: Comparison of sites of action of prostaglandin and leucocyte pyrogen in brain. In: Lomax, P., Schönbaum, G., Jacob, J. (Eds.): Temperature Regulation and Drug Action, pp. 218—226. Basel: Karger 1975

Veale, W.L., Whishaw, I.: Temperature responses produced in the rat by PGE_1 and NE microinjected into the brain (1974). Quoted from Veale and Cooper (1974b)

Villablanca, J., Myers, R.D.: Fever produced by microinjection of typhoid vaccine into hypothalamus of cats. Amer. J. Physiol. **208**, 703—707 (1965)

Viswanathan, C.T., Rudy, T.A.: Modulation of central cholinergic function as a possible basis for prostaglandin-evoked hyperthermia in the rat. Fed. Proc. **33**, 286 (1974)

Waller, M.B., Myers, R.D.: Hyperthermia and operant responding for heat evoked in the monkey by intrahypothalamic prostaglandin. Paper presented at the Society for Neuroscience Meeting, San Diego, Calif. 1973

Weeks, J.R., Wingerson, F.: Cardiovascular action of prostaglandin E_1 evaluated using unanaesthetized relatively unrestrained rats. Fed. Proc. **23**, 327 (1964)

Westphal, O.: Pyrogen. In: Springer, G.F. (Ed.): Polysaccharides in Biology, p. 115. New York: Macy 1957

Westphal, O.: Bacterial endotoxins. Int. Arch. Allergy **49**, 1—43 (1975)

Willis, A.L., Davison, P., Ramwell, P.W., Brocklehurst, W.E., Smith, B.: Release and actions or prostaglandins in inflammation and fever: inhibition by anti-inflammatory and antipyretic drugs. In: Ramwell, P.W., Pharris, B.B. (Eds.): Prostaglandins in Cellular Biology, pp. 227—259. New York: Plenum Press 1972

Wit, A., Wang, S. C.: Temperature-sensitive neurons in pre-optic/anterior hypothalamic region: actions of pyrogens and acetylsalicylate. Amer. J. Physiol. **215**, 1160—1169 (1968)
Woolf, C. J., Willis, G. H., Laburn, H., Rosendorff, C.: Pyrogen and prostaglandin fever in the rabbit. I. Effects of salicylate and the role of cyclic AMP. Neuropharmacology **14**, 397—403 (1975)
Work, E.: Production, chemistry and properties of bacterial pyrogen and endotoxins. In: Wolstenholme, G. E. W., Birch, J. (Eds.): Pyrogens and Fever, pp. 23—47. London: Churchill Livingston 1971

Author Index

Page numbers in *italics* refer to bibliography

Subject Index

Handbuch der experimentellen Pharmakologie/ Handbook of Experimental Pharmacology

Heffter-Heubner, New Series

Springer-Verlag
Berlin
Heidelberg
New York

MIX
Papier aus verantwortungsvollen Quellen
Paper from responsible sources
FSC® C105338

If you have any concerns about our products,
you can contact us on
ProductSafety@springernature.com

In case Publisher is established outside the EU,
the EU authorized representative is:
Springer Nature Customer Service Center GmbH
Europaplatz 3, 69115 Heidelberg, Germany

Printed by Libri Plureos GmbH
in Hamburg, Germany